Nobel Laureate	Country*	Year of Award	Accomplishment
Gerald M. Edelman Rodney R. Porter	United States United Kingdom	1972	Elucidation of the nature and structure of antibody molecules
David Baltimore Howard Temin Renato Dulbecco	United States United States United States (Italy)	1975	Studies on the transformation of cells by tumor viruses
Baruch Blumberg D. Carleton Gajdusek	United States United States	1976	Discovery of Australia antigen Description of slow virus disease
Rosalyn Yalow	United States	1977	Development of the radioimmunoassay procedure
Robert C.L. Guillemin Andrew V. Schally	United States (France) United States (Poland)		Synthesis of peptide hormones
Daniel Nathans Hamilton Smith Werner Arber	United States United States Switzerland	1978	Studies on restriction enzymes and their use in genetic engineering
Baruj Benacerral George D. Snell Jean Dausser	United States United States France	1980	Discovery of the histocompatibility antigens used in tissue typing
Barbara McClintock	United States	1983	Studies on transposable genetic elements
Cesar Milstein Georges J.F. Köhler	United Kingdom (Argentina) Switzerland (Germany)	1984	Development of monoclonal antibody technique
Niels K. Jerne	Switzerland (Denmark)		Research in immunology
Susumu Tonegawa	United States (Japan)	1987	Discovery of the genetic principle of antibody diversity
James W. Black Gertrude B. Elion George H. Hitchings	United Kingdom United States United States	1988	Elucidation of important principles of drug therapy for disease
J. Michael Bishop Harold Varmus	United States United States	1989	Studies on the genetic basis of cancer
Joseph E. Murray E. Donnall Thomas	United States United States	1990	Research into transplantation methods
Erwin Neher Bert Sakmann	Germany Germany	1991	Discovery of ion channels in biological membranes
Philip Sharp Richard Roberts	United States United States	1993	Identification of exons and introns in mRNA synthesis
Alfred G. Gilman Martin Rodbell	United States United States	1994	Discovery of G-proteins and their function in signal transduction
Peter C. Doherty Rolf Zinkernagel	Australia Switzerland	1996	Studies on MHC proteins and antigen recognition in defense processes
Stanley B. Prusiner	United States	1997	Research on prions
Günter Blobel	United States (Germany)	1999	Research on mechanisms for protein movement and localization in cells

* Indicates country in which work was performed; country of birth in parentheses.

Fundamentals of Microbiology

SIXTH EDITION

I. EDWARD ALCAMO, Ph.D.

Professor of Microbiology
State University of New York at Farmingdale

JONES AND BARTLETT PUBLISHERS
Sudbury, Massachusetts
BOSTON   TORONTO   LONDON   SINGAPORE

http://microbiology.jbpub.com

Jones and Bartlett Publishers is pleased to introduce our **Microbiology** web site, developed exclusively for this Sixth Edition of *Fundamentals of Microbiology*. This site, http://microbiology.jbpub.com, offers a variety of resources designed to enhance the learning process. With this site, you will soon discover how the Internet can enrich your learning experience.

The **Fundamentals of Microbiology** web page offers unparalleled quality and reliability:

- All of the Internet resources are reviewed or handpicked by the author.

- Descriptive information is provided on each linked outside site, so you know how the site relates to the chapter you've been reading.

- The web page is maintained by Jones and Bartlett Publishers, so any broken links are quickly repaired or replaced.

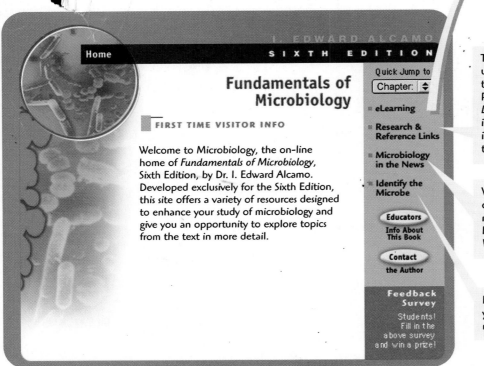

These links offer reliable and up-to-date information from sites like the Centers for Disease Control and Prevention, *The Emerging Infectious Disease Journal,* and many other independent sites that provide more in-depth coverage of microbiology topics.

We've linked to useful sites that report on news and research in the field of microbiology. You'll also find a direct link to *The Morbidity and Mortality Weekly Report* here.

Identify the Microbe exercises allow you to test your knowledge of the microorganisms you've studied.

Dr. Vilma Yuzbasiyan-Gurkan

eLearning

eLearning is a study tool with a variety of interactive activities designed to help you review your class material. You will find study quizzes, virtual flash cards, chapter outlines, and chapter objectives.

Chapter outlines guide you through your review of each chapter by focusing on the material point by point.

Chapter objectives help you focus your studying on the most important aspects of each chapter.

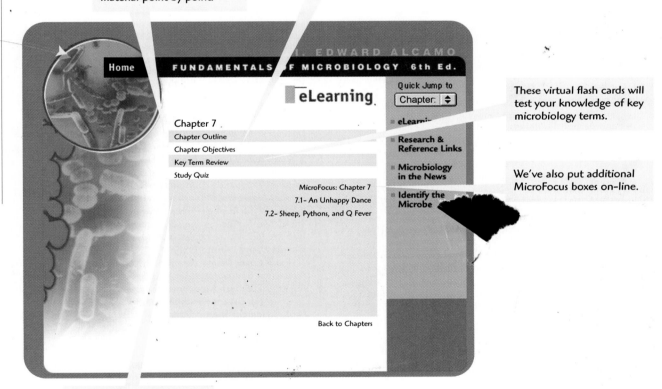

EDWARD ALCAMO

Home | FUNDAMENTALS OF MICROBIOLOGY 6th Ed.

eLearning

Quick Jump to
Chapter:

Chapter 7
Chapter Outline
Chapter Objectives
Key Term Review
Study Quiz

MicroFocus: Chapter 7
7.1- An Unhappy Dance
7.2- Sheep, Pythons, and Q Fever

Back to Chapters

- eLearning
- Research & Reference Links
- Microbiology in the News
- Identify the Microbe

These virtual flash cards will test your knowledge of key microbiology terms.

We've also put additional MicroFocus boxes on-line.

The study quizzes test your knowledge of important concepts and applications in each chapter.

To find out more about the **Microbiology** web site, please e-mail microbiology@jbpub.com or call your Jones and Bartlett Publisher's Representative at 800-832-0034.

DEDICATION

To my wife Charlene Alice,
As we celebrate the first
anniversary of our marriage.

I love you dearly

World Headquarters
Jones and Bartlett Publishers
40 Tall Pine Drive
Sudbury, MA 01776
978-443-5000
info@jbpub.com
www.jbpub.com

Jones and Bartlett Publishers Canada
2406 Nikanna Road
Mississauga, ON L5C 2W6 Canada

Jones and Bartlett Publishers International
Barb House, Barb Mews
London W6 7PA UK

COPYRIGHT © 2001 BY JON̶E̶ TT PUBLISHERS, INC.

All rights reserved. No part of the material protected by this
copyright notice may be reproduced or utilized in any form,
electronic or mechanical, including photocopying, recording,
or by any information storage and retrieval system, without
written permission from the copyright owner.

Library of Congress Cataloging-in-Publication Data
Alcamo, I. Edward.
    Fundamentals of microbiology / I. Edward Alcamo.—6th ed.
      p. cm.
    Includes index.
    ISBN 0-7637-1067-9 (hardcover : alk. paper)
    1. Microbiology. 2. Medical microbiology. I. Title.
QR41.2 .A43 2000
579—dc21
                           00-024358
                           CIP

Printed in the United States of America

04 03 02 01 00 10 9 8 7 6 5 4 3 2

CREDITS

Chief Executive Officer: Clayton Jones
Chief Operating Officer: Don W. Jones, Jr.
Executive Vice President and Publisher: Tom Manning
V.P., Managing Editor: Judith H. Hauck
V.P., College Editorial Director: Brian L. McKean
V.P., Design and Production: Anne Spencer
V.P., Sales and Marketing: Paul Shepardson
Director of Manufacturing and Inventory: Therese Bräuer
Senior Development Editor: Dean DeChambeau
Special Projects Editor: Mary Hill
Assistant Production Editor: Jennifer Angel
Editorial/Production Assistant: Anne Trafton
Product Marketing Manager: Elizabeth Pearson
Interactive Technology Product Manager: W. Scott Smith
Interactive Technology Project Editor: Nicole Healey
Web Product Manager: Adam Alboyadjian
Website Design: Kristin Ohlin
Text and Cover Design: Seventeenth Street Studios
Production and Editorial Services: Seventeenth Street Studios
Artwork: Elizabeth Morales (technical art)
            Jim Bryant (Textbook Cases)
Photo Research: Sharon Donahue
Copy Editor: Betsy Dilernia
Indexing: Kathy Pitcoff
Cover Manufacture: Lehigh Press
Book Manufacture: Courier Kendallville

Brief Contents

Contents

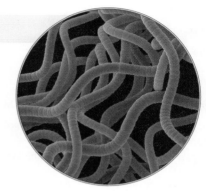

PART TWO

THE BACTERIA

4 Bacterial Structure and Growth

5 Bacterial Metabolism

6 Bacterial Genetics

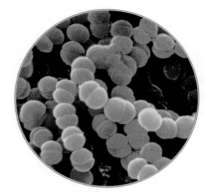

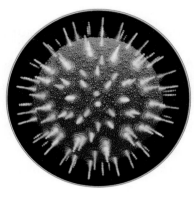

16 The Multicellular Parasites 509

PART FIVE
DISEASE AND RESISTANCE 530

17 Infection and Disease 533

18 Resistance and the Immune System 567

23 Chemotherapeutic Agents and Antibiotics 722

24 Microbiology of Foods 755

Preface

"A NEW EDITION FOR A NEW CENTURY"

I was here last century. I saw the emergence of AIDS, the development of genetic engineering, and the increasing interest in biofilms. I remember when Lyme disease came on the scene, when antibiotic resistance surfaced in bacteria, and when health officials implemented new standards for food safety. I was here when bioremediation was developed, when the role of RNA in protein synthesis was solidified, and when the reputation of normally benign *E. coli* was tarnished.

And I am going to share with you what I know about these and numerous other topics so you can be an enlightened and knowledgeable citizen of your community. I am going to bring you up to speed in microbiology so you can read a newspaper with understanding, talk to your doctor with confidence, and mix smoothly with other members of the health community. I am also going to give you a feel for what it was like to live in the 20th century.

But this is a book for the 21st century, so I will be giving you a glimpse of the future by exploring where microbiology is going in the years ahead. For example, it is becoming increasingly clear that microorganisms communicate among themselves, that viruses are far more complex than researchers ever imagined, and that new forms of defense against disease are waiting to be discovered on the other side of the hill. We'll see why knowing the human genome is important, why researchers believe a vaccine for tooth decay may soon be possible, and why epidemics of new diseases are probably around the corner. Hop aboard for the ride. I think you'll find it exhilarating.

Up-to-date content is only one of the new things in this book. The book has a new publisher and a new commitment to be the best microbiology text in today's bookstores. It is presented in rich and absorbing color, with completely new artwork and an abundance of new photographs, both macroscopic and microscopic. It contains a new series of "Textbook Cases" and many other new features. And the book retains the friendly accessibility that has endeared it to readers since it first appeared in 1983, a generation ago. Let me tell you more.

AUDIENCE

Fundamentals of Microbiology, Sixth Edition is written for introductory microbiology courses having an emphasis on the biology of human disease. It is geared toward students in health and allied health science curricula such as nursing, dental hygiene, medical assistance, sanitary science, and medical laboratory technology. It will also be an asset to students studying food science, agriculture, environmental science, and health administration. In addition, the text should provide a firm foundation for advanced programs in biological sciences, as well as medicine, dentistry, and other health professions.

OBJECTIVES

Fundamentals of Microbiology is an ambitious title for a book, because it suggests a broad coverage of microorganisms. I have attempted to fulfill that promise by conveying the multiple dimensions of microbiology and by showing that knowledge of microorganisms has enriched all segments of daily life. For example, the book contains numerous discussions of the roles microorganisms play in food production, mineral ecology, sewage disposal, and the emerging technologies of our time. Various sections also explain the abundance of life forms within the microbial world, the novel genetic features seen in microorganisms, and the basic patterns of infectious disease and resistance.

One of my most important objectives has always been accessibility. We both know that a book can be long on fact and information, but short on the ability to communicate. I have tried to guide you through the world of microorganisms by telling lots of stories (that was how people learned in past centuries); by focusing on the men and women who worked to make our knowledge base possible; by telling you *why* something is important, not just *that* it is important; and by sharing my fascination with the microbial world. I hope you will find the reading friendly and comfortable.

ORGANIZATION

Fundamentals of Microbiology, Sixth Edition is divided into seven major areas of concentration. These areas use basic principles as frameworks to provide the unity and diversity of microbiology. Among the principles explored are the variations in structure and growth of microorganisms, the basis for infectious disease and resistance, and the beneficial effects microorganisms have on our lives.

Part 1 deals with foundations of microbiology. It includes chapters on the origins of microbiology and the universal concepts that underpin the science. Part 2 then concentrates on the bacteria, since these are the microorganisms most of us think of when we say "germs." The discussions carry over to Part 3, where the spectrum of bacterial diseases is surveyed. Part 4 then looks at the significance of other microorganisms, including viruses, fungi, and protozoa.

In Part 5 of the text, the emphasis turns to infectious disease and the body's resistance through the immune system. Here, we study the reasons for disease and the means for surviving it. A logical segue is in Part 6, which presents various mechanisms for controlling microorganisms using such things as heat, radiations, disinfectants, and antibiotics. Part 7 closes the text with brief discussions of how public health measures interrupt epidemics. Some key insights are also given on the positive effects microorganisms exert through biotechnology.

WHY PATHOGENS?

Microorganisms perform many useful services for humans when they produce food products, manufacture organic materials in industrial plants, and recycle such elements as carbon and nitrogen. The emphasis of this book, however, is on the tiny, but important percentage of microorganisms that cause human disease, the so-called pathogens. Why do we emphasize pathogens? Here are several reasons:

■ Pathogens have regularly altered the course of human history.

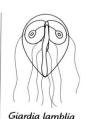

Giardia lamblia

- Pathogens are familiar to audiences of microbiology.

- Pathogens add drama to an invisible world of microorganisms.

- Pathogens illustrate ecological relationships between humans and micro-organisms.

- Pathogens point up the diversity of microorganisms.

Moreover, the study of pathogens makes basic science relevant and shows how microbiology interfaces with other disciplines such as sociology, economics, history, politics, and geography. Finally, the study of pathogens helps us to understand contemporary newspaper articles, magazine headlines, and stories on the late news. And in the end, that makes us better citizens. Indeed, the famous essayist Thomas Mann has written, "All interest in disease is only another expression of interest in life."

SPECIAL FEATURES

To help you achieve your learning goals and to reduce the anxiety that comes with approaching a new subject, the publisher and I have incorporated several features into this book. We hope that these features will enhance the accessibility of the key concepts and generate real enthusiasm for microbiology.

Introductions provide a stimulating thought or historical perspective to set the tone for the chapter.

Career Essays, titled "Microbiology Pathways," discuss various career options available.

Mid-Chapter Summaries, titled "To This Point," allow you to pause and summarize the previous few pages and preview the next few pages.

Boldface Terms highlight important terms and phrases in the text.

Marginal Pronunciations encourage you to learn the pronunciations of difficult terms as they are encountered in the text.

Marginal Definitions present succinct definitions of notable terms as they enter the discussion or recall them from previous uses.

MicroFocus Boxes explore stimulating topics of microbiological interest.

sit-ah-ko′sis

Serotypes:
variants of organisms that differ according to the antibodies they elicit from the immune system.

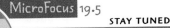

MicroFocus 19.5

STAY TUNED

Just when you thought you had seen it all, something new pops onto the radar screen. This time it's plantibodies. That's right, plantibodies—corn plants that produce human antibodies.

The proud parents are scientists from Agracetus Inc., a biotechnology company in Wisconsin. Using a secret gene-delivery system, the researchers force genes that encode human antibodies into the genome of corn seeds. Then they plant the latter in an unpretentious cornfield. When harvested by conven-

tional agricultural methods, ' kernels yield human antibod' be used to ferry radioisotop tumor cells and destroy ther 1999, the researchers were p' clinical trials of their new isot ery system.

But there's more. Alrea the fields are soybeans that herpes simplex antibodies (to genital herpes), and tobacco , manufacture streptococcal a The latter might be added to a

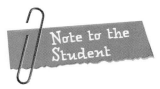

Summary Tables pull together the similarities and differences of topics discussed in the chapter.

Notes to the Student at the end of each chapter present an editorial comment within the framework of the chapter.

Questions for Thought and Discussion encourage you to use the text to resolve thought-provoking problems with contemporary relevance.

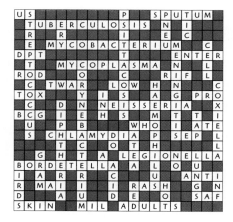

Chapter Reviews contain questions of a somewhat unconventional type to assist review of the chapter contents.

The **Glossary** lists over a thousand words used in the text together with a concise definition, pronunciation, and chapter location.

A postage-paid **Questionnaire** at the back of the text encourages you to express your views of the text and suggest improvements.

Textbook Cases present contemporary disease outbreaks in pictorial format.

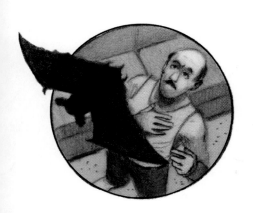

SUPPLEMENTS TO THE TEXT

We have developed a number of ancillaries that further amplify the concepts of this text:

The web site we have developed exclusively for this text, http://microbiology. jbpub.com, offers a variety of resources to enhance understanding of microbiology. The site contains eLearning, a free on-line study guide with review questions, chapter outlines, key term reviews, chapter objectives, and additional MicroFocus boxes.

Laboratory Fundamentals of Microbiology Sixth Edition is a series of 30 multipart laboratory exercises that provide basic training in the handling of microorganisms and help you understand the properties and uses of microorganisms.

The *Study Guide* that accompanies this textbook contains over 3000 practice exercises and study questions of various types to help you learn and retain the information in the text.

An anthology called *Encounters with Microbiology* brings together "Vital Signs" articles from *Discover* Magazine in which health professionals use their knowledge of microbiology in their medical cases.

The *Instructor's ToolKit CD-ROM* contains complete text files of the Instructor's Manual and Test Bank, an electronic test bank and test-generating software, full-color figures from the text for computer projection, and PowerPoint™ Lecture Outline slides.

The *Instructor's Manual and Test Bank* lists 2000 questions suitable for testing purposes, provides outlines for classroom lectures, summarizes each chapter, and provides answers to all the Questions for Thought and Discussion.

A set of *Acetate Overhead Transparencies* includes 100 color figures and 75 electron micrographs from the textbook.

Acknowledgments

Though authors traditionally receive credit (or vilification) for textbooks, the truth is that many talented people contribute their expertise to the final product. At Jones and Bartlett Publishers, the driving force behind this book has been Brian McKean, Vice-President and College Editorial Director. Brian signed me up, then took on various roles as supervising editor, drill sergeant, taskmaster, and make-it-happen person. Suffice to say that the publishing world needs more Brian McKeans.

I was particularly fortunate to work with some of the world's finest production professionals. Mary Hill supervised the production process with a firm but gentle and wise touch (Mary could sell refrigerators to Eskimos). Judy Hauck and Dean DeChambeau contributed their insightful and creative juices to the project and helped transform this book from the ordinary to something special. Betsy Dilernia was the copy editor *par excellence*; Lorrie Fink and the staff at Seventeenth Street Studios designed each page with elegance and care; Elizabeth Morales and Jim Bryant lent their considerable experience to the imaginative and sparkling artwork; Anne Trafton and Sharon Donahue hunted down many of the great photos that dress the pages; and Karen Bonura expertly typed much of the manuscript.

But the real hero was Jennifer Angel. Jenny was the Times Square of *Fundamentals*, the hub through which all the spokes of the wheel passed. She managed the never-ending series of day-to-day challenges and ensured that all the square pegs found their way to the square holes, and the round pegs to the round holes. I'll not forget Jenny's boundless drive to create the best book in the marketplace. To her and the countless other professionals who contributed their talents to this project, I extend a heartfelt word of thanks.

The book also benefited from the wisdom of my fellow microbiologists who have reviewed this edition. Reviewers for the Sixth Edition included Professors Katharine Gregg of West Virginia Wesleyan College; Fred A. Rosenberg of Northeastern University; Derald Smith of the University of Central Arkansas; Clifford W. Bond of Montana State University; Joseph Gauthier of the University of Alabama, Birmingham; Ruth E. Beattie of the University of Kentucky; Robert Alico of Indiana University of Pennsylvania; and David Filmer of Purdue University.

I am also indebted to the students and instructors like yourself who have written to me since the first edition was published in 1983. You've told me how to make this book more useful to your needs—what to add and what to eliminate—and you have encouraged me to take some unusual (and occasionally, light-hearted) steps to write a book that you can learn from. Microbiology is an imposing subject, but you have spurred me to present it so it can be understood. I thank you, and I hope you will continue to keep me on the straight-and-narrow path. In addition, I express my appreciation to the FedEx couriers who visited daily and broke the monotony with their spirited comments on Jets football and Yankees baseball.

I could not finish without acknowledging four of my favorite people: my children Michael, Tracey, Elizabeth, and Patricia. As I punch this out on my trusty PC, Michael is a successful attorney in New York City; Tracey is a computer whiz who keeps me current on emerging technologies; Elizabeth has just completed her doctoral degree (in molecular biology) at MIT and is now pursuing postdoctoral research at Stanford University; and Patricia has graduated from Princeton and is enjoying a rewarding career in business, with travels that take her nationally and internationally. No father could be prouder of his brood.

And I have saved the best for last. On April 11, 1999, the former Charlene Alice McPherson became my wife. Charlene and I met three years ago at an outing with our local hiking club. We fell in love, and we have walked in each other's footsteps ever since. Her love takes me to places I've not seen before and inspires me to accept the day-to-day challenges of writing a textbook. The poet put it this way: "We see ourselves best in the reflected love of another." This book is for her.

— E. Alcamo
Farmingdale, NY
Spring, 2000

To the Student

When I was a student, I hardly ever read the "To the Student" sections of my textbooks, and I only discovered later in my years what they contain. Therefore, I am encouraged that you are reading this, and I welcome the opportunity to let you know what *Fundamentals of Microbiology* is all about.

Let me begin by saying I have yet to meet a student who picked up a microbiology textbook for the sheer joy of it. I am assuming, therefore, that this book has been assigned as part of your microbiology program, and I have worked hard to make it your friend, and relieve some of the stress that comes with learning microbiology. Let me tell you how.

I have kept the chapters to approximately the same length so you can estimate the time necessary for each and plan your study accordingly. I have also avoided lengthy presentations and instead have focused on smaller sections, each with its own heading. These should accommodate short study periods, while providing flexibility for your instructor.

As you proceed, you will find many historical narratives within the chapters. All too often, significant events and the names of key investigators fall into obscurity. I have tried to resurrect these events and names to show that real people like ourselves pondered, experimented, and sometimes gave their lives to make the knowledge of microbiology possible. I have also tried to use current research trends to show you the direction microbiology is moving in the future.

They say the hardest part is the beginning, so I've tried to give careful attention to chapter introductions to usher you into the reading, and I have written midchapter summaries to let you reorient yourself before getting too deeply into the material—I hope these pauses will help you to see the forest for the trees. Several chapters contain stories of local disease outbreaks expressed as pictorial representations, a medium that may help you remember them better. We call them "Textbook Cases."

At the end of each chapter you will find a Note to the Student. This is where I have an opportunity to do a bit of soapboxing and present an editorial opinion relative to the chapter. A textbook writer has to be objective, and one soon gets tired of "just the facts." I have therefore added a personal thought or two, which I offer for your consideration. The end of the chapter also contains a Summary of the major principles of that chapter. It is a good idea to read the summary before delving into the chapter. That way you will have a framework of the chapter before filling in the nitty-gritty information.

I really enjoyed writing the thought questions, and I trust you will see them as challenging applications of microbiology. Perhaps they may even precipitate a classroom discussion or two, in which case they will fulfill my hope that you understand the relevance of microbiology. The review questions are a bit unconventional and should provide a refreshing alternative to the traditional type of short-answer questions. The traditional questions asking you to select, list, match, agree or disagree, summarize, and so forth can be found in the *Study Guide* that accompanies this text. Traditional questions can also be found on the eLearning page at this text's web site, http://microbiology.jbpub.com. Incidentally, there are more than 3000 questions in the *Study Guide* (plus more puzzles). That translates to over 100 questions per chapter at a cost of around one dollar per chapter. I think it is a good investment, and I hope you will agree.

As you leaf through the pages, you will note that the pronunciations of difficult words are presented alongside the word. Learning the correct pronunciations should increase your familiarity with the terms, make you more confident in using them, and add to your knowledge of microbiology. The pages also contain a running glossary of important terms. These definitions are culled from the neighboring text or from other places in the book where explanations are more complete. They should provide quick reviews and refreshers. It's also a good idea to frequently check the word's definition in the Glossary at the back of the book.

I'd like to say I'm taking a vacation after this book is published, but the truth of the matter is that I am already thinking about the Seventh Edition. I have no idea what it will contain, but that goes with the territory, for microbiology is like the everchanging sand on a beach. Indeed, keeping up with the microorganisms is a never-ending job.

And so, I'd like to close with an invitation: Please write and let me know what is good about this book so I can build on it and what is bad so I can change or eliminate it. To help you along, we've included a postage-paid Questionnaire at the back of the book. Simply clip it out, staple or tape it, and drop it in the mailbox—you don't even need a stamp. Also, I would be pleased to hear about any news of microbiology in your community, and I'd be happy to help you locate any information not covered in the text. I can be reached at the Department of Microbiology; State University of New York; Farmingdale, New York 11735. My phone number is 631-420-2423; or you can email me at alcamoie@farmingdale.edu.

Please accept my best wishes for a successful experience in microbiology. And welcome to the wild and wonderful world of microorganisms.

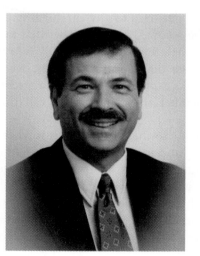

— *E. Alcamo*

Fundamentals
of Microbiology

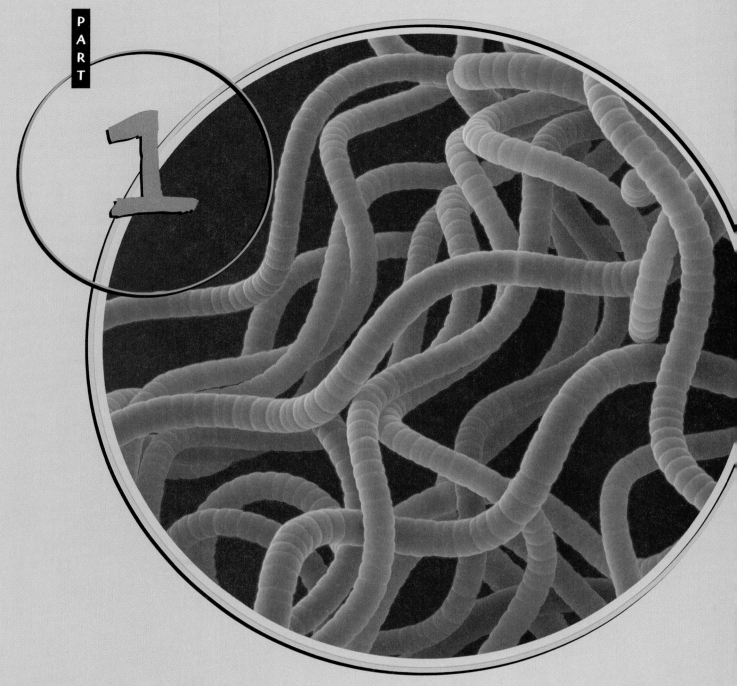

PART

1

Foundations of Microbiology

In 1676, a century before the Declaration of Independence, a Dutch merchant named Anton van Leeuwenhoek sent a noteworthy letter to the Royal Society of London. Writing in the vernacular of his home in the Netherlands, van Leeuwenhoek described how he used a primitive microscope to observe vast populations of minute creatures. His report opened a chapter of science that would evolve into the study of microscopic organisms and the discipline of microbiology. At that time, few people, including van Leeuwenhoek, attached any practical significance to the microorganisms, but during the next three centuries, scientists learned how profoundly they influence the quality of our lives.

We shall begin our study of the microorganisms by exploring the grass-roots developments that led to the establishment of microbiology as a science. These developments are surveyed in Chapter 1, where we focus on the individuals who stood at the forefront of discovery. You will note that Chapter 1 only goes as far as the early 1900s because the remaining chapters of this book describe the discoveries of microbiology since that time. Indeed, our understanding of microorganisms continues to grow even as you read this book.

Part 1 also contains a chapter on basic chemistry, inasmuch as microorganisms are chemical machines. Moreover, their activities are all related to chemistry. The third and final chapter in Part 1 will set down some basic concepts that apply to all microorganisms, much as the alphabet applies to word development. In succeeding chapters, we shall formulate words into sentences and sentences into ideas, as we survey the types of microorganisms and concentrate on their importance to public health and human welfare.

BEING A SCIENTIST

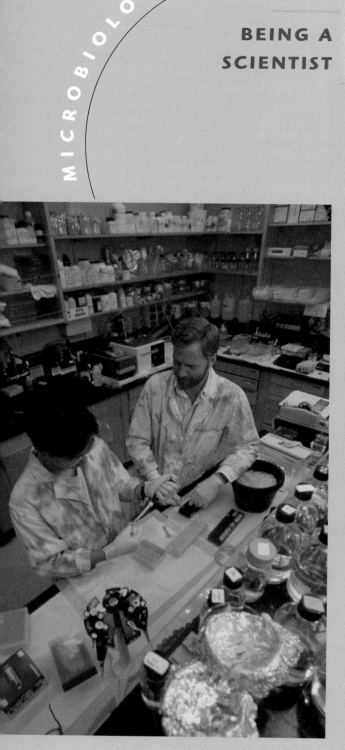

As you read the next chapter and those beyond, you might wonder why certain individuals have the good fortune to make key discoveries while others are not even mentioned in the pages of textbooks. To be sure, it is sometimes the luck of the draw, but in other cases individuals have a set of characteristics that put them on the trail to success.

Robert S. Root–Bernstein attempted to identify some of these characteristics in an article published in *The Sciences* (May/June 1988). Root–Bernstein points out that many prominent scientists like to goof around, play games, and surround themselves with a type of chaos aimed at revealing the unexpected. Their labs may appear to be a disorderly mess, but they know exactly where every tube or bottle belongs. Scientists also identify intimately with the things or creatures they study (it is said that Louis Pasteur actually dreamed about microorganisms), and this identification brings on an intuition, a sense about what an organism will do. Plus, there is the ability to recognize patterns that might eventually reveal hidden truths. (Pasteur had studied art as a teenager, and therefore he had an appreciation of patterns.)

In 1992, I received a letter from a student at Red Deer College in Alberta, Canada, asking why I became a microbiologist. Essentially, I answered, it was because I enjoyed my undergraduate microbiology course (thanks, Dr. Marazzella), and when I needed to select a graduate major, microbiology seemed like a good idea. I also think I had some of the characteristics described by Root–Bernstein: I loved to try out different projects; my corner of the world qualified as disaster area; still I was a nut on organization, insisting that all the square pegs fit into the square holes. If all this sounds familiar, then maybe you fit the mold of a scientist. Why not consider pursuing a career in microbiology? Some possibilities are listed in this book, but you should also visit with your instructor. Simply stop by the cafeteria, buy two cups of coffee, and you're on your way.

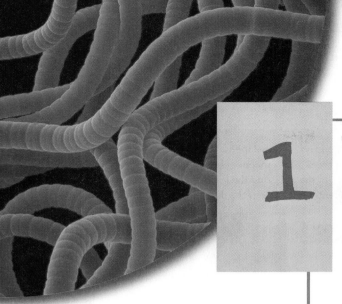

1 The Development of Microbiology

"There are science and the applications of science, separate yet bound together as the fruit of the tree."

—Louis Pasteur, describing how pure and practical science are related

DURING WORLD WAR II, a U.S. Navy fighting ship was cruising off the coast of California. One evening, the galley served baked ham without apparent consequences (except for the usual complaints). However, the leftovers remained overnight at room temperatures, and by morning, the ham was contaminated with staphylococci, the bacteria that cause food poisoning. Ham and eggs were on the morning's menu, and within hours, hundreds of sailors were severely indisposed.

staf'i-lo-kok'si

As the situation worsened, a senior officer radioed the Los Angeles Department of Health and asked advice on how to deal with the developing problem. When little assistance was forthcoming, he became exasperated and exclaimed, "What do we do if the Japanese fleet appears on the horizon?" Equally exasperated, the department director replied "Shoot over the damned ham!"

As we know, the Japanese fleet did not materialize that morning, nor did microorganisms have the opportunity to alter the course of history that particular time. But such was not the case in other instances. For example, the great plague of the 1300s changed the course of Western civilization so profoundly that it hastened the end of feudalism, encouraged the founding of the Protestant church, and spurred the invention of the clock (MicroFocus 1.1). A fungus may have precipitated the French Revolution, a bacterium put firepower into British guns during World War I, and a microscopic worm apparently interrupted the invasion of Taiwan during World War II.

Microorganisms: microscopic forms of life studied in microbiology.

MicroFocus 1.1

THE TRAGEDY OF EYAM

Each year a group of English pilgrims gather in the English countryside outside the village of Eyam, to pay homage to the townsfolk who gave their lives three centuries before so that others might live. The pilgrims pause, bow their heads, and remember.

Bubonic plague erupted in Eyam in the spring of 1666. The rich were the first to flee the town, and soon the commonfolk also considered leaving. However, they knew that by doing so they would probably spread the disease to nearby communities. At this point, the village rector made a passionate plea that they stay. After some deep soul-searching, most resolved to remain. They marked off a circle of stones outside the village limits, and people from the adjacent towns nervously brought food and supplies to the barrier, leaving it there for the self-quarantined villagers. In the end, 259 of the town's 350 residents succumbed to the plague.

The memorial service has a poignant moment as the pilgrims somberly recite a rhyme traced to that period:

Ring-a-ring of rosies
A pocketful of posies
Achoo! Achoo!
We all fall down.

There is no laughter in the group; indeed, some are moved to tears. The ring of rosies refers to the rose-shaped splotches on the chest and armpits of plague victims. Posies were tiny flowers the people hoped would ward off the evil spirits. "Achoo!" refers to the fits of sneezing that accompanied the disease. And the last line, the saddest of all, suggests the death that befell so many.

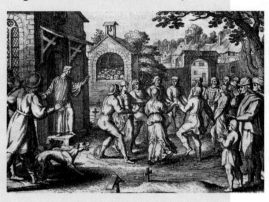

■ *A dance in a graveyard to ward off the plague.*

Smallpox:
a fatal viral disease of the skin, accompanied by extensive lesions.

Engaging as these stories are (and we shall explore all of them in this book), none is so profound as the involvement of microorganisms in disease. Microorganisms have carved out great swatches of humanity as epidemics passed over the land. Some diseases—such as typhoid fever, cholera, and smallpox—have become known as "slate-wipers," a reference to the barren towns they left in their wake; others—such as AIDS, measles, and polio—have been more insidious in their progress but no less dangerous.

Indeed, infectious disease has always left people thunderstruck with terror. Up to the 1850s, the fear of disease was compounded by ignorance because no one knew the cause of diseases, much less how to deal with them. Many strange brews and potions were offered as cures, but few were reliable, and some made an already bad situation even worse.

In the late 1800s, Louis Pasteur, Robert Koch, and their contemporaries forged the link between disease and microorganisms. Neither saw the connection in a blinding flash of light; instead both worked long, arduous hours to prove a germ theory of disease they believed to be true. And once their methods were established, scientists flocked to them from all corners of the world. Indeed, the explosion of research and discovery led to an understanding and control of many diseases, a dream anticipated for centuries.

The work of Pasteur, Koch, and their fellow scientists is a major theme of this chapter. But Pasteur and Koch were not the first to report microorganisms (by the 1800s, microorganisms were well established in the menageries of biologists). Thus, to begin our story, we reach back to the 1600s, where we encounter some equally inquisitive figures.

The Beginnings of Microbiology

An interest in microorganisms was developing almost 200 years before the time of Pasteur and Koch. In 1665, in England, a scientist named **Robert Hooke** published a work called *Micrographie*. The book contained a miscellany of his thoughts on chemistry, as well as a description of the microscope and its uses. Hooke did not invent the microscope (that distinction is generally attributed to Zacharias Janssen, a spectacles-maker from Middleburg, the Netherlands), but he did give it respectability.

Hooke's writings awakened the learned of Europe to the world of the very small. His illustrations included the eye of a fly, stinger of a bee, structure of a feather, shell of a protozoan, and plantlike form of a mold. He also described a slice of cork and suggested that it was composed of compartments, which he called "cells." By this account, he secured a place in the history of cell biology.

Mold:
a type of microorganism composed of threadlike filaments.
Protozoa:
animal-like microorganisms, often large and motile.

Other scientists were quick to follow Hooke's lead: The Dutch naturalist Jan Swammerdam described tiny bodies, the red blood cells, in blood. Another Dutchman, Regnier de Graaf, discovered cell clusters called follicles (known today as Graafian follicles) in the animal ovary. And the Italian physiologist Marcello Malpighi described the tiny capillaries of an animal's cardiovascular system.

ren'yā

mal-píg'ē

The discoveries by Hooke, Swammerdam, and others showed the microscope to be an important tool for unlocking the secrets of nature. It is not surprising, therefore, that scientists were interested when Anton van Leeuwenhoek revealed his descriptions of microorganisms in the 1670s. MicroFocus 1.2 discusses what life was like at that time.

MicroFocus 1.2

THAT WAS THEN . . .

Warning: Do not read this box if you are squeamish, if you've just finished eating, or if you get upset easily. We are going to tell you what life was like in Anton van Leeuwenhoek's time when no one had any inkling that microorganisms are the agents of infectious disease.

At that period in history, it was customary for a person to be bathed three times during his or her life: at birth, on getting married, and after death. This applied to people of nobility as well as peasants. Skin boils and abscesses were common.

There was no indoor plumbing, and chamber pots were often emptied out the window. The contents landed on the street below and remained there. In other places, flies moved easily from outdoor cesspools to the surfaces of foods, and when the cesspool flooded, its runoff mixed with the community drinking water. Typhoid fever, cholera, and dysentery were rampant.

There were no refrigerators, so food decomposed almost overnight. This left people the choice of either eating rotten food or starving. Food poisoning and botulism broke out often.

Rats patrolled the streets and were everywhere, carrying their fleas to all corners of the community. No one was without lice, and during the hot months, mosquitoes were as thick as fog. Epidemics of malaria, plague, and typhus fever occurred regularly.

As of the year 2000, the life expectancy of an average American was estimated to be roughly 78 years. In Europe, during van Leeuwenhoek's time (1775), the life expectancy was 42. Small wonder.

ANTON VAN LEEUWENHOEK

van-lu'en-hōk'

Anton van Leeuwenhoek (FIGURE 1.1a) was a draper and haberdasher and the owner of a dry goods business in Delft, the Netherlands. He enjoyed a comfortable living selling silk, wool, cotton, buttons, and baskets used to pack Delft china off to world markets. He was head of the City Council, inspector of weights and measures, and court surveyor. In his spare time, he ground pieces of glass into fine lenses, placing them between two silver or brass plates riveted together, as shown in FIGURE 1.1b. Gradually, he developed a skill that would remain unmatched for many generations.

Van Leeuwenhoek's lenses were no larger than the head of a pin, but by most accounts they could magnify an object over 200 times. Initially he used the lenses to inspect the quality of cloth, but as his fascination with microscopic objects developed, he examined hair fibers, skin scales, blood cells, and even samples of his own feces. At one point, van Leeuwenhoek observed tiny sperm cells and speculated that they contain microscopic embryos. As one anonymous writer penned:

> *He worked instead of tending store,*
> *At grinding special lenses for*
> *A microscope. Some of the things*
> *He looked at were: mosquito wings,*
> *The hairs of sheep, the legs of lice,*
> *The skin of people, dogs, and mice.*

FIGURE 1.1

Anton van Leeuwenhoek

(a) Van Leeuwenhoek at work in his study. Using a primitive microscope, van Leeuwenhoek was able to achieve magnifications of over 200 times and describe various biological specimens, including numerous types of microorganisms. (b) Details of van Leeuwenhoek's lens system. The object is placed on the point of the specimen mount. The mount is adjusted by turning the focusing screw and the elevating screw. Light is reflected from the specimen through the lens, thereby magnifying the specimen.

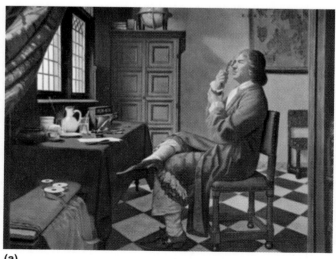

(a)

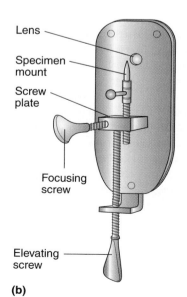

Lens

Specimen mount

Screw plate

Focusing screw

Elevating screw

(b)

Van Leeuwenhoek's work did not go unnoticed. Probably the only scientific group of that period was the Royal Society of London, but correspondence with this group was tenuous because England and the Netherlands were bitter rivals for commercial treasures of the East Indies. Nevertheless, in 1673 Regnier de Graaf, a fellow of the Royal Society, urged members to contact van Leeuwenhoek. They did so, and van Leeuwenhoek was soon sending along his illustrations and observations.

In September 1674, van Leeuwenhoek filled a glass with greenish, cloudy water from a marshy lake outside Delft and placed a sample under his lens. The water teemed with tiny microorganisms, which he called **animalcules.** His curiosity aroused, van Leeuwenhoek soon located animalcules in rainwater, in material from his own teeth and feces, and eventually in most specimens he examined. The creatures astonished him at first, then delighted and perplexed him as he pondered their origin and purpose.

In 1676, van Leeuwenhoek sent his eighth letter to the Royal Society. This letter, published the next year, has special significance to microbiology because it contains his first description of microorganisms:

> *May the 26th, I took about ⅓ of an ounce of whole pepper and having pounded it small, I put it into a Thea-cup with 2½ ounces of Rainwater upon it, stirring it about, the better to mingle the pepper with it, and then suffering the pepper to fall to the bottom. After it had stood an hour or two, I took some of the water, before spoken of, wherein the whole pepper lay, and wherein were so many several sorts of little animals; and mingled it with this water, wherein the pounded pepper had lain an hour or two, and observed that, when there was much of the water of the pounded pepper, with that other, the said animals soon died, but when little they remained alive.*

> *June 2, in the morning, after I had made divers observations since the 26th of May, I could not discover any living thing, but saw some creatures, which tho they had the figures of little animals, yet could I perceive no life in them how attentively I beheld them. . . .*

Van Leeuwenhoek's sketches were elegant in detail and clarity. In succeeding letters, he outlined structural details of the familiar protozoa *Paramecium* and *Amoeba,* and he described the threadlike fungi, as well as certain microscopic algae. A particularly noteworthy letter, written in 1683, included drawings of what are now believed to be bacterial rods, spheres, and spirals. FIGURE 1.2 illustrates how van Leeuwenhoek perceived them. His work, performed exclusively with single-lens microscopes, opened the door to a completely new concept of the makeup of all living things.

Royal Society:
an English scientific society of physicists, chemists, and biologists founded in the 1660s and in existence today.

an-i-mal'cules
Animalcules:
Anton van Leeuwenhoek's term for microorganisms.

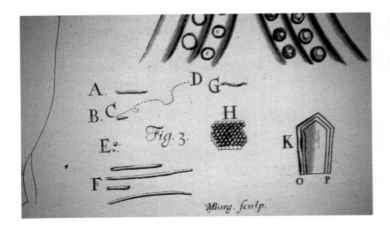

FIGURE 1.2

Van Leeuwenhoek's Drawings of Bacteria

Examples from a letter written by van Leeuwenhoek to the Royal Society dated September 17, 1683. Both A and B represent rod forms, with C and D indicating the pathway of motion. A spherical form is shown in E and longer types are depicted in F. The type shown in G appears to be a spiral form, and a cluster of spheres is shown in H. Van Leeuwenhoek found many of these organisms between his teeth.

In 1680, van Leeuwenhoek was elected to fellowship in the Royal Society, and, with Isaac Newton and Robert Boyle, he became one of the most famous men of his time. Peter the Great of Russia and the Queen of England came to peer into his microscopes. His technique was so fastidious that when some of his slides were discovered 300 years later, scientists found perfectly preserved specimens of cotton seeds, slices of cork, and the optic nerve of a cow. In all, van Leeuwenhoek bombarded the Royal Society with over 200 letters about his findings. He died in 1723 at the age of 90 (his longevity a notable achievement in itself).

Van Leeuwenhoek was a very suspicious and secretive person. He invited no one to work with him, nor did he show anyone how to grind lenses or construct a microscope. This is one reason why interest in the microorganisms waned after his death. Another reason, and perhaps of more significance, is that scientists of the day saw the microorganisms as curiosities of nature. In the 1700s, disease was still shrouded in magic and mysticism, and few people believed that microorganisms could cause disease in so lofty a creature as the human being. Thus, the development of microbiology would be delayed until the technology for an efficient microscope emerged and an association was drawn between microorganisms and disease. This would not happen until the late 1800s.

1.2 The Transition Period

Biology in the 1700s was a body of knowledge without a focus. Basically, it consisted of observations of plant and animal life and attempts to place the organisms in some logical order. New World explorers returned to Europe regularly with specimens to be described and catalogued, and interest in the variety of life forms grew. The dominant figure of the era was **Carolus Linnaeus,** a Swedish botanist who brought the plants and animals together under one great classification scheme (Chapter 3).

A few scientists continued to explore the microscopic world. In 1718, for example, Louis Joblot published a review of protozoa, and in 1725 Abraham Tremblay described the simple animal known as the hydra. However, scientists did not believe that microscopic organisms could cause infection. Rather, they theorized that infectious disease spread by an altered chemical quality of the atmosphere, an entity called **miasma.** Miasma arose from decaying or diseased bodies known as miasms. The **miasma theory** figured prominently in medical thinking well into the 1800s.

As the years unfolded, some biologists began to scrutinize the laws of nature and to question the origin of living things as they exist today. The resulting controversy surrounding spontaneous generation could be answered only by experimentation. Explorations of this type reached to the very essence of biology and bridged the gap between van Leeuwenhoek's time and the mid-1800s.

SPONTANEOUS GENERATION

In the fourth century B.C., Aristotle wrote that flies, worms, and other small animals arise from decaying matter (i.e., without the need of parent organisms). His observations laid the basis for the doctrine of **spontaneous generation,** a belief that lifeless substances could give rise to living creatures. Indeed, in the early 1600s, the eminent Flemish physician Jan Baptista van Helmont lent credence to the belief when he observed that rats "originate" from wheat bran and old rags. Common peo-

lin-ā'us

job-lo'
Hydra:
a multicellular aquatic animal having long fingerlike projections.

mi-az'mah

Spontaneous generation:
the doctrine that held that lifeless objects give rise to living organisms.

ple embraced the idea, for even they could see slime "breeding" toads and meat "generating" wormlike maggots.

Among the first to dispute the theory of spontaneous generation was the Florentine scientist **Francesco Redi.** Noting van Leeuwenhoek's complex descriptions of tiny animals, Redi reasoned that flies had reproductive organs. He suggested that flies land on pieces of exposed meat and lay their eggs, which then hatch to maggots. In the 1670s, Redi performed a series of tests in which he covered jars of meat with fine lace, thereby preventing the entry of flies. So protected, the meat would not produce maggots. Redi temporarily put to rest the notion of spontaneous generation. His work was one of history's first experiments in biology (FIGURE 1.3).

Although Redi's work became widely known, science in the 1700s had theological overtones, and some radical philosophers found spontaneous generation to be useful in showing that God had no place in creation. Reports of microorganisms were becoming widespread during that period, and in 1748 a British clergyman named **John Needham** suggested that microorganisms arise spontaneously in flasks of mutton gravy. Needham even boiled several flasks of gravy and sealed the flasks with corks, as Redi had sealed his jars. Still, the microorganisms appeared. The Royal Society of London was duly impressed and elected Needham to membership.

However, an Italian cleric and scientist, **Abbé Lazzaro Spallanzani,** criticized Needham's work. In 1767, Spallanzani boiled meat and vegetable broths for long periods of time and then sealed the necks by melting the glass. As control experiments, he left some flasks open to the air, stoppered some loosely with corks, and boiled some briefly, as Needham had done. After two days, he found the control flasks swarming with organisms, but the sealed flasks contained none. Spallanzani's

Maggots: wormlike larvae of certain insects, such as houseflies.

red′ē

nēd′am

spa′lan-zan′e

FIGURE 1.3

Francesco Redi: Disputing Spontaneous Generation

In the 1670s, Francesco Redi (a) attempted to disprove the belief that maggots (fly larvae) arise from decaying meat. (b) He placed a piece of meat in an open jar and showed that maggots originate as eggs laid by flies. People of that period believed that the maggots arose spontaneously from the decaying meat. He then placed a second meat sample in a jar covered with lace. The flies could not reach the meat, and maggots did not appear on the surface. This relatively simple experiment disproved spontaneous generation and was among the first ever performed in biology.

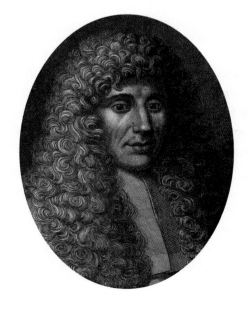

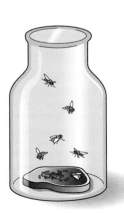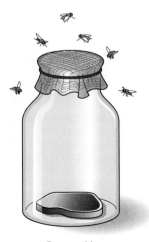

Open jar—maggots appear on meat

Covered jar— no maggots

(a)   **(b)**

experiment did not settle the issue, though. Needham countered that Spallanzani had destroyed the "vital force" of life with excessive amounts heat. Other scientists suggested that the air necessary for life had been excluded.

The controversy over spontaneous generation was no closer to being resolved as the 1800s began. However, the debate focused attention on the fundamental nature of life and encouraged scientists to experiment in biology.

DISEASE TRANSMISSION

fra′cos-tor′o

While spontaneous generation was being debated, other scientists studied how disease was transmitted. As early as 1546, the Italian poet and scientist **Girolamo Fracostoro** wrote: "Contagion is an infection that passes from one thing to another." Fracostoro recognized three forms of passage: contact, lifeless objects, and air (TABLE 1.1). His ideas were later interwoven with the miasma theory.

kir′ker

The notion that microorganisms were the substance of contagion received little credibility, however. Thus, Athanasius Kircher was paid little attention when he reported "microscopic worms" in the blood of plague victims; nor was Christian Fabricius taken seriously in the 1700s when he suggested that fungi cause rust and smut diseases in plants. On the contrary, Edward Jenner was accorded many honors in 1798 when he discovered immunization for smallpox (MicroFocus 1.3), despite his inability to explain the cause of the disease.

sem′el-vīse

Blood poisoning:
a colloquial expression for infectious disease of the blood.

By the mid-1800s enough knowledge had accumulated to convince physicians that disease could be transmitted among individuals, and that the transmission could be interrupted. The works of two investigators, **Ignaz Semmelweis** and **John Snow,** intensified this belief. Semmelweis was a Hungarian physician who, in 1847, reported that the agent of blood poisoning was transmitted to maternity patients by physicians fresh from performing autopsies in the mortuary. Semmelweis showed that hand washing in chlorine water could stop the spread of disease (Chapter 22). Snow, a British physician, traced the source of cholera to the municipal water supply of London during an 1854 outbreak. He reasoned that by avoiding the contam-

TABLE 1.1

Some Early Observations in Microbiology

INVESTIGATOR	TIME FRAME	OBSERVATIONS/CONCLUSIONS
Aristotle	Fourth century B.C.	Living things do not need parents; spontaneous generation apparently occurs
Fracostoro	Mid-1500s	"Contagion" passes among individuals, objects, and air
Kircher	Mid-1600s	"Microscopic worms" are present in blood of plague victims
Redi	Mid-1600s	Fly larvae do not arise by spontaneous generation
Van Leeuwenhoek	Late 1600s	Microscopic organisms are present in numerous environments
Fabricius	Early 1700s	Fungi cause plant disease
Joblot	Early 1700s	Various forms of protozoa exist
Needham	Mid-1700s	Microorganisms in broth arise by spontaneous generation
Spallanzani	Mid-1700s	Heat destroys microorganisms in broth
Jenner	Late 1700s	Recoverers from cowpox do not contract smallpox
Semmelweis	Mid-1800s	Chlorine disinfection prevents disease spread
Snow	Mid-1800s	Water is involved in disease transmission

MicroFocus 1.3

AHEAD OF HIS TIME

In the 1700s, smallpox was hardly ever absent from Europe. In England, epidemics were so severe that one-third of the children died before reaching the age of three. Many victims were blinded by smallpox, and most people were left pockmarked for life.

But for those who survived the pox, immunity lasted forever. People therefore sought a way of contracting a mild form of the disease. From the Far East came word of inoculation parties. A doctor would make a small wound in the arm and insert a few drops of pus from a smallpox skin lesion. A walnut was then tied over the area. Though mild smallpox often resulted, there was the danger of developing a deadly form.

Then came Edward Jenner. In the 1700s, while apprenticed to a country surgeon, Jenner learned that people who experienced cowpox were apparently immune to smallpox. Cowpox was a disease of the udders of cows. It was common in farmers and milkmaids, and it expressed itself as a mild, smallpoxlike disease.

For years, Jenner pondered whether intentionally giving cowpox to people would protect them against smallpox.

He finally decided to put the matter to the test. In 1796, a dairy maid named Sarah Nelmes came to his office, the lesions of cowpox evident on her hand. Jenner took material from her lesions and scratched it into the skin of a boy named James Phipps. Several weeks later he inoculated young Phipps with material from a smallpox lesion. Within days, the boy developed a reaction at the site but failed to show any sign of smallpox.

Jenner continued his experiments for two years, switching to infected cows as a source of cowpox material. In 1798, he published an historic pamphlet on his work that generated considerable interest. Prominent physicians confirmed his findings, and within a few years, Jenner's method of "vaccination" spread through the world (*vacca* is Latin for "cow"). It is estimated that by 1801, some 100,000 people in England were vaccinated. In Russia, the first child vaccinated was renamed Vaccinor and was educated by the state. And President Thomas Jefferson wrote to Jenner: "You have erased from the calendar of human afflictions one of its

greatest. Yours is the comfortable reflection that mankind can never forget that you have lived."

A hundred years passed before scientists realized that the milder cowpox viruses were setting up a defensive mechanism in the body against the deadlier smallpox viruses. It is thus remarkable that Jenner accomplished what he did. His experimentation methods and interpretation of the vaccination results might well serve as models for accurate and careful laboratory work in modern microbiology.

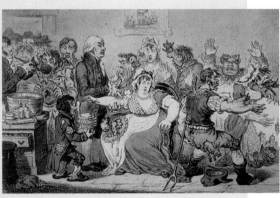

■ *A cartoon from Jenner's time showing skepticism for his new method.*

inated water source, people could avoid the disease (Chapter 17). In their work, both Semmelweis and Snow also drew attention to the fact that a poison or unseen object in the environment, not a miasma, was responsible for disease (**FIGURE 1.4**). Proof, however, was still lacking.

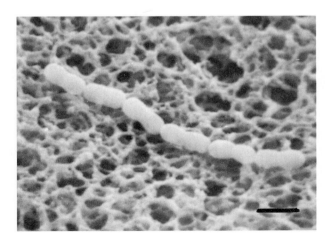

FIGURE 1.4

A Streptococcus

An electron microscopic view of a bacterium known as a streptococcus. The bacterium has been caught on the rough surface of a filter, and the cells appear in chains typical of a streptococcus. A species of streptococcus is now known to be one of the causes of the "blood poisoning" studied by Semmelweis. The bar represents a length of one micrometer (1 μm) or 0.001 millimeter.

To this point . . .

We have explored the development of microbiology by focusing on the work of Anton van Leeuwenhoek and illustrating how he called attention to a previously invisible world of microorganisms. In the late 1600s, van Leeuwenhoek communicated with the Royal Society of London and portrayed many commonly recognized microorganisms, including protozoa, fungi, and bacteria. After his death, however, there was little interest in microbiology because microscopes were unavailable and because people simply could not conceive that organisms so tiny could bring on something so overpowering as sickness and death.

We then described spontaneous generation and showed how the controversy surrounding this doctrine stirred people to question the nature of living things and take heed of the existence of microorganisms. Redi, Needham, and Spallanzani achieved distinction during the controversy. We next focussed on disease transmission. We explored the works of Semmelweis and Snow to show how scientists were coming to believe that something tangible in nature was causing disease. This specific agent contrasted with the miasma theory, which pointed to a vague, intangible disease cause.

In the next section we shall see how Louis Pasteur and Robert Koch sought to establish the principle that microorganisms cause infectious disease. We shall discuss their experiments in depth and observe how the proofs for the germ theory of disease evolved. As the foundations of microbiology were strengthened, many other scientists expanded the work of Pasteur and Koch, and worldwide interest in microorganisms emerged. Modern microbiology is a product of that interest.

1.3

The Golden Age of Microbiology

Microbiology blossomed during a period of about 60 years referred to as the **Golden Age of Microbiology.** The period began in 1857 with the work of Louis Pasteur and continued into the twentieth century until the advent of World War I. During these years, numerous branches of microbiology were established, and the foundations were laid for the maturing process that has led to modern microbiology.

LOUIS PASTEUR

dif-thē′rē-ah
Diphtheria:
a bacterial disease, accompanied by clogging of the respiratory passageways, especially in children

In a world ravaged by plague, tuberculosis, typhoid fever, and diphtheria, a large family was often necessary to ensure the next generation. Neither royalty nor commonfolk were immune to disease. There were virtually no cures for disease. Indeed, no one was really sure what caused it.

Such were the times in which **Louis Pasteur** (FIGURE 1.5) studied at the French school, the *École Normale Supérieure.* In 1848, he achieved distinction in organic chemistry for his discovery that tartaric acid, a four-carbon organic compound, forms two different types of crystals. Using a microscope, Pasteur successfully separated the crystals and developed a skill that aided his later studies of microorganisms. In 1854, at the age of 32, he was appointed Professor of Chemistry at the University of Lille in northern France.

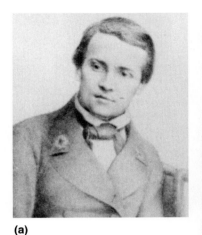

(a)

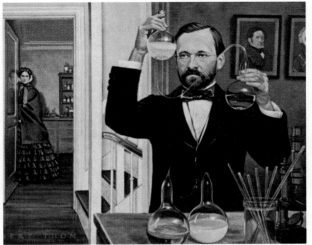

(b)

FIGURE 1.5

Louis Pasteur

Two portraits of Louis Pasteur, one of the founders of the science of microbiology. (a) As a young man while studying chemistry at the *École Normale Supérieure.* (b) As a scientist working in a makeshift laboratory in his home. In his right hand, Pasteur holds a flask of broth previously exposed to the air and now cloudy with growth. In his left hand, he is holding a swan-neck flask that is clear because microscopic organisms cannot enter through the flask's neck.

Pasteur believed that the discoveries of science should have practical applications. He therefore grasped the opportunity in 1857 to try and unravel the mystery of why local wines were turning sour. The prevailing theory held that wine fermentation results from the chemical breakdown of grape juice to alcohol. No living thing seemed to be involved. But Pasteur's microscope consistently revealed large numbers of tiny **yeast cells** overlooked by other scientists. Moreover, he noticed that sour wines contained populations of barely visible sticks and rods, known then and now as **bacteria.**

Yeast cells: oval or round microorganisms important in fermentation, baking, and other industrial processes.

In a classic series of experiments, Pasteur clarified the role of yeasts in fermentation and showed that bacteria were responsible for sour wine. First he removed all traces of yeasts from a flask of grape juice and set the juice aside to ferment. Nothing happened. Next he added back the yeasts, and soon the fermentation was proceeding normally. He then found that if he could remove all bacteria from the grape juice, the wine would not turn sour.

Pasteur's work shook the scientific community. His results demonstrated that yeast cells and bacteria are tiny, living factories where important chemical changes take place. His work also drew attention to microorganisms as agents of change, because bacteria appeared to make the wine "sick." For years, physicians had interpreted bacteria as an *effect* of disease; that is, they were thought to arise in the body during illness. Pasteur's work appeared to indicate that they could be a *cause* of disease, for if they could sour the wine, perhaps they could also make people sick. In 1857, Pasteur published a short paper on souring by bacteria. In the paper, he implied that microorganisms were related to human illness and set down the foundation for the **germ theory of disease.** Essentially, this theory holds that microorganisms are responsible for infectious diseases.

Germ: a common word for a microorganism.

Pasteur also recommended a practical solution to the sour wine problem. He suggested that grape juice be heated to destroy all the evidence of life, after which yeasts should be added to begin the fermentation. An alternative was to heat the wine after fermentation and before aging, when the bacteria soured it. Acceptance of his technique, known as **pasteurization,** gradually ended the problem and made Pasteur famous. His elation was tempered with sadness, however. In 1859, his daughter Jeanne died of typhoid fever.

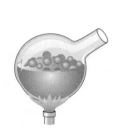

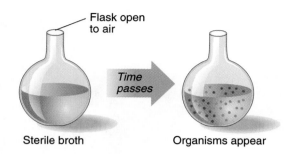

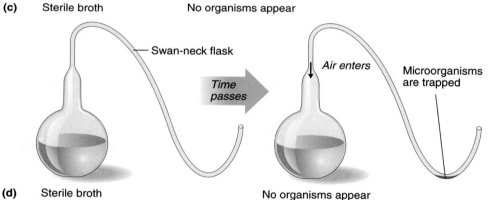

Each experiment begins with sterilized broth. Any living things the broth may have contained have been destroyed by heat.

(a) Sterile broth — Organisms appear

Pasteur: The broth provides a nutrient medium for the growth of unseen organisms in the air: life comes from other life.

His critics: A sterilized broth gives rise to life: spontaneous generation.

(b) Sterile broth — No organisms appear

Pasteur: The heat has killed the microorganisms in the air.

His critics: Sealing the flask prevents entry of the "life force."

(c) Sterile broth — No organisms appear

Pasteur: The heat has killed the microorganisms in the air.

His critics: Sterilizing the air kills the "life force."

(d) Sterile broth — No organisms appear

Pasteur: No living thing will appear in the flask because microorganisms will not be able to reach the broth.

His critics: If the "life force" has free access to the flask, life will appear, given enough time.

Some days later the flask is still free of any living thing. Pasteur has disproved the doctrine of spontaneous generation.

FIGURE 1.6

Pasteur and the Spontaneous Generation Controversy

(a) When a flask of sterilized broth is left open to the air, organisms appear.
(b) When a flask of sterilized broth is boiled and sealed, no living things appear.
(c) When air entering a flask of sterilized broth is heated with a flame, no living things appear. (d) Broth sterilized in a swan-neck flask is left open to the air. The curvature of the neck traps dust particles and microorganisms, preventing them from reaching the broth.

PASTEUR AND DISEASE

Pasteur's interest in microorganisms rose as he learned more about them. He found bacteria in soil, water, air, and the blood of disease victims. Extending his germ theory of disease, he reasoned that if microorganisms were acquired from the environment, their spread could be controlled. If so, perhaps the chain of disease transmission could be broken. However, many scientists stubbornly stuck to the notion that bacteria arise spontaneously from organic matter and that disease is inevitable as long as the "life force" is present. Pasteur was therefore drawn into the lingering debate on spontaneous generation, and he sought to discredit the doctrine in order to salvage his own germ theory of disease.

Pasteur first showed that where disease was rampant, the air was full of microorganisms, but where disease was uncommon, the air was clean. He opened flasks of nutrient-rich broth to air from the crowded city, then from the countryside, and next from a high mountain. In each succeeding experiment, fewer flasks became contaminated with microorganisms. Still, his critics were vocal. When he boiled broths and showed that they remained free of life, the critics argued that boiling destroyed the "life force" believed to reside in the air.

Finally, in an elegant series of experiments, Pasteur silenced all but the most extreme supporters of spontaneous generation. He prepared broth in a series of **swan-neck flasks,** so named because their S-shaped necks resembled a swan's. Pasteur boiled the flasks, then left them open to the air and any "life force." However, the S-shaped curvature of the neck trapped airborne microorganisms and prevented their entry to the flask. No microorganisms grew in the broth. When the neck was cut off, however, airborne organisms quickly fell into the broth, and growth appeared within hours. Pasteur's classic experiment is outlined in FIGURE 1.6.

Pasteur's work brought to an end the long and tenacious debate on spontaneous generation begun two centuries earlier. By now he was a national celebrity. Once more, however, tragedy entered his life; in 1865, his 2-year-old daughter Camille developed a tumor and died of blood poisoning. Pasteur realized that he was no closer to solving the riddle of disease.

That same year, 1865, **cholera** engulfed Paris, killing 200 people a day. Pasteur attempted to capture the responsible bacterium by filtering the hospital air and trapping the bacteria in cotton. Unfortunately, Pasteur was unable to cultivate one bacterium apart from the others because he was using broth. (In later experiments, Koch would use solid culture media instead of broth media.) Although Pasteur demonstrated that bacterial inoculations made animals ill, he could not pinpoint an exact cause. Some of his critics claimed that a poison, or toxin, in the broth was responsible for the disease.

In an effort to help French industry, Pasteur turned his attention to **pébrine,** the disease of **silkworms.** Late in 1865, he identified a protozoan infesting the silkworms and the mulberry leaves fed to them. Next he separated the healthy silkworms from the diseased silkworms and their food, and he managed to quell the spread of disease. The achievement strengthened the germ theory of disease. For Pasteur, however, it was another time of grief. Cecille, his third daughter, died of typhoid fever in 1866 (at the age of 12). Again he returned to the study of human disease.

ROBERT KOCH

Although Pasteur failed to relate a specific organism to a specific human disease, his work stimulated others to investigate the nature of microorganisms and to ponder

Organic matter:
chemical substances associated with living things.

Swan-neck flasks:
broth flasks having an S-shaped curvature to trap dust and microorganisms.

Cholera:
a bacterial disease of the intestines, accompanied by loss of large volumes of fluid.

Toxin:
a chemical substance poisonous to the body tissues.

pa-brēn

FIGURE 1.7

Joseph Lister and Robert Koch

(a) Joseph Lister was a British physician who was impressed with the work of Pasteur and who promulgated the germ theory of disease. In the 1860s, Lister introduced the principles of sterile surgery to his practice. (b) Koch was one of the first to relate a specific organism to a specific disease, and thus verify the germ theory of disease.

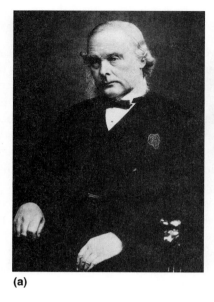

(a)

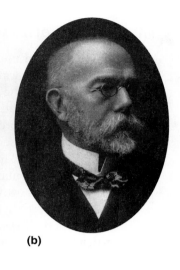

(b)

Relapsing fever:
a bacterial disease, accompanied by recurring periods of fever.

koke

Aqueous humor:
the sterile gel-like fluid behind the lens of the eye.
Spore:
a highly resistant oval body formed by certain types of bacteria.

Koch's postulates:
a series of procedures by which a specific microorganism can be related to a specific infectious disease.

their association with disease. For example, Gerhard Hansen, a Norwegian physician, identified bacteria in the tissues of leprosy patients in 1871, and Otto Obermeier of Germany described bacteria in the blood of relapsing fever patients in 1873. Another German bacteriologist, Ferdinand J. Cohn, discovered that bacteria multiply by dividing into two cells. In England, **Joseph Lister** (FIGURE 1.7a) was sufficiently impressed with Pasteur's writings on disease to begin applying antiseptics to wound infections.

The definitive verification of the germ theory of disease was offered by **Robert Koch** (FIGURE 1.7b), a country doctor from East Prussia (now part of Germany). Koch's primary interest was **anthrax,** a deadly blood disease in cattle and sheep. Anthrax was a threat to farmers because it ravaged their herds periodically and seemed to reappear time and again in the same district without warning.

Koch was determined to learn more about anthrax. In 1875, in a makeshift laboratory in his home, he injected mice with the blood of diseased sheep and cattle. He then performed meticulous autopsies and noted the same symptoms appearing regularly. Next, he isolated a few rod-shaped bacilli from the blood in the sterile aqueous humor of an ox's eye. Koch watched for hours as the bacilli multiplied, formed tangled threads, and finally reverted to highly resistant spores. At this point, he took several spores on a sliver of wood and injected them into healthy mice. The symptoms of anthrax appeared within hours. Koch autopsied the animals and found their blood swarming with bacilli. He reisolated the bacilli in fresh aqueous humor. The cycle was now complete.

A year later Koch presented his work at the University of Breslau. Scientists there were astonished. Here was the verification of the germ theory of disease that had eluded Pasteur and for which many scientists were waiting. Koch's procedures came to be known as **Koch's postulates.** These techniques, illustrated in FIGURE 1.8, were adopted as a guide for relating specific organisms to specific diseases. The postulates state that the same microorganism must be identified in all cases of the disease, the microorganism must be isolated and cultivated in pure culture, and the disease must be reproduced in experimental animals inoculated with these pure cultures. The same microorganism must then be recovered. (Originally the postulates had been outlined in 1840 by Jakob Henle, a German researcher. One of his students was Robert Koch.)

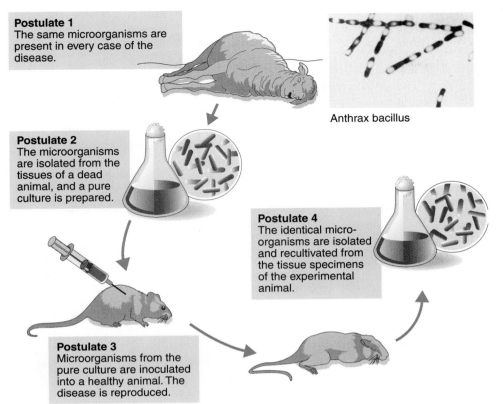

Postulate 1
The same microorganisms are present in every case of the disease.

Anthrax bacillus

Postulate 2
The microorganisms are isolated from the tissues of a dead animal, and a pure culture is prepared.

Postulate 4
The identical microorganisms are isolated and recultivated from the tissue specimens of the experimental animal.

Postulate 3
Microorganisms from the pure culture are inoculated into a healthy animal. The disease is reproduced.

FIGURE 1.8

A Demonstration of Koch's Postulates

Koch's postulates are used to relate a single microorganism to a single disease. The photo shows the rods of the anthrax bacillus as Koch observed them. Many rods are swollen with spores.

KOCH AND PURE CULTURE TECHNIQUES

After the sensation at Breslau subsided, Koch returned to his laboratory and developed numerous staining methods for bacteria. In 1880 he accepted an appointment to the Imperial Health Office, and while there he happened upon the **cultivation techniques** that sparked the further development of microbiology.

Koch chanced to observe that a slice of potato contained small masses of bacteria, which he termed **colonies.** Colonies contained millions of only one kind of bacterium. Seeing that bacteria could grow and multiply on solid surfaces, Koch added gelatin to his broth to prepare a **solid culture medium.** He then inoculated bacteria to the surface and set the medium aside to incubate. Next morning, visible colonies were present on the surface. When the colonies grew together, a **pure culture** formed. Koch could now inoculate laboratory animals with a pure culture of bacteria and be certain that only one species of bacterium was involved. His work proved that bacteria, not toxins in the broth, were the cause of disease. MicroFocus 1.4 details a further advance in cultivation techniques.

In 1881, Koch demonstrated his pure culture techniques to the International Medical Congress, meeting at Lister's laboratory in London. Pasteur and several of his co-workers were present as Koch outlined his methods. Several days later, Koch received a personal letter of congratulations from Pasteur.

Colony:
a visible mass of microorganisms, usually of a single type.

Pure culture:
an accumulation of one type of microorganism formed by the growth of colonies of that organism.

THE COMPETITION PERIOD

At another point in history, Pasteur and Koch might have become friends and colleagues in their search for the agents of disease. However, the years following the 1870 Franco-Prussian war were accompanied by fierce national pride. Both France and Germany were undergoing unification, and heroes played an important role in

MicroFocus 1.4

JAMS, JELLIES, AND MICROORGANISMS

One of the major developments in microbiology was Robert Koch's use of a solid culture medium on which bacteria would grow. He accomplished this by solidifying beef broth with gelatin. When inoculated onto the surface of the nutritious medium, bacteria grew vigorously at room temperature and produced discrete, visible mounds of cells.

On occasion, however, Koch was dismayed to find that the gelatin turned to liquid. It appeared that certain types of bacteria were producing a chemical substance to digest the gelatin. Moreover, gelatin liquefied at the high incubator temperatures commonly used to cultivate certain bacteria.

Walther Hesse, an associate of Koch's, mentioned the problem to his wife and laboratory assistant, Fanny Eilshemius. She had a possible solution. For years, she had been using a seaweed-derived powder called agar (pronounced ahg'ar) to solidify her jams and jellies. The formula had been passed to her by her mother, who learned it from Dutch friends living in Java. Agar was valuable because it mixed easily with most liquids and once gelled, it did not liquefy, even at high temperatures.

Hesse was sufficiently impressed to recommend agar to Koch. Soon Koch was using it routinely in his culture media, and in 1884 he first mentioned agar in his paper on the isolation of the tubercle bacillus. It is noteworthy that Fanny Eilshemius may have been among the first Americans to make a significant contribution to microbiology (she was originally from New Jersey).

Another point of interest: The common Petri dish was also invented about this time by Julius Petri, another of Koch's assistants.

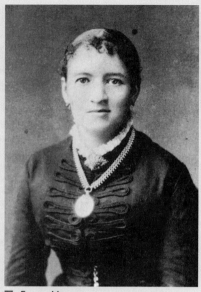
■ *Fanny Hesse.*

the spirit of nationalism. Pasteur became a symbol of French achievement and Koch, his German rival. A competition sprung up that would last into the next century (TABLE 1.2).

Koch's verification of the germ theory was presented in 1876. Within 2 years, Pasteur had verified the proof and gone a step further. He reported that bacteria were temperature-sensitive because chickens did not acquire anthrax at their normal body temperature of 42°C but did so when the animals were cooled down to 37°C. He also recovered anthrax spores from the soil and suggested that dead animals be burned or buried deeply in soil unfit for grazing.

One of Pasteur's more remarkable discoveries was made in 1880. For months he had been working on ways to enfeeble the bacteria of chicken cholera using heat, different growth media, successive inoculations in animals, and virtually anything that might weaken them. Finally, he developed a weak strain of bacteria. The trick, according to his notebooks, was to suspend the bacteria in a mildly acidic medium and allow the culture to remain undisturbed for a long period of time. When the bacteria were inoculated to chickens and later followed by a dose of lethal bacilli, the animals did not develop cholera. This principle is the basis for many **vaccines** for immunity. Pasteur applied the principle to anthrax in 1881 (FIGURE 1.9) and found he could protect sheep against the disease.

Pasteur's experiments put France in the forefront of science. However, Koch's 1881 announcement of pure culture techniques drew attention back to Germany, and within a year Koch isolated the bacillus that causes tuberculosis. In 1884 his associate, **Georg Gaffky**, cultivated the typhoid bacillus, and that same year another coworker, **Friederich Löeffler,** isolated the diphtheria bacillus. Soon, news was forthcoming from France that **Emile Roux** and **Alexandre Yersin** of Pasteur's group

Vaccine:
a preparation of modified microorganisms, treated toxins, or parts of microorganisms used for immunization purposes.

lef'ler

roo

TABLE 1.2

A Comparison of Louis Pasteur and Robert Koch

CHARACTERISTIC	LOUIS PASTEUR	ROBERT KOCH
Country of origin	France	Germany (Prussia)
Preparatory education	Chemistry	Medicine
Initial investigations	Milk souring; beer, wine fermentations	Cause of anthrax
Accomplishments	Proposed germ theory of disease	Verified germ theory of disease
	Disproved theory of spontaneous generation	Developed cultivation methods for bacteria
	Developed immunization techniques	Isolated bacterium that causes tuberculosis
	Resolved pébrine problem of silkworms	Developed staining methods for bacteria
	Developed rabies vaccine	Investigated cholera, malaria, sleeping sickness
Associates	Roux, Yersin, Metchnikoff	Gaffky, Löeffler, von Behring, Kitasato
Nobel Prize	No	Yes

had linked diphtheria to a toxin produced in the body. In later years, Koch's co-worker **Emil von Behring** successfully treated diphtheria by injecting antitoxin, a preparation of antibodies obtained from animals immunized against diphtheria. For his work, von Behring was awarded the first Nobel Prize in Physiology or Medicine.

There was also an international flavor in the French and German laboratories. **Shibasaburo Kitasato** of Japan studied with Koch and successfully cultivated the tetanus bacillus, an organism that grows only in the absence of oxygen. One of Pasteur's associates was **Elie Metchnikoff**, a native of the Ukraine. In 1884, Metchnikoff

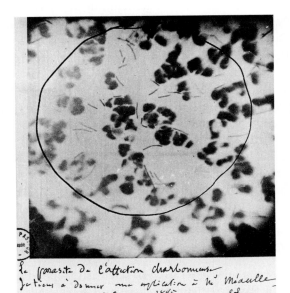

FIGURE 1.9

The Anthrax Bacillus as Photographed by Pasteur

A photomicrograph of the anthrax bacillus taken by Louis Pasteur. Pasteur circled the bacilli in tissue and annotated the photograph "the parasite of Charbonneuse." (Charbonneuse is the French equivalent of anthrax.) He requested that the photograph be brought to the attention of Monsieur Méderlle, dated it 20 March, 1885, and initialed it in the lower right.

MicroFocus 1.5

THE PRIVATE PASTEUR

The notebooks of Louis Pasteur had been an enduring mystery of science ever since the scientist himself requested his family not to show them to anyone. But in 1964, Pasteur's last surviving grandson donated the notebooks to the National Library in Paris, and after soul-searching for a decade, the directors made them available to a select group of scholars. Among the group was Gerald Geison of Princeton University. What Geison found stripped away part of the veneration conferred on Pasteur and showed another side to his work.

In 1881, Pasteur conducted a trial of his new anthrax vaccine by inoculating half a flock of animals with the vaccine, then exposing the entire flock to the disease. When the vaccinated half survived, Pasteur was showered with accolades. However, Pasteur's notebooks, according to Geison, reveal that he had prepared the vaccine not by his own method, but by a competitor's. (Coincidentally, the competitor suffered a nervous breakdown and died a month after the experiment ended.)

Pasteur also apparently sidestepped established protocols when he inoculated two boys with a rabies vaccine before it was tested on animals. Fortunately, the two boys survived, possibly because they were not actually infected or because the vaccine was, indeed, safe and effective. Nevertheless, the untested treatment should not have been used, says Geison. His book, *The Private Science of Louis Pasteur*, places the scientist in a more realistic light and shows that today's pressures to succeed in research are little different than they were a century ago.

---

fag'o-sī-to'sis

published an account of **phagocytosis,** a defensive process in which the body's white blood cells engulf and destroy microorganisms.

This period also witnessed two technical improvements in microscopy, both attributed to the German physicist **Ernst Karl Abbé** and both enhancing the study of microorganisms. In 1878, Abbé introduced the **oil-immersion lens,** a standard feature of modern microscopes. Eight years later he invented the system of lenses and mirrors known as the **Abbé condenser.** This apparatus concentrates light on objects being viewed and makes increased magnification feasible.

Rabies:
a deadly viral disease, accompanied by paralysis and usually acquired by animal bites.

In 1885, Pasteur reached the zenith of his career when he successfully immunized young Joseph Meister against the dreaded disease **rabies.** Although he never saw the causative agent of rabies, Pasteur was able to cultivate it in the brain of animals and inject the boy with bits of the tissue (**MicroFocus 1.5**). The experiment was a triumph because it fulfilled his dream of applying the principles of science to practical problems. Many monetary rewards followed, including a generous gift from the Russian government after Pasteur immunized 20 peasants against rabies. The funds helped establish the Pasteur Institute in Paris, one of the world's foremost scientific establishments. Pasteur presided over the Institute until his death in 1895.

Koch also reached the height of his influence in the 1880s. In 1883, he interrupted his work on tuberculosis to lead groups studying cholera in Egypt and India. In both countries, Koch isolated a comma-shaped bacillus and confirmed the suspicion first raised by John Snow 30 years earlier that water is the key to transmission. In 1891, he became Director of Berlin's Institute for Infectious Diseases. At various times, Koch studied malaria, plague, and sleeping sickness, but his work with tuberculosis ultimately gained him the 1905 Nobel Prize in Physiology or Medicine (**MicroFocus 1.6**). He died of a stroke in 1910 at the age of 66.

Typhus fever:
a louseborne bacterial disease of the blood, characterized by a skin rash and high fever.

OTHER PIONEERS OF MICROBIOLOGY

With the aging of Pasteur and Koch, a new generation of scientists stepped in to expand their work. For example, a Pasteur Institute scientist, **Charles Nicolle,**

MicroFocus 1.6

THE NOBEL PRIZE

The Nobel Prizes are among the world's most venerated awards. They were first conceived as a gesture of peace by a man whose discovery had unintentionally added to the destructive forces of warfare.

Alfred Bernhard Nobel was the third son of a Swedish munitions expert. As a young engineer, he developed an interest in nitroglycerine, the oily substance 25 times more explosive than gunpowder. In 1863, Nobel obtained a patent for a detonator of mercury fulminate, and within 4 years he used it with solid nitroglycerine mixed with a type of sandy clay. The mixture was called dynamite, from the Greek *dynamis* meaning "power."

Dynamite had a clear advantage over other explosives because it could be transported easily and handled without fear. It became an overnight success and was adapted to applications in mining,

tunnel construction, and bridge and road building. Before long, it was being used in armaments on the battlefield.

Nobel soon amassed a fortune through the control of several European companies that produced dynamite. However, toward the end of his life he became a pacifist and began speaking out against the use of dynamite in warfare. In 26 lines of his handwritten will, Nobel directed that the bulk of his estate should be used to award prizes that would promote peace, friendship, and service to humanity.

After his death in 1896, the governments of Sweden and Norway established Nobel Prizes in five categories: chemistry, physics, physiology or medicine, literature, and peace. A sixth category, economics, was added in 1969. Every year, Nobel laureates assemble in Oslo or Stockholm on December 10, the

anniversary of Nobel's death. Each laureate receives a medallion, a scroll, and all or part of a cash award currently valued at about $1 million per category.

The first Nobel Prize winners were announced in 1901. Among the recipients were Wilhelm K. Roentgen, the discoverer of X rays; Jean Henri Durant, the founder of the Red Cross; and Emil von Behring, the developer of the diphtheria antitoxin.

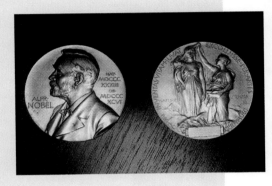

proved that typhus fever was transmitted by lice. **Albert Calmette**, also of the Institute, developed a harmless strain of the tubercle bacillus used for immunization. And **Jules Bordet**, another French scientist, isolated the bacillus of pertussis (whooping cough).

Koch's successors included Emil von Behring and **Richard Pfeiffer**, who isolated one of several organisms that cause meningitis. Another coworker was **Paul Ehrlich**, a chemist who explored the mechanisms of immunity and synthesized the "magic bullet," an arsenic compound that would seek out and destroy syphilis organisms in the human body.

By the turn of the century, microbiology had moved far beyond the boundaries of France and Germany. **Ronald Ross**, an English physician working in the Far East, proved that mosquitoes are the vital link in malaria transmission. The discovery earned him the 1902 Nobel Prize. Another Englishman, **David Bruce**, showed that tsetse flies transmit sleeping sickness. The control of this insect opened the African continent to British colonization. A third British subject, **Almroth Wright**, described opsonins, the chemical substances that assist phagocytosis in the body. Thirty years later, his student Alexander Fleming discovered the antibiotic penicillin.

Several Japanese investigators also achieved distinction. In 1897, **Masaki Ogata** reported that rat fleas transmit bubonic plague, thereby solving a centuries-old mystery of how plague spread. A year later, **Kiyoshi Shiga** isolated the bacterium that causes bacterial dysentery, an important intestinal disease. The organism was later named *Shigella*. A third Japanese investigator is profiled in *MicroFocus 1.7*.

kal'met

bor-dā'

Meningitis:
disease of the coverings of the spinal cord and brain.
Syphilis:
a bacterial disease of multiple body organs, transmitted by sexual contact.

MicroFocus 1.7

OF MICROORGANISMS AND CHERRY TREES

In the 1880s, while medical microbiologists were searching out the causes of infectious disease, a Japanese biochemist was busy acquiring enormous experience and wealth as one of the first industrial microbiologists. His name was Jokichi Takamini.

In the 1870s, Takamini left his native Japan to study engineering in the West. By the 1890s, he had married an American girl and was an expert on the enzymes of a common mold named *Aspergillus* (as-per-jil'us). Having isolated and purified a certain *Aspergillus* enzyme, he used it to help make whiskey at his fermentation plant in Peoria, Illinois. Local brewers turned against his innovative methods, however, so he patented the enzyme and licensed it to a pharmaceutical company. The company mixed it with peppermint and sold it as a digestive aid. Marketed as "takadiastase," the enzyme became the Alka-Seltzer of the 1890s.

Takamini was also one of the first biotechnologists. After moving to New York, he and an assistant set out to iso-

late the active principle (the hormone) in adrenal glands. For months they separated, precipitated, dissolved, purified, repurified, and hunted for the elusive substance. Then one night, his assistant, too tired to wash the glassware, left it for the morning and went home. The next day, a glass that had contained extract solution was lined with crystals of epinephrine (adrenalin). The isolation was a success, and Takamini's patent rights to epinephrine yielded wealth beyond his imagination.

In later years, Takamini became a patron of the arts and a philanthropist. Then, on August 30, 1909, the city of Tokyo announced a gift to the people of the United States: The city would be honored to adorn the Tidal Basin in Washington, D.C. with dozens of Japanese cherry trees. In the decades that followed, the cherry trees grew to become a splendid attraction in the nation's capital and an annual harbinger of spring. What few people know is that the gift was funded anonymously by Jokichi Takamini.

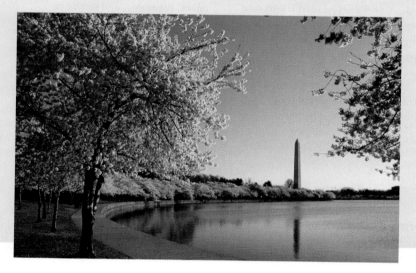

The American group of microbiologists was represented by **Daniel E. Salmon** and **Theobald Smith**. Salmon studied swine plague and lent his name to *Salmonella*, the cause of typhoid fever. Smith showed that Texas fever, a disease of cattle, was transmitted by ticks. In addition, the University of Chicago pathologist **Howard Taylor Ricketts** located the agent of Rocky Mountain spotted fever in the human bloodstream and demonstrated its transmission via ticks. Another American, **William Welch,** isolated the gas gangrene bacillus. And **Walter Reed** led a contingent to Cuba, where he pinpointed mosquitoes as the insects that transmit yellow fever. His discovery led to the mosquito eradication programs that made possible the building of the Panama Canal.

Amid the burgeoning interest in medical microbiology, other scientists devoted their research to the environmental importance of microorganisms. The Russian scientist **Sergius Winogradsky**, for example, discovered that certain bacteria utilize carbon dioxide to synthesize carbohydrates, much as plants do in photosynthesis (Chapter 5). And **Martinus Beijerinck**, a Dutch investigator, isolated bacteria that trap nitrogen in the soil and make it available to plants for use in constructing amino

Rocky Mountain spotted fever: a tickborne bacterial disease of the blood, characterized by high fever and skin rash.

win-o-grad'sky

bi'jer-ink

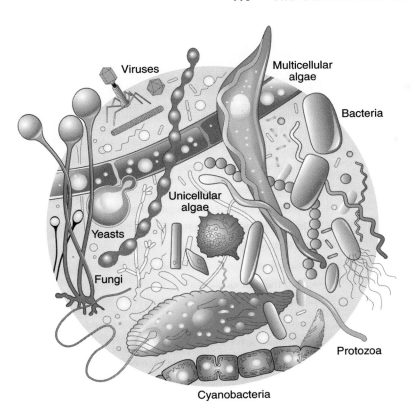

Viruses
Multicellular algae
Bacteria
Unicellular algae
Yeasts
Fungi
Protozoa
Cyanobacteria

FIGURE 1.10

A Microbial Menagerie

A menagerie of microorganisms as conceived by an artist. Many of these organisms were studied for the first time during the Golden Age of Microbiology. The notable exception are the viruses, which awaited the electron microscope for visualization. All of these microorganisms are discussed in later chapters of the text.

acids (Chapter 26). He also devoted much of his time to the properties of viruses (Chapter 11). Together with Winogradsky, he developed many of the laboratory media essential for the study of environmental microbiology, while adding to the developing menagerie of microorganisms (FIGURE 1.10).

THE END OF THE GOLDEN AGE

The advent of World War I in 1914 signaled a dramatic pause in microbiology research and brought to an end the Golden Age of Microbiology. The Pasteur Institute was closed as Paris came under siege, and the German laboratories focused on producing antibacterial serums for treating war-related diseases.

The Golden Age witnessed a series of discoveries unparalleled in medicine (TABLE 1.3). Although cures for established diseases would not come until the 1940s, scientists became aware that infectious disease is caused by microorganisms and that the chains of transmission can be broken. Their discoveries led to calls for sterile practices in hospitals, the pasteurization of milk, purification of water, control of insects, and care in the preparation of food for consumption. Together with improved sanitation and careful personal hygiene, these measures brought about a substantial reduction in the incidence of bacterial disease.

However, the agents of such diseases as measles, mumps, smallpox, yellow fever, and polio continued to elude microbiologists. As the 1920s and 1930s passed, the belief developed that some sort of "virus" was to blame and that discovering the virus was simply a matter of time. When viruses were finally visualized in the 1940s, they were unlike anything that scientists had imagined. We shall explore how this took place in Chapter 11.

Virus:
an infectious particle, composed of nucleic acid and protein, that replicates within living cells.

TABLE 1.3

Some Notable Figures and Their Accomplishments During the Golden Age of Microbiology, 1857–1914

INVESTIGATOR	COUNTRY	ACCOMPLISHMENT
Gerhard Hansen	Norway	Observed bacteria in leprosy patients
Otto F. H. Obermeier	Germany	Observed bacteria in relapsing fever patients
Ferdinand J. Cohn	Germany	Described life cycle of certain bacteria
Joseph Lister	Great Britain	Developed the principles of aseptic surgery
Georg Gaffky	Germany	Cultivated the typhoid bacillus
Emile Roux and Alexandre Yersin	France	Identified the diphtheria toxin
Emil von Behring	Germany	Developed the diphtheria antitoxin
Shibasaburo Kitasato	Japan	Isolated the tetanus bacillus
Elie Metchnikoff	Ukraine	Described phagocytosis
Ernst Karl Abbé	Germany	Developed the oil-immersion lens and Abbé condenser
Charles Nicolle	France	Proved that lice transmit typhus fever
Albert Calmette	France	Developed immunization process for tuberculosis
Jules Bordet	France	Isolated the pertussis bacillus
Richard Pfeiffer	Germany	Identified a cause of meningitis
Paul Ehrlich	Germany	Synthesized a "magic bullet" for syphilis
Ronald Ross	Great Britain	Showed that mosquitoes transmit malaria
David Bruce	Great Britain	Proved that tsetse flies transmit sleeping sickness
Almroth Wright	Great Britain	Described opsonins to assist phagocytosis
Masaki Ogata	Japan	Discovered that rat fleas transmit plague
Kiyoshi Shiga	Japan	Isolated a cause of bacterial dysentery
Daniel E. Salmon	United States	Studied swine plague
Theobald Smith	United States	Proved that ticks transmit Texas fever
Howard T. Ricketts	United States	Showed that ticks transmit Rocky Mountain spotted fever
William Welch	United States	Isolated the gas gangrene bacillus
Walter Reed	United States	Proved that mosquitoes transmit yellow fever
Sergius Winogradsky	Russia	Studied the biochemistry of soil bacteria
Martinus Beijerinck	Netherlands	Developed the discipline of environmental microbiology

In our era, many viral diseases are coming under control, much as many bacterial diseases did at the turn of the century. Smallpox has not occurred in the world since 1977, and polio, rubella, and measles are on a rapid decline. As this trend continues to take place, we shall be watching for the diseases of the future. In this generation, the lexicon of microbiology already has added such terms as Legionnaires' disease, Ebola fever, Kawasaki disease, toxic shock syndrome, and acquired immune deficiency syndrome (AIDS). Illnesses such as these represent the challenges for tomorrow's pioneers of microbiology.

It would be overly simplistic to believe that Pasteur and Koch were the only ones of their era to think that microorganisms cause infectious disease. Quite the contrary, a substantial number of scientists sensed that different diseases were due to microbial agents, but few were bold enough to say it publicly without proof. Blaming disease on microorganisms was breaking with centuries-old traditions rooted in beliefs and dogmas. That is why the works of Pasteur and Koch are so special: Pasteur's studies brought microorganisms to the public eye, and Koch provided proof of their involvement in disease. There followed a veritable explosion in research that was worldwide in scope. I have tried to highlight some of the excitement of the times and the variety of studies taking place.

You will note that we have focused on the development of microbiology in Europe. This chapter says little about medical discoveries taking place in other parts of the world, simply because historians are not really sure what was happening there. However, we know that Eastern people were far ahead of Europeans in certain areas. For instance, people in China practiced vaccination against smallpox long before Jenner introduced it in Europe. Perhaps when the history of microbiology in the East is better known, it will be necessary to rewrite this chapter substantially.

We have largely ignored twentieth-century microbiology because the remaining chapters in this text cover it in depth. Most of what you will learn is a product of research in the 1900s. Witness, for example, how measles has come under control during our lifetime. If you watch the newspapers, magazines, and other media, you will see the history of microbiology unfolding. Perhaps your grandchildren will be surprised to learn that you once had measles, a disease they could read about in a textbook but would never experience firsthand.

Note to the Student

Summary

In the late 1600s, Anton van Leeuwenhoek reported the existence of microorganisms and sparked interest in a previously unknown world of microscopic life. Although strong interest in the microbial world did not continue after his death in 1723, the controversy concerning spontaneous generation drew scientists to explore the origin and nature of living things. In the 1860s, scientists such as Snow and Semmelweis believed that infectious disease could be caused by something transmitted from the environment and that the transmission could be interrupted.

The fermentation experiments of Louis Pasteur, begun in the 1850s, were innovative and imaginative because they focused attention on the chemical changes that microorganisms induce. Gradually, Pasteur was led to the possibility that human disease could be due to chemical changes brought about by microorganisms in the body, and he proposed a germ theory of disease.

However, Pasteur was unable to cultivate microorganisms in pure culture and verify his germ theory, and it fell to Robert Koch to set down the methods for relating a single microorganism to a single disease. Soon an intense rivalry developed between the associates of Pasteur and Koch as they hunted down the microorganisms of infectious disease. Scientists throughout the world continued and developed the research in microbiology, and they instituted a Golden Age of Microbiology, a period that lasted until the advent of World War I. The science of microbiology has developed from that research.

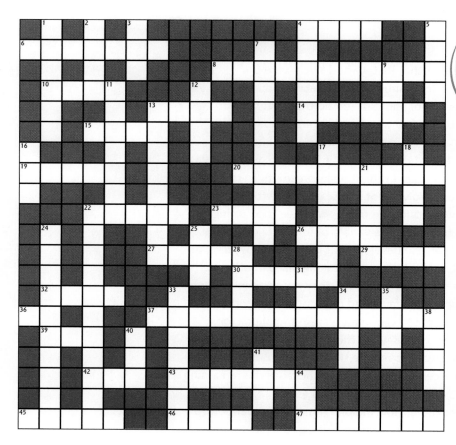

This chapter has explored the development of microbiology up through the period of World War I. To test your knowledge of the chapter contents, complete the following crossword puzzle. The answers are listed in Appendix D.

■ ACROSS

4. Arthropod that transmits plague
6. Microorganisms poorly studied during the Golden Age
8. Van Leeuwenhoek's term for microorganisms
10. Pasteur's flasks had the neck of a _____
13. Related diphtheria to a toxin
14. Mass of bacteria isolated by Koch
15. Attempted to disprove spontaneous generation by covering meat
19. Isolated the gas gangrene bacillus
20. Used chlorine water for hand disinfection in hospital
22. Related a specific arthropod to Texas fever

Questions for Thought and Discussion

1. Abu-Bakr Muhammed al-Razi, better known to history as Rhazes, was a famous Arabic doctor during the 900s. On moving to Baghdad to establish a hospital, he picked a site by hanging pieces of meat throughout the city and choosing the place where the last piece of meat turned rotten. How does this insight show an early appreciation of the relationship between disease and something present in the air?

2. In her biography of Louis Pasteur, Patrice Debré describes Pasteur's 1857 paper on lactose fermentation of milk as "the birth certificate of microbiology." Why do you suppose she thinks so highly of the paper? Further, she writes that as a result of the "Pasteurian revolution," medicine could no longer do without science, and hospitals could no longer be mere hospices. What does she have in mind?

3. Suppose you were a research microbiologist in the year 1900 and you had a consuming interest in the organism that causes measles. What direction would your research be taking, and what would be its fate?

4. Controversy in scientific thought often generates what one author has described as "dueling experiments." In this model, a scientific experiment is conducted to counter or refute another experiment. How many examples of dueling experiments can you find in this chapter?

5. Many people are fond of pinpointing events that alter the course of history. In your mind, which single event in this chapter had the greatest influence on the development of microbiology? What event would be in second place?

23. Environment where anthrax spores are located
26. Souring attracted attention of Pasteur
27. Isolated the bacterium that causes dysentery
29. Believed by Pasteur to be the cause of spoilage in wine
30. Proved that tsetse flies transmit African sleeping sickness
32. First described by Robert Hooke
36. Tetanus bacilli grow where there is _____ oxygen
37. Dutch investigator who reported the existence of microorganisms
39. Pasteur was the _____ of a French tanner
42. In the Golden _____ , microbiology experienced substantial growth
43. Searched for a magic bullet to treat syphilis
45. Produced by the bacterium in cases of diphtheria
46. Studied the role of mosquitoes in yellow fever epidemics
47. Causative agent studied by Kitasato

■ DOWN
1. Vague airborne principle believed to cause disease
2. Country in which Reed performed his studies
3. Insect whose stinger was described by Hooke
4. Pasteur's country
5. Fungal disease of plants
7. Disease agent isolated by Löeffler
9. Van Leeuwenhoek's microscope had a single _____
11. His broth experiments supported spontaneous generation
12. Type of culture obtained by Koch
13. Related ticks to Rocky Mountain spotted fever
16. Van Leeuwenhoek's letters number over _____ hundred
17. Disease of silkworms studied by Pasteur
18. Arthropod that can transmit Texas fever
21. Environment in which van Leeuwenhoek observed microorganisms

22. Broth experiments opposed spontaneous generation
24. Recognized three forms by which contagion passed
25. Believed by Pasteur to be a source of disease microorganisms
28. Developed the condenser for use in microscopy
31. Animal infected by anthrax bacillus
33. One of the founders of the science of microbiology
34. Studied cholera during an outbreak in London
35. Won the Nobel Prize for work on malaria and mosquitoes
38. Proved that a specific microorganism causes a specific disease
40. Source of aqueous humor used by Koch
41. Used by Abbé to increase microscope magnification
44. Article of clothing sold by van Leeuwenhoek

6. Suppose spontaneous generation were an accepted tenet of medicine and science. How would our view of infectious disease be affected? Now consider how our view is affected by belief in the germ theory of disease.

7. In 1911, the Polish chemist Casimir Funk isolated an active substance from rice husks and proposed that it prevents beriberi, a disease of the muscular and nervous systems. "Nonsense," he was told. "Spend your time more profitably—look for a microorganism!" Today we know that Funk was correct: Beriberi is a nutritional disease caused by a vitamin deficiency. But at that time, the scientific community scoffed at his idea. Why do you think that happened?

8. In 1878, after studying bacteriology in Germany, William Welch returned to the United States, eager to apply the principles he had learned to his medical practice. Welch approached administrators at New York's Bellevue Hospital Medical College for space and money to conduct research, and he was awarded a paltry $25 for three kitchen tables to serve as laboratory benches. Why do you believe Welch was rebuffed?

9. The year 1884 was a particularly fruitful one in microbiology. For example, the Danish physician Christian Gram developed the Gram stain technique, which is used to differentiate bacteria into two major groups. In the same year, the German physician Albert Frankel identified an important cause of bacterial pneumonia. How many other events or pieces of research can you locate that occurred or were ongoing that year?

10. The word *microbe* was coined in 1879 by the French investigator Charles E. Sedillot as a term for a microscopic creature. Today the word is sometimes used

interchangeably with *microorganism*. Do you think Sedillot had something else in mind over 100 years ago? If so, what?

11. Suppose uncooked hamburger meat became smelly after some days in the refrigerator, and imagine that you brought a sample to the laboratory, where microorganisms were revealed. How could you prove that the organisms did not arise by spontaneous generation?

12. Abbé's development of oil-immersion microscopy and his invention of the microscope condenser appeared to parallel the interest in microorganisms in the 1880s. Some maintain that the availability of new technologies made the discovery and study of microorganisms possible, but others assert that the intense interest in microorganisms demanded that the technologies be developed. Which argument would you favor? Why?

13. Anton van Leeuwenhoek's letters to the Royal Society were laced with crotchety asides about the inanities of his neighbors and the state of his own health. But the august members of the Royal Society recognized the diamond in the rough. They increasingly relished the acuity of his scientific observations, and van Leeuwenhoek's fame spread. In the end, van Leeuwenhoek opened the door to a completely new concept of the makeup of living things. Why is this so?

14. Why do you suppose there was no follow-up work on smallpox after Edward Jenner's development of a smallpox vaccine? And why might you enjoy learning the art of persuasion from Jenner?

15. In downtown Mexico City, at the crossroads of Insurgents Avenue and Paseo de la Reforma, there is an area called Plaza Louis Pasteur. In the plaza stands an elegant statue of Pasteur given to Mexico City by the French residents of Mexico in 1910. That year marked the centennial of the start of the Mexican War of Independence. What connection can you see among these facts and events?

http://microbiology.jbpub.com

The site features **eLearning,** an on-line review area that provides quizzes and other tools to help you study for your class. You can also follow useful links for in-depth information, read more MicroFocus stories, or just find out the latest microbiology news.

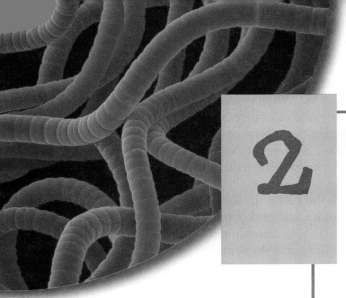

2 Principles of Chemistry

Organic chemistry is the chemistry of carbon compounds. Biochemistry is the study of carbon compounds that crawl.

—Mike Adams

THE WORDS "MICROBIAL LIFE" often bring to mind images of microorganisms cavorting in a droplet of pond water, or molds growing on a piece of stale bread, or bacteria multiplying in a festering wound. But microbiologists generally go a step beyond. They commonly ask *why* microorganisms act as they do, *how* they are organized, and *what* they are made of. Their questions reflect a curiosity about aspects of microbial life that are less visible, but perhaps more fundamental.

Untold generations ago, humans first pondered the composition of living things. They reasoned that because living things differ so greatly from nonliving things, there must be a corresponding difference in their construction. Then, during the early 1800s, chemists identified a group of basic substances found in the earth and atmosphere, including carbon, hydrogen, and oxygen. Surprisingly, the cells of living things proved to be made of the same materials; the only apparent difference was how the substances were organized. Chemists began referring to the materials associated with living things as "organic substances," while all others were termed "inorganic substances." Organic substances could be converted to inorganic substances easily enough, but the reverse appeared impossible. Living things seemed to be unique.

In 1821, an important discovery was made by the German chemist Friedrich Wöhler. Wöhler was investigating the properties of cyanides, a group of chemicals generally accepted as inorganic. While heating ammonium cyanate,

u–rē′ah

he found, to his amazement, that crystals of urea were forming. Urea is a major component of urine and an organic compound. Wöhler's work showed that an inorganic substance could be converted to an organic substance. More fundamentally, it indicated that it was possible to synthesize the substances of living things. His work encouraged other scientists to tackle the synthesis of the organic substances of living things, and soon scientists realized that knowledge of the chemicals of life was within their grasp.

During the late 1800s and through the 1900s, the distinction between living and nonliving things continued to evaporate as chemists produced numerous organic compounds and began to understand life processes in terms of chemical reactions. Today it is clear that all biology, including microbiology, has a chemical basis. Biology and chemistry are inseparable if scientists are to find answers to the questions of *why, how,* and *what.*

Organic compounds: compounds associated with living things.

In this chapter, we shall review the fundamental concepts of chemistry in order to lay a foundation for the chapters ahead. We shall enumerate the elements that make up all known substances and show how these elements combine to form the components of living things. Four major groups of organic substances found in virtually all forms of life will be studied in depth. An understanding of chemistry is vital if we are to comprehend the principles of living systems that researchers are uncovering in our era.

2.1

The Elements of the Physical Universe

As far as scientists know, all matter in the physical universe is composed of a number of basic substances called **elements.** Ninety-two naturally occurring elements have been discovered and characterized. Each is designated by one or two letters standing for its English or Latin name. For example, H is the symbol for hydrogen, O for oxygen, Cl for chlorine, and Mg for magnesium. Some Latin abbreviations include Na from *natrium* (which translates to sodium), K from *kalium* (which is Latin for potassium), and Fe from *ferrum* (the Latin word for iron).

Element: any of 92 naturally occurring basic substances that make up the physical universe.

TABLE 2.1 lists some of the major elements in living things. Note that only six elements—carbon, hydrogen, nitrogen, oxygen, phosphorus, and sulfur—make up 99 percent of the dry weight of a bacterium. (The acronym CHNOPS is helpful in remembering these.)

THE STRUCTURE OF ATOMS

The matter in elements cannot be subdivided without limit. Eventually, the subdivisions lead to units indivisible by ordinary chemical means. These units are called **atoms.** Although sophisticated devices are beginning to visualize atoms, their existence has been assured by reams of experimental evidence. An atom cannot be broken down further without losing the quality of the element: Chlorine consists of chlorine atoms, carbon of carbon atoms, and so forth.

Atom: a unit of an element that cannot be further subdivided without losing the quality of the element.

As early as 1808, the English chemist John Dalton conceived that in matter, atoms combine to form more complex substances. For the next century, the atom was considered to be solid and indivisible. However, in 1911, Ernest Rutherford proposed that every atom consists of a positively charged **nucleus** surrounded by a negatively

TABLE 2.1

The Major Elements of Living Organisms

ELEMENT	SYMBOL	PERCENTAGE BY WEIGHT IN BODY	ATOMIC NUMBER	ATOMIC WEIGHT
Oxygen	O	65%	8	16
Carbon	C	18	6	12
Hydrogen	H	10	1	1
Nitrogen	N	3	7	14
Calcium	Ca	2	20	40
Phosphorus	P	1	15	31
Potassium	K	0.9	19	39
Sulfur	S	0.9	16	32
Chlorine	Cl	0.9	17	35
Sodium	Na	0.9	11	23
Magnesium	Mg	0.9	12	24
Iron	Fe	0.9	26	56
Manganese	Mn	0.1	25	55
Copper	Cu	0.1	29	64
Iodine	I	0.1	53	127
Cobalt	Co	0.1	27	59
Zinc	Zn	0.1	30	65
Boron	B	0.1	5	11

THE MAJOR ELEMENTS OF A BACTERIUM

ELEMENT	SYMBOL	PERCENTAGE BY WEIGHT IN BODY	ATOMIC NUMBER	ATOMIC WEIGHT
Carbon	C	12.14%		
Hydrogen	H	9.94		
Nitrogen	N	3.04		
Oxygen	O	73.68		
Phosphorus	P	0.60		
Sulfur	S	0.32		

charged system of **electrons.** In the ensuing years, scientists found that the nucleus contains most of the atom's mass and is composed of two kinds of particles called **protons** and **neutrons.** These two particles have about the same mass. Protons bear a positive electrical charge, while neutrons have no charge. Electrons, by contrast, have a negative charge. In any atom, the electrons are equal in number to the protons, but each electron has only $\frac{1}{1835}$ of the mass of a proton.

The number of protons in an atom is the determining factor in the physical and chemical properties of the atom and, therefore, of the element. For example, carbon atoms have six protons, and nitrogen atoms have seven. The number of protons is the **atomic number** of the atom. Thus, carbon with six protons has an atomic number

Atomic number: the number of protons in an atom.

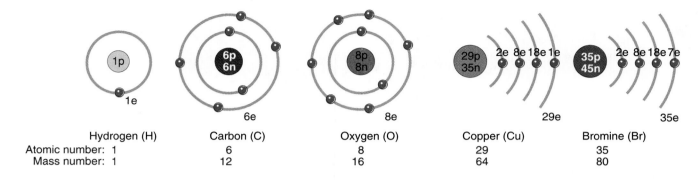

Hydrogen (H)	Carbon (C)	Oxygen (O)	Copper (Cu)	Bromine (Br)
Atomic number: 1	6	8	29	35
Mass number: 1	12	16	64	80

FIGURE 2.1

The Atomic Structure of Five Important Elements

Note that the number of protons is equal to the number of electrons (though not necessarily equal to the number of neutrons). Also note that the electrons are arranged in concentric shells about the nucleus. The atomic number is the proton number, and the mass number is the sum of the numbers of protons and neutrons.

of 6. The **mass number** is the number of protons and neutrons combined. Since carbon atoms have six protons and six neutrons in their nucleus, the mass number of carbon is 12. FIGURE 2.1 provides a simple diagram of the structures, atomic numbers, and mass numbers of various atoms.

In chemistry it is often helpful to express the relative size of a chemical substance. In such instances, scientists use the term **atomic weight.** The atomic weight of an atom is nearly the same as its mass number. Atomic weights are determined by adding together the weights of the protons, neutrons, and electrons in the atom. These are not the real weights of the particles, but relative weights. Physicists assign the value of 12 to the weight of a carbon atom and determine the weights of other atoms relative to carbon. For example, a hydrogen atom actually weighs 1.67×10^{-24} g, but relative to carbon its weight is 1.008. Therefore the atomic weight of a hydrogen atom is regarded as 1 and, in this case, it is close enough to be the same as the mass number.

Atomic weight:
the sum of the relative weights of the protons, neutrons, and electrons of an atom.

ISOTOPES AND IONS

Although the number of protons is the same for all atoms in an element, the number of neutrons may vary. Consequently, the mass number of atoms of an element may vary. For example, most carbon atoms have a mass number of 12, but some atoms of carbon have eight neutrons in the nucleus and, hence, a mass number of 14. Atoms of the same element that have different numbers of neutrons are called **isotopes.** For example, carbon-12 and carbon-14 (symbolized as ^{12}C and ^{14}C) are isotopes of carbon. Carbon-14 is especially important because it gives off energy and is useful as a radioactive tracer. By attaching it to organic substances, biologists can use carbon-14 to follow the fate of the substance.

Atoms are uncharged when they contain equal numbers of electrons and protons. Atoms do not gain or lose protons, but a gain or loss of electrons is possible. When this takes place, the atom is converted to a charged atom, or **ion.** For example, the addition of one electron adds a negative electrical charge to the atom and converts it to a negatively charged ion. By contrast, the loss of one electron leaves the atom

Isotopes:
atoms of an element that vary in the number of neutrons they possess.

i'on
Ion:
an atom with an electrical charge due to the acquisition or loss of one or more electrons.

with one extra proton and yields a positively charged ion. Ion formation is important in ionic bonding in atoms.

Groups of atoms often join together to form complex ions. Some of the important ions in microbiology are the ammonium ion (NH_4^+), the carbonate ion ($CO_3^=$), the hydrogen ion (H^+), the hydroxyl ion (OH^-), the nitrate ion (NO_3^-), the phosphate ion ($PO_4^=$), and the sulfate ion ($SO_4^=$). They will occur often in our discussions and an appreciation of their elemental composition is of value.

ELECTRON PLACEMENT

In 1913, the Danish physicist Niels Bohr suggested one of the first models of the atom. In his model the atom is perceived as a miniature solar system, with Rutherford's system of electrons revolving around the nucleus in concentric orbits (FIGURE 2.2). This simplified model has been greatly modified by contemporary physicists. Definite electron pathways have been eliminated, and the location of electrons is now regarded as a three-dimensional region of space around the nucleus, as shown in Figure 2.2. This cloudlike area is referred to as an **orbital**, to distinguish it from Bohr's orbit.

> **Orbital:**
> the cloudlike area describing a three-dimensional region where an electron is located.

The distance of an electron from the nucleus is a function of the electron's energy. Electrons with higher energy are probably farther from the nucleus than those with lower energy. Therefore, while physicists cannot say precisely where an electron is, they can make a statistical estimate of where it is likely to be. The energy level in which an electron is found most often is called the **shell** of the electron. In illustrations of the atom, the shell and the orbital are commonly represented by a ring, with the electron shown as a spot on the ring, as done in Figure 2.1. The model, though technically wrong, is useful for interpreting chemical phenomena.

> **Shell:**
> the energy level of an atom in which a particular electron will most likely be found.

The number of concentric electron shells in an atom varies with the atom. Each shell can hold a maximum number of electrons. The first shell next to the nucleus can accommodate two electrons, while the second shell can hold eight. Other shells also have maximum numbers, but no atom can have more than eight electrons in its outermost shell. Inner shells are filled first and, if there are not enough electrons to fill all the shells, the outer one is left incomplete.

The shells of atoms of certain elements are filled completely, and the elements do not enter into any chemical reactions. Such an element is said to be an **inert element.** Neon is an inert element because its outer shell contains the maximum eight electrons. By contrast, a carbon atom, with six electrons, has two electrons in its first shell and only four in the second. For this reason, carbon is extremely active and forms innumerable combinations with other elements.

> **Inert element:**
> an element whose atoms have an outer shell filled with electrons.

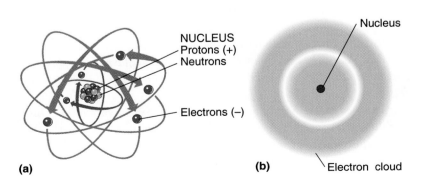

NUCLEUS
Protons (+)
Neutrons

Electrons (−)

Nucleus

Electron cloud

(a)   **(b)**

FIGURE 2.2

Two Models of the Atom's Structure

(a) An early model of the atom shows electrons "in orbit" about the nucleus. (b) A modern view of the atom has electrons occupying distinct cloudlike areas of three-dimensional space around the nucleus.

COMPOUNDS AND MOLECULES

Compound:
a substance composed of two or more elements.

Molecule:
the smallest unit of a compound that retains the properties of the compound and cannot be further subdivided without losing the quality of the compound.

Molecular weight:
the sum of the atomic weights of the atoms in a molecule.

Antibodies:
protein molecules produced by the immune system as a defensive measure against certain substances.

When atoms of two or more elements interact with one another to achieve stability, they form a substance called a **compound.** In a compound, the atoms of different elements combine in specific proportions with a particular pattern of linkages called **chemical bonds.** Each compound, like each element, has a definite formula and set of properties that distinguish it from its components. For example, both hydrogen and oxygen are gases, but the compound they form is water.

The smallest part of a compound that retains the properties of the compound is termed a **molecule.** The compound and molecule are analogous to the element and atom. Molecules may be composed of only one kind of atom, as in oxygen gas (O_2), or they may consist of different kinds of atoms in such things as water (H_2O), ammonia (NH_3), and the simple sugar glucose ($C_6H_{12}O_6$). The kinds and amounts of atoms in a molecule are symbolized by a designation called the **molecular formula.**

To appreciate the relative size of a molecule, it is valuable to know its **molecular weight.** This is determined by adding together the atomic weights of the atoms in the molecule and expressing the sum in units called **daltons.** (A dalton is equal to the mass of one hydrogen atom.) The molecular weight of a water molecule is 18 daltons, while the molecular weight of a glucose molecule is 180 daltons. Some molecular weights reach astonishing proportions. For instance, the antibodies produced by the body's immune system may have a molecular weight of 150,000 daltons, and the toxic poison secreted by the bacterium of botulism has a molecular weight of over 900,000 daltons.

The term **mole** is used to express the quantity of a substance whose weight in grams is numerically equivalent to its molecular weight: A mole of water weighs 18 grams, a mole of glucose weighs 180 grams, and a mole of a typical antibody weighs 150,000 grams. The mole concept is important in Chapter 5, where the energy content of a mole of certain substances is discussed.

To this point . . .

We began studying the principles of chemistry by noting why chemistry is essential to the study of living things. We then outlined the elements of the physical universe and reduced the elements to the level of atoms, because atoms join together to form the chemical substances of life. To understand how the joining takes place, we explored atomic structure, emphasizing electrons and their placement in the atom. As we shall see in the next section, atoms may combine in a number of ways to yield the familiar substances of all living things—be they bacteria, trees, or humans.

The section also reviewed some important concepts of chemistry that will recur in many of the later chapters. For example, isotopes are commonly used in diagnostic procedures for disease, and ions are participants in the chemical processes of most microorganisms. We shall also encounter molecules and compounds in the chemistry of life processes, and, in many places, the molecular formula and molecular weight of a compound will be mentioned. It is therefore essential to grasp the meaning of these terms as a prelude to later use.

We shall now turn to the types of bonding that occur in chemical compounds. This is where we construct the substances of living things, including microorganisms. We shall examine chemical reactions from a general standpoint and learn the basis for the chemical processes that go on in all life forms. A short explanation of acids and bases is included because they are very significant in biological chemistry.

2.2

Chemical Bonding

Molecules form when atoms interact with one another and link together. Linkage requires that two atoms come close enough for their electron orbitals to overlap. At this point an energy exchange takes place, and each of the participating atoms assumes an electron configuration more stable than its original configuration. The rearrangement can occur in two major ways: One atom can give up some of its electrons to the other, or each atom can share electrons with the other. When two or more atoms are linked together, the force that holds them is called a **chemical bond.** Chemical bonds usually form in order to complete the outer electron shell. FIGURE 2.3 and TABLE 2.2 compare different types of chemical bonds.

Chemical bond: the force that holds atoms together in molecules.

IONIC BONDING

In **ionic bonding,** one atom gives up its outermost electrons to another. The reaction between sodium and chlorine is illustrative. Sodium has an atomic number of 11, with electrons arranged in groups of 2, 8, and 1, as shown in Figure 2.3a. Chlorine,

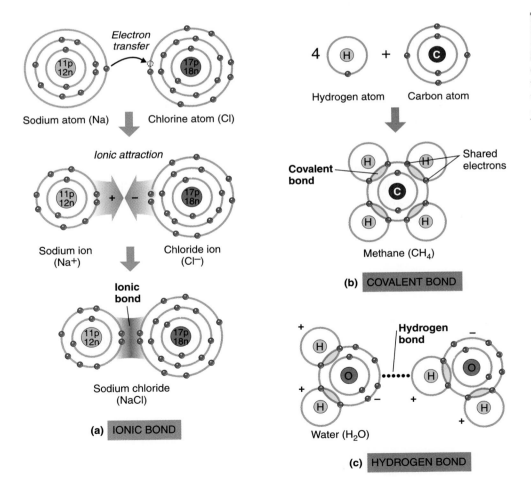

Sodium atom (Na)   Chlorine atom (Cl)

Sodium ion (Na+)   Chloride ion (Cl−)

Sodium chloride (NaCl)

(a)   IONIC BOND

Hydrogen atom   Carbon atom

Covalent bond   Shared electrons

Methane (CH₄)

(b)   COVALENT BOND

Hydrogen bond

Water (H₂O)

(c)   HYDROGEN BOND

FIGURE 2.3

Chemical Bonding

(a) The transfer of an electron from an atom of sodium to an atom of chlorine creates oppositely charged ions. The electrical attraction between these ions creates an ionic bond. The resulting molecule is sodium chloride. (b) A covalent bond involves the sharing of electrons between atoms, the example shown here being the simple organic compound methane. (c) Hydrogen bonds form when uneven sharing of electrons creates polarized "ends" within a molecule. Hydrogen atoms are typicaly involved, as is the case with the hydrogen bonding that occurs between water molecues.

TABLE 2.2

Three Types of Chemical Bonds in Organic Molecules

TYPE	CHEMICAL BASIS	STRENGTH	EXAMPLE
Ionic	Attraction between oppositely charged ions	Strong	Sodium chloride
Covalent	Sharing of electron pairs between atoms	Strong	Carbon-to-carbon bonds
Hydrogen	Attraction of a hydrogen nucleus (a proton) to negatively charged atoms in neighboring molecules	Weak	Cohesiveness of water

with an atomic number of 17, has its electrons in groups of 2, 8, and 7. To achieve stability, sodium atoms need only lose one electron and chlorine atoms need only gain one. Thus when atoms of the two elements are brought together, the sodium atoms donate one electron to the chlorine atoms.

The transfer of electrons leads to ion formation. By acquiring one electron, chlorine atoms become chloride ions (Cl^-). By contrast, sodium atoms now have an extra proton and therefore are sodium ions (Na^+). Since opposite electrical charges attract each other, the chloride ions and sodium ions come together to form sodium chloride (NaCl) molecules, or table salt. The force that holds the ions together in a molecule is called an **ionic bond.**

Ionic bond:
the force that holds ions together in a molecule.

COVALENT BONDING

Atoms can also achieve stability by sharing their electrons, a process called **covalent bonding.** Such bonds are very important in biology because the major elements of life (carbon, oxygen, nitrogen, and hydrogen) almost always enter into covalent bonds with one another.

The bonding in water molecules is typical of covalent bonding. Oxygen atoms are not strong enough to attract the electrons from hydrogen atoms, nor is a hydrogen atom sufficiently weak to give up its electron. Therefore, the oxygen and hydrogen atoms share their electrons and form a **covalent bond** in water. The electrons circle both the oxygen and the hydrogen.

Scientists use one or more lines between chemical symbols to represent covalent bonds. Water is represented as $H-O-H$. If two pairs of electrons are shared, as in carbon dioxide (CO_2), then two lines are used to indicate the double bond: $O=C=O$.

Covalent bonding occurs frequently in carbon because this element has four electrons in its outer shell (Figure 2.3b). The carbon atom is not strong enough to acquire four additional electrons, but it is sufficiently strong to retain the four that it has. It therefore enters into a huge variety of covalent bonds with four other atoms, ions, or groups of atoms. So vast is the array of carbon compounds that **organic chemistry,** the chemistry of living things, is basically the chemistry of carbon.

The simplest derivatives of carbon are the **hydrocarbons,** so named because they consist solely of hydrogen and carbon. Methane, or natural gas, is the most fundamental hydrocarbon. It contains one carbon atom and four hydrogen atoms. Other hydrocarbons consist of chains of carbon atoms and, in some cases, the chains may be closed to form a cyclic molecule.

Some carbon compounds consist of carbon atoms covalently bonded to a group of atoms operating as a unit. Such a group is called a **functional group.** In microbi-

Covalent bond:
the force resulting from the sharing of electrons among the atoms in a molecule.

Organic chemistry:
the chemistry of living things.

Hydrocarbons:
a group of organic substances consisting solely of carbon and hydrogen.

ology, the important functional groups include the hydroxyl group (−OH), the amino group (−NH$_2$), the acid or carboxyl group (−COOH), the sulfhydryl group (−SH), and the aldehyde group (−CHO). When a molecule containing any of these groups reacts with another molecule, the groups generally function as a single entity and may be exchanged for another group.

hi-drox'ill

kar-box'ill

sulf-hi'drill

HYDROGEN BONDING

When atoms bond together to form a molecule, they establish a definite geometric relationship determined largely by the electron configuration. This leads to an uneven distribution of electrical charge. In water, the two hydrogen atoms are attached on one side of the oxygen atom. As a result, the protons gather at this side and give the molecule a slightly positive charge. By contrast, the other side of the molecule carries a slightly negative charge owing to the accumulation of electrons. The water molecule therefore has poles and is said to be polar. When attractions develop between the poles of adjacent molecules, a weak polar bond is formed (Figure 2.3c). Such a bond is called a **hydrogen bond** because it generally involves hydrogen.

Hydrogen bonds may last only a brief instant, but they are strong enough to prevent water from easily becoming ice or steam. Also, the hydrogen bonds are important in shaping the structures of proteins and nucleic acids, two of the major components of all living things.

Hydrogen bond:
the force resulting from the attractions between oppositely charged poles of adjacent molecules.

CHEMICAL REACTIONS

A **chemical reaction** is a process in which atoms or molecules interact and form new bonds, thereby undergoing a change through electron rearrangement. Different combinations of atoms or molecules result from the reaction.

Chemists use an arrow to separate the original and final substances in a chemical reaction. The atoms or molecules to the left of the arrow are the **reactants,** and those to the right are the **products.** In some reactions, two reactants combine to form a molecule:

$$Na^+ \quad + \quad Cl^- \quad \rightarrow \quad NaCl$$

Sodium ion   Chloride ion   Sodium chloride

In other cases, reactions involve a switch of reactants:

$$HCl \quad + \quad NaOH \quad \rightarrow \quad H_2O \quad + \quad NaCl$$

Hydrochloric   Sodium   Water   Sodium
acid   hydroxide   chloride

Other reactions involve a decomposition in which water functions as a reactant. Such reactions are called **hydrolysis** reactions:

$$C_{12}H_{22}O_{11} \quad + \quad H_2O \quad \rightarrow \quad C_6H_{12}O_6 \quad + \quad C_6H_{12}O_6$$

Sucrose   Water   Glucose   Fructose

Hydrolysis:
a decomposition chemical reaction in which water functions as an intermediary.

In certain reactions, an oxidation and a reduction take place. In an **oxidation,** one reactant loses electrons. In a **reduction,** a reactant gains electrons. Energy transfer is often involved in such a reaction:

$$Cytochrome—A—Fe^{++} \quad + \quad Cytochrome—B—Fe^{+++} \quad \xrightarrow{\text{electron transfer}}$$

$$Cytochrome—A—Fe^{+++} \quad + \quad Cytochrome—B—Fe^{++}$$
$$\text{\textit{reduction}} \qquad\qquad\qquad\qquad \text{\textit{oxidation}}$$

Cytochrome:
a cellular pigment that functions in energy reactions in a living cell.

In this reaction, cytochrome A has lost an electron to cytochrome B. Note that by losing an electron, cytochrome A is left with an additional positive charge, while cytochrome B gains the electron that neutralizes one of its positive charges. This type of reaction is essential to bacterial metabolism, as we shall see in Chapter 5.

ACIDS AND BASES

Acid:
a chemical substance that adds hydrogen ions (protons) to a solution.
Base:
a chemical substance that removes hydrogen ions from a solution and thereby increases the number of hydroxyl ions.

There are many possible definitions for acids and bases. For our purposes, an **acid** is a chemical substance that donates protons, or hydrogen ions (H^+), to water or other solution. By contrast, a **base** (or **alkali**) is a substance that accepts hydrogen ions in solution. Since the acceptance of a hydrogen ion increases the concentration of hydroxyl ions (OH^-) in solution, a base may also be considered a substance that increases the amount of hydroxyl ions.

Acids are distinguished by their sour taste. Some common examples are acetic acid in vinegar, citric acid in citrus fruits, and lactic acid in sour milk products. Strong acids are those that donate large numbers of hydrogen ions to a solution. Hydrochloric acid (HCl), sulfuric acid (H_2SO_4), and nitric acid (HNO_3) are examples. Weak acids, typified by carbonic acid (H_2CO_3), donate a small number of hydrogen ions.

Bases have a bitter taste. Strong bases take up numerous hydrogen ions from a solution and leave it with a high concentration of hydroxyl ions. Potassium hydroxide (KOH), a material used to make soap, is among them. Weak bases take up smaller amounts of hydrogen ions and are illustrated by compounds containing amino ($-NH_2$) groups.

Because of their opposing chemical characteristics, acids and bases frequently react with each other. Such a reaction neutralizes both the acid and the base to form water and a salt. For example, when hydrochloric acid (HCl) and sodium hydroxide ($NaOH$) react, the result is water (H_2O) and ordinary table salt ($NaCl$).

pH:
a measure of the acidity or alkalinity of a substance.

In 1909, the Danish chemist Søren P. L. Sørensen introduced the symbol pH and the **pH scale** to refer to the strength of an acid or base. The scale extends from 0 to 14 and is based on actual calculations of the number of hydrogen ions present when a substance mixes with water. The strongest acid has a pH of 0; the strongest base has a pH of 14. A substance with a pH of 7, such as water, is said to be neutral. Most known bacteria live at neutral pH environments, but many fungi tolerate a more acidic environment. Thus fungi are often found in sour cream, yogurt, and citrus fruit products. FIGURE 2.4 summarizes the pH values of several substances.

FIGURE 2.4

A Sample of pH Values

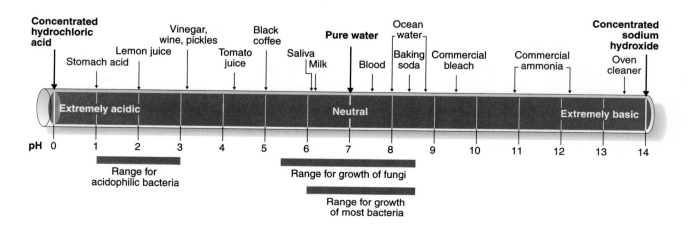

To this point . . .

We have studied atoms as the fundamental units of elements and noted that they achieve stability when their electron shells are complete. We then moved on to discuss how atoms combine with one another in three types of bonding. Ionic bonding, the first type, involves a transfer of electrons between atoms and an attraction of ions. Covalent bonding, by comparison, is based on a sharing of electrons. Hydrogen bonding, the third method, involves the linking of groups of atoms in a molecule by weak forces developing from the polarity of the components. Virtually all chemical reactions are based on the interactions of the chemical forces in bonding.

We also reviewed the various types of chemical reactions in which bonds are broken and reconstituted. The reaction may involve a combining of two reactants, a switch among reactants, a hydrolysis, or an oxidation-reduction reaction. The discussion closed with a brief review of acids and bases. Acids are hydrogen ion donors, while bases are hydrogen ion acceptors. By taking up hydrogen ions, bases also increase the level of hydroxyl ions in a solution. We reviewed the pH scale used to measure the relative strength or weakness of an acid or base.

In this final section, we shall focus on four important classes of organic compounds: carbohydrates, lipids, proteins, and nucleic acids. We shall examine the structures and functions of these compounds and touch on their importance in microbiology. All living things, including microorganisms, are composed of these substances. The discussions in this chapter's first two sections were largely designed to prepare us for this study.

2.3

Major Organic Compounds of Living Things

Living things are composed of numerous organic compounds, most of which belong to four distinct classes having different chemical compositions and properties. Organic compounds also provide a nutritious environment in which microorganisms grow, as FIGURE 2.5 illustrates.

CARBOHYDRATES

Carbohydrates are organic compounds of carbon, hydrogen, and oxygen. In simple carbohydrates, the ratio of hydrogen to oxygen is 2 to 1, the same as in water. For this reason, the carbohydrates are often considered "hydrated carbon," hence their name. However, the atoms are not present as water molecules bound to carbon, but rather in H—C—OH configurations. This combination occurs frequently in carbohydrate structures.

Carbohydrates function as energy sources in cells. They are also found in several microbial structures, such as bacterial capsules. Carbohydrates are synthesized from water and carbon dioxide through the process of photosynthesis (Chapter 5). Certain bacteria and other microorganisms have the necessary chemical machinery for this process. Often the carbohydrates are termed **saccharides** from the Latin word *saccharon*, meaning "sugar." The word *sugar* is applied to simple carbohydrates.

Photosynthesis:
a chemical process in which light energy is used to form the chemical bonds in carbohydrate molecules.

TEXTBOOK CASES

FIGURE 2.5

A Case of Salmonella Food Poisoning

This outbreak occurred at a restaurant during October, 1991. *Salmonella enteritidis* was isolated from stools of all 13 patrons of the restaurant who sought medical attention.

1. During the morning of October 17, a restaurant employee prepared dressing for Caesar salad, cracking fresh eggs into a large bowl containing olive oil. The eggs were probably contaminated with *Salmonella* bacteria.

3. The warm water raised the temperature of the mixture slightly and encouraged bacteria to grow. Although the dressing was placed in the refrigerator, the bacteria probably had an opportunity to grow before the dressing cooled.

2. Anchovies, garlic, and warm water were then mixed into the egg and oil.

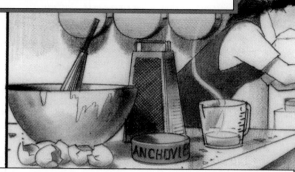

4. Later that day, the Caesar dressing was placed at the salad bar in a cooled compartment having a temperature of about 60°F (comfortable room temperature is a slightly higher 70–75°F). There the dressing remained until the restaurant closed, a period of 8 to 10 hours. During that time, Many patrons helped themselves to the Caesar salad.

5. Within three days, fifteen restaurant patrons fell ill with diarrhea, fever, abdominal cramps, nausea, and chills. Thirteen sought medical care, and eight required intravenous rehydration.

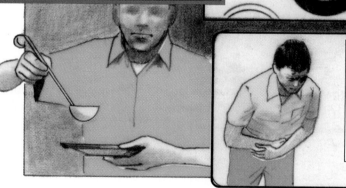

Carbohydrates are generally divided into three classes: monosaccharides, disaccharides, and polysaccharides (FIGURE 2.6). **Monosaccharides** are the simplest carbohydrates; they represent the building blocks for disaccharides and polysaccharides. Some monosaccharides, such as glyceraldehyde, have three carbon atoms; others have four, five, six, or more carbon atoms.

Glucose and fructose are among the most widely encountered monosaccharides. Both have a molecular formula typical of carbohydrates: $C_6H_{12}O_6$. However, their structural formulas are different. Such molecules are called **isomers.** Isomers react differently and usually have different properties. For example, fructose is much sweeter than glucose. Glucose serves as the basic supply of energy in the world. Estimates vary,

gli-cer-al'de-hyde

i'so-mer
Isomers:
chemical molecules with the same molecular formulas but different structural formulas.

but many scientists suggest that half the world's carbon exists as glucose. Chapter 5 is devoted to the production of glucose in microorganisms and its use for energy.

Disaccharides are double sugars. They are composed of two monosaccharides held together by covalent bonds. Maltose is an example. This disaccharide is constructed from glucose molecules by **dehydration synthesis**. In dehydration synthesis, the products of water are removed during the formation of covalent bonds. Maltose occurs in cereal grains such as barley and is fermented by yeasts to form the alcohol in beer. Another disaccharide, lactose, is composed of the monosaccharides glucose and galactose. Lactose is known as milk sugar because it is the principal carbohydrate in milk. Under controlled industrial conditions, microorganisms digest the lactose to form acid in yogurt, sour cream, and other sour dairy products.

Dehydration synthesis: a chemical process in which the products of water are removed during the synthesis of a molecule.

FIGURE 2.6

Structural Formulas for Monosaccharides, Disaccharides, and a Polysaccharide

Note that in the synthesis of the disaccharides, the products of water are removed from the reactants. This is dehydration synthesis. The polysaccharide starch is pictured as a very complex arrangement of glucose molecules covalently bonded to one another.

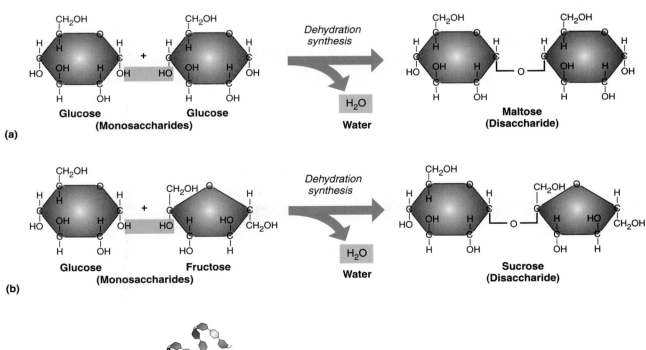

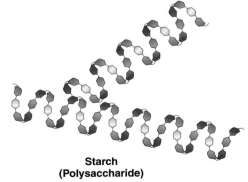

Sucrose, or table sugar, is a third disaccharide. It is a starting point in wine fermentations, and it is often involved in tooth decay (MicroFocus 2.1).

Complex sugars are called **polysaccharides.** These carbohydrates are generally large compounds formed by joining together hundreds or thousands of glucose units. Covalent bonds resulting from dehydration synthesis link the units. Starch, a common polysaccharide, is used by many bacteria as an energy source. Cellulose, another polysaccharide, is a component of the cell walls of plants and certain fungi.

pol'i-sak'a-rides

LIPIDS

The **lipids** are a broad group of organic compounds that dissolve in organic solvents such as ether or benzene but generally do not dissolve in water. Like carbohydrates, lipids are composed of carbon, hydrogen, and oxygen, but the proportion of oxygen is much lower. Lipids may also contain other elements, such as sulfur or phosphorus.

The best-known lipids are the **fats.** Fats serve living organisms as important energy sources. They are located in the granules of bacteria and are components of the cell membrane in most microorganisms. As shown in FIGURE 2.7, fats consist of a three-carbon glycerol molecule and up to three long-chain fatty acids. Each fatty

Fatty acid:
a long chain of carbon atoms with multiple hydrogen atoms and an acid group.

MicroFocus 2.1

THE REAL CAUSE OF CAVITIES

How many times were we told as children to avoid sweets because they cause cavities? Probably more times than we could count. The advice was good because sweets do indeed contribute to cavities, but only in an indirect way. The real culprits are the bacteria.

What happens in a cavity is this. As bacteria pass through the mouth, certain ones are trapped in the plaque. Plaque is a gummy layer of protein and carbohydrate materials formed from saliva and food particles. It accumulates between the teeth and at the gum line. Ironically, plaque is an oxygen-free environment in a part of the body where air is plentiful. Bacteria that accumulate in the plaque must be able to survive under oxygen-free conditions. Such bacteria are said to be anaerobic.

As the bacteria multiply, they digest the sucrose and other carbohydrates in sweets, producing large amounts of acid. The acid eats away at the tooth enamel, and soon a depression, or cavity, forms.

When the soft dental tissues underneath are reached, the bacteria penetrate to this area. Toothache pain results from the exposure of the sensitive nerve endings in the soft tissues, and part of the throb is due to bacterial gases that press against the nerves. When the dentist finally drills through to this area, the foul-smelling gas is released, and the pain subsides.

Sweets do not present serious problems so long as the acid-producing bacteria are eliminated. This is where conscientious brushing and flossing enter the picture. Tooth decay is really a disease. It is so widespread that it is considered one of the most prevalent diseases in the world.

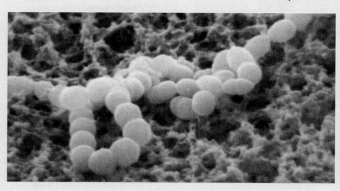

■ *A highly magnified view of streptococci from the surface of the teeth (×2500). Organisms such as these exist in the plaque and produce the acid that leads to cavities.*

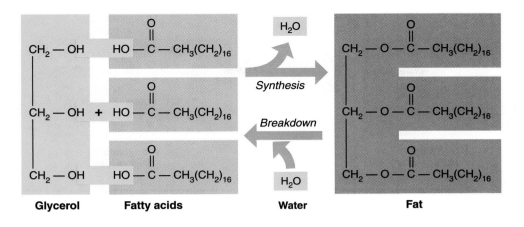

Glycerol   **Fatty acids**   **Water**   **Fat**

FIGURE 2.7

The Molecular Structures of Fat Components and the Synthesis and Breakdown of a Fat

Fats consist of fatty acids and glycerol. Each fatty acid contains numerous carbon and hydrogen atoms. Fat formation occurs by dehydration synthesis, as the components of water are removed from the reactants and covalent bonds are formed. During breakdown, the opposite occurs.

acid generally has between 16 and 18 carbon atoms in the chain. Bonding to the glycerol molecule occurs by dehydration synthesis.

There are two major types of fatty acids. **Saturated fatty acids** contain the maximum possible number of hydrogen atoms, while unsaturated fatty acids contain less than the maximum. **Unsaturated fatty acids** appear to be a factor in good health for humans because they lower the levels of cholesterol in the blood, thereby reducing the likelihood of clogged blood vessels.

Other types of lipids are the waxes, phospholipids, and steroids. Waxes are composed of long chains of fatty acids, while phospholipids are lipids that contain a phosphate group. Steroids, such as cholesterol, are composed of several rings of carbon atoms with side chains.

Cholesterol:
a sterol fat that accumulates in blood vessels and impedes blood flow.

PROTEINS

Proteins are by far the most abundant organic components of microorganisms and other living things. They function as structural materials as well as **enzymes,** a group of biological compounds that catalyze chemical reactions. Destruction of the proteins in an organism, such as with heat or chemicals, usually spells death for the organism.

Proteins consist essentially of chains of nitrogen-containing compounds called **amino acids.** At the root of each amino acid is a carbon atom. Attached to this atom are an amino group ($-NH_2$), an organic acid group ($-COOH$), and another side group. The side group determines the nature of the amino acid. There are approximately 20 different amino acids in proteins.

In protein formation, amino acids are joined together by covalent bonds when the amino groups are linked to the acid groups by dehydration synthesis (FIGURE 2.8). The chain that results is known as a peptide, and the bond is therefore called a **peptide bond.** In some cases the peptide is the total protein, but in other situations, one

Enzymes:
a group of proteins that regulate the rates of many biochemical reactions while themselves remaining unchanged.

Amino acid:
a building block of proteins that consists of an amino group, an organic acid group, and a specified side group.

Peptide:
a relatively small chain of amino acids.

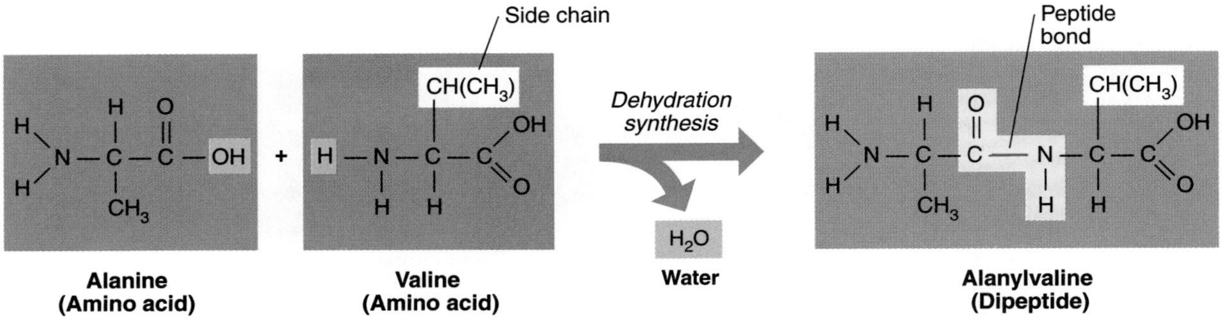

FIGURE 2.8

The Formation of a Small Protein (a Dipeptide) by Dehydration Synthesis

The amino acids alanine and valine are shown, with the differences shaded. The —OH group from the acid group of alanine combines with the —H ion from the amino group of valine to form water. The open bonds then link together, yielding a peptide bond. The dipeptide in this example is called alanylvaline.

or more chemical groups are added to constitute the complete protein. How the amino acids are slotted into position in peptide synthesis is a complex process discussed in Chapter 5. It should be noted that the sequence of amino acids is of the utmost importance because a single amino acid improperly positioned may change the character of the protein.

The chain of amino acids in the protein represents the **primary structure** of the protein. Many simple proteins, such as the human hormone oxytocin, occur in this form. Numerous proteins have a **secondary structure** that forms when the amino acid chain twists itself into a corkscrewlike pattern. Hydrogen bonds between nearby amino acids and sulfur-to-sulfur (disulfide) linkages help maintain this structure. A secondary structure may also form when amino acid chains line up alongside one another, as in the animal hormone insulin.

In addition, many proteins have a **tertiary structure.** In this case, the protein is folded back on itself much like a spiral telephone cord folded on a table. Hydrogen bonds maintain the protein in its tertiary structure. When subjected to heat or chemicals, the bonds break easily and the protein reverts to its secondary structure. This process is referred to as **denaturation.** Since most enzymes are tertiary proteins, heat or chemicals may be used to denature them and thus interrupt the important chemical reactions they control. Death of the organism usually follows. Viruses may also be destroyed by denaturing the tertiary proteins found in the outer viral surfaces. The white of a boiled egg is denatured egg protein; cottage cheese is denatured milk protein. In the human body, the cornea of the eye is composed primarily of protein, and, as such, it may supply nutrients to encourage the growth of disease-causing (pathogenic) bacteria, as FIGURE 2.9 indicates.

NUCLEIC ACIDS

The **nucleic acids** are among the largest molecules found in organisms. Two types function in all living things: **deoxyribonucleic acid (DNA)** and **ribonucleic acid (RNA).** DNA is the genetic material of the chromosome, while RNA functions in the construction of proteins (TABLE 2.3).

Oxytocin:
the hormone that stimulates uterine contractions during menstruation and childbirth.

Denaturation:
a chemical process in which the tertiary structure of a protein is destroyed and the protein often solidifies.

Nucleic acid:
a major organic substance composed of a carbohydrate (ribose or deoxyribose), a phosphate group, and five nitrogenous bases.

de-ox'e-ri-bo-new-klay'ik

FIGURE 2.9

A Case of Corneal Infection Caused by a Pathogenic Bacterium

This incident happened in Georgia during the winter of 1989.

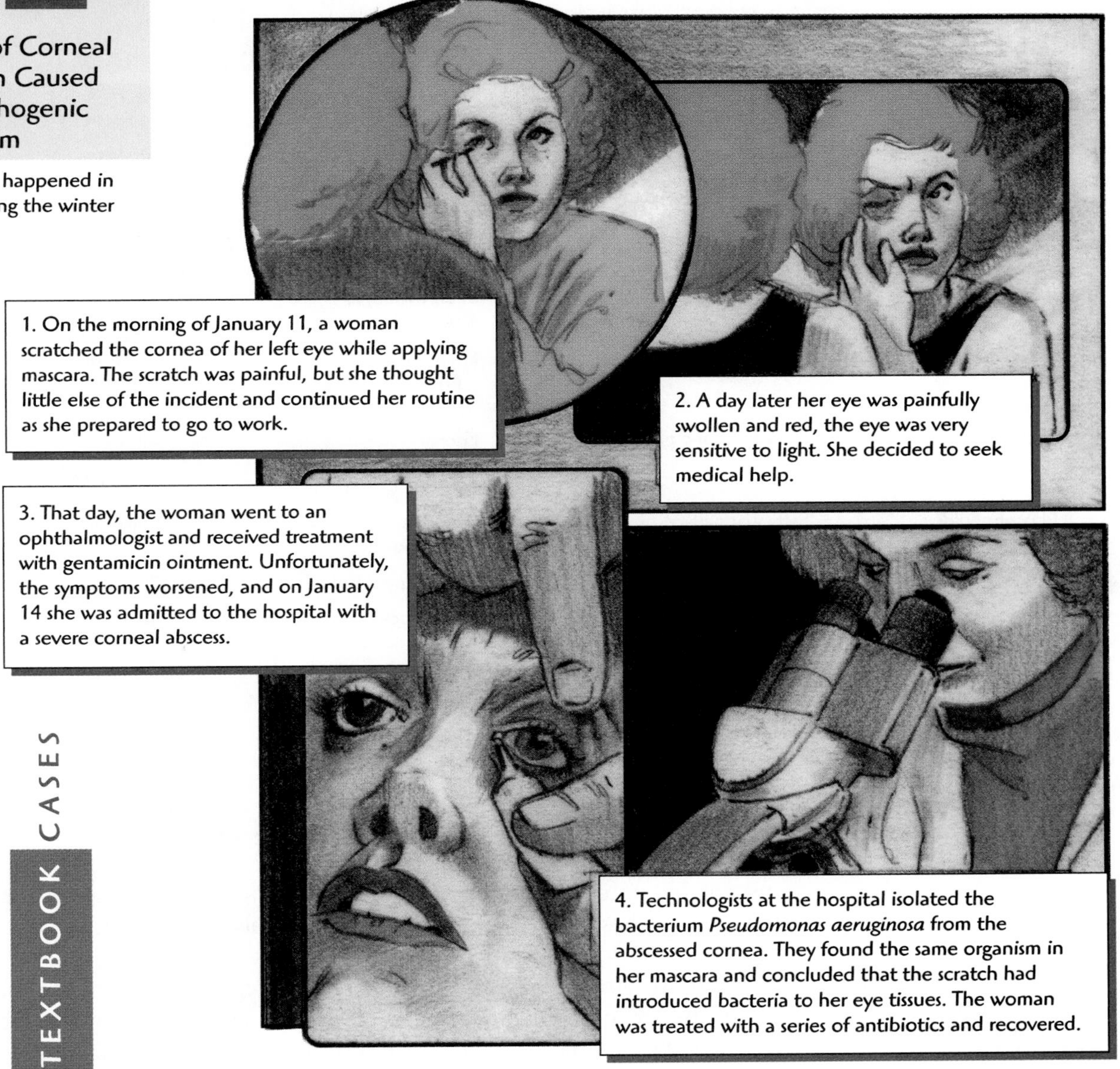

TEXTBOOK CASES

1. On the morning of January 11, a woman scratched the cornea of her left eye while applying mascara. The scratch was painful, but she thought little else of the incident and continued her routine as she prepared to go to work.

2. A day later her eye was painfully swollen and red, the eye was very sensitive to light. She decided to seek medical help.

3. That day, the woman went to an ophthalmologist and received treatment with gentamicin ointment. Unfortunately, the symptoms worsened, and on January 14 she was admitted to the hospital with a severe corneal abscess.

4. Technologists at the hospital isolated the bacterium *Pseudomonas aeruginosa* from the abscessed cornea. They found the same organism in her mascara and concluded that the scratch had introduced bacteria to her eye tissues. The woman was treated with a series of antibiotics and recovered.

Both DNA and RNA are composed of repeating units called **nucleotides.** Each nucleotide has three components: a carbohydrate molecule, a phosphate group, and a nitrogenous base. The carbohydrate molecule in RNA is ribose, while in DNA it is the closely related compound deoxyribose. The phosphate group is an organic ion formed by the loss of hydrogen ions from phosphoric acid. **Nitrogenous bases** are any of five nitrogen-containing compounds that have large numbers of amino groups and therefore act as bases. In DNA, the bases are adenine, guanine, cytosine, and thymine. In RNA, adenine, guanine, and cytosine are also

Nucleotide: a building block of nucleic acids consisting of a carbohydrate molecule, a phosphate group, and a nitrogenous base.

ni-troj'en-us

gwan'een

TABLE 2.3

Major Organic Compounds of Living Things

ORGANIC COMPOUND	BUILDING BLOCK	SOME MAJOR FUNCTIONS	EXAMPLES
Carbohydrate: Monosaccharide	—	Energy storage; physical structure	Glucose, galactose, fructose
Disaccharide	Monosaccharides	Energy storage; physical structure	Lactose, maltose, sucrose
Polysaccharide	Monosaccharides	Energy storage; physical structure	Starch, cellulose, chitin, glycogen
Protein	Amino acids	Enzymes; toxins; physical structures	Antibodies; viral surface; flagella; pili
Lipid: Triglycerides	Fatty acids and glycerol	Energy storage; thermal insulation; shock absorption	Fat; oil
Phospholipids	Fatty acids, glycerol, phosphate, and an R group[a]	Foundation for cell membranes	Cell membranes
Steroids	Four-ringed structure[b]	Membrane stability	Cholesterol
Nucleic acid	Ribonucleotides; deoxyribonucleotides	Inheritance; instructions for protein synthesis	DNA, RNA

[a]R group = a variable portion of a molecule.
[b]Technically, steroids are neither polymers nor macromolecules.

Chromosome:
a molecule containing DNA, which encodes the hereditary information of the cell.

present, but uracil is found instead of thymine. FIGURE 2.10 displays the structural formulas of these bases. The nucleotides are joined by covalent bonds to form the nucleic acids.

The most familiar location of DNA is in the chromosome of the cell, where it constitutes genetic information and directs the synthesis of protein. To form the complete DNA molecule, two single strands of DNA oppose each other in a ladderlike arrangement. Guanine and cytosine line up opposite one another, and thymine and adenine oppose each other. This forms a double strand of DNA. The double strand then twists to form a spiral arrangement called the **double helix,** shown in Chapter 6.

As with proteins, the nucleic acids cannot be altered without injuring the organism or killing it. Ultraviolet light damages DNA, and thus it can be used to control bacteria on an environmental surface. Chemicals such as formaldehyde alter the nucleic acids of viruses and can be used in the preparation of vaccines. Certain antibiotics interfere with RNA function and thereby kill bacteria. We shall encounter other instances where tampering with nucleic acids is the basis for controlling microorganisms. An entire chapter, Chapter 6, is devoted to the role of nucleic acids in the genetics of bacteria. Together with proteins, carbohydrates, and lipids, the nucleic acids form the chemical bases for all living things, including microorganisms. The major organic compounds are summarized in Table 2.3.

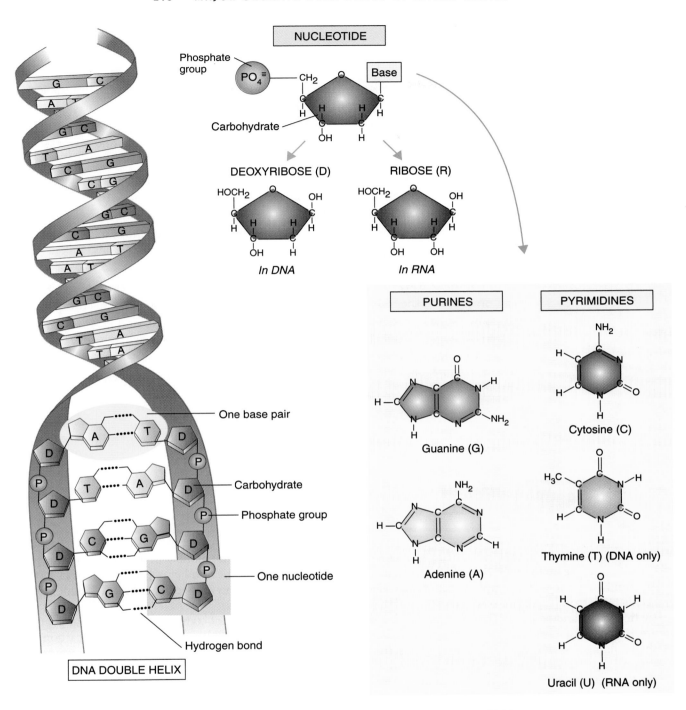

FIGURE 2.10

The Molecular Structures of Nucleotide Components and the Construction of a Nucleic Acid

The carbohydrates (pentose sugars) in nucleotides are ribose and deoxyribose. These two small compounds are identical except at one carbon atom. The nitrogenous bases include adenine and guanine, which are large purine molecules, and thymine, cytosine, and uracil, which are smaller pyrimidine molecules. Note the similarities in the structures of these bases and the differences in the side groups.

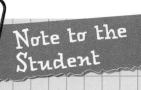

Note to the Student

You might well ask at this point whether this is going to be a chemistry book or a microbiology book. In a sense, it is going to be both.

In past centuries, biology was the study of nature. Biologists described natural phenomena, classified plants and animals, performed dissections, and marveled at the world of microscopic creatures. Then, in 1828, Friedrich Wöhler synthesized urea and showed that the substances of living things could be produced by scientists. Later, in the 1850s, Pasteur announced his observations about fermentation and pointed out that microorganisms were tiny, chemical factories in which sugar was converted to alcohol. As a result of these and other advances, microbiology became irrevocably bound to chemistry.

In future chapters, we shall discuss such topics as the metabolism of microorganisms, the activity of antibodies, the mechanisms of disease, the action of antibiotics on bacteria, the replication of viruses, and the chemical control of microorganisms. None of these processes was understood 100 years ago, partly because knowledge of their chemical bases was lacking. Such is not the case today.

The chemicals are the nuts and bolts of all living things. I recommend that you give this chapter a careful reading. In succeeding chapters, I shall try to make your time investment worthwhile.

Summary

Ninety-two naturally occurring elements make up the substance of all known living and nonliving things. The simplest unit of these elements is the atom, a particle consisting of a nucleus (with protons and neutrons) and electrons. Electrons are arranged outside the nucleus in shells, with each shell holding a maximum number of electrons. Interactions occur between atoms to fill the shells with electrons. These interactions can consist of a transfer of electrons between two atoms to form an ionic bond, or a sharing of electrons between two atoms to form a covalent bond. The interactions between atoms result in molecules. A mass of molecules is a compound.

Among the important compounds in living things are acids and bases. Acids are compounds that donate hydrogen ions to a solution; bases are compounds that remove hydrogen ions from a solution and, in so doing, increase the number of hydroxyl ions. The pH scale indicates the number of hydrogen ions in a solution and indicates how acidic or basic (alkaline) the solution is.

Other important compounds in living things are carbohydrates. These compounds contain carbon, hydrogen, and oxygen. They are used primarily as energy sources for life processes, and they include monosaccharides such as glucose and fructose, disaccharides such as lactose and maltose, and polysaccharides such as starch and cellulose. Lipids have the same types of atoms as carbohydrates, but the proportion of oxygen is much lower. Like carbohydrates, lipids serve as energy sources, but they are also used in structural materials. Fats are types of lipids.

The compounds of living things also include proteins. These are chains of amino acids connected by peptide bonds, a type of covalent bond. Proteins are used as enzymes and as structural components of cells. Primary, secondary, and tertiary structures are found in many proteins. The genetic instructions for living things are located in compounds called nucleic acids. A nucleic acid is composed of carbohydrate molecules, phosphate ions, and a series of nitrogenous bases. Two nucleic acids are important in biological systems: ribonucleic acid (RNA) and deoxyribonucleic acid (DNA). With the other organic compounds, nucleic acids form the chemical bases of all living things.

Questions for Thought and Discussion

1. Calcium atoms have two electrons in their outer shells; magnesium atoms also have two. Do you expect that good "chemistry" will occur between these elements when their atoms are brought together? Why or why not?

2. Some individuals unable to drink milk are said to suffer "lactose intolerance." What chemistry do you think their digestive tracts are unable to perform?

3. Certain detergent disinfectants are known to dissolve lipids. How would this activity encourage the destruction of bacterial cells?

4. Why do you think organic molecules tend to be so large?

5. An atom of carbon is an almost incomprehensible one ten-billionth of a meter in diameter. Put another way, 10 billion carbon atoms could line up along the length of a meter stick. Suppose you were to count each carbon atom along the length of the meter stick at a rate of one atom per second. How long would it take to complete your counting?

6. Why is Wöhler's synthesis of urea in 1828 considered to be a landmark achievement in bridging the gap between biology and chemistry?

7. Bacteria do not grow on bars of soap even though the soap is wet and covered with bacteria after one has washed. Can you surmise why this is so?

8. The area occupied by the nucleus of an atom relative to the entire atom is similar to the area occupied by a raisin sitting on the 50-yard line of a football stadium relative to the stadium. What takes up the remainder of the space in the atom?

9. Oxygen comprises about 65 percent of the weight of a living organism. This means that a 120-pound person contains 78 pounds of oxygen. How can this be so?

10. Suppose you had the choice of destroying one group of chemical substances in bacteria in order to prevent their spread. Which would you choose? Why?

11. Two bottles of acid are taken from the shelf. One is labeled pH 1.5, the other pH 6.78. Which bottle should be handled more carefully? Why?

12. Carbon is so common in living things that the chemistry of carbon is often said to be the chemistry of life. What property of carbon is responsible for its ability to enter a wide variety of chemical combinations?

13. The toxin associated with the foodborne disease botulism is a protein. To avoid botulism, home canners are advised to heat preserved foods to boiling for at least 12 minutes before tasting or consuming them. How does the heat help?

14. Water is generally considered to be the universal solvent of life. In how many places in this chapter does water live up to its reputation?

15. Proteins are made up of chains of amino acids, yet the proteins themselves are not acidic. Why do you think this is so?

Review

This chapter has focused on the elements of living things, how the elements combine to form molecules, and the major compounds of microorganisms and other life forms. To test your knowledge of the chapter contents, rearrange the scrambled letters to spell out the correct word for the available space. The answers are listed in Appendix D.

1. During _____ bonding, an electron or a series of electrons are transferred between atoms.

   O   C   I   I   N

2. The chemistry of living things is _____ chemistry.

   R   N   C   I   O   G   A

3. An acid is a chemical substance that donates _____ ions to a solution such as water.

   Y   R   N   H   G   O   D   E

4. The carbohydrate _____ contains the basic supply of the world's energy to living things.

   U   C   E   S   L   G   O

5. The best known lipids are the _____.

   A   S   T   F

6. In all living organisms, proteins function both as structural materials and as _____.

   E   E   S   Y   M   N   Z

7. Both DNA and RNA are composed of repeating units called _____.

   U   L   S   T   E   N   I   E   C   O   D

8. The _____ structure of a protein consists of the amino acid chain.

   I   A   M   R   Y   P   R

9. In _____ synthesis, the products of water are removed during the formation of covalent bonds.

   Y   D   A   I   R   E   O   D   H   T   N

10. The pH scale relates the measure of _____ of a chemical substance.

    A   D   Y   T   I   C   I

11. The smallest part of a compound that retains the property of the compound is a _____.

    L   U   C   O   E   L   E   M

12. _____ are atoms of the same element that have different numbers of neutrons.

    T   I   P   E   S   S   O   O

13. A functional group designated —COOH is known as an acid group or a _____ group.

    A   B   X   C   R   O   L   Y

14. Examples of disaccharides include lactose, sucrose, and _____.

    T   A   M   E   O   L   S

15. The _____ bond is a weak bond that exists between poles of adjacent molecules.

    G   R   N   H   E   O   D   Y

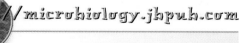

http://microbiology.jbpub.com

The site features **eLearning,** an on-line review area that provides quizzes and other tools to help you study for your class. You can also follow useful links for in-depth information, read more MicroFocus stories, or just find out the latest microbiology news.

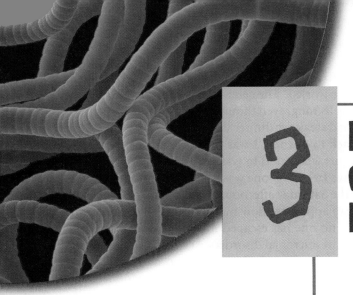

3 Basic Concepts of Microbiology

"It's as if [he] lifted a whole submerged continent out of the ocean."

—A prominent biologist speaking of Carl Woese, whose work led to the three-domain vision of living things

I N THE SPRING OF 1954, I was a lad of thirteen growing up in the Bronx and looking forward to a carefree summer. But I could feel the tension in my parents' voices as they anticipated the months ahead, for summer was the dreaded polio season.

And sure enough, by early July the tension had turned to outright fear. I was told to avoid the public pool and the lusciously cool air-conditioned movie house. I had to report any cough or stiff neck promptly. "Stick with your old friends," my father told me. "You've already got their germs." Most of the time I was indoors, and the only baseball I got to play was in my imagination, as I listened to the Yankees every afternoon on my portable radio.

Our family was one of the lucky few to have a television, and each night we watched row upon row of iron lungs, and we saw the faces of the kids whose bodies were captured forever in their iron prisons. (Iron lungs, I was told, help you breathe when paralysis affects the respiratory muscles.) We heard and read about the daily toll from polio, where the victims lived, and how many kids had died.

But there was hope. My mom and her friends were out collecting dimes to fight polio (they called it the Mothers' March Against Polio), and the National Foundation of Infantile Paralysis said it had 75 million dimes to help fund the tests of a new vaccine—Dr. Salk's vaccine. Two million children would be getting shots. Maybe next year would be different.

Polio:
a viral disease affecting the nervous system and often causing paralysis.

Boy, was next year ever different! On April 12, 1955, at a televised news conference, Dr. Jonas Salk declared: "The vaccine works!" The celebration was wild. Our school closed for the day. And the church bells rang, even though it was a Thursday. I could tell my mother was relieved—we had steak for dinner that night.

By summertime, things were back to normal. I was now fourteen and eager to show off my baseball skills to any girl who cared to watch. Down at the neighborhood pool I was learning how to dive (when no one was watching). And for a quarter, I got to cheer for the cavalry at the Saturday afternoon movie. Summer was back.

So it was that once again I came to appreciate how microorganisms influence the way people think and act. Virtually no one has escaped infectious disease, and the search continues daily for the causes of microbial disorders, as well as for their treatment and prevention (MicroFocus 3.1). In the quality-control laboratory, inspectors are on constant alert to interrupt disease transmission in food and dairy products, and in water-purification and sewage-treatment facilities, highly sophisticated technologies are used to prevent the spread of microorganisms through the fluids we drink.

But microbiology also has many positive aspects. Ecologists study microbiology to understand the natural recycling of minerals such as carbon and nitrogen. Evolutionary biologists look to the microorganisms to learn more about the ancestors of contemporary forms, and biochemists use microorganisms as miniature laboratories to discover the chemical systems that underlie all living things. Geneticists observe hereditary material at work in microscopic forms and then apply what they have learned to more complex organisms. Even behavioral psychologists find value in studying how certain microorganisms respond to environmental stimuli.

MicroFocus 3.1

EPIDEMIC

Patrons of fast food restaurants are usually safe from infectious disease, surprisingly safe in view of the huge volume of food served and the speed of preparation.

But, occasionally things go wrong, and in the winter of 1993 things went very wrong. That January, close to 500 people in several northwestern states became seriously ill after eating at their local Jack-in-the-Box restaurants. Three children died during the epidemic, and many others required hospitalization, including some who needed kidney dialysis.

The problem came to light when several patrons in Washington State called their physicians to report the onset of bloody diarrhea. Most were experiencing gut-wrenching stomach cramps, and many were sick with fever. Similar reports were soon received from patients in Nevada, Oregon, Idaho, and California.

Local health departments moved quickly and contacted the Centers for Disease Control and Prevention, the federal agency for dealing with problems of this magnitude. Health officials were soon on the scene, taking food samples at several restaurants and sending the samples to laboratories for bacterial testing. Within days, the laboratories reported isolations of a common bacterium called *Escherichia coli*. Normally a benign inhabitant of the human and animal intestines, this particular strain of *E. coli* was the notorious toxin-producing strain O157:H7. The toxin was destroying cells of the intestinal lining, which led to the bleeding; and it was causing hemorrhages in the kidneys. All signs pointed to the hamburger meat as the source. Most likely, it had been contaminated with feces from the intestines of cattle during slaughter.

Decisive action followed. The management of Jack-in-the-Box restaurants ordered its employees to increase the cooking time for hamburgers by 12.5 percent. Federal guidelines were instituted requiring ground beef to be cooked at 155 degrees Fahrenheit (instead of the usual 140 degrees). Physicians throughout the country were alerted to watch for additional cases, and infected children were not permitted to return to day-care centers until two successive tests proved they had no residual bacteria in their intestine. Consumers were warned to avoid rare hamburgers. The operative expression became: "If it's gray, it's OK."

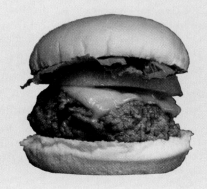

Our study of microbiology begins with a review of the position microorganisms occupy in the world of living things. We present thumbnail sketches of the major groups of microorganisms, after which we explore the methods used to classify microorganisms. Discussions follow on the origin of their names, their sizes and shapes, and the techniques used to view them. These basic considerations provide a foundation for studying the microorganisms in detail in future chapters.

3.1

A Brief Survey of Microorganisms

Despite their microscopic size, microorganisms exhibit numerous features also found in more complex cells. For example, DNA is the hereditary material in microorganisms as it is in all other living things, and many of the biochemical patterns of growth are identical. However, a number of significant differences set microorganisms apart. Before we explore these differences and unique features, we shall examine the total spectrum of living things by distinguishing two broad groups of organisms, the prokaryotes and eukaryotes. Once the characteristics of these groups are defined, we shall see how microorganisms fit into the pattern.

DNA:
deoxyribonucleic acid, the organic substance that contains the hereditary information of the cell.

PROKARYOTES AND EUKARYOTES

One of the most important generalizations to emerge in recent decades is that all organisms may be categorized as either **prokaryotes** or **eukaryotes** (terms first proposed in 1937 by Edward Chatton). Both terms are derived from the Greek word *karyon* meaning "nut," a reference to the nucleus of the cell. Prokaryotes lack a nucleus (*pro* implies primitive), whereas eukaryotes possess a well-defined nucleus (*eu* means "true"). In some texts, the words are spelled procaryote and eucaryote, but we shall retain the original spelling.

pro-kar′e-ōt
u-kar′e-ōt

Prokaryotes:
organisms whose cells lack nuclei and organelles and have other characteristics distinguishing them from eukaryotes.

According to modern biologists, bacteria and cyanobacteria ("blue-green algae") are prokaryotes, while fungi, protozoa, plants, and animals (including humans) are eukaryotes. Knowing this can have practical significance because we can define an organism's characteristics by knowing whether its cells are prokaryotic or eukaryotic.

Indeed, scientists have found that the distinctions between prokaryotes and eukaryotes go deeper than the nucleus. The cells of prokaryotes and eukaryotes both have a gel-like cytoplasm (sometimes called cytosol), but eukaryotic cells have a variety of membrane-enclosed components absent in prokaryotes (FIGURE 3.1). These components are called **organelles.** They include the **endoplasmic reticulum,** a series of membranes extending throughout the cytoplasm; the **Golgi body,** a number of flattened sacs where the cell's proteins and lipids are processed and packaged before release; the **lysosome,** a somewhat circular, droplike sac of digestive enzymes within the cytoplasm; and the **mitochondrion,** the organelle where much chemical energy is released for cell use (which is why mitochondria are called the "powerhouses of the cells").

Organelles:
membrane-enclosed compartments in eukaryotic cells.

mi′to-chon′dri-on

Certain microorganisms, such as simple algae and green-sulfur bacteria, possess chlorophyll, a pigmented substance used in photosynthesis. The chlorophyll is dissolved in membranes in prokaryotic cells, but in eukaryotic microorganisms (such as the protozoan *Euglena*), it is contained in an organelle called the **chloroplast.** Still another organelle within the eukaryotic cell is the **cytoskeleton,** an interconnected

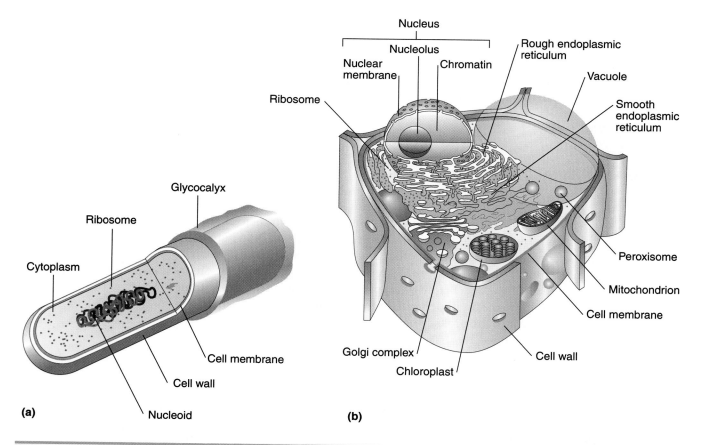

FIGURE 3.1

A Comparison of Prokaryotic and Eukaryotic Cells

(a) A stylized bacterial cell as an example of a prokaryotic cell. Relatively few structures are seen. (b) A plant cell as a typical eukaryotic cell. Note the variety and large size of the cellular features, many of which are discussed in the text. The presence of a nucleus is the primary feature distinguishing the eukaryotic cell from the prokaryotic cell.

Ribosomes:
ultramicroscopic bodies of RNA and protein where protein synthesis takes place in cells.

Cilia:
cellular organs of motion found in protozoa such as *Paramecium.*

system of fibers, threads, and interwoven molecules that give structure to the cell. The main components of the cytoskeleton are microtubules, microfilaments, and intermediate filaments, all assembled from subunits of protein. Another organelle called the **centriole** is a cylinderlike structure occurring in pairs and functioning in the formation of motility structures (flagella and cilia) and, possibly, in cell division.

All prokaryotes and eukaryotes possess **ribosomes,** the RNA-protein bodies that participate in protein synthesis (Chapter 5). Prokaryotic ribosomes (70S ribosomes) are smaller than their counterparts (80S ribosomes) in eukaryotic cells. Moreover, prokaryotic ribosomes exist free in the cytoplasm, while eukaryotic ribosomes can be free, but are usually bound to membranes of the endoplasmic reticulum.

Many prokaryotic and eukaryotic cells contain organelles called flagella and cilia. **Flagella** are long and hairlike and extend from the cell to provide cell movement. In prokaryotic cells, such as bacteria, the flagella rotate like the propeller of a motorboat (Chapter 4). In eukaryotic cells, such as certain protozoa and sperm cells, the flagella whip about. **Cilia** are shorter and more numerous than flagella. In moving cells, they wave in synchrony and propel the cell forward. *Paramecium* is a well-known ciliated protozoan.

Both prokaryotic and eukaryotic cells have their hereditary characteristics stored in molecules of deoxyribonucleic acid (DNA) organized in **chromosomes.** In prokaryotic cells, the chromosome consists of a single DNA molecule in a closed loop, while in eukaryotic cells, the DNA occurs in multiple chromosomes arranged in the nucleus. Eukaryotic chromosomes contain histone proteins; prokaryotic chromosomes do not. However, prokaryotic chromosomes have some protein in the form of topoisomerases, a group of enzyme proteins that prevent excessive coiling of the DNA molecule.

to′po-i-som′er-ase

The **cell membrane** (also known as the **plasma membrane**) lies at the border of all cells. Like other membranes of the cell, it is composed primarily of proteins and lipids, especially phospholipids. The lipid occurs in two layers, referred to as a bilayer, and protein globules appear to float within the lipid. Therefore, the membrane is constantly in flux and is referred to as a **fluid mosaic structure.** Within the fluid mosaic, proteins carry out most of the transport functions of the membrane.

Many prokaryotic and eukaryotic cells contain a structure outside the cell membrane called the **cell wall.** With only a few exceptions, all bacteria have a thick, rigid cell wall. Among the eukaryotes, the algae, fungi, and plants have cell walls. The cell walls are not identical in these organisms, however. In fungi, the cell wall contains a polysaccharide called chitin (Chapter 14), while bacteria possess a different polysaccharide, one called peptidoglycan (Chapter 4). The primary cell wall component of plants and algae is cellulose, along with pectins, lignins, and other substances. Cell walls provide support for the cells, give them shape, and help them resist mechanical pressures. A summary of the many differences between prokaryotes and eukaryotes is presented in TABLE 3.1.

al′jē
Algae:
plantlike organisms that perform photosynthesis and differ structurally from other land plants.

TABLE 3.1

A Comparison of Prokaryotes and Eukaryotes

CHARACTERISTIC	PROKARYOTES	EUKARYOTES
Nucleus	Absent	Present with nuclear membrane
Organelles	Absent	Present in a variety of forms
DNA structure	Single closed loop Almost naked strand with very little protein	Multiple chromosomes in nucleus Structural protein (histone) associated with DNA
Chlorophyll	When present, dissolved in cytoplasmic membranes	When present, dissolved in chloroplast membranes
Ribosomes	Smaller than eukaryotic ribosomes Free in cytoplasm	Larger than prokaryotic ribosomes Free or bound to membranes
Cell walls	Generally present Complex chemical composition	Present in some types, absent in others Complex chemical composition
Flagella	Rotating movement	Whipping movement
Cilia	Absent	In some cells
Reproduction	Usually by fission Sexual reproduction unusual	By mitosis Sexual reproduction usual
Examples	Bacteria, rickettsiae, chlamydiae, cyanobacteria	Fungi, protozoa, plants, animals, humans (all other organisms)

It is important to remember that all living things are either prokaryotes or eukaryotes. Note, however, that viruses are neither, since they are not living organisms. Viruses are fragments of nucleic acid packaged in a protein shell. Nevertheless we consider them "microorganisms" because of their infectious nature. In the following sections, we shall summarize other significant properties of the major groups of microorganisms.

BACTERIA

The term **bacteria** is a plural form of the Latin *bacterium,* meaning "staff" or "rod." Bacteria are prokaryotes and are among the most abundant organisms on Earth. The vast majority play a positive role in nature: They digest sewage into simple chemicals, they extract nitrogen from the air and make it available to plants for protein production, they break down the remains of all that die and recycle the carbon and other elements, and they produce foods for human consumption and products for industrial technology. Many biologists believe that life as we know it would be impossible without the bacteria.

Of course, some bacteria are harmful. Certain species multiply within the human body, where they digest the tissues or produce toxins that result in disease. Other bacteria infect plant crops and animal herds. Disease-causing bacteria (i.e., pathogenic bacteria) are a global threat to all forms of life.

Bacteria have adapted to more different living conditions than any other group of organisms. They inhabit the air, soil, and water, and they exist in enormous numbers on the surfaces of virtually all plants and animals. They can be isolated from Arctic ice, thermal hot springs, the fringes of space, and the tissues of animals (FIGURE 3.2). Some can withstand the searing acid in volcanic ash, the crushing pressures of ocean trenches, and the powerful activity of digestive enzymes. Other bacteria sur-

Toxin:
a chemical substance poisonous to body tissues.

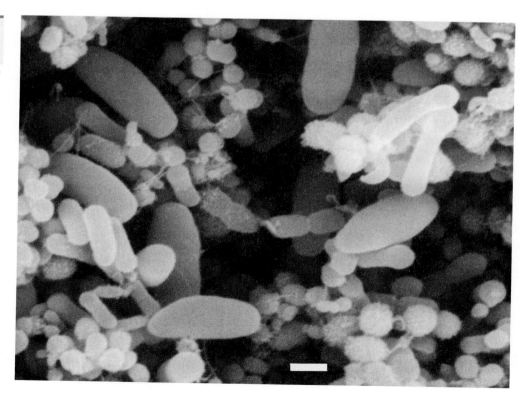

FIGURE 3.2

Mixed Bacteria

An electron microscopic view of mixed bacteria from the gastrointestinal tract of a lamb. Rod and spherical forms in various sizes and shapes are visible. (Bar = 1 μm.)

MicroFocus 3.2

AN UNKNOWN WORLD

Practically everyone is familiar with the word *bacteria*, but it may surprise you that hardly anyone really knows the bacteria. Yes, bacteria have been thoroughly studied in medicine, ecology, and molecular genetics, but the vast majority of bacteria remain unknown to science.

Hold a pinch of rich soil in the palm of your hand. You are now face to face with an estimated billion bacteria representing some 10,000 different species. If you were to try cultivating them using the most sophisticated methods available, perhaps 500 species might grow. That leaves 9500 species unknown until the right combinations of nutrients and environmental conditions are established in the laboratory.

Traditionally, *Bergey's Manual* has been the most authoritative guide to bacterial species. About 4000 species are listed in this book, a far cry from the thousands more believed to exist. Those who believe there are no more worlds to conquer should take note.

vive in oxygen-free environments, boiling water, and extremely dry locations. Bacteria have so completely invaded every part of the Earth that the mass of bacterial cells is estimated to outweigh the mass of all plants and animals combined (**Micro-Focus 3.2**). Chapters 4, 5, and 6 are devoted to the structure, growth, biochemistry, and genetics of bacteria, and Chapters 7 through 10 discuss the diseases they cause.

RICKETTSIAE, CHLAMYDIAE, AND MYCOPLASMAS

Rickettsiae (sing., rickettsia), chlamydiae, and mycoplasmas are also prokaryotes. Until the early 1970s these microorganisms were considered apart from the bacteria, but contemporary microbiologists now classify them as "small bacteria." Unfortunately, old habits linger and some microbiologists still think of them as distinct groups, which is why we separate them here.

Rickettsiae were first described by Howard Taylor Ricketts in 1909. These tiny bacteria can barely be seen with the most sophisticated light microscope and they are transmitted among humans primarily by arthropods such as ticks and lice. They are cultivated only in living tissues such as fertilized eggs, and different species cause a number of important diseases, including Rocky Mountain spotted fever and typhus fever. Chapter 9 contains a more thorough description of their properties.

rik-et'se-e

Arthropods:
animals with jointed appendages and a hard outer skeleton; examples are mosquitoes, ticks, and fleas.

Chlamydiae (sing., chlamydia) are roughly half the size of the rickettsiae and are so small that they cannot be seen with the light microscope. The chlamydiae can be cultivated within living cells, and one species causes the gonorrhealike disease known as chlamydia. This and several other chlamydial diseases are described in Chapters 7 and 10.

klah-mid'e-a

Mycoplasmas are another notch smaller than chlamydiae and are possibly the smallest known bacteria (**TABLE 3.2**). They can be cultivated outside living tissues in artificial laboratory media, and, although they are prokaryotes, they do not have cell walls like other bacteria. One form of pneumonia is caused by a mycoplasma (Chapter 7) and one sexually transmitted disease (Chapter 10) is a mycoplasmal illness.

CYANOBACTERIA

In older textbooks, **cyanobacteria** were known as blue-green algae. Today these microorganisms are considered bacteria because structural and biochemical properties are similar. However, cyanobacteria are not unique because of fundamental differences in how they form carbohydrates in photosynthesis (Chapter 5).

si'ah-no-bak-ter'e-ah

TABLE 3.2

An Overview of the Microorganisms

MICROORGANISMS	CLASSIFICATION	DISTINGUISHING CHARACTERISTICS
Bacteria	Prokaryotic	Extremely abundant; microscopic; many positive roles in nature; some cause disease; all microscopic
Rickettsiae Chlamydiae Mycoplasmas	Prokaryotic	Types of "small bacteria"; many involved in disease; rickettsiae and chlamydiae multiply only in host cells; mycoplasmas have no cell walls
Cyanobacteria	Prokaryotic	Pigmented organisms; formerly "blue-green algae"; similar to true bacteria
Protozoa	Eukaryotic	Animal-like; classified by type of motion; no cell walls; usually not photosynthetic
Fungi	Eukaryotic	Molds, yeasts, and other forms; usually filamentous; plantlike but not photosynthetic; unique cell walls
Unicellular algae	Eukaryotic	Plantlike; photosynthetic; most marine forms; include diatoms and dinoflagellates
Viruses	(Nonliving)	Fragment of nucleic acid (RNA or DNA) enclosed in protein; envelope in some; noncellular inert particles; replicate only in living host cells; ultramicroscopic

Photosynthesis:
a chemical process in which light energy is used to form chemical bonds in carbohydrate molecules.

Cyanobacteria are prokaryotes. They possess light-trapping pigments that function in photosynthesis taking place in the cell. Many of the pigments are blue, but some are black, yellow, green, or red. The periodic redness of the Red Sea, for example, is due to a species of cyanobacteria whose members contain large amounts of red pigment.

Cyanobacteria may occur as unicellular or filamentous organisms. Many species are able to incorporate atmospheric nitrogen (they "fix" nitrogen) into organic compounds useful to plants, thereby filling an important ecological niche. Cyanobacteria inhabit freshwater as well as marine environments. When ponds or lakes contain a rich supply of nutrients, the organisms may "bloom" and convert the water to a pea-soup green with a foul odor. Swimming pools and aquaria experience this problem if algicide is not used regularly.

PROTOZOA

Cellulose:
a polysaccharide of plant cell walls normally indigestible by humans.

Protozoa (sing., protozoan) are single-celled eukaryotes, most of which lack cell walls, ingest food particles, and move about freely. Many protozoal species join with other microorganisms to decompose dead organisms and recycle nutrients. Indeed, numerous species are important links in the food chain as they convert nutritionally inaccessible materials into protozoal substances easily digested by other organisms. In some plant-eating animals (e.g., cattle, goats, and other ruminants), protozoa live in the digestive tract and, along with bacteria, enable the animals to use grass and other high-cellulose foods they could not otherwise digest.

Protozoa exhibit a bewildering assortment of shapes, sizes, and structural components (FIGURE 3.3). A few species have the necessary pigments for photosynthesis and can therefore synthesize their own foods. Most protozoal species, however, must obtain nutrients from preformed organic matter. Protozoa are classified into groups according to how they move. Some have whiplike flagella, others possess hairlike cilia, and still others move by means of cytoplasmic extensions called pseudopodia ("false feet").

soo'do-po'de-ah

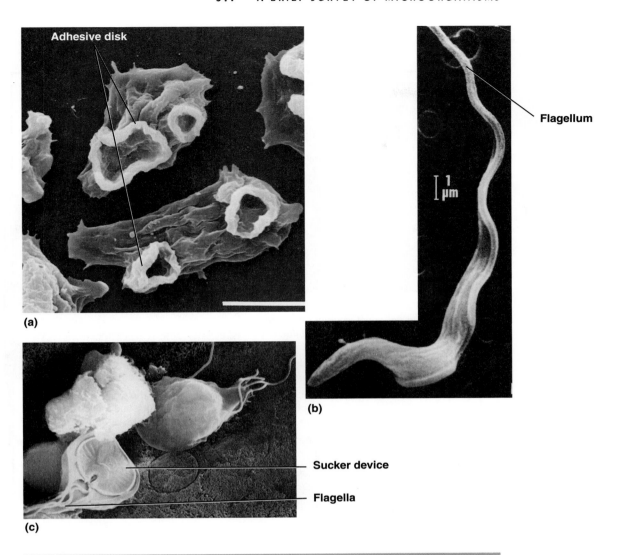

FIGURE 3.3

Three Species of Protozoa

Electron micrographs of three species of protozoa illustrating differences in shape and size. (a) The amoeba *Naegleria fowleri*, a cause of meningitis in humans. Note the irregular shape of this organism. (Bar = 5 μm.) (b) A protozoan called a trypanosome. The elongated shape and hairlike appendage (flagellum) are apparent. This organism causes African sleeping sickness. (c) Another flagellated protozoan, *Giardia lamblia* (×8026). The organism has a flat shape with multiple flagella extending toward the rear. The protozoan on the left shows the sucker device on its lower surface for holding fast to tissue. *Giardia* causes diarrhea in humans.

Although most protozoa are harmless to humans, some species are feared because they are pathogenic. Among the more notorious protozoal species are those that cause malaria of the blood and sleeping sickness in the nervous system. Other species are waterborne and cause such diseases as giardiasis, amoebic dysentery, and cryptosporidiosis (FIGURE 3.4). In recent years, the protozoan *Pneumocystis carinii* has been thrust into the headlines as a major cause of death in people with AIDS. We shall study protozoal diseases in depth in Chapter 15.

Malaria:
a mosquitoborne blood disease in which protozoa multiply within and destroy red blood cells.

ji-ar-di'a-sis

nu'mo-sis'tis car-in'i-i

FIGURE 3.4

An Outbreak of Intestinal Disease at a Summer Day Camp

This outbreak occurred in Florida during July and August 1996. Health officials recommended measures to restrict access to the hose believed to be the source of the outbreak.

TEXTBOOK CASES

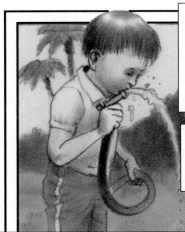
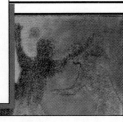
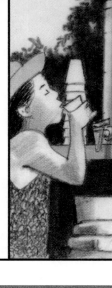

1. During the summer, a group of 98 children and 6 counselors attended a day camp in Alachua County, Florida, on the grounds of a public elementary school. The attendees ranged in age from 4 to 12 years.

2. The days were hot, and occasionally the children took a break from play to take a drink from a nearby hose with a spray nozzle. There was also water available from coolers, refilled often from the same garden hose.

3. The hose was also used to clean the garbage cans. Occasionally, camp personnel would leave the hose lying on the ground unattended. Feces of unknown origin were sometimes seen near the hose.

4. That summer, 72 children and 5 of the 6 counselors reported symptoms of intestinal disease, including abdominal pain, nausea, vomiting, and three or more watery stools each day.

5. Health officials visited the camp and obtained samples from various food and water sources. The outdoor faucet, its hose, and the spray nozzle were found to harbor *Cryptosporidium parvum,* a protozoan that causes intestinal illness.

FUNGI

fun'jī

kī'tin
Chitin:
a carbohydrate substance found in the cell wall of fungi.

Because of their distinctive cell walls, **fungi** were once considered members of the plant kingdom (indeed, many botany books and courses still discuss the fungi in detail). However, researchers have found the carbohydrate chitin in the fungal cell wall but not in the plant cell wall. Moreover, fungi do not synthesize nutrients by photosynthesis; instead they use preformed organic matter from the environment as a nutritional strategy. These characteristics, among others, separate them from plants.

Fungi are eukaryotic organisms often spoken of in two broad groups: the yeasts and the molds (FIGURE 3.5). **Yeasts** are unicellular organisms larger than bacteria. They play a vital role in the fermentation of wine and beer and the production of bread. **Molds** are long chains of cells often seen as fuzzy or fluffy masses on bread and other food products, especially acidic products. Commonly the molds assume vivid colors from the pigments in spores they produce for reproductive purposes. The chains of cells are called hyphae (sing., hypha). Cells of the hypha are highly efficient exploiters of available nutrients—during periods of peak growth, a mold can grow more than a half-mile of new hyphae in a single day. (Incidentally, the word *mold* has no technical significance, but we use it because it is ingrained in the English language.)

hi'fā

Fungi are among the major decomposers of organic matter in the world. Yet a few fungal species do not wait for an organism to die before they start consuming it. These are the pathogenic fungi, which cause some of the most common and persistent challenges to modern medicine. More than 20 percent of the world's population suffers from fungal disease, ranging from irritating maladies of the skin and mucous membranes (e.g., athlete's foot and yeast infection) to life-threatening diseases such as cryptococcosis. Chapter 14 discusses these diseases in more detail.

krip'to-kok-o'sis

UNICELLULAR ALGAE

The word **algae** (sing., alga) refers to any plantlike organisms that practice photosynthesis and differ structurally from typical land plants such as mosses, ferns, and seed plants. Two types of unicellular algae, the diatoms and the dinoflagellates, are important in microbiology.

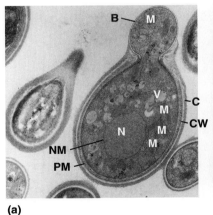
(a)

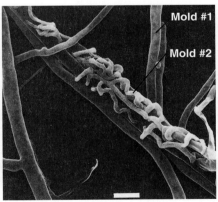
(b)

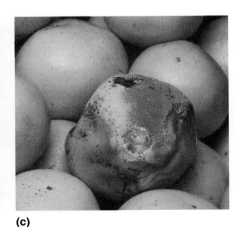
(c)

FIGURE 3.5

Three Views of Fungi

(a) A transmission electron micrograph of a yeast cell showing typical eukaryotic features. Note the cell wall (CW), capsule (C), and plasma membrane (PM) on the cell surface. In the cytoplasm, clear bodies called vacuoles (V) and mitochondria (M) may be seen. The nucleus (N) is surrounded by a nuclear membrane (NM). In the upper portion of the photograph, a reproductive structure, the bud (B), is growing out from the parent cell. (b) Two molds, one wrapped around the other, in a parasitic relationship. The long filamentous form of each mold and the many branches are visible (Bar = 10 μm.) (c) A mold growing on a grapefruit.

di'ah-tomz

Diatoms are eukaryotic microorganisms and an important source of food in the world's oceans. Through photosynthesis, they trap the sun's energy and manufacture carbohydrates, which are passed on to other marine organisms as food. The cell walls of diatoms are impregnated with silicon dioxide, a glasslike substance. When diatoms die, their remains accumulate on the seafloor as diatomaceous earth. The latter is gathered and used to produce filters. **Dinoflagellates** are a group of photosynthetic eukaryotes composed of amoebas encased in hard shells (hence the name *dino*). Dinoflagellates are important members of the world's food chains. They also cause the periodic red tides occurring in the oceans. Both diatoms and dinoflagellates are discussed in Chapter 25.

Diatomaceous earth:
the remains of diatoms used in filtering materials.

VIRUSES

Viruses are neither prokaryotes nor eukaryotes, as we noted previously. Many microbiologists even question whether viruses are living organisms because they are noncellular. They do not grow, nor do they display any nutritional patterns. Viruses have no observable activity except replication, and they accomplish this function only within living cells. Indeed, outside a living cell, a virus is no more alive than a grain of sand.

Viruses are smaller than the tiniest bacteria, so small that an electron microscope is necessary to see them. The simplest forms consist of nothing more than nucleic acid and protein. The nucleic acid is either DNA or RNA, but not both. Constituting as few as seven genes, the nucleic acid is packed inside the protein, and it is released when the virus penetrates its host cell. By commandeering the host cell's structures and enzymes, the virus then replicates itself many hundreds of times, often destroying the cell in the process. As nearby cells are penetrated and destroyed, the tissues disintegrate. Tissue disintegration is common to all viral diseases, including influenza, AIDS, hepatitis, chickenpox, herpes simplex, and rabies (FIGURE 3.6). We shall pay considerable attention to the structure and physiology of viruses in Chapter 11 and survey their diseases in Chapters 12 and 13.

Nucleic acid:
a major organic substance composed of a carbohydrate (ribose or deoxyribose), a phosphate group, and any of five nitrogenous bases.

To this point . . .

We have begun our study of microbiology by placing microorganisms into the panorama of living things as prokaryotes or eukaryotes. Knowing whether an organism is a prokaryote or a eukaryote is important because it enables us to see microorganisms in relation to plants and animals, while giving us a glimpse of their properties. We then developed brief sketches of different microorganisms to observe the spectrum of forms studied in the chapters ahead. Viruses were included because they are important agents of disease, even though they are neither prokaryotes nor eukaryotes.

We shall now focus on some general properties that apply to all microorganisms. Included here are such properties as classification, nomenclature, and size. This study will serve as a prelude to studying individual characteristics of the groups of microorganisms in other chapters.

FIGURE 3.6

A Case of Rabies Occurring in Warren County, New Jersey, in October 1997

This was the first case of human rabies in New Jersey since 1971.

TEXTBOOK CASES

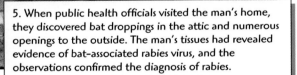

1. During early July, a man spotted a bat in the living room of his apartment in New Jersey. The apartment was on the second floor of an old wooden house in poor repair. Above the apartment was the attic, also in disrepair. After some minutes, the man captured the bat by isolating it in a corner. He grabbed the bat with a cloth and carried it to the doorway, where he released it outside. This was the second time the man had captured a bat in the house.

2. On October 12, the man developed an aching sensation in his right shoulder and neck, and he became restless. The symptoms worsened, and the next day, with chills and a sore throat, he visited a hospital emergency room.

3. The man was given an anesthetic throat spray for the pain and antibiotics by oral administration. He was sent home with other recommendations on how to care for a respiratory ailment.

4. The symptoms became more acute, and the man was admitted to the hospital with hallucinations, high fever, and terrible muscle aches. Within days, he developed shock and kidney failure, and he died on October 23.

5. When public health officials visited the man's home, they discovered bat droppings in the attic and numerous openings to the outside. The man's tissues had revealed evidence of bat-associated rabies virus, and the observations confirmed the diagnosis of rabies.

3.2

General Properties of Microorganisms

The basic concepts of microbiology include a number of properties that apply to all microorganisms. For example, all microorganisms have scientific names, and all have certain sizes. In addition, there are classification schemes into which most fit. In this section, we shall explore the principles on which these properties are based.

ORIGINS OF CLASSIFICATION

Taxonomy:
the study of the logical arrangement of living things into categories.

The science of classification, or **taxonomy,** deals with the systematized arrangements of related microorganisms and other living things into logical categories. Derived from Greek roots meaning "law of arrangements," taxonomy is essential to an understanding of relationships among living things. Taxonomy focuses on unifying concepts among organisms, while providing a basis for communication among biologists.

One of the first taxonomists was the Greek philosopher **Aristotle.** In the fourth century B.C., Aristotle categorized living forms in the world around him and described over 500 species of plants and animals according to their appearance and habits. Without reference books or instruments to help him, Aristotle made some key observations, including the fact that the whale is more like a mammal than a fish.

lin-ā'us

plant'ā
an-i-mal'ē-ah

The modern basis of taxonomy was devised by the Swedish botanist Carl von Linné, better known to history as **Carolus Linnaeus.** In his *Systema Naturae,* published in several editions between 1735 and 1759, Linnaeus named thousands of plants and animals and classified them in the kingdoms **Plantae** and **Animalia.** He inspired an unprecedented worldwide program of specimen hunting and sent his students around the globe in search of new life forms. He also popularized the binomial scheme of nomenclature, thus resurrecting the use of Latin as a language of the learned (MicroFocus 3.3). In his otherwise exacting system, Linnaeus reflected the scant knowledge of microorganisms and his general disinterest in them by grouping them separately under the heading of Vermes (as in vermin) in the category Chaos (confusion). In the years after Linnaeus, however, some microorganisms came to be considered plants while others were categorized as animals.

hek'el

In 1866, the German naturalist **Ernst H. Haeckel** disturbed the tidiness of the plant and animal kingdoms by proposing a new system to separate the microorganisms. Haeckel was unsatisfied placing mushrooms with plants because mushrooms have no chlorophyll, and by his time, there was a plethora of newly described "in-

MicroFocus 3.3

"WHAT WAS THAT NAME?"

The binomial system of nomenclature appears to be so obvious that it hardly needed to be invented. However, before Carolus Linnaeus popularized the scheme in 1735, scientists could not agree on scientific names for the organisms they studied. Different names were invented by different writers to serve as both designation and description. Confusion was rampant.

Linnaeus' great simplifying decision was to use the genus name and a modifying adjective for the label and description of an organism. He had to work quickly lest other naturalists use the same name for different organisms. In a monumental task of linguistic invention, Linnaeus ransacked his Latin for enough

terms to make up thousands of labels. Some names he took from an organism's manner of growth, others from the discoverer, others from classical heroes, and still others from vernacular names. Any parent who has had to name a child can appreciate what he was up against.

In a 1753 book on plants, Linnaeus supplied binomial names for over 5900 plant species known at that time. In his tenth edition of *Systema Naturae* (1759), he extended the scheme to animals. Within decades, his binomial names were adopted by European scientists and were reaching across the world. And just in time, because explorers were returning to Europe from distant corners of the globe with newly discovered life

forms (penguins, tobacco, potato, manatees, kangaroos, and others).

How important is the binomial system of nomenclature? It is clear that, to be understood, scientists must avoid ambiguity, and this is what the binomial system accomplishes. In the United States, for example, corn refers to a tall plant that produces yellow kernels on a cob. However, in England, the same plant is called maize. English "corn" is any number of different cereal grains, such as wheat, rye, and barley. Thus, to eliminate confusion, scientists use the term *Zea mays* when they refer to American corn or English maize. For scientists, the binomial system contains more than a grain of truth.

between" organisms, including many forms of protozoa, microscopic algae, and bacteria. Haeckel therefore coined the term **protist** for a microorganism, and he placed all protists in the new kingdom **Protista**. Protista came to include fungi, protozoa, bacteria, and virtually all organisms that share plant and animal characteristics but are not plants or animals. Some microbiologists, however, were not eager to accepts Haeckel's view, and they continued to classify bacteria and fungi with plants because all three have cell walls, while placing protozoa with the animals (TABLE 3.3).

Protist:
a name coined by Haeckel to refer to microorganisms; now used for a specific group of microorganisms.

THE FIVE KINGDOMS

During the twentieth century, advances in cell biology and interest in evolutionary biology led scientists to question the two- or three-kingdom classification schemes. In 1969, Robert H. Whittaker of Cornell University proposed a system that has gained wide acceptance in the scientific community. Further expanded in succeeding years by Lynn Margulis of the University of Massachusetts, the system recognizes five kingdoms of living things: Monera, Protista (also known as Protoctista by Margulis' supporters), Fungi, Animalia, and Plantae (FIGURE 3.7).

pro'toc-tist'ah

In the five-kingdom system, bacteria (including cyanobacteria) are classified together in the kingdom **Monera**, also called **Procaryotae**. These organisms are the only true prokaryotes. They differ significantly from members of the other four kingdoms in the cellular details described earlier. The second kingdom, **Protista**, includes unicellular and colonial eukaryotes such as protozoa, slime molds, and primitive algae. Members of the kingdom generally have flagella at some time in their lives, and even though there are some larger forms (e.g., complex algae), the tissue level of organization is absent. Many members of the kingdom are "taxonomic misfits" because they do no appear to fit in other kingdoms. However, they share certain characteristics with plants and animals, and some species appear to be plant and animal ancestors.

pro-kary-o'tā

In Whittaker's system, the kingdom **Fungi** includes nongreen, nonphotosynthetic eukaryotic organisms (i.e., fungi) whose cell walls differ chemically from those in bacteria or plants. Also, there is a mingling of cytoplasms of adjacent cells in the fungus, so true multicellularity does not exist, as in plants and animals. Fungi absorb

---

TABLE 3.3

A Summary of Microbial "Classifiers"

INVESTIGATOR	TIME FRAME	PROPOSAL
Aristotle	Fourth century B.C.	Described 500 species of plants and animals
Carolus Linnaeus	1750s	Devised plant and animal kingdoms Developed classification system for plants and animals Grouped microorganisms as "Chaos"
Ernst Haeckel	1860s	Separated microorganisms into third kingdom (Protista)
Ferdinand Cohn	1880s	Placed bacteria with plants because of presence of cell wall
David Bergey	1923	Developed a classification of bacteria in *Bergey's Manual*
Robert Whittaker	1969	Devised five-kingdom classification; microorganisms occupy kingdoms Monera, Protista, and Fungi
Carl Woese	1976	Devised three-domain classification system with Archaea, Eubacteria, and Eukarya

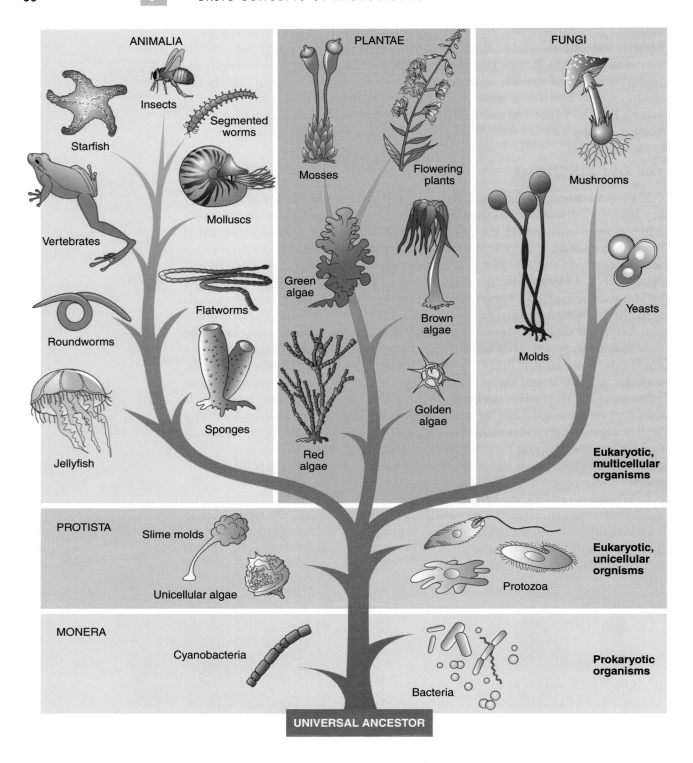

FIGURE 3.7

The Five-Kingdom System of Classification

Devised by Robert H. Whittaker, this system implies an evolutionary lineage, beginning with the Monera and extending to the Protista. Certain of the Protista are believed to be ancestors of the Plantae, Fungi, and Animalia. Divergence at each level is based on the three modes of nutrition: photosynthesis, absorption, and ingestion. Unicellular and multicellular organization are also key features in the system, although the fungi are not truly multicellular.

dissolved organic matter. It appears that fungi are not ancestors of plants or animals, so inclusion with the protists is not appropriate.

The final two kingdoms **Plantae** and **Animalia** are the traditional multicellular plants and animals. Plants use photosynthesis to synthesize their organic molecules; animals ingest their food through some form of mouth, then use digestive enzymes to break food particles into absorbable fragments.

The mechanics of the classification system have remained consistent since first outlined by Linnaeus. The fundamental rank is the **species** (pl., species). For microorganisms, the members of a species have 70 percent biochemical similarity and they differ significantly from other species. (For plants and animals, a species is a group of individuals in a population that can breed with one another). Two or more species are grouped together as a **genus** (pl., genera). A collection of genera make up a **family,** and families with similar characteristics make up an **order.** Orders are placed together as a **class,** and classes are assembled into a **phylum** (or **division,** in bacteriology and botany). Two or more phyla are grouped as a **kingdom.** TABLE 3.4 outlines the classification schemes for three organisms in the five-kingdom system.

In bacteriology, a microorganism may belong to a rank below the species level to indicate that a special characteristic exists within a subgroup of the species. Such ranks have no official standing in nomenclature, but they have practical usefulness in helping further to identify an organism. For example, two biotypes of the cholera bacillus, *Vibrio cholerae,* are known to exist: *Vibrio cholerae* classical biotype and *Vibrio cholerae* El tor biotype. Other designations of ranks include subspecies, serotype, strain, morphotype, and variety. Some bacteriologists recommend changing all these subspecies ranks to "varieties" and then using names such as biovar and serovar.

Species:
the fundamental rank in the classification system.

Genus:
a collection of two or more species of organisms.

Cholera:
a bacterial disease of the intestines, characterized by extreme diarrhea.

THE THREE DOMAINS

The view that five kingdoms alone represent the natural lines of division among living things has been further modified by the development of the three domains, or superkingdoms. First proposed in the 1970s by **Carl Woese** and his coworkers at the University of Illinois, the three-domain system is based on new techniques in molecular biology and biochemistry. It also encompasses new knowledge about a

woes

TABLE 3.4

The Taxonomy of Three Common Species of Organisms

	HOMO SAPIENS (HUMAN BEING)	*FELIS DOMESTICA* (HOUSE CAT)	*LEPTOSPIRA INTERROGANS* (BACTERIUM)
Kingdom	Animalia	Animalia	Procaryotae
Phylum (Division)	Chordata	Chordata	Gracilicutes
Class	Mammalia	Mammalia	Scotobacteria
Order	Primata	Carnivora	Spirochaetales
Family	Homindae	Felidae	Leptospiraceae
Genus	*Homo*	*Felis*	*Leptospira*
Species	*H. sapiens*	*F. domestica*	*L. interrogans*

group of bacteria called archaebacteria (also known as archaea). Archaebacteria (archaea) are bacterial forms known for their ability to live under extremely harsh environments (Chapter 4).

In Woese's **three-domain system**, the first domain includes the archaebacteria (archaea) and is called **Archaea**, the second encompasses all the remaining true bacteria and is called **Eubacteria** (similar to Monera but without archaebacteria), and the third includes the remaining four kingdoms of Whittaker and is called **Eukarya** (FIGURE 3.8). Archaea and Eubacteria differ significantly in the base sequence of the RNA in their ribosomes, the composition of their cell walls, the types of lipids in their membranes, and their sensitivity to certain antibiotics.

Scientists were initially reluctant to accept the three-domain system of classification, and many deemed it a threat to the tenet that all living things are either prokaryotes or eukaryotes. Then in 1996, **Craig Venter** and his coworkers deciphered the nitrogenous base sequence of the DNA of the archaebacterium *Methanococcus jannaschii* and showed that the genes are almost two-thirds different from those of a common eubacterium. They also found that proteins replicating the DNA and involved in the RNA synthesis of archaea have no counterpart in the Eubacteria. With persuasive evidence as this, the three-domain system has won new converts.

ar-ka'-a-bac-ter'i-a
ar-ka'ah
u-bac-ter'i-a

meth-an-o-kok'us jan'a-shi

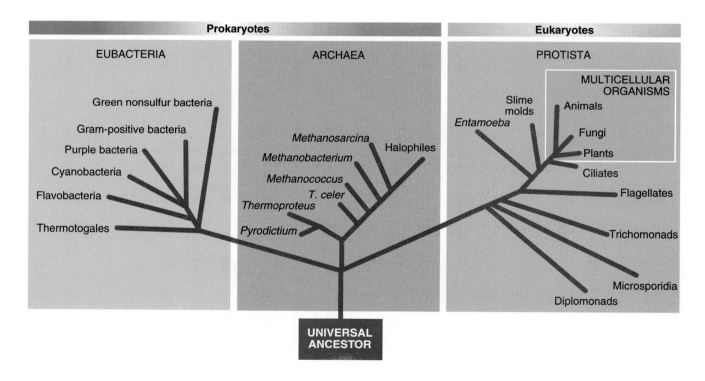

FIGURE 3.8

The Three-Domain System

Fundamental differences in genetic endowments are the basis for the three domains of all organisms on Earth. The relationships are determined from the sequences of nitrogenous bases in ribosomal RNA. The line length between any two groups is proportional to their genetic differences.

BACTERIAL TAXONOMY

We shall consider the taxonomy of most groups of microorganisms in their respective chapters. Bacterial taxonomy, however, merits special attention because bacteria occupy an important position in microbiology and have a complex system of taxonomy. We shall therefore discuss it here to show how a classification system develops. Also, we shall use bacterial classification as a prelude to Chapter 4.

One of the first systems of classification for the bacteria was devised in 1923 by David Hendricks Bergey. His book *Bergey's Manual of Determinative Bacteriology* was updated and greatly expanded in the decades that followed and exists today as the four-volume ***Bergey's Manual of Systematic Bacteriology.*** The first volume of the first edition of this later work was published in 1984, and three succeeding volumes appeared in following years. *Bergey's Manual,* as it is commonly known, is considered the official listing of all recognized bacteria. It is also intended to be a guide to identification.

Bergey's Manual: the official listing of all recognized bacteria.

In 1984, the editors of *Bergey's Manual* noted that there is no "official" classification of bacteria and that the closest approximation to an official classification is the one most widely accepted by the community of microbiologists. They stated that a comprehensive classification may one day be possible, but that a general scheme cannot currently be perceived because of the volume and complexity of available information.

Nevertheless, volume I of *Bergey's Manual* contains an interim classification scheme during the years of transition. The editors propose that bacteria be placed in the kingdom **Procaryotae** and that the kingdom be further broken down to four divisions. Three divisions of the kingdom Procaryotae consist of the traditional bacteria, and the fourth encompasses the archaebacteria. Microbiologists are currently studying how the divisions can be worked into kingdoms to fit the three-domain system coming into widespread use. For the time being, the four divisions are subdivided into a total of 33 sections encompassing seven classes of bacteria. Each section is described by a number of experts in that area, and decisions on further classification are left to them. No further classification is offered beyond the division level, but instead the bacteria are separated into sections. Each section is described by a number of experts in that area, and decisions on further classification are left to the experts.

Procaryotae: the kingdom name used by bacteriologists for bacteria.

The criteria used in the **identification** and classification of bacteria are rigorous and thorough. For example, the organism's shape and size; its oxygen, pH, and temperature requirements; and its laboratory characteristics are considered. Staining reactions, sporeforming ability, and type of movement are other important determinants. Pathogenic effects on animals are also noted. The biochemistry of the organism, including its photosynthetic nature and ability to digest certain organic substances, yields additional data. Tests are also performed to see whether it interacts with known antibodies. Even a laser beam can be used to identify an organism. In 1993, for example, researchers discovered that each species of bacterium has an "optical fingerprint" and reflects or absorbs laser light in its own characteristic way.

Antibodies: protein molecule produced by the immune system that react specifically with organisms or chemical substances.

In the 1970s, scientists found that the DNA of bacteria could be isolated rather easily and that purified DNA could be centrifuged at a high speed to measure its density, which was found to vary according to the relative amounts of the four nitrogenous bases in DNA. Scientists could then estimate the proportion of guanine and cytosine relative to the total amount of bases in DNA and derive a so-called **GC ratio** for numerous species of bacteria. While this procedure added another criterion for classification, it also caused some consternation because bacteria thought to be

Guanine, cytosine: two of the four nitrogenous bases found in DNA.

related were found to have very different GC ratios. The current trend is to assume a close relationship between two species of bacteria only if their GC ratios differ by less than 10 percent.

NOMENCLATURE

In addition to giving the descriptions and properties of microorganisms, taxonomies like the one in *Bergey's Manual* provide the genus name by which scientists refer to specific microorganisms. All microorganisms have a double name, usually from Latin or Greek stems. The name consists of the **genus** to which the organism belongs and a **species modifier** (a descriptive adjective) that further describes the genus name. This system of nomenclature is called the **binomial system**, from the Latin for "two names." First suggested by Linnaeus, the binomial system gives biologists throughout the world an international language for life forms and eliminates incalculable amounts of confusion.

When the genus and species modifier of an organism are written, only the first letter of the genus name is capitalized. The remainder of the genus name and species modifier are written in lowercase letters. Both words should be printed in italics, but if this is not possible, they should be underlined. For example, the species of intestinal rod discovered in 1888 by Theodor Escherich is written as *Escherichia coli* or Escherichia coli.

esh'er-ik

esh'er-ik'e-a

Scientists often abbreviate binomial names by writing the first letter of the genus name, or some accepted substitution, together with the full species modifier. The abbreviation should also be italicized or underlined. Thus, *Escherichia coli* becomes *E. coli,* and *Bacillus subtilis* is written *B. subtilis.* Where similarities occur, international committees on nomenclature have intervened.

The rules for assigning names to protozoa are listed in the *International Code of Zoological Nomenclature,* for fungi in the *International Code for Botanical Nomenclature,* and for bacteria in the *Bacteriological Code.* Viruses have no universally accepted binomial names as yet. (Note: A single volume entitled *Bergey's Manual of Determinative Bacteriology* is still available for use as a quick, handy guide to identifying bacteria.)

SIZE RELATIONSHIPS

Another important property of a microorganism is its size. In microbiology, the unit of length most often used is the **micrometer.** This unit is equivalent to a millionth (micro-) of a meter. The abbreviation for micrometer is **μm**, a combination of the Greek letter μ (pronounced "mue") and the abbreviation m for meter. To appreciate how small a micrometer is, consider this: Comparing a micrometer to an inch is like comparing a housefly to New York City's Empire State Building, 1472 feet high.

Micrometer:
a unit of measurement equal to a millionth of a meter.

Microorganisms range in size from the relatively large, almost visible protozoa (100 μm) down to the incredibly tiny viruses (0.01 μm), ten-thousand times smaller (FIGURE 3.9). Molds consist of intertwined filaments so long and twisted that they are visible, but the individual mold cells measure only about 40 μm by 10 μm. One group of fungi, the yeasts, are commonly about 8 μm in diameter. Most bacteria are about 1 μm to 5 μm in length, but the largest ones reach approximately 20 μm in length, although in 1993 a notable addition to the microbial world appeared in print (MicroFocus 3.4). The smaller bacteria known as the rickettsiae may be only about 0.4 μm long. Chlamydiae, among the smallest bacteria, are a scant 0.25 μm in length.

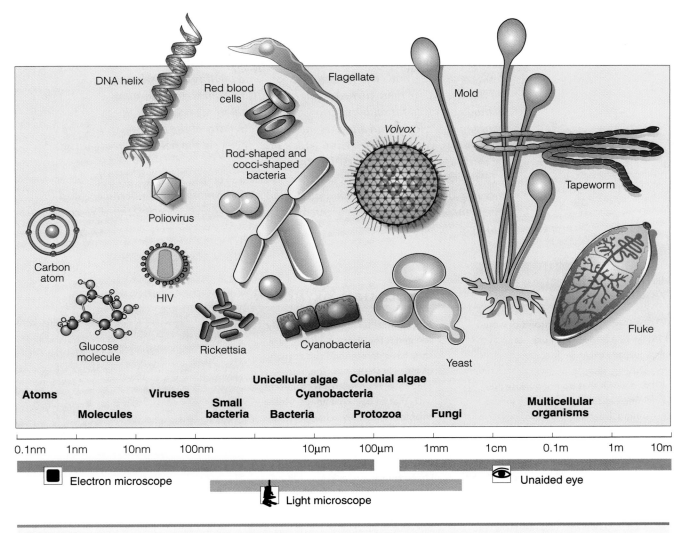

Atoms
Molecules
Viruses
Small bacteria
Bacteria
Unicellular algae
Cyanobacteria
Colonial algae
Cyanobacteria
Protozoa
Fungi
Multicellular organisms

0.1nm   1nm   10nm   100nm   10μm   100μm   1mm   1cm   0.1m   1m   10m

■ Electron microscope

Light microscope

👁 Unaided eye

FIGURE 3.9

Size Comparisons Among Various Living Things

To avoid decimals of micrometers, scientists often express the size of viruses in **nanometers**. The nanometer, abbreviated as **nm**, is equivalent to a billionth (nano-) of a meter. Using nanometers, the size of a smallpox virus may be written as 250 nm, rather than 0.25 mm. The poliovirus, among the smaller viruses, measures 20 nm in diameter. Other objects measured in nanometers include the wavelength of radiant energy, such as visible or ultraviolet light, and the size of certain large molecules.

Nanometer:
a unit of measurement equal to a billionth of a meter.
nm:
the abbreviation for nanometer, a billionth of a meter.

To this point . . .

We have discussed the spectrum of microorganisms and focused on some of their properties. One such property, classification, has been studied by Linnaeus and Haeckel, but the currently accepted system is the one devised by Whittaker then modified by Woese. Microorganisms occupy three of the five kingdoms in Whittaker's system and two of the three domains in Woese's. We noted that the classification systems for different microbial groups are handled in more specific textbooks on the groups (e.g., fungi, protozoa, and viruses). For bacteria, the classification system is complex and is outlined in four volumes of Bergey's Manual of Systematic Bacteriology. *To provide a glimpse of the taxonomist's work, we listed several criteria used to classify and identify a bacterium.*

The discussion then turned to nomenclature, where the binomial system is the method employed for all living things. A binomial name consists of the genus to which an organism belongs and a species modifier. Both parts of the binomial name are written in italics. We closed the section with a brief review of the size of microorganisms and the units used to measure their length.

In the final section of this chapter, we shall survey the methods used for observing microorganisms. We open with a discussion of the common light microscope and then review three specialized types of microscopy. Some remarks on electron microscopy will complete the chapter.

MicroFocus 3.4

A BIOLOGICAL OXYMORON

An English professor would define an oxymoron as two mutually exclusive juxtaposed terms. To ordinary people, an oxymoron is simply two words that do not go together. Some typical oxymorons are jumbo shrimp, holy war, old news, negative attraction, and sweet sorrow.

In 1993, researchers at Indiana University reported their discovery of a visible bacterium, and headlines proclaimed it a biological oxymoron. Why? Because a bacterium, by definition, is an invisible organism. And yet, here was a visible bacterium, an organism so large that a microscope was not needed to see it. The spectacular giant measures over 0.6 mm in length (that's 600 µm compared to 2 µm for *E. coli*) and dwarfs a *Paramecium*. Found in the gut of the surgeonfish near Australian reefs, the bacterium is the largest ever observed.

But is it really a bacterium? Its discoverers maintain it is. They have used biochemical techniques to amplify the genes for ribosomal RNA, and they have determined the sequence of bases in the genes. The base sequence, they report, is consistent with that of bacterial genes. Moreover, cellular analysis has failed to reveal a nucleus or nuclear membrane or subcellular compartmentalization, all of which bacteria characteristically lack. In addition, the DNA analysis of the organism's chromosome has indicated its relationship to the bacteria of the genera *Epulopiscium* and *Clostridium*.

Will the data stand the scrutiny of time and additional research? If they do not, then the definition of the bacterium is safe. If, however, this giant is indeed a bacterium, then the definition of a bacterium will have to change lest microbiologists be accused of spreading an oxymoron—and no one wants that to happen.

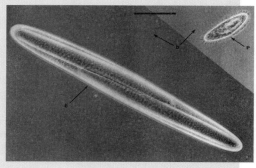

■ *A scanning electron micrograph of an immense bacterium isolated from the gut of a marine surgeonfish in 1993. the organism is labeled E because its name is* Epulopiscium fishelsoni. *Over 0.61 mm (610 µm) long, the bacterium can be compared to* Paramecium *(P), a relatively large protozoan at the upper right. The arrows from b point to typical bacteria added to the mixture for reference. (Bar = 0.1 mm.)*

3-3

Microscopy

Modern technologists have made available to microbiologists a broad range of instruments for viewing microorganisms. These instruments include the common light microscope, as well as a number of specialized instruments and the highly sophisticated electron microscopes. All operate on the same basic principle: Energy is projected toward an object, such as a microorganism. The energy bounces off the object and creates an impression on a sensing device. This device may be a television screen, a photographic film, or the human eye. The image reveals the form, shape, size, and other structural features of the object.

LIGHT MICROSCOPY

The basic microscopic system used in the microbiology laboratory is the **light microscope** (FIGURE 3.10). This instrument is also called a **bright-field microscope** because visible light passes directly through its lenses until it reaches the eye. Another common name is **compound microscope** because of its two-lens system, with the objective lens nearer the object and the ocular lens nearer the eye.

In light microscopy, visible light is projected through a substage condenser, which focuses the light into a sharp cone. The light then passes through the opening in the stage, into the slide, and bounces off the object. Next, it enters the objective lens to form a magnified image darker than the background. This image is called a **real image** because it can be projected onto a screen. However, the image is not seen by the microscopist. Instead, the image becomes an object for the ocular lens, which magnifies the image a second time to create a **virtual image** in space. Only the observer can see this image. It appears about as distant from the eye as this page is from your eye. FIGURE 3.11 traces the pathway of light and the formation of the virtual image.

A light microscope usually has three objective lenses: the low-power, high-power, and oil-immersion lenses. In general, these lenses magnify an object 10, 40, and 100 times, respectively. The magnification is represented by the multiplication sign, ×. The real image is then remagnified by the ocular lens, as noted above. With a 10× ocular, the total magnifications achieved are 100×, 400×, and 1000×, respectively.

For an object to be seen distinctly, the lens system must have good **resolving power;** that is, it must transmit light without variation and allow closely spaced objects to be clearly distinguished. For example, a car seen in the distance at night may appear to have a single headlight because the eyes lack resolving power. However, as the car comes closer, the two headlights can be seen clearly as the resolving power of the eye increases. The headlights now have resolution or clarity.

Objective lens:
the lens of a compound microscope nearest the object.

Ocular lens:
the lens of a compound microscope nearest the eye.

Resolving power:
the ability of a lens system to transmit light without variation and permit nearby objects to be clearly distinguished.

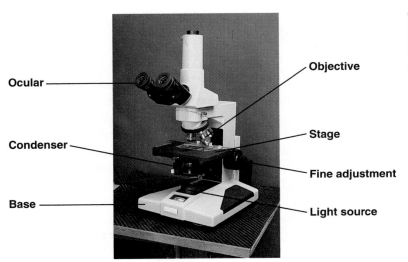

Ocular

Condenser

Base

Objective

Stage

Fine adjustment

Light source

FIGURE 3.10

The Light Microscope

This is the familiar light microscope used in many instructional and clinical laboratories. Note the important features of the microscope that contribute to the visualization of the object.

FIGURE 3.11

Image Formation in Light Microscopy

Light passes through the objective lens, forming an inverted real image A. This image serves as an object for the ocular lens, which remagnifies the image and forms the virtual image B. The lens system of the eye perceives this image and captures it on the retina.

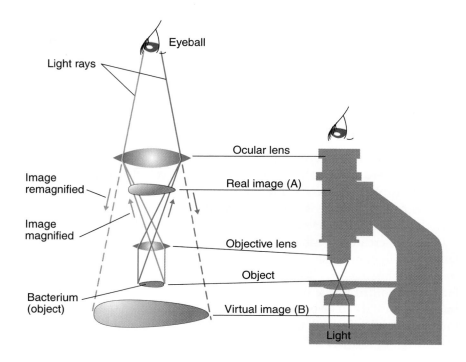

The resolving power (RP) of a lens system is important in microscopy because it denotes the size of the smallest object that can be seen clearly. Resolving powers vary for each objective lens and are calculated using the following formula:

$$RP = \frac{\lambda}{2 \times NA}$$

In this formula, the Greek letter λ (lambda) represents the wavelength of light and is usually set at 550 nm, the halfway point between the limits of visible light. The symbol NA stands for the **numerical aperture** of the lens. This number is generally printed on the side of the objective lens. It refers to the size of the cone of light that enters the objective and the medium in which the lens is suspended, usually air. For a low-power objective with an NA of 0.25, the resolving power may be calculated as follows:

$$RP = \frac{550 \text{ nm}}{2 \times 0.25} = \frac{550}{0.50} = 1100 \text{ nm or } 1.1 \text{ } \mu m$$

Since the resolving power for this lens system is 1.1 μm, any object smaller than 1.1 μm could not be seen, but an object larger than 1.1 μm would be visible.

Another factor of the compound microscope is the **working distance,** the amount of clearance between the slide and the bottom of the objective lens. Working distance is related to where the object comes into focus. For the low-power objective, a common working distance is 6.8 millimeters (mm); for the oil-immersion objective, it is a scant 0.12 mm, almost 60 times closer.

When switching from the low-power lens to the oil-immersion lens, one quickly finds that the image has become fuzzy. The object lacks resolution, and the resolving power of the lens system appears to be poor. This is because the objective lens

Working distance:
the amount of clearance between the slide and the bottom of the objective lens.

should be used with immersion oil. The system's resolving power is calculated with the lens suspended in oil rather than air, a factor that increases the numerical aperture to 1.25.

Oil is needed for **oil-immersion microscopy** because light bends abruptly as it leaves the glass slide and enters the air (FIGURE 3.12). Both low-power and high-power objectives are wide enough to capture sufficient light for viewing, but the oil-immersion objective is so narrow that most light bends away and would miss the objective if oil were not used. The **index of refraction** (or refractive index) is a measure of the light-bending ability of a medium. Immersion oil has an index of refraction of 1.5, which is almost identical to the index of refraction of glass. Because the refractive index is the same for oil and glass, the light does not bend as it passes from the glass slide into the oil. By comparison, air has an index of refraction of 1.0, which accounts for the abrupt bending as light enters it. The oil thus provides a homogeneous pathway for light from the slide to the objective, and the resolution of the object increases.

Index of refraction: a measure of the light-bending ability of a medium.

STAINING TECHNIQUES

When preparing for light microscopy, microbiologists commonly stain bacteria because the cytoplasm of bacteria lacks color. Several techniques have been developed for this purpose.

To perform the **simple stain technique,** a small amount of bacteria is placed in a droplet of water on a glass slide, and the slide is air-dried. Next, the slide is passed through a flame in a process called **heat fixing.** This bonds the cells to the slide, kills many organisms that may still be alive, and prepares them for staining. Now the slide is flooded with a **basic dye** such as crystal violet or methylene blue. Cytoplasm generally has a negative charge, and since basic dyes have a positive

Heat fixing: a procedure in which a slide containing bacteria is subjected to a moment of heat from a flame.

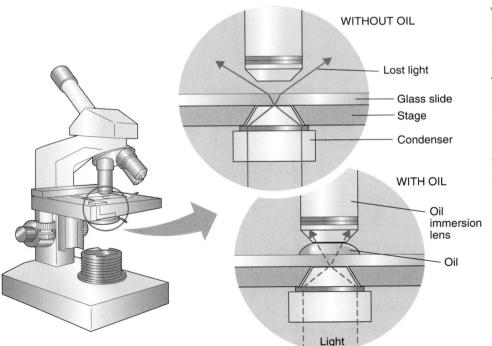

WITHOUT OIL

Lost light
Glass slide
Stage
Condenser

WITH OIL

Oil immersion lens
Oil

Light

FIGURE 3.12

Aspects of Oil-Immersion Microscopy

When light rays enter the air (solid arrow), they miss the objective lens. However, they remain on a straight line (dashed arrow) in the oil. This pathway leads them directly into the lens. The resolution increases with increased light.

charge, the dye is attracted to the cytoplasm, where staining takes place. FIGURE 3.13 illustrates this principle.

The **negative stain technique** works in the opposite manner (Figure 3.13). Bacteria are mixed on a slide with an **acidic dye** such as nigrosin (a black stain) or Congo red (a red dye). The mixture is then smeared across the face of the slide and allowed to air-dry. Because the acidic dye carries a negative charge, it is repelled by the cytoplasm. The stain gathers around the negatively charged cells, and the microscopist observes clear or white cells on a colored background. Since this technique avoids chemical reactions and heat fixing, the cells appear less shriveled and less distorted and are closer to their natural condition.

The **Gram stain technique** allows us to view stained cells while learning something about them. The technique is named for Christian Gram, the Danish physician who first suggested its use in 1884. It is a differential technique because it differen-

> **Gram stain technique:**
> a staining procedure that differentiates bacteria into two separate groups, Gram-positive and Gram-negative.

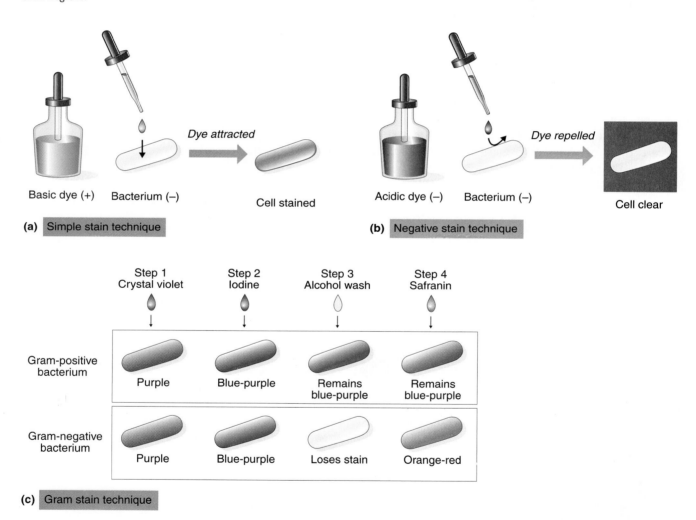

(a) Simple stain technique

Basic dye (+)   Bacterium (–)   Dye attracted   Cell stained

(b) Negative stain technique

Acidic dye (–)   Bacterium (–)   Dye repelled   Cell clear

(c) Gram stain technique

	Step 1 Crystal violet	Step 2 Iodine	Step 3 Alcohol wash	Step 4 Safranin
Gram-positive bacterium	Purple	Blue-purple	Remains blue-purple	Remains blue-purple
Gram-negative bacterium	Purple	Blue-purple	Loses stain	Orange-red

FIGURE 3.13

Important Staining Reactions in Microbiology

(a) In the simple stain technique, the positive-charged stain is attracted to the negative-charged bacteria, and staining takes place.
(b) With the negative stain technique, negative-charged dye is repelled by the bacteria, and the cells remain clear on a dark background.
(c) The Gram stain technique is a differential procedure. All bacteria stain with the crystal violet and iodine, but only Gram-negative bacteria lose the color when alcohol is applied. Subsequently, these bacteria stain with the safranin dye. Gram-positive bacteria remain blue-purple.

MicroFocus 3.5

"A.O. MEANS WHAT?"

In modern bacteriology laboratories, the crystal violet solution used for Gram staining is prepared by mixing solid dye particles with ammonium oxalate. This procedure has not changed since 1929, when a graduate student named Thomas Hucker introduced it. How this "Hucker modification" came about is part of the folklore of microbiology.

Hucker was studying bacteriology at Yale University. Early in 1929, his advisor suggested that he contact several hospital and university laboratories to see how they were performing the Gram stain technique. Hucker was to report his findings in a paper presentation at an upcoming scientific meeting in Philadelphia. He dutifully sent out a series of

letters and learned that the standard procedures were being used at all laboratories—all, that is, except Dartmouth's.

The reply from Dartmouth College piqued his interest. At the time, the usual procedure was to dissolve crystal violet in aniline oil. But Dartmouth bacteriologists apparently were using ammonium oxalate. Hucker tried ammonium oxalate and found that the stain improved with age and gave clearer results. He prepared his paper for the Philadelphia meeting and sent a draft to Dartmouth's biology department with a note of thanks. Soon thereafter he received a phone call from Dartmouth— they had never heard of ammonium oxalate for Gram staining. Hucker was perplexed.

In the days that followed, Hucker learned that a chemist had intercepted his survey letter and sent the reply. In writing out the method for crystal violet preparation, the chemist had read "A.O." on the bottle of stain and assumed that it meant the dye was dissolved in ammonium oxalate. Aniline oil simply did not occur to him. Moreover, he had not bothered to check with the biology department because it was inventory time and other things were on his mind. Thus, a case of badly interpreted bacteriological shorthand led to the Hucker modification. Hucker became famous; the chemist remained anonymous.

tiates bacteria into two groups depending on the results. Certain bacteria are called Gram-positive bacteria; others are Gram-negative.

The first two steps of the technique are straightforward. Air-dried heat-fixed smears are stained with crystal violet (MicroFocus 3.5), then with a special Gram's iodine solution. All bacteria become blue-purple. Next the smear is rinsed with a decolorizer such as 95 percent alcohol or an alcohol-acetone mixture. At this point, certain bacteria lose their color and become transparent. These are the **Gram-negative bacteria.** Other bacteria retain the blue-purple stain. These are the **Gram-positive bacteria.** When safranin, a red dye, is applied to the slide, only the Gram-negative organisms accept the stain. Thus at the technique's conclusion, Gram-positive bacteria are blue-purple while Gram-negative organisms appear orange or red (Figure 3.13). By observing the color of the cells at the conclusion of the process, one may decide the group to which the bacteria belong.

It is not totally clear why bacteria respond differently to the Gram stain technique. One theory suggests that crystal violet and iodine form a chemical complex in the bacterial cytoplasm. Since Gram-negative bacteria have a high lipid content in their cell walls, some microbiologists maintain that the alcohol dissolves the lipid and allows the crystal violet-iodine complex to leak out of the cytoplasm. Gram-positive bacteria, with less cell wall lipid, are less susceptible to the alcohol's effects. Another theory points to the heavy concentration of peptidoglycan in the cell wall of Gram-positive bacteria. Peptidoglycan, a complex carbohydrate, is thought to trap the crystal violet-iodine complex in its many cross-linkages. Gram-negative bacteria have considerably less peptidoglycan in their cell walls, hence they would trap less of the complex. Note that the words "positive" and "negative" are nothing more than convenient expressions and that electrical charges play a minimal role in Gram staining.

Knowing whether an organism is Gram-positive or Gram-negative is important for several reasons. For instance, microbiologists use results from the Gram stain

Safranin:
a basic dye with a red color, used in Gram staining.

pep'ti-do-gli'kan
Peptidoglycan:
a complex carbohydrate present in the cell walls of bacteria.

technique to identify an unknown organism and classify it in *Bergey's Manual.* Gram-positive and Gram-negative bacteria differ in their susceptibility to chemical substances such as antibiotics (Gram-positive bacteria are more susceptible to penicillin, Gram-negatives to tetracycline), and they have different structural components (Gram-negative bacteria have more complex cell walls, with an outer membrane). They produce different types of toxic poisons as well.

One other differential technique, the **acid-fast technique,** deserves mention. This technique is used to identify members of the genus *Mycobacterium,* one species of which causes **tuberculosis.** These bacteria are normally difficult to stain, but they stain red when treated with carbolfuchsin and heat (or lipid solubilizer). Then they retain their color when washed with a dilute acid-alcohol solution. Other bacteria lose their color easily during the acid-alcohol wash. The *Mycobacterium* species is therefore said to be acid-resistant or "acid-fast." (A blue counterstain is used to give color to nonacid-fast bacteria.) Because they stain red and break sharply when they reproduce, *Mycobacterium* species are euphemistically referred to as "red snappers."

> **Acid-fast technique:**
> a staining technique in which stain is forced into bacteria, then retained by the cells even on treatment with a dilute acid-alcohol solution; used to identify *Mycobacterium* species.

DARK-FIELD AND PHASE-CONTRAST MICROSCOPY

In **dark-field microscopy,** the background remains dark, and the object is illuminated (FIGURE 3.14). A special condenser mounted under the stage of the dark-field microscope scatters the light and causes it to hit the object from different angles. Some light bounces off the object into the lens to make the object visible, but the surrounding area appears dark because it lacks background light. The effect is similar to seeing the moon at night. In this case, sunlight from behind the Earth reflects off the moon and we can see it, but the sky appears dark because the sun is hidden.

> **Condenser:**
> a series of lenses mounted under the stage of a microscope.

Dark-field microscopy helps in the diagnosis of diseases caused by spiral bacteria because these organisms are near the limit of resolution and do not stain well. For example, **syphilis** is caused by *Treponema palladum,* a spiral bacterium with a diameter of about 0.15 μm. This bacterium may be observed in scrapings taken from a lesion of a person who has the disease.

> trep'o-nē-mah pal'e-dum

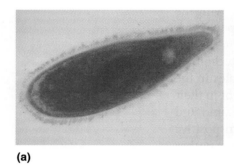 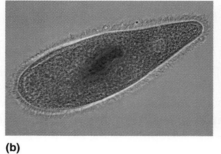 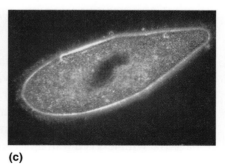

(a)   (b)   (c)

FIGURE 3.14

Variations in Microscopy

The same organism seen under three different microscopes (400×). The paramecium is visualized under (a) the light microscope , (b) the phase-contrast microscope, and (c) the dark-field microscope. Note the different view that each microscope affords.

Special microscope parts are also used in **phase-contrast microscopy.** A series of special condensers and filters split a light beam and throw the light rays slightly out of phase. The separated beams of light then pass through and around microscopic objects, and small differences in the densities of the objects show up as different degrees of brightness and contrast. With the phase-contrast microscope, microbiologists can see organisms alive and unstained. The fine structures of yeasts, molds, and protozoa are studied with this instrument. The various types of microscopes are compared in TABLE 3.5.

Phase-contrast microscope: a microscope in which light rays are thrown out of phase by condensers, then used to illuminate details of living cells.

FLUORESCENCE AND ELECTRON MICROSCOPY

During the past generation, **fluorescence microscopy** has emerged to become a major asset to diagnostic and research laboratories. The technique has been applied to the identification of many microorganisms and is a mainstay of modern microbiology, especially in health-related issues (MicroFocus 3.6). Microorganisms are coated with a fluorescent dye, such as **fluorescein,** then illuminated with ultraviolet light energy. The energy excites electrons in the dye, and they move to higher energy levels. However, the electrons quickly drop back to their original energy levels and give off the excess energy as visible light. The coated microorganisms appear to fluoresce.

An important application of fluorescence microscopy is in the **fluorescent antibody technique** used to identify an unknown organism. In one variation of this procedure, fluorescein is chemically united with antibodies, the protein molecules produced by the body's immune system when stimulated by a specific organism.

Ultraviolet light: a type of energy with a wavelength shorter than that of visible light.

TABLE 3.5

A Comparison of Various Types of Microscopy

TYPE OF MICROSCOPE	SPECIAL FEATURE	APPEARANCE OF OBJECT	MAGNIFICATION	OBJECTS OBSERVED
Light (compound)	Visible light illuminates object	Stained microorganisms on clear background	1000×	Form, shape, and size of killed microorganisms (except viruses, spirochetes)
Dark-field	Special condenser scatters light	Unstained microorganisms on dark background	1000×	Live, unstained microorganisms (e.g., spirochetes)
Phase-contrast	Special condenser throws light rays "out of phase"	Unstained microorganisms on dark background	1000×	Internal structures of live, unstained eukaryotic microorganisms
Fluorescence	UV light illuminates fluorescent-coated objects	Fluorescing microorganisms on dark background	1000×	Outline of microorganisms coated with fluorescent-tagged antibodies
Transmission electron microscope (TEM)	Short-wavelength electron beam penetrates sections	Alternating light and dark areas reflecting internal cell structures	20 million×	Ultrathin slices of microorganisms and internal components of eukaryotic cells
Scanning electron microscope (SEM)	Short-wavelength electron beam knocks loose electron showers	Microbial surfaces	100,000×	Surfaces and textures of microorganisms and cell components

MicroFocus 3.6

THE CENTERS FOR DISEASE CONTROL AND PREVENTION

The Centers for Disease Control and Prevention (CDC) has its headquarters in Atlanta, Georgia, and is one of six major agencies of the U.S. Public Health Service. Originally established as the Communicable Disease Center in 1946, the CDC was the first governmental health organization ever set up to coordinate a national control program against infectious diseases. At first, it was concerned with diseases spread from person to person, from animals to people, or from the environment to humans. Eventually, though, all communicable diseases came under its aegis. Atlanta was selected as the site for the CDC because it was a convenient central point for the study of malaria, which was then common in the South.

In April 1955, two weeks after release of the Salk vaccine for polio, the CDC received reports of six cases of polio in vaccinated children. Two days later, it established the Polio Surveillance Unit and began collecting data on polio occurrence and summarizing it for health professionals. More than 80 percent of vaccine-associated polio cases were related to a single manufacturer, and its vaccine was withdrawn at once. This incident established the role of the CDC in health emergencies, and soon it became a national resource for the development and dissemination of information on communicable disease. In 1960, the CDC moved to a new headquarters complex adjoining Emory University. The unassuming appearance of the facility belies its importance.

Reorganized with its current name in 1980 (the words "and Prevention" were added in 1992 but the CDC acronym was retained), the CDC is charged with protecting the public health of the United States populace by providing leadership and direction in the prevention and control of infectious disease and other preventable conditions, such as cancer. It is concerned with urban rat control, quarantine measures, health education, and the upgrading and licensing of clinical laboratories. The CDC also provides international consultation on disease and participates with other nations in the control and eradication of communicable infections. It employs 3500 physicians and scientists, the largest group in the world, and processes 170,000 samples of tissue annually. Its publication *The Morbidity and Mortality Weekly Report* is distributed each week to over 100,000 health professionals.

"Tagged" antibodies result. Next, these antibodies are mixed with a sample of the unknown organism. If the antibodies are specific for that organism, they will bind to it and coat the cells with the dye. When subjected to ultraviolet light, the organisms will fluoresce. If the organisms fail to fluoresce, antibodies for a different organism are tried.

Electron microscope:
a microscope in which a beam of electrons substitutes for the light energy used in other microscopes.

The **electron microscope** grew out of an engineering design made in 1933 by German physicist Ernst Ruska (winner of the 1986 Nobel Prize in Physics). Ruska showed that electrons flow in a sealed tube if a vacuum is maintained to prevent electron wandering. Magnets pinpoint the flow onto an object, where the electrons are absorbed or deflected, depending on the density of structures within the object. When projected onto a screen underneath, the electrons form an image that outlines the structures.

The key to electron microscopy is the extraordinarily short wavelength of the beam of electrons. Measured at 0.005 nm (compared to 550 nm for visible light), the short wavelength dramatically increases the resolving power of the system and makes possible the visualization of viruses, fine cellular structures, and large molecules such as DNA (FIGURE 3.15).

Transmission electron microscope:
a microscope in which an electron beam passes through an ultrathin slice of an object.

Two types of electron microscopes are currently in use. The first type, the **transmission electron microscope (TEM)**, is used to photograph detailed structures within cells. Ultrathin sections of the object must be prepared because the electron beam can penetrate matter only a short distance. After embedding the specimen in a suitable mounting medium or freezing it, scientists cut the specimen into sections with a diamond knife. In this manner, a single bacterium can be sliced the long way into a hundred or more sections. It is also possible to fracture the cells after freezing with a special knife, and then view the cast rather than the cell itself. The cast allows the observation of surfaces outside the cell as well as within it. This technique is called freeze-fracturing (FIGURE 3.16).

Once sectioned, the portions of the object are stained with a heavy metal such as gold or palladium to make certain parts dense. Next, the microscopist inserts the sections into the vacuum chamber of the instrument and focuses a 10,000-volt electron beam on them using magnetic lenses. An image forms below. A photograph prepared from the image may be enlarged with enough resolution to achieve a total magnification of over 20 million times. Objects as small as 2.0 nm can be seen.

The second type is the **scanning electron microscope (SEM).** This instrument, developed in the late 1960s, enables researchers to see the surfaces of objects in the natural state and without sectioning. The specimens are placed in the vacuum chamber and covered with a thin coat of gold to increase electrical conductivity and decrease blurring. The electron beam then sweeps across the object and knocks loose showers of electrons that are captured by a detector. An image builds line by line, as in a television receiver. Electrons that strike a sloping surface yield fewer electrons, thereby producing a darker contrasting spot and a sense of three dimensions. Magnifications with the SEM are limited to about 75,000 to 100,000 times, but the instrument is relatively easy to operate and gives vivid and undistorted views of an organism's surface details. FIGURE 3.17 shows the same organism viewed with the two different forms of electron microscopy.

The electron microscope has added immeasurably to our understanding of the structure and function of microorganisms by letting us penetrate their innermost secrets. In the chapters ahead, we shall study myriad fine structures displayed by the electron microscope, and we will better appreciate microbial physiology as it is defined by microbial structures.

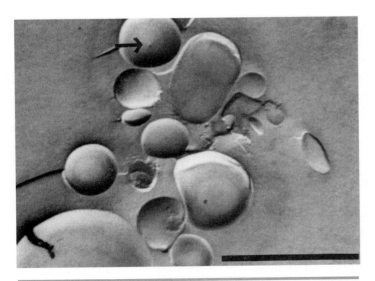

FIGURE 3.16

Freeze-Fracturing

An electron micrograph of casts of the outer membrane from the syphilis organism *Treponema pallidum*. Note that we are looking into cavities made by submicroscopic extensions of the membrane. The arrow points to a protein particle in the fracture face. (Bar = 0.5 μm.)

Scanning electron microscope: a microscope in which an electron beam sweeps across the surface of an object.

FIGURE 3.15

Improving Object Resolution

How the energy of shorter wavelength increases the resolution of an observed object. In diagrams 1 to 4, successively smaller circles outline the figure and the figure becomes clearer. In the same way, energies of decreasing wavelengths (e.g., visible light–ultraviolet light–electron beam) outline an object more precisely and give an instrument better resolving power and the object better resolution.

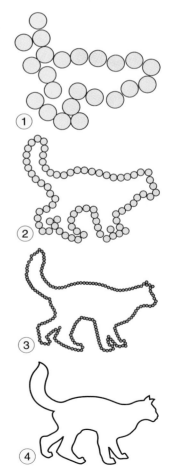

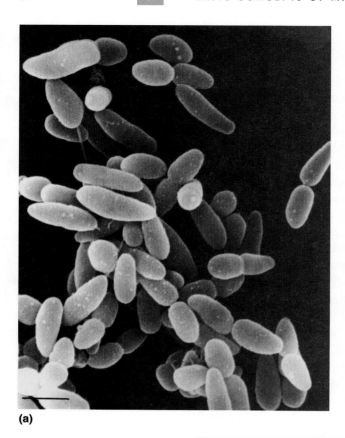

(a)

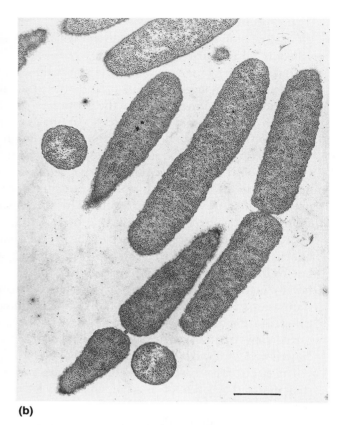

(b)

FIGURE 3.17

Scanning and Transmission Electron Microscopy Compared

The bacterium *Pseudomonas aeruginosa* as seen with two types of electron microscopy. (a) A view of whole cells seen with the scanning electron microscope. (Bar = 1.0 μm.) (b) A view of sectioned cells seen with the transmission electron microscope. (Bar = 0.5 μm.) The difference in perspective with the two microscopes is clear.

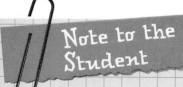

Note to the Student

As microbiology continues to capture headlines in the public media, it becomes more and more common to see microbial names in print. And all too often the name is misspelled, miswritten, or misinterpreted. For example, I once read in a newspaper that *Staphylococcus aureus*, a well-known cause of skin infections, was a recurring problem in a local hospital. In the vernacular of our times, the disease is often called a "staph infection." However, the newspaper reported it as a "staff infection."

I believe that if one is to write or speak microbiology, one should try to do it correctly. I would recommend, therefore, that you pay particular attention to the microbial names as we encounter them and that you develop the habit of pronouncing them and writing them correctly. You should also insist that magazines and newspapers follow the accepted standards for writing the names of microorganisms, A letter to the editor does much to improve the publication's awareness of its error. You should not be reluctant to send one.

Summary

Some characteristics applied to all microorganisms are surveyed in this chapter. For example, microorganisms fit the pattern wherein all living things are categorized as prokaryotes or eukaryotes, the distinguishing hallmarks being cellular features such as the nucleus, ribosomes, and organelles, as well as patterns such as reproductive methods. Bacteria are prokaryotes, while fungi and protozoa are eukaryotes. Brief sketches of microorganisms give insight into microbial structure and physiology, and they point to the importance of microorganisms in the natural world and in medical microbiology.

Many systems of classification for living things have been devised. The efforts of Aristotle, Linnaeus, and Haeckel are notable. The currently accepted system is the five-kingdom system proposed by Robert H. Whittaker in 1969. In Whittaker's classification, bacteria are placed in the kingdom Monera, protozoa in Protista, and fungi in a kingdom with the same name, Fungi. The three-domain system of Woese is also gaining acceptance. Part of an organism's binomial name is the genus name; the remaining part is an adjective that describes the genus name. Another criterion of a microorganism is its size, a characteristic that varies among members of different groups. The micrometer, a millionth of a meter, is used to measure the dimensions of bacteria, protozoa, and fungi. The nanometer, a billionth of a meter, is commonly used to express viral measurements.

The instrument most widely used to observe microorganisms is the light microscope. For bacteria, staining generally precedes observation. The simple, negative, Gram, and other staining techniques can be used to impart color to bacteria and determine structural or physiological properties. Microscopes such as the dark-field, phase-contrast, and fluorescence microscopes have specialized uses in microbiology. To increase resolution and achieve extremely high magnification, the electron microscope employs a beam of electrons instead of a beam of light. To see whole objects, the scanning electron microscope is useful; to observe internal details, the transmission electron microscope is most often used. The various microscopes help us visualize and conceptualize microorganisms, and understanding their basic properties helps us see their place in the scheme of living things.

Questions for Thought and Discussion

1. A student is asked on an examination to write a description of the protozoa. She blanks out. However, she remembers that protozoa are eukaryotes, and she recalls the properties of eukaryotes. How can she use this information to answer the question?

2. A local newspaper once contained an article about "the famous bacteria eecoli." How many things can you find wrong in this phrase?

3. Microorganisms have been described as the most chemically diverse, the most adaptable, and the most ubiquitous organisms on Earth. Although your knowledge of microorganisms still may be limited at this point, try to add to this list of "mosts."

4. A student is performing the Gram stain technique in the laboratory. In reaching for the alcohol bottle in step 3, he inadvertently takes the water bottle and proceeds with the technique. What will be the colors of Gram-positive and Gram-negative bacteria at the conclusion of the technique?

5. In older textbooks the words *micron* and *millimicron* are used where we now use the terms *micrometer* and *nanometer*. Why is current terminology preferable?

6. In 1997, a writer from *The New York Times* described microorganisms as the "New Yorkers of the living world: irrepressible, vilified, and able to reproduce in wildly inhospitable environments." From your general knowledge of microorganisms, what characteristics do they have in common with the residents of the city where you live?

7. While working in the lab, a student notices that there is no applicator in the bottle of immersion oil. But then she unscrews the cap and, as she lifts it from the oil, a glass applicator appears. Why did the applicator escape her ability to see it?

8. A new bacteriology laboratory is opening in your community. What is one of the first books that the laboratory director will want to purchase?

9. While scanning a menu in an Italian restaurant, you notice an entire section entitled Fungi. Among the choices are spaghetti with fungi, stuffed fungi, and fungi parmigiana. What will you receive if you order any of these?

10. A car parked along the street displays a license plate that reads E. COLI. What do you suppose the owner does for a living?

11. Christian Gram, developer of the Gram stain technique, originally intended his technique for use in distinguishing bacteria from cellular nuclei in slides of patients' tissues. Develop a scenario in which he might have realized that it would be more useful for separating bacteria into groups.

12. In 1987, in a respected journal of science, an author wrote, "Linnaeus gave each life form two Latin names, the first denoting its genus and the second its species." A few lines later, the author wrote, "Man was given his own genus and species *Homo sapiens*." What is conceptually and technically wrong with both statements?

13. A student of general biology observes a microbiology student using immersion oil and asks why the oil is used. "To increase the magnification of the microscope" is the reply. Would you agree? Why?

14. Assume that a small spherical bacterium has a diameter of 1 micrometer. A million of these bacteria would therefore fit in the space occupied by a meter (39.39 inches, or slightly more than 3 feet). Suppose you were to count each bacterium in this space at a rate of one bacterium per second. How long would it take you to count all the bacteria? Does this help you conceptualize how small a bacterium truly is?

15. A 1980s *Far Side* cartoon by Gary Larson was entitled Single Cell Bar. Assuming you were the artist, how many different cell shapes and sizes would you include in your drawing?

http://microbiology.jbpub.com

The site features **eLearning,** an on-line review area that provides quizzes and other tools to help you study for your class. You can also follow useful links for in-depth information, read more MicroFocus stories, or just find out the latest microbiology news.

Review

The types of microorganisms; their classification, nomenclature, and size; and the methods for observing microorganisms were the major themes of this chapter. To test your understanding of these themes, match the statement on the left to the term on the right by placing the letter of the term in the available space. Appendix D contains the correct answers.

_____ 1. System of nomenclature used for microorganisms and other living things.

_____ 2. Unit of measurement used for viruses and equal to a billionth of a meter.

_____ 3. Major group of organisms whose cells have no nucleus or organelles in the cytoplasm.

_____ 4. Once known as blue-green algae.

_____ 5. Devised the five-kingdom system of classification in which microorganisms are placed.

_____ 6. Type of microscope that uses a special condenser to split the light beam.

_____ 7. Type of electron microscope for which cell sectioning is not required.

_____ 8. Eukaryotes classified into groups according to how they move.

_____ 9. Prokaryotic microorganisms that have no cell wall.

_____ 10. Neither prokaryotes nor eukaryotes.

_____ 11. Kingdom in which the bacteria are classified.

_____ 12. Staining technique that differentiates bacteria into two groups.

_____ 13. Author of an early system of classification for bacteria.

_____ 14. Category into which two or more species of bacteria are grouped.

_____ 15. Coined the name Protista for microorganisms.

_____ 16. Considered to be unicellular algae.

_____ 17. Used to write the binomial name of microorganisms.

_____ 18. Unit of measurement for bacteria and equal to a millionth of a meter.

_____ 19. Type of unspecialized laboratory microscope having a two-lens system.

_____ 20. Staining technique in which the background is colored and the cells are clear.

A. Viruses

B. Italics

C. Gram

D. Mycoplasmas

E. Simple

F. Genus

G. Binomial

H. Boldface

I. Diatoms

J. Micrometer

K. Prokaryotes

L. Cyanobacteria

M. Dark-field

N. Scanning

O. Haeckel

P. Bergey

Q. Negative

R. Protista

S. Eukaryote

T. Nanometer

U. Phase-contrast

V. Monera

W. Protozoa

X. Whittaker

Y. Chlamydia

Z. Compound

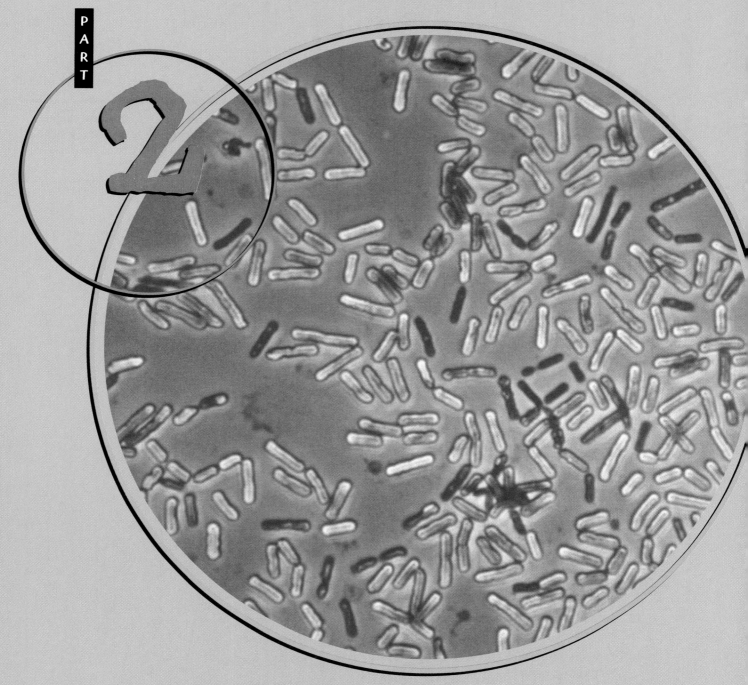

PART

2

The Bacteria

We live at the center of a microbial universe. On all sides, microscopic organisms surround us and make their presence felt—for good or ill. The useful species outnumber the harmful ones by thousands and are so valuable we could not live without them. The remaining species are agents of disease and death.

Only since the mid–1800s have scientists linked microorganisms to events of human importance (not surprisingly, because microorganisms can be seen only with a microscope). Before then, disease processes now attributed to microorganisms seemed to happen almost spontaneously and without apparent cause. Even thinking about disease in terms of microorganisms could be dangerous because it was heresy to consider disease as anything other than supernatural.

In Part 2 of this text, we shall focus on one group of microorganisms, the bacteria. These microorganisms have traditionally occupied an important niche in microbiology because scientists probably know more about bacteria than any other organisms. Bacteria have been involved in the great plagues of history, and for centuries their effects have captured the imagination of scientists and writers. Bacteria are easily studied in the laboratory, and their chemical activities have been charted and well documented. Also, many helpful ones play key roles in industrial processes. We often mean bacteria when we talk about "germs," and we need only consider how often we use that word to appreciate the significance of bacteria in our lives.

Small as they are, bacteria are endowed with the ability to perform certain acts characteristic of all living things. They take in food, grow, excrete waste products, reproduce, and die. In addition, bacteria are sensitive to external agents and stimuli, and they respond in some fashion. In Chapter 4, we shall survey their structural frameworks and growth patterns, and in Chapter 5, we examine their biochemical activities. Chapter 6 is devoted to the genetics of bacteria and includes some of the key findings of modern biotechnology. The discussions in Part 2 have broad significance not only in medicine, research, and industry, but also in our daily lives.

BIOTECHNOLOGY

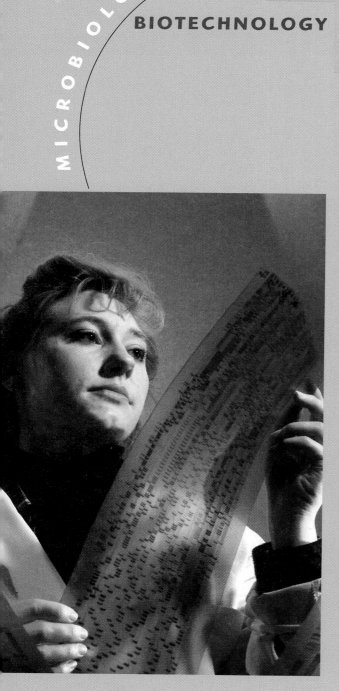

During the 1980s, the editors of *Time Magazine* referred to DNA technology as "the most awesome skill acquired by man since the splitting of the atom." Indeed, the work with DNA, begun in the 1950s and continuing today, has opened vistas previously unimagined. Scientists can now remove bits of DNA from organisms, snip and rearrange the genes, and insert them into fresh organisms, where the genes will express themselves. Practical results of these experiments have led to the mass production of hormones, clotting factors, and other pharmaceutical products. They have also given us diagnostic methods based on DNA fingerprinting; advances in gene therapy; a revolution in agricultural research; barnyard animals producing human hemo-globin; and a colossal attempt to map the entire human genome.

If you would like to be part of what promises to be this century's great technology, then microbiology is the place to be. You would be well advised to take a course in biochemistry, as well as one in genetics. Courses in physiology and neurobiology are also helpful. Employers will be looking for individuals with good laboratory skills, so be sure to take as many lab courses as you can. And don't be afraid to become a "lab-rat" (the scientific equivalent of basketball's "gym-rat").

You may enter the biotechnology field with an associate's, bachelor's, master's, or doctoral degree. This is because there are so many levels at which individuals are hired. An employer will be looking for work experience, which you can obtain by assisting a senior scientist, doing an internship, or working summers in a biotech firm (usually for slave wages). The campus research lab is another good place to obtain work experience. It might also be a good idea to sharpen your writing skills, since you will be preparing numerous reports. As Chapter 6 explains, the novel and imaginative research that established biotechnology was founded in micro-biology, and it continues to call on microbiology for its continuing growth.

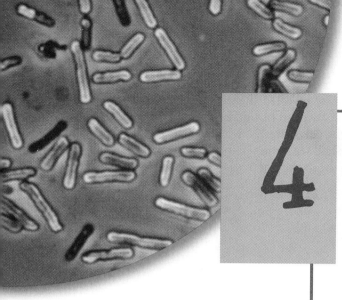

4

Bacterial Structure and Growth

> Our planet has always been in the "Age of Bacteria," ever since the first fossils—bacteria of course—were entombed in rocks more than 3 billion years ago. On any possible, reasonable criterion, bacteria are—and always have been—the dominant forms of life on Earth.
>
> —Paleontologist Stephen Jay Gould writing in a popular magazine

I N A 1683 LETTER TO THE Royal Society of London, Anton van Leeuwenhoek described microscopic "streaks and threads" among his tiny animals. The streaks and threads remained nameless until 1773, when the Danish scientist Otto Frederick Müller christened them "bacilli." Bacilli is the plural form of the Latin *bacillus*, meaning "little rod."

van-lu'en-hōk'

myu'ler

But not all bacilli were rods. Some were spiral and some were circular, and the word *bacilli* would not do. Therefore, in the 1850s, the French investigator Casimir Davaine began calling the microscopic creatures "bacteria," even though this derivative of the Greek *bacterion* also means rod. Time has a way of sorting out confusion, and in the next few decades "bacteria" came to refer to all the microorganisms in that group, and the word "bacillus" was reserved for rod forms only.

da-vane'

The terminology problem was resolved just in time because, in the 1850s, bacteria were attracting considerable attention. At that time, Pasteur's work showed that bacteria are chemical factories capable of bringing about significant changes in nature, and in the 1870s, Koch's experiments verified their link to infectious disease. In the late 1800s, the rush to locate and isolate the bacterial causes of infectious disease was unlike anything previously experienced in medical science.

As it happened, neither van Leeuwenhoek, nor Davaine, nor Pasteur, nor Koch could see what lay ahead. As the twentieth century unfolded, scientists found that bacteria have structures and growth patterns far beyond what had been imagined in the years before. With the

91

development of the electron microscope in the 1940s and the revelations of biochemistry during that period, bacteria revealed themselves as more than simple sticks and rods. Scientists uncovered a wealth of microscopic and submicroscopic details in bacteria and showed how the very minute bacteria can be as complex as the very large, visible organisms. As we shall see in this chapter, a study of the structural features of bacteria provides a window to their activities and illustrates how bacteria relate to other living things.

4.1

The Structure of Bacteria

The structure of an organism refers to its size and shape and the physical features that make it distinctive. Structure is an inherited trait derived from information stored in the chromosomal DNA. This trait is passed from generation to generation in the genes.

Viewed with the light microscope, most clinically significant bacteria appear in variations of three different shapes: the rod, the sphere, and the spiral. As suggested by Müller, the rod is known as a **bacillus** (pl., bacilli). In various species of bacteria, a bacillus may be as long as 20 μm or as short as 0.5 μm. Certain rods, such as those that cause typhoid fever, are slender; others, such as the agents of anthrax, are rectangular with squared ends; still others, such as diphtheria bacilli, are club-shaped. Most rods occur singly, but some form long chains called **streptobacilli**. FIGURE 4.1 illustrates this diversity. It should be noted that the word *bacillus* is used two ways in microbiology: to denote a rod form, and as a genus name. The organism of anthrax, for instance, is a bacillus having the name *Bacillus anthracis*.

A bacterial sphere is known as a **coccus** (pl., cocci), a term derived from the Greek *kokkos*, meaning "berry." Cocci are approximately 0.5 μm to 1.0 μm in diameter. They are usually round, but they may also be oval, elongated, or indented on one side. Those cocci remaining together in pairs after reproducing are called **diplococci**. The organisms that cause gonorrhea and one type of bacterial meningitis are examples. Those cocci consisting of chains of diplococci are called **streptococci**

Genes:
segments of DNA that provide the biochemical code for inherited traits.

μm:
the abbreviation for micrometer, a millionth of a meter.

dif-the're-ah

Streptobacillus:
a chain of bacterial rods.

kok'us
kok'si

FIGURE 4.1

Variations in Bacterial Structure

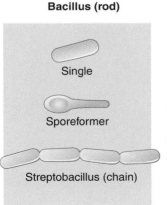

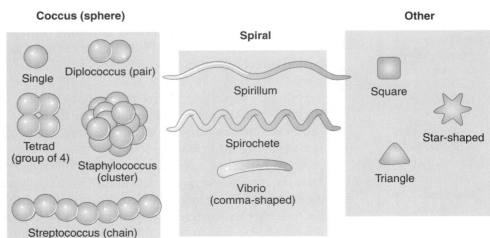

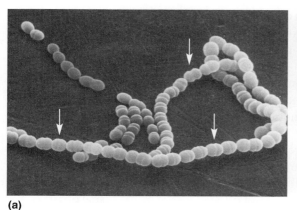
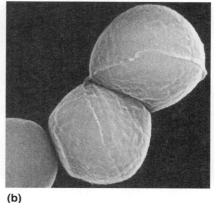
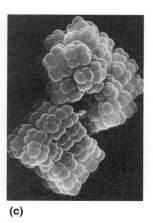

(a)

(b)

(c)

FIGURE 4.2

Scanning Electron Micrographs of Three Variations of Cocci

(a) A streptococcus such as is found in the intestine. Note the characteristic string-of-beads appearance of diplococci in the chain. The arrows indicate three of the many positions at which the cocci are undergoing division. (b) Two cocci from a cluster of *Staphylococcus aureus* cells (×49,000). (c) Clusters of sarcinae in cubelike packets of eight.

(FIGURE 4.2a). Certain species of streptococci are involved in strep throat and tooth decay, but some species are harmless enough to be used for producing dairy products such as yogurt. Lactobacilli are also used in yogurt production.

Another variation of cocci is the **sarcina**, a cubelike packet of eight cocci *(sarcina* is Latin for "bundle"). One species, *Micrococcus luteus*, is a common inhabitant of the skin. Certain cocci divide randomly and form an irregular grapelike cluster of cells called a **staphylococcus** (FIGURE 4.2b), from *staphyle*, the Greek word for "grape." A well-known example, *Staphylococcus aureus*, is a widespread cause of food poisoning as well as toxic shock syndrome and numerous skin infections. The latter are known in the modern vernacular as "staph" infections.

The third important shape of bacterial organisms is the **spiral**. Certain spiral bacteria called **vibrios** are curved rods that resemble commas. The cholera organism is typical. Other spiral bacteria called **spirilla** (sing., spirillum) have a corkscrew shape with a rigid cell wall and hairlike projections called flagella that assist movement

Streptococcus:
a chain of bacterial diplococci.

sar-cē'nah

staf'i-lo-kok'us au're-us

Cholera:
a serious bacterial disease of the intestines, characterized by the loss of large volumes of water.

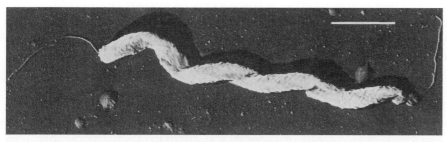

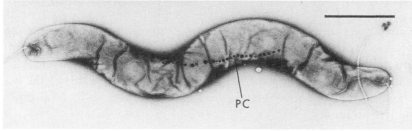

PC

FIGURE 4.3

Electron Micrographs of a Freshwater Spirillum

(a) The spiral shape is seen clearly in this cell, and flagella are visible at the poles of the cell. (b) In this cell, the background is enhanced by negative staining to enable viewing of the cell interior. An electron-dense particle chain (PC) is visible in the cytoplasm. This chain of particles gives magnetic properties to the spirillum. In the 1980 publication where these photographs first appeared, the researchers proposed that the chain be called a "magnetosome." (Bar = 1.0 μm.)

spi'ro-kēt

caul-o-bak'ter

(FIGURE 4.3). Still others, known as **spirochetes**, have a flexible cell wall but no flagella in the traditional sense. Movement in these organisms occurs by contractions of long filaments (axial flagella) that run the length of the cell. The organism of syphilis typifies a spirochete.

In addition to these shapes, some other variations exist. In the genus *Caulobacter*, for example, there are appendaged bacteria; members of the genus *Nocardia* consist of branching filaments; and some archaebacteria (archaea) have square and star shapes.

Variations in bacterial structure are readily visible when the organisms are magnified 1000 times under the light microscope. When the electron microscope is used, however, a magnification of 1 million times or more is achieved, and scientists can observe a world of fine bacterial details not otherwise seen by the casual observer. We shall examine some of these details next.

FLAGELLA

Numerous species of bacterial rods and spirilla and a limited number of species of cocci are capable of independent motion. To achieve motion, they use **flagella** (sing., flagellum). Flagella are composed of long, rigid strands of protein subunits called **flagellin**. Within the strands, the protein exists in ultrathin fibers permanently bent like a coil or helix. This structure enables the flagellum to rotate. By contrast, in eukaryotic cells such as protozoa, the flagella whip about (*flagellum* is Latin for "whip"). In eukaryotic cells, the strands are flexible, and the fibers are elongated and slide past one another.

Flagellin:
the protein of which flagella are composed.

Electron microscopy reveals that the bacterial flagellum is anchored at the cell membrane by a basal region consisting of a hooklike structure and basal body. The **basal body** has a central rod and set of enclosing rings. Gram-positive bacteria have one ring embedded in the cell membrane and one in the cell wall, while Gram-negative bacteria have a pair of rings embedded in the cell membrane and another pair associated with chemical components of the cell wall (FIGURE 4.4).

Gram-positive bacteria:
bacteria that retain the primary stain when subjected to an alcohol wash during Gram staining.

Most bacterial flagella rotate like L-shaped hooks, as one ring in the membrane rotates, while the other remains stationary. When the flagellum rotates counterclockwise, the organism moves straight ahead; it "runs." But when the flagellum rotates clockwise, the bacterium "tumbles" without direction. These movements require a considerable amount of energy. Often the movements are stimulated by a chemical attraction or repulsion called **chemotaxis**. Movement toward an attractant is characterized by lengthened runs and shortened tumbles. Movement away from a chemical repellent is accompanied by the reverse.

Chemotaxis:
a chemical attraction or repulsion.

Flagella can vary in number and placement. A **monotrichous** bacterium (a monotrichaete) possesses a single flagellum, while a **lophotrichous** organism (a lophotrichaete) has a group of two or more flagella at one pole of the cell. An **amphitrichous** bacterium (an amphitrichaete) has groups of flagella at both ends, and a **peritrichous** bacterium (a peritrichaete) is covered with flagella. The arrangement of flagella is characteristic of a species and useful in classifying the species in a taxonomic scheme.

mon'o-trik'us

loff'o-trik'us

am'fi-trik'us

The flagellum ranges in length from 10 μm to 20 μm and is many times the length of the cell, as Figure 4.4d shows. However, the flagellum is only about 0.2 μm thick and cannot be seen with the light microscope unless coated with dye. In the human body, flagella enable bacteria such as cholera bacilli to move among the tissues and escape phagocytes. Some bacteria are known to travel up to 2000 times their own length in an hour.

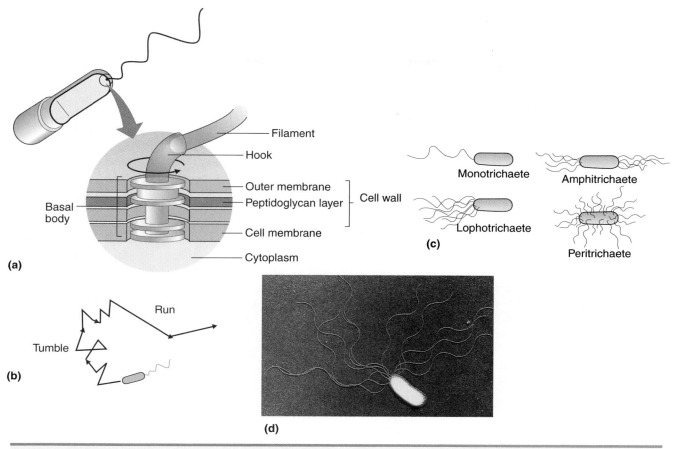

(a)

(b)

Tumble

Run

Filament
Hook

Outer membrane
Peptidoglycan layer — Cell wall
Cell membrane

Basal body

Cytoplasm

Monotrichaete Amphitrichaete

Lophotrichaete

Peritrichaete

(c)

(d)

FIGURE 4.4

Details of the Bacterial Flagellum

(a) In a Gram–negative bacterium, shown here, the flagellum is attached to the cell wall and membrane by a complex mechanism of structures. (In a Gram-positive bactium, the arrangement is slightly different.) (b) Rotation of the flagellum in one direction causes the bacterium to "run," while rotation of the flagellum in the opposite direction causes the bacterium to "tumble," as shown. (c) Various configurations of flagella occur among bacteria. Monotrichous bacteria possess a single flagellum, amphitrichous bacteria have flagella at both poles of the cell, and lophotrichous organisms have them at one end. Peritrichous bacteria are surrounded by flagella. (d) A transmission electron micrograph of *Pseudomonas marginalis* showing polar flagella (×38,800). Note that the flagella are many times the length of the bacillus and appear in a characteristic wavy format. This bacterium is lophotrichous.

PILI

Pili (sing., pilus) are bacterial appendages that appear as short straight hairlike fibers (**FIGURE 4.5**). Certain **sex pili** aid the transfer of genetic material among bacteria (Chapter 6), while other pili anchor bacteria to surfaces such as living tissue. These latter pili contain at their tips proteins called **adhesins**, which stick to a surface molecule of the tissue, thereby enhancing an organism's ability to cause disease (**MicroFocus 4.1**). In 1997, researchers identified an adhesin of *E. coli* and used it to produce a vaccine. When injected into healthy mice, the adhesin induced the animal's immune system to produce antibodies, which united with the adhesin and prevented the *E. coli* from attaching. Without the chemical mooring line lashing it to the cells, the bacterium could not infect the tissue.

Pili are comprised primarily of protein subunits called **pilin**. They are often found on Gram-negative bacteria such as *Neisseria gonorhoeae*, the cause of gonorrhea. Antibodies produced against the pilin would discourage attachment, as noted

pĭ'lus

ad-hēs'in

nī-se're-ah

Gonorrhea:
a sexually transmitted bacterial disease, characterized by colonization of the reproductive and urinary tract tissues.

MicroFocus 4.1

DIARRHEA DOOZIES

They gathered at the clinical research center at Stanford University to do their part for the advancement of science (and earn a few dollars as well). They were the "sensational sixty"—sixty young men and women who would spend three days and nights and earn $300 to help determine whether hairlike structures called pili have a significant place in disease.

A number of nurses and doctors were on hand to help them through their ordeal. The students would drink a fruit-flavored cocktail containing a special diarrhea-causing strain of *Escherichia coli (E. coli)*. Thirty cocktails had *E. coli* with normal pili, while thirty had *E. coli* with pili mutated beyond repair. Bacteria with the threadlike pili should latch onto intestinal tissue and cause diarrhea, while those with mutated pili should be swept away by the rush of intestinal movements and not cause intestinal distress. At least that's what the sensational sixty would either verify or prove false.

On that fateful day in 1997, the experiment began. Neither the students nor the health professionals knew who was drinking the diarrhea cocktail and who was getting the "free pass"; it was a double-blind experiment. Then came the waiting. Some experienced no symptoms, but others felt the bacterial onslaught and clutched at their last remaining vestiges of dignity. For some it was three days of hell, with nausea, abdominal cramps, and numerous bathroom trips; for others, luck was on their side, and investing in a lottery ticket seemed like a good idea.

When it was all over, the numbers appeared to bear out the theory: The great majority of volunteers with mutated bacteria experienced no diarrhea, while the great majority of those with normal bacteria had attacks of diarrhea, in some cases real doozies. All appeared to profit from the experience: The scientists had some real-life evidence that pili contribute to infection; the students made their sacrifice to science and pocketed $300 each; and the local supermarket had a surge of profits from unexpected sales of toilet paper, Pepto-Bismol, and Immodium.

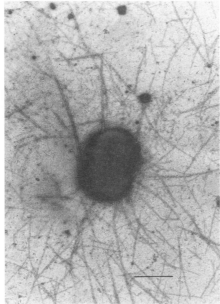

(a)   (b)

FIGURE 4.5

Two Examples of Pili in Bacteria

(a) A heavily piliated cell of *Neisseria gonorrhoeae*, the agent of gonorrhea. The stain has obscured the diplococcus form of the organism, but you can see two cocci if you look closely. (Bar = 1 μm.) (b) Numerous *Klebsiella pneumoniae* cells displaying pili ($\times 20,300$). Both organisms shown are pathogens, and the pili enhance pathogenicity by enabling the organism to adhere to the tissue.

TABLE 4.1

A Comparison of Flagella and Pili

CHARACTERISTIC	FLAGELLA	PILI
Composition	Flagellin, a protein	Pilin, a protein
Size	0.01–0.05 µm width; 10–20 µm length	0.007–0.008 µm width; 0.5–2 µm length
Occurrence	Many bacterial rods but few cocci	Many Gram-negative rods and cocci
Structure	Adjacent fibrils with no regular pattern	Wound fibers with a hollow center
Number	Varies according to the organism; one to several hundred	Varies according to the organism; one to several hundred
Function	Motion	Attachment, conjugation
Origin	Hooklike insertion to basal body inside cell wall	Cell cytoplasm, through cell membrane, wall, and glycocalyx

above, and might be used together with antibiotics, especially since resistance to antibiotics is an ongoing concern in gonorrhea therapy. It should be noted that some microbiologists use the word **fimbria** (pl., fimbriae) for bacterial structures used for attachment and reserve the word *pili* for structures functioning in genetic transfers. Pili are also known to be receptors for some bacteriophages, the viruses that multiply in bacteria. TABLE 4.1 compares the characteristics of flagella and pili.

fim'bre-ah (s)
fim'bre-ā (pl)

THE GLYCOCALYX

Many species of bacteria secrete an adhering layer of polysaccharides and small proteins called the **glycocalyx**, as shown in FIGURE 4.6. The layer can be thick and tightly bound to the cell, in which case it is known as a **capsule**. When thinner, flowing, and less tightly bound, it is referred to as a **slime layer**.

gli'ko-kay'liks

FIGURE 4.6

A Hypothetical Bacterial Cell

The structural features of this composite, "idealized" bacterium are drawn in a way that shows their relationships. Such a bacterium probably does not exist.

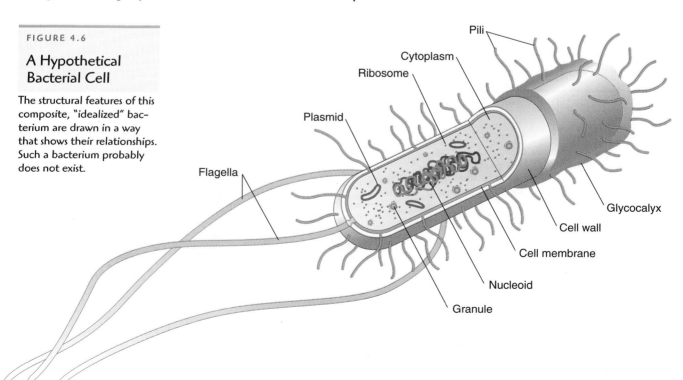

The glycocalyx (meaning "sweet coat")is formed by various bacterial rods and cocci, but not by spiral bacteria. It serves as a buffer between the cell and its external environment, and because of its high water content, it prevents nutrients from flowing away. The glycocalyx also contributes to the disease process because encapsulated bacteria such as *Streptococcus pneumoniae* (a principal cause of pneumonia) cannot be easily engulfed by white blood cells during phagocytosis. When the capsule is experimentally removed, the organism is harmless. Scientists believe that the repulsion between bacterium and white blood cell is due to strong negative charges in the capsule and white blood cell. The glycocalyx of *E. coli* is shown in FIGURE 4.7.

The slime layer usually contains a mass of tangled fibers of a polysaccharide called **dextran**. The fibers attach the bacterium to tissue surfaces. A case in point is *Streptococcus mutans*, an important cause of tooth decay. This bacterium attaches itself to the surface of the teeth using the dextran it synthesizes from sucrose (table sugar). Soon a layer of dental plaque has formed, and the streptococci begin breaking down dietary carbohydrates to the acids that dissolve tooth enamel.

Slime layers and capsules are key elements in the formation of **biofilms**. The latter are a series of encased microcolonies of bacteria attached to such surfaces as industrial pipelines, medical instruments, sewage-treatment systems, and body tissues (dental plaque is an example). A slime layer about 10 µm thick lies at the base of the biofilm and attaches the bacteria to the surface. Biofilms exist wherever a fluid meets a solid surface, and one researcher has estimated that most bacteria live within the layer's microscopic community. A carbohydrate matrix binds the microcolonies together, and surrounding water channels deliver nutrients and remove waste. Dental caries (cavities) and urinary tract infections both are consequences of biofilms (Chapter 10). Living within a biofilm effectively shields bacteria from the body's immune defenses, as well as from antibiotics and other therapies. FIGURE 4.8 details a medical consequence of a biofilm.

In food products, the slime-producing bacteria may cause an unsightly and distasteful experience. For instance, the gluelike slime of *Alcaligenes viscolactis* accumulates in milk, causing it to become thick and stringy. The result is **ropy milk**. Bread may also become ropy if contaminated with slime-producing *Bacillus subtilis*.

Phagocytosis:
a defensive measure of the body in which white blood cells engulf and destroy microorganisms.

al'kah-lij'ĕ-nēz

Ropy milk:
thick, stringy milk that contains the gluelike slime of capsule-producing bacteria.

FIGURE 4.7

The Glycocalyx of *Escherichia coli*

An electron micrograph of *Escherichia coli* from the intestine of an animal. Each bacillus is surrounded by a glycocalyx. (Bar = 0.1 µm.)

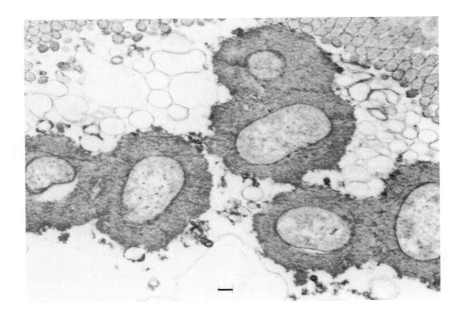

FIGURE 4.8

FIGURE 4.8

An Outbreak of
Enterobacter cloacae
Infection Associated
with Biofilms in the
Waste Drainpipe of
a Hemodialysis
Machine

The incident points up the
need for the correct maintenance of machines through
which fluid flows.

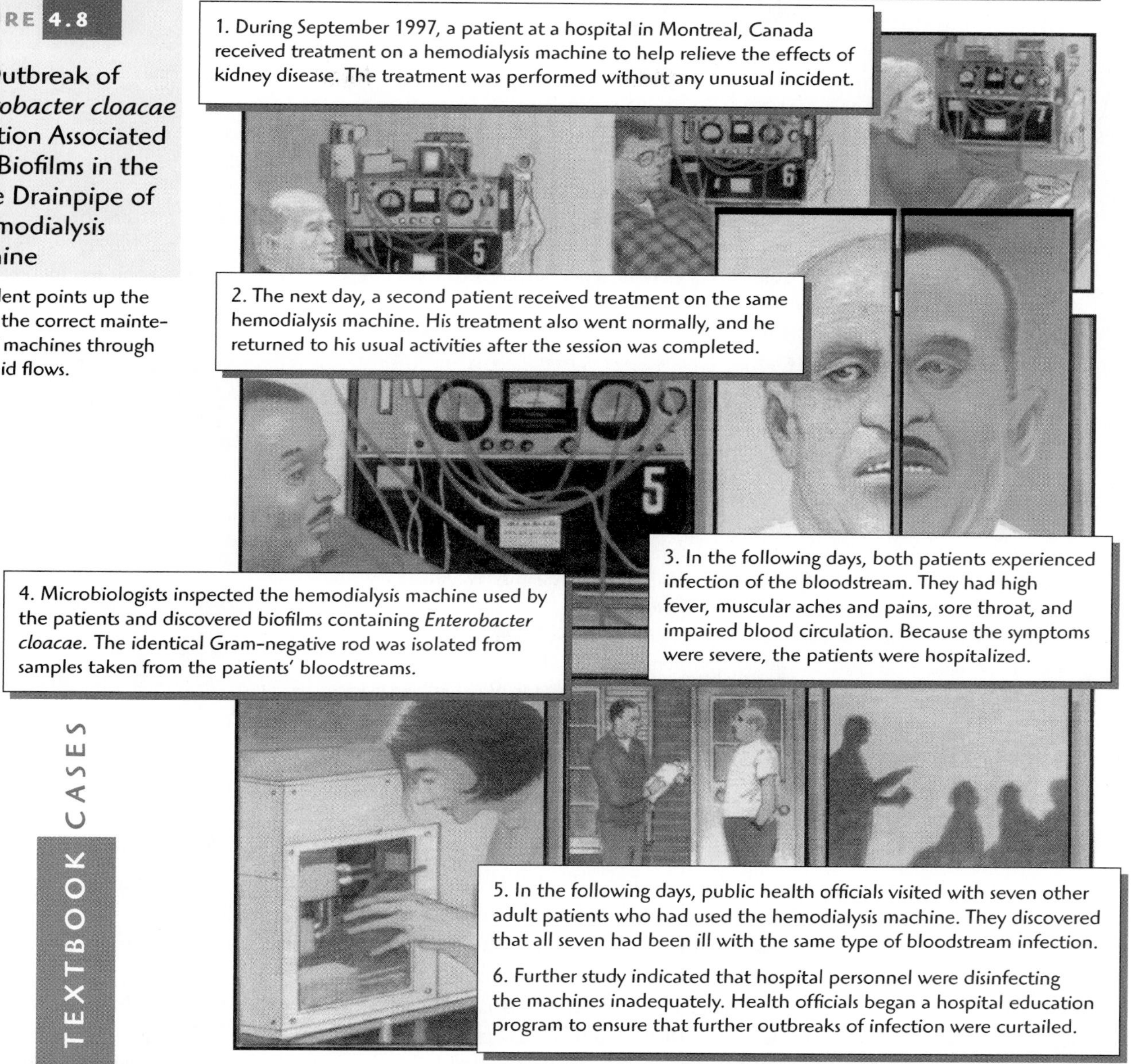

TEXTBOOK CASES

1. During September 1997, a patient at a hospital in Montreal, Canada received treatment on a hemodialysis machine to help relieve the effects of kidney disease. The treatment was performed without any unusual incident.

2. The next day, a second patient received treatment on the same hemodialysis machine. His treatment also went normally, and he returned to his usual activities after the session was completed.

4. Microbiologists inspected the hemodialysis machine used by the patients and discovered biofilms containing *Enterobacter cloacae*. The identical Gram-negative rod was isolated from samples taken from the patients' bloodstreams.

3. In the following days, both patients experienced infection of the bloodstream. They had high fever, muscular aches and pains, sore throat, and impaired blood circulation. Because the symptoms were severe, the patients were hospitalized.

5. In the following days, public health officials visited with seven other adult patients who had used the hemodialysis machine. They discovered that all seven had been ill with the same type of bloodstream infection.

6. Further study indicated that hospital personnel were disinfecting the machines inadequately. Health officials began a hospital education program to ensure that further outbreaks of infection were curtailed.

THE CELL WALL

With the notable exception of mycoplasmas, all bacteria have a **cell wall**. This structure protects the cell and enhances its survival (**MicroFocus 4.2**). To a large extent, it also determines cell shape. A century ago, taxonomists classified bacteria as plants because of the presence of a cell wall, but modern biochemists have established that the chemical composition of the bacterial cell wall differs markedly from that of plants.

MicroFocus 4.2

ASLEEP FOR 11,000 YEARS

It was 2 feet long, reddish-brown, and tube-shaped. It could have been a piece of rusted pipe, but it smelled so bad and had such a convoluted shape that the pipe theory was quickly discarded. Workers had found the object while building a new fourteenth hole at the Burning Tree Golf Course near Columbus, Ohio. While digging a mere 5 feet into the soil, they hit upon the skeletal remains of a mastodon, an elephantlike animal that lived 11,000 years ago. This tube-shaped object was near the animal's rib cage.

Paleontologists theorized that the object was probably part of the mastodon's intestinal tract. It so happened that Gerald Goldstein of Ohio Wesleyan University was visiting the site at the invitation of a friend involved in the excavation. He half-jokingly suggested that something might still be alive in the intestinal contents, and he

was given a small bag of the smelly material. Back at his laboratory, he placed a sample of the intestinal contents on ordinary bacteriological medium and surprise, surprise . . . the next day the medium teemed with bacteria. The organism was *Enterobacter cloacae*, a well-known resident of the mammalian intestine.

In 1991, Goldstein announced his discovery to a skeptical scientific community. He determined that the *E. cloacae* was not a contaminant from the surrounding soil by searching for the organism in 12 samples from nearby sites. All 12 samples failed to yield *E. cloacae*. An independent "blind" analysis, in which scientists were not told the sources of the samples, confirmed the results.

Assuming Goldstein's discovery remains intact, the bacteria he cultivated would be the oldest known living

bacteria recovered from nature (bacterial spores excluded). A 3-foot cap of clay had apparently sealed the site, and the chilly 45°F temperature probably contributed to placing the bacteria in a state of suspended animation. As one writer suggested, "Move over Rip van Winkle. There's a new record for slumber time."

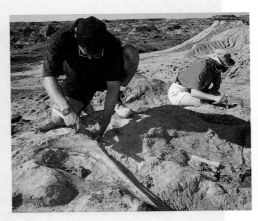

---

pep′tī-do-gly′kan

acetyl-glucose-amine
acetyl-muramic

nm:
the abbreviation for nanometer, a billionth of a meter.

Gram stain technique:
a four-part staining procedure that differentiates bacteria into two groups, Gram-positive and Gram-negative.

lip′o-pol-i-sak′a-ride

Endotoxin:
a toxin retained in the outer membrane of certain Gram-negative bacteria and released when they disintegrate.

An important chemical constituent of the cell wall in eubacteria is **peptidoglycan** (archaebacteria have none). This is a very large molecule composed of alternating units of two amino-containing carbohydrates, *N*-acetylglucosamine (NAG) and *N*-acetylmuramic acid (NAM), joined by cross-bridges of amino acids. Peptidoglycan occurs in multiple layers connected by side chains of four amino acids, as illustrated in FIGURE 4.9. Therefore, the many layers comprise one extremely large molecule, somewhat similar in structure to a fence of chicken wire.

The cell walls of Gram-positive and Gram-negative bacteria differ considerably. In Gram-positive bacteria, the peptidoglycan layer is about 25 nm wide and contains an additional polysaccharide called **teichoic acid**. About 60 to 90 percent of the cell wall is peptidoglycan, and the material is so abundant that Gram-positive bacteria are able to retain the crystal violet–iodine complex in Gram staining (Chapter 3).

By contrast, the cell wall of Gram-negative bacteria has no teichoic acid, and its peptidoglycan layer is only about 3 nm thick; this is probably why it loses the stain components in Gram staining. The wall is enclosed by an **outer membrane** not found in Gram-positive bacteria. The membrane consists of two rows of molecules: an inner row of phospholipid; and an outer row of **lipopolysaccharide (LPS)** not found in any other living thing. In this unique molecule, the lipid portion (known as lipid A) occurs at one end and functions as an endotoxin, causing fever and circulatory collapse when it is released in the bloodstream or digestive system of a host organism. The polysaccharide portion of the LPS (O polysaccharide) elicits antibody production and is used to identify variants of a species (e.g., strain O157:H7 of *E. coli*). The membrane's two rows provide protection against certain antimicrobial agents, dyes, disinfectants, and digestive enzymes.

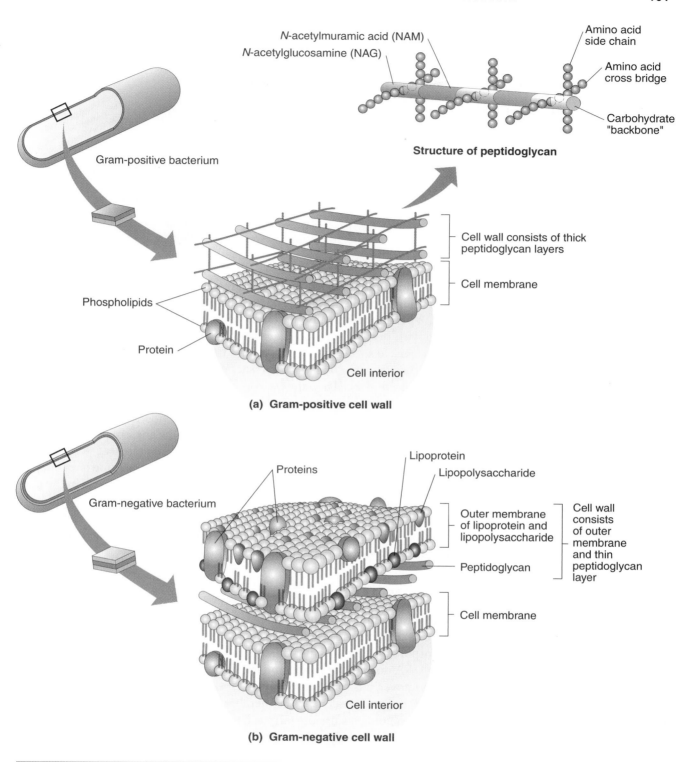

N-acetylmuramic acid (NAM)

N-acetylglucosamine (NAG)

Amino acid side chain

Amino acid cross bridge

Carbohydrate "backbone"

Structure of peptidoglycan

Gram-positive bacterium

Cell wall consists of thick peptidoglycan layers

Cell membrane

Phospholipids

Protein

Cell interior

(a) Gram-positive cell wall

Gram-negative bacterium

Proteins

Lipoprotein

Lipopolysaccharide

Outer membrane of lipoprotein and lipopolysaccharide

Cell wall consists of outer membrane and thin peptidoglycan layer

Peptidoglycan

Cell membrane

Cell interior

(b) Gram-negative cell wall

FIGURE 4.9

A Comparison of the Cell Walls of Gram-Positive and Gram-Negative Bacteria

(a) The cell wall of a Gram-positive bacterium is composed of peptidoglycan layers combined with teichoic acid molecules (not shown). The structure of peptidoglycan is shown as units of NAG and NAM joined laterally by amino acid cross-bridges and vertically by side chains of four amino acids. (b) In the Gram-negative cell wall, the peptidoglycan layer is much thinner, and there is no teichoic acid. Moreover, an outer membrane closely overlies the peptidoglycan layer so that the membrane and layer comprise the cell wall. Note the structure of the cell membrane in this figure. The bacterial membrane conforms to the fluid mosaic model found in most eukaryotic membranes.

FIGURE 4.10

The Effect of Penicillin

A photomicrograph of a *Staphylococcus aureus* cell exploding on exposure to penicillin (×150,000). The antibiotic has prevented construction of the peptidoglycan layer of the cell wall, and internal pressures have led to weakening and disruption of the cell membrane.

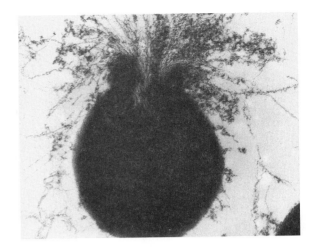

per'i-plas-m

Antibiotic:
the naturally occurring or synthetic product of a micro-organism that inhibits the growth of other microorganisms.

Penicillin:
a mold-derived antibiotic that prevents the construction of the cell wall, especially in Gram-positive bacteria.

li'so-zīm

The outer membrane also contains proteins acting as channels for molecular thoroughfare. The proteins, known as **porins**, allow the passage of nutrients and vitamins into the **periplasmic region** between the outer membrane and cell wall. This area is filled with **periplasm**, a gel-like material containing digestive enzymes and transport proteins to speed entry to the cell wall and membrane. The porins are also sites where viruses attach when these particles unite with Gram-negative bacteria.

The cell wall holds the cell together. It also prevents the cell from bursting because the internal pressure may be up to 20 times the external pressure due to the high concentration of inorganic salts, carbohydrates, amino acids, and other small molecules within the cell. The antibiotic **penicillin** prevents the construction of the peptidoglycan of the cell wall in new cells, and they quickly burst (FIGURE 4.10). Where penicillin acts on new cells, lysozyme destroys existing cells. **Lysozyme** is an enzyme in human tears and saliva. It attacks the linkages between carbohydrates in the peptidoglycan layer, thus causing the cell wall to break down and the cell to explode. In both cases, the effect is more dramatic in Gram-positive bacteria because these organisms have more peptidoglycan. Moreover, the outer membrane plays a protective role in Gram-negative organisms.

THE CELL MEMBRANE

The **cell membrane** (also called the **plasma membrane**) is the boundary layer between the bacterium and its environment. It exists inside the cell wall and functions in transporting nutrients into the cell and waste materials out of the cell. It also anchors the DNA during replication and is a site for enzymes functioning in cell wall synthesis. Moreover, it is the location of enzymes used in energy metabolism, a factor that makes it the equivalent of the membranes of mitochondria in a eukaryotic cell. Some microbiologists use the term **cell envelope** to refer collectively to the cell membrane, cell wall, and glycocalyx (if present).

Approximately 60 percent of the cell membrane is composed of protein and about 40 percent of lipid, mainly phospholipid. The phospholipid molecules are arranged in two parallel layers (a phospholipid bilayer), one at the outside and the other at the inside of the membrane. In contrast, the proteins exist as globules floating like icebergs at or near the inner and outer surfaces of the membrane, and some globules extend from one surface of the membrane to the other. This model of the membrane, called the **fluid mosaic model**, accounts for the membrane's appearance when viewed with the electron microscope and helps explain how it allows the passage of certain substances. For example, lipid-soluble materials dissolve in the phospholipid layer

Mitochondria:
organelles of eukaryotic cells in which energy-yielding biochemical reactions occur.

Phospholipids:
molecules of lipids that contain a large number of phosphate groups.

MicroFocus 4.3

A (NOT SO) FATAL ATTRACTION

To get from place to place, humans usually require the assistance of maps, compasses, and gas station attendants. In the microbial world, life is generally more simple, and traveling is no exception.

Consider the bacteria, for example. In the early 1980s, Richard P. Blakmore and his colleagues at the University of New Hampshire observed that certain mud-dwelling bacteria tend to gather at the north end of water droplets. On further study, they found that each bacterium had a chain of magnetic particles acting as a kind of bacterial dipole directing the organism's movements. Bacteria possessing the particles swim toward the north in the Northern Hemisphere and toward the south in the Southern Hemisphere. Indeed, when genetic mutations are caused in

the bacteria, they head in the wrong direction—and wind up in a hostile environment and die.

This last observation is particularly noteworthy because it appears to give rhyme and reason to the particles. The conventional wisdom is that the so-called magnetotactic bacteria use their traveling skills to locate a favorable environment. In 1992, Dennis A. Bazylinski of Iowa State University theorized how this hypothesis might work in nature. Certain magnetotactic bacteria are anaerobic; that is, they live in an oxygen-free environment. While swimming toward a pole (north or south), the bacteria are also oriented downward by Earth's magnetic field. The downward tilt pulls them away from the oxygen-rich water and toward the oxygen-poor mud below. On

reaching their type of optimum environment, the bacteria reach a sort of biological nirvana and settle in for a life of anaerobic bliss.

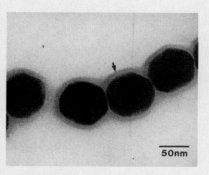

■ *Magnetite-containing magnetosomes extracted from a magnetotactic bacterium. Note the membrane (at arrow) surrounding the magnetic particles.*

and pass through the membrane, while amino acids and nitrogenous bases, which do not dissolve in lipids, move through the protein passageways.

When antimicrobial substances act on the cell membrane, bacterial death usually follows. Certain detergents, for instance, dissolve the phospholipid layers and cause the cytoplasmic contents to leak out. Ethyl alcohol and some antibiotics such as polymyxin work similarly.

Detergents:
synthetic chemicals used as antiseptics and disinfectants to kill bacteria by altering the structure of the cell membrane.

pol-e-mix'in

THE CYTOPLASM

Inside the cell membrane lies the **cytoplasm**, a gelatinous mass of proteins, carbohydrates, lipids, nucleic acids, salts, and inorganic ions, all dissolved in water. Cytoplasm is the foundation substance of a cell and the center of its growth and biochemistry. It is thick, semitransparent, and elastic.

Several cytoplasmic bodies are of interest. **Ribosomes** are bodies of RNA and protein associated with the synthesis of protein (Chapter 5). Other bodies found in various species of bacteria include granules of starch, glycogen, sulfur, or lipid. Often referred to collectively as **inclusion bodies**, these granules store nutrients for later use during periods of starvation. Certain other bodies serve as phosphate depots. Commonly known as **metachromatic granules**, or volutin, these bodies stain deeply with dyes such as methylene blue. Their presence in diphtheria bacilli assists identification procedures. A recently discovered body, the **magnetosome**, helps certain bacteria orient themselves to the environment (MicroFocus 4.3). Crystals of an iron-containing compound called magnetite fill the magnetosome and align themselves with the local magnetic field. Scientists believe that the magnetite directs bacteria toward their preferred habitat.

vol'u-tin

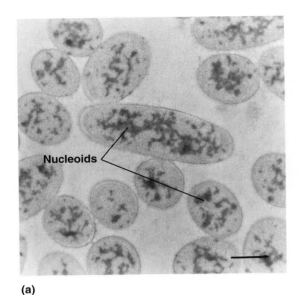

(a)

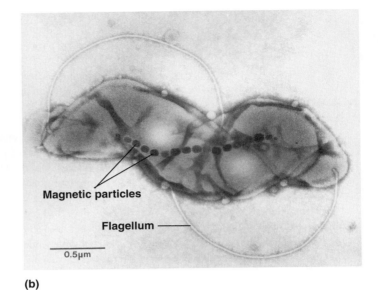

(b)

FIGURE 4.11

The Nucleoids and Magnetosome of Bacteria

(a) In this transmission electron micrograph of *Escherichia coli,* nucleoids are seen in irregular coralline (coral–shaped) forms. Nucleoids can be observed occupying a large area in a bacterium, which indicates how far the DNA of the bacterium is spread out. Both longitudinal and cross sections of *E. coli* are visible. (Bar = 0.5 μm.) (b) The bacterial magnetosome is seen in this remarkable electron micrograph of a magnetotactic marine spirillum. Particles of magnetite in the magnetosome apparently influence the direction the bacteria move in the environment. The flagella of the spirillum are clearly visible.

Nucleoid:
the chromosome region of a bacterial cell.

The cytoplasm is also the site of the bacterial **chromosome**. This closed loop of DNA contains the hereditary information of the cell. It is suspended in the cytoplasm without a covering or membrane and is not associated with histone protein (as in eukaryotic cells). The term **nucleoid** is often applied to the chromosome region (FIGURE 4.11).

Smaller molecules of DNA (about a tenth the size of chromosomes) exist apart from the chromosome in closed loops called **plasmids**. Although they contain few genes and are not essential for bacterial growth, plasmids are significant because some have genes for toxicity and many carry genes for drug resistance. For this reason they are often called **R factors** (R for resistance). Plasmids may be transferred between cells during recombination processes (Chapter 6) and are known to multiply independently during cell reproduction. They are a focus of attention in industrial technologies that utilize genetic engineering.

Recombination:
a process in which the genetic material of a bacterium changes in response to the incorporation of new DNA.

TABLE 4.2 summarizes the structural features of bacterial cells.

SPORES

Certain Gram-positive bacteria are able to produce highly resistant structures called **endospores** or, simply, **spores**. Members of the genera *Bacillus* and *Clostridium* are among the best-known sporeformers (FIGURE 4.12). These bacteria grow, mature, and reproduce for several hours as **vegetative cells**. When nutrients are exhausted, or other environmental pressures exist, spore formation begins. The bacterial chromosome replicates, a small amount of cytoplasm gathers with it, and

klo-strid'e-um

Vegetative cell:
a cell that is growing, maturing, and reproducing.

TABLE 4.2

A Summary of the Structural Features of Bacteria

STRUCTURE	CHEMICAL COMPOSITION	FUNCTION	COMMENT
Flagella	Protein	Movement	Present in many rods and spirilla; few cocci; vary in number and placement
Pili	Protein	Attachment to surfaces Genetic transfers	Found in many Gram-negative bacteria Stimulate immune system
Glycocalyx	Polysaccharides and small proteins	Buffer to environment Contributes to disease Cell protection Attachment to surfaces	Source of ropy milk and bread Found in plaque bacteria and biofilms Capsule and slime layer
Cell wall	Gram-positives have much peptidoglycan, with teichoic acid Gram-negatives have little peptidoglycan and an outer membrane	Cell protection Shape determination	Site of activity of penicillin and lysozyme Absent in mycoplasmas Multiple layers in Gram-negatives
Cell membrane	Protein Phospholipid	Cell boundary Transport into/out of cell Site of enzymatic reactions	Conforms to fluid mosaic model Susceptible to detergents, alcohols, and some antibiotics
Cytoplasm	Water, proteins, lipids, carbohydrates, nucleic acids	Foundation substance of cell	Center of biochemistry and growth Semitransparent, thick
Ribosomes	RNA and protein	Protein synthesis	Inhibited by certain antibiotics
Inclusion bodies	Starch, glycogen, or lipid	Nutrient storage	Used as nutrients during starvation periods
Metachromatic granules	Polyphosphate	Storage for ATP and nucleic acid synthesis	Found in diphtheria bacilli
Magnetosome	Magnetite	Cell orientation	Helps locate preferred habitat
Chromosome	DNA	Site of genetic code Site of inheritance	Exists as single, closed loop Located at nucleoid
Plasmids	DNA	Site of some genes	Contains R factors
Spores	Complex chemical composition with dipicolinic acid	Resistance to environment	Produced by *Bacillus* and *Clostridium* species Probably the most resistant living thing known

the cell membrane grows in to seal off the developing spore. Thick layers of peptidoglycan form, and a series of protein coats are synthesized to protect the contents further. The cell wall of the vegetative cell then disintegrates, and the spore is freed.

Endospores may develop at the end of the cell, near the end, or at the center of the cell, depending on the species (the position is useful for identification purposes). They contain little water (which increases heat resistance) and exhibit very few chemical reactions. However, they do have a large amount of **dipicolinic acid**, a unique organic substance that helps stabilize their proteins, as well as

di'pik-o-lin'ik

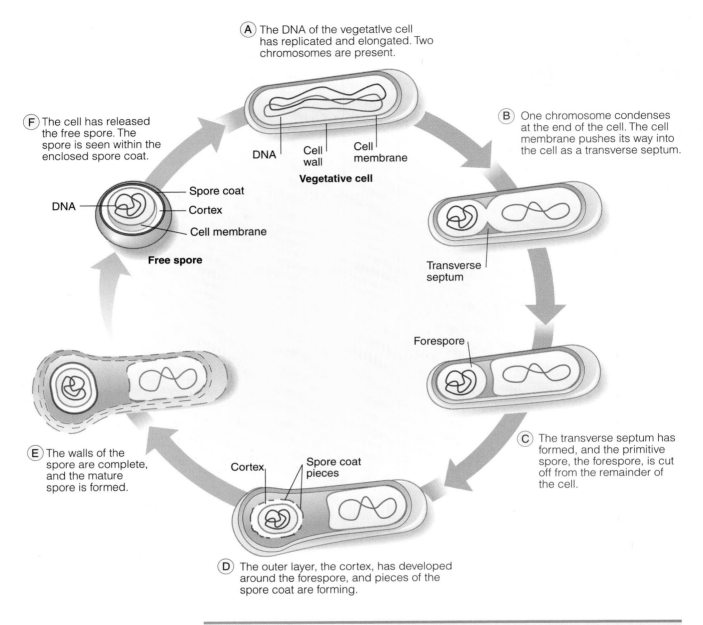

(A) The DNA of the vegetative cell has replicated and elongated. Two chromosomes are present.

DNA
Cell wall
Cell membrane

Vegetative cell

(B) One chromosome condenses at the end of the cell. The cell membrane pushes its way into the cell as a transverse septum.

(F) The cell has released the free spore. The spore is seen within the enclosed spore coat.

DNA
Spore coat
Cortex
Cell membrane

Free spore

Transverse septum

Forespore

(C) The transverse septum has formed, and the primitive spore, the forespore, is cut off from the remainder of the cell.

(E) The walls of the spore are complete, and the mature spore is formed.

Cortex
Spore coat pieces

(D) The outer layer, the cortex, has developed around the forespore, and pieces of the spore coat are forming.

FIGURE 4.12

The Formation of a Bacterial Spore

The cell metabolizes nutrients and multiplies for many generations as a vegetative cell. After some time, the cell enters the sporulation cycle shown here.

some ribosomes and enzymes. When the external environment is favorable, the protective layers break down and the spores germinate to vegetative cells (FIGURE 4.13). It should be noted that spore formation is not a reproductive process; a vegetative cell forms a single spore, and later the spore germinates to one vegetative cell.

Bacterial spores are probably the most resistant living things known. For example, most vegetative bacteria die quickly in water over 80°C, but bacterial spores may remain alive in boiling water (100°C) for 2 hours or more. When placed in 70 per-

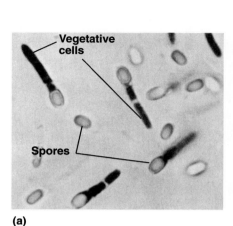
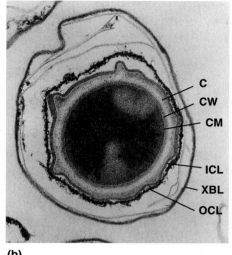
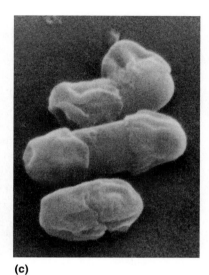

(a) (b) (c)

FIGURE 4.13

Three Different Views of Bacterial Spores

(a) A view of *Clostridium* with the light microscope, showing terminal spore formation. Note the characteristic drumstick appearance of the cells. (b) The fine structure of a *Bacillus thuringiensis* spore seen using the transmission electron microscope. The visible spore structures include the core membrane (CM), core wall (CW), cortex (C), inner coat layer (ICL), outer coat layer (OCL), and exosporium basal layer (XBL). These layers contribute to spore resistance. (c) A scanning electron microscope view of a germinating spore (×30,000). Note that the spore coat divides equatorially along the long axis, and as it separates, the vegetative cell emerges.

cent ethyl alcohol, spores have survived for 20 years. Humans can barely withstand 500 rems of radiation, but spores can survive 1 million rems. Drying has little effect on spores; living spores have been recovered from the intestines of Egyptian mummies. In 1983, archaeologists found spores alive in sediment lining Minnesota's Elk Lake. The sediment was 7518 years old.

But all the records pale in comparison to the controversial discovery reported in 1996 by researcher **Raul Cano** of California Polytechnic State University. Cano found bacterial spores in the stomach of a fossilized bee caught in the resin flowing from a tree in the Dominican Republic (when the resin hardens it becomes amber). The fossilized bee was about 20 million years old. The equally ancient spores from its gut germinated when placed in laboratory nutrients and produced a culture strikingly similar to *Bacillus sphaericus*, which is found today in Dominican bees.

Only a few serious diseases in humans are known to be caused by sporeformers. The first, anthrax, is caused by *Bacillus anthracis* (Chapter 9). This deadly blood disease was studied by Koch and Pasteur. The periodic recurrence of anthrax in the countryside was due to spores remaining alive in the soil where they could be ingested by animals. Another *Bacillus* species, *B. cereus*, is a cause of foodborne infection.

Other diseases are botulism, gas gangrene, and tetanus. These diseases are caused by species of *Clostridium*. Clostridial spores are often found in soil, as well as in human and animal intestines. For the spores to germinate to vegetative cells, the environment must be free of oxygen. The dead tissue in a wound provides such an environment for the sporeforming bacteria that cause tetanus and gas gangrene (Chapter 9), and a vacuum-sealed can of food is suitable for the sporeforming bacteria of botulism (Chapter 8). Some imaginative scientists envision spores as visitors to Earth from a distant galaxy (**MicroFocus** 4.4).

Ethyl alcohol: a two-carbon alcohol compound used as a disinfectant and antiseptic.

spher'i-cus

Gas gangrene: a bacterial disease of the muscles accompanied by large amounts of gas.

MicroFocus 4.4

VISITORS?

In 1901, the Swedish chemist Svante Arrhenius (Ar-ren'e-us) proposed that the first form of life on Earth may have been bacterial spores drifting from some distant planet. In the ensuing decades, Arrhenius' suggestion formed the basis for the panspermia theory. This theory argues that primitive life began with biological substances raining down from space.

In the 1970s, two scientists from the University of Leiden, The Netherlands, took a closer look at Arrhenius' proposal (and by inference, the panspermia theory). They subjected bacterial spores to laboratory conditions that mimicked conditions found in outer space. The scientists, Peter Weber and J. Mayo Greenberg, found that *Bacillus subtilis* spores could survive in a vacuum chamber made extremely cold by helium. Moreover, the spores would survive when subjected to irradiation by mercury and hydrogen lamps simulating the sun's ultraviolet rays. Their results intrigued the scientific community.

But the ability to survive a spacelike environment would not matter unless transport to Earth was possible. Arrhenius suggested that biological objects must be lifted into space from a source. Weber and Greenberg answered that concern by theorizing that a comet or meteorites striking a planet could create the necessary updraft. During space transport, they postulated, a molecular cloud of dust and gas could protect spores against radiation during the in-drift. Arrhenius also wondered how living things could survive for thousands of years. The Dutch scientists projected a 0.1 percent survival of spores for as long as 2500 years within a molecular cloud.

Finally, Arrhenius reasoned that the spores would have to enter Earth's environment and land. This was difficult for Weber and Greenberg to explain, because radiation pressures tend to prevent small particles from entering Earth's environment and solar winds push particles away from the planet.

The prospects for visitations by extraterrestrial spores do not appear bright, according to current thinking. Such a scenario would require several coinciding events, which at present do not appear possible. Still . . .

To this point . . .

We have explored the structural features of bacteria and have noted the three major shapes that a bacterium can take: bacillus, coccus, and spiral. We then analyzed the fine details of a bacterium and discussed how bacterial structures are related to bacterial functions. For example, flagella assist movement in many bacterial rods and spirilla, while pili are used as organs of attachment and in genetic transfers. The bacterial glycocalyx is a sticky, gelatinous structure serving as a protective buffer between the bacterium and its environment.

All bacteria, except mycoplasmas, have a rigid cell wall that gives shape to the organism and prevents its disruption by internal pressure. Penicillin prevents cell wall synthesis and lysozyme breaks the cell wall down, both substances contributing to bacterial destruction. The cell membrane conforms to the fluid mosaic model of a membrane and functions primarily in nutrient and waste transport and as an anchor for DNA and a site for key enzymes. The cytoplasm is the center of cell growth and the ground substance in which several structures, such as chromosomes, are located. The final structure discussed was the bacterial spore, an ultraresistant body formed by species of Bacillus and Clostridium.

In the second half of this chapter, we turn to the growth patterns exhibited by bacteria. We shall study how bacteria reproduce and then explore the dynamics that attend the growth of a bacterial population. Next we shall outline some of the conditions that encourage bacterial growth and discuss certain nutritional patterns. We shall also see how bacteria are cultivated in the laboratory, describe their relationships with other organisms, and focus on an entirely separate domain of bacteria. You might take note of the broad variety of environmental conditions under which bacteria grow. For this reason they can be located in virtually any environment on Earth.

4.2

Bacterial Reproduction and Growth

Most bacteria reproduce by an asexual process called **binary fission**. In this sequence of events, the chromosome duplicates, the cell elongates, and the plasma membrane pinches inward at the center of the cell. When the nuclear material has been evenly distributed, the cell wall thickens and expands inward to separate the dividing cell. No mitotic structures (e.g., spindle, aster) are present as in eukaryotic cells. However, in 1997, researchers demonstrated that two different proteins appear to guide the two chromosomes to opposite poles of the cell.

Reproduction by binary fission lends a certain immortality to bacteria because there is never a moment at which the first bacterium has died. Bacteria mature, undergo binary fission, and are young again. It is conceivable that the original bacterium, though billions of years old, is still among us.

Once the division is complete, bacteria grow and develop the features that make each species unique. The interval of time until the completion of the next division is known as the **generation time** (or **doubling time**). In some bacteria, the generation time is very short; for others, it is quite long. For example, for *Staphylococcus aureus*, the generation time is about 30 minutes; for *Mycobacterium tuberculosis*, the agent of tuberculosis, it is approximately 18 hours; and for the syphilis spirochete, *Treponema pallidum*, it is a long 33 hours. The generation time helps determine the amount of time that passes before disease symptoms appear in an infected individual.

> **Generation time:** the time period that passes between binary fissions in bacteria.

One of the most remarkable generation times is the 20 minutes for *Escherichia coli* growing under optimal conditions. If you were to begin with a single rod at 8:00 A.M. this morning, two would be present by 8:20, four by 8:40, and eight by 9:00 A.M. You would have sixty-four rods by 10:00 A.M. and 512 by 11:00 A.M. By 6:00 tonight, the culture would contain just over a billion rods. Indeed, one enterprising mathematician has calculated that if binary fission were to continue for 36 hours, or until 8:00 tomorrow night, there would be enough bacteria to cover the face of the Earth!

> esh'er-ik'e-a

Fortunately, the reproductive potential of a bacterium is never realized because of the limitations of the external environment. Thus, we need never worry about being smothered with bacteria. Apparently bacteria are subject to the same controls as all other organisms on Earth, as we shall see next.

THE BACTERIAL GROWTH CURVE

A typical **growth curve** for a population of bacterial cells (FIGURE 4.14) illustrates some of the dynamics that affect the population over the course of time. The population's history may begin when several bacteria enter the human respiratory tract or are transferred to a tube of growth medium in the laboratory. Four distinct phases of the curve are recognized: the lag phase, the logarithmic phase, the stationary phase, and the decline phase.

> **Growth medium:** material for the cultivation of microorganisms.

The **lag phase** encompasses the first few hours of the curve. During this time, bacteria adapt to their new environment. In the respiratory tract, scavenging white blood cells may engulf and destroy some bacteria; in growth media, some organisms may die from the shock of transfer or the inability to adapt to the new environment. However, the biochemical activity in the remaining bacteria is intense as they store nutrients, synthesize enzymes, and prepare for binary fission. The curve remains at a plateau, balanced by reproduction in some cells and death in others.

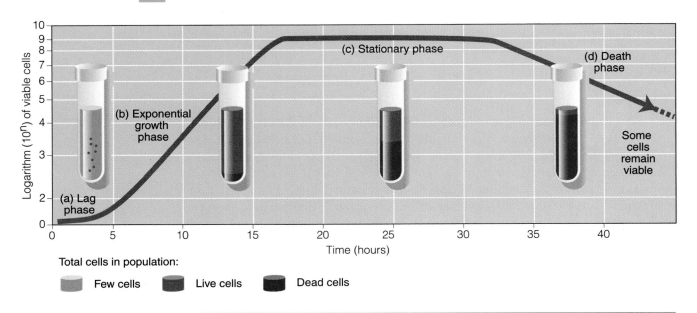

Total cells in population:

Few cells   Live cells   Dead cells

FIGURE 4.14

The Growth Curve for a Bacterial Population

(a) During the lag phase, the population numbers remain stable as bacteria prepare for division. (b) During the logarithmic (exponential growth) phase, the numbers double with each generation time. Environmental factors later lead to cell death, and (c) the stationary phase shows a stabilizing population. (d) The decline phase is the period during which cell death becomes substantial.

Logarithmic phase:
the phase of a bacterial growth curve at which reproduction and growth are at their highest rates.

Stationary phase:
the phase of a bacterial growth curve at which the reproduction rate equals the death rate.

The population then enters an active stage of growth called the **logarithmic phase** (or log phase); the term **exponential growth phase** is also used. The mass of each cell increases rapidly, and reproduction follows. As each generation time passes, the number of bacteria doubles, and the graph rises in a straight line if logarithms (powers of 10) of the numbers are used for the curve. However, a J-shaped curve develops if the actual numbers are used (FIGURE 4.15).

In humans, disease symptoms usually develop during the log phase because the bacteria and their toxins are causing tissue damage. Coughing or fever may occur, and fluid may enter the lungs if the air sacs are damaged. If the bacteria produce toxins, tissue destruction may become apparent. But vulnerability to antibiotics is also highest at this stage. In the laboratory, the population growth may be so vigorous that visible colonies appear on solid media, each colony consisting of millions of organisms (FIGURE 4.16). Broth media may become cloudy with growth. Because the population is at its biochemical optimum, research experiments are generally performed during the log phase.

After some hours or days, the vigor of the population changes and, as the reproductive and death rates equalize, the population enters another plateau, the **stationary phase**. In the respiratory tract, antibodies from the immune system are attacking the bacteria, and phagocytosis by white blood cells adds to their destruction. Perhaps the person was given an antibiotic to supplement the body's defensive measures. In the culture tube, nutrients have become scarce, waste products have accumulated, and factors such as oxygen and water are in short supply.

If these conditions continue, the external environment will exert its limiting powers on the population and the **decline phase** (or **exponential death phase**) will

FIGURE 4.15

A Skyrocketing Bacterial Population

The number of bacteria progresses from 1 cell to 2 million cells in a mere 7 hours. The J-shaped growth curve gets steeper and steeper as the hours pass. Only a depletion of food, buildup of waste, or some other limitation will halt the progress of the curve.

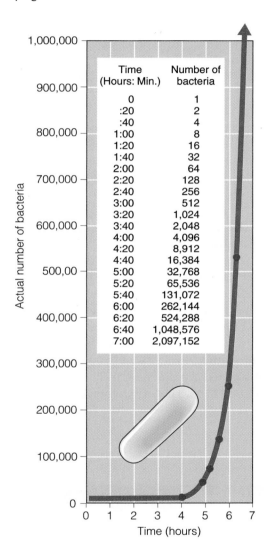

Time (Hours: Min.)	Number of bacteria
0	1
:20	2
:40	4
1:00	8
1:20	16
1:40	32
2:00	64
2:20	128
2:40	256
3:00	512
3:20	1,024
3:40	2,048
4:00	4,096
4:20	8,912
4:40	16,384
5:00	32,768
5:20	65,536
5:40	131,072
6:00	262,144
6:20	524,288
6:40	1,048,576
7:00	2,097,152

FIGURE 4.16

Two Views of Bacterial Colonies

(a) Colonies of *Bacillus macerans* isolated from sewage and growing in a medium of solidified soybean meal and casein peptone. These colonies are several millimeters in height; they have been euphemistically called "Rockies in a Petri dish." (b) A scanning electron micrograph of the surface of a colony of *Staphylococcus aureus* on a solid medium ($\times$6000). Note the irregular nature of the surface of the colony, with numerous conical pits.

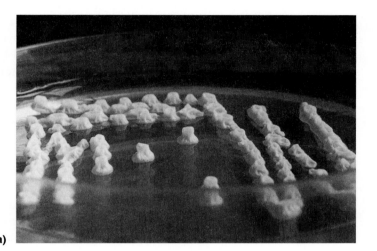

(a)

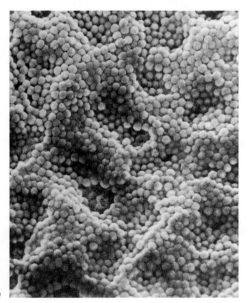

(b)

ensue. Now the number of dying cells exceeds the number of new cells formed. A bacterial glycocalyx may forestall death by acting as a buffer to the environment, and flagella may enable organisms to move to a new location. If the organism is a species of *Bacillus* or *Clostridium*, the vegetative cells will revert to spores, and the stationary phase may extend for months or years. For many species, though, the history of the population comes to an end with the death of the last cell.

TEMPERATURE

Bacteria inhabit almost every environment on Earth because different species can tolerate the myriad conditions found on the planet. For example, different bacterial species grow at different temperatures. Certain bacteria have their shortest generation times at temperatures in the range of 0°C to 20°C; these bacteria are called **psychrophiles**. Other bacteria, the **mesophiles**, thrive at the middle range of 20°C to 40°C; and **thermophiles** (FIGURE 4.17) multiply best at temperatures of 40°C to 90°C or higher.

si'kro-filz

Most bacteria are mesophiles. This is especially true of pathogenic bacteria growing in the human body, where the temperature is 37°C. It should be noted that pathogenic bacteria usually grow over a 35°C to 42°C range. Thus, when the body temperature rises to 40°C (104°F), there is a negligible "cooking effect" on bacteria. The common laboratory incubator is set at 37°C to provide the proper environment for mesophiles.

Pathogenic bacteria: bacteria that can cause disease in plants and animals.

Some mesophiles can grow at temperatures substantially below their normal range. Certain species, for instance, grow in refrigerated foods at 5°C when they are left there for long periods of time. Then they may produce waste products and cause food spoilage. For example, staphylococci deposit their toxins in cold cuts, salads, and various leftovers. When such foods are consumed without heating, the toxins may cause food poisoning. Other examples of mesophiles growing in the cold are *Campylobacter* species, which can be infectious (FIGURE 4.18), and *Proteus vulgaris*, which causes blackening of eggs accompanied by a characteristic rotten odor. Since these organisms are not truly psychrophilic, some microbiologists prefer to describe them as **psychrotrophic** or **psychrotolerant**. True psychrophiles live in the ocean depths and in Arctic and Antarctic regions where no other form of life is known to exist.

si'kro-troph'ik

Thermophiles are present in compost heaps and hot springs, and are important contaminants in dairy products because they survive pasteurization temperatures. However, thermophiles pose little threat to human health because they do not grow well at the cooler temperature of the body. In the 1980s, scientists isolated thermophilic bacteria from seawater brought up from hot-water vents along rifts on the floor of the Pacific Ocean. Using high pressure to keep the water from boiling, they found that the bacteria grew at an astonishing 113°C. The term **hyperthermophile** is used for forms such as these.

FIGURE 4.17

A Thermophile

An electron micrograph of a thermophilic bacterium isolated from a compost heap where the temperature was 80°C (176°F). This organism was identified as a strain of *Thermus* closely related to *T. thermophilus*. Growing at a temperature close to that of boiling water, this organism has adapted to the conditions in the hot-compost ecosystem, and it is a factor in the degradation of kitchen and garden waste.

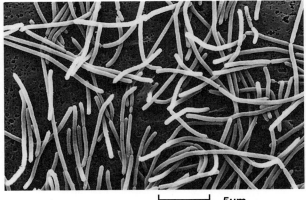

5μm

TEXTBOOK CASES

FIGURE 4.18

An Outbreak of Campylobacteriosis Caused by *Campylobacter jejuni* Occurring in Oklahoma

This outbreak occurred between August 16 and 20, 1996.

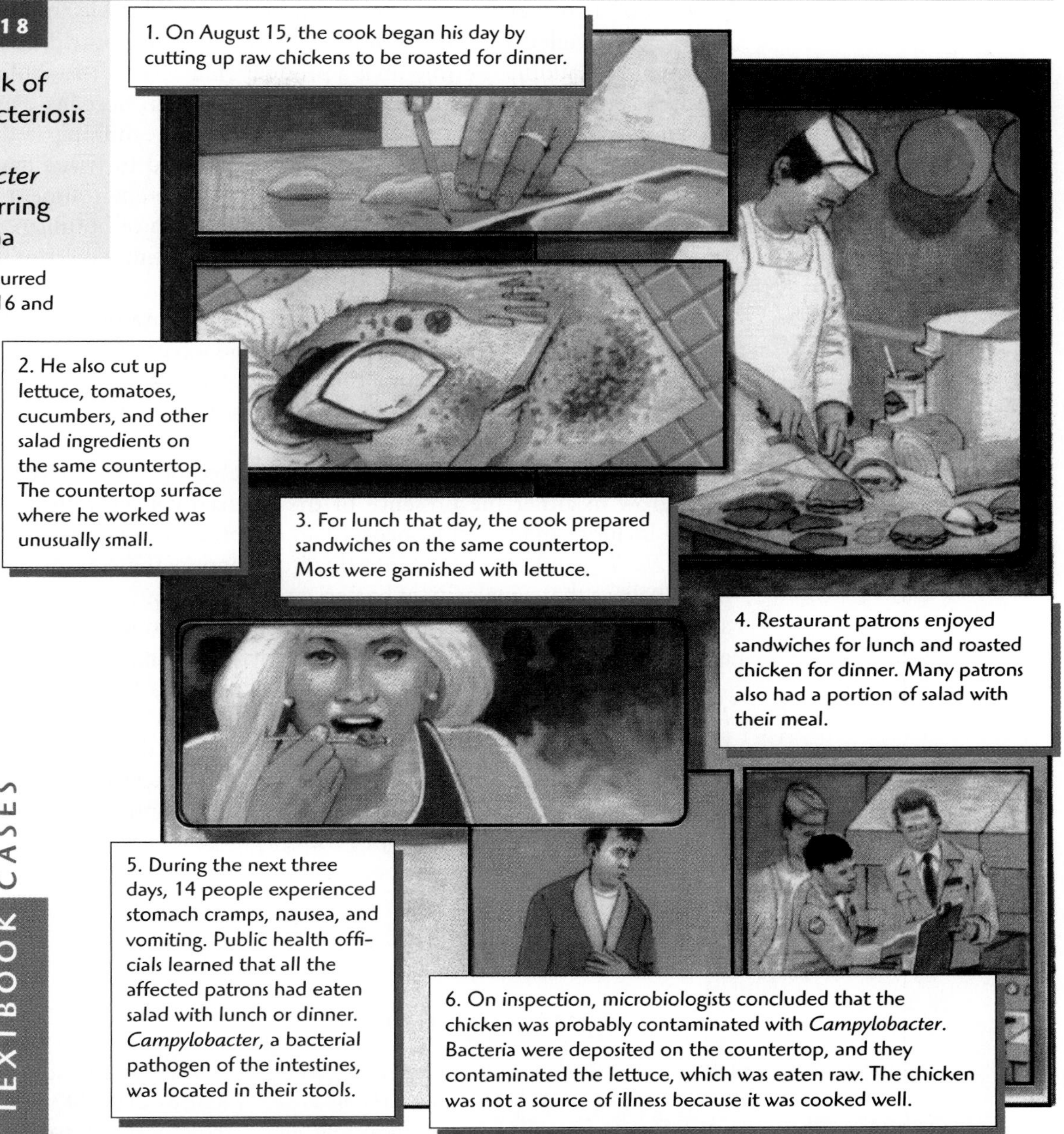

1. On August 15, the cook began his day by cutting up raw chickens to be roasted for dinner.

2. He also cut up lettuce, tomatoes, cucumbers, and other salad ingredients on the same countertop. The countertop surface where he worked was unusually small.

3. For lunch that day, the cook prepared sandwiches on the same countertop. Most were garnished with lettuce.

4. Restaurant patrons enjoyed sandwiches for lunch and roasted chicken for dinner. Many patrons also had a portion of salad with their meal.

5. During the next three days, 14 people experienced stomach cramps, nausea, and vomiting. Public health officials learned that all the affected patrons had eaten salad with lunch or dinner. *Campylobacter*, a bacterial pathogen of the intestines, was located in their stools.

6. On inspection, microbiologists concluded that the chicken was probably contaminated with *Campylobacter*. Bacteria were deposited on the countertop, and they contaminated the lettuce, which was eaten raw. The chicken was not a source of illness because it was cooked well.

OXYGEN

The growth of many bacteria also depends on a plentiful supply of oxygen, and in this respect, **aerobic** bacteria are similar to more complex organisms. **Anaerobic** bacteria, by contrast, live in an oxygen-free environment. Some anaerobic bacteria actually die if oxygen is present, while others fail to grow and multiply. Certain anaerobic bacteria use sulfur in their metabolic activities instead of oxygen, and therefore they produce hydrogen sulfide (H_2S) rather than water (H_2O) as a waste product of their metabolism. Others synthesize considerable amounts of methane (CH_4), often called swamp gas. Both of these gases give putrid odors to marshes, swamps, and landfills. Petroleum is a product of anaerobic metabolism.

Some species of anaerobic bacteria cause disease in humans. For example, the *Clostridium* species that cause tetanus and gas gangrene multiply in the dead, anaerobic tissue of a wound and produce toxins that lead to tissue damage. Another species of *Clostridium* multiplies in the oxygen-free environment of a vacuum-sealed can of food, where it produces the lethal toxin of botulism. In one bizarre incident, a restaurant owner died of botulism after tasting a piece of fish marinating under a layer of oil (MicroFocus 4.5).

Anaerobic conditions may be established in the laboratory by a number of methods. One method uses thioglycollic acid to bind oxygen in thioglycollate medium. Among the most widely used methods is the GasPak system, in which hydrogen reacts with oxygen in the presence of a catalyst to form water, thereby creating an oxygen-free atmosphere (FIGURE 4.19).

Some bacteria are neither aerobic nor anaerobic, but **facultative**. Facultative bacteria grow in either the presence or the reduced concentration of oxygen. This group includes many staphylococci and streptococci, as well as members of the genus *Bacillus* and a variety of intestinal rods, among them *E. coli*. Some microbiologists believe that a majority of bacteria may be facultative organisms. A facultative aerobe prefers anaerobic conditions (but grows aerobically), while a facultative anaerobe prefers oxygen-rich conditions (but grows anaerobically).

Still another group is the **microaerophilic** bacteria typified by *Treponema pallidum*, the agent of syphilis. These organisms require a low concentration of oxygen for growth. In the body, certain microaerophiles cause disease of the oral cavity, urinary tract, and gastrointestinal tract. Some species of bacteria, said to be **capnophilic**, require an atmosphere low in oxygen but rich in carbon dioxide. The CO_2 content can be increased in the laboratory by using a gas-generating apparatus or by burning a candle in a closed jar with the bacteria. Members of the genera *Neisseria* and *Streptococcus* are capnophiles.

Anaerobic bacteria: bacteria that grow in the absence of oxygen.

thi'o-gli'ko-lāt

Facultative bacteria: bacteria that grow in the presence or absence of oxygen.

mi'kro-a-ro-fil'ik

cap-no-fil'ik

MicroFocus 4.5

OF MARINATED FISH

It was September 1978, and the man was in serious condition. He had come to the hospital emergency room in Puerto Rico complaining of blurred vision, difficulty swallowing, erratic breathing, and numbness in his fingers and arms. Now the ER personnel were frantically trying to save his life. He owned a restaurant, he gasped. No, there were no other sick members in his house. No, he hadn't done anything unusual that he could remember. Slowly he was slipping away. By morning, he was gone.

Before long, the investigation was in progress. Public health officials visited the man's restaurant and spoke with his wife. She was fond of marinating fish, and occasionally she would leave some in the restaurant to cure. Normally the fish cured in wide, shallow trays, but this time, she had no trays available so she used narrow-mouthed, screw-capped jars. Officials noted that a thick layer of oil had formed over the fish, and they surmised that the oil created anaerobic conditions underneath. (The narrow mouth of the jar also contributed to the lack of air movement.)

Now their suspicions were aroused. A sample of the fish was taken back to the laboratory for bacteriological testing. At the same time, in another part of the lab, the man's tissues were being studied for evidence of bacterial toxins. The results came back almost simultaneously. The organism was *Clostridium botulinum*; the disease was botulism. The man had probably tasted the fish to see how it was coming along. He could not have foreseen what lay ahead.

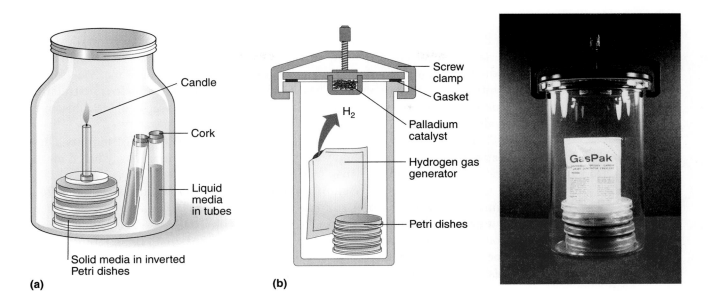

(a)

- Candle
- Cork
- Liquid media in tubes
- Solid media in inverted Petri dishes

(b)

- Screw clamp
- Gasket
- Palladium catalyst
- Hydrogen gas generator
- Petri dishes
- H₂

GasPak

FIGURE 4.19

Bacterial Cultivation in Different Gas Environments

Two types of cultivation methods are shown for bacteria that grow poorly in an oxygen–rich environment. (a) A candle jar, in which micro-aerophilic bacteria grow in an atmosphere where the oxygen is reduced by the burning candle. (b) An anaerobic jar, in which hydrogen is released from a generator and then combines with oxygen to form water and create an anaerobic environment.

ACIDITY/ALKALINITY

Because the internal environment of most bacteria has a pH of about 7.0, the majority of species grow best under neutral pH conditions. Although most growth media for laboratory cultivation are set at pH 7.0, bacteria tolerate acidic conditions as low as pH 2.0 and alkaline conditions as high as pH 9.5. (*Vibrio cholerae*, the agent of cholera, is an example of the latter.) Human blood and tissues, with a pH of approximately 7.2 to 7.4, provide a suitable environment for the proliferation of disease-causing bacteria.

Acid-tolerant bacteria called **acidophiles** are valuable in the food and dairy industries. For example, certain species of *Lactobacillus* and *Streptococcus* produce the acid that converts milk to buttermilk and cream to sour cream. These species pose no threat to good health even when consumed in large amounts. The "active cultures" in a cup of yogurt are actually acid-tolerant (acidophilic) bacteria. Extreme acidophiles are found among the archaea (archaeabacteria).

The majority of known bacterial species, however, do not grow well under acidic conditions. Thus, the acidic environment of the stomach helps deter disease in this organ, while providing a natural barrier to the organs beyond. In addition, you may have noted that certain acidic foods are hardly ever contaminated with bacteria. Examples are lemons, oranges, and other citrus fruits, as well as such vegetables as cabbage and rhubarb. Traditionally, tomatoes were too acidic to support bacterial growth. However, modern technologists have developed the "neutral tomato," along with a host of new problems for consumers, especially those who grow and can their own tomatoes.

pH:
a measure of the acidity or alkalinity of a substance or solution.

PATTERNS OF NUTRITION

Bacteria must meet certain nutritional requirements in order to grow. Most bacteria have relatively simple requirements, with water an absolute necessity. In addition, bacteria need foods that can serve as energy sources and raw materials for the synthesis of cell components. These foods generally include proteins for structural compounds and enzymes, carbohydrates for energy, and a series of vitamins, minerals, and inorganic salts.

Two different patterns exist for satisfying an organism's nutritional needs. These patterns are called autotrophy and heterotrophy. They are primarily based on the source of carbon used for making cell components.

Organisms that practice **autotrophy** are able to synthesize their own foods from simple inorganic carbon sources (Chapter 5). The organisms are said to be autotrophic (literally "self-feeding"). Autotrophs obtain their carbon from inorganic compounds such as carbon dioxide and ions such as carbonate. Energy for food synthesis may come from the sun or from chemical reactions taking place in the cytoplasm, as Chapter 5 explains.

The second pattern, **heterotrophy**, is practiced by heterotrophic organisms (literally "other-feeders"). These organisms obtain preformed organic molecules from the environment and use them for structural components and energy. The heterotrophic bacteria that feed exclusively on dead organic matter, such as rotting wood, are commonly called **saprobes**. For many years these organisms were known as saprophytes, from Greek stems meaning "rotten" and "plant," but the name has been changed to saprobes to reflect feeding on both plants and animals. Heterotrophs that feed on living organic matter, such as human tissues, are commonly known as **parasites**. The word **pathogen** (from the Greek *pathos* for "suffering") is used if the parasite causes disease in its host organism.

BACTERIAL CULTIVATION

Since the time of Pasteur and Koch, microbiologists have used media such as beef broth for the laboratory cultivation of bacteria. The modern form of this liquid medium, called **nutrient broth**, consists of water, beef extract, and peptone, a protein supplement from plant or animal sources. When agar is added to solidify the medium, the product is called **nutrient agar**. Agar is a polysaccharide derived from marine red algae. It adds no nutrients to the medium but only serves to make it solid so that bacteria can be cultivated on the surface. Sometimes it is valuable to use a semisolid medium, such as when testing bacterial motility. In this case, a small portion of agar is added to the medium to make it stiff but not as solid as nutrient agar.

Most common bacteria grow well in nutrient broth and nutrient agar, but certain fastidious bacteria may require **enriched media** containing special nutrients. For example, the streptococci that cause strep throat grow well when washed human red blood cells are added to the nutrient medium. In this instance, the medium is called blood agar. To encourage the growth of *Neisseria* species, agar with whole human blood is heated before solidification, a process that disrupts the red blood cells and releases the hemoglobin. The medium is now termed chocolate agar because of its charred brown appearance.

Selective media contain ingredients to inhibit the growth of certain bacteria in a mixture while allowing the growth of others. For example, certain staphylococci are cultivated on mannitol salt agar. This medium contains mannitol, an alcoholic car-

aw'to-trōph'e
Autotroph:
an organism that synthesizes its foods from simple inorganic carbon compounds.

het'er-o-trōph'e
Heterotroph:
an organism that obtains its foods from preformed organic carbon compounds.

Medium:
a substance used to support the growth of microorganisms (e.g., nutrient agar).

ahg'ar

Fastidious:
having special requirements.

ni-se're-ah

TABLE 4.3

A Comparison of Bacterial Media

NAME	COMPONENTS	USES	EXAMPLES
Nutrient broth	Water, beef extract, peptone	General use	—
Nutrient agar	Water, beef extract, peptone, agar	General use	—
Enriched medium	Growth stimulants	Cultivating fastidious bacteria	Blood agar for streptococci; chocolate agar for *Neisseria* species
Selective medium	Growth stimulants Growth inhibitors	Selecting certain bacteria out of mixture	Mannitol salt agar for staphylococci
Differential medium	Dyes Growth stimulants Growth inhibitors	Distinguishing different bacteria in a mixture	MacConkey agar for Gram-negative bacteria

bohydrate fermented by staphylococci, as well as a high salt concentration that inhibits most other bacteria.

Another type of medium is the **differential medium**. This medium makes it easy to distinguish colonies of one organism from colonies of other organisms on the same plate. MacConkey agar is typical. It contains the dyes neutral red and crystal violet as well as the carbohydrate lactose. Those bacteria that ferment the lactose take up the dyes and form red colonies; other bacteria show up as colorless colonies. In addition, MacConkey agar contains bile salts to inhibit the growth of Gram-positive bacteria. This medium is thus selective as well as differential. (For a summary of the various media, see TABLE 4.3.)

Differential medium: a medium in which colonies of different bacteria can be distinguished.

The bacterial media just described represent nonchemically defined media, or **natural media**. This is because one cannot be certain of the exact components or their quantity. Another type of medium is the chemically defined, or **synthetic medium**. In this case, the nature and amount of each component are known. Such a medium might contain glucose, ammonium phosphate, potassium phosphate, magnesium sulfate, and sodium chloride. Each component fills a need. For example, glucose supplies energy to the cell, ammonium ions are a source of nitrogen for amino acid and nucleic acid formation, and phosphate is used in DNA and RNA synthesis.

Synthetic medium: a medium in which the nature and quantity of each component are known.

ISOLATION AND MEASUREMENT

Bacteria rarely occur in nature alone. In virtually all cases, they are mixed with species of other bacteria, a so-called **mixed culture** (a swab from the gum area is an example). But to work with bacteria, the laboratory technologist must use a **pure culture**—that is, a population of only one bacterial species. This is particularly important when identifying a pathogen.

Pure culture: a population containing only one species.

For isolating bacteria from mixed cultures, two standard methods are available. The first method, called the **streak plate isolation method**, uses a single plate of bacteriological medium (FIGURE 4.20). An inoculum from a culture is taken with a loop or needle, and a series of streaks is made in one area of the plate. The instrument is

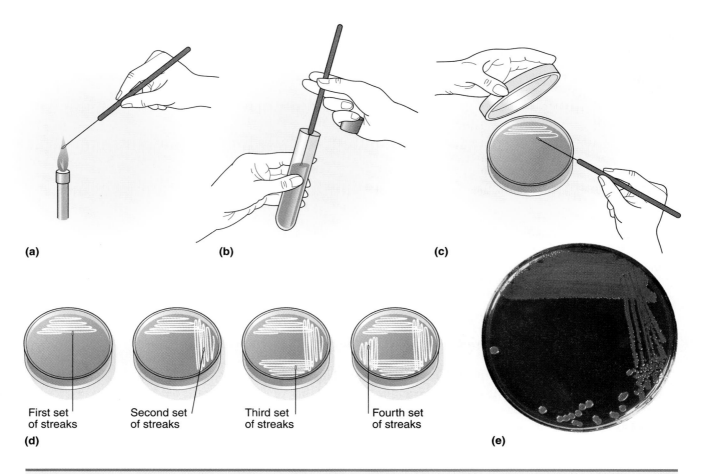

(a)   **(b)**   **(c)**

First set of streaks   Second set of streaks   Third set of streaks   Fourth set of streaks

(d)   **(e)**

FIGURE 4.20

The Streak Plate Isolation Method

A loop is sterilized, and a sample of bacteria is obtained and streaked along one edge of the plate of medium. Successive streaks are performed, and the plate is incubated. Well-isolated and defined colonies illustrate a successful isolation.

flamed, touched to the first area, and a second series is made in a second area. Similarly, streaks are made in the third and fourth areas, thereby spreading out the different bacteria so they can form discrete colonies on incubation. The second method is the **pour plate isolation method**. Here, a sample of bacteria is diluted in several tubes of melted, cooled agar medium. The agar is then poured into sterile Petri dishes and allowed to harden. During incubation, the bacteria will form discrete colonies where they have been diluted the most. The technologist can then pick samples of the colonies for further testing.

To measure the amount of bacterial growth in a medium, there are numerous methods. For example, the cloudiness, or **turbidity**, of a liquid culture may be used to estimate the number of bacteria it contains. The scientist may wish to perform a **direct microscopic count** using a known sample of the culture on a specially prepared slide (a Petroff-Hausser counting chamber). The **dry weight** of the bacteria gives an indication of the cell mass, and the **oxygen uptake** in metabolism can be measured as an indication of the bacterial number.

It is also possible to perform a **most probable number test** (Chapter 25) or a **standard plate count procedure** (Chapter 25). In the former test, samples of bacteria are added to numerous lactose broth tubes, and the presence or absence of gas formed in fermentation gives a rough estimation of the bacterial number. In the latter test, a bacterial culture is diluted, and samples of dilutions are placed in agar plates. The number of colonies appearing after incubation reflects the number of bacteria originally present. This test is desirable because it gives the **viable count** of bacteria (the living bacteria only), compared to a microscopic count or dry weight test that gives the **total bacterial count** (the living as well as dead bacteria).

Some bacteria are impossible to cultivate on artificial laboratory media, but instead require a living tissue medium. Most rickettsiae and chlamydiae are examples of such bacteria. They must be grown in fertilized eggs, tissue cultures, animals, or other environments where living cells are found. The difficulty in cultivation often makes detection and study of these organisms a challenge.

INTERMICROBIAL RELATIONSHIPS

Closely allied to the nutritional needs of bacteria is their relationship with other organisms and with each other (MicroFocus 4.6). The term **symbiosis** (literally, "living together") is applied to the relationship. Symbiosis implies a situation in which two populations of organisms interact in a close and permanent association. The benefits obtained through this interaction may involve food, protection, support, or other life-sustaining factors. *sim'bi-o'sis*

If a symbiosis between two populations of organisms benefits both populations, the relationship is termed **mutualism** (FIGURE 4.21). For example, bacteria live on the roots of pod-bearing plants such as peas and beans, where they trap nitrogen from the atmosphere and convert it to ammonium ions. The plant then uses the ammonium ions to synthesize amino acids. The plant, in turn, provides a stable environment for the bacteria and supplies them with essential growth factors. The significance of this relationship is explored more fully in Chapter 25.

MicroFocus 4.6

TEAM PLAYERS

In the traditional view, bacteria are rugged individuals with a self-reliant way of life centering on growth and reproduction. But that view may be changing, as scientists observe coalitions of bacteria performing feats not achieved by individual cells. Apparently, a mass of bacteria must mobilize before the feat is accomplished.

The concept of single-celled organisms communicating and exhibiting complex behavior is new to science. Apparently, though, it is real. For the past several years, microbiologists have been studying *Vibrio fischeri*, a bacterium that inhabits squid and produces light, but only when the population reaches a high density and the cells are nutritionally challenged. The light results

from the action of an enzyme on a luminescent compound. Normally the bacteria produce too little enzyme to light up the area. But then a mass of organisms cooperate, and the bacteria produce a signaling compound that accumulates and unites with a protein in the local environment. The signal-protein combination binds to a section of DNA on the bacterial chromosome and switches on the genes that encode the light-producing enzymes. The enzyme molecules build up rapidly, and as they break down the luminescent compound, the area glows with an eerie green light.

Scientists remain unsure about the benefit of turning on the lights. Armchair speculators might hypothesize, for

example, that the light helps the colony find food. Another outlook is that signaling molecules are used in competition among various types of microorganisms. Simple algae, for example, produce substances that inhibit bacterial signals and thereby prevent bacterial overgrowth. This lesson is not lost on scientists who seek new antibacterial drugs.

The phenomenon of microbial communication has been termed *quorum sensing*, meaning that organisms can sense when a crowd has gathered and can prepare for a change in the environment. Sounds like something a crowd of humans would do. But maybe the bacteria were doing it long before the NFL or NBA came into existence.

Legionella
pneumophila

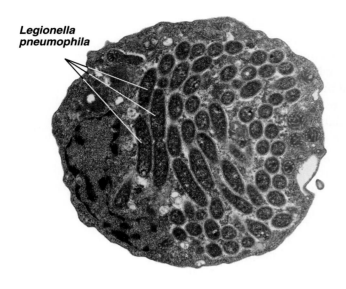

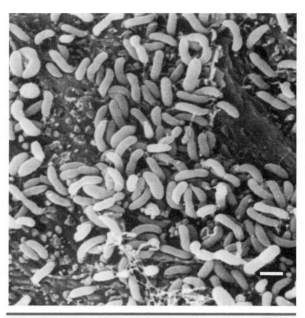

FIGURE 4.21

Mutualism Among Microorganisms

The bacterium *Legionella pneumophila* is the cause of Legionnaires' disease. In nature, this organism lives within various types of protozoa. In this electron micrograph, the bacilli can be seen in a *Hartmanella* cell. Living within a protozoan helps the bacterium survive environmental extremes.

FIGURE 4.22

Commensalism

A scanning electron micrograph of a section from the gastrointestinal tract of a young sheep, showing an area inhabited by a mass of curved rods. These organisms are probably commensals because the animal exhibited no signs of disease. (Bar = 1.0 μm.)

Commensalism:
a symbiotic relationship in which one population receives benefit while the other receives neither benefit nor harm.

sin'er-jizm

Trench mouth:
a disease of the dental tissues, accompanied by bleeding ulcers, foul odor, and bad taste.

Another type of symbiosis is **commensalism**. This relationship occurs when one population receives benefit from the relationship while the other receives neither benefit nor harm (**FIGURE 4.22**). An example is found in some populations of bacteria (commensals) inhabiting the human skin. Another commensal is *Escherichia coli*, the Gram-negative rod that thrives in the human intestine but usually causes no damage. To some investigators this relationship is more symbolic of mutualism, because it appears that *E. coli* provides certain vitamins for human nutrition and breaks down otherwise indigestible foodstuffs, while keeping pathogens in check.

A third type of symbiosis is **synergism**. In this case, two populations of organisms live together and accomplish what neither population could accomplish alone. In trench mouth, for example, at least two populations of bacteria must be present for infection of the oral cavity to occur. Usually one population consists of rods, the other of spirochetes.

When a symbiosis is beneficial to one organism but harmful to the other, the result is **parasitism**. In this situation, the organism that benefits is the parasite, and the one that suffers injury is the host. The bacteria of human disease are typical parasites. Many microbiologists believe that severe injury to the host is probably not in the best interest of the parasite, because if the host were to die, the parasite might also die. A relationship such as this is explored more completely in Chapter 17.

ARCHAEBACTERIA (ARCHAEA)

We shall close our discussion of bacterial structure and growth with a discussion about a unique type of prokaryote called **archaebacteria** (sometimes spelled archaeobacteria). These organisms are also known as **archaea**, to distinguish them as a separate group from traditional bacteria. Microbiologists are in two camps regarding the correct nomenclature. Thus, we shall express the organisms as archaebacteria (archaea). In future editions, you may see the organisms expressed as "archaea (archaebacteria)"; then just "archaea," as the issue continues to be sorted out.

ar′ka-a-bac-ter′i-a
ar-ka′ah

The reason for the nomenclature conflict is the gradually emerging agreement that archaebacteria (archaea) are not bacteria in the traditional sense. Although the organisms resemble traditional bacteria when viewed microscopically, they have several distinguishing features: (1) their cell walls do not contain peptidoglycan, (2) their cell membranes have unusual lipid compositions, and (3) they have unique nucleotide sequences in the RNA of their ribosomes. Moreover, when the nucleotide base sequence of an archaebacterium (archaeon) was determined in 1996, the genes were found to be over 50 percent different than the genes of traditional bacteria and eukaryotes, as Chapter 3 notes.

Largely for these reasons, **Carl Woese, George Fox,** and their colleagues have recommended that the organisms be placed in a **domain** (or **superkingdom**) called **Archaea**. Traditional bacteria would occupy a separate domain called Eubacteria (*eu* means "true"), and all remaining organisms would be Eukarya. (Chapter 3 discusses this concept in more detail.)

woes

Another reason for separating archaebacteria (archaea) from other prokaryotes is the extremely harsh environments in which they live (**MicroFocus 4.7**). Indeed, the

MicroFocus 4.7

OUR NEIGHBORS ON THE RED PLANET

Among the more engaging stories of 1996 was the notion of possible life on Mars. In August, David E. McKay and his colleagues at the National Aeronautics and Space Administration (NASA) raised eyebrows with their announcement that a 4.3 pound, potato-sized meteorite from space apparently contains fossilized microorganisms.

Scientists agree that the meteorite (named ALH84001) is from Mars because, on heating, it gives off a mixture of gases unique to the Martian atmosphere; they agree that crystals in the meteorite look like crystals produced by Earth's bacteria; and they agree that the meteorite contains polycyclic aromatic hydrocarbons, a group of chemical compounds found on Earth (such as in diesel exhaust) and often

associated with living things. But they sharply disagree about the "microbial fossils" in ALH84001.

The electron microscope views of the fossils (Figure 1) transfixed researchers throughout the world. The wormy, tubular shapes with rounded edges are about 20 nm long and resemble photos of microorganisms from Earth, but in miniature. Wishing to avoid the term "breakthrough," McKay and his colleagues exercised cautious optimism about their discovery.

And well they did, for within 15 months, scientists had answered most of McKay's observations with reasonable alternatives. New images of the Martian meteorite indicated that the microfossils could be narrow ledges of mineral protruding from the underlying rock (Figure 2). And, scientists concluded, 20 nm of

space is simply too small for even the most basic chemical machinery of life to exist. Further, the hydrocarbons might have come from inorganic chemicals just as plausibly as from life-associated substances (the possibility of contamination from Earth was raised). Even if the hydrocarbons were of Martian origin, they could be from a primordial soup that never achieved life.

Is the controversy over? Not as of this writing (although the McKay team has withdrawn some of its evidence). NASA is scheduled to send a probe to our distant neighbor and return it in the year 2008 with soil samples for more careful study. For the moment, "the hypothesis has not fared well," as a Harvard paleontologist understated in 1999.

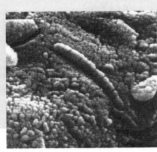

■ *Figure 1.*
A wormlike microfossil observed in meteorite ALH84001 and proposed as evidence of bacterial life on Mars.

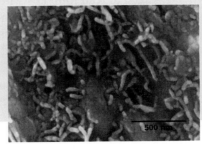

■ *Figure 2.*
Narrow mineral ledges from meteorite ALH84001 resembling microfossils.

FIGURE 4.23

The Habitat of Extremophiles

A view of the effluent channel of an alkaline spring in Yellowstone Park showing a mat of cyanobacteria in the foreground. The temperature in the channel is about 75°C (37°C is body temperature).

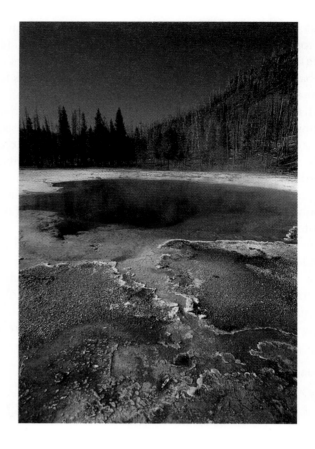

ex-trēm′o-files

ther′mo-a-cid′o-files

sul-fo-lo′bus
a′cid-o-cal-dar′e-us

pi-ro-lo′bus fum-ar′e-i

meth-an′-o-gen

Halophiles:
bacteria living in high-salt environments.

new word **extremophiles** has been coined for organisms such as these. One group of archaebacteria (archaea) are the **thermoacidophiles**. These organisms live under extremely acidic and extremely high temperature conditions (FIGURE 4.23). One organism *Sulfolobus acidocaldarius*, grows well at temperatures of 85°C (about 185°F) in soil with a pH of 1.0. The most heat-resistant organism isolated to date is *Pyrolobus fumarii*, found in a hydrothermal vent at the bottom of the ocean. This remarkable hyperthermophile grows at a temperature of 113°C, well above the boiling point of water. The waxy molecules in its cell membrane and the many disulfide linkages in the proteins help protect it from the heat.

Another group of archaebacteria (archaea) are the **methanogens**. These prokaryotes are autotrophs that live on carbon dioxide, nitrogen, and water. They produce methane under anaerobic conditions and have been found in volcanic rock, marshes, lake bottoms, and animal feces (and hence, in their intestines). A third group are the **extreme halophiles**, which thrive in high-salt environments such as Utah's Great Salt Lake. These organisms account for the redness in salt collection ponds near California's San Francisco Bay. Those who are fascinated by life at the extremes are encouraged to read John Postgate's book, *The Outer Reaches of Life* (1996).

Archaebacteria (archaea) are so-named because molecular paleontologists believe the organisms were in existence under primitive Earth conditions. Indeed, they are believed to predate traditional bacteria and possibly to evolve to them. That notion has come under scrutiny, however, with recent evidence. Some researchers postulate that a universal ancestor gave rise to both groups of prokaryotes. It is conceivable that traces of that ancestor are waiting to be discovered somewhere in a primordial swamp.

Note to the Student

It is fairly common to read in biology books about the "higher" and "lower" forms of life, Typically, humans are cast as higher forms, while insects, worms, microorganisms, and similar creatures are considered "lower" forms.

Discerning biologists would probably disagree with this concept. They would point out that each species of organism is a product of evolution and, as such, each is exquisitely adapted to its environment and way of life. Indeed, it is probable that a cockroach is better equipped to survive the rigors of this world than a human being.

Now consider the bacteria. Bacterial species thrive in environments ranging from ice to boiling-hot springs. Many species can live with or without oxygen. A large percentage make their own foods from chemicals in the soil. Bacteria have no built-in death age, and they double in number every hour or so. We humans, by contrast, must maintain a constant body temperature; we suffocate without oxygen; we eat complex foods; we reach a certain age, then die; and it takes a full 25 years to produce a generation.

It is difficult to believe that microorganisms are "lower" than any other forms of living things. Certainly they are not "lower" than humans. Bacteria were here long before we humans came on the scene, and they will undoubtedly be here long after we "higher" forms have vanished.

Summary

Bacteria occur in variations of three shapes: the rod (bacillus), the sphere (coccus), and the spiral (vibrio, spirochete, or spirillum). Viewed with the microscope, rods and spirals generally appear singly, but cocci occur in a number of configurations, including the diplococcus, streptococcus, and staphylococcus.

The electron microscope reveals a number of bacterial structures that give insight into bacterial functions. Flagella, for example, occur on many rods and provide motion. Pili are short hairlike appendages that permit attachment to a surface. The glycocalyx is a sticky layer of polysaccharides that buffers a bacterium against the external environment. The cell wall provides rigidity and structure to the cell, while the cell membrane is a site of transfer into and out of the cell as well as an enzyme site. Various bodies exist in the cell cytoplasm, but there is no bacterial nucleus. A highly resistant structure called the spore is produced by members of the genera *Bacillus* and *Clostridium*.

The reproduction of bacteria takes place by binary fission, a process wherein chromosomal duplication and cytoplasmic separation are major events. Binary fissions occur at intervals called the generation time, which for bacteria may be as short as 20 minutes. Although the potential for incalculable masses of bacteria is great, the dynamics of the growth curve show how a population reaches a certain peak and then levels off and declines.

Bacterial species are able to grow over a vast array of conditions. Certain species, for example, grow at temperatures as low as 0°C, others at 90°C. Bacteria may grow with or without oxygen, depending on the species, and most grow over a range of pH. Different species have different nutritional patterns, such as autotrophy and heterotrophy, and laboratory media are devised to reflect these patterns. In nature, bacterial populations interact with other populations of living things in certain recognizable ways. These interrelationships fit the bacteria into the scheme of living things on Earth. The (archaebacteria) archaea live at extreme environments and are among the more interesting bacteria because they give us insights about the beginning of life.

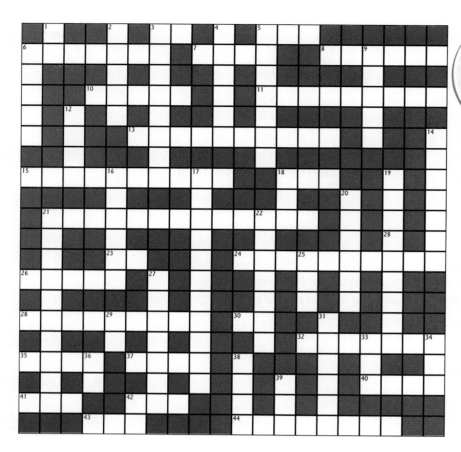

One of the major topics of this chapter has been a survey of microscopic bacterial structures seen through the light and electron microscopes. To test your recall of these structures, fill in the following crossword puzzle. The answers to the puzzle are in Appendix D.

■ **ACROSS**

3. Glycocalyx-producing bacterial species (initials)
5. The genetic material of a bacterium
6. A cluster of four or eight cocci
7. The ____ structure of a bacterium is visible with the electron microscope
8. Contains the enzyme lysozyme for bacterial destruction
10. The ____ mosaic model describes the structure of the cell membrane
11. The cell membrane is the structure of ____ into the cell cytoplasm
13. A bacterial capsule having a loose consistency

Questions for Thought and Discussion

1. Suppose a bacterium had the opportunity to form a capsule, a flagellum, a pilus, or a spore. Which do you think it might choose? Why?

2. The glycocalyx is a structure associated with many bacterial species. The term is relatively new to microbiology and is derived from the Greek words *glykos* for "sweet" and *kalyx,* referring to the cup of a flower. What do you think microbiologists had in mind when they conceived the word?

3. Consumers are advised to avoid stuffing a turkey the night before cooking, even though the turkey is refrigerated. A homemaker questions this advice and points out that the bacteria of human disease grow mainly at warm temperatures, not in the refrigerator. What explanation might you offer to counter this argument?

4. Extremophiles are of interest to industrial corporations, who see the bacteria as important sources of enzymes that function at temperatures of 100°C and pH levels of 10 (the enzymes have been dubbed "extremozymes"). What practical uses can you foresee for these enzymes?

5. In the fall of 1993, public health officials found that the water in a midwestern town was contaminated with sewage bacteria. The officials suggested that homeowners boil their water for a couple of minutes before drinking it. Would this treatment sterilize the water? Why?

6. An organism is described as a peritrichous, anaerobic, heterotrophic, mesophilic streptococcus. How might you translate this complex bacteriological language into a description of the organism?

15. Closed loop of DNA having the bacterial inheritance characteristics
18. Nucleic acid not found in plasmids
21. The important chemical constituent of the bacterial cell wall
23. Unit of measurement (abbr) for width of cell wall
24. Bacterial spiral with a flexible cell wall
26. A short hairlike projection for attachment and genetic transfers
28. Bodies of RNA and protein that function in protein synthesis
30. Bacterium (initials) that occurs as a sarcina
32. Closed loop of DNA apart from the chromosome in the cytoplasm
35. The slime of the capsule of *A. viscolactis* resembles _____
37. Teichoic acid is present in the cell walls of ___-positive bacteria
40. Flagella permit a bacterium to _____
41. A monotrichaete has only _____ flagellum
42. A component (abbr) of the principal layer of the bacterial cell wall
43. The cell membrane has _____ important organic constituents

44. The name for the chromosomal region of a bacterium

■ **DOWN**
1. Bacterium (initials) that appears as a grapelike cluster
2. A pair of bacterial cocci is a _____-coccus
3. A bacterial rod
4. A curved rod that resembles a comma under the microscope
5. A polysaccharide existing as tangled fibers in the glycocalyx
6. Another name for the glycocalyx is the _____ layer
9. About 40 percent of the cell membrane consists of _____
12. The side chains of peptidoglycan consist of _____ amino acids
14. The presence of a capsule contributes to the ability to cause _____
16. A capsule-containing cause of tooth decay is *Streptococcus* _____
17. A cytoplasmic body that helps a bacterium orient itself
18. Nucleic acid not found in plasmids
19. Many times the length of a bacterium but extremely thin; used for motility

20. A bacterial sphere
21. Antibiotic that interrupts construction of bacterial cell wall
22. Serves as a buffer between bacterium and external environment
25. Form displayed by typhoid, anthrax, and diphtheria bacilli
27. Alternative name for pilus
29. Bacterium (initials) well-known for its capsule
31. Layer of bacteria and other materials on tooth surface
33. Microscope (abbr) used to visualize ultrasmall bacterial structures
34. Used to stain metachromatic granules in cytoplasm
36. Unlike ___-karyotic cells, bacteria have no nuclei
38. Common site of infection by staphylococci
39. Type of cell (abbr) that does not engulf bacteria if capsule present
36. Pili have _____ function in mobility despite their location and appearance.

7. Researchers have estimated that, in broad terms, about one-third of human feces are composed of bacteria. That being the case, about how much bacteria do we "produce" in a week? In a year? How can this be possible?

8. This chapter points out that some bacteria can travel a distance of up to 2000 times their own length in an hour. There is another interesting creature that can travel the same distance in the same time. Can you guess its name?

9. Suppose this chapter on the structure and growth of bacteria had been written in 1940, before the electron microscope became available. Which parts of the chapter would probably be missing?

10. Bacterium X has been identified as a cause of human disease. Knowing that it is a pathogen, can you guess what structures it might have? Explain your reasons for each choice.

11. Many people believe that bacteria do little more than cause human illness and infectious disease. How does the information in this chapter help you correct that misconception?

12. During the filming of the movie *Titanic*, researchers discovered at least 20 different species of bacteria literally consuming the ship, especially a rather large piece of the midsection. What type of bacteria would you expect were at work on the ship?

13. Although thermophilic bacteria are presumably harmless because they do not grow at body temperatures, they may still present a hazard to good health. Can you think of a situation in which this might occur?

14. To prevent decay by bacteria and to display the mummified remains of ancient peoples, museum officials place the mummies in glass cases where oxygen has been replaced with nitrogen gas. Why do you think nitrogen is used? Will any bacteria-related decay occur in this environment?

15. Every state has an official animal, flower, or tree, but only Oregon has a bacterium named in its honor: *Methanohalophilus oregonese*. The species modifier *oregonese* is obvious, but can you decipher the meaning of the genus name?

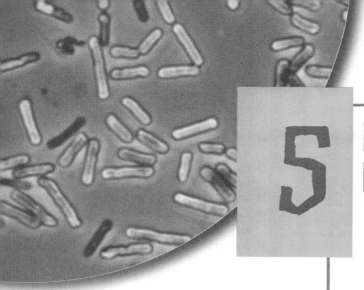

5 Bacterial Metabolism

Life is like a fire; it begins in smoke and ends in ashes.

—Ancient Arab proverb connecting energy to life

CHARLIE SWAART HAD BEEN a social drinker for years, but in 1945 he began a nightmare that would make medical history. One October day, while stationed in Tokyo after World War II, Swaart suddenly became drunk for no apparent reason. For years thereafter, the episodes continued—bouts of drunkenness and monumental hangovers without drinking so much as a beer. Doctors warned him not to drink for fear of damaging his liver. Swaart followed their advice to the letter; still, he got drunk.

Twenty years passed before Swaart learned of a similar case in Japan. A Japanese businessman had endured years of social and professional disgrace before doctors found a yeastlike fungus fermenting carbohydrates to alcohol right there in his intestine. An antibiotic had worked to kill the yeast (known as *Candida albicans*). With this knowledge in hand, Swaart approached his doctor. Sure enough, lab tests showed massive colonies of *Candida albicans* in Swaart's intestine. Having *Candida* in one's intestine is not uncommon; but finding a fermenting *Candida* was historic. The sugar in a cup of coffee or any carbohydrate in pasta, cake, or candy could bring on drunkenness.

Swaart's doctor prescribed an antibiotic, but the initial result was disappointing. After several tries, however, an effective antibiotic was found. Researchers believe that the atomic blasts of Hiroshima and Nagasaki may have caused a normal *Candida* to

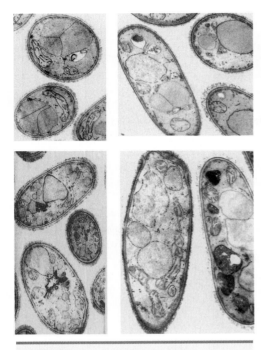

FIGURE 5.1

Candida albicans

Transmission electron micrographs of the yeast–like fungus *Candida albicans*. Mutant strains of this organism may ferment carbohydrates to ethyl alcohol. Note the typically oval structure of the yeasts.

TABLE 5.1

A Comparison of Two Key Aspects of Cellular Metabolism

CATABOLISM	ANABOLISM
Breakdown of large molecules	Buildup of small molecules
Energy is generally released	Energy is generally required
Products are small molecules	Products are large molecules
Glycolysis, Krebs cycle, electron transport, chemiosmosis	Photosynthesis, protein synthesis
Mediated by enzymes	Mediated by enzymes
Reactions converge to major pathways	Reactions diverge from basic pathways

mutate to a fermenting *Candida* (FIGURE 5.1). Perhaps there are thousands of other individuals whose intestines are indwelling fermentation vats. For Charlie Swaart, though, the nightmare was over.

The process of fermentation is but one aspect of the broad topic of microbial metabolism. **Metabolism** refers to the sum total of all biochemical processes taking place in living cells. Metabolic processes may be divided into two general categories: **anabolism,** or the synthesis of chemical compounds; and **catabolism,** or the digestion of chemical compounds. (TABLE 5.1 compares anabolism and catabolism.)

Metabolism:
the sum total of all biochemical processes taking place in living cells.

5.1

Enzymes and Energy in Metabolism

In order for metabolic processes to take place, living cells such as bacteria must have an adequate supply of enzymes. We shall therefore begin our study of metabolism with a detailed discussion of these substances, which have been known only since the early 1900s (MicroFocus 5.1). In addition, this section will contain some general concepts relating to energy, because the chemical reactions of anabolism generally utilize energy, while those in catabolism often liberate energy. Since the discussions will deal with proteins, carbohydrates, and lipids, you may wish to review Chapter 2 as a refresher.

MicroFocus 5.1

"HANS, DU WIRST DAS NICHT GLAUBEN!"

Louis Pasteur's discovery of the role of yeast cells in fermentation heralded the beginnings of microbiology because it showed that tiny organisms could bring about important chemical changes. However, it also opened debate on how yeasts accomplish fermentation. Soon, a lively controversy evolved among scientists. Some thought that sugars from grape juice enter yeast cells to be fermented; others believed that fermentation occurs outside the cells. The question would not be resolved until a fortunate accident happened in the late 1890s.

In 1897, two German chemists, Eduard and Hans Buchner, were preparing yeast as a nutritional supplement for medicinal purposes. They ground yeast cells with sand and collected the cell-free juice. To preserve the juice, they added a large quantity of sugar (as was commonly done at that time) and set the mixture aside. Several days later Eduard noticed an unusual alcoholic aroma coming from the mixture. Excitedly, he called to his brother. One taste confirmed their suspicion: The sugar had fermented to alcohol.

The discovery of the Buchner brothers was momentous because it demonstrated that a chemical substance inside yeast cells brings about fermentation, and that fermentation can occur without living cells. The chemical substance came to be known as an "enzyme," meaning "in yeast." In 1905, the English chemist Arthur Haden expanded the Buchner study by showing that "enzyme" is really a multitude of chemical compounds and should better be termed "enzymes." Thus, he added to the belief that fermentation is a chemical process. Soon, many chemists became biochemists, and biochemistry gradually emerged as a new scientific discipline.

ENZYMES

Enzyme:
an organic molecule (usually protein) that brings about a chemical change while *itself* remaining unchanged.

Enzymes are a group of organic molecules (usually proteins) that bring about chemical changes while themselves remaining unchanged. They catalyze, or speed up, chemical processes by accomplishing in seconds what otherwise might take hours, days, or longer to happen spontaneously. This is especially true during the bonding of large organic molecules, where the concentration of the molecules is generally low and the reaction areas are often hidden. Random collisions between large molecules are unlikely to occur, and bonding may not otherwise take place. Thus, the reaction rate would be very low were it not for the activity of enzymes.

Enzymes are reusable. Once a chemical reaction has occurred, the enzyme is released to participate in another reaction, as illustrated in FIGURE 5.2. The number of enzymes in a bacterium is therefore quite small compared to the hundreds of thousands of chemical reactions taking place. Enzyme activity is also highly specific; an enzyme that functions in one chemical reaction usually will not participate in another type. The substance acted upon is called the **substrate,** and the products are appropriately termed **end-products.** Since the reactions are usually reversible, enzymes may bring about syntheses as well as digestions. This factor is important in metabolism because anabolism often occurs by a reversal of many steps in catabolism.

Substrate:
the substance acted upon by an enzyme molecule.

Basically, enzymes function by aligning molecules in such a way that a reaction can take place. In a synthesis reaction, for example, the jagged surface of an enzyme molecule holds the substrates so their electron clouds overlap in the spot where the chemical bond should form. In a digestion reaction, by contrast, the enzyme binds to the substrate and pushes it slightly out of shape so that the bond breaks.

In order for synthesis or digestion to take place, certain critical areas called **active sites** must be present and available on the enzyme molecule. Active sites often contain sulfhydryl groups ($-SH$), so any substance reacting with sulfhydryl groups will tie up the groups and prevent enzyme activity. A heavy metal such as silver acts in this fashion, and, consequently, it is useful as a disinfectant in such forms as silver nitrate. Another way of inactivating an enzyme is by blocking its active site with a

sul-fi′dril
Heavy metal:
an element whose atoms have a large atomic weight and are electron donors.

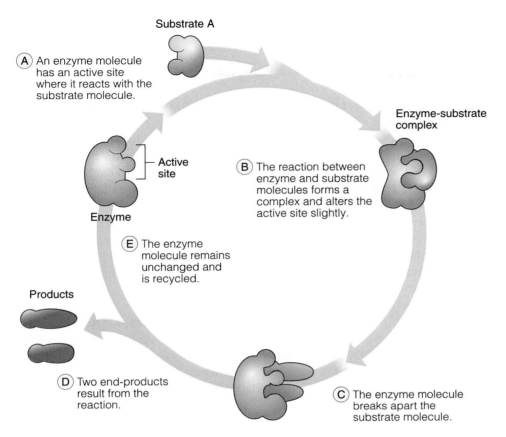

Substrate A

(A) An enzyme molecule has an active site where it reacts with the substrate molecule.

Active site

Enzyme

Enzyme-substrate complex

(B) The reaction between enzyme and substrate molecules forms a complex and alters the active site slightly.

(E) The enzyme molecule remains unchanged and is recycled.

Products

(D) Two end-products result from the reaction.

(C) The enzyme molecule breaks apart the substrate molecule.

FIGURE 5.2

The Mechanism of Enzyme Action

compound closely related to the normal substrate. **Sulfonamide drugs** operate in this way (Chapter 23).

Enzymes were originally named for the chemical reactions they catalyze. For instance, pepsin (from the Greek *pepsis,* for "digestion") refers to the protein-digesting enzyme of the human gastrointestinal tract. Modern biochemists have adopted the *-ase* ending for enzymes, and many enzymes are currently named for the substrate on which they act. Lactase, for example, is the enzyme that digests lactose, sucrase breaks down sucrose, and ribonuclease digests ribonucleic acid. Some groups of enzymes carry names corresponding to their activity. For example, the **hydrolases** operate in hydrolysis reactions in which hydroxyl and hydrogen ions (the products of water) are added to the end-products. Hydrolases include lipase, which breaks down lipids, and peptidase, which digests peptides to amino acids.

Since most enzymes are protein molecules, they are sensitive to any physical or chemical agents that injure proteins. Heat can be used to kill bacteria because heat alters the tertiary structure of enzyme proteins. Certain chemicals, such as alcohol and phenol, precipitate enzyme proteins and therefore act as disinfectants. And any antibiotic that interferes with protein synthesis automatically interferes with enzyme production.

Some enzymes are made up entirely of protein. An example is **lysozyme,** the enzyme in human tears and saliva that digests the cell walls of Gram-positive bacteria. Lysozyme is composed of 129 amino acids. Other enzymes contain a nonprotein part such as an ion of magnesium, iron, or zinc. Ions such as these are called **cofactors.** When the nonprotein part is an organic molecule, biochemists refer to it as a **coenzyme.** Examples of coenzymes are nicotinamide adenine dinucleotide (NAD)

sul-fon'ah-mid
Sulfonamides:
a group of antimicrobial drugs that contain sulfur and amino groups.

Hydrolysis:
a chemical reaction in which a major reactant is split into two products, with the addition of H to one product and OH to the other.

li'so-zī m

nik'o-tin'ah-mid
di-new'kle-o-tide

Coenzyme:
an organic molecule that is the nonprotein part of an enzyme.

and flavin adenine dinucleotide (FAD). These coenzymes play a significant role as electron carriers in metabolism, and we shall encounter them in our ensuing study.

ENERGY AND ATP

In bacteria and other living cells, molecules are constantly moving about, a factor that often leads to chemical reactions. Certain chemical reactions yield energy, but in many cases, energy (i.e., "activation energy") must be supplied for reactions to take place. This is because covalent bonds are forced apart into new combinations. Once a reaction has begun, however, it often gives off enough energy to keep itself going. It may even liberate excess energy in the form of heat or light, or the energy may cause another chemical reaction to occur.

Covalent bond:
the force resulting from the sharing of electrons among the atoms in a molecule.

Enzymes play a key role in metabolism because they lower the amount of activation energy required for a reaction to take place. They assist in the destruction of chemical bonds and the creation of new ones by separating or joining atoms in a carefully orchestrated fashion. The reaction could probably occur without enzymes, but much more slowly and far less efficiently.

ATP:
adenosine triphosphate, a high-energy molecule that serves as an immediate energy source for cells.

In the biochemical reactions of metabolism, enzymes often require the chemical energy available in a compound called **adenosine triphosphate,** or simply **ATP** (FIGURE 5.3 illustrates this molecule). A molecule of ATP, which is similar to a nucleotide, acts like a portable battery. It moves to any part of the cell where an energy-consuming reaction is taking place and provides energy. In a bacterium, ATP supplies energy for binary fission, flagellar motion, and spore formation. On a more

FIGURE 5.3

Adenosine Triphosphate

Adenosine triphosphate (ATP) is a key immediate energy source for bacteria and other living things. (a) The ATP molecule is composed of adenine and ribose bonded to one another and to three phosphate groups, as shown. (b) When the molecule breaks down (right), it releases a phosphate group and 7300 calories of energy per mole; it becomes adenosine diphosphate (ADP). For the synthesis of ATP (left), energy and a phosphate group must be supplied to an ADP molecule.

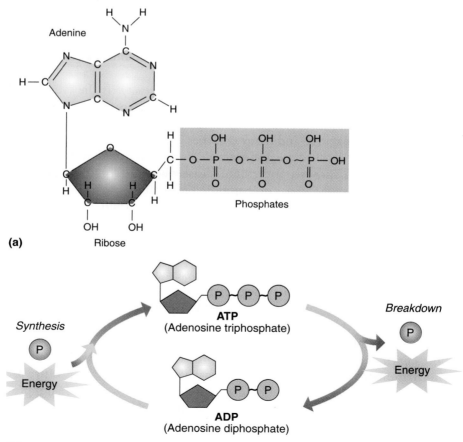

chemical level, it fuels protein synthesis and carbohydrate breakdown. Scientists believe that a major share of bacterial functions depend on a supply of ATP. When the supply is exhausted, the cell usually dies.

The energy in ATP molecules is released by breaking the high-energy bond holding the last phosphate group onto the molecule, thereby producing adenosine diphosphate (ADP) and a phosphate group. An enzyme called **adenosine triphosphatase (ATPase)** catalyzes this reaction. The energy formerly locked up in the bond is now set free to do work. A single mole of ATP releases 7300 calories of energy when its bonds are broken. (A mole of ATP weighs 507 grams.)

Although ATP molecules are used everywhere in a bacterium to meet energy needs, they are not suitable for storing energy. The molecules are unstable, and any significant surplus takes up too much space in a cell. Therefore, cells synthesize or obtain small molecules such as glucose or lipids for energy storage. Later, the energy in these molecules can be released in catabolism and used to reform ATP from adenosine diphosphate (ADP) and phosphate. The new ATP is then used to drive the reactions of metabolism and any other activities of the bacterium. This principle is the basis for much of the chemistry in the discussion to follow.

Mole:
the quantity of a substance whose weight in grams is numerically equivalent to its molecular weight.

To this point . . .

We have introduced the concept of metabolism as the sum total of all the biochemical processes taking place in bacteria and other living cells. Metabolism is subdivided into two major categories: anabolism, the synthesis of organic compounds, and catabolism, the breakdown of these compounds. For anabolism and catabolism to take place, enzymes must be available. We therefore explored these vital molecules in depth, with emphasis on their activity, specificity, inhibition, and chemical makeup.

We also discussed the importance of energy as a governing factor in metabolism. Energy is required to assist the construction and destruction of chemical bonds. For the reactions of metabolism to take place, the most important energy source is adenosine triphosphate (ATP). This compound is not stored in the cell; as it is used up, it must be resynthesized, using the energy present in molecules such as glucose and lipid. In the next section, we shall follow the chemical events in which glucose energy is released and converted to ATP energy. As we proceed through this involved biochemistry, try to keep in mind that the ultimate goal of the process is to form ATP molecules.

5.2

The Catabolism of Glucose

One of the most thoroughly studied and best-understood aspects of metabolism is the catabolism of **glucose.** Since the early part of the twentieth century, the chemistry of glucose catabolism has been the subject of intense investigation by biochemists because glucose is a key source of energy for ATP production. Moreover, the process of glucose catabolism is essentially similar in myriad living things—bacterium, plant, animal, or human being. This "metabolic interlock" is one feature that unites bacteria in a population. We shall therefore give close scrutiny to the process.

A mole of glucose (180 g) contains about 686,000 cal of energy. This fact can be demonstrated in the laboratory by setting fire to a mole of glucose and measuring the energy released. In a bacterium, however, not all the energy is set free from glucose,

Glucose:
a 6-carbon carbohydrate important in energy metabolism.

Calorie:
a unit of energy defined as the amount of heat required to raise one kilogram of water 1°C.

nor can the bacterium trap all that is released. Instead, a bacterium traps 277,400 cal of the energy in 38 moles of ATP formed during glucose catabolism (38 moles of ATP × 7300 cal per mole = 277,400 cal). In the discussions that follow, we shall see how these 38 moles of ATP emerge. The process accounts for the transfer of about 40 percent of the glucose energy to ATP energy. To simplify matters, we shall use the word *molecule* instead of *mole* and follow the fate of a "glucose molecule."

The catabolism of a glucose molecule does not take place in one chemical reaction, nor do 38 molecules of ATP form all at once. Instead, the process involves one or more metabolic pathways. A **metabolic pathway** is a sequence of chemical reactions, usually catalyzed by enzymes, in which the product of one reaction serves as a substrate for the next reaction. Should a reaction in the sequence require energy, then a coupled reaction often takes place to supply the energy. Also, if a reaction happens to yield excess energy, then a coupled reaction may take place to trap and preserve the energy. Thus, a metabolic pathway involves a sequence of reactions, many of which are associated with coupled reactions.

Respiration is a series of biochemical reactions in which energy is liberated. Therefore glucose catabolism is a form of respiration. In this text we shall use the terms *respiration* and *catabolism* interchangeably. Respiration may occur in the presence of oxygen, in which case it is **aerobic respiration**. In other instances, it may take place in the absence of oxygen, in which case it is called **anaerobic respiration** or, in a special form, **fermentation**. Glucose catabolism is known to take place by both methods.

To begin our study of glucose catabolism, we shall follow the process of aerobic respiration as it occurs in bacteria. There are numerous metabolic pathways for aerobic respiration, but the one we shall discuss is represented by the following chemical formula:

$$C_6H_{12}O_6 + 6\,O_2 + 38\,ADP + 38\,P \rightarrow 6\,CO_2 + 6\,H_2O + 38\,ATP$$

Glucose   Oxygen   Carbon dioxide   Water

This straightforward equation summarizes a complex series of metabolic reactions conveniently divided into three processes: glycolysis, the Krebs cycle, and oxidative phosphorylation. We shall examine each in turn.

THE GLYCOLYSIS

The chemical breakdown of glucose is called **glycolysis**, from *glyco-*, referring to glucose, and *lysis*, meaning "to break." Several metabolic pathways for this breakdown exist. The best known pathway, and the one we shall follow, is called the **Embden–Meyerhof pathway**, after **Gustav Embden** and **Otto Meyerhof**, two German biochemists who described many of its details in the 1930s. The process occurs in the cytoplasm of bacteria and involves the conversion of glucose to a 3-carbon organic acid called pyruvic acid (also called pyruvate because the sodium salt forms in living cytoplasm). Between glucose and pyruvic acid there are nine chemical reactions. Each reaction, or step in the process, is catalyzed by a specific enzyme. Even though glycolysis is part of the overall scheme of aerobic respiration, it takes place in the absence of oxygen. FIGURE 5.4 illustrates the process. For easy referral, parenthetical numbers in the figure identify each reaction, and it would be helpful to refer to the figure as the discussion proceeds.

In glycolysis, one 6-carbon glucose molecule is eventually converted into two 3-carbon **pyruvic acid** molecules. For the conversion to take place, two molecules of ATP must be supplied. Note in Figure 5.4 that one molecule of ATP is used up in

Metabolic pathway:
a sequence of chemical reactions in which the product of one reaction serves as the substrate for the next reaction.

Respiration:
a series of biochemical reactions in which energy is liberated.

Fermentation:
an anaerobic form of metabolism in which an intermediary in the process acts as an electron acceptor.

fos'for-ĭ-la'shum

gli-kol'ĭ-sis

Pyruvic acid:
a 3-carbon molecule that results from the breakdown of glucose in glycolysis.

pi'roo-vic

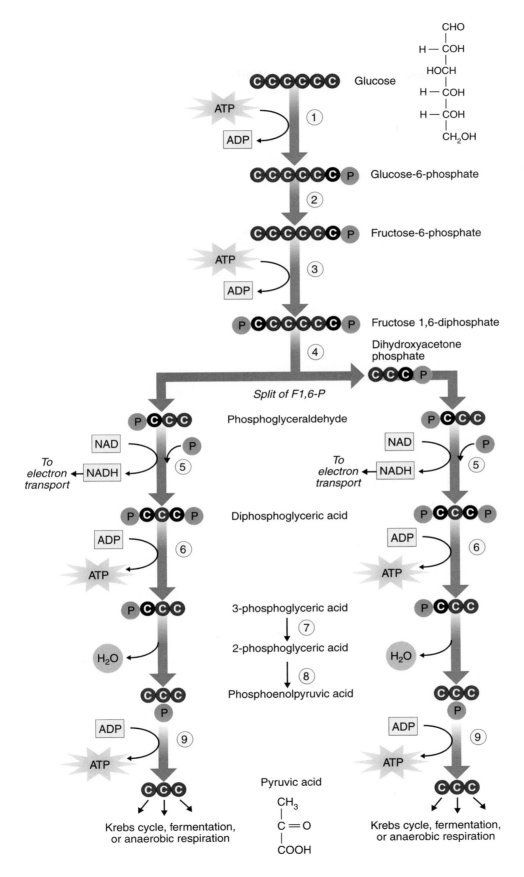

FIGURE 5.4

Glycolysis by the Embden–Meyerhof Pathway

Carbon atoms are represented by circles. The dark circles represent carbon atoms bonded to phosphate groups. ATP is supplied to glucose in reaction (1) and to fructose-6-phosphate in reaction (3). The splitting of F–1–6–diphosphate in reaction (4) yields PGAL and DHAP. DHAP then converts to another PGAL molecule. Both PGAL molecules proceed through reactions (5) to (9) and yield two molecules of pyruvic acid. Two ATP molecules are generated in reaction (6) and two more in reaction (9). The total ATP produced is four molecules and, since two are used up in glycolysis, the net gain is two molecules of ATP. Also, in reaction (5), high–energy electrons and protons are captured by an NAD molecule. Note that the original six carbon atoms of glucose exist in two pyruvic acid molecules.

reaction (1) at the beginning of glycolysis and that a second ATP molecule is needed for reaction (3). In both cases, the phosphate group from ATP attaches to the substrate molecule. Thus, reaction (1) gives us glucose-6-phosphate, and reaction (3) yields fructose 1-6-diphosphate (*di* means "two"; two phosphate molecules).

An important split occurs in reaction (4). The fructose 1-6-diphosphate molecule breaks apart to yield two molecules, each with three carbons. One is dihydroxyacetone phosphate (DHAP); the other is **phosphoglyceraldehyde (PGAL)**. Note that an enzyme converts the DHAP molecule to another PGAL molecule. This is important because we now have two molecules of PGAL.

In the next series of reactions, each PGAL molecule passes through a series of conversions and ultimately forms pyruvic acid (Figure 5.4). These conversions occur in reactions (5) through (9). A significant event takes place in reaction (6). As the enzyme conversion proceeds, enough energy is released to synthesize an ATP molecule from ADP and phosphate in a coupled reaction. This chemistry happens again in reaction (9). Thus, each time a PGAL molecule is broken down to pyruvic acid through the sequence, two ATP molecules are formed. But two PGAL molecules are available. Therefore as the second PGAL molecule breaks down, two more ATP molecules result. The total is four molecules of ATP. Considering that we "invested" two ATP molecules in reactions (1) and (3) and received back four molecules, the net gain from glycolysis is two molecules of ATP.

Before we proceed, take note of reaction (5). In this reaction, two high-energy electrons and two protons are released and shuttled to NAD. This event will have great significance shortly. Also of interest is the fact that, as a result of glycolysis, the cell has gained two ATP molecules for use in its metabolism even though no oxygen has been utilized. This has importance in fermentation reactions to be outlined later. For the moment, we shall follow the fate of pyruvic acid.

THE KREBS CYCLE

The **Krebs cycle** is a series of chemical reactions named for **Hans A. Krebs**, who won the 1953 Nobel Prize for the discovery of several participating substances. It is referred to as a cycle because the substance formed at the end of the sequence is identical to the substance at the beginning. All the reactions are catalyzed by enzymes, and all take place along the cell membranes of bacteria. In eukaryotic organisms such as protozoa and fungi, the reactions occur in the mitochondria.

The Krebs cycle is somewhat like a wheel constantly turning. Each time the wheel comes back to the starting point, something must be added to spin it for another rotation. That something is a pyruvic acid molecule derived from glycolysis. FIGURE 5.5 shows the Krebs cycle. Capital letters in parentheses are used to identify the reactions and guide us through the cycle.

Before a pyruvic acid molecule enters the Krebs cycle it undergoes a change, indicated in reaction (A). An enzyme removes a carbon atom from the pyruvic acid molecule and releases the carbon as carbon dioxide (CO_2). The remaining two carbon atoms are then combined with a substance called coenzyme A to form acetyl-coenzyme A, or simply **acetyl-CoA**. The discovery of coenzyme A by **Fritz A. Lipmann** provided a key to the understanding of the Krebs cycle. For his work, Lipmann shared the 1953 Nobel Prize in Physiology or Medicine with Krebs. Coenzyme A contains the vitamin pantothenic acid.

The two remaining carbons from pyruvic acid are now ready to enter the Krebs cycle. In reaction (B), acetyl-CoA unites with the 4-carbon substance oxaloacetic acid to form **citric acid**, a 6-carbon organic acid. (Citric acid may be familiar to you as a component of soft drinks.) The citric acid molecule changes in reaction (C) to

fos′fo-glis′er-al′dĕ-hīd

Proton:
the positively charged nucleus of a hydrogen atom.

ox-ah′lo-acetic

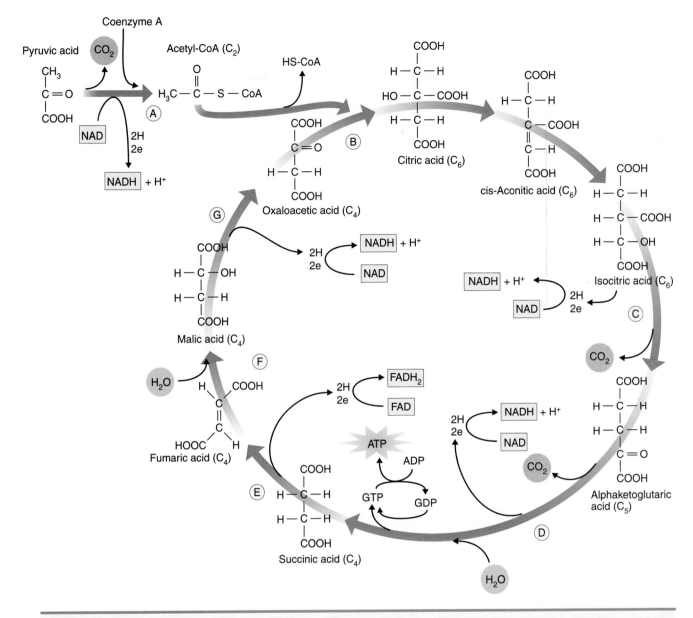

FIGURE 5.5

The Krebs Cycle

Pyruvic acid from glycolysis combines with coenzyme A to form acetyl–CoA in reaction (A). This molecule then condenses with oxaloacetic acid to form citric acid (B). In reactions (C) through (F), citric acid is converted to alphaketoglutaric acid and then to succinic, fumaric, and malic acids in succession. Malic acid regenerates oxaloacetic acid in the last reaction, (G). During the process, the three carbons of pyruvic acid are liberated as three molecules of carbon dioxide. ATP is formed in reaction (D) via GTP, and high-energy electrons and protons are liberated during certain of the reactions. These are captured by NAD or FAD molecules, and the electrons are utilized for oxidative phosphorylation.

a substance called **alphaketoglutaric acid.** Note in Figure 5.5 that alphaketoglutaric acid has only five carbon atoms. The sixth atom has been lost as CO_2. In the next step, reaction (D), alphaketoglutaric acid is converted by an enzyme to **succinic acid,** which has four carbon atoms. The fifth carbon atom is lost as CO_2. Succinic acid then is converted to **fumaric acid,** which then converts to **malic acid,** and malic acid converts to **oxaloacetic acid** (reactions E, F, and G). The cycle is now complete, and oxaloacetic acid is ready to unite with another molecule of acetyl-CoA.

al′fah-ke′to-gloo-tar′ik

suk-sĭ′nik

Several features of the Krebs cycle merit closer scrutiny. First we shall follow the carbon. Pyruvic acid, with three carbon atoms, emerged from glycolysis, but after one turn of the cycle, its carbon atoms exist in three molecules of CO_2. There were two molecules of pyruvic acid from glycolysis, so when the second molecule enters the Krebs cycle, its carbon atoms will also form three CO_2 molecules. Remember that we began with a 6-carbon glucose molecule; six CO_2 molecules have now been produced. This fulfills part of the equation for aerobic respiration:

$$C_6H_{12}O_6 + 6\,O_2 + 38\,ADP + 38\,P \rightarrow 6\,CO_2 + 6\,H_2O + 38\,ATP$$

The second feature of the Krebs cycle that draws our attention is reaction (D). Here a molecule of guanosine triphosphate (GTP) forms in the conversion to succinic acid because the reaction is an energy-yielding conversion. Its energy is immediately used to form an ATP molecule. Since we have two pyruvic acid molecules entering the cycle (per molecule of glucose), a second ATP molecule will form from GTP when the second pyruvic acid passes through the cycle. Combining the two ATPs with the net gain of two ATPs from glycolysis, the total gain rises to four ATPs. Impressive as this is, the major gain of ATP is still to come.

OXIDATIVE PHOSPHORYLATION

fos'for-ĭ-la'shun

Oxidative phosphorylation refers to a sequence of reactions in which two events happen: Pairs of electrons are passed from one chemical substance to another, and the energy released during the passage is used to combine phosphate with ADP to form ATP. The adjective **oxidative** is derived from the term *oxidation*, which refers to the loss of electron pairs from chemical molecules in the sequence. The noun **phosphorylation** implies the union of phosphate with ADP (to phosphorylate a molecule is to add phosphate to it). Like the Krebs cycle, oxidative phosphorylation takes place at the cell membrane in bacteria and in the mitochondria of eukaryotic cells.

Oxidation:
a chemical reaction in which electrons are lost from the reactant.

Oxidative phosphorylation is the process in which most of the ATP molecules form. Indeed, 34 of the 38 molecules produced during glucose catabolism are manufactured here. The overall sequence begins with glycolysis and the Krebs cycle. In these processes, high-energy electrons and protons are released during several reactions. During **oxidative phosphorylation**, the electrons pass along a series of chemical molecules, and the energy in the electrons is gradually lost. But the energy is not lost in the sense that it is gone forever. Instead, the energy is used to combine ADP molecules with phosphate molecules to yield ATP molecules. Each time a pair of electrons passes through the system, enough energy is released to generate up to three ATP molecules.

NAD:
an acronym for the coenzyme nicotinamide adenine dinucleotide.
FAD:
an acronym for the coenzyme flavin adenine dinucleotide.

Two important coenzymes that function in oxidative phosphorylation are NAD and FAD (NAD is also written as NAD^+ because it has positive charge). Another important group of molecules are the **cytochromes.** Cytochromes are a set of protein cellular pigments (*cyto-* for "cell"; *chrome* for "color") containing iron ions that accept and release electrons during the sequence. Cytochromes are designated by letters (cytochrome A, A_3, B, C). The last link in the chain is oxygen (MicroFocus 5.2). Because oxidative phosphorylation involves the passage of electrons, the process is often called **electron transport.**

When oxidative phosphorylation is in operation (as in Figure 5.5), two electrons and one proton are released and accepted by NAD during selected metabolic reactions. The NAD now becomes NADH. (A second proton is liberated to the cytoplasm.) The electron pair then passes to a flavoprotein (a protein attached to a flavin molecule) and then to an FAD molecule, which also takes on two protons to become FADH$_2$. This molecule passes the electron pair to the cytochrome chain and releases the protons to the cytoplasm. The release regenerates FAD, which can then accept more electrons. The cytochromes now pass the electron pair along to one another until the electron pair is finally accepted by an oxygen atom, as **FIGURE 5.6** illustrates. Now the **oxygen atom** acquires two protons (2 H$^+$) from the cytoplasm and becomes water (H$_2$O). Oxygen's role is of great significance because if oxygen were not present, there would be no way for cytochromes to unload their electrons, and the entire system would soon come to a halt. This role is also reflected in the equation for aerobic respiration:

$$C_6H_{12}O_6 + \mathbf{6\,O_2} + 38\,ADP + 38\,P \rightarrow 6\,CO_2 + \mathbf{6\,H_2O} + 38\,ATP$$

We have noted that for every transport of an electron pair along the sequence, up to three ATP molecules are formed. The actual mechanism for ATP formation is called **chemiosmosis** because it involves both chemical and transport (*osmosis*) processes (Figure 5.6). First proposed by Nobel Prize winner **Peter Mitchell**,

kem'e-os-mo'sis

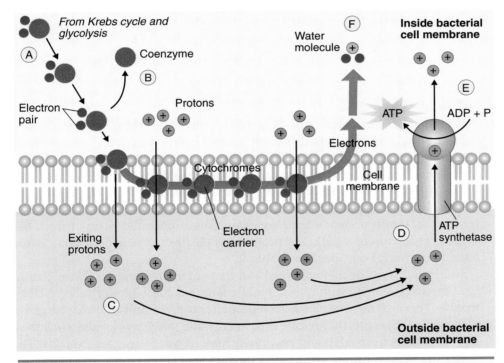

FIGURE 5.6

Chemiosmosis in Bacteria

(a) Originating in glycolysis or the Krebs cycle, a coenzyme (e.g., NADH or FADH$_2$) transports electron pairs to cytochromes in the cell membrane. (b) The NAD or FAD coenzyme is regenerated for reuse. (c) As cytochromes transport the electron pairs among themselves, they release energy, which fuels the transport of protons across the cell membrane at three points. (d) Each set of protons then reenters the cytoplasm of the cell through a protein channel lined with ATP synthetase. (e) An ADP molecule is joined with a phosphate each time a set of protons moves through the channel, thereby accounting for three ATP molecules produced for each electron pair. (f) The electrons combine with other protons to form water molecules.

MicroFocus 5.2

"IT'S NOT TOXIC TO US!"

It's hard to think of oxygen as a poisonous gas, but billions of years ago, oxygen was as toxic as cyanide. One whiff by an organism, and a cascade of highly destructive oxidation reactions was set into motion. Death followed quickly.

Difficult to believe? Not if you realize that ancient organisms relied on fermentation and anaerobic chemistry for their energy needs. They took organic materials from the environment and digested them to release the available energy. The atmosphere was full of methane, hydrogen, ammonia, carbon dioxide, and other gases. But no oxygen. And it was that way for hundreds of millions of years.

Then came the cyanobacteria and their ability to perform photosynthesis. Chlorophyll and chlorophyll-like pigments evolved, and organisms could now trap radiant energy from the sun and convert it to chemical energy in carbohydrate. But there was a down side: Oxygen was a waste product of the process—and it was deadly.

Except to those organisms that could adapt. As millions of species died off in the toxic oceans and atmosphere, a few species survived because they had the enzymes to safely tuck away oxygen atoms in a nontoxic form. And then, surprise, some species even evolved the ability to recycle the oxygen for a beneficial purpose (Mother Nature really had

to work overtime on this one). They used oxygen as a final electron acceptor in an electron transport system to tap foods for large amounts of energy. And so the Krebs cycle and oxidative phosphorylation came into existence.

Also coming into existence were millions of new species, some merely surviving, others thriving in the oxygen-rich environment. The face of planet Earth was changing as anaerobic and fermenting species declined and aerobic species proliferated. A couple of billion years would pass before one particularly well-known species of oxygen-breathing creature evolved: *Homo sapiens*.

Chemiosmosis:
a biochemical process in which energy from electrons powers the movement of protons across the bacterial membrane, a process that leads to ATP formation.

chemiosmosis uses the power of proton motion across a membrane to conserve energy for ATP synthesis.

What happens in chemiosmosis is this: As electrons move between the coenzymes and cytochromes, significant amounts of energy are released at three transition points (shown in Figure 5.6). The energy powers the pumping of protons from the bacterial cytoplasm across the cell membrane to the area outside of the membrane (the energy is the so-called "proton motive force"). Soon a large number of protons have built up outside the membrane, and because they cannot easily reenter the cell, they represent a large concentration of potential energy (much like a boulder at the top of a hill). The protons are positively charged, so there is also a buildup of charges outside the membrane.

Suddenly a series of channels open and the proton flow reverses. Each "channel" is a protein pore lined with molecules of a large enzyme complex called ATP synthetase. This enzyme complex has binding sites for ATP and ADP. As the protons rush through the pore, they release their energy, and the energy is used to synthesize ATP molecules from ADP and phosphate ions, as MicroFocus 5.3 explains. Three molecules of ATP can be synthesized for each pair of electrons originating from NADH and two molecules, for each pair from $FADH_2$.

Chemiosmosis occurs only in structurally intact membranes. Indeed, if the membrane is damaged so proton movement cannot take place, the synthesis of ATP ceases even though electron transport through the cytochrome system continues. With the end of ATP production, the organism rapidly dies. This is one reason why damage to the bacterial membrane, such as with antibiotics or detergent disinfectants, is so harmful to a bacterium.

Disinfectant:
a chemical substance used to control microorganisms on a lifeless object.

At this point we shall see how the electron pairs are supplied for oxidative phosphorylation and chemiosmosis. Referring to the figures for glycolysis (Figure 5.4) and the Krebs cycle (Figure 5.5) will be helpful.

Note in the Krebs cycle that reactions (B) and (C) yield electron pairs and protons to NAD and that reactions (D) and (G) do likewise. In each case, oxidative phosphorylation takes place. At a rate of three ATPs per reaction, the four reactions (B, C, D, and G) give us a total of 12 ATPs. In reaction (E), the electron pair and protons are passed to FAD directly. In this situation, only two ATPs result by oxidative phosphorylation. This brings the total to 14 ATPs per turn of the Krebs cycle.

But there are two turns of the cycle because two molecules of pyruvic acid come from glucose in glycolysis. Therefore we gain another 14 ATPs as the second turn of the cycle takes place. We thus arrive at a total of 28 ATPs from the Krebs cycle.

Our attention now turns to glycolysis (Figure 5.4). Reaction (5) of this process was highlighted previously. The reaction yields an electron pair and a proton that proceed to NAD. Oxidative phosphorylation takes place, and the result is three more ATPs. But reaction (5) takes place two times because two PGAL molecules are formed. Therefore with the second reaction, another oxidative phosphorylation occurs and three more ATPs form. This gives us a total of six from the reactions originating in glycolysis.

MicroFocus 5.3

"CELL MACHINERY"

Every day, an adult human weighing 160 pounds uses up about 80 pounds of ATP (about half his or her weight). The ATP is changed to its two breakdown products, ADP and phosphate, and huge amounts of energy are released.

But the body's weight does not go down, nor does it change perceptibly because the cells are constantly regenerating stores of ATP from the breakdown products. Discovering how this is accomplished and how the recycling works were the seminal achievements of 1997's Nobel Prize winners in Chemistry.

One of the three winners was Paul D. Boyer at the University of California at Los Angeles. Boyer's work expanded the pioneering work of Peter Mitchell, who developed the concept of chemiosmosis. Central to this concept is the enzyme ATP synthetase. Operating in the membranes of all cells, ATP synthetase uses the energy liberated by rapidly streaming hydrogen ions (the proton motive force) to put together ADP and phosphate and form ATP molecules.

But how? Researchers knew that ATP synthetase has a wheel-like protein lodged in the membrane. Extending from one end of the protein "wheel" is a protein rod. And the enzyme has a protein cylinder that wraps around the rod and extends out from the membrane. (Research evidence shows that ATP molecules are synthesized at the cylinder surface.) Boyer took the pieces and made a chemical machine (as shown in the figure). His exhaustive and meticulous research indicated that hydrogen ions cause the wheel to spin as they stream by (somewhat reminiscent of a turning waterwheel). The rod spins with the wheel, but the cylinder remains stationary and exposes its ADP and phosphate at three sites. The spinning rod alters the cylinder protein slightly, and the alteration brings the ADP and phosphate together to form an ATP molecule. Since there are three reaction sites, three ATP molecules are produced each time the rod makes a complete revolution.

Is the mechanism complete? Not quite yet. Researchers want to know, for example, how do the hydrogen ions spin the wheel? Nevertheless, the Nobel committee was sufficiently impressed with Boyer's set of molecular gears, and it concluded that "cell machinery" is just that.

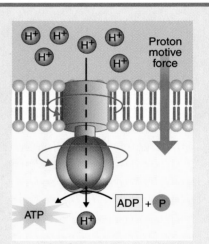

■ ATP synthetase, the "cell machine" of ATP synthesis. The rod of ATP synthetase spins as hydrogen ions pass through, but the cylinder remains stationary and exposes its ADP and phosphate molecules. The spinning rod alters the cylinder and brings ADP and phosphate together to form an ATP molecule.

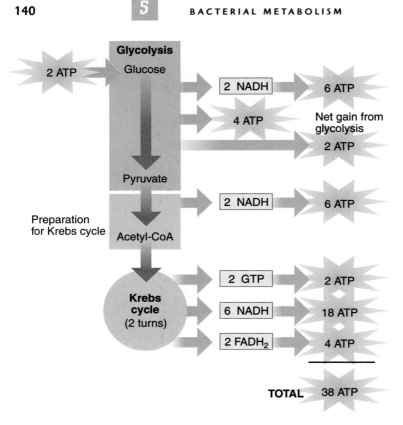

FIGURE 5.7

The ATP Yield From Aerobic Respiration

In a bacterial cell, 38 molecules of ATP normally result from the metabolism of a molecule of glucose. Each NADH molecule accounts for the formation of three molecules of ATP; each molecule of $FADH_2$ accounts for two ATP molecules.

We may summarize the ATP yield as follows:

6 ATPs from reaction (5) in glycolysis via 2 NADHs
2 ATPs from the net gain in glycolysis
6 ATPs from preparation for the Krebs cycle
2 ATPs from reaction (D) in the Krebs cycle via GTP
18 ATPs from 6 NADH from the Krebs cycle
4 ATPs from 2 $FADH_2$ from the Krebs cycle

The grand total of ATPs is therefore 38 molecules of ATP, as FIGURE 5.7 illustrates. At 7300 calories per mole of ATP, this yields 277,400 cal of energy preserved from the energy in glucose. It also completes the equation for aerobic respiration:

$$C_6H_{12}O_6 + 6\,O_2 + \mathbf{38\,ADP} + \mathbf{38\,P} \rightarrow 6\,CO_2 + 6\,H_2O + \mathbf{38\,ATP}$$

To this point . . .

We have discussed the catabolism of glucose by exploring the biochemical reactions of glycolysis, the Krebs cycle, and oxidative phosphorylation. In these processes, glucose is first converted to pyruvic acid, which then feeds into the Krebs cycle. The carbon of glucose is ultimately released as carbon dioxide. In addition, ATP molecules are formed from reactions that accompany the main metabolic pathway. The major percentage of ATP, however, results from oxidative phosphorylation and chemiosmosis, as electrons from glycolysis and Krebs cycle reactions pass among coenzymes and cytochromes and eventually wind up in oxygen atoms. The energy released during the passages is used to form ATP. We saw that a total of 38 ATP molecules can be formed from the energy in a single glucose molecule through the reactions in metabolism.

Glucose is fundamental to the life of a bacterium because it provides the energy for chemical activities. However, glucose is not the only chemical substance used for energy. Modern biochemists have found that numerous other carbohydrates, as well as proteins and fats, contribute to the energy metabolism of bacteria. In the next section, we shall see how these compounds are processed. In addition, we shall study mechanisms by which certain microorganisms obtain their energy even though oxygen is not available as an electron acceptor.

Other Aspects of Catabolism

The catabolism of glucose is a complex process and, for the student of microbiology, it is a demanding aspect of biochemistry to learn and understand. However, the process is central to the metabolism of bacteria, as well as a great many other living things, and it provides a glimpse of how living things obtain energy for life. Moreover, the process of glucose catabolism is a main thoroughfare to which many other biochemical pathways lead and from which numerous pathways extend. In this section, we shall examine how cells obtain energy from various other organic substances by incorporating the substances into the process of glucose catabolism. We shall also see how modifications of the basic scheme account for the utilization of glucose in the absence of oxygen. The use of one major pathway with multiple offshoots lends a modicum of economy to the metabolism of a cell.

THE CATABOLISM OF OTHER CARBOHYDRATES

A wide variety of monosaccharides, disaccharides, and polysaccharides serve as useful energy sources for bacteria and other living cells. All of these carbohydrates undergo a series of preparatory conversions before they are processed in glycolysis, the Krebs cycle, and oxidative phosphorylation.

In preparation for entry into the scheme of metabolism, different carbohydrates utilize different pathways. **Sucrose**, for example, is first digested by the enzyme sucrase into its constituent molecules, glucose and fructose. The glucose molecule enters the glycolysis pathway directly, but the fructose molecule is first converted to fructose-1-phosphate. The latter then undergoes further conversions and a molecular split before it enters the scheme as dihydroxyacetone phosphate (DHAP). **Lactose**, another disaccharide, is broken in two by the enzyme lactase to glucose and galactose. Glucose enters the pathway, as before, but galactose undergoes a series of changes before it is ready to enter glycolysis in the form of glucose-6-phosphate.

Polysaccharides also undergo a system of changes before entering the mainstream of glycolysis. Starch and glycogen are metabolized as enzymes remove one glucose unit at a time and convert it to glucose-1-phosphate. An enzyme converts this compound to glucose-6-phosphate, ready for entry to the glycolysis pathway. We shall not examine the intricate details of these processes, but most biochemistry books explain the conversions. The point is that carbohydrates other than glucose can be used just as glucose is used as an energy source.

Lactose:
a disaccharide composed of glucose and galactose units.
Galactose:
an isomer of glucose bound to glucose in lactose.
Polysaccharide:
a carbohydrate composed of multiple units of monosaccharides.
Glycogen:
an animal tissue polysaccharide composed of glucose units.

THE CATABOLISM OF PROTEINS AND FATS

The economy of metabolism is further demonstrated when we consider protein and fat catabolism. Although proteins are generally not considered energy sources, cells utilize them for energy when carbohydrates and fats are in short supply. Fats, by contrast, are extremely valuable energy sources because their chemical bonds contain enormous amounts of chemical energy. There is so much energy, in fact, that when a bacterium has excessive amounts of carbohydrates, its enzymes convert the carbohydrates to fats to store the energy for later use. Human metabolism is similar.

Both proteins and fats are broken down through the pathway of glucose catabolism as well as many other smaller pathways. Basically, the proteins and fats undergo a series of enzyme-catalyzed conversions and form components normally occurring in carbohydrate metabolism. These components then continue along the scheme as if they originated from carbohydrates. **Proteins**, for example, are broken down to amino acids. Enzymes then convert many amino acids to pathway components by removing the amino group and substituting a carbonyl group. This process is called **deamination.** Alanine is converted to pyruvic acid, and aspartic acid is converted to oxaloacetic acid. For certain amino acids the process is more complex, but the end result is the same: The amino acids become pathway intermediaries and are metabolized to conserve energy in ATP.

Fats consist of one or more fatty acids bonded to a glycerol molecule. To be useful for energy purposes, the fatty acids are separated from the glycerol by the enzyme lipase. Once this has taken place, the glycerol portion is converted to DHAP. For fatty acids, there is a complex series of conversions called **beta oxidation**. In this process, each long-chain fatty acid is broken by enzymes into 2-carbon units, and enzymes convert each unit to a molecule of acetyl-CoA ready for the Krebs cycle. We previously noted that for each turn of the Krebs cycle, 14 molecules of ATP are derived. A quick calculation should illustrate the substantial energy output from a 16-carbon fatty acid (eight 2-carbon units).

> de-am'ĭ-na'shun

> Beta oxidation:
> a series of biochemical reactions in which fatty acids are converted to 2-carbon units.

ANAEROBIC RESPIRATION

Certain bacteria metabolize carbohydrates through **anaerobic respiration,** a process in which oxygen is not used as an electron acceptor. But even without oxygen, the mechanism of electron transport takes place by oxidative phosphorylation. Instead of oxygen, anaerobic bacteria use an inorganic molecule as a final electron acceptor. For example, *Escherichia coli* uses **nitrate ions** (NO_3^-) at the end of the cytochrome chain. Electrons combine with the nitrate ions and convert the latter into nitrite ions (NO_2^-). Microbiologists take advantage of this chemistry in a laboratory diagnostic test for identifying nitrite producers, such as *E. coli.*

Members of the genus *Desulfovibrio* use **sulfate ions** ($SO_4^=$) for anaerobic respiration. The sulfate combines with electrons and changes to hydrogen sulfide (H_2S). This gas gives a rotten egg smell to the environment (as in a tightly compacted landfill). A final example is exhibited by members of the genera *Methanobacterium* and *Methanococcus.* These archaea use **carbon dioxide** as an electron acceptor, and, with hydrogen nuclei, they form large amounts of methane (CH_4). Some scientists believe that because of this chemistry, methane-producing bacteria existed on Earth when the only available gas was carbon dioxide. They postulate that methane may actually have entered the atmosphere for the first time through the activity of these bacteria.

> esh'er-i'ke-a

> de-sul'fo-vib're-o

> meth-an'o-bak-te're-um
> meth-an'o-kok'us

FERMENTATION

The chemical process of **fermentation** may be considered a type of anaerobic respiration because it does not use oxygen as a final electron acceptor (FIGURE 5.8). Fermentation is a unique process because an organic molecule, usually an intermediary in a metabolic pathway, accepts the electrons. For example, in the fermentation of glucose by certain bacteria and yeasts, an intermediary molecule accepts the electrons and proton from NADH formed in reaction (5) of glycolysis. This regenerates NAD molecules for reuse as electron acceptors. NAD exists in limited supply

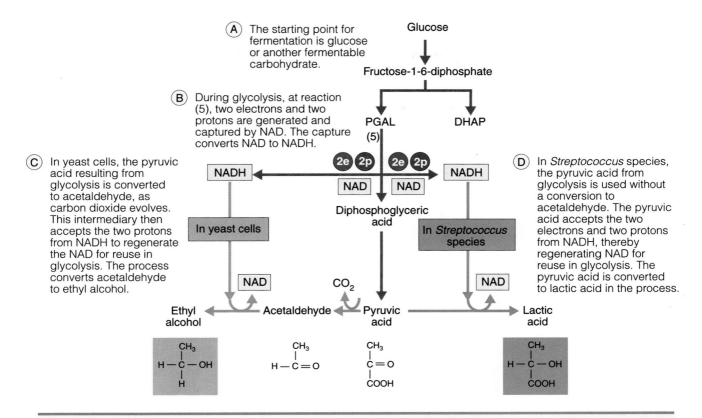

(A) The starting point for fermentation is glucose or another fermentable carbohydrate.

(B) During glycolysis, at reaction (5), two electrons and two protons are generated and captured by NAD. The capture converts NAD to NADH.

(C) In yeast cells, the pyruvic acid resulting from glycolysis is converted to acetaldehyde, as carbon dioxide evolves. This intermediary then accepts the two protons from NADH to regenerate the NAD for reuse in glycolysis. The process converts acetaldehyde to ethyl alcohol.

(D) In *Streptococcus* species, the pyruvic acid from glycolysis is used without a conversion to acetaldehyde. The pyruvic acid accepts the two electrons and two protons from NADH, thereby regenerating NAD for reuse in glycolysis. The pyruvic acid is converted to lactic acid in the process.

FIGURE 5.8

The Relationship of Fermentation to Glycolysis

in the cytoplasm and must be continually regenerated so that glycolysis may proceed. (When oxidative phosphorylation is taking place, the NAD is regenerated by giving up its electrons and proton to the electron transport chain.)

The bacterium *Streptococcus lactis* practices fermentation by using pyruvic acid to accept the electrons and proton from NADH. An enzyme reaction converts the pyruvic acid to lactic acid in the process. In a dairy plant, the metabolism is carefully controlled to make buttermilk from fresh milk. (FIGURE 5.9 shows the bacterium.)

The fermentation chemistry in **yeasts** such as *Saccharomyces* is somewhat different because yeasts contain a different enzyme. In these cells the pyruvic acid is first converted to acetaldehyde, a process in which carbon dioxide evolves. Acetaldehyde then serves as an acceptor for the electrons and proton of NADH, and the acetaldehyde converts to ethyl alcohol. The liquor industry uses the ethyl alcohol produced in fermentation to make alcoholic beverages such as beer and wine (Chapter 26).

sak'ah-ro-mi'sēz

as'et-al'dĕ-hīd

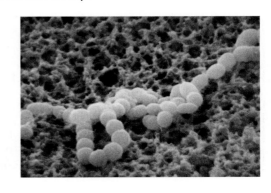

FIGURE 5.9

A Species of *Streptococcus*

This species of *Streptococcus* is *S. lactis*. It is used in industrial processes to produce lactic acid in dairy products through the fermentation of milk.

Yeast fermentation of carbohydrates to alcohol may also take place in the human body, as explained in the opening of this chapter.

The energy benefits to *Streptococcus lactis* and yeasts are far less in fermentation than in aerobic respiration. The only ATP that evolves are the net two molecules resulting from glycolysis. This is in sharp contrast to the 38 molecules evolving in aerobic respiration. It is clear that aerobic respiration is the better choice for energy conservation, but under the circumstances of an oxygen-free environment, there is little alternative if life for *Streptococcus lactis* or *Saccharomyces* (yeast) is to continue.

In the food industry, fermentation results in a broad variety of useful products. Swiss cheese, for instance, develops its flavor partly from propionic acid resulting from fermentation and gets its holes from fermentation gases. Pickles and sauerkraut are sour because bacteria ferment the carbohydrates in cucumbers and cabbage, respectively. Sausage tastes like sausage because bacteria ferment the meat proteins. Thus, fermentation is useful not only to the microorganisms but also to consumers who enjoy its products.

To this point . . .

We have surveyed the process of aerobic respiration in glucose, and we saw how numerous carbohydrates, proteins, and fats can be metabolized by bacterial cells through modifications of the scheme. In the latter cases, enzymes first convert the organic molecules to intermediary compounds of the process. The intermediates then proceed along the metabolic pathway and give up their energy to yield ATP. This chemistry illustrates a basic economy in cell metabolism because a centralized process is used, and various organic molecules fit into it.

The discussion then shifted gears to explore how energy may be obtained when oxygen is not available as a final electron acceptor. We described how inorganic molecules are used as electron acceptors under anaerobic conditions so that the metabolism can continue. Some time was spent with fermentation, a unique process that utilizes an organic intermediary as an electron acceptor. Fermentation has great significance in the food and liquor industries.

We shall now turn our attention to anabolism and discuss the methods by which carbohydrates and proteins are synthesized in bacterial cells. Fats will not be considered because they are formed essentially by a reversal of catabolism. The anabolism of carbohydrates and that of proteins are complex processes, and both are essential to an appreciation of bacterial metabolism. Our discussions will be relatively brief because we are more interested in an overview than in specific details. The processes of anabolism, together with those of catabolism, provide a window to the fundamental biochemistry of bacterial life.

5.4

The Anabolism of Carbohydrates

Although the anabolism of carbohydrates takes place through various mechanisms in bacteria, the unifying feature is the requirement for energy. In many bacteria, energy comes from sunlight, but in several species, energy is derived from chemical reactions. On these bases, two general patterns of bacterial anabolism exist: photosynthesis and chemosynthesis. In addition, bacteria obtain the carbon for carbohydrate synthesis from either of two different sources, as we shall see.

PHOTOSYNTHESIS

Photosynthesis is a process in which light energy is converted to chemical energy, which is then used to synthesize organic compounds from carbon dioxide. The process takes place in organisms having chlorophyll and chlorophyll-like pigments. Adenosine triphosphate (ATP) is a key intermediary compound in the process, and glucose is a major end-product.

Photosynthesis occurs in the cell membranes of both eukaryotic and prokaryotic microorganisms. Among eukaryotes, it takes place in such organisms as diatoms, dinoflagellates, and algae. Among prokaryotes, photosynthesis occurs in the cyanobacteria (formerly called blue-green algae), the green sulfur bacteria, and the purple sulfur bacteria. Our discussion will focus on the prokaryotes.

Cyanobacteria practice photosynthesis in much the same manner as eukaryotic microorganisms and green plants (FIGURE 5.10). The cyanobacteria absorb light energy in their green pigment **chlorophyll a,** a magnesium-containing, lipid-soluble compound. The light excites pigment molecules, and each molecule loses one electron. Dislodged electrons are then accepted by a compound called **phaeophytin,** which is a chlorophyll molecule missing its magnesium atom. Phaeophytin passes electrons to a series of cytochromes, and eventually the electrons are taken up by a new series of chlorophyll molecules. When these molecules are excited by light energy, the electrons are again boosted out of the pigment molecules to a molecule of ferredoxin and then to another series of cytochrome molecules, and finally to a molecule of **nicotinamide adenine dinucleotide phosphate (NADP)**. The latter receives hydrogen ions from water molecules and becomes **NADPH$_2$**.

During the electron transfer in cytochromes, a proton motive force develops in the cell membrane of the cyanobacterium, and chemiosmosis takes place. As described previously, **ATP** is formed when protons pass back across the membrane and release their energy. Hence, two major products, ATP and NADPH$_2$, result from this phase of photosynthesis. The phase is termed the **energy-fixing reaction** because light energy is trapped and converted to (or "fixed" as) chemical energy. It is important to note that electrons are replaced in the chlorophyll molecules by electrons from **water molecules** (which also supply hydrogen ions, as noted above). The residual portions of the water molecules recombine with one another and yield oxygen, the **oxygen** that fills the atmosphere and is used by living creatures in respiration. Organisms that produce oxygen in photosynthesis are said to be **oxygenic**.

In the next step, carbohydrate is formed. The process is known as the **carbon-fixing reaction** because the carbon in carbon dioxide is trapped. Using the energy stored in ATP from the light reaction, an enzyme bonds carbon dioxide to a 5-carbon organic substance called ribulose-1,5-bisphosphate. (The enzyme is called ribulose phosphate carboxylase.) The resulting 6-carbon molecule then splits to form two molecules of phosphoglyceraldehyde

Photosynthesis: carbohydrate anabolism using light as an energy source.

Prokaryotes: simple organisms such as bacteria that lack a nucleus and organelles, and reproduce by fission.

Cyanobacteria: prokaryotic aquatic microorganisms, formerly called blue-green algae.

pha'o-fi'tin

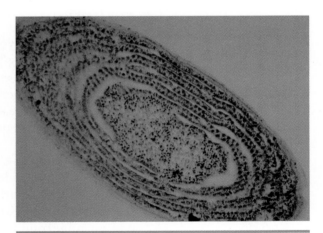

FIGURE 5.10

Cyanobacterial Membranes

An electron micrograph of a cyanobacterium (blue-green alga), displaying the membranes along which photosynthetic pigments are located. These membranes are analogous to thylakoid membranes in the chloroplasts of complex plant cells.

(PGAL). This is identical to the substance formed in reaction (4) of glycolysis. Hydrogen ions for the reaction are obtained from $NADPH_2$, which also supplies electrons to the process. The two molecules of PGAL then condense with each other. Now a reversal of glycolysis reactions take place, and a molecule of glucose eventually forms. Thus, the overall formula for photosynthesis may be expressed as:

$$6 \, CO_2 + 6 \, H_2O + ATP \rightarrow C_6H_{12}O_6 + 6 \, O_2 + ADP + P$$

You may correctly note that this equation is the reverse of the equation for aerobic respiration. The fundamental difference is that aerobic respiration is an energy-yielding process, while photosynthesis is an energy-trapping process. Photosynthesis for cyanobacteria is summarized in FIGURE 5.11.

In addition to the cyanobacteria, several other groups of prokaryotes trap energy by photosynthesis. Two such groups are the **green sulfur bacteria** and **purple sulfur bacteria**, so-named because of the colors imparted by their pigments. These bacteria have chlorophyll-like pigments known as **bacteriochlorophylls,** to distinguish them from other chlorophylls. Bacteriochlorophylls a and b are found in purple sulfur bacteria. In the production of carbohydrate in the carbon-fixing reaction, the organisms do not use water as a source of hydrogen ions. Consequently, no oxygen is liberated, and the bacteria are said to be **anoxygenic.** Instead of water, a series of organic or inorganic substances are utilized as a source of hydrogen ions. Certain species of green sulfur bacteria use **hydrogen sulfide (H_2S)** as a hydrogen ion source and convert it to elemental sulfur. Species of purple sulfur bacteria use small fatty acids as hydrogen ion donors. The green and purple sulfur bacteria commonly live under anaerobic conditions in environments such as sulfur springs and stagnant ponds.

Another variation of bacterial photosynthesis occurs in the archaebacteria (archaea). Instead of the usual chlorophylls, the extreme halophiles of this group contain a pigment called **bacteriorhodopsin** (which is similar to the rhodopsin of the human eye). In the presence of oxygen, extreme halophiles can synthesize ATP with the aid of this pigment.

Bacteriochlorophyll: a type of chlorophyll found in certain species of bacteria.

bak-te're-o-ro-dop'sin

Halophiles: bacteria that live in high-salt environments.

CHEMOSYNTHESIS

Bacteria of the type we have discussed are commonly known as **photoautotrophs**, meaning "light self-feeders." This name derives from the observation that they utilize light energy to synthesize foods in photosynthesis. Another group of bacteria are the **chemoautotrophs**. During carbohydrate synthesis, these organisms use chemical reactions to obtain energy from inorganic compounds. The process of carbohydrate anabolism is therefore called **chemosynthesis** rather than photosynthesis.

Chemoautotrophs can survive in environments rich in inorganic substances, as long as carbon dioxide and oxygen are available. Certain bacteria obtain energy from ATP formed during reactions taking place in their cytoplasm. For example, species of *Nitrosomonas* convert ammonium ions (NH_4^+) into nitrite ions (NO_2^-) under aerobic conditions, thereby obtaining ATP. Bacteria of the genus *Nitrobacter* then convert the nitrite ions into nitrate ions (NO_3^-), also as an ATP-generating mechanism. In addition to providing energy to both species of bacteria, these reactions have great significance in the environment because they preserve nitrogen in the soil in the form of nitrate. The nitrate may then be used by green plants to form amino acids in the **nitrogen cycle** (Chapter 25). Other bacteria living near ocean

fo'to-aw'to-troph

ke'mo-aw'to-troph

Chemosynthesis: carbohydrate anabolism using chemical reactions as energy sources.

ni-tro'so-mon'as

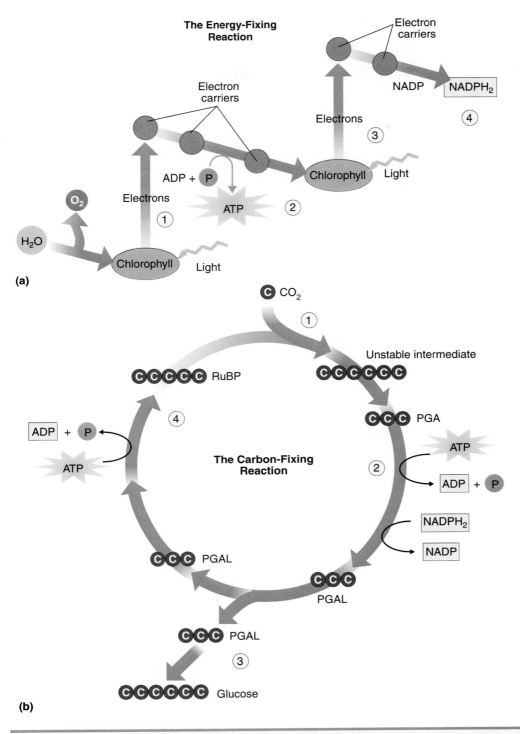

FIGURE 5.11

Photosynthesis in Microorganisms

(a) The energy-fixing reaction occurring along the membranes of a cyanobacterium. (1) Electrons in chlorophyll receive a boost in energy from light and (2) ATP is synthesized as the electrons pass among electron carriers. (3) In noncyclic photosynthesis, the electrons receive a second boost, and (4) the energy is used to form high-energy $NADPH_2$. The ATP and $NADPH_2$ are used in the carbon-fixing reactions. (b) The carbon-fixing reaction. (1) Carbon dioxide unites with ribulose bisphosphate (RuBP) to form an unstable 6-carbon molecule. (2) The latter splits to form two molecules of phosphoglyceric acid (PGA) then phosphoglyceraldehyde (PGAL). ATP and $NADPH_2$ from the light-fixing reaction are used in the conversion. (3) Condensations of two 3-carbon PGAL molecules yields glucose, and (4) the remainder is used to form RuBP to continue the process. ATP is used in the latter reaction.

FIGURE 5.12

Chemoautotrophs

(a) A scanning electron micrograph of bacteria and other microorganisms attached to natural surfaces near cracks in the floor of the Pacific Ocean. These samples were retrieved from a depth of 2550 meters (about 1.68 miles) near vents where the temperature was over 400°F. Hydrogen sulfide from the vent is a major source of energy for these marine bacteria. (Bar = 5 μm.) (b) The typical habitat of chemo-autotrophic bacteria includes a diversity of other organisms, including red-tipped tube-worms, shown here.

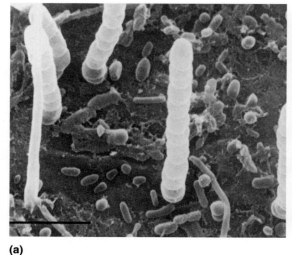

(a)

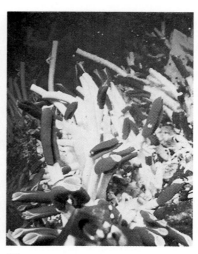

(b)

vents can obtain their energy from hydrogen sulfide (FIGURE 5.12). Marine bacteria can also use other electron acceptors.

CARBON SOURCES

fo′to-het′er-o-troph
ke′mo-het′er-o-troph

Photoheterotroph:
a microorganism that uses light as an energy source and organic compounds as carbon sources.

In addition to their classification as photoautotrophs and chemoautotrophs, bacteria can also be categorized as **photoheterotrophs** or **chemoheterotrophs.** The prefix *photo-* or *chemo-* refers to whether light or chemical reactions are used for energy. The stem *hetero* refers to "other" substances, implying that photoheterotrophs and chemoheterotrophs use organic compounds instead of carbon dioxide to obtain the carbon for carbohydrates. Alcohols, fatty acids, and other organic acids are examples of the organic compounds that may supply the carbon. Photoheterotrophs include certain green nonsulfur and purple nonsulfur bacteria in nature, while chemoheterotrophs include the vast majority of bacteria, as well as all fungi, protozoa, and animals. The "chemos" and "photos" can be difficult to remember, but TABLE 5.2 may help.

TABLE 5.2

A Nutritional Classification of Microorganisms

NUTRITIONAL TYPE	ENERGY SOURCE	CARBON SOURCE	EXAMPLES
Photoautotroph	Light	Carbon dioxide (CO_2)	Photosynthetic bacteria (green sulfur and purple sulfur bacteria), cyanobacteria, extreme halophiles
Photoheterotroph	Light	Organic compounds	Purple nonsulfur and green nonsulfur bacteria
Chemoautotroph	Chemical reactions	Carbon dioxide (CO_2)	*Nitrosomonas, Nitrobacter*
Chemoheterotroph	Chemical reactions	Organic compounds	Most bacteria, and all fungi, protozoa, and animals

5-5

The Anabolism of Proteins (Protein Synthesis)

The anabolism (synthesis) of proteins stands in stark contrast to the anabolism of carbohydrates, and we must reorder our thinking because there is no glycolysis, Krebs cycle, photosynthesis, or "trophs" in this aspect of metabolism. Instead, protein anabolism, or **protein synthesis** as it is more commonly known, is a process in which amino acids are precisely bound together in a sequence determined by the hereditary information in the cell. The compounds resulting from protein synthesis are utilized as cellular enzymes, structural components, toxins, or other forms.

Before the 1950s, scientists were perplexed by how proteins are assembled from amino acids. Early on, they suggested that the amino acid chain of a protein serves

MicroFocus 5.4

THE THIRD MAN

The names James D. Watson and Francis H.C. Crick are familiar to students of biology as the scientists who first proposed the structure of DNA. In doing so, they constructed a model of how hereditary material makes replicas of itself and showed how genes could encode the synthesis of protein in a cell. In 1962, Watson and Crick received the Nobel Prize in Physiology or Medicine for their work.

Also cited that year was their co-worker, a British scientist named Maurice Hugh Frederick Wilkins. Working with his colleague Rosalind Franklin, Wilkins made available the data that permitted construction of the Watson-Crick model.

Wilkins was originally a physicist of New Zealand heritage. Educated in England, he came to the United States during World War II to work on uranium separation for the Manhattan Project, which produced the first atomic bomb. Partly because of the destructive effects of the bomb, his interest turned from the atomic nucleus to the cell nucleus. Returning to England in the late 1940s, he assumed a research position at King's College.

Wilkins' forte was X-ray crystallography. Using a special camera, he placed crystals of DNA before a beam of X rays and charted their patterns of deflection. When substances crystallize, their atoms line up in a lattice-work of repeating units. These units deflect X rays in a regular pattern, and by studying the patterns, a scientist can determine the distances between different components of the latticework. (The effect is much like determining the structure of monkeybars by analyzing the shadow they cast when hit by the sun at various angles.) Wilkins theorized that DNA molecules form a helix, a pattern resembling a corkscrew wrapped around a cylinder.

In 1951, Watson arrived in Cambridge, England, on a research fellowship to learn about molecular structures. There, at the Cavendish Laboratory, he met Francis Crick. Both were intensely interested in DNA's structure, and they immediately set to work to solve the puzzle. Watson and Crick did no experiments in the usual sense. They worked entirely with other people's material, including the X-ray photographs of Wilkins and Franklin. Carefully they

moved around the nucleotide components with jigsaw models so that DNA would conform to the helical pattern shown by the X rays. Finally, in the April 25, 1953 issue of *Nature*, a British scientific journal, Watson and Crick made their historic suggestion about the structure of DNA . . . but not before checking with Wilkins.

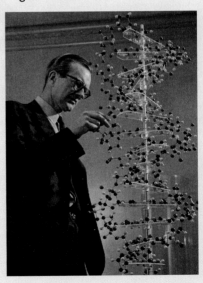

■ *Maurice H.F. Wilkins, the co-laureate with Watson and Crick of the 1962 Nobel Prize in Physiology or Medicine. This photograph was taken on October 18, 1962.*

Deoxyribonucleic acid:
DNA, the nucleic acid that forms
the hereditary information of the
cell and provides the genetic
code for protein synthesis.

as a template for the construction of new proteins. However, the transformation experiments of Griffith and the work of Avery and his coworkers (Chapter 6) focused attention on the deoxyribonucleic acid (DNA) of a cell. Then, in 1953, the determination of DNA's double helix structure by **James D. Watson** and **Francis H.C. Crick** provided a glimpse into how DNA encodes the manufacture of proteins. Their work was based in large measure on X-ray diffraction studies by **Rosalind Franklin** and **Maurice Wilkins** (MicroFocus 5.4). The work on DNA did not displace anything in science. Rather, it filled a critical gap in understanding how a cell produces protein. Watson, Crick, and Wilkins shared the 1962 Nobel Prize in Physiology or Medicine for their insight. Although Franklin died of cancer before the award was made (Nobel Prizes are not awarded posthumously), her contributions to the work are universally accepted.

Today it is recognized that protein synthesis requires not only DNA of the chromosome but also ribonucleic acid (RNA). Both DNA and RNA are described in Chapter 2. A review of their structure is recommended if their functions are to be fully comprehended. Protein synthesis also utilizes ATP and GTP as energy sources, as well as a series of important enzymes. Amino acids must likewise be available. A refresher on their structure and the peptide bonds that hold them together in a protein (Chapter 2) may be of value.

Genes:
segments of DNA that provide
the biochemical code for protein
synthesis.

The central theme of protein synthesis holds that segments of DNA on the chromosome, known as **genes**, provide a code for the production of molecules of RNA (as shown in FIGURE 5.13). The genetic code of DNA is expressed in RNA by a process called **transcription**. One type of RNA then functions as a messenger by car-

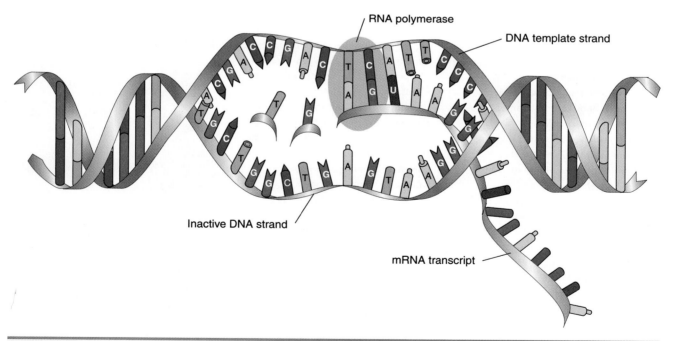

FIGURE 5.13

A DNA Molecule and Its Activity

DNA in action in the process of transcription. The enzyme RNA polymerase moves along one strand of the DNA double helix and synthesizes a complementary molecule of RNA using the nitrogenous base code as a guide. The mRNA transcript will carry the genetic message of DNA into the cytoplasm, where protein synthesis occurs. Note that the remaining strand of DNA is not transcribed.

rying the code to other areas of the cytoplasm, where amino acids are fitted together in a precise sequence to form the protein. This sequencing process, called **translation**, reflects the genetic code in the DNA. The overall process is summarized as follows:

$$\text{DNA} \xrightarrow{\text{Transcription}} \text{RNA} \xrightarrow{\text{Translation}} \text{Protein}$$

The following paragraphs describe transcription and translation in detail. It should be noted that RNA can also act alone in certain circumstances (MicroFocus 5.5).

TRANSCRIPTION

In **transcription,** various types of RNA are produced according to the code of nitrogenous bases in the DNA molecule. (TABLE 5.3 compares DNA and RNA.) The DNA thus serves as a template for new RNA molecules. The process begins with an uncoupling of the two DNA strands as the hydrogen bonds between opposing bases break down. The DNA double helix then unwinds at certain internal regions.

At this point, RNA nucleotides containing ribose, phosphate groups, and nitrogenous bases are aligned along one strand of DNA. Enzymes position the bases of the RNA to complement the DNA bases. For example, guanine stands opposite cytosine, cytosine opposes guanine, and adenine opposes thymine. Because RNA contains no thymine, an adenine base on the DNA stands opposite a uracil base. The RNA components are then linked together, beginning at a specific site, by an enzyme called **RNA polymerase**. This enzyme was first described by **Severo Ochoa**, who shared the 1959 Nobel Prize in Physiology or Medicine. The sequence of bases in

Hydrogen bonds: weak bonds between protons and adjacent pairs of electrons.

o-cho'ah

MicroFocus 5.5

OUT WITH THE OLD

Until the 1980s, one of the bedrock principles of biochemistry was the division of labor in cells: Nucleic acids (DNA and RNA) hold the information for directing the biochemical reaction in the cell; proteins serve as the functional molecules (the enzymes) that catalyze the thousands of chemical reactions taking place. But chemistry research in the late 1970s and early 1980s helped overturn this principle. Contemporary scientists now believe that RNA acting by itself can trigger certain chemical reactions.

The seminal research on RNA was performed independently by Thomas R. Cech of the University of Colorado and Sidney Altman of Yale University. In the late 1970s, Altman found an unusual enzyme in bacteria, an enzyme composed of RNA and protein. Initially, he thought the RNA was a contaminant, but when he separated the RNA from the protein, the enzyme could not func-

tion. After several years, Altman and his colleagues showed that RNA was the enzyme's key component because under carefully controlled laboratory conditions, it could act alone. At about the same time, Cech discovered that RNA molecules from protozoa could catalyze certain reactions under laboratory conditions. He went further and showed that a molecule of RNA could cut internal segments out of itself and splice together the remaining segments.

Many biologists responded to the findings of Cech and Altman with disbelief. The implication of the research was that proteins and nucleic acids are not necessarily interdependent, as had been assumed. The research also opened the possibility that RNA could have evolved on Earth without protein and that a self-catalyzing form of RNA could have been the first primitive molecule able to reproduce itself. Perhaps, scientists reasoned, the biochemical machinery for

translating the DNA-based genetic code in modern cells evolved much later. In essence, there arose a whole new way of imagining how life might have begun on Earth. The Nobel Prize committee was equally impressed. In 1989, it awarded the Nobel Prize in Chemistry to Cech and Altman.

By 1990, the self-reproducing molecule of RNA had a name—ribozyme. Biochemists at Massachusetts General Hospital soon modified a ribozyme by removing its internal segments. Then they showed that the new ribozyme could join together separate short nucleotide segments aligned on specially designed, external templates. The research was a step toward designing a completely self-copying RNA molecule. Would such a ribozyme enclosed in a membrane constitute a primitive cell? If so, the cell would be quite different from what most scientists have imagined the first cells to be.

TABLE 5.3

A Comparison of DNA and RNA

DNA (DEOXYRIBONUCLEIC ACID)	RNA (RIBONUCLEIC ACID)
In prokaryotes, found in the nucleoid and plasmids; in eukaryotes, found in the nucleus and in some extranuclear organelles	In prokaryotes and eukaryotes, found dissolved in the cytoplasm and at ribosomes; in eukaryotes, found in the nucleolus
Always associated with chromosome (genes); each chromosome has a fixed amount of DNA	Found mainly in combinations with proteins in ribosomes in the cytoplasm, as messenger RNA, and as transfer RNA
Contains a pentose (5-carbon) sugar called deoxyribose	Contains a pentose (5-carbon) sugar called ribose
Contains bases adenine, guanine, cytosine, thymine	Contains bases adenine, guanine, cytosine, uracil
Contains phosphorus (in phosphate groups) that connects various sugars with one another	Contains phosphorus (in phosphate groups) that connects various sugars with one another
Functions as the molecule of inheritance	Functions in protein synthesis
Double-stranded	Usually single-stranded
Larger size	Smaller size

Ribosomes:
submicroscopic particles of RNA and protein that function in protein synthesis.

Transfer RNA:
the RNA molecule that unites with amino acids in the cytoplasm and transports them to the ribosomes for assembly into proteins.

Codon:
a three-base code on an mRNA molecule that is specific for an amino acid.

DNA thus forms a complementary image of itself in the RNA. The language, or genetic code, of DNA has been transcribed.

Three types of RNA result from transcription. One type, **ribosomal RNA (rRNA)**, forms from certain regions of the DNA. Together with protein, this RNA serves as the basic framework of submicroscopic particles called **ribosomes**. Over 30,000 ribosomes are present in each bacterial cell. They are sites at which amino acids assemble into protein.

A second type of RNA is **transfer RNA**, or simply **tRNA**. Transfer RNA is the smallest RNA molecule, with a molecular mass of about 25,000 daltons and containing approximately 75 nucleotides. The molecule is shaped roughly like a cloverleaf, with one point exhibiting a sequence of three nitrogenous bases (a triplet) that functions as a code. At least one type of tRNA exists for each of the 20 amino acids, and a high degree of specificity exists between the tRNA and its amino acid. For example, the amino acid alanine binds only to the tRNA specialized to transport alanine. Transfer RNA molecules deliver amino acids to the ribosome for assembly into proteins, as we shall see presently.

Both ribosomal RNA and transfer RNA are produced at irregular intervals and remain for long periods of time in the cytoplasm. The third form of RNA appears each time a protein is manufactured. This RNA is called **messenger RNA (mRNA)** because it carries the genetic message for protein synthesis. Discovered by **Sol Spiegelman** and his coworkers, mRNA provides the template that indicates the sequence the amino acids have in the protein. Its message consists of a series of three-base codes or **codons.** Each codon specifies an individual amino acid to be slotted into position.

One of the startling discoveries of biochemistry is that one or more three-base codes exist for each amino acid. Since there are four nitrogenous bases available to work with, mathematics tells us that 64 possible combinations can be made of the bases, using three at a time. But there are only 20 amino acids for which a code must be supplied. How do scientists, then, account for the remaining 44 codes? It is now known that 61 of the 64 codes are used for an amino acid and that most amino acids have multiple codons (as shown in TABLE 5.4). For example, GCU, GCC, GCA, and GCG all code for alanine. The three remaining codons act like punctuation marks and stop the addition of amino acids to a growing chain of protein.

The genetic code of bases is nearly universal for all species, be they prokaryotic or eukaryotic. Thus, the GCU code for alanine in bacteria is also the code for alanine in animal cells. However, the complete set of codes varies in sequence among species, thereby providing a constancy as well as a variation in all living things.

There is an important difference between use of the codes in prokaryotes and eukaryotes. In prokaryotes, all the codes appear to be transcribed to an mRNA molecule during protein synthesis, but in eukaryotes, some are left out when the final mRNA is produced. In 1977, **Philip Sharp** and his associates at the Massachusetts Institute of Technology found that certain portions of eukaryotic DNA are not transcribed to the final mRNA. Apparently these portions are a type of "genetic gibberish" that must be removed from the mRNA before the molecule is able to function. The DNA segments were promptly labeled **introns** because they are *intragenic* ("between the genes") segments, while the functioning genes were called **exons** because they are *ex*pressed. Bacteria do not have introns; the genes are entirely sensible. Sharp became a Nobel laureate in 1993.

Exons: segments of DNA that are expressed as a genetic code in protein synthesis.

TRANSLATION

In the process of **translation,** the genetic code (expressed in mRNA) translates into a sequence of amino acids in a molecule of peptide. The process takes place at the ribosome, where the mRNA molecule meets tRNA molecules bound to their

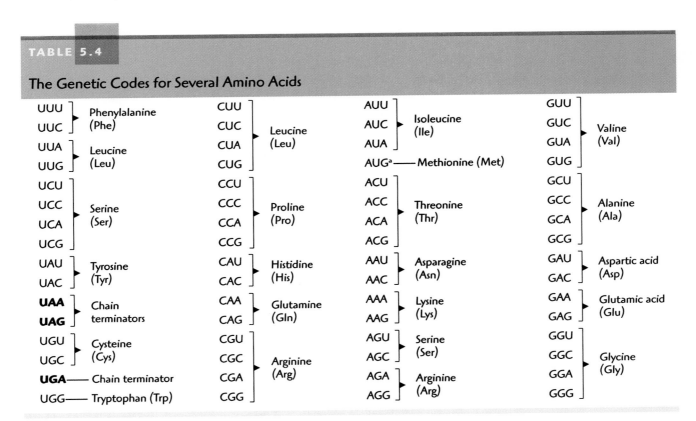

TABLE 5.4

The Genetic Codes for Several Amino Acids

UUU ⎤ Phenylalanine UUC ⎦ (Phe)	CUU ⎤ CUC ⎥ Leucine CUA ⎥ (Leu) CUG ⎦	AUU ⎤ AUC ⎥ Isoleucine AUA ⎦ (Ile) AUGª —— Methionine (Met)	GUU ⎤ GUC ⎥ Valine GUA ⎥ (Val) GUG ⎦
UUA ⎤ Leucine UUG ⎦ (Leu)			
UCU ⎤ UCC ⎥ Serine UCA ⎥ (Ser) UCG ⎦	CCU ⎤ CCC ⎥ Proline CCA ⎥ (Pro) CCG ⎦	ACU ⎤ ACC ⎥ Threonine ACA ⎥ (Thr) ACG ⎦	GCU ⎤ GCC ⎥ Alanine GCA ⎥ (Ala) GCG ⎦
UAU ⎤ Tyrosine UAC ⎦ (Tyr)	CAU ⎤ Histidine CAC ⎦ (His)	AAU ⎤ Asparagine AAC ⎦ (Asn)	GAU ⎤ Aspartic acid GAC ⎦ (Asp)
UAA ⎤ Chain **UAG** ⎦ terminators	CAA ⎤ Glutamine CAG ⎦ (Gln)	AAA ⎤ Lysine AAG ⎦ (Lys)	GAA ⎤ Glutamic acid GAG ⎦ (Glu)
UGU ⎤ Cysteine UGC ⎦ (Cys)	CGU ⎤ CGC ⎥ Arginine CGA ⎥ (Arg) CGG ⎦	AGU ⎤ Serine AGC ⎦ (Ser)	GGU ⎤ GGC ⎥ Glycine GGA ⎥ (Gly) GGG ⎦
UGA —— Chain terminator		AGA ⎤ Arginine AGG ⎦ (Arg)	
UGG —— Tryptophan (Trp)			

Boldface codes are chain terminators.

ªAUG encodes formyl methionine in bacteria.

Anticodon:
a three-base code on a tRNA
molecule that complements the
codon on an mRNA molecule.

amino acids (as illustrated in FIGURE 5.14). The amino acids were bonded to their individual tRNA molecules using energy from ATP and specific enzymes. Now they are ready to be assembled into a peptide (also known as a polypeptide, because numerous amino acids are often involved in its formation).

Translation takes place as the ribosome moves along the mRNA, with the codons in mRNA exposed. The three-base sequences of the tRNA molecules are called **anticodons.** The anticodons match themselves with the complementary codons, and the tRNAs thus bring their amino acids into a carefully ordered position. For example, the codon of GCC on the mRNA will match with a complementary anticodon of CGG on the tRNA carrying alanine. Alanine will then be placed into position. Hydrogen bonds between the codon and anticodon bases momentarily hold the tRNA in position, while an enzyme forms a peptide bond between alanine and the adjacent amino acid. **Guanosine triphosphate (GTP)** supplies energy for the reaction. The tRNA then breaks free, leaving its alanine molecule on the amino acid chain. The next codon attracts a tRNA with its amino acid, and the process continues. When a codon on the mRNA signals the end of chain formation, the process comes to a halt and the peptide (or polypeptide) falls away from the ribosome. This termination code may be UAA, UAG, or UGA.

In practice, a single mRNA molecule may provide the code for several identical peptides at a time. This is because other ribosomes can attach to the mRNA and begin translating the code while the first ribosome is still there. After synthesis, the linear peptide breaks away and twists into its secondary form. As the peptide folds into a tertiary structure, other groups may be added to form the complete protein. (TABLE 5.5 places protein synthesis in context with other metabolic pathways of bacterial metabolism.)

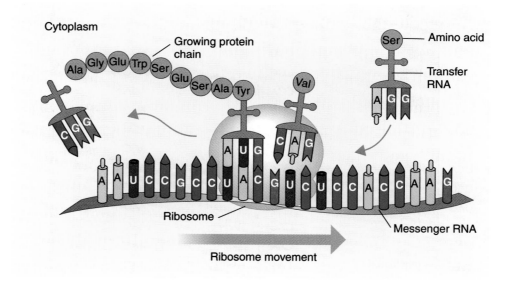

FIGURE 5.14

The Translation Process in Protein Synthesis

The messenger RNA moves to the ribosome, where it is met by transfer RNA molecules bonded to different amino acids. The tRNA molecules align themselves opposite the mRNA molecule and bring the amino acids into position. A peptide bond forms between adjacent amino acids on the growing protein chain, after which the amino acid leaves the tRNA. The tRNA returns to the cytoplasm to bond with another molecule of the same amino acid.

TABLE 5.5

Some Characteristics of Major Pathways of Bacterial Metabolism

FORM	PATHWAY	LOCATIONS	REACTANTS	PRODUCTS
Glycolysis	Embden-Meyerhoff pathway	Cytoplasm	Glucose	2 pyruvic acid, 8 ATP (if oxygen present) 2 ATP (if not present)
Aerobic respiration	Acetyl CoA formation Krebs cycle (2 turns) Electron transport and chemiosmosis	Bacterial membranes Bacterial membranes Bacterial membranes	Pyruvic acid Acetyl CoA 10 NADH, 2 FADH$_2$	NADH, CO$_2$, acetyl CoA 2 ATP, 6 NADH, 4 CO$_2$, FADH$_2$ 28 ATP, H$_2$O
Anaerobic respiration	Electron transport	Bacterial membranes	Nitrate or sulfate or carbon dioxide	Nitrite or H$_2$S or methane
Fermentation	Alcoholic (yeast) Lactic acid (bacteria)	Cytoplasm Cytoplasm	Pyruvic acid Pyruvic acid	Ethanol, CO$_2$ Lactic acid
Photosynthesis (cyanobacteria)	1. Energy-fixing reaction 2. Carbon-fixing reaction	Bacterial membranes Cytoplasm	Energy + 6 H$_2$O 6 CO$_2$, ATP, NADPH	Oxygen gas, ATP, NADPH Glucose, H$_2$O
Chemosynthesis (green sulfur bacteria)	Energy metabolism	Bacterial membranes	H$_2$S	Elemental sulfur
Protein synthesis	1. Transcription	Nucleoid	DNA	Messenger RNA, transfer RNA, ribosomal RNA
	2. Translation	Ribosomes	Amino acids	Protein

5.6

The Control of Protein Synthesis

As biochemical knowledge increased, scientists questioned how cells regulate the complex machinery of protein synthesis. They reasoned that the continuous synthesis of all enzymes for all possible nutrients would probably represent a waste of energy for the cells, as well as a storage problem. They asked what would prevent a cell from running at full throttle all the time, and they pondered how bacteria could economize the synthesis of protein. Their experiments indicated that certain enzymes appear only when their substrates are present, and that a delicate and flexible regulation of metabolism is the rule rather than the exception.

In 1961, two Pasteur Institute scientists, **François Jacob** and **Jacques Monod**, proposed a mechanism for controlling protein synthesis. Jacob and Monod suggested that bacterial genes fall into several groups: **structural genes**, which provide genetic codes for proteins in the process we have discussed; an adjacent **operator gene**, which stimulates and controls the expression of structural genes; and a distant **repressor gene**, which controls the operator gene. Jacob and Monod named the entire unit for expressing a particular trait an **operon**. In 1965 they won the Nobel Prize in Physiology or Medicine for their work. In recent years, scientists have identified a **promoter region** next to the operator gene.

The operon theory helps explain the control of protein synthesis. When a nutrient is absent from the cytoplasmic environment, the repressor gene codes for mRNA, and a **repressor protein** forms (FIGURE 5.15). In 1965, **Mark Ptashne** of Harvard University first isolated a repressor protein. The repressor protein binds to

zhah-kōb'
mo-no'

Operon:
a unit of various genes that control the synthesis of protein.

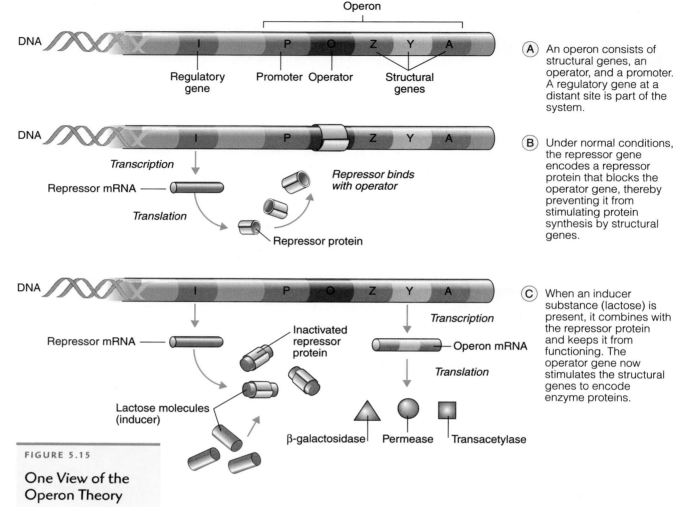

Operon

A An operon consists of structural genes, an operator, and a promoter. A regulatory gene at a distant site is part of the system.

B Under normal conditions, the repressor gene encodes a repressor protein that blocks the operator gene, thereby preventing it from stimulating protein synthesis by structural genes.

C When an inducer substance (lactose) is present, it combines with the repressor protein and keeps it from functioning. The operator gene now stimulates the structural genes to encode enzyme proteins.

FIGURE 5.15

One View of the Operon Theory

Tryptophan:
a ring–containing amino acid.

the operator gene and overlaps the adjacent promoter region. This action prevents RNA polymerase from stimulating the transcription at the structural genes, and the cell cannot produce enzyme proteins.

At some later point, a nutrient enters the environment. This nutrient, known as an **inducer,** binds to the repressor protein and inactivates it. With the repressor protein no longer free, the operator gene and promoter region can stimulate the structural genes to encode protein. This system was first worked out in *E. coli*. It explains why a lactose-digesting enzyme forms only when lactose (the inducer) is present in the bacterial cytoplasm.

A second type of control mechanism, also traced to the operon, explains how enzyme production can be shut down when products of gene activity accumulate in the environment. For instance, bacteria such as *E. coli* cease their production of a tryptophan-synthesizing enzyme when tryptophan accumulates in the cytoplasm. The tryptophan itself does not cause the enzyme production to stop, nor does a repressor protein shut down the mechanism. Instead, tryptophan molecules unite with the repressor protein, and the tryptophan-repressor complex links to the operator gene. As the operator gene is inhibited, the structural genes cease producing tryptophan-synthesizing enzyme. In this way, tryptophan helps control its own synthesis.

The control of protein synthesis is an intricate series of recognitions, regulations, and biochemical changes at the very core of protein anabolism. Indeed, an understanding of control mechanisms is essential to an understanding of gene activity, and before microbial genetics or DNA technology could emerge as disciplines of science, the complexity of control systems had to be worked out. Though they are involved and quite complex to the beginning student of biochemistry, the operations of control systems in bacteria are relatively simple compared to the control systems in eukaryotic cells (if for no other reason than a human cell has 100,000 genes compared to 4000 in an *E. coli* cell).

Nor is the control of protein synthesis confined to the level of transcription. Indeed, molecular biologists have identified control measures in the manner by which mRNA molecules are processed before leaving the DNA area, where mRNA molecules bind to the ribosome, and how the protein is modified to its final form.

Scientists continue to grapple with the intricacies of control mechanisms, for the latter are as important to protein synthesis as transcription and translation. And a thorough understanding of protein synthesis was to have broad ramifications in the 1980s and 1990s, when scientists learned how to manage the process to improve the quality of life. We shall explore the research that led to this breakthrough in Chapter 6.

Note to the Student

This chapter contains some of the most difficult concepts you will encounter in microbiology. The concepts are also among the most fundamental because the biochemistry applies to all life, be it bacterial life, plant life, or human life. I hope you can step back and see the forest as well as the trees. Virtually all living things obtain their energy by glucose digestion, all creatures depend ultimately on the carbohydrate produced in photosynthesis, and all protein in the world is produced essentially as we have described it.

One of the corollary benefits of studying the biochemistry of microorganisms is that you come away with a better understanding of living things in general. Nowhere is this more apparent than in this chapter. Bacteria and other microorganisms are mere tools used to discover the biochemical foundations that govern all living things. Beyond the window dressing of variation, there is an underlying kinship among all forms of life. To understand one form is to understand them all.

Summary

The two major themes of bacterial metabolism are catabolism (the breakdown of organic molecules) and anabolism (the synthesis of organic molecules). For either of these two processes to occur, bacteria and other living things utilize enzymes, a series of protein molecules that speed up a chemical change while themselves remaining unchanged. The activity of enzymes often requires chemical energy, usually supplied by adenosine triphosphate (ATP). Since ATP molecules are constantly being used in living cells, they must be resynthesized to maintain the reactions of metabolism.

One of the principal objectives of catabolism is to release the energy in organic molecules for the synthesis of ATP. Such a reaction series in which energy is released is a process called respiration. The aerobic respiration of glucose molecules is a multistep procedure including the step-by-step conversion of glucose to pyruvic acid (glycolysis), the release of energy and carbon dioxide from pyruvic acid (the Krebs cycle), and the use of the energy to form ATP molecules (oxidative phosphorylation). Other carbohydrates, as well as proteins and fats, also are metabolized through this reaction series. The anaerobic respiration of glucose molecules involves a conversion to pyruvic acid, after which an inorganic molecule of an intermediary of the process is used as an electron acceptor to produce ions, gases, or acids and alcohols (fermentation). Less energy is conserved in the anaerobic process.

The anabolism of carbohydrates occurs by photosynthesis. In this process, light energy is used to synthesize ATP, and the latter is then used to fix atmospheric carbon dioxide into carbohydrate molecules. Pigments such as chlorophyll and bacteriorhodopsin can be used by various bacteria, and chemical energy can be used instead of light energy. Even the carbon can come from different sources.

The anabolism of proteins takes place by a complex mechanism in which the genetic information in DNA is first transcribed to a genetic message in RNA, then translated to a sequence of amino acids in the protein. Various forms of RNA, including mRNA, tRNA, and ribosomal RNA, function in the process, and a careful ordering of codons and anticodons is essential to successful completion of the process. Different control factors influence the mechanism and provide balance to the overall scheme of metabolism.

Questions for Thought and Discussion

1. Some years ago, a magazine cartoon pictured newspapers being carried into a "conversion plant" and beef cattle coming out. The cartoonist envisioned that bacteria in the plant would convert the cellulose of the newspapers into the protein of beef cattle. Can you explain the chemistry behind this look into the future?

2. Citrase is the enzyme that converts citric acid to alphaketoglutaric acid in the Krebs cycle. A chemical company has located a mutant microorganism that cannot produce this enzyme and proposes to use the microorganism to manufacture a particular product. What do you suppose the product is? How might this product be useful?

3. A student observes that during the process of respiration, a bacterium exhales before it inhales. What is he thinking?

4. A microbiology professor from a California college maintains that the most abundant enzyme in the world is ribulose phosphate carboxylase. What do you think this enzyme accomplishes? On what basis does she make her claim?

5. One of the most important steps in the evolution of life on Earth was the appearance of certain organisms in which photosynthesis takes place. Why was this critical?

6. If ATP is such an important energy source in bacteria, why do you think it is not added routinely to the growth medium for these organisms?

7. One student maintains that organisms use proteins to synthesize enzymes. A second student counters that organisms use enzymes to synthesize proteins. Which student is right? Why?

8. A major pharmaceutical company has developed a new pesticide for controlling mosquitoes. However, laboratory tests indicate that the pesticide combines with and alters chlorophyll molecules. What horror story would occur if this chemical were sprayed in the environment?

9. A microbiology professor from Virginia writes: "In the fall when the apples were ripe in our farm orchard, we had a cow who could not be stopped by any fence (shades of the old nursery rhyme). Topsy would stagger home to the barn every night doing a very good imitation of a drunken sailor. . . ." What two possibilities might you offer for this observation?

10. The formula for a growth medium for a particular bacterium stipulates that riboflavin must be added for the synthesis of a certain chemical compound of the catabolism process. Can you guess which compound? What would be the effect of omitting riboflavin?

11. A stagnant pond usually has a putrid odor because hydrogen sulfide has accumulated in the water. A microbiologist recommends that tons of green sulfur bacteria be added to remove the smell. What chemical process does the microbiologist have in mind? Do you think it will work?

12. Certain antibiotics, such as streptomycin, are known to bind to the ribosome, causing a misreading of messenger RNA molecules. What effect will this have on the metabolism of a bacterium?

13. Suppose glycolysis came to a halt in a bacterial cell. Would this mean that the Krebs cycle would also stop? Why?

14. An essential factor in the growth media for bacteria is phosphate. How many places can you cite where it is needed?

15. When the author was completing his doctorate degree, he was required to sit for an 8-hour compre-hensive examination on each of three successive Sat-urdays. The biochemistry portion consisted of a sin-gle-line question: "Discuss the interrelationships between anabolism and catabolism." How might you have answered this question?

Review

When you have completed your study of bacterial metabolism, test your knowledge of its important facts and concepts by circling the choices that best complete each of the following statements. The answers are listed in Appendix D.

1. The sum total of all a bacterium's biochemical reac-tions is known as (catabolism, metabolism); it includes all the (synthesis, digestion) reactions called anabolism and all the breakdown reactions known as (inactivation, catabolism).

2. Enzymes are a group of (carbohydrate, protein) molecules that generally (slow down, speed up) a chemical reaction by converting the (substrate, sub-start) to end-products.

3. The aerobic respiration of glucose begins with the process of (oxidative phosphorylation, glycolysis) and requires that (amino acids, energy) be supplied by (ATP, GTP) molecules.

4. The process of (fermentation, Krebs cycle) takes place in the absence of (oxygen, magnesium) and begins with a molecule of (glucose, protein) and ends with molecules of (amino acid, alcohol).

5. In oxidative phosphorylation, pairs of (neutrons, electrons) are passed among a series of (chromo-somes, cytochromes) with the result that (oxygen, energy) is released for (NAD, ATP) synthesis.

6. In the Krebs cycle, (glucose, pyruvic acid) undergoes a series of changes and releases its (carbon, nitrogen) as (nitrous oxide, carbon dioxide) and its electrons to (NAD, TPA).

7. For use as energy compounds, proteins are first digested to (hydrochloric, amino) acids, which then lose their (carboxyl, amino) groups in the process of (fermentation, deamination) and become interme-diates of respiration.

8. Ribulose phosphate receives (carbon monoxide, car-bon dioxide) molecules in the process of (fermenta-tion, photosynthesis), a process that ultimately results in molecules of (gluconic acid, glucose).

9. Chemoautotrophs use energy from (light, chemical reactions) to synthesize (carbohydrates, proteins) and are typified by species of (*Staphylococcus, Nitrosomonas*).

10. The synthesis of proteins begins with the (respira-tory, genetic) code in molecules of (DNA, RNA), and that code is transferred to molecules of (rRNA, mRNA) in the process called (transamination, transcription).

11. At the (lysosome, ribosome) of the cell, the codon in an mRNA molecule is used to attract the (anticodon, supercodon) of the tRNA molecule in order to bring (a carbohydrate, an amino acid) molecule into posi-tion for protein synthesis.

12. The control of protein synthesis can be exerted by a (repressor, detractor) protein that binds to the (stimulator, operator) gene and prevents this gene from stimulating the (protein, structural) gene.

http://microbiology.jbpub.com

The site features **eLearning,** an on-line review area that provides quizzes and other tools to help you study for your class. You can also follow useful links for in-depth information, read more MicroFocus stories, or just find out the latest microbiology news.

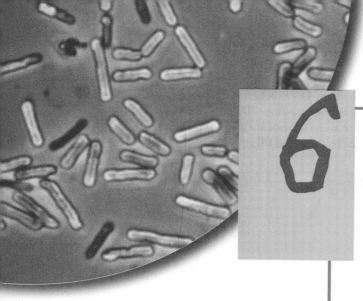

6 Bacterial Genetics

Genetic engineering is the most powerful and awesome skill acquired by man since the splitting of the atom.

—The editors of *Time* magazine describing the potential for genetic engineering

N THE MODERN ERA, when time is measured in minutes and seconds, our minds find it difficult to imagine the colossal 4.5 *billion* years that the Earth has been in existence. It may help, however, to think of Earth's history as a single year. In our "historic" year, the Earth was a Marslike, lifeless ball of rock until mid-July when bacteria, or something akin to bacteria, first appeared. These were the only creatures on Earth until mid-October, when multicellular organisms emerged. Not until the end of November did the first land plants come into being, and not until early December did animals move out of the sea onto the land. The dinosaurs were in existence from December 19 to December 25, and by December 27, the Earth bore a resemblance to modern Earth. Finally, on December 31, close to midnight, humans appeared.

We take this trek through geologic time to help us appreciate why bacteria have prospered genetically and in evolutionary terms. They have been successful primarily because they have been around the longest and have adapted well. Bacteria have been on Earth about 3.5 billion years (versus about 200,000 years for humans), as FIGURE 6.1 shows. During this time, gene changes have been occurring regularly and nature has used the bacteria to test its newest genetic traits. The "bad" traits have been eliminated (together with the bacteria unlucky enough to have them), while the "good" traits have thrived and have moved onto the next generation—and onto the present day.

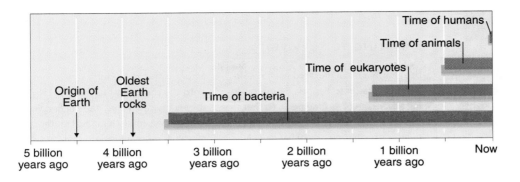

FIGURE 6.1

The Bacteria on Earth

This timeline shows the relative amounts of time that various groups of organisms have existed on Earth. The bacteria have been in existence for a notably longer period than any other group, particularly humans. They have adapted well to Earth simply because they have had the longest opportunity to adapt.

Modern bacteria, therefore, enjoy the fruits of genetic changes. Because of their diverse genes, bacteria can thrive everywhere, whether it be the snows of the Arctic or the boiling hot vents of the oceans. No other organism can compare to bacteria in sheer numbers—a pinch of rich soil has more bacteria than all the people living in the United States today. Finally, consider a bacterium's multiplication rate—a new generation every half hour—and it is easy to see how a useful genetic change (such as drug resistance) can be propagated quickly in a stressful environment (one containing a drug).

Any one of these factors—time on Earth, sheer numbers, multiplication rate—would be sufficient to explain how bacteria have evolved to their current form. When taken together, the factors help us appreciate why bacteria have done very well in the evolutionary lottery—very well, indeed.

In this chapter we shall study mutation and recombination, the two processes that have brought ancient bacteria to the myriad forms we observe on Earth today. **Mutation** (MicroFocus 6.1) is an alteration in the bacterial chromosome by a change in its DNA, whereas **recombination** is a chromosomal alteration by the acquisition of new DNA from another organism. The two processes are the major subdivisions of bacterial genetics.

Included under the umbrella of bacterial genetics is the topic of **genetic engineering** and **biotechnology**, collectively one of the most extraordinary technological advances of all time. Genetic engineering enables molecular biologists to treat genes almost as playthings—isolating them, altering them, inserting them into fresh organisms, and watching to see what they will do. The fruits of this technology have been awe-inspiring, and we have only begun to see what is possible. Thus, we shall devote a substantial portion of the chapter to exploring the accomplishments and future of genetic engineering. It is but one of the many practical applications of bacterial genetics.

Genes: segments of DNA that provide the biochemical code for protein synthesis.

Mutation: a permanent change for good or ill in the DNA of an organism.

Recombination: a change in an organism's DNA resulting from the acquisition and incorporation of another organism's genes.

MicroFocus 6.1

MUTATING TO SURVIVE?

Giraffes got their long necks by stretching into treetops for food when they were starving. Right? "Of course not," you say. "That's the theory of acquired characteristics. It was suggested by Lamarck long before Charles Darwin explained how evolution really works. According to Darwin, long-necked animals just happen to exist in a mixed population, and when food at ground level is scarce, they survive because they can feed higher up in the trees. And everyone knows Darwin was right."

Well, maybe not everyone. Many scientists believe that mutations (and hence, evolution) are not passive Darwinian events. Instead, they point to evidence indicating that bacteria undergo mutations when they are confronted with a stressful situation, and when mutation is in their own self-interest. For example, researchers suggest that antibiotic-resistant bacteria do not simply exist by random chance in a cell population; rather, they spring into being when the population finds itself immersed in an antibiotic. Taken to the extreme, this theory would hold that

the giraffe is not a mutated animal waiting for a disaster to happen before taking advantage of its long neck. Rather, the giraffe did not even exist until the disaster struck; then an animal quickly underwent a mutation to lengthen its neck and become a giraffe.

This is not easy stuff for a biologist to accept, and admittedly, the evidence is not overwhelming. But for bacteria, the body of support is mounting. In 1988, John Cairns at the Harvard School of Public Health performed experiments in which he altered the genes of *E. coli* so it could not use lactose as an energy source. Then he placed the bacteria in a starvation medium where they needed lactose to survive and reproduce. Cairns found that some bacteria corrected the alteration and mutated back to the original form so they could use the lactose. And they passed the beneficial gene on to their descendents.

Cairns' experiments were expanded in 1995 by university researchers who pinpointed the lactose gene mutation on the F-plasmid used in bacterial conjugation. This discovery provides a glimpse of how the mutated gene passes

among different bacteria and latches onto the chromosome. Then, in 1997, studies indicated that starving *E. coli* cells can accumulate survival mutations, as well as other mutations that provide no apparent survival advantages. In other words, the bacteria mutate to meet the threat of starvation and, almost as a bonus, mutate to form genes for other, unrelated situations. These results contradict the purest definition of the adaptive mutation theory (i.e., that stressed cells accumulate useful mutations), but they reinforce the idea that under stress, bacteria undergo mutations to boost their chances of survival. (They also show how chance mutations can indeed exist in a population—the Darwinian idea.)

So, did the starving giraffe really get its long neck by mutating when a disaster struck? And are we on the threshold of a radically new idea about evolution? Will the molecular system observed in bacteria hold true for more complex organisms? Stay tuned. This fascinating story can only get better.

6.1

The Bacterial Chromosome

esh'er-ik'e-a

Most of the genetic information in a bacterial (or prokaryotic) cell is contained within the **chromosome**, a single molecule of DNA arranged as a double helix, usually in a closed loop. The chromosome exists freely in the cytoplasm in a space called the **nucleoid**, without the surrounding membrane or histone protein support found in eukaryotic cells (FIGURE 6.2). In *Escherichia coli*, it occupies about half of the total volume of a bacterial cell, and when extended its full length, it is about 1.5 millimeters (mm) long. This is approximately 1500 times the length of the bacterium that contains it. The tight packing accounts in part for the explosive release of DNA when the membrane of the cell is broken. The eukaryotic chromosome is compared to the bacterial (prokaryotic) chromosome in TABLE 6.1. It would be helpful to review the chemical structure of DNA in Chapter 2 before proceeding too far in this chapter.

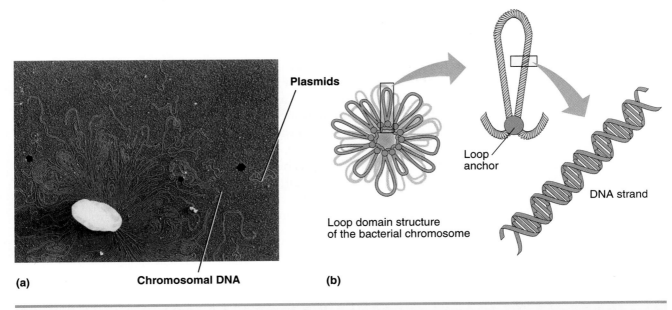

Plasmids

Chromosomal DNA

(a)

Loop anchor

DNA strand

Loop domain structure of the bacterial chromosome

(b)

FIGURE 6.2

Bacterial DNA

(a) An electron micrograph of an *E. coli* cell immediately after disruption. The tangled mass is the organism's DNA. Changes in the DNA occurring through mutation and recombination have helped the bacteria adapt to most environments on Earth. (b) The loop domain structure of the chromosome, as seen head-on. The loops in DNA help account for the compacting of a large amount of DNA in a relatively small bacterial cell.

TABLE 6.1

Characteristics of Prokaryotic (Bacterial) and Eukaryotic Chromosomes

PROKARYOTIC (BACTERIAL) CHROMOSOME	EUKARYOTIC CHROMOSOME
Replicates just prior to binary fission	Replicates just prior to mitosis
Single molecule of DNA per genetic trait (haploid)	Two molecules of DNA per genetic trait (diploid); some organisms haploid
Closed loop	Linear
No protein present	Histone protein present
No dominance or recessiveness in genes	Genes may be dominant or recessive or codominant
Organized at the nucleoid	Organized in the nucleus with a nuclear membrane
No introns present	Introns present
DNA also in plasmids	DNA also in mitochondria and other organelles
Mutations occur in DNA	Mutations occur in DNA
Genetic recombinations occur	No genetic recombinations occur
4000 genes in *E. coli* chromosome	100,000 genes in total of human chromosomes
About 1 mm in length	Tens or hundreds of millimeters in length
Replicates by semiconservative method Rolling circle method occurs	Replicates by semiconservative method No evidence of rolling circle method

The chromosome of the intestinal bacterium *E. coli* has probably been studied more thoroughly than any other single chromosome. Distributed around the chromosome are individual sites to which genetic activity can be traced. Each site, called a **locus** (pl., loci), consists of one or several genes for that activity. The chromosome of *E. coli* has about 4000 genes. Some viruses, by contrast, have as few as seven genes, while human chromosomes have a total of over 100,000.

How a 1.5 mm long chromosome could fit into a 1.0 μm *E. coli* cell was poorly understood until 1998, when scientists reported that the chromosome exists in a **loop domain structure**. In this structure, chromosomal regions attach to one another at anchorage points existing at intervals of about 50,000 bases. An overall "flower" structure results, as shown in Figure 6.2b. At present, the elements forming the anchors of the loops remain unknown. This structure is quite different than the histone-containing nucleosome structure associated with eukaryotic chromosomes.

REPLICATION OF THE CHROMOSOME

The bacterial chromosome replicates just prior to the process of binary fission. At the beginning of the replication sequence, the DNA is usually anchored to a particular point on the cell membrane. The double helix then unwinds, and enzymes synthesize a new strand of DNA for each of the original strands. This is accomplished by joining together nucleotides whose bases complement bases in the original strand. One of the important enzymes, **DNA polymerase**, was discovered by **Arthur Kornberg**, a corecipient of the 1959 Nobel Prize in Physiology or Medicine. Each new strand then combines with a parent strand, and the replicated DNA twists to reform the double helix. This combination of new and parent strands was first observed in *E. coli* in 1958 by **Matthew J. Meselson** and **Franklin W. Stahl**. It is called the **semiconservative method of replication** because one strand of the parent DNA is conserved in the new DNA molecule and one strand is newly synthesized. Unfortunately, if a mutation has occurred and is not corrected, the replication process will propagate the mutation.

The semiconservative method accounts for DNA replication, but it does not shed light on how a closed loop chromosome replicates. This problem perplexed microbiologists until 1962, when **John Cairns** and his coworkers clarified some of the details of the process.

Cairns' experiments showed that DNA unwinds at a fixed point, whereupon an enzyme nicks the closed loop at a site called the **origin of replication**. The two strands now separate, or "unzip," to establish a V-shaped replicating fork, as FIGURE 6.3 shows. Synthesis of DNA then occurs along the sides of the fork. In later years microbiologists established that along one side, DNA is manufactured by the continuous assembly of nucleotides, beginning at the origin. However, along the other side, synthesis begins at the point of forking and proceeds in a discontinuous fashion (Figure 6.3). Here the DNA is synthesized in a series of segments that later join with the help of an enzyme called DNA ligase. The segments came to be known as **Okazaki fragments**, after Reiji Okazaki, who discovered them in 1968. Each of the new DNA strands then combines with a parent strand, as Meselson and Stahl postulated.

A second type of DNA replication is called the **rolling circle mechanism**. This process takes place in bacteria undergoing the mating process of conjugation. While one strand of DNA remains in a closed loop, an enzyme nicks the other strand. The broken strand then "rolls off" the loop and serves as a template for synthesis of a DNA strand complementary to itself. When the two strands combine, a double helix

DNA polymerase:
an enzyme used in the synthesis of DNA from a series of nucleotides.

o-ka-zak'-e

Conjugation:
a mating process in which DNA passes from one bacterium to another after they have joined together.

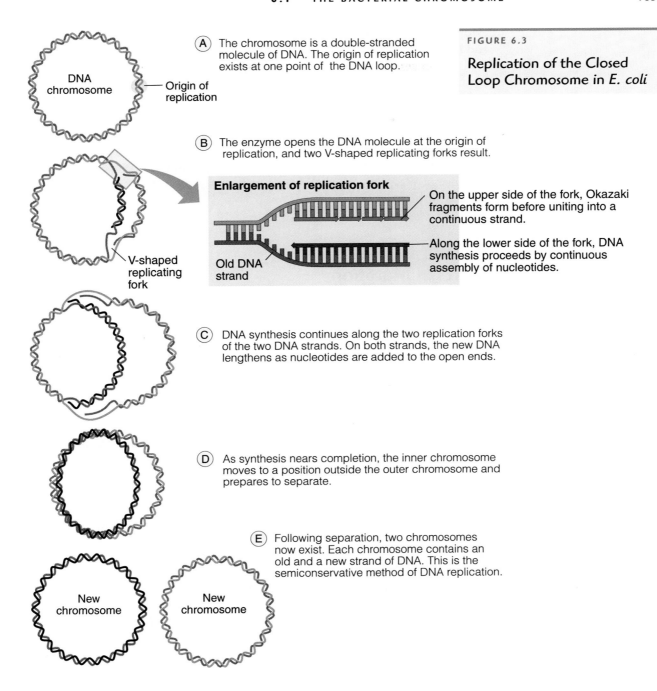

FIGURE 6.3

Replication of the Closed Loop Chromosome in *E. coli*

(A) The chromosome is a double-stranded molecule of DNA. The origin of replication exists at one point of the DNA loop.

DNA chromosome

Origin of replication

(B) The enzyme opens the DNA molecule at the origin of replication, and two V-shaped replicating forks result.

Enlargement of replication fork

On the upper side of the fork, Okazaki fragments form before uniting into a continuous strand.

Along the lower side of the fork, DNA synthesis proceeds by continuous assembly of nucleotides.

Old DNA strand

V-shaped replicating fork

(C) DNA synthesis continues along the two replication forks of the two DNA strands. On both strands, the new DNA lengthens as nucleotides are added to the open ends.

(D) As synthesis nears completion, the inner chromosome moves to a position outside the outer chromosome and prepares to separate.

(E) Following separation, two chromosomes now exist. Each chromosome contains an old and a new strand of DNA. This is the semiconservative method of DNA replication.

New chromosome

New chromosome

reforms. Meanwhile the intact loop revolves 360 degrees and serves as a template for a strand of DNA complementary to itself. The loop combines with its new strand to form a second double helix. The bacterium now has two chromosomes, one of which will be used in mating.

PLASMIDS

Some microorganisms contain genetic material in closed loops of DNA called **plasmids**. Plasmids exist apart from the chromosome as independent units in the

Plasmid:
a self–replicating closed loop of DNA in the cytoplasm of a cell.

cytoplasm. They contain about 2 percent of the total genetic information of the cell and multiply independently of the chromosome.

Plasmids are not essential to the life of the cell, but they may confer selective advantages for those organisms that have them. For example, some plasmids called **R factors** ("resistance" factors) carry genes for antibiotic resistance, while other plasmids allow bacteria to transfer their genetic material to receptive cells in recombination processes. Still other plasmids contain genes for the production of **bacteriocins**, a group of proteins toxic to other bacteria, and other genes code for toxins that affect human cells and processes. Gram-negative bacteria are notable for the presence of plasmids. We shall have much to say about these extrachromosomal units as we proceed in this chapter.

R factors:
plasmids that carry genes, which confer antibiotic resistance on a bacterium.

bak-te're-o'sinz

6.2

Bacterial Mutation

The information in a bacterial chromosome may be altered through a permanent change in the DNA called a **mutation**. In most cases a mutation involves a disruption of the nitrogenous base sequence in the DNA molecule or the loss of significant parts of a gene. Often this leads to the production of a miscoded messenger RNA molecule (Chapter 5) and the insertion of one or more incorrect amino acids into protein molecules during synthesis. Since proteins govern virtually all activities of a cell, it follows that a mutation will alter the cell's biochemical functions. Some alterations have little effect, but others may be significant, such as when a bacterium loses its ability to produce a toxin or changes its chemistry. Micro-Focus 6.2 explains such an instance.

MicroFocus 6.2

THREE GENES

Could the Black Death of the fourteenth century have resulted from three defective genes? Could 25 million Europeans have succumbed to plague because of three genes? Could the entire course of Western civilization have turned on three genes?

Possibly so, maintain researchers from the federal Rocky Mountain laboratory in Montana. In 1996, a research group led by Joseph Hinnebush reported that three genes in the plague bacillus are not present in a harmless form of the organism. And it is possible that the entire story of plague's pathogenicity revolves around these three genes.

The scenario goes like this: Bubonic, septicemic, and pneumonic plague are caused by *Yersinia pestis*, a rod-shaped bacterium transmitted by the rat flea. When the flea is infected, the bacteria amass in its foregut and obstruct its gastrointestinal tract. Soon the flea is starving, and it starts biting humans and rodents uncontrollably and feeding on their blood. During the bite, the flea regurgitates the mass of bacteria in the bloodstream and spreads the plague.

The three genes enter the picture at the very beginning. It appears that nonpathogenic plague bacilli have genes encouraging them to remain harmlessly in the midgut of the flea

(although scientists are not sure why this happens). Pathogenic plague bacilli, by contrast, do not have the genes, and they migrate to the foregut and form a plug of packed bacilli; these are the organisms that pass on to the next plague victim.

Sometimes it is dangerous to oversimplify matters, and this may be one of those times. Still, scientists are inclined to reduce concepts to their least common denominators. And if the tragic Black Death reduces to three genes, then so be it.

SPONTANEOUS MUTATIONS

Spontaneous mutations are mutations that take place in nature without human intervention or identifiable cause. It has been estimated that one such mutation may occur for every 10^6 to 10^{10} replications of a bacterium. This implies that in a colony of a billion (10^9) bacteria, at least one mutant may be present.

Spontaneous mutation: a mutation that takes place in nature without an identifiable cause.

In the normal course of events, cells arising from a spontaneous mutation are masked by normal cells. However, should a selective agent be introduced, the mutant may survive, multiply, and emerge. For many decades, for example, doctors have used penicillin to treat gonorrhea. Since 1976, however, a penicillin-resistant strain of *Neisseria gonorrhoeae*, the gonorrhea organism, has been emerging in human populations. Many investigators believe that the resistant strain arose by spontaneous mutation at some unknown time, perhaps centuries ago, and as penicillin gradually eliminated susceptible strains, the resistant strain filled the niche. An equally disturbing problem has been encountered with antibiotic-resistant *Salmonella* strains.

ni-se're-ah

INDUCED MUTATIONS

Most of the information gathered on mutation has come from **induced mutations**, where the cause can be identified. Occasionally these mutations occur by accident. More often they result from planned experiments in which laboratory scientists subject bacteria to chemical or physical agents. The agents are referred to as **mutagens**. Experiments in molecular genetics reveal that a broad variety of induced mutations may arise, depending on the type of mutagen used.

Induced mutation: an experimental mutation in which a cause can be identified.

Mutations arising from treatment with **ultraviolet light** are among the best understood (FIGURE 6.4). Ultraviolet light is a form of energy not perceived by the human eye. When this energy is absorbed by DNA, it induces adjacent thymine (or cytosine) molecules to link together. The DNA thus loses its ability to insert adenine

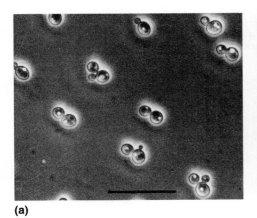
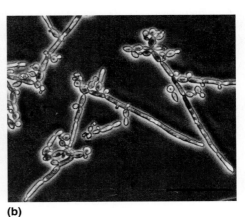

(a)   (b)

FIGURE 6.4

Two Morphological Forms of *Candida albicans*

Phase-contrast micrographs of the agent of yeast infections in humans. (a) The oval yeast form commonly seen in vaginal infections. (b) The filamentous moldlike form often observed in invaded tissue. (Bar = 40 μm.) In 1990, investigators demonstrated that the yeast form of *C. albicans* could be converted to the moldlike form by treating the organism with nitrous acid and ultraviolet light, thereby mutating its genetic material.

ser-a'she-ah mar-ses'ens

hi'po-zan'thēn

(or guanine) bases in mRNA molecules during protein synthesis. Ultraviolet light is sometimes used for disinfection purposes because it quickly kills bacteria. In the Gram-negative rod *Serratia marcescens*, ultraviolet light induces mutations that prevent the organism from forming its normal red pigment.

Nitrous acid, another mutagen, converts DNA's adenine molecules to hypoxanthine molecules. Adenine will normally be complemented by thymine during DNA replication, but hypoxanthine is complemented by cytosine. Later, when protein synthesis takes place, the new DNA codes for guanine in the mRNA instead of the normal adenine (FIGURE 6.5a).

Mutations can also be induced by a series of **base analogs**. These are substances bearing a chemical resemblance to nitrogenous bases. One example, 5-bromouracil, is taken up by cells and incorporated into DNA where thymine should be positioned (FIGURE 6.5b). The new DNA functions poorly with the analog in place. In the treatment of diseases caused by DNA viruses, a base analog is valuable because nucleic acid directs viral replication, and a virus with a functionless DNA molecule cannot replicate. The drug acyclovir is a base analog that works against herpesviruses.

Other mutations involve the **deletion** or **insertion** of a nucleotide into the DNA molecule. Such a mutation is caused by benzopyrene, which is present in industrial soot and smoke, and aflatoxin, a fungal toxin found in certain animal products and foods. Substances such as benzopyrene and aflatoxin do not themselves become part of the DNA molecule, but they cause the deletion or insertion of extra nucleotides during replication. This may lead to a **frameshift mutation** because the genetic code

FIGURE 6.5

Mutations in Bacteria

(a) Nitrous acid causes induced mutations in bacteria. (b) Base analogs induce mutations by substituting for nitrogenous bases in the synthesis of DNA. Note the similarity in chemical structure between thymine and the base analog 5-bromouracil.

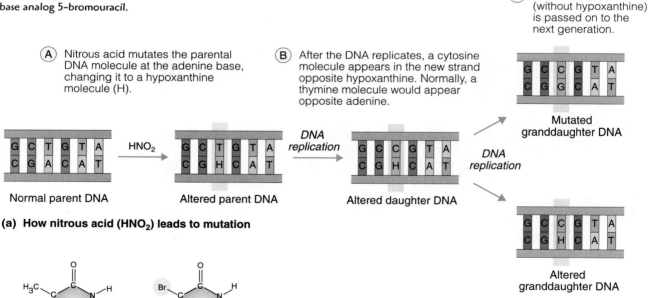

Ⓐ Nitrous acid mutates the parental DNA molecule at the adenine base, changing it to a hypoxanthine molecule (H).

Ⓑ After the DNA replicates, a cytosine molecule appears in the new strand opposite hypoxanthine. Normally, a thymine molecule would appear opposite adenine.

Ⓒ The mutated DNA (without hypoxanthine) is passed on to the next generation.

Ⓓ The mutated DNA (with hypoxanthine) is also passed on.

Normal parent DNA → HNO₂ → Altered parent DNA → DNA replication → Altered daughter DNA

Mutated granddaughter DNA

Altered granddaughter DNA

(a) How nitrous acid (HNO₂) leads to mutation

Thymine   5-bromouracil

(b) A nitrogenous base and its mutation-causing analog

MicroFocus 6.3

"MAKE THOSE REPAIRS—PLEASE!"

As any homeowner knows, failure to repair the plumbing or fix the electrical wiring or patch the roof can make a day miserable. One would imagine that the same holds true for a bacterium. Unfortunately, the misery is often inflicted on its host.

Consider *Escherichia coli*. Before 1982, *E. coli* O157:H7 apparently was not recognized. Then this pathogenic strain emerged, and ever since, it has been a source of intestinal nightmares: the Jack-in-the-Box outbreak of 1993 (Chapter 3), thousands of Japanese people sick in 1996 from eating contaminated radish sprouts, and several recent incidents of severe diarrhea traced to unpasteurized apple cider.

Scientists believe that the new strain of *E. coli* can invade tissues and produce toxins unlike the traditionally harmless

E. coli. To do so, it must have genes that the traditional *E. coli* does not have. It is reasonably safe to assume that mutations in the chromosomal DNA brought about these new genes. But, scientists have wondered, why weren't the mutations corrected or discarded?

Researchers from the U.S. Food and Drug Administration (FDA) think they have an answer. It all goes back to the repair mechanism, they say. Led by Thomas Cebula, FDA microbiologists examined numerous "new" strains of pathogens and compared their proteins to nonpathogenic strains of the same organism. In 1996, the researchers reported their findings: The new pathogens lack the repair enzymes available in harmless strains. They simply cannot repair the faulty DNA sometimes produced during DNA replication.

Ordinarily, the new DNA would be corrected, but if the repair enzymes are lacking, the defective DNA remains. And, if the DNA encodes a toxin or protein that encourages tissue invasion, then the harmless bacterium becomes a pathogen.

For many years, health officials believed that microbial pathogens had been brought under control, but their thinking has changed. Indeed, emerging pathogens such as *E. coli* O157:H7 are humbling reminders that bacteria can reinvent themselves and undergo a swift evolution as they adapt to new hosts, new conditions, and new pharmaceutical countermeasures. Something to think about as you figure out how to repair the plumbing.

is modified, and the wrong mRNA is encoded beyond the point of mutation. A protein with an incorrect amino acid sequence results.

REPAIR MECHANISMS

Over the course of its existence, the DNA of a bacterial cell (indeed, of every prokaryotic and eukaryotic cell) undergoes a form of molecular punishment. Thousands of bases are lost regularly, and mutations occur during replication processes and on exposure to the environment. The cell maintains its DNA by using a diverse array of **DNA repair enzymes** that literally patrol the DNA, locating and repairing alterations and distortions. (It's somewhat like driving with a mechanic in the back seat.) MicroFocus 6.3 explains what may happen if repair is not effected.

One type of repair mechanism is called **mismatch repair**. In this case, a repair enzyme called DNA polymerase "proofreads" the DNA synthesis it has just catalyzed and removes nucleotides that it incorrectly placed in the new DNA strand. Scientists estimate that about 1 in 10,000 bases is incorrectly placed and subject to replacement.

When DNA is damaged by physical or chemical mutagens, an enzyme known as nuclease performs **damage repair**. Almost 100 different forms of nuclease are known to exist in *E. coli* cells. They cut out (excise) the damaged DNA and insert nucleotides that properly complement nucleotides in the undamaged strand. Damage repair is alternately known as **excision repair**. In 1998, Texas A&M researchers reported that plasmids are apparently the site of genes that encode excision repair enzymes. They discovered that when the number of plasmids increases, the damage due to ultraviolet light is repaired significantly faster.

TRANSPOSABLE GENETIC ELEMENTS

Insertion sequence:
a segment of DNA that forms copies that move elsewhere on the chromosome.

Mutations of a different nature may be caused by fragments of DNA called **transposable genetic elements**. Two types are known: insertion sequences and transposons. **Insertion sequences** are small segments of DNA with about 1000 base pairs. They are found at one or more sites on the bacterial chromosome and appear to have no genetic information other than for the ability to insert into a chromosome (as we shall see during our discussion of conjugation). Insertion sequences form copies of themselves, and the copies move into other areas of the chromosome. Here they interrupt the coding sequence, thereby inducing the wrong protein or no protein to form. Insertion sequences may be a prime force behind spontaneous mutation.

Transposon:
a segment of DNA that carries functional genes from one chromosomal location to another.

Within recent decades, scientists have learned much about the second type of transposable genetic elements—**transposons**. These are the so-called "jumping genes" for which **Barbara McClintock** won the 1983 Nobel Prize in Physiology or Medicine (MicroFocus 6.4). First identified and named in 1974 by British microbiologists R.W. Hedges and A.E. Jacobs, transposons are larger than insertion sequences and carry information for protein synthesis. Like insertion sequences, they interrupt the genetic code.

MicroFocus 6.4

JUMPING GENES

In the early 1950s, scientists assumed that genes were fixed elements, always found in the same position on the same chromosome. But in 1951, Barbara McClintock unveiled her research with corn plants at a symposium at Cold Spring Harbor Laboratory on Long Island, New York. McClintock described genes that apparently move from one chromosome to another. The audience listened in respectful silence. There were no questions after her talk, and only three people requested copies of her paper.

Like Gregor Mendel 100 years before, McClintock kept close watch over color changes in her plants. Whereas Mendel cultivated peas, however, McClintock grew Indian corn, or maize. In the 1940s she noticed curious patterns of pigmentation on the kernels. Other scientists might have missed the patterns as random variations of nature, but McClintock's record-keeping and careful analysis revealed a method to nature's madness. The pigment genes causing the splotches of color appeared to be switched on or off in particular generations. Still more remarkable, the

"switches" seemed to occur in a later generation at different places along the same chromosome. Some switches even showed up in different chromosomes. Such "controlling elements," as McClintock called them, were available whenever needed to turn the genes on or off.

In the modern lexicon of molecular genetics, McClintock's elements are recognized as a two-gene system. One is an activator gene, the other a dissociation gene. The activator gene, for reasons unknown, can direct a dissociation gene to "jump" along the arm of the ninth chromosome in maize plants where color is regulated. When the jumping gene reinserts itself, it turns off the neighboring pigmentation genes, thereby altering the color of the kernel.

The jumping gene is identical to the transposon found in bacteria. It may cause important mutations and gene rearrangements. Many scientists suspect that jumping genes play significant roles in the development of a fertilized egg into a mature organism, while serving as a driving force in evolution.

For Barbara McClintock, recognition came 30 years after that symposium at

Cold Spring Harbor. In 1981 (at the age of 79) she received eight awards, among them a $60,000-a-year lifetime grant from the MacArthur Foundation and the $15,000 Lasker prize. In 1983, she was awarded the Nobel Prize in Physiology or Medicine. When informed of the Nobel award, she replied to an interviewer's question that "it seemed unfair to reward a person for having so much pleasure over the years, asking the maize plants to solve specific problems and then watching their response."

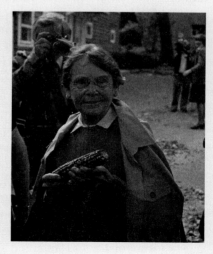

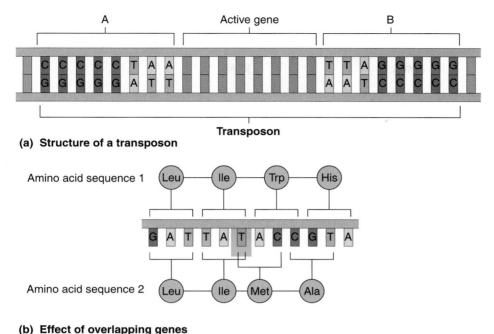

(a) Structure of a transposon

(b) Effect of overlapping genes

FIGURE 6.6

Stimulants of Mutation

(a) The structure of a typical transposon. This transposon contains one or more active genes bordered by inverted repetitive sequences. Note that the base sequence in A is the reverse and complement of the base sequence in B. Such a situation is called a palindrome. Also note the presence of inverted repetitive base sequences (C–G and G–C) at the ends of the transposon. (b) The effect of overlapping genes. The single-stranded DNA provides the genetic code for two amino acid sequences. Below the DNA strand, the base sequence for the third amino acid (Met) includes thymine, a base from the previous base sequence. A mutation at the thymine (shaded) would thus change two base codes.

The movement of transposons appears to be nonreciprocal, meaning that an element moves away from its location and nothing takes its place. (This contrasts with insertion sequences, where copies move.) Transposons move from plasmid to plasmid, from plasmid to chromosome, or from chromosome to plasmid. The presence of inverted repetitive base sequences at the ends of the element (FIGURE 6.6a) appears to be important in establishing the ability to move.

Of particular significance is the finding that many transposons contain genes for antibiotic resistance. If the plasmid containing the transposon moves from one bacterium to the next, as plasmids are known to do, the transposon will move along with it, thus spreading the genes for antibiotic resistance among bacteria. Moreover, the movement of transposons among plasmids help explain how a single plasmid acquires numerous genes for resistance to different antibiotics.

OVERLAPPING GENES

For years scientists assumed that a mutation in a gene affects the production of a single protein. However, **Frederick Sanger**'s 1977 work indicated otherwise. Sanger determined the entire nucleotide sequence of a viral DNA molecule and mapped its 5386 bases. Analysis of the DNA by Sanger's coworkers showed that at least four of the genes are overlapping, as shown in FIGURE 6.6b. This implies that an individual triplet of bases might code for two different amino acids. Thus, a mutation at a base could affect not one amino acid but two, and, in effect, not one protein, but two. In 1958, Sanger had won the Nobel Prize in Chemistry for sequencing the amino acids in insulin. In 1980, he shared a second Nobel Prize in Chemistry for mapping the bases of the viral DNA.

THE AMES TEST

Some years ago, scientists observed that about 90 percent of the agents causing cancer in humans also induce mutations in bacteria. Working on this premise,

Cancer:
a condition characterized by the uncontrolled growth and multiplication of cells.

FIGURE 6.7

Using the Ames Test

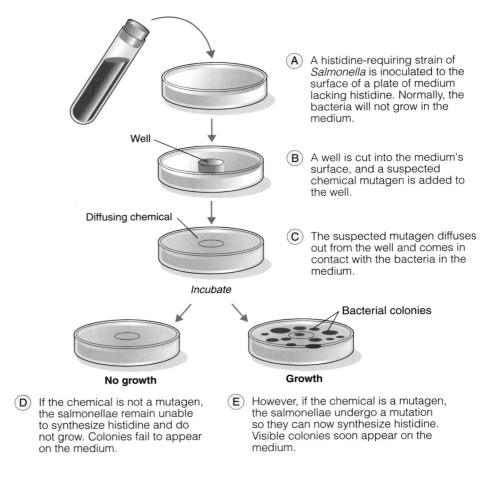

(A) A histidine-requiring strain of *Salmonella* is inoculated to the surface of a plate of medium lacking histidine. Normally, the bacteria will not grow in the medium.

Well

(B) A well is cut into the medium's surface, and a suspected chemical mutagen is added to the well.

Diffusing chemical

(C) The suspected mutagen diffuses out from the well and comes in contact with the bacteria in the medium.

Incubate

Bacterial colonies

No growth

Growth

(D) If the chemical is not a mutagen, the salmonellae remain unable to synthesize histidine and do not grow. Colonies fail to appear on the medium.

(E) However, if the chemical is a mutagen, the salmonellae undergo a mutation so they can now synthesize histidine. Visible colonies soon appear on the medium.

Histidine:
one of 20 amino acids found in proteins.

Bruce Ames of the University of California developed a procedure to help identify an agent of cancer by determining whether it can mutate bacteria. The procedure, called the **Ames test**, is a widely used, relatively inexpensive, rapid, and accurate screening test.

To perform the Ames test, a technician inoculates a histidine-requiring strain of *Salmonella typhimurium* onto a plate of bacteriological medium lacking histidine. Normally this strain of *Salmonella* will not grow in the medium because the gene inducing histidine synthesis is mutated and hence not active. Now the potential cancer agent is added to the medium, and the plate is incubated. If bacterial colonies appear, one may conclude that the agent mutated the bacterial gene so it could encode the enzyme needed for histidine synthesis. Because the agent is a mutagen, it is therefore a possible cause of cancer. If bacterial colonies fail to appear, one assumes that no mutation took place (FIGURE 6.7). However, it is possible that a mutation occurred, then was repaired by a DNA repair enzyme.

To this point . . .

We have surveyed the bacterial chromosome, a single molecule of DNA arranged as a closed loop, which exists free in the cytoplasm without a surrounding membrane or protein support. The chromosome replicates by the semiconservative method when the bacterium is undergoing binary fission, or by the rolling circle method when conjugation is taking place. Small loops of DNA called plasmids exist apart from the DNA and are key players in conjugation and genetic engineering, as we shall see presently.

The discussion then turned to mutation, a process in which the chromosome is altered through a permanent change in the DNA. We compared spontaneous mutations, which take place in nature without human intervention, to induced mutations, which usually occur under laboratory conditions. Various types of induced mutations illustrated how changes in DNA can be brought about by different mutagens. Possible mutagens include insertion sequences and transposons. These fragments of DNA slot into areas of gene activity, thereby changing the genetic code and inducing a chromosome or plasmid alteration. The concept of overlapping genes was mentioned to show how a mutation may affect more than one gene, and the Ames test was discussed to illustrate how mutations are used for practical benefit.

We shall now turn our attention to bacterial recombination. In this remarkable process of bacterial genetics, two organisms are involved in the transfer of DNA, and an alteration of the genetic material occurs. We shall examine three processes: transformation, conjugation, and transduction. In transformation, an organism acquires DNA from its extracellular environment; in conjugation, two organisms come together and DNA passes from one bacterium to the other; and in transduction, a virus transports DNA between bacteria. Research in this area has many applications to clinical medicine. Moreover, an understanding of bacterial recombination led to the process of genetic engineering, as we shall see later in the chapter.

6.3

Bacterial Recombination

The second general method for altering the genetic material of a bacterium is through the process of **recombination**. Although some scientists consider mutation a form of recombination, we shall use recombination in the more restricted sense to mean the genetic process in which two organisms are involved: a **donor cell** and a **recipient cell**. The donor cell contributes chromosomal DNA or plasmid DNA to the recipient cell. If plasmids are obtained, they exist independently in the recipient's cytoplasm and begin to multiply and encode proteins immediately. If the recipient obtains chromosomal DNA, the new DNA pairs with a complementary region of recipient DNA and replaces it. Thus, there is no change in quantity of the recipient's DNA, but there may be a substantial change in its quality.

Microbiologists have identified three methods for bacterial recombination: transformation, conjugation, and transduction. We shall examine each in turn.

TRANSFORMATION

In 1928, an English bacteriologist named **Frederick Griffith** published the results of an interesting set of experiments with *Streptococcus pneumoniae*. This organism is a major cause of bacterial pneumonia; the bacterium is often referred to as a pneumococcus (pl., pneumococci). At Griffith's time, the experimental results were considered unusual, but in retrospect, microbiologists note that they gave some of the first clues to gene activity.

Pneumococci occur in different strains. There are encapsulated strains, designated S, because the organisms grow in smooth colonies. These strains cause pneumonia.

Pneumonia:
an infectious disease of the lungs, due to several types of microorganisms, including bacteria.

S strain pneumococci:
those that form smooth colonies and are pathogenic.

R strain pneumococci:
those that form rough colonies and are nonpathogenic.

Pathogenic:
able to cause disease.

There is also an unencapsulated strain, designated R, because the colonies are rough. Organisms in this strain are harmless. In an early experiment, Griffith showed that mice injected with living S strain pneumococci die, while those injected with living R strain pneumococci live. This was what he expected. Also, he showed that mice injected with dead S strain organisms live (FIGURE 6.8). Again, this result was not unusual.

What happened next puzzled Griffith. He mixed heat-killed, dead **S strain** bacteria with live **R strain** bacteria and let the mixture incubate; then he injected the mixture into mice. The mice died. Griffith wondered how a mixture of live harmless bacteria (R) and debris from pathogenic bacteria (S) could kill the mice. His answer came when he autopsied the animals: they were full of live S strain pneumococci. Apparently the live R strain bacteria had been transformed to live S strain bacteria. Though he could not understand how this happened, he published his results and continued his research.

Five years later (1933), James L. Alloway of the Rockefeller Institute in New York confirmed Griffith's work. Alloway used fragments and debris from the dead S strain cells to transform the R strain cells. However, it was not until 1944 that

---

FIGURE 6.8

The Transformation Experiments of Griffith

Griffith's experiments were among the first to demonstrate bacterial transformation and the transfer of genetic information.

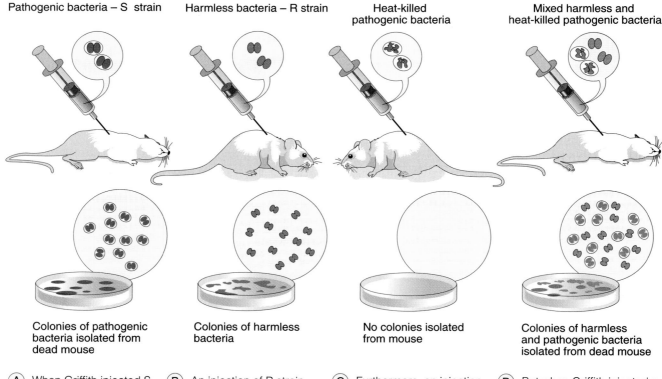

Pathogenic bacteria – S strain   Harmless bacteria – R strain   Heat-killed pathogenic bacteria   Mixed harmless and heat-killed pathogenic bacteria

Colonies of pathogenic bacteria isolated from dead mouse   Colonies of harmless bacteria   No colonies isolated from mouse   Colonies of harmless and pathogenic bacteria isolated from dead mouse

(A) When Griffith injected S strain (encapsulated, pathogenic) bacteria into the mouse, it developed pneumonia and died.

(B) An injection of R strain (unencapsulated, harmless) bacteria did no harm to the mouse. This was as Griffith anticipated.

(C) Furthermore, an injection of heat-killed S strain bacteria did no harm because the bacteria were dead.

(D) But when Griffith injected a mixture of live R strain and heat-killed S strain bacteria into the mouse, it died. When Griffith cultivated bacteria from the blood, he found live S strain bacteria.

Oswald T. Avery and his associates **Colin M. MacLeod** and **Maclyn N. McCarty**, also of the Rockefeller Institute, purified and identified the transforming substance. These investigators found that the substance was not protein, as had been anticipated, but a then-obscure organic compound called **deoxyribonucleic acid (DNA)**.

The majority of scientists were blind to Avery's discovery and were reluctant to accept DNA as a hereditary substance. Geneticists of that period were not trained as chemists, and Avery's experiments were difficult to repeat. Also, many scientists believed that experimental results from bacteria could not necessarily be applied to eukaryotes. Moreover, preoccupation with World War II had restricted the dissemination and flow of scientific knowledge. Not until the 1950s was DNA widely accepted as the molecule of heredity and transformation as a concept of bacterial recombination.

Modern scientists regard **transformation** as an important recombination method even though it takes place in less than 1 percent of a bacterial population. In transformation, a number of donor cells break apart and explosively release fragments of DNA. A segment of double-stranded DNA containing about 10 to 20 genes then passes through the cell wall and membrane of a **recipient cell**, as shown in FIGURE 6.9. After entry to the recipient cell, an enzyme degrades one strand of the DNA,

Eukaryotes:
complex organisms such as plants and animals whose cells have a nucleus and organelles.

Transformation:
the uptake of DNA from the local environment by a competent recipient bacterium.

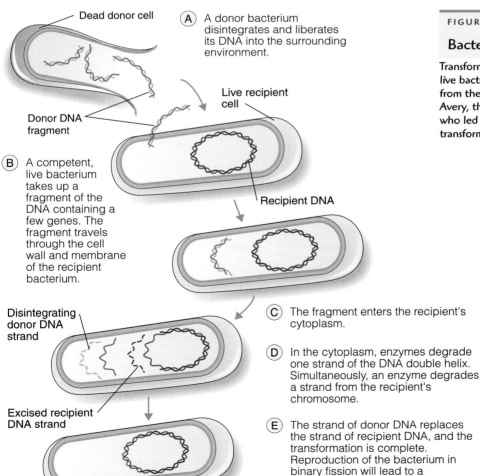

A donor bacterium disintegrates and liberates its DNA into the surrounding environment.

(A) **Dead donor cell** — **Live recipient cell** — **Donor DNA fragment**

(B) A competent, live bacterium takes up a fragment of the DNA containing a few genes. The fragment travels through the cell wall and membrane of the recipient bacterium. — **Recipient DNA**

(C) The fragment enters the recipient's cytoplasm. — **Disintegrating donor DNA strand** — **Excised recipient DNA strand**

(D) In the cytoplasm, enzymes degrade one strand of the DNA double helix. Simultaneously, an enzyme degrades a strand from the recipient's chromosome.

(E) The strand of donor DNA replaces the strand of recipient DNA, and the transformation is complete. Reproduction of the bacterium in binary fission will lead to a population of transformed bacteria.

Transformed recombinant cell

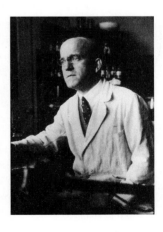

FIGURE 6.9

Bacterial Transformation

Transformation is the process in which a live bacterium acquires DNA fragments from the environment. Pictured is Oswald Avery, the Rockefeller Institute investigator who led the effort to identify DNA as the transforming principle.

leaving the second strand to displace a segment of DNA from the recipient's chromosome. The displaced DNA is degraded by another enzyme in the cell. Transformation may also take place by the reception of plasmids, in which case no chromosomal DNA is displaced. MicroFocus 6.5 describes experiments that precisely located the insertion point for the new DNA.

Competence:
the ability of a bacterium to take up DNA from the extracellular environment.

The ability of a cell to be transformed depends on its **competence**, defined as the ability of a recipient bacterium to take up DNA from the environment. Competence is an intriguing property that varies among bacteria. For example, in *Streptococcus pneumoniae*, competence is displayed in the entire cell population late in the logarithmic phase of growth when a competence-provoking factor is produced. By contrast, *Bacillus* species exhibit competence during the early events leading to spore formation. Sometimes competence does not develop at all.

Factors affecting the cell surface are important to competence, particularly changes in **membrane permeability** or **surface receptors**. The uptake of DNA by *E. coli*, for example, can be induced in the laboratory by chilling bacteria to 4°C in the presence of calcium chloride, then quickly heating them to 42°C. This treatment apparently alters the membrane and encourages the passage of DNA strands. Competent streptococci and *Bacillus* cells have approximately 50 surface receptors where DNA can bind before uptake.

Under natural conditions, transformation takes place in organisms whose DNA is very similar to the DNA being received, which generally implies cells of the same species. The process has been observed in the species mentioned above, as well as in *Haemophilus*, *Neisseria*, and *Azotobacter* species.

he-mof'il-us
ah-zo'to-bak'ter

One of the effects of transformation is to increase an organism's pathogenicity. In pneumococci, for example, the acquisition of genes for capsule formation

---

MicroFocus 6.5

PROGRAMMING YOUR VCR

To the great majority of people, VCR stands for video cassette recorder. But to Julian Davies and his coworkers at the University of British Columbia, VCR has a much more scientific meaning—*Vibrio cholerae* repeating sequences.

Davies is a molecular microbiologist. In 1998, he reported his research on the repeating sequences in DNA of the cholera bacillus *Vibrio cholerae*. Repeating sequences are a type of genetic stutter; that is, stretches of DNA whose nitrogenous bases follow an identifiable pattern of repetition (e.g., note the five-base repeat in GTGGAGTGGAG-TGGA . . .). Scientists have long known that repeating sequences border the genes for antibiotic resistance that insert into transformed bacteria. But Davies

and his group performed experiments demonstrating that the sequences flank locations where other acquired genes insert as well. They extracted a *Vibrio cholerae* gene and its adjacent repeating sequences and inserted the combination (a VCR cassette) into a plasmid. Then they forced the plasmid into *E. coli* cells and noted that the gene inserted into the recipient's DNA at a predetermined site. Soon the *V. cholerae* gene was expressing itself by encoding an identifiable protein.

The research evidence points up the possibility that acquired genes wind up at the same location in a recipient bacterium, regardless of whether they are antibiotic-resistance genes, toxin genes, adhesion genes, or any other genes. If so, the findings would improve the working

model for how bacteria acquire genes to enhance their virulence (virulent *E. coli* strains are an example); or how bacteria acquire resistance to numerous antibiotics (multidrug resistant *Staphylococcus aureus*, for instance); or how transformations in general take place.

Molecular geneticists have a name for the insertion site: the integron. They also have a name for the enzyme that inserts genes into the integron: integrase. Now they have an idea of where to find the integron and the site of integrase activity for all genes acquired by the cell: Just look for repeating sequences flanking the insertion site.

For Davies, the work with VCR was fruitful and significant. Finally he could go home and catch a good movie. Where? On his VCR, of course.

allows an organism to avoid body defenses and cause disease, as Griffith showed. Microbiologists have also demonstrated that when mildly pathogenic strains of bacteria take up DNA from other mildly pathogenic strains, there is a cumulative effect, and the degree of pathogenicity increases. Observations such as these may help explain why very aggressive strains of bacteria appear from time to time. Transformed bacteria may also display enhanced drug resistance as a result of the acquisition of R factors. Pigment production may be another characteristic derived through transformation.

How significant is transformation as a means of genetic recombination under natural conditions? No one knows for sure, but it appears certain that transformation occurs regularly where bacteria exist in crowded conditions, such as in rich soil or the human intestinal tract.

CONJUGATION

In the recombination process called **conjugation**, two live bacteria come together, and the donor cell transfers genetic material to the recipient cell. This process was first observed in 1946 by **Joshua Lederberg** and **Edward Tatum** in a series of experiments with *E. coli*. Lederberg and Tatum mixed two different strains of bacteria and found that genetic traits could be transferred among them if contact occurred. The investigators shared the 1958 Nobel Prize in Physiology or Medicine for their work.

Experiments in the 1950s by **William Hayes, François Jacob**, and **Elie L. Wollman** established that conjugating bacteria are of two mating types. Certain "male" types donate their DNA. These are designated **F⁺ cells**. Other "female" types receive the DNA and are known as **F⁻ cells**. Jacob and Wollman found that F⁻ cells (recipients) became F⁺ cells (donors) when they acquire a small amount of DNA. Their work eventually led Hayes to discover the **F (fertility) factors** present in the donor cell. Although the male and female nomenclature is occasionally used today, the process of bacterial conjugation is fundamentally different from sexual mating, since the mechanisms of DNA incorporation are very different.

zhah-kob'

In contemporary microbiology, the donor's F factors are known to be **plasmids**, the double-stranded loops of DNA existing apart from the chromosome. The factors (plasmids) contain about 20 to 30 genes, most of which are associated with conjugation. These genes encode enzymes that replicate DNA during conjugation and structural proteins needed to synthesize special pili at the cell surface. Known as **F pili** or **sex pili**, these hairlike fibers contact the recipient bacteria, then retract so that the surfaces of donor and recipient are very close or touching one another. At the area of contact, a channel or conjugation bridge is believed to form.

F factor:
a plasmid that functions in conjugations among bacteria.

Once contact via sex pili has been made, the F factor (plasmid) begins replicating by the rolling circle mechanism discussed earlier. A single strand of the factor then passes over or through the channel to the recipient. When it arrives, enzymes synthesize a complementary strand, and a double helix forms. The double helix bends to a loop and reforms an F factor (plasmid), thereby completing the conversion of the recipient from F⁻ cell to F⁺ cell. Meanwhile, back in the donor cell, a new strand of DNA forms to complement the leftover strand of the F plasmid.

F pili:
short hairlike fibers of protein that connect donor and recipient cells during conjugation.

The transfer of F factors involves no activity of the bacterial chromosome; therefore, the recipient does not acquire new genes other than those on the F factor. A type of conjugation that accounts for the passage of chromosomal material does exist in bacteria, however. Strains of bacteria that exhibit the ability to donate chromosomal genes are called **high frequency of recombination**, or **Hfr strains**. Such strains were discovered in the 1950s by William Hayes in *E. coli*.

Hfr strain:
a strain of bacteria in which chromosomal material passes to a recipient during conjugation.

In Hfr strains, the F factor attaches to the chromosome. This attachment is a rare event that requires an insertion sequence to recognize the F factor. At the attachment point, the chromosome opens and one strand replicates itself by the rolling circle mechanism. A portion of the new DNA then passes into the recipient cell, where it replaces a similar region in the recipient chromosome, as **FIGURE 6.10** illustrates.

During conjugation, the first genes to enter the recipient are the F factor genes. But these are not the ones that determine whether the organism is a donor or recipient. Rather, the last genes control the donor state, and these rarely enter the recipient, partly because conjugation is usually interrupted by movements that break the attachment. Indeed, an estimated 100 minutes is required for the transfer of a complete *E. coli* chromosome. Thus, the F⁻ cell usually remains a recipient, although it now has new genes from the donor.

FIGURE 6.10

Conjugation in Bacteria

The conjugation shown here is between an Hfr cell and a recipient cell.

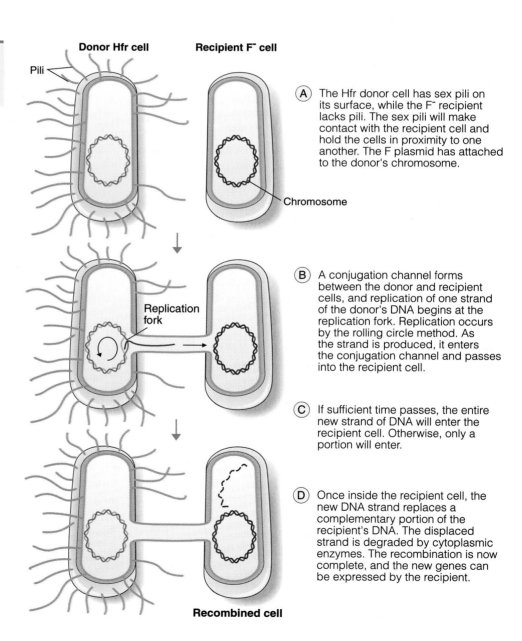

Donor Hfr cell   **Recipient F⁻ cell**

Pili

Chromosome

(A) The Hfr donor cell has sex pili on its surface, while the F⁻ recipient lacks pili. The sex pili will make contact with the recipient cell and hold the cells in proximity to one another. The F plasmid has attached to the donor's chromosome.

Replication fork

(B) A conjugation channel forms between the donor and recipient cells, and replication of one strand of the donor's DNA begins at the replication fork. Replication occurs by the rolling circle method. As the strand is produced, it enters the conjugation channel and passes into the recipient cell.

(C) If sufficient time passes, the entire new strand of DNA will enter the recipient cell. Otherwise, only a portion will enter.

(D) Once inside the recipient cell, the new DNA strand replaces a complementary portion of the recipient's DNA. The displaced strand is degraded by cytoplasmic enzymes. The recombination is now complete, and the new genes can be expressed by the recipient.

Recombined cell

But in certain cases, the entire chromosome is transferred to the recipient. When this happens, the F factor usually detaches from the chromosome, and enzymes synthesize a strand of complementary DNA. The F factor now forms a loop to assume an existence as a plasmid, and the recipient becomes a donor cell (an F$^+$ cell).

Occasionally, in an Hfr cell, the F factor breaks free from the chromosome and resumes an independent status. The Hfr cell then reverts to an F$^+$ cell. Sometimes when the F factor leaves the chromosome, it takes along a fragment of chromosomal DNA. The factor with its extra DNA is now called an **F′ factor** (pronounced "F-prime"). When the F′ factor is transferred during a subsequent conjugation, the recipient acquires some chromosomal genes excised from the donor. This process, known as **sexduction**, results in a recipient with its own genes for a particular process, as well as additional genes from the donor for that same process. In the genetic sense, the recipient is a partially diploid organism because there are two genes for a given function.

Conjugation has been demonstrated to occur between cells of various genera of bacteria (in contrast to transformation, which appears to occur only among cells of the same species). For example, conjugation occurs between such Gram-negative bacteria as *Escherichia* and *Shigella*, *Salmonella* and *Serratia*, and *Escherichia* and *Salmonella*. **Intergenic transfer**, as the process is known, has great significance in the transfer of antibiotic-resistance genes carried on plasmids. (MicroFocus 6.6 describes one case with serious medical overtones.) Moreover, when the genes are attached to

Diploid:
having two sets of genes for a particular trait.

ser-a'she-ah

MicroFocus 6.6

TRANSFERABLE DRUG RESISTANCE

In 1968, an extremely serious form of bacterial dysentery broke out in Guatemala. Dysentery is a disease of the human intestine characterized by tissue erosion and considerable fluid loss. The responsible bacterium, *Shigella dysenteriae*, resisted treatment with chloramphenicol, tetracycline, streptomycin, and sulfanilamide, any one of which is normally used in therapy. In the three years that the epidemic raged, 100,000 people were infected and 12,000 died.

This particular outbreak of drug-resistant dysentery points up the consequences of what could happen when antibiotic treatment is stifled by resistant bacteria. How *Shigella* may have acquired the resistance was first shown in the 1950s in a remarkable set of experiments by a Japanese team of investigators.

The story began in 1955 when a Japanese woman suffered a case of

dysentery caused by bacteria resistant to the same quartet of drugs observed years later in Guatemala. Doctors at Tokyo University, led by Tomoichiro Akiba, investigated the case and found that drug-resistant *Shigella* strains were fairly widespread in Japan. They also noted a surprising coincidence: Patients with drug-resistant *Shigella* also had in their intestine a strain of *Escherichia coli* with resistance to the same four drugs. Since simultaneous mutations were highly unlikely, researchers postulated that the resistance had been transferred between organisms.

Akiba and his colleagues devised a series of experiments to test this hypothesis. They mixed liquid suspensions of drug-resistant *E. coli* with laboratory-reared drug-sensitive *Shigella dysenteriae*. Then they carefully isolated and tested the *Shigella*. The results were startling: *Shigella* was now resistant to

the same drugs as *E. coli*. A transfer had indeed taken place.

In the following years, numerous studies verified transferable drug resistance, and R factor plasmids were identified as the medium of transfer. Epidemics such as that in Guatemala soon broke out elsewhere, as drug-resistant bacteria began appearing in different human populations. By the 1990s, microbiologists had identified resistance in such diverse organisms as streptococci, gonococci, leprosy and tuberculosis bacilli, and malaria parasites. In the 1980s, an article in *Discover* magazine described a Detroit epidemic caused by a drug-resistant strain of *Staphylococcus aureus*. The strain was quickly dubbed "super staph," and the headline was an eye-grabbing "Bugs That Won't Die." Transferable drug resistance had made the popular media.

transposons, the transposons may "jump" from ordinary plasmids to F factors, after which transfer may occur.

Gram-positive bacteria also appear capable of conjugation. Microbiologists have experimented extensively with *Streptococcus mutans*, a common cause of dental caries. In this organism, conjugation appears to involve only plasmids, particularly those carrying genes for antibiotic resistance. Moreover, the conjugation does not involve pili. Rather, the recipient cell apparently secretes substances encouraging the donor cell to produce **clumping factors** composed of protein. The factors bring the donor and recipient cells together, and pores form between the cells to permit plasmid transfer. Similar observations have been made in *Bacteroides* and *Clostridium* species. To this point, chromosomal transfer has not been demonstrated. (TABLE 6.2 compares conjugation to the other two types of recombination.)

bak'ter-oi'dez
klo-strid'e-um

TRANSDUCTION

Bacterial recombination by the process of **transduction** was first reported in 1952 by **Joshua Lederberg** and **Norton Zinder**. While working with *Salmonella* cells, Lederberg and Zinder observed recombination, but ruled out conjugation and transformation because the cells were separated by a thin membrane and DNA was absent in the extracellular fluid. Eventually, they discovered a **virus** in the fluid and uncovered the details of what was taking place.

bak-te're-o-faj'
Bacteriophage:
a virus that attacks bacteria.

The virus that participates in transduction is called a **bacteriophage**, or simply **phage** (FIGURE 6.11). Though invisible at the time, the activity of a bacteriophage (literally "bacteria-eater") was described in 1915 by Frederick Twort and two years later by Felix d'Herelle. Bacteriophages (phages) were originally assumed to be a type of poison because they dissolve bacteria (Chapter 11). Today scientists recognize them as viruses composed of a core of DNA or RNA surrounded by a coat of protein. Phages that participate in transduction are called **transducing phages**. All the latter contain DNA. Figure 6.11 contains electron micrographs of phage particles.

Lytic cycle:
the process in which a phage replicates within a bacterium, thereby destroying the bacterium.

In the replication cycle of a bacteriophage, the phage interacts with bacteria in either of two ways. In one way, the phage invades the bacterium, then replicates itself and destroys the bacterium as new phages are released. This cycle is called the **lytic cycle** of infection because at its conclusion the invaded bacteria lyse, or rupture. Phages that cause lysis are known as **virulent phages**.

TABLE 6.2

A Comparison of Transformation, Conjugation, and Transduction

CHARACTERISTIC	TRANSFORMATION	CONJUGATION	TRANSDUCTION
Method of DNA transfer	Movement across wall and membrane of recipient	Through channel after cell-to-cell contact	By an intermediary virus
Amount of DNA transferred	Few genes	Few genes to entire chromosome	Few genes
Plasmid transferred	Yes	Yes	Not likely
Entire chromosome transferred	No	Sometimes	No
Virus required	No	No	Yes
Live bacteria required	Yes	Yes	Yes
Cell debris required	Yes	No	No
Used to acquire antibiotic resistance	Yes	Yes	Not likely

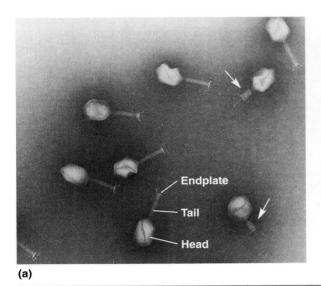

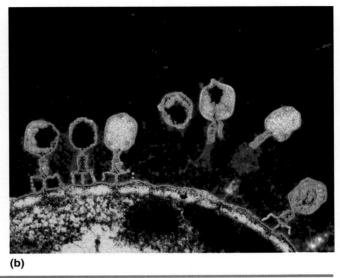

(a)   **(b)**

FIGURE 6.11

Bacteriophages

(a) A transmission electron microscope view of a T2 bacteriophage. Note that each bacteriophage is composed of a head and a tail with a complex endplate. In two cases (arrows), the tail is contracted and a core may be seen protruding. This structure penetrates the bacterial cell wall and membrane during viral replication. (b) Bacteriophages adsorbed to receptor sites on a bacterial cell. Note the relative sizes of the viruses and the bacterium.

The second way that phages interact with bacteria also involves invasion of the bacterium. In this case, however, the phage DNA encodes a repressor protein that inhibits replication. The phage DNA may remain in the cytoplasm as a plasmid, or it may form a closed circle, align next to the bacterial chromosome, and integrate into the bacterial chromosome (as the F factor does in Hfr strains). This process is called **lysogeny**. The phage that participates in lysogeny is known as a **temperate phage**, and the integrated viral DNA is called a **prophage**. Because there are two forms of phage interaction with bacteria, there are two ways in which phages can be involved in the transfer of bacterial genes: generalized transduction and specialized transduction.

Generalized transduction is carried out by virulent phages that have a lytic cycle of infection (**FIGURE 6.12**). During phage replication a long, linear chain of DNA is first produced. It is then enzymatically cut into fragments that will become phage DNAs. During this process, segments of bacterial DNA may accidentally get caught up in the cutting process, and bacterial segments may end up in phages where phage fragments should be. This event is considered rare (1 in every 100,000 new phages may have bacterial DNA). Such a phage is fully formed but carries no phage genes. It cannot encode its own replication.

Now the transduction takes place. The transducing phage is released along with all the other normal phages, and it attaches to a new (recipient) bacterium and injects its bacterial DNA. Once released in the recipient, the new genes pair with a section of the recipient's DNA and replace the section. The recipient has now been transduced (changed) using genes from the donor bacterium and the phage intermediary. Two examples of transducing phages are phage P1, which infects *E. coli*, and P22 which infects *Salmonella typhimurium*.

Specialized transduction occurs as a result of **lysogeny**, the process in which DNA from the phage incorporates into the chromosomal DNA of the bacterium (**FIGURE 6.13**). The site of incorporation (insertion site) may vary for different

Lysogeny:
the process in which a phage incorporates into a bacterium and does not replicate itself or destroy the bacterium.
Prophage:
viral genes integrated into a bacterial chromosome.
Generalized transduction:
transduction in which phages carry random fragments of donor DNA into a recipient cell.

Specialized transduction:
transduction in which phages carry selected segments of DNA from the chromosome of a donor cell into a recipient cell.

ti'fe-mur'e-um

FIGURE 6.12

Generalized Transduction

During generalized transduction, a virus carries random DNA fragments from a donor bacterium to a recipient bacterium. The latter is thus recombined.

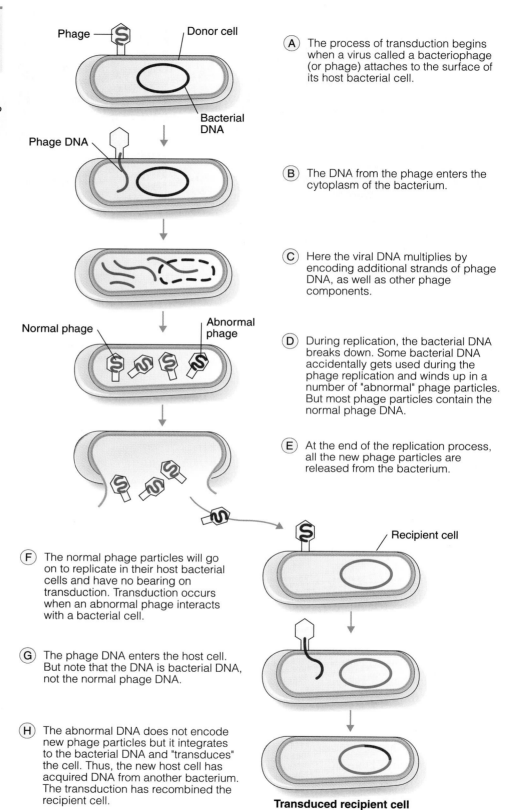

(A) The process of transduction begins when a virus called a bacteriophage (or phage) attaches to the surface of its host bacterial cell.

(B) The DNA from the phage enters the cytoplasm of the bacterium.

(C) Here the viral DNA multiplies by encoding additional strands of phage DNA, as well as other phage components.

(D) During replication, the bacterial DNA breaks down. Some bacterial DNA accidentally gets used during the phage replication and winds up in a number of "abnormal" phage particles. But most phage particles contain the normal phage DNA.

(E) At the end of the replication process, all the new phage particles are released from the bacterium.

(F) The normal phage particles will go on to replicate in their host bacterial cells and have no bearing on transduction. Transduction occurs when an abnormal phage interacts with a bacterial cell.

(G) The phage DNA enters the host cell. But note that the DNA is bacterial DNA, not the normal phage DNA.

(H) The abnormal DNA does not encode new phage particles but it integrates to the bacterial DNA and "transduces" the cell. Thus, the new host cell has acquired DNA from another bacterium. The transduction has recombined the recipient cell.

Transduced recipient cell

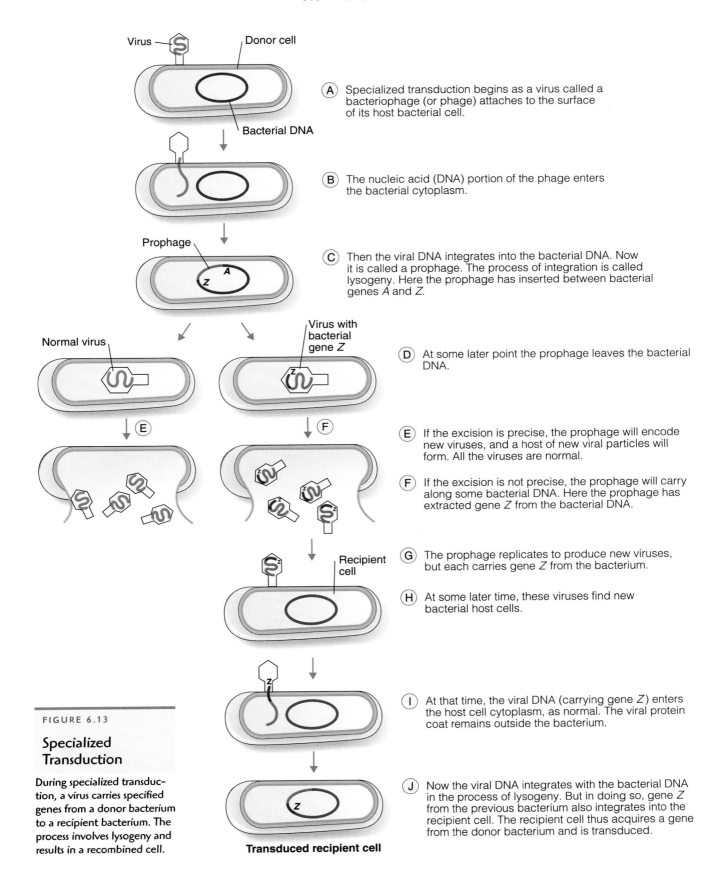

A   Specialized transduction begins as a virus called a bacteriophage (or phage) attaches to the surface of its host bacterial cell.

B   The nucleic acid (DNA) portion of the phage enters the bacterial cytoplasm.

C   Then the viral DNA integrates into the bacterial DNA. Now it is called a prophage. The process of integration is called lysogeny. Here the prophage has inserted between bacterial genes *A* and *Z*.

D   At some later point the prophage leaves the bacterial DNA.

E   If the excision is precise, the prophage will encode new viruses, and a host of new viral particles will form. All the viruses are normal.

F   If the excision is not precise, the prophage will carry along some bacterial DNA. Here the prophage has extracted gene *Z* from the bacterial DNA.

G   The prophage replicates to produce new viruses, but each carries gene *Z* from the bacterium.

H   At some later time, these viruses find new bacterial host cells.

I   At that time, the viral DNA (carrying gene *Z*) enters the host cell cytoplasm, as normal. The viral protein coat remains outside the bacterium.

J   Now the viral DNA integrates with the bacterial DNA in the process of lysogeny. But in doing so, gene *Z* from the previous bacterium also integrates into the recipient cell. The recipient cell thus acquires a gene from the donor bacterium and is transduced.

FIGURE 6.13

Specialized Transduction

During specialized transduction, a virus carries specified genes from a donor bacterium to a recipient bacterium. The process involves lysogeny and results in a recombined cell.

phages and is often a region where an insertion sequence is located. In this situation, phage genes are actually integrating into the sequence of bacterial genes rather than replacing bacterial genes (as in transformation). In the integrated state, the set of phage genes is called a **prophage**, as noted previously, and the bacterium carrying the prophage is said to be **lysogenic**.

At some time in the future, a mutagen such as UV light or a DNA inhibitor activates an enzyme complex that excises the prophage out of the bacterial chromosome and causes it to reenter the lytic cycle. Most of the time the excision occurs precisely and an intact set of phage genes (prophage) is released. Sometimes, however, an imprecise excision occurs, and the excised prophage takes along bacterial genes while leaving behind some phage genes. At the conclusion of the replication, multiple copies of the phage, each with some bacterial genes, are produced.

Because the phage nucleic acid is missing some essential genes, the phage resulting from the lytic cycle is defective. It can infect another bacterium and transfer its genes to a recipient, but the genes cannot encode a lytic cycle. Instead, the genes integrate into the bacterial chromosome, carrying the donor's bacterial genes with them. As before, the recipient bacterium has acquired genes from the original bacterium and the recipient is now considered transduced, as Figure 6.13 shows.

Generalized transduction and specialized transduction are summarized and compared in TABLE 6.3.

Specialized transduction is an extremely rare event in comparison to the generalized form, because genes do not easily break free from the bacterial chromosome. However, the potential for recombination is substantial because lysogeny with prophages has been well established in clinical microbiology. For example, the diphtheria bacillus, *Corynebacterium diphtheriae* harbors a prophage that provides the genetic code for a toxin that destroys human cells. Other toxins encoded by prophages include staphylococcal enterotoxins in food poisoning, clostridial toxins in some forms of botulism, and streptococcal toxins in scarlet fever. Also, *Salmonella* cells carry prophages that encode lipopolysaccharides in the outer membrane. These lipopolysaccharides provide the basis for separating *Salmonella* into serological types (serotypes) rather than species.

ko-ri'ne-bac-te're-um
dif-the're-a

Lipopolysaccharides: polysaccharides with lipid component.

TABLE 6.3

Generalized Transduction Compared to Specialized Transduction

GENERALIZED TRANSDUCTION	SPECIALIZED TRANSDUCTION
1. Viruses (phages) penetrate bacterial cell and enter lytic cycle.	1. Viruses (phages) penetrate bacterial cell and enter lysogenic cycle.
2. Viral DNA begins to replicate immediately in the bacterial cytoplasm.	2. Viral DNA incorporates into the DNA of the bacterium. Replication begins at a later time.
3. During replication, enzymes accidentally use some bacterial DNA to make new viruses.	3. During release from chromosome in replication, viral DNA accidentally excises some bacterial DNA to make new viruses.
4. Any bacterial genes are randomly packaged into new viruses.	4. Bacterial genes adjacent to previously incorporated virus are packaged into new viruses.
5. Some new viruses have bacterial DNA and no viral DNA.	5. Some new viruses have both viral DNA and bacterial DNA.
6. Transducing viruses enter recipient bacterium.	6. Transducing viruses enter recipient bacterium.
7. Donor bacterial genes are incorporated into chromosome of new bacterium.	7. Donor bacterial genes are incorporated into chromosome of new bacterium together with transducing viruses.

Certain viruses are known to remain in human body cells for years, expressing themselves at unspecified intervals. The viruses of herpes simplex, infectious mononucleosis, and chickenpox are examples. In addition, many tumor viruses are believed to associate with human chromosomes and transform the normal cell to a tumor cell. Such viruses may be considered types of prophages, and the ability to transduce human cells under clinical conditions may be analogous to what is taking place in bacterial recombination.

To this point . . .

We have described how the genetic material of a bacterium may be altered by mutation and by three forms of recombination processes. Our study of the first form, transformation, began with Griffith's classic experiment that revealed a genetic alteration, and followed with Avery's isolation of DNA. We then moved to the modern era and described the conditions under which competent cells obtain DNA from the local environment and incorporate it into the bacterial chromosome. In the second method, conjugation, we observed how two organisms come together and enable DNA to move from the donor cell to the recipient cell. The importance of the F factor was highlighted, and the Hfr strain was described. Plasmid transfer is common in conjugation, but chromosomal transfer is a rare event.

In the third type of recombination, transduction, a virus functions as an intermediary between cells. We began by describing the lytic cycle of viral replication and contrasted this with lysogeny. We then explained how in generalized transduction, the virus may randomly incorporate segments of bacterial DNA to itself and carry the genes to the next cell when lysogeny is established. This process contrasts with specialized transduction, where bacterial genes are excised from the chromosome with the prophage and replicated along with the virus. Some practical applications of transduction were noted.

In the final section, we shall focus on experiments that alter bacterial DNA in the process of genetic engineering. This is where the knowledge from bacterial genetics is applied to the insertion of foreign genes to bacteria. We shall see how the process emerged and how the modern applications of genetic engineering yield products to enhance the quality of life.

6.4

Genetic Engineering

Experiments in bacterial recombination entered a new dimension in the late 1970s, when it became possible to insert genes into bacterial DNA and thereby establish a cell line that would produce proteins according to the instructions of microbiologists. The use of basic research to solve practical problems had far-reaching ramifications, and an entirely new industry, **genetic engineering**, emerged.

THE HISTORY OF GENETIC ENGINEERING

The first glimmer of interest in genetic engineering surfaced in the 1960s with the discovery and isolation of a group of bacterial enzymes called **endonucleases**. These enzymes, also called **restriction enzymes**, cleave phosphate-sugar bonds in the backbone of nucleic acids, and they could be used to open a bacterial chromosome. Their existence was first postulated by **Werner Arber** when he noted bacterial

Endonucleases: enzymes that cleave sugar-phosphate bonds in nucleic acids. Restriction enzymes: endonucleases that act at restricted sites on a DNA molecule.

enzymes scissoring the DNA of a virus at selected spots. **Hamilton Smith** subsequently isolated a restriction enzyme from Gram-negative rod *Haemophilus influenzae.* In 1971, **Daniel Nathans** used Smith's enzyme to split the DNA of simian virus 40 (SV40), a cause of tumors in monkeys. In 1978, the Nobel Prize in Physiology or Medicine was awarded to the three scientists. By that time, over 100 different restriction enzymes had been isolated and characterized.

Among the first scientists to attempt a genetic manipulation was **Paul Berg** of Stanford University. In 1971, Berg and his coworkers opened the DNA molecule from the SV40 virus and spliced it to a bacterial chromosome. In doing so, they constructed the first **recombinant DNA molecule**. However, the process was extremely tedious because the bacterial and viral DNAs had blunt ends. Berg therefore had to utilize exhaustive enzyme chemistry to form staggered ends that would combine easily. Nevertheless, he achieved a momentous first and was later honored as a co-recipient (with Sanger and Walter Gilbert) of the 1980 Nobel Prize in Chemistry.

While Berg was performing his experiments in 1971, an important development came from **Herbert Boyer** and his group at the University of California. Boyer isolated a restriction enzyme that nicks a chromosome and leaves it with mortiselike staggered ends. The bits of single-stranded DNA extending out from the chromosome easily attached to a new fragment of DNA in recombinant experiments. Scientists quickly dubbed the single-stranded extensions "sticky ends."

During that same period, **Stanley Cohen,** also at Stanford University, was accumulating data on the plasmids of *Escherichia coli* (FIGURE 6.14). Cohen found that he could isolate plasmids from the bacterium and insert them into fresh bacteria by suspending the organisms in calcium chloride and heating them suddenly to achieve a transformation. Once inside *E. coli* cells, the plasmids multiply independently and produce copies of themselves. Cohen's data indicated that scientists need not work with the larger, less manageable chromosome.

The final link to the process was provided by the **DNA ligases**. These enzymes, known since the 1960s, function during the replication of DNA and the repair of broken DNA molecules. Essentially, they operate in a manner opposite that of endonucleases; they seal together DNA fragments.

Progress came rapidly. Working together, Boyer and Cohen isolated plasmids from *E. coli* and opened them with restriction enzymes (MicroFocus 6.7). Next they

Recombinant DNA:
a DNA molecule resulting from an alteration of its structure, such as the insertion of a DNA segment.

DNA ligase:
an enzyme that combines fragments of DNA.

MicroFocus 6.7

OF CORNED BEEF AND PLASMIDS

In 1972, they met at a scientific conference in Hawaii—Stanley Cohen and Herbert Boyer. Cohen was there to lecture about his work with plasmids, the submicroscopic loops of DNA in the bacterial cytoplasm. Boyer was an expert on a restriction enzyme that could cut DNA—any DNA—at a precise point. As he sat in the audience and listened to Cohen, Boyer's mind stirred. Could his enzyme cut Cohen's plasmid and allow a foreign piece of DNA to attach?

Scientific conferences are the last place to talk about science, so Boyer invited Cohen to lunch at a local delicatessen in Waikiki. The corned beef was good that day, and the sandwiches hit the spot. The deli mustard was biting hot, and the beer was ice cold. The time was ripe to talk history—and talk history they did. They would collaborate on a set of genetic engineering experiments, the ones that, in retrospect, revolutionized the science of molecular genetics. As the afternoon wore on, the ideas flowed and

the friendship took root. Only one thing about that historic lunch has remained a mystery: Who picked up the tab?

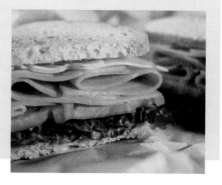

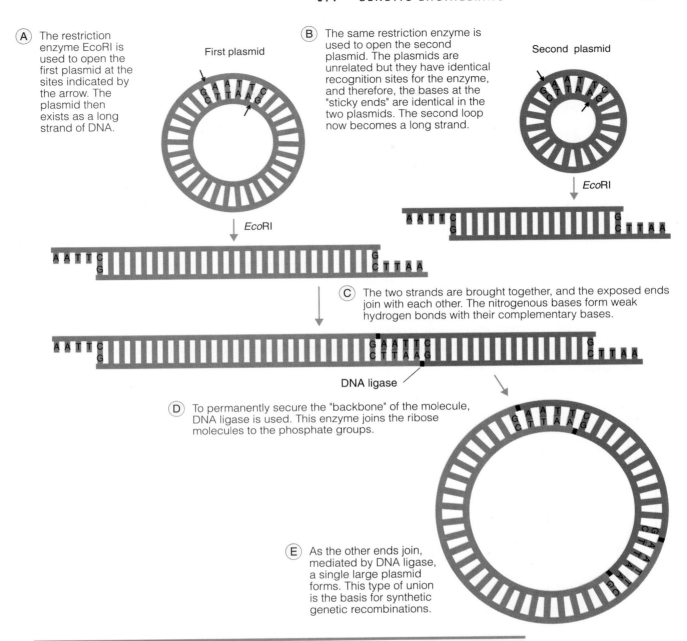

(A) The restriction enzyme EcoRI is used to open the first plasmid at the sites indicated by the arrow. The plasmid then exists as a long strand of DNA.

First plasmid

(B) The same restriction enzyme is used to open the second plasmid. The plasmids are unrelated but they have identical recognition sites for the enzyme, and therefore, the bases at the "sticky ends" are identical in the two plasmids. The second loop now becomes a long strand.

Second plasmid

*Eco*RI

*Eco*RI

(C) The two strands are brought together, and the exposed ends join with each other. The nitrogenous bases form weak hydrogen bonds with their complementary bases.

DNA ligase

(D) To permanently secure the "backbone" of the molecule, DNA ligase is used. This enzyme joins the ribose molecules to the phosphate groups.

(E) As the other ends join, mediated by DNA ligase, a single large plasmid forms. This type of union is the basis for synthetic genetic recombinations.

FIGURE 6.14

Construction of a Recombinant DNA Molecule

In this construction, two unrelated plasmids (loops of DNA) are united to form a single plasmid.

inserted a segment of foreign DNA using DNA ligase. Then they implanted the plasmids into fresh *E. coli*. By 1973, they had successfully spliced genes from *Staphylococcus aureus* into *E. coli*. The recombined plasmids were termed **chimeras** from the mythical lion-goat-serpent monster of Greek literature.

Genetic engineering experiments intrigued the scientific community because genes from widely divergent species could be spliced together. But there was the legal problem of who owns genetically altered bacteria. In the late 1970s, researchers engineered a strain of *Pseudomonas* to dissolve oil rapidly. They hoped to use the new bacteria to clean up oil spills. The question arose as to whether a patent could be obtained for the organism. Testimony was presented in the courts. Finally, in 1980, the U.S. Supreme Court ruled by a 5-to-4 vote that a patent could, indeed, be issued for the new organism.

MODERN APPLICATIONS

By the year 2000, thousands of companies worldwide were working on the industrial applications of genetic engineering and DNA technology, spurred in part by new technologies (**MicroFocus 6.8**). Some were research companies with special units for these studies, while others were established solely to pursue and develop new products by gene-splicing techniques.

PHARMACEUTICAL APPLICATIONS

Insulin:
a pancreatic hormone that assists the passage of glucose molecules from the blood into the cells, thereby preventing diabetes.

in'ter-fer'on
Interferon:
a naturally produced human protein that interferes with viral replication.

The pharmaceutical products of DNA are numerous and diverse. In 1986, the Eli Lilly company began marketing Humulin, a bacteria-produced form of human **insulin**. For decades, insulin had been obtained from the pancreas tissues of animals, a factor that accounted for occasional allergic reactions. With the advent of genetic engineering, the insulin could be produced by inserting "insulin genes" to bacterial plasmids and using bacteria such as *E. coli* as chemical factories (**FIGURE 6.15**).

Also during the 1980s, a genetically engineered form of **interferon** came into use. This antiviral drug (Chapter 11) is produced by genetically altered *E. coli* cells. Interferon has been approved for use against Kaposi's sarcoma (a type of cancer common in AIDS patients), malignant myeloma, and multiple myeloma. Research is continuing on the use of **antisense molecules** as therapeutic agents. Antisense molecules are fragments of nucleic acids that unite with and neutralize mRNA molecules carrying the genetic message for protein synthesis. To treat AIDS, for example, an antisense molecule would block the mRNA used for synthesis of new HIV particles (Chapter 13).

MicroFocus 6.8

CUSTOMIZED PROTEINS

Before chemist Michael Smith began tinkering with genes, mutation studies were hit-and-miss. Scientists would expose cells to a mutagen such as ultraviolet light, then forage among a crowd of mutated proteins, hoping to find a clue on where the mutation occurred. But Smith had a better idea: He would control the mutation at a particular site and see what the organism produced.

Smith began by splicing the single-stranded DNA of a gene into the single-stranded DNA of a virus. (The viral DNA would later act as a carrier for the gene DNA to transport it into a cell.) Then he synthesized a short strand of DNA complementary to the gene DNA, except at just one amino acid coding site (i.e.,

the mutation site). Next he combined this mutated strand with the normal gene. The new, short strand bound tightly to the gene, except at the one site where the mutation existed. (The effect is somewhat like having a zipper with a small opening in the middle .) Then Smith used an enzyme to complete the second strand—that is, the DNA complementary to the viral DNA. This formed a complete double-stranded DNA molecule.

Now the DNA molecule was inserted into fresh bacteria to see what would happen. Smith was pleased to note that the normal version of the gene was encoding a normal protein, while the mutated version of the gene encoded a mutated protein. A customized gene

was encoding a customized protein. He then set to work comparing the normal and new proteins.

Smith's work opened many new doors to microbial geneticists. For example, researchers could now determine whether a single amino acid mutation could induce a change in the function of the protein. In effect, does one amino acid influence a protein's activity? And if so, how? Moreover, they now could tailor enzyme proteins simply by adjusting the genetic code. Scientists were excited. They called the process site-directed mutagenesis. The Nobel Prize Committee had a better expression: Class A science. They awarded Smith a share of the 1993 Nobel Prize in Chemistry.

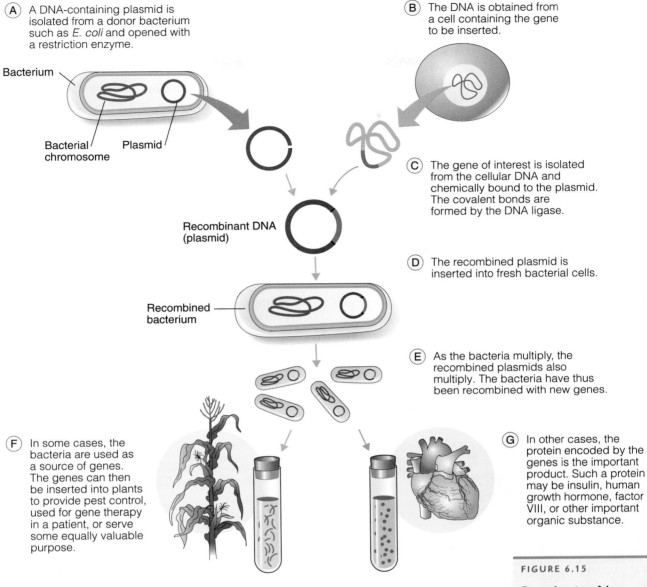

(A) A DNA-containing plasmid is isolated from a donor bacterium such as *E. coli* and opened with a restriction enzyme.

Bacterium

Bacterial chromosome   Plasmid

(B) The DNA is obtained from a cell containing the gene to be inserted.

(C) The gene of interest is isolated from the cellular DNA and chemically bound to the plasmid. The covalent bonds are formed by the DNA ligase.

Recombinant DNA (plasmid)

(D) The recombined plasmid is inserted into fresh bacterial cells.

Recombined bacterium

(E) As the bacteria multiply, the recombined plasmids also multiply. The bacteria have thus been recombined with new genes.

(F) In some cases, the bacteria are used as a source of genes. The genes can then be inserted into plants to provide pest control, used for gene therapy in a patient, or serve some equally valuable purpose.

(G) In other cases, the protein encoded by the genes is the important product. Such a protein may be insulin, human growth hormone, factor VIII, or other important organic substance.

FIGURE 6.15

Developing New Products Using Genetic Engineering

Genetic engineering is a method for inserting foreign genes into a bacterium and obtaining chemically useful products.

Gene engineers have also used the new biochemical methods to produce **human growth hormone**. In 1986, the genetically engineered form of this hormone became available as Protropin to treat pituitary dwarfism. (One child suffering from this disease grew five inches in a year.) By 1994, a type of synthetic **Factor VIII** was available for patients with hemophilia, and a protein called **tissue plasminogen activator (TPA)** was in use to dissolve blood clots. To prevent infectious diseases, physicians have a genetically engineered **vaccine** for hepatitis B, and research continues today on an AIDS vaccine using components produced in bacterial cells. Optimism is also high for innovative vaccines for cholera, malaria, and herpes simplex.

■ **AGRICULTURAL APPLICATIONS**   Genetic engineering has extended into many realms of science. In agriculture, for example, genes for herbicide resistance have been transplanted from bacteria into tobacco plants, demonstrating that plants can

Herbicide: a plant-killing chemical, often used to control weeds.

be engineered to better tolerate the herbicides used for weed control. For tomato growers, a notable advance was made in 1988 when researchers at Washington University spliced genes from a pathogenic virus into tomato plant cells and demonstrated that the cells would produce viral proteins at their surface. The viral proteins blocked viral encroachment and lent resistance to the tomato plants.

For gene transfer experiments in plants, the mechanism often used for transfer is a plasmid from *Agrobacterium tumefaciens*. This organism causes a plant tumor called crown gall, which develops when DNA from the bacterium inserts itself into the plant cell's chromosomes (**FIGURE 6.16**). Researchers remove the tumor-inducing gene, then splice the desired gene into the plasmid and allow the bacterium to infect the plant.

The **dairy industry** was the first to feel the dramatic effect of the new DNA technology. In the 1980s, for example, researchers at Cornell University injected dairy cows with bacteria-produced **bovine growth hormone** and reported a 41 percent increase in milk from the experimental cows. Also being researched is a pig with more meat and less fat, a product of genetically engineered porcine growth hormone. And in 1989, scientists at Auburn University endowed young carp with extra copies of activated growth hormone genes, hoping to enable the fish to grow more efficiently in aquacultural surroundings.

ag'ro-bak-te're-um
toom-e-fa'shens

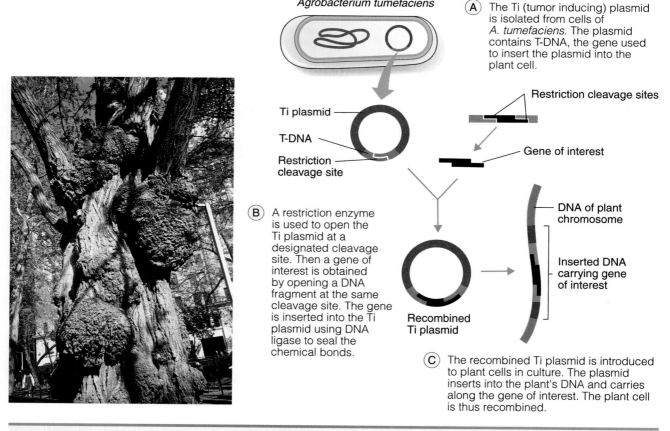

Agrobacterium tumefaciens

(A) The Ti (tumor inducing) plasmid is isolated from cells of *A. tumefaciens*. The plasmid contains T-DNA, the gene used to insert the plasmid into the plant cell.

Ti plasmid
T-DNA
Restriction cleavage site

Restriction cleavage sites
Gene of interest

(B) A restriction enzyme is used to open the Ti plasmid at a designated cleavage site. Then a gene of interest is obtained by opening a DNA fragment at the same cleavage site. The gene is inserted into the Ti plasmid using DNA ligase to seal the chemical bonds.

Recombined Ti plasmid

DNA of plant chromosome
Inserted DNA carrying gene of interest

(C) The recombined Ti plasmid is introduced to plant cells in culture. The plasmid inserts into the plant's DNA and carries along the gene of interest. The plant cell is thus recombined.

FIGURE 6.16

Agrobacterium tumefaciens as a Vector in Genetic Engineering

A. tumefaciens induces tumors in plants and causes a disease called crown gall. A lump of tumor tissue forms at the infection site, as the photograph shows. The catalyst for infection is a plasmid carrying DNA. This plasmid is used to carry a gene of interest into plant cells.

■ **DETECTION AND DIAGNOSIS**   In the **medical laboratory**, diagnosticians are optimistic about the use of **gene probes**, a set of single-stranded DNA molecules that can recognize and bind to certain DNA sites in a host cell's chromosome. The probe hybridizes to its complementary nucleic acid sequence, much like strips of Velcro® stick together. To make a probe, scientists must first identify the DNA segment (or gene) that will be the object of a probe. Using this segment, they synthetically construct an mRNA fragment, then use the enzyme reverse transcriptase to synthesize a complementary fragment of DNA. This newly formed segment of DNA is the probe (Chapter 19 explains further).

Gene probe:
a segment of single-stranded DNA that binds with a complementary single-stranded segment during diagnostic procedures.

When diagnostic information is necessary, cells are obtained and the DNA is isolated. Now the DNA is treated to open all the strands, and a radioactive gene probe is added. The probe "searches" among the thousands of genes and ultimately binds to the complementary gene. In doing so, it concentrates radioactivity at that site and indicates that a match has been made. Gene probes are currently used to detect a variety of genetic disorders as well as to locate and identify the bacteria, viruses, and other pathogens of numerous human diseases.

Detection of a different sort can be accomplished through **DNA fingerprinting**, a technology derived from observations reported by Alec J. Jeffreys in 1985. Jeffreys noted that short, repetitive segments of DNA of unknown function exist between the body's functional genes. He found that the segments appear in all people, but the number of times they are repeated changes per person.

DNA fingerprint:
the presence of certain identifiable segments of DNA in the chromosomal material of an individual.

To make a DNA fingerprint, human cells are obtained, the DNA is extracted, and restriction enzymes scissor the DNA into fragments. The fragments are then separated according to size by a process called electrophoresis, in which an electric current drives the fragments through a gel in a narrow channel. Radioactive gene probes are then used to seek out the fragments and mark them with radiation. In this way the fragment positions can be revealed as dark bands, looking similar to a bar code. DNA fingerprinting was introduced to the legal system in 1987.

e-lec'tro-for-e'sis

■ **GENOME DETERMINATIONS**   One of the most ambitious projects in the history of molecular genetics—indeed, the history of biology—was launched in January 1989. That month a group of biologists, ethicists, industrial scientists, computer experts, and engineers began a monumental effort to map the **human genome**—to identify all the nitrogenous bases and their sequence in the 100,000 human genes. Their goal: to spell out for the world the entire genetic message hidden in the code of bases in human DNA.

je'nōm
Human genome:
all the nitrogenous bases and their sequence in the full set of human genes.

With the U.S. federal government supporting the project, a staggering $3 billion will be expended during the 15 years estimated for completion. There are about 3 billion pairs of bases that need to be sequenced, so the project is costing $1 per base pair. Most genes consist of about 10,000 to 150,000 base pairs, and between them are endless stretches of bases that appear to have no meaning, at least in the views of contemporary scientists. The human genome to be deciphered has been equated to a rope 2 inches in diameter and 32,000 miles long, all neatly arranged in a structure (the nucleus) about the size of a domed stadium.

Determining the nature of the human genome requires a multistep approach, beginning with assigning genes to particular chromosomes, continuing with locating genes on a chromosome, and ending with determining the sequence of base pairs in the DNA chain. Already a number of successes have been achieved. History was made in May 1995, when J. Craig Venter and his associates at The Institute for Genomic Research (TIGR) won the race to provide the first complete

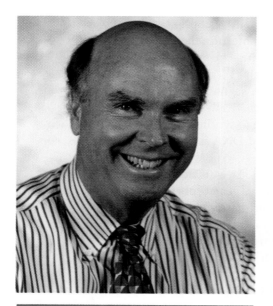

FIGURE 6.17

A Contemporary Gene Engineer

J. Craig Venter. Venter and his research team worked with Hamilton Smith and his group to decipher the first complete genetic code for a prokaryote, the bacterium *Haemophilus influenzae*. Their report was published in 1995.

sak-a-ro-mī'cĕz cer-e-vis'e-a

Streptococcus pneumoniae: a Gram-positive chain of diplococci that causes pneumonia, usually in immunocompromised individuals.

genome of a free-living organism (FIGURE 6.17). Working with Hamilton Smith and his coworkers at Johns Hopkins University, Venter unveiled the sequence of the 1.8 million base pairs in the genome of the bacterium *Haemophilus influenzae*, a Gram-negative rod whose strain b causes bacterial meningitis in young children. The genome consists of 1749 genes and contains the entire information needed to sustain life. The Venter-Smith team fragmented the bacterial genome with ultrasonic (high-pitch) vibrations, then sequenced the fragments, and arranged them in order using innovative computer software and sequence overlap information. In a few short months they were able to decipher the genome for a second organism, *Mycoplasma genitalium*. This reproductive tract pathogen is among the smallest bacteria known, having only 580,000 base pairs and about 250 genes.

By 1996, the Venter group had completed the sequencing of the bacterium *Methanococcus jannaschii*. This organism represents the Archaea (discussed in Chapter 3). Venter's research solidified Carl Woese's proposal of a third domain by showing that the genes of *M. jannaschii* are considerably different than those of traditional bacteria. The genome sequences for another bacterium and a virus were also announced in 1996. In March, scientists published the sequence of 2.8 million base pairs in the 2400 genes of *Staphylococcus aureus*. (Strains of this organism cause food poisoning, skin infections, and toxic shock syndrome.) The virus sequenced was the molluscum contagiosum virus, a cause of benign skin tumors. Its relatively small genome contains only 163 genes. The virus is discussed in Chapter 12.

But the big news of 1996 was the completion of the genome for the yeast *Saccharomyces cerevisiae*. In a field already littered with milestones, the sequencing of *S. cerevisiae* marked the first insight into the eukaryotic genome. Sixteen chromosomes were analyzed, 12 million bases were sequenced, and 6000 genes were identified. The sequencing revealed many genes wholly new to biology. It also showed a high degree of redundancy in the genome; that is, many genes are repeated over and over again, the significance of which remains unexplained. Moreover, the knowledge provides an opportunity to study genes that regulate the fermentation process.

In 1997, the science of whole genome sequencing took off. Among the bacterial genomes sequenced were those of *Helicobacter pylori*, a cause of gastric ulcers (FIGURE 6.18); *Borrelia burgdorferi*, the agent of Lyme disease; and *Streptococcus pneumoniae*, among the most serious causes of bacterial pneumonia. These successes gave biologists new starting points from which to develop diagnostic tests and vaccines.

That same year, European and Japanese biochemists determined the sequence of bases in the genome of *Bacillus subtilis*. This organism is familiar to most students of microbiology because it is widely used as a laboratory test organism. It is also familiar to industrial microbiologists because of its value as a source of enzymes for the production of vitamins, detergents, and food products. Another genome completed in 1997 was that of the archaeon *Archaeglobus fulgidus*. Information from this genome verified the uniqueness of the Archaea.

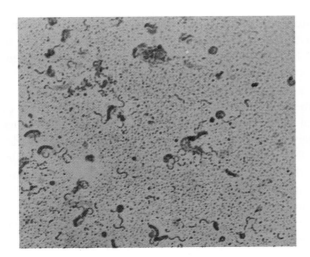

FIGURE 6.18

A Genome Decoded

A light micrograph of *Helicobacter pylori*, widely regarded as the major cause of gastric ulcers. The genome for this organism was decoded in 1997. The organisms have been stained by the Liefson method to highlight their flagella, which appear as tails extending from the curved cells (×1250).

But probably the outstanding achievement of 1997 was the complete sequencing of *Escherichia coli*. The long-awaited announcement was made by Frederick R. Blattner of the University of Wisconsin-Madison. Studied for decades and a regular on the pages of this book, *E. coli* is the organism of choice for studying how bacteria work. Because there is an enormous biological literature on the organism, a gene and its gene product can be fit into the vast understanding of its biology. Blattner's research group identified 4,638,858 base pairs in the 4288 genes of the *E. coli* genome. Over half bear no strong resemblance to any known genes, but 1827 genes were previously characterized.

The Institute for Genomic Research was back in the news in 1997, having participated in the sequencing for the genome of *Treponema pallidum*, the cause of syphilis. Analysis of the genome revealed that the organism cannot encode various enzymes and complex molecules normally required for independent living. It thus has a strong reliance on its host organism. Another pathogen, *Mycobacterium tuberculosis*, was also sequenced in 1997. This agent of tuberculosis has a complex cell wall that protects it against body defenses and antibiotics. The newly identified genes will help scientists understand this defense.

Mycobacterium tuberculosis: an acid-fast bacterial rod that causes tuberculosis.

By 1998, genome sequencing of microorganisms was reaching unprecedented heights. The typhus fever microbe *Rickettsia prowazekii* was sequenced that year, all 97 million bases of the worm *Caenorhabditis elegans* were finally decoded, and botanists were eagerly awaiting genomic information on the small plant *Arabidopsis thaliana*. By the end of the century, the genomes of over 50 organisms were known.

The publication of prokaryotic and eukaryotic genomes presented scientists with great volumes of data, and, for the first time in history, made available the entire genetic content of a living organism. But it also created the dilemma of what to do with the data. As studies continued and years passed, there emerged the new science of **genomics**, referring to the mapping, sequencing, and study of genomes.

For the microbiologist, the field of medical genomics offers fresh insights about the disease process. From genome analysis, for example, scientists can deduce the importance of a specific function. *Mycoplasma genitalium*, for instance, uses a full 5 percent of its gene content to encode a gene allowing it to adhere to the reproductive tissue. Research directed toward altering these genes might be a useful starting point for therapy. Furthermore, *Haemophilus influenzae* lacks the genes for three Krebs cycle enzymes, a fact that may help microbiologists understand its ability to thrive in the human body. And by comparing the genomes of virulent and avirulent strains, a window should open to the pathogenic process.

Some researchers see the genes as mechanisms for diagnosing disease, and they envision DNA as molecular snippets they can use to send patients home cured of their illness. In that sense, all the DNA knowledge uncovered in the past half-century is merely a preamble to the startling discoveries waiting to be made in the decades ahead. For many physicians, DNA will be a pharmacological substance of extraordinary potency that can be used to treat disease and its symptoms, while correcting the imperfections that make patients susceptible to disease.

James Watson, the Nobel laureate cited for deducing the structure of DNA, has written: "We used to think our fate was in the stars. We know now that, in large measure, our fate is in our genes."

Note to the Student

Louis Pasteur once wrote, "There are science and the applications of science, separate yet bound together as the fruit to the tree which bears it." The truth of this statement is particularly apparent in genetic engineering. Genetic engineering represents an apex in microbiology research. It is the equivalent of the engineer's dream of landing on the moon and the physicist's vision of peaceful uses of nuclear power.

The capabilities of genetic engineering have turned microbiology from an analytical science into a synthetic science. By extracting genes from one species and inserting them into another, microbiologists have acquired the ability to make large quantities of proteins previously available only in minute amounts. Triumph has followed triumph. Rarely in scientific history have the discoveries of pure research had such immediate applications and implications upon the society of their time.

I would recommend that you browse through this chapter and try to visualize the growth of molecular genetics beginning with Griffith's puzzling observations in 1928, and continuing with Avery's work in 1944 and the discoveries in bacterial genetics in the 1950s. It was during this period that the idea of gene manipulations arose. Watch for daily announcements in the press of new products that are derived from genetic engineering. It is a historic time for microbiology—a second Golden Age of Microbiology; and we should all share the excitement. Louis Pasteur would have been proud to see this day.

Summary

Bacterial genetics is concerned with the gene changes that take place in a bacterium's chromosome and plasmids, changes that reflect themselves in the morphology, physiology, and pathology of the organism. The changes can take place by mutation and by recombination.

Mutation is a permanent change in the cellular DNA, occurring spontaneously in nature or by induced methods in the laboratory. Such things as ultraviolet light, chemicals, and base analogs may induce mutations. Deletions or insertions involving the chromosome, as well as transposons and insertion sequences, may also be mutagenic.

Recombinations imply a transfer of DNA between bacteria and thus, an acquisition of genes. In one form of recombination called transformation, a "competent" bacterium takes up DNA from the local environment; this DNA has been left behind by a disrupted bacterium. The new DNA displaces a segment of equivalent DNA in the recipient cell, and new genetic characteristics are assumed. In another form, conjugation, a live donor cell contributes a portion of its DNA to a recipient cell. Plasmids are commonly transferred, but chromosomal DNA may also be contributed. In the third form of recombination, transduction, a virus enters a bacterium and later replicates within it. During replication, the virus incorporates some bacterial DNA to its protein coat and transports that DNA to a new bacterium. In the specialized form of transduction, the virus first attaches to, then detaches from, the bacterial chromosome, taking a segment of bacterial DNA with it. Thus, all three forms of recombination are characterized by the introduction of new genes to a recipient bacterium.

Genetic engineering is an outgrowth of studies in bacterial genetics. In one type of this technology, plasmids are isolated from a bacterium, spliced with foreign genes, then inserted into fresh bacteria where the foreign genes are expressed as protein. Bacteria are thus used as the biochemical factories for the synthesis of such proteins as insulin, interferon, human growth hormone, and others. But genetic engineering is only one branch of modern biotechnology. This technology utilizes DNA-based techniques to perform diagnoses, identify individuals in forensic medicine, detect and treat genetic diseases, and spark innovative approaches to agriculture. The practical benefits of research in bacterial genetics have helped revolutionize myriad fields of human endeavor.

http://microbiology.jbpub.com

The site features **eLearning,** an on-line review area that provides quizzes and other tools to help you study for your class. You can also follow useful links for in-depth information, read more MicroFocus stories, or just find out the latest microbiology news.

Questions for Thought and Discussion

1. Try to put yourself in Griffith's position in 1928. Genetics is poorly understood, DNA is virtually unknown, and bacterial biochemistry has not been clearly defined. How would you explain transformation?

2. In hospitals, it is common practice to clear the air bubble from a syringe by expelling a small amount of the syringe contents into the air. One microbiologist estimates that this practice results in the release of up to 30 liters of antibiotic into a typical hospital's environment annually. How might this lead to the appearance of antibiotic-resistant mutants in hospitals?

3. Some geneticists maintain that the movement of transposons in a bacterial cell is a form of recombination—specifically, "illegitimate recombination." What arguments can be made for and against calling the movement a recombination, and why do you suppose it is labeled "illegitimate"?

4. Which of the recombination processes (transformation, conjugation, or transduction) would be most likely to occur in the natural environment? What factors would encourage or discourage your choice from taking place?

5. The author of a general biology textbook writes in reference to the development of antibiotic resistance: "The speed at which bacteria reproduce ensures that sooner or later a mutant bacterium will appear that is able to resist the poison." How might this mutant bacterium appear? Do you agree with the statement? Does this bode ill for the future use of antibiotics?

6. William Hayes and his colleagues established and outlined the method of bacterial conjugation in which DNA passes from a donor cell to a recipient cell. But it didn't have to be that way. What other methods can you propose to explain the results of the bacterial recombination we now call conjugation?

7. Certain developments, such as Koch's cultivation methods for bacteria, are pivotal because they open the door to other discoveries and spark research in other areas. Which discoveries in bacterial genetics do you believe to be pivotal?

8. Some scientists suggest that mutation is the single most important event in evolution. Do you agree? Why or why not?

9. In 1976, an outbreak of pulmonary infections among participants at an American Legion convention in Philadelphia led to the identification of a new disease, Legionnaires' disease. The bacterium responsible for the disease had never before been known to be pathogenic. From your knowledge of bacterial genetics, can you postulate how it might have acquired the ability to cause disease?

10. At this writing, the smallest known bacterium whose genome has been deciphered is the submicroscopic organism *Mycoplasma genitalium* (a possible cause of a sexually transmitted disease). This bacterium is able to survive on about 470 genes. (A human cell, by comparison, has about 100,000 genes.) What do you suppose are some of the proteins encoded by the genes in this minimal genome?

11. The development of genetic engineering has been hailed as the beginning of a second Industrial Revolution. Do you believe this label is justified? How many products of genetic engineering or applications of the process can you think of?

12. In 1994, the CDC reported that the percentage of antibiotic-resistant isolates of *Haemophilus influenzae* had risen from 4.5 percent to 28 percent over the previous 5 years. What factors might have accounted for this change?

13. Since the 1950s, the world has been plagued by a broad series of influenza viruses that differ genetically from one another. For example, we have heard of swine flu, Hong Kong flu, Bangkok flu, and Victoria flu. How might the process of transduction help explain this variability?

14. It is not uncommon for students of microbiology to confuse the terms *reproduction* and *recombination*. How do the terms differ?

15. In modern medicine, physicians are strongly urged to prescribe an antibiotic that is specifically geared to the organism causing the present disease, rather than a broad-spectrum antibiotic that kills many different bacteria including the present organism. Why?

Review

Use the following syllables to compose the term that answers each of the clues below from bacterial genetics. The number of letters in each term is indicated by the blank lines, and the number of syllables is shown by the number in parentheses. Each syllable is used only once, and the answers are listed in Appendix D.

A ASE BAC CHI CHROM CLE COC COM CON CUS DO DUC EN FER FER FITH GA GASE GE GEN GRIF I I IN JU LA LENT LI LI LY MER MIDS MO MO MU MU NEL NU NY O O ON PE PHAGE PI PLAS PNEU PO SAL SEX SO SOME SON TA TA TENCE TER TER TIL TION TION TION TRANS TY U VIR

1. Closed loops of DNA   (2) __ __ __ __ __ __ __ __

2. Type of conjugation   (3) __ __ __ __ __ __ __ __ __ __

3. Genetic change   (3) __ __ __ __ __ __ __ __ __

4. Used in Ames test   (4) __ __ __ __ __ __ __ __ __ __

5. Transforming property   (3) __ __ __ __ __ __ __ __ __ __

6. Factor for conjugation   (4) __ __ __ __ __ __ __ __ __ __

7. Transduction virus   (5) __ __ __ __ __ __ __ __ __ __ __ __ __

8. Recombinant DNA enzyme   (5) __ __ __ __ __ __ __ __ __ __ __ __

9. Transformed bacterium   (4) __ __ __ __ __ __ __ __ __ __ __

10. Conjugation structures   (2) __ __ __ __

11. Viral nonreplication   (4) __ __ __ __ __ __ __ __ __

12. Recombined plasmid   (3) __ __ __ __ __ __ __ __

13. DNA linking enzyme   (2) __ __ __ __ __

14. Gene engineered drug   (4) __ __ __ __ __ __ __ __ __ __ __

15. Movable genetic element   (3) __ __ __ __ __ __ __ __ __

16. Discovered transformation (2) __ __ __ __ __ __

17. Type of recombination   (4) __ __ __ __ __ __ __ __ __ __ __

18. Induces genetic change   (3) __ __ __ __ __ __ __

19. Phage that causes lysis   (3) __ __ __ __ __ __ __ __ __

20. Only one per bacterium   (3) __ __ __ __ __ __ __ __ __ __

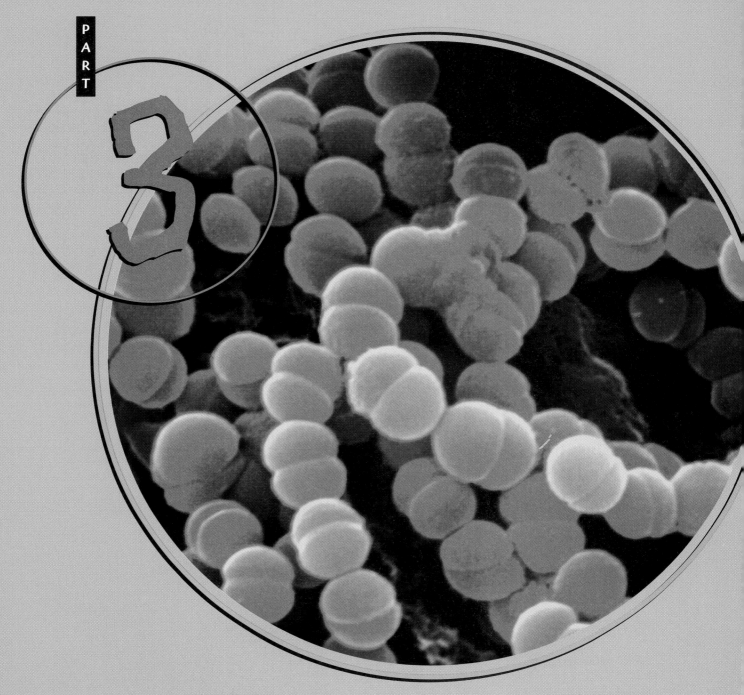

PART 3

Bacterial Diseases of Humans

Throughout history, bacterial diseases have posed a formidable challenge to humans and have often swept through populations virtually unchecked. In the eighteenth century, for example, the first European visitors to the South Pacific found the islanders robust, happy, and well adapted to their environment. But the explorers introduced syphilis, tuberculosis, and pertussis (whooping cough), and soon these diseases spread like wildfire. Hawaii was struck with unusually terrible force. The population of the islands was about 300,000 when Captain Cook landed there in 1778; by 1860, it had been reduced to fewer than 37,000 people.

With equally devastating results, the Great Plague came to Europe from the Orient, and cholera spread eastward from India. Together with tuberculosis, diphtheria, and dysentery, these bacterial diseases ravaged European populations for centuries and insidiously wove themselves into the pattern of life. Infant mortality was particularly shocking: England's Queen Anne, who reigned in the early 1700s, lost 16 of her 17 babies to disease; and until the mid–1800s, only half the children born in the United States reached their fifth year.

Today, humans are better able to cope with bacterial diseases. Though credit is often given to wonder drugs, the major health gains have resulted from understanding disease and the body's resistance mechanisms, coupled with modern sanitary methods that prevent microorganisms from reaching their targets. Immunization has also played a key role in preventing disease. Indeed, very few people in our society die of the bacterial diseases that once accounted for the majority of all deaths.

In Part 3 of this text, we shall study the bacterial diseases of humans over the course of four chapters. The diseases have been grouped according to their major mode of transmission. Airborne diseases are discussed in Chapter 7; foodborne and waterborne diseases in Chapter 8; soilborne and arthropodborne diseases in Chapter 9; and sexually transmitted, contact, and miscellaneous diseases in Chapter 10. Many of the diseases we shall study are of historical interest and are currently under control. But just as the garden always faces new onslaughts of weeds and pests, so, too, the human body is continually confronted with newly emerging diseases. In this regard, the modern era is no different than Europe or the South Pacific islands of past centuries. On the fundamental level, disease has not changed. Only the pattern of disease has changed.

CLINICAL MICROBIOLOGY

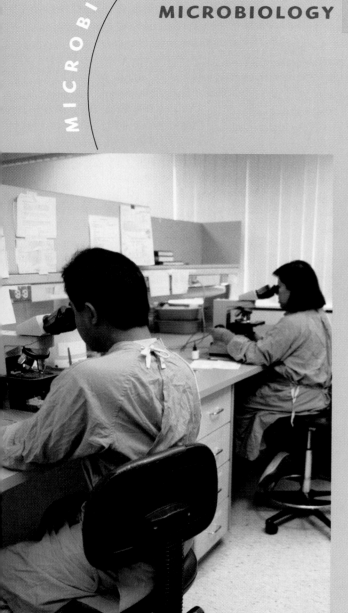

One of the most famous books of the 20th century was *Microbe Hunters* by Paul de Kruif. In his book, first published in the 1920s, de Kruif describes the joys and frustrations of Pasteur, Koch, Ehrlich, von Behring, and many of the original microbe hunters. The exploits of these scientists make for fascinating reading and help us understand how the concepts of microbiology were formulated. I would urge you to leaf through the book at your leisure.

Microbe hunters did not come to an end with Pasteur, Koch, and their contemporaries, nor did the stories of microbe hunters end with the publication of de Kruif's book. The men and women working in hospital, public, and private laboratories are today's detectives of microbiology. These individuals search for the pathogens of disease. Many travel to far corners of the world studying organisms, and many more remain close to home, identifying the pathogens in samples sent by physicians. Microbiologists even work in dental clinical labs, since many bacteria are involved in tooth decay and periodontal disease.

Clinical microbiology also offers an outlet for the talents of those who prefer to tinker with machinery. New instruments and laboratory procedures are constantly being researched in an effort to shorten the time between detection and identification of microorganisms. Many tests reflect human ingenuity. For example, there is a test that detects bacteria by its interference with the passage of light and its ability to scatter light at peculiar angles. Such modern devices as laser beams are used in this kind of instrumentation.

The microbe hunters have not changed materially in the past 100 years. The objectives of the search may be different, but the fundamental principles of the detective work remain the same. The clinical microbiologist is today's version of the great masters of a bygone era.

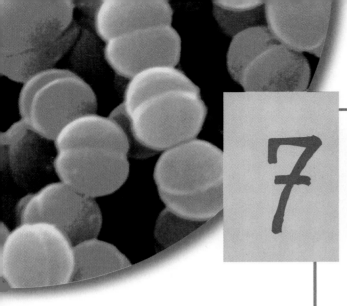

7 Airborne Bacterial Diseases

The captain of all these men of death that came against him to take him away was the Consumption, for it was that that brought him down to the grave.

—John Bunyam describing tuberculosis in *The Life and Death of Mr. Badman* (1680)

THE PRODUCE LOOKED GOOD THAT DAY. The lettuce was green and crisp, and the carrots just seemed to ring out with good health. The broccoli was a deep, forest green and the cauliflower a lily white. It was probably due to the ultrasonic humidifier spraying its cool mist over the vegetable section. The fresh, clean mist made everything look terrific.

So it was in Bogaloosa, Louisiana, that November morning when officials from the local Department of Health walked into the supermarket. They had a disturbing story: 28 people were sick with Legionnaires' disease, and 2 had already died of pneumonia. Most of the patients, it seemed, had been in the grocery store within the previous 10 days.

The investigators were friendly but firm. How long, they asked, did the air conditioner run each day? Were the vegetables washed before putting them out, and if so, for how long and where? Had any of the employees been sick recently? Who was the supermarket's supplier? And that humidifier—how long had it been there?

Three days later, the investigators were back with an answer. It was the humidifier! The lab had found *Legionella pneumophila* (**FIGURE 7.1**) in the water in its reservoir. Could the owner please remove the humidifier from the store and clean it out with disinfectant before reusing it? Within a day, the humidifier was gone. The broccoli didn't look quite as good any more, and the lettuce leaves seemed to droop a bit. But at least the air was safer to breathe, and that was important.

Though known only since 1976, Legionnaires' disease is recognized today throughout the world, and outbreaks,

Pneumonia:
an often serious microbial disease of the bronchi and lungs.

le'gion-el'lah nu-mof'i-lah

Legionnaires' disease:
a bacterial disease of the respiratory tract transmitted by the air and often accompanied by pneumonia; named for an outbreak at a convention of the American Legion in 1976.

FIGURE 7.1

Legionella pneumophila

A scanning electron micrograph of *Legionella pneumophila*, the agent of Legionnaires' disease. The rod-shaped bacillus is attached to a cytoplasmic extension of an amoeba in the first stage leading to engulfment by the amoeba.

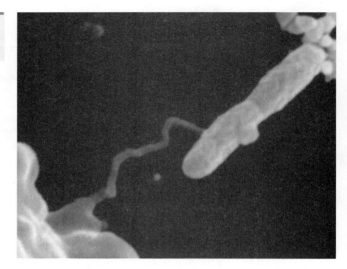

such as this 1989 incident in Louisiana, are reported regularly to the Centers for Disease Control and Prevention (CDC). In the United States alone, microbiologists estimate that between 25,000 and 50,000 cases occur annually, though most go unreported (13,306 cases were reported in 1999). Legionnaires' disease is one of the contemporary airborne bacterial diseases that we shall discuss in this chapter. Such diseases are generally spread by airborne droplets where people crowd together.

We shall divide the airborne bacterial diseases into two general categories. The first category will include diseases of the upper respiratory tract, such as strep throat, scarlet fever, diphtheria, pertussis, and several forms of meningitis. The second category will include diseases of the lower respiratory tract: tuberculosis, pneumococcal pneumonia, primary atypical pneumonia, Legionnaires' disease, and others. As we proceed, note how the initial focus of infection is followed by spread to other organs. Also note that antibiotics are available for treating these diseases and that immunizations are used for protecting the community at large.

dif-the're-ah

7.1 Diseases of the Upper Respiratory Tract

The diseases of the upper respiratory tract can be severe, as several diseases in this section illustrate. One reason is that the respiratory tract is a portal of entry to the blood, and from there, the disease can affect the more sensitive internal organs.

STREPTOCOCCAL DISEASES

Streptococci are a large and diverse group of encapsulated Gram-positive bacteria. They cause streptococcal sore throat (strep throat), scarlet fever, and several other diseases in humans. The bacteria divide in one plane and cling together to form chains of various lengths. This observation is apparent in streptococci grown in liquid media, but it may not be obvious in streptococci from solid media (FIGURE 7.2).

Microbiologists classify the streptococci by several systems, two of which are widely accepted. The first system, developed by J. H. Brown in 1919, divides strep-

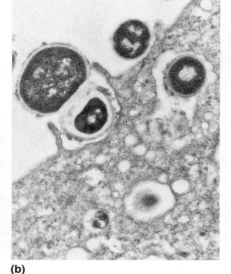

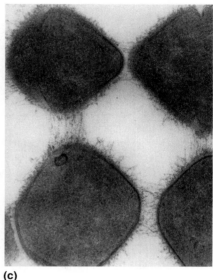

(a) (b) (c)

FIGURE 7.2

Streptococci and Their Host Cell

(a) A scanning electron micrograph of *Streptococcus mutans*, a species that causes many cases of tooth decay. (b) A transmission electron micrograph of *Streptococcus pyogenes* attaching to cells cultured from the human pharynx. The bacteria associate with microvilli of the cells. Surface proteins, especially the streptococcal M protein, function in this association. A streptococcal cell has been internalized and is seen within the cytoplasm of the pharyngeal cell (×24,300). (c) A closeup view of *S. pyogenes* cells showing strands of M protein. The M protein enhances virulence by encouraging attachment to the host cell (×50,000).

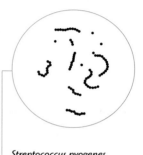

Streptococcus pyogenes

tococci into hemolytic ("blood-digesting") groups, depending on how they affect red blood cells in blood agar. **Alpha-hemolytic streptococci** turn blood agar an olive-green color as they partially destroy red blood cells in the medium; colonies of **beta-hemolytic streptococci** are surrounded by clear, colorless zones due to the complete destruction of red blood cells; and **gamma-hemolytic streptococci** have no effect on red blood cells and thus cause no change in blood agar.

he′mo-lit′ik

The second classification system, suggested by Rebecca Lancefield in 1935, is based on variants of a specific carbohydrate, the C substance, in cell walls of streptococci. Groups A through O streptococci have been distinguished. Most streptococcal diseases in humans are caused by species of group A streptococci; ***Streptococcus pyogenes*** is the most common species. This beta-hemolytic organism is generally implied when physicians refer to "group A beta-hemolytic streptococci."

C substance:
a specific carbohydrate in the cell walls of streptococci.

pi–oj′ĕ-nez

Streptococcus pyogenes causes streptococcal sore throat, popularly known as **strep throat.** The streptococci reach the upper respiratory tract within airborne **droplets,** the tiny particles of mucus expelled during coughing and sneezing. Patients experience a high fever, coughing, swollen lymph nodes and tonsils, and a fiery red "beefy" appearance to pharyngeal tissues owing to tissue erosion. About 500,000 Americans suffer strep throat annually, many cases complicated by an infection of the middle ear, **otitis media.**

Lymph nodes:
bean-shaped pockets of tissue containing white blood cells that respond to disease organisms.

The pathogenicity of *Streptococcus pyogenes* is enhanced by a substance called **M protein** (Figure 7.2c). This protein, located in the cell wall and pili, encourages adherence to the pharyngeal tissue and retards phagocytosis. Over 60 specific types

MicroFocus 7·1

DANGER ON THE FARM

It's called tilapia (ti-lap'i-ah), and it's one of fish-farming's more popular products. Raised in huge tanks by modern methods of aquaculture, tilapia is appearing more and more in restaurants and supermarkets—but so are the bacteria that infect tilapia.

The lesson was driven home in 1996 when several people in Ontario, Canada became ill after handling fresh tilapia. One patient punctured his hand with a fish bone while cutting the fish into filets; another punctured her finger with the dorsal fin of the fish while scaling it; yet another suffered a skin wound from a knife used to cut the fish. In all cases,

the patients developed infection with *Streptococcus iniae*, a known fish pathogen. The patients exhibited the symptoms of various diseases, including meningitis, transient arthritis, and endocarditis. All received antibiotic therapy and recovered successfully.

The outbreak underscores the possibility that fish pathogens can adapt to human tissues—in effect, jumping from one species to another. Health officials are concerend by this because it means a new human pathogen may emerge. Furthermore, aquaculture is a fast-growing industry and a promising source of foods for the future. However, it also represents

possible human exposure to new bacteria, and, as the cases in Canada illustrate, that can pose a formidable danger.

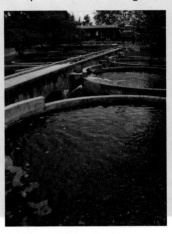

Antibodies:
highly specific protein molecules produced by the immune system in response to microorganisms and chemical substances.

Antitoxins:
highly specific antibodies that react with toxins.

Bacteriophages:
viruses that penetrate bacteria and often remain within them.

Antigen:
a chemical substance that stimulates a response by the immune system.
glo-mer'u-lo-nĕ-fri'tis

er'ĭ-sip'e-las

nec'ro-tiz'ing fas-i-i'tis

pu-er'per-al

---

of M protein have been identified, and complete immunity to streptococcal disease requires that a person produce antibodies against all 60 types.

Scarlet fever is strep throat accompanied by a skin rash. The rash develops as a pink-red blush, apparent on the neck, chest, and soft-skin areas of the arms. It results from blood leaking through the walls of capillaries damaged by a toxin. This toxin, called an **erythrogenic** ("red-forming") **toxin**, is produced only by certain strains of *S. pyogenes*. Normally an individual experiences only one case of scarlet fever in a lifetime because the immune system produces special antibodies, called **antitoxins**, which circulate in the bloodstream and neutralize the toxins during succeeding episodes.

Treatment of streptococcal diseases is generally successful with antibiotics such as penicillin and erythromycin (MicroFocus 7.1). However, widespread resistance to antibiotics has been noted since the early 1970s, and research indicates that many strains of *S. pyogenes* carry bacteriophages having antibiotic-resistance genes.

An important complication of streptococcal disease is **rheumatic fever**. This condition is characterized by fever and inflammations of the small blood vessels. Joint pain is common, but the most significant long-range effect is permanent scarring and distortion of the heart valves, a condition called **rheumatic heart disease**. The damage arises from a reaction of the body's antibodies with streptococcal antigens bound to the heart tissue. Another manifestation of this reaction may develop in the kidneys, where the condition is called **glomerulonephritis**.

S. pyogenes is commonly present in the human nose and throat, and transmission to many other tissues is possible. For example, streptococci may cause disease in open wounds or skin abrasions, resulting in **erysipelas**. If invasive group A streptococci invade and infect the fascia over the muscles and beneath the skin, their toxins cause a condition called **necrotizing fasciitis** and an unsightly degeneration and dissolving of the skin tissues, as shown in FIGURE 7.3. (Tabloid newspapers and TV programs had a field day with this disease in 1994 as they heralded an outbreak of the "flesh-eating bacteria"; see MicroFocus 7.2.) If the tissue of the uterus becomes infected during the birth process, the mother may suffer **puerperal sepsis**, also

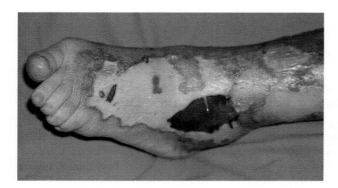

FIGURE 7.3

Necrotizing Fasciitis

This patient shows the symptoms of necrotizing fasciitis. This disease is caused by a species of *Streptococcus*. It affects the fascia surrounding the muscle tissues and results in tissue degeneration as powerful toxins interfere with cell metabolism. The disease has been known since ancient times but has attracted interest since 1994.

known as **childbed fever**. Moreover, streptococci may infect the lower respiratory tract and cause streptococcal pneumonia as a complication to viral disease. In past generations, many died of **septicemia** or "blood poisoning," a disease now known to be due to several organisms, including streptococci. One of Louis Pasteur's daughters was a victim of this disease.

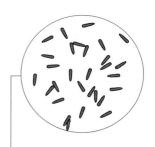

Corynebacterium diphtheriae

DIPHTHERIA

Diphtheria was first recognized as a clinical entity in 1826 by French pathologist Pierre F. Bretonneau. Bretonneau named the disease *la diphtherite,* from the Greek *diphthera* for "membrane," a reference to the membranes that appear in the throats of patients. In 1883, Edwin Klebs observed a bacterium in material from a patient's throat, and the next year, Friederich Löeffler successfully cultivated the organism. The so-called Klebs-Löeffler bacillus has the scientific name *Corynebacterium diphtheriae* because it resembles a club (*coryne* is Greek for "club") and forms membranes.

Corynebacterium diphtheriae is a Gram-positive bacillus containing numerous **metachromatic granules** that show up with special stains as cytoplasmic dots. The

dif-the're-ah

bret-o-no'

Lef'ler

ko-ri'ne-bac-te're-um
dif-the're-ā

MicroFocus 7.2

TOO GOOD TO BE TRUE

They needed a story for their tabloid newspaper. It had to be attention-grabbing, current, just slightly scientific, and health-related. Then they heard about the man in southwest England. It was too good to be true.

"A flesh-eating bug ate my face!"—the tabloid screamed. Soon the stories rolled in: Limbs were rotting before people's eyes; facial features were melting away; doctors were making emergency amputations to save lives. It wasn't Armageddon—it was the flesh-eating bacteria!

The medical community scoffed. The "bug," they said, was a species of *Streptococcus* called *Streptococcus pyogenes,* a group A streptococcus, and the "new"

disease already had a name: necrotizing fasciitis. (Necrotizing is from the Greek *nekros* for "dead"; and fasciitis refers to the fascia that surrounds muscle tissue and attracts the streptococci.) There was nothing new about the disease—hospital physicians had seen it in contaminated wounds as early as the Civil War; and it was common in nursing home patients. They knew it as "hospital gangrene," "putrid ulcer," and by other descriptive expressions. Some even called it the Second Disease, since the skin often turned a deep red (see the discussion of Fifth Disease in Chapter 12).

But why was it flaring up now? Was it a publicity stunt, as some physicians sus-

pected? Apparently not, said the researchers. They presented evidence that the streptococci had become more virulent. They also linked contemporary cases to the new nonsteroidal anti-inflammatory drugs, such as ibuprofen. They pointed out that a significant number of patients were taking the drugs at the time of disease.

Whatever the source, the flesh-eating bacteria were here to stay. The tabloid had scored its coup, and the editors were ecstatic. Newspapers were selling faster than ever, and even the late news had picked up the story. Now, what would next week's story be?

MicroFocus 7.3

A PREDICTION FULFILLED

It was the early eighteen-eighties, and diphtheria—which several times each hundred years seems to have violent ups and downs of viciousness—diphtheria was particularly murderous then. The wards of the hospitals for sick children were melancholy with a forlorn wailing; there were gurgling coughs foretelling suffocation; on the sad rows of narrow beds were white pillows framing small faces blue with the strangling grip of an unknown hand.

—Paul de Kruif,
Microbe Hunters, 1925

So it was. Five of every ten cots sent their tenants to the morgue, and there in the morgue, Friederich Löeffler (pronounced "lef'ler") searched for the organisms of diphtheria.

Löeffler, the student of Robert Koch, worked tirelessly. Finally, in 1884, he was sure he had the culprit: a club-shaped rod isolated from the throats of children. But the rods were nowhere else in the body. It was inconceivable that these few organisms, staying in the throat, could kill a human or animal so huge. Yet it was happening, time and again. Perhaps there was a poison, a toxin that leaked out of the bacilli and spread to other parts of the body.

Four years later, Löeffler's prediction came true in an outrageous experiment performed by Louis Pasteur's young assistant, Emile Roux (pronounced "roo"). Roux was smitten by the toxin theory. Although no one had ever separated a toxin from bacteria, he was determined to try. Carefully he inoculated large quantities of broth with diphtheria bacilli. After four days, he separated the bacilli from the broth using a porcelain filter and injected the broth into animals. Nothing happened. He tried a larger dose, again without success. Still larger doses brought more failure.

Now came the experiment that would change the medical view of diphtheria. It was born of frustration, desperation, and a touch of insight. Roux injected a huge 35 milliliters of the broth into a guinea pig and an equal amount into a rabbit. This was equivalent to injecting a bucketful of fluid into a human. Privately he scoffed at his own experiment and speculated whether the sheer volume of broth would kill the animals. But they survived the injection, and 48 hours later, both the guinea pig and rabbit showed unmistakable signs of diphtheria. The toxin was there, but the amount was infinitesimal.

Next came refinement. Roux found that if he cultivated the bacilli for weeks instead of days, the amount of toxin increased dramatically. Soon he could show that an unbelievably tiny amount of toxin caused diphtheria. The door was now open to an understanding of the disease. Löeffler had been right after all!

In the years thereafter, another Emil (spelled the German way), Emil von Behring, found a way to cure diphtheria by administering antitoxins. Deaths from diphtheria soon declined, and with the development of the diphtheria vaccine in the 1920s, the incidence of disease dropped dramatically. The strangling grip of diphtheria was finally loosened.

bacteria remain close to one another after multiplying and form a palisade layer, a picket-fence arrangement. Diphtheria is acquired by inhaling respiratory droplets into the upper respiratory tract near the tonsils. The bacteria produce a potent **exotoxin** that interferes with protein synthesis in epithelial cells, the cubelike cells that line the skin and body cavities such as the respiratory tract. (MicroFocus 7.3 describes the toxin's discovery.) As dead tissue accumulates with mucus, white blood cells, and fibrous material, a leathery **pseudomembrane** forms ("pseudo" because it does not fit the definition of a true membrane). Respiratory blockage and death may follow, especially in children. In adults, the toxin often spreads to the bloodstream, where it causes neck swelling ("bullneck"), heart damage, and destruction of the fatty sheaths surrounding nerves. Treatment requires both antibiotics for the bacteria and antitoxins to neutralize the toxins.

At present, the number of cases of diphtheria in the United States is less than a dozen annually, but the disease remains a health problem in many regions of the world, especially parts of Asia. From 1990 to 1995, for example, a major outbreak occurred in 13 of the 14 new states of the former Soviet Union; it affected almost 50,000 people, with about 4000 deaths.

Immunization against diphtheria may be rendered by an injection of diphtheria **toxoid** contained in the diphtheria-tetanus-acellular pertussis (DTaP) vaccine. A toxoid consists of toxin molecules treated with formaldehyde or heat to destroy their toxic qualities. The toxoid induces the immune system to produce antitoxins that circulate in the bloodstream throughout the person's life.

In 1961, V. J. Freeman discovered that a virus attached to the bacterial chromosome contains the genetic code for exotoxin production. The virus, termed a **corynephage**, exists in a lysogenic relationship with the bacterium (Chapter 6). Strains of *C. diphtheriae* lacking the virus are harmless, but they may become pathogenic if the virus infects them. The same phage is carried by cells of *C. ulcerans*, a related species found primarily in cattle. In 1997, a woman was diagnosed with diphtheria due to this organism.

PERTUSSIS (WHOOPING COUGH)

Pertussis, also known as **whooping cough**, is one of the more dangerous diseases of childhood years. Although the incidence of this disease has declined substantially from the 250,000 annual cases reported during the 1930s, the number of cases in the United States still remains significant. For example, the CDC recorded about 6500 cases in 1997, and the numbers were growing. Almost half occurred in children under 6 months of age. Recent studies also show that about 20 percent of adults with a persistent cough have undiagnosed pertussis.

Pertussis is caused by ***Bordetella pertussis***, a small Gram-negative rod first isolated by Jules Bordet and Octave Gengou in 1906, and commonly known as the Bordet-Gengou bacillus. The bacillus is spread by droplets and uses its pili to adhere to the cilia of epithelial cells in the upper respiratory tract. No tissue invasion occurs, but the ciliated cells are destroyed and mucus movement is impaired.

Typical cases of pertussis occur in three stages. The initial stage is marked by general malaise, low-grade fever, and increasingly severe cough. During the next stage, disintegrating cells and mucus accumulate in the airways and cause labored breathing. Patients experience multiple paroxysms (violent spells) of rapid-fire **staccato coughs** all in one exhalation, followed by a forced inhalation over a partially closed glottis. The rapid inhalation results in the characteristic "whoop" (hence, the name whooping cough). Ten to fifteen paroxysms may occur daily, and exhaustion usually follows each. During the third stage, sporadic coughing continues for several weeks, even after the bacteria have vanished. (Doctors call it the "100-day cough.")

Treatment of pertussis is generally successful when penicillin or erythromycin is administered before the respiratory passageways become blocked. Diagnosis is performed by obtaining swabs from the posterior pharyngeal wall and identifying *B. pertussis* on selective media. A fluorescent antibody test (Chapter 19) is also used. Although several toxins have been observed, no one toxin is considered the prime factor in the disease.

As with diphtheria, the declining incidence of pertussis stems partly from use of a pertussis vaccine. The older vaccine (diphtheria-pertussis-tetanus, or DPT) contained Merthiolate-killed *B. pertussis* cells (the "P" component) and was considered risky because about one in 300,000 vaccinees suffered high fevers and seizures. As of 1993, public health officials were recommending the newer acellular pertussis vaccine prepared from *Bordetella pertussis* chemical extracts. Combined with diphtheria and tetanus toxoids, the triple vaccine is given the acronym DTaP. Commercially, it is known as Tripedia.

Toxoid:
a preparation of altered toxin molecules used for immunization purposes.

Exotoxin:
a poisonous chemical substance produced by bacteria and immediately excreted.
ko-ri'ne-faj
li'so-gen'ik

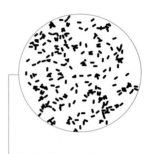

Bordetella pertussis

bor-da', zhan-goo'

par-oks'ism
Paroxysm:
a severe attack.
Glottis:
the slitlike opening to the respiratory tract.

Erythromycin:
an antibiotic that inhibits protein synthesis in various types of bacteria.

Merthiolate:
a heavy metal compound often used as an antiseptic and preservative.

MENINGOCOCCAL MENINGITIS

The term **meningitis** refers to several diseases of the meninges, the three membranous coverings of the brain and spinal cord. Meningitis may be caused by viruses, fungi, protozoa, or bacteria, and different forms of the disease have different mortality rates. In all forms, the meninges become inflamed, causing pressure on the spinal cord and brain. Patients experience headaches, neckaches, and lower backaches.

A particularly dangerous form of meningitis is **meningococcal meningitis**. This disease is caused by *Neisseria meningitidis*, a small Gram-negative, encapsulated diplococcus commonly called the **meningococcus**. Meningococci enter the body by droplets, often from a reservoir. In most cases, the disease consists of an influenza-like upper respiratory infection. However, the infection sometimes spreads to the bloodstream (**FIGURE 7.4**), where bacterial toxins may overwhelm the body in as little as 2 hours and cause death. This condition is called **meningococcemia**. In survivors, the meninges become inflamed, and patients experience a characteristic stiff, arched neck and pounding headache. A rash also appears on the skin, beginning as bright-red patches, which progress to blue-black spots. Fifty percent of untreated cases may be fatal.

Early diagnosis and treatment of meningococcal meningitis can prevent irreversible nerve damage or death. A principal criterion for diagnosis is the observation and/or cultivation of Gram-negative diplococci in samples of spinal fluid obtained by a spinal tap. Treatment with rifampin, penicillin, or sulfonamide drugs is usually recommended. A vaccine containing capsular polysaccharides from sev-

Mortality rate:
the rate of death in a population from infectious disease.

men'in-go-coc'cal
ni-se're-ah men'in-gi-ti'dis

me-ning'go-kok-se'me-ah

Rifampin:
an antibiotic that interferes with RNA synthesis in various types of bacteria.
sul-fon'a-mid

FIGURE 7.4

Meningococcal Meningitis

Meningococcal meningitis is caused by the Gram-negative diplococcus *Neisseria meningitidis*. (a) The bacteria colonize the nasopharynx, then invade the epithelium causing respiratory distress. They pass into the bloodstream, where they induce meningococcemia. Finally, they disseminate to tissues near the spinal cord, causing inflammation and meningitis. (b) A scanning electron micrograph of *N. meningitidis* at the surface of epithelial cells of the respiratory tract. Numerous hairlike pili can be seen. The pili bind the meningococci to the epithelial cells and encourage infection.

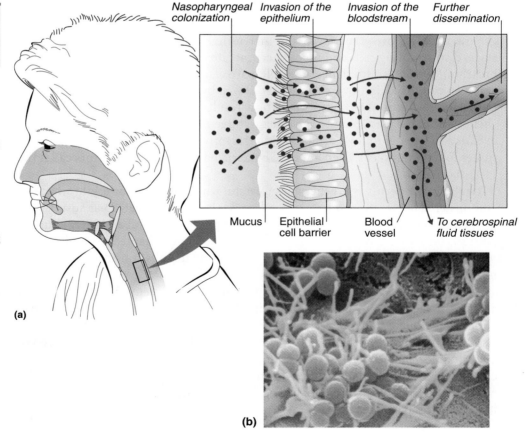

Nasopharyngeal colonization | Invasion of the epithelium | Invasion of the bloodstream | Further dissemination

Mucus | Epithelial cell barrier | Blood vessel | *To cerebrospinal fluid tissues*

(a)

(b)

eral groups of meningococci is available for immunization but it is used only under special circumstances.

Cases of meningococcal meningitis are sometimes complicated by the formation of lesions in the adrenal glands and accompanying hormone imbalances. This condition, called the **Waterhouse-Friderichsen syndrome**, may be a manifestation of a hypersensitivity reaction taking place in the body (Chapter 20).

Neisseria meningitidis is a fragile organism that does not survive easily in the environment and must be maintained in nature by person-to-person transfer. Meningococcal meningitis is therefore prevalent where people are in close proximity for long periods of time. Grade-school classrooms, military camps, and prisons are examples. Though most people suffer nothing worse than a respiratory disease, the CDC reported about 3300 cases of *Neisseria*-linked meningitis in 1997.

TABLE 7.1 compares meningococcal meningitis and *Haemophilus* meningitis, which is discussed below.

Adrenal glands: endocrine glands located atop the kidneys that produce multiple hormones.

HAEMOPHILUS MENINGITIS

In 1892, Richard Pfeiffer isolated a small, Gram-negative encapsulated rod he thought was the cause of influenza. Because of this relationship and due to its attraction to blood ("hemo-philus"), he named the organism *Haemophilus influenzae*. However, during the great influenza epidemic of 1918 to 1919, Pfeiffer's bacillus was identified as a secondary cause of disease, and influenza was attributed to a virus rather than a bacterium (Chapter 12).

fi-fer

he-mof'ĭ-lus

Haemophilus influenzae is now regarded as a cause of respiratory tract infections, occurring primarily as a complication to a previous disease. Moreover, *H. influenzae* **type b** has attracted widespread attention as a cause of meningitis in children between the ages of 6 months and 2 years. (The disease is sometimes called **Hib disease**.) The organism moves from the respiratory tract to the blood and then to the meninges, where it causes ***Haemophilus* meningitis**. Symptoms of disease include stiff neck, severe headache, and other evidence of neurological involvement such as listlessness, drowsiness, and irritability. Combinations of

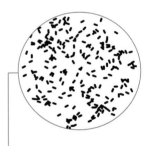

Haemophilus influenzae b

TABLE 7.1

A Comparison of Meningococcal Meningitis and *Haemophilus* Meningitis

CHARACTERISTIC	MENINGOCOCCAL MENINGITIS	*HAEMOPHILUS* MENINGITIS
Agent	*Neisseria meningitidis*	*Haemophilus influenzae* b
Description	Gram-negative diplococcus	Gram-negative rod
Transmission	Respiratory droplets	Respiratory droplets
Early symptoms	Respiratory disease	Respiratory disease
Blood symptoms	Meningococcemia, serious fever, malaise	Few symptoms
Nervous symptoms	Stiff, arched neck; headache	Stiff, arched neck; headache
Skin rash	Red to blue-black spots	Rare
Age group affected	All	Children primarily
Mortality rate	High	Low
Vaccine available	Not to general public	Available to all
Complications	Waterhouse-Friderichsen syndrome	Few

rif-am'pin

Polysaccharides:
complex carbohydrate molecules, each consisting of multiple units of a monosaccharide.

drugs, including rifampin, are used for treatment. The disease has a mortality rate of about 5 percent.

In 1986, about 18,000 cases of *Haemophilus* meningitis were occurring in the United States annually, and *H. influenzae* type b was named the most common cause of bacterial meningitis. By that time, however, a vaccine had been licensed by the FDA and the epidemic had peaked (FIGURE 7.5). The vaccine consists of polysaccharides from the organism's capsule and is thus an acellular vaccine. As of 1993, the vaccine was combined with the DTaP vaccine for distribution to children as Tetramune, and by 1996, the number of annual cases in the United States was down to 254. This disease and other airborne bacterial diseases of the upper respiratory tract are summarized in TABLE 7.2.

To this point . . .

We have studied a number of airborne bacterial diseases in which the initial focus of infection is in the upper respiratory tract. Symptoms generally include coughing, inflammation of the throat tissues, and the accumulation of mucus in the respiratory passageways. In diseases such as pertussis, this is the extent of disease, but in other diseases, bacteria invade the blood and cause serious damage elsewhere. This spread is evident in scarlet fever, diphtheria, and two forms of bacterial meningitis.

The next group of diseases involve the lower respiratory tract. Infection takes place in the lung tissue, and as the breathing capacity is reduced, a life-threatening situation is established. We shall see that lung damage occurs in tuberculosis, pneumococcal pneumonia, Legionnaires' disease, and other diseases surveyed. We shall also examine a number of respiratory diseases that do not spread easily from person to person, but develop from organisms already in the patient's respiratory tract. Our survey will conclude with diseases of the lower respiratory tract caused by rickettsiae, a group of small bacteria.

TABLE 7.2

A Summary of Airborne Bacterial Diseases of the Upper Respiratory Tract

DISEASE	CAUSATIVE AGENT	DESCRIPTION OF AGENT	ORGANS AFFECTED	CHARACTERISTIC SIGNS
Strep throat Scarlet fever	*Streptococcus pyogenes*	Gram-positive encapsulated streptococcus	Upper resp. tract Blood Skin	Sore throat Skin rash Septicemia
Diphtheria	*Corynebacterium diphtheriae*	Gram-positive rod	Upper resp. tract Heart, nerve fibers	Pseudomembrane
Pertussis (whooping cough)	*Bordetella pertussis*	Gram-negative rod	Upper resp. tract	Mucous plugs Paroxysms of cough with "whoop"
Meningococcal meningitis	*Neisseria meningitidis*	Gram-negative encapsulated diplococcus	Upper resp. tract Blood Meninges	Toxemia Paralysis Skin spots
Haemophilus meningitis	*Haemophilus influenzae* b	Gram-negative encapsulated rod	Upper resp. tract Meninges	Respiratory symptoms Paralysis

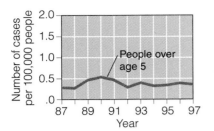

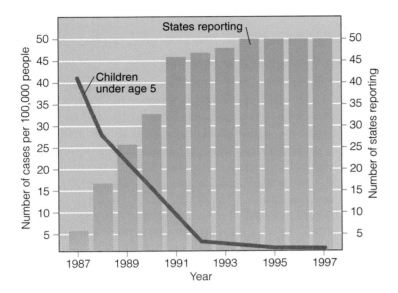

FIGURE 7.5

The Decline of *Haemophilus* Meningitis

This graph illustrates the declining number of cases of *Haemophilus* meningitis in the United States between 1987 and 1997 in children under age 5. The decline is set against the increased number of states participating in the reporting mechanism. The graph indicates that the decline is due in part to the surveillance mechanism set up in the states. Note that the number of cases in people over age 5 (small box) has remained constant in this period. A very small number of cases occur in this group.

TOXIN INVOLVED	TREATMENT ADMINISTERED	IMMUNIZATION AVAILABLE	COMMENT
Erythrogenic toxin	Penicillin Erythromycin	None	Rheumatic fever or glomerulonephritis possible Beta-hemolytic strains
Yes	Penicillin Antitoxin	Toxoid in DTaP	Corynephage involved Metachromatic granules
Not established	Penicillin Erythromycin	Acellular vaccine available as DTaP	Vaccine may cause side effects 2500 cases annually Mucus movement impaired
Yes	Rifampin Penicillin Sulfonamides	Polysaccharide vaccine	Possibly fatal Adrenal gland involvement
Not established	Rifampin	Polysaccharide vaccine to type b only	Occurs in young children Six bacterial types known

7.2

Diseases of the Lower Respiratory Tract

In the lower respiratory tract, a number of bacterial diseases affect the lung tissues. As the latter are destroyed, fluid builds up in the lung cavity, and the space for obtaining oxygen and eliminating carbon dioxide is reduced. This is the basis for a possibly fatal pneumonia.

TUBERCULOSIS

At the turn of the century, **tuberculosis** was the world's leading cause of death from all causes, accounting for one fatality in every seven cases. Today's statistics, though improved, are still very high. In developing countries, public health officials report more deaths from tuberculosis than from any other bacterial disease. In the United States, about 20,000 new cases are identified annually, with almost 3000 fatalities, most among individuals from minority groups. The World Health Organization (WHO) has referred to the global situation as a scandal and estimates that 1.7 billion people are infected. In 1997, an estimated 3 million died of the disease. MicroFocus 7.4 recounts its existence in the Americas.

Tuberculosis is caused by ***Mycobacterium tuberculosis***, the "tubercle" bacillus first isolated by Robert Koch in 1882. It is a small rod that enters the respiratory tract in droplets (multiple exposures are generally necessary). People who live in urban ghettoes often contract tuberculosis because malnutrition and a generally poor quality of life contribute to the establishment of disease, and overcrowding increases the concentration of bacilli in the air.

About 10 percent of people who contract tuberculosis become ill within 3 months (FIGURE 7.6). They experience chronic cough, chest pain, and high fever, and they expel sputum, the thick matter accumulating in the lower respiratory tract. (Often the sputum is rust-colored, signaling that blood has entered the lung cavity.) The remaining 90 percent exhibit mild symptoms, including malaise, fever, and weight loss. In these cases the body responds to the disease by forming a wall of white blood cells, calcium salts, and fibrous materials around the organisms. As

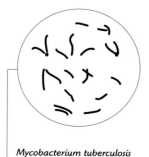

Mycobacterium tuberculosis

spu'tum

MicroFocus 7.4

"NOT GUILTY!"

Poor Christopher Columbus! Historians have accused you of bringing smallpox to the New World—and measles, whooping cough, tuberculosis, and almost every other conceivable disease. One can almost imagine that the stately *Santa María* was a hospital ship!

Well, rest easy, Chris, for scientists have cleared you of bringing at least one disease—tuberculosis. Your defense is based on 1995 research by Arthur

Aufderheide (pronounced off'der-hide) from the University of Minnesota. Some years before, Aufderheide was studying the remains of a mummified woman from Peru when he noticed in her lung tissues several lumps reminiscent of tuberculosis. He enlisted the help of a molecular biologist to extract DNA from the lumps and amplify it so there was enough to identify. The DNA turned out to be identical to that of *Mycobac-*

terium tuberculosis, the tubercle bacillus.

Why was that important? Well, Chris, the mummy was a thousand years old—that's right, one thousand years. Apparently both the woman and the tuberculosis were already here hundreds of years before you arrived. It's even possible you might have taken some back with you to Europe. . . . Oops! Sorry!

FIGURE 7.6

The Progress of Tuberculosis

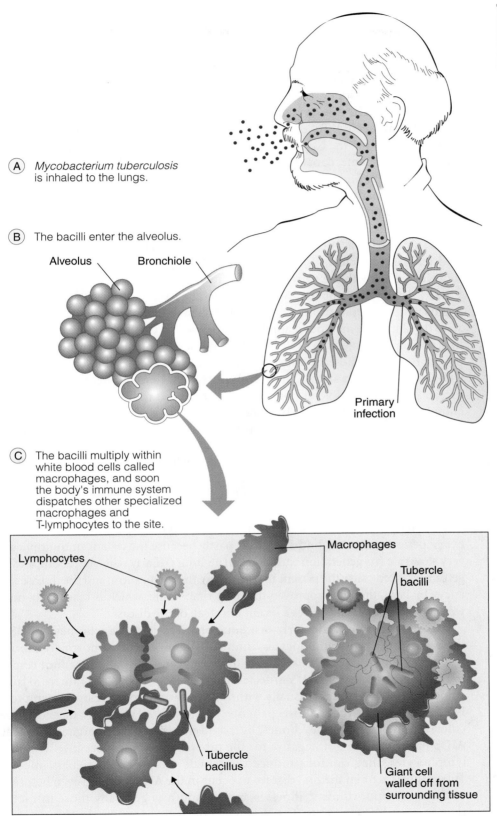

(A) *Mycobacterium tuberculosis* is inhaled to the lungs.

(B) The bacilli enter the alveolus.

Alveolus   Bronchiole

Primary infection

(C) The bacilli multiply within white blood cells called macrophages, and soon the body's immune system dispatches other specialized macrophages and T-lymphocytes to the site.

Lymphocytes

Macrophages

Tubercle bacilli

Tubercle bacillus

Giant cell walled off from surrounding tissue

(D) Multinucleated giant cells develop as the cells join together.

(E) A wall of cells, calcium salts, and fibrous materials eventually form around the giant cell. This is the tubercle.

Tubercle:
a hard nodule consisting of mycobacteria surrounded by white blood cells, salts, and fibrous material.

these materials accumulate in the lung, a hard nodule called a **tubercle** arises (hence the name tuberculosis). This tubercle may be visible in a chest X ray. Unfortunately, the bacilli are not killed, and the tubercle may expand as the lung tissue progressively deteriorates.

In many instances, the tubercle breaks apart and bacteria spread to other organs such as the liver, kidney, meninges, and bone. (Tuberculosis of the spine is called **Pott's disease**.) The disease is now called **miliary tuberculosis** (from the Latin *milium*, meaning "seed"). Tubercle bacilli produce no discernible toxins, but growth is so unrelenting that the tissues are literally consumed, a factor that gave tuberculosis its alternate name, **consumption**.

In its cell wall, *Mycobacterium tuberculosis* contains a layer of fatty waxy material that greatly enhances resistance to environmental pressures. In the laboratory, stain must be accompanied by heat to penetrate this barrier, or a lipid-dissolving material must be used. Once stained, however, the organisms resist decolorization, even when subjected to a 5 percent acid-alcohol solution. Thus, the bacilli are said to be acid-resistant, or **acid-fast**. The acid-fast test (Chapter 3) is an important screening tool when used with the patient's sputum.

Tuberculin test:
a rapid screening procedure for tuberculosis performed by applying PPD to the skin and noting a characteristic reaction.

man-too'

Early detection of tuberculosis is aided by the **tuberculin test**, a procedure that begins with the application of a purified protein derivative (PPD) of *M. tuberculosis* to the skin. One method of application, devised by Charles Mantoux in 1910, utilizes a superficial injection of PPD to the outer skin layers (the **Mantoux test**). If the patient has been exposed to tubercle bacilli, the skin becomes thick, and a raised, red welt develops within 48 to 72 hours. A positive test does not necessarily reflect the presence of tuberculosis but may indicate a recent immunization, previous tuberculin test, or past exposure to the disease. It suggests a need for further tests.

i'so-ni'ah-zid

pi'ra-zin'-ah-mid

eth'i-on'ah-mid
si'clo-ser'ēn

Tuberculosis is an extremely stubborn disease. Physicians once recommended fresh air (as MicroFocus 7.5 indicates), but now they treat it with such drugs as isoniazid (INH), pyrazinamide, rifampin, and, to a lesser extent, ethambutol and streptomycin. Alternatives include ethionamide, viomycin, and cycloserine. Unfortunately, these drugs have toxic side effects. The recent appearance of **multi-drug-resistant *Mycobacterium tuberculosis* (MDR-TB)** has necessitated the use of two or more drugs to help delay the emergence of resistant strains. In addition, drug therapy is intensive and must be extended over a period of 6 to 9 months or more, partly because the organism multiplies at a very slow rate (its generation time is about 18 hours). Early relief, boredom, and forgetfulness often cause the patient to stop taking the medication, and the disease flares anew. In 1998, the FDA approved the drug rifapentine, which is taken only once a week. MicroFocus 7.6 describes a recent outbreak of the disease.

Tuberculosis is a particularly insidious problem to those who have **AIDS**. In these patients, the T-lymphocytes, immune system cells that normally mount a response to *M. tuberculosis*, are being destroyed, and the patient cannot respond to the bacterial infection. HIV-infected patients face a mortality rate from tuberculosis of 70 to 90 percent, usually within 1 to 4 months of developing symptoms. Unlike most other tuberculosis patients, those with HIV usually develop tuberculosis in the lymph nodes, bones, liver, and numerous other organs. Ironically, AIDS patients often test negative for the tuberculin skin test because without T-lymphocytes, they cannot produce the telltale red welt that signals infection. Tuberculosis is often the first disease to occur in the AIDS patient, even before any of the other opportunistic illnesses appear, and it is generally more intractable than in non-AIDS patients. The WHO estimates that worldwide, about 4.4 million people are coinfected with HIV and *M. tuberculosis*. AIDS is discussed in more detail in Chapter 13.

A BREATH OF FRESH AIR

Edward Livingston Trudeau, an American physician, understood the danger in nursing his brother, who was suffering from tuberculosis. It was 1865. Scientists believed that tuberculosis was passed among individuals, but the cause of the disease remained unknown. In Europe, Louis Pasteur was busy with his swan-neck flask experiments, and Robert Koch was still in medical school.

Several years later, Trudeau's worst fears became reality when he developed tuberculosis. His left lung was almost completely involved, and the disease had begun to appear in his right lung. Trudeau's doctor advised him to go South and exercise; hopefully, he would survive a few months. Instead, Trudeau resolved to spend his last days in the Adirondack Mountains of New York. In 1873, he left for Saranac Lake and a

precious last opportunity to hunt and fish in the mountains he loved.

However, death was not yet ready to claim Trudeau. While in the mountains, he found his tuberculosis slowly but steadily going into remission, and within months, his recovery was complete. Trudeau became a strong advocate for the open-air treatment of tuberculosis, and in 1884 he built two small cottages and established the sanatarium at Saranac Lake to care for tuberculosis

patients. Death did eventually come, but not until 1915—a full 42 years after he was told to expect it.

Today the Trudeau Institute at Saranac Lake remains a research facility for the study of human disease. And it continues to be watched over by a Trudeau—the latest director, Francis Trudeau, is the grandson of Edward. (Francis Trudeau's son, incidentally, is Gary Trudeau, author of the comic strip *Doonesbury*.)

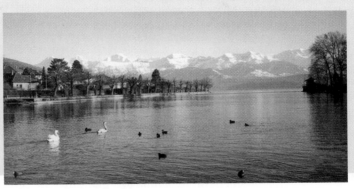

Immunization to tuberculosis may be rendered by injections of an attenuated (weakened) strain of ***Mycobacterium bovis***. This species causes tuberculosis in cows as well as humans. The attenuated strain is called **bacille Calmette Guérin,** or **BCG**, after Albert Calmette and Camille Guérin, the two French investigators who developed it in the 1920s (Chapter 19). Though the vaccine is utilized in other parts of the world, many scientists oppose its use in the United States because they point to the success of early detection and treatment and to the vaccine's occasional side effects. New vaccines consisting of subunits, molecules of DNA, and attenuated strains of mycobacteria are currently being developed, as Chapter 19 explores. In 1989, the CDC announced a strategic plan to eliminate tuberculosis from the United States by the year 2010. The plan emphasized more effective use of existing prevention and control methods and the development of new technologies for diagnosis and treatment. As of 1998, the WHO considered tuberculosis the number-one killer of humans.

Several other species of *Mycobacterium* deserve a brief mention. The first, ***Mycobacterium cheloni***, is an acid-fast rod frequently found in soil and water. During the 1980s, microbiologists first recognized this bacillus as a cause of lung diseases, wound infections, arthritis, and skin abscesses. ***Mycobacterium haemophilum*** surfaced as a pathogen in 1991 when 13 cases occurred in immunocompromised individuals in New York City hospitals. Cutaneous ulcerating lesions and respiratory symptoms were observed in the patients. ***Mycobacterium abscessus*** caused an outbreak of abscesses at injection sites when it contaminated a hormone extract administered to 47 patients in Colorado in 1996. Another notable species is

Attenuated:
weakened by chemical or cultural processes.
bah-cil'ap kal'met ga-ran'

ki-lōn'e

he-mof'i-lum

MicroFocus 7.6

TRAGIC ENDING

In the early 1990s, a powerful strain of drug-resistant *Mycobacterium tuberculosis* emerged in New York City. Affecting hundreds of people in hospitals and prisons, tuberculosis killed 80 percent of the patients. The city responded with direct-observation therapy (DOT); that is, it dispatched health-care workers to stand and watch people take their medication. The DOT seemed to work, and the epidemic subsided.

But not for long. In 1997, it was back, this time in South Carolina. What happened was this: During the interim period, a New York patient had moved to South Carolina. His tuberculosis had lingered, and he infected three family members in his new community. Soon, another six members of the community were sick with tuberculosis. However, they had not had contact with the family; in fact they did not even know the family.

Investigators from the CDC were soon on hand. They learned that one family member had been in the hospital, where he was examined with a bronchoscope (a lighted tube extended into the air passageways). Unfortunately, the bronchoscope was not disinfected properly after his examination. The contaminated instrument apparently passed the strain of *M. tuberculosis* to the six new patients.

Many stories have happy endings, but this is not one of them. The six patients were infected with a highly dangerous, drug-resistant strain of *M. tuberculosis*. Two of the six died from the tuberculosis; three died from other causes while battling the tuberculosis. Only one recovered.

Mycobacterium avium-intracellulare. This acid-fast rod may be the cause of lung disease, especially in people who have AIDS. The disease is commonly called **mycobacteriosis,** or **MAI disease**.

skrof'u-la'ce-um

skrof'u-lah

Another organism we shall mention is *Mycobacterium scrofulaceum.* This rod causes tuberculosis of the neck tissues, a disease commonly known as **scrofula** (from the Latin *scrophula* for "glandular swelling"). Scrofula is characterized by the growth of mycobacteria in the lymph nodes of the neck and substantial swelling of the tissues. Its prevalence in the Elizabethan era may have influenced people to wear the high-neck collars characteristic of that period. FIGURE 7.7 shows an example.

PNEUMOCOCCAL PNEUMONIA

The term **pneumonia** refers to microbial disease of the bronchial tubes and lungs. A wide spectrum of organisms, including many different viruses and bacteria, may cause pneumonia. Over 80 percent of bacterial cases are due to *Streptococcus pneumoniae*, a Gram-positive, encapsulated chain of diplococci traditionally known as the **pneumococcus**. The disease is commonly called **pneumococcal pneumonia**.

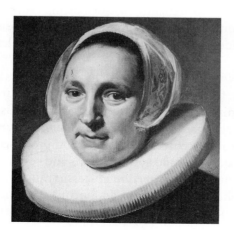

FIGURE 7.7

Scrofula and Fashion

Portrait of a Woman by Franz Hals, a painting that demonstrates the high-collar fashions of Elizabethan Europe of the late 1600s. The prevalence of scrofula is believed to have influenced the popularity of high collars, or ruffs, because they hid the swollen neck glands.

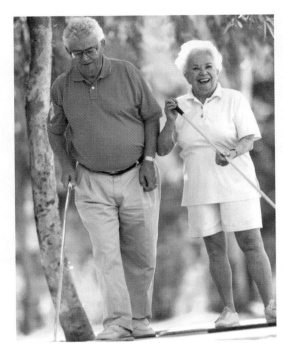

FIGURE 7.8

At Risk for Pneumonia

As people age, the immune system becomes less efficient, and individuals become more susceptible to opportunistic diseases such as pneumococcal pneumonia. Protection can be enhanced through use of the pneumonia vaccine, which contains antigens against numerous strains of the bacteria.

Pneumococcal pneumonia exists in all age groups, but the mortality rate is highest among the elderly (FIGURE 7.8) and those with underlying medical conditions. *Streptococcus pneumoniae* is usually acquired by droplets or contact, and the pneumococci exist in the respiratory tract of the majority of Americans. However, the natural resistance of the body is high, and disease usually does not develop until the defenses are compromised. Malnutrition, smoking, viral infections, and treatment with immune-suppressing drugs are typical conditions that may precede pneumonia.

Patients with pneumococcal pneumonia experience high fever, sharp chest pains, difficulty breathing, and rust-colored sputum. The color results from blood seeping into the alveolar sacs of the lung as bacteria multiply and cause the tissues to deteriorate. The involvement of an entire lobe of the lung is called **lobar pneumonia**. If both left and right lungs are involved, the condition is called **double pneumonia**. Scattered patches of infection in the respiratory passageways are referred to as **bronchopneumonia**.

The traditional drug of choice for pneumococcal pneumonia has been penicillin, with tetracycline and chloramphenicol as alternatives for allergic people. To their chagrin, public health microbiologists have noted an increasing incidence of resistant strains of *S. pneumoniae*, and as early as 1981, the first bacterial strain resistant to all three antibiotics was reported. In such cases, erythromycin is useful.

Microbiologists have identified over 80 strains of *S. pneumoniae*, based on the presence of different capsule components. Unfortunately, recovery from one strain confers immunity to that strain alone. In 1983, the FDA licensed a vaccine for immunization to 23 strains of the organism. Since these strains are responsible for 87 percent of cases, there is hope that pneumococcal pneumonia may be controlled in high-risk patients.

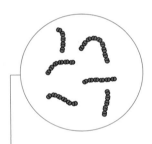

Streptococcus pneumoniae

Alveolar sacs:
millions of microscopic air sacs that make up the human lung.

klo′ram-fen′ĭ-kol

PRIMARY ATYPICAL PNEUMONIA

During the 1940s, a sudden increase in the number of cases of pneumonia prompted a search for a new infectious agent. At Harvard University, Monroe Eaton isolated a tiny agent from the respiratory tracts of patients and cultivated it

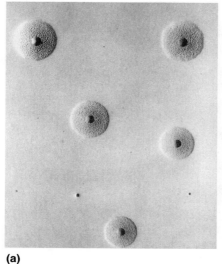

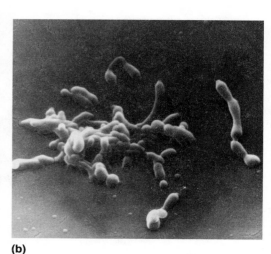

(a)   (b)

FIGURE 7.9

Mycoplasma pneumoniae

Two views of *Mycoplasma pneumoniae*, the agent of primary atypical pneumonia. (a) Colonies of *M. pneumoniae* on solid culture medium, showing the typical "fried egg" appearance. (b) A scanning electron micrograph of *M. pneumoniae*, demonstrating the pleomorphism exhibited by mycoplasmas. Note that the cells appear in multiple shapes, many in filamentous forms.

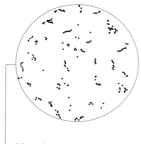

Mycoplasma pneumoniae

ple'o-mor'fic
Pleomorphic:
occurring in a variety of shapes.

Walking pneumonia:
a colloquial expression for a relatively mild case of pneumonia.

Agglutinate:
an alternate expression for clump.

on media supplemented with blood (as shown in FIGURE 7.9a). The organism was subsequently named *Mycoplasma pneumoniae*, the Eaton agent. Its disease came to be known as **primary atypical pneumonia (PAP)**—"primary" because it occurs in previously healthy individuals (pneumococcal pneumonia is usually a secondary disease); "atypical" because the organism differs from the typical pneumococcus and because symptoms are unlike those in pneumococcal disease.

Mycoplasma pneumoniae is recognized as one of the smallest bacteria causing human disease. Mycoplasmas measure about 0.2 μm in size and are **pleomorphic**; that is, they assume a variety of shapes (FIGURE 7.9b). Because they have no cell wall, they have no Gram reaction or sensitivity to penicillin. *M. pneumoniae* is very fragile and does not survive for long outside the human or animal host. Therefore it is maintained in nature by passage in droplets from host to host.

The symptoms of PAP resemble those of viral pneumonia (Chapter 12). The patient experiences fever, fatigue, and a characteristic dry, hacking cough. Research indicates that the organisms attach to and destroy the ciliated cells lining the respiratory tract. Blood invasion does not occur, and the disease is rarely fatal. Often it is called ***Mycoplasma* pneumonia** or **walking pneumonia** (even though the latter term has no clinical significance). Epidemics are common where crowded conditions exist, such as in college dormitories, military bases, and urban ghettoes. Erythromycin and tetracycline are commonly used as treatments.

Research in the 1940s established that antibodies produced against *Mycoplasma pneumoniae* agglutinate type O human red blood cells at 4°C but not at 37°C. This observation was used to develop the **cold agglutinin screening test (CAST)**: A patient's serum is combined with red blood cells at cold temperatures, and the red cells are observed for clumping. Diagnosis is also assisted by isolation of the organism on blood agar and observation of a distinctive "fried-egg" colony appearance (Figure 7.9a).

KLEBSIELLA PNEUMONIA

In 1882, Carl Friedländer isolated *Klebsiella pneumoniae,* an important cause of bacterial pneumonia. In the years thereafter, Friedländer's bacillus was related to about 5 percent of cases.

Klebsiella pneumoniae is a Gram-negative encapsulated rod, shown in FIGURE 7.10. The bacillus is acquired by droplets, and often it occurs naturally in the respiratory tracts of humans. *Klebsiella* pneumonia may be a primary disease or a secondary disease. As a primary pneumonia, it is characterized by sudden onset and a gelatinous reddish-brown sputum. The organisms grow over the lung surface and rapidly destroy the tissue, often causing death. In its secondary form, *Klebsiella* pneumonia occurs in already ill individuals and is a nosocomial, or hospital-acquired, disease spread by such routes as clothing, intravenous solutions, foods, and the hands of health-care workers.

kleb'se-el'lah

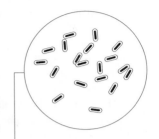

Klebsiella pneumoniae

nos'o-ko'me-al

SERRATIA PNEUMONIA

For many decades, microbiologists considered *Serratia marcescens* a nonpathogenic bacillus and often used it as a test organism in their experiments (MicroFocus 7.7 describes an example.) Today they view this Gram-negative rod as a cause of respiratory disease in compromised patients. A patient may be predisposed to infection by such conditions as chronic illness, impaired immunity due to immunosuppressive therapy, radiation, or surgical treatments such as urinary catheterization, lumbar puncture, or blood transfusion.

se-ra'she-ah mar-ses'ens

Serratia pneumonia is accompanied by patches of bronchopneumonia and, in some cases, substantial tissue destruction in the lungs. The major clinical problem in treating the disease is resistance to antibiotic therapy, apparently due to R factors (Chapter 6). The literature of the 1990s has also cited *Serratia marcescens* as a cause

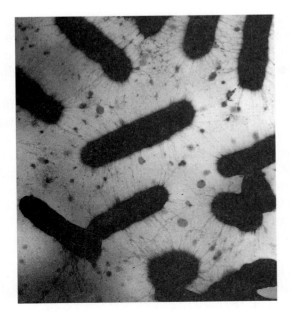

FIGURE 7.10

Klebsiella pneumoniae

A transmission electron micrograph of *Klebsiella pneumoniae,* one of the agents of bacterial pneumonia. Note that the bacilli have pili, a series of hair-like appendages that assist attachment to the tissue (×24,400).

MicroFocus 7·7

"KEEP IT SHORT, PLEASE!"

Defining, developing, and proving the germ theory of disease was one of the great triumphs of scientists in the late 1800s. Applying the theory to practical problems was another matter, however, because people were reluctant to change their ways. It would take some rather persuasive evidence to move them.

In the summer of 1904, influenza struck with terrible force among members of Britain's House of Commons. Soon the members began wondering aloud whether they should ventilate their crowded chamber. They decided to hire British bacteriologist Mervyn Henry Gordon to determine whether "germs" were being transferred through the air and whether ventilation would help the situation.

Gordon devised an ingenious (and, by today's standards, hazardous) experiment. He selected as his test organism *Serratia marcescens*, a bacterium that forms bright red colonies in Petri dishes of nutrient agar. Gordon prepared a liquid suspension of the bacteria and gargled with it. (*S. marcescens* is now considered a pathogen in some individuals.) Gordon then stood in the chamber and delivered a 2-hour oration consisting of selections from Shakespeare's *Julius Caesar* and *Henry V*. His audience was hundreds of open Petri dishes. The theory was simple: If bacteria were transferred during Gordon's long-winded speeches, then they would land on the agar plates and form red colonies.

And land they did. After several days, red colonies appeared on plates placed right in front of Gordon, as well as in distant reaches of the chamber. The members were impressed. They proposed a more constant flow of fresh air to the chamber, as well as shorter speeches. No one was about to object to either solution, especially the latter.

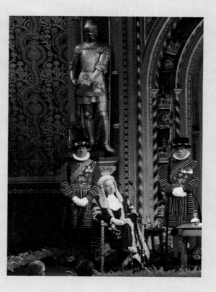

Conjunctivitis:
infection of the membrane that covers the cornea and lines the inner eyelid.

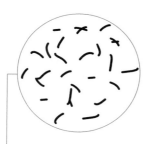

Legionella pnuemophila

of eye infections, conjunctivitis, bone disease, arthritis, and meningitis. In addition, it is an agent of urinary tract diseases.

LEGIONNAIRES' DISEASE (LEGIONELLOSIS)

From July 21 to July 24, 1976, the Bellevue-Stratford Hotel in Philadelphia was the site of the 58th annual convention of Pennsylvania's chapter of the American Legion. Toward the end of the convention, 140 conventioneers and 72 other people in or near the hotel became ill with fever, coughing, and pneumonia. Eventually, 34 individuals died of the disease and its complications.

Initially some scientists suspected that the outbreak was the first wave of a swine flu epidemic predicted for that year, but as the weeks wore on, it became apparent that an unknown microorganism was responsible. By early December, the mystery had deepened to the point that a writer from the respected journal *Science* described the "investigation that failed." But finally, in January 1977, CDC investigators announced the isolation of a bacterium from the lung tissue of one of the patients. The organism appeared responsible not only for the Legionnaires' disease (as the disease had come to be known) but also for a number of other unresolved pneumonialike diseases. The writer from *Science* swallowed hard and acknowledged "the investigation may be successful after all."

le'gion-el-lo'sis

le'gion-el'lah nu-mof'ĭ-lah

In contemporary microbiology, **Legionnaires' disease** (also called **legionellosis**) is known to be caused by the organism isolated in 1977, a Gram-negative rod named ***Legionella pneumophila*** (FIGURE 7.11). The bacillus exists where water collects, and

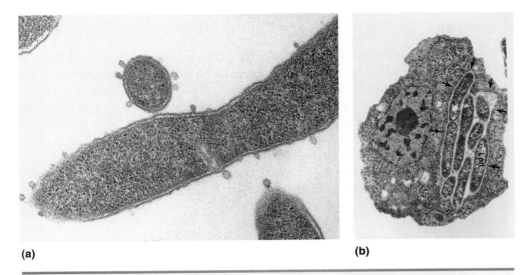

(a) (b)

FIGURE 7.11

Legionella pneumophila

Two views of *Legionella pneumophila*, the agent of Legionnaires' disease. (a) A transmission electron micrograph of *Legionella pneumophila*. Both inner (cytoplasmic) and outer membranes can be seen, as well as several evaginations (blebs) at the outer membrane. ($\times$105,000.) (b) A transmission electron micrograph of the protozoan *Hartmanella vermiformis* infected with several cells of *Legionella pneumophila*. The arrows mark the boundary membrane of the vacuole enclosing the bacilli. Legionellae are now known to sequester themselves in protozoa like these and thereby escape environmental extremes ($\times$15,000).

apparently it becomes airborne in wind gusts and breezes. Cooling towers, industrial air-conditioning units, lakes, stagnant pools, and puddles of water have been identified as sources of bacteria. Humans breathe the contaminated droplets into the respiratory tract, and disease develops a few days later (recall the chapter opening).

The symptoms of Legionnaires' disease include fever, a dry cough with little sputum, and some diarrhea and vomiting. In addition, chest X rays show a characteristic pattern of lung involvement, and pneumonia is the most dangerous effect of the disease. Erythromycin is effective for treatment, and person-to-person transmission is uncommon.

After *L. pneumophila* was isolated in early 1977, microbiologists found that the organism was responsible for many epidemics of pneumonia in previous years. One such outbreak, called **Pontiac fever**, took place in Michigan in 1968. In the years after 1977, reports of Legionnaires' disease occurred throughout the world, and invariably, water was involved. For example, 66 cases in Sweden were linked to water collecting on the rooftop of a shopping center, and 23 cases in Italy were traced to well water used for bathing. In 1990 in South Dakota, 26 cases and 10 deaths were linked to the water in showers at a particular hospital, and in 1994, a notable outbreak occurred on a cruise ship (FIGURE 7.12).

Since the discovery of *Legionella* in water, microbiologists have been perplexed as to how such fastidious bacilli could survive in an aquatic environment that is often hostile. An answer was suggested by studies showing that the bacilli could live and grow within the protective confines of waterborne protozoa. In the South Dakota episode cited above, amoebas were found in abundance in the hospital's water supply. The water was treated by heating and adding chlorine to help quell the spread of legionellae.

Fastidious:
having special nutritional requirements for growth.

Q FEVER

rik-et'se-e

Q fever is one of several diseases caused by a group of bacteria known as **rickettsiae** (sing., rickettsia). Once regarded as an intermediate type of organism between bacteria and viruses, the rickettsiae are now recognized as "small bacteria" below the resolving power of the normal light microscope and measuring about 0.45 μm. They have no flagella, pili, or capsules, and they reproduce by binary fission. With a few exceptions, rickettsiae are cultivated in the laboratory only within living tissue cultures such as fertilized eggs or animals. Arthropods are usually involved in their transmission.

The term **Q fever** was first used by E. H. Derrick in 1937 to describe an illness that broke out among workers at a meat-packing plant in Australia. The "Q" may have

TEXTBOOK CASES

FIGURE 7.12

Legionnaires' Disease on a Cruise Ship

This outbreak demonstrates how warm water can provide an incubator for infectious microorganisms.

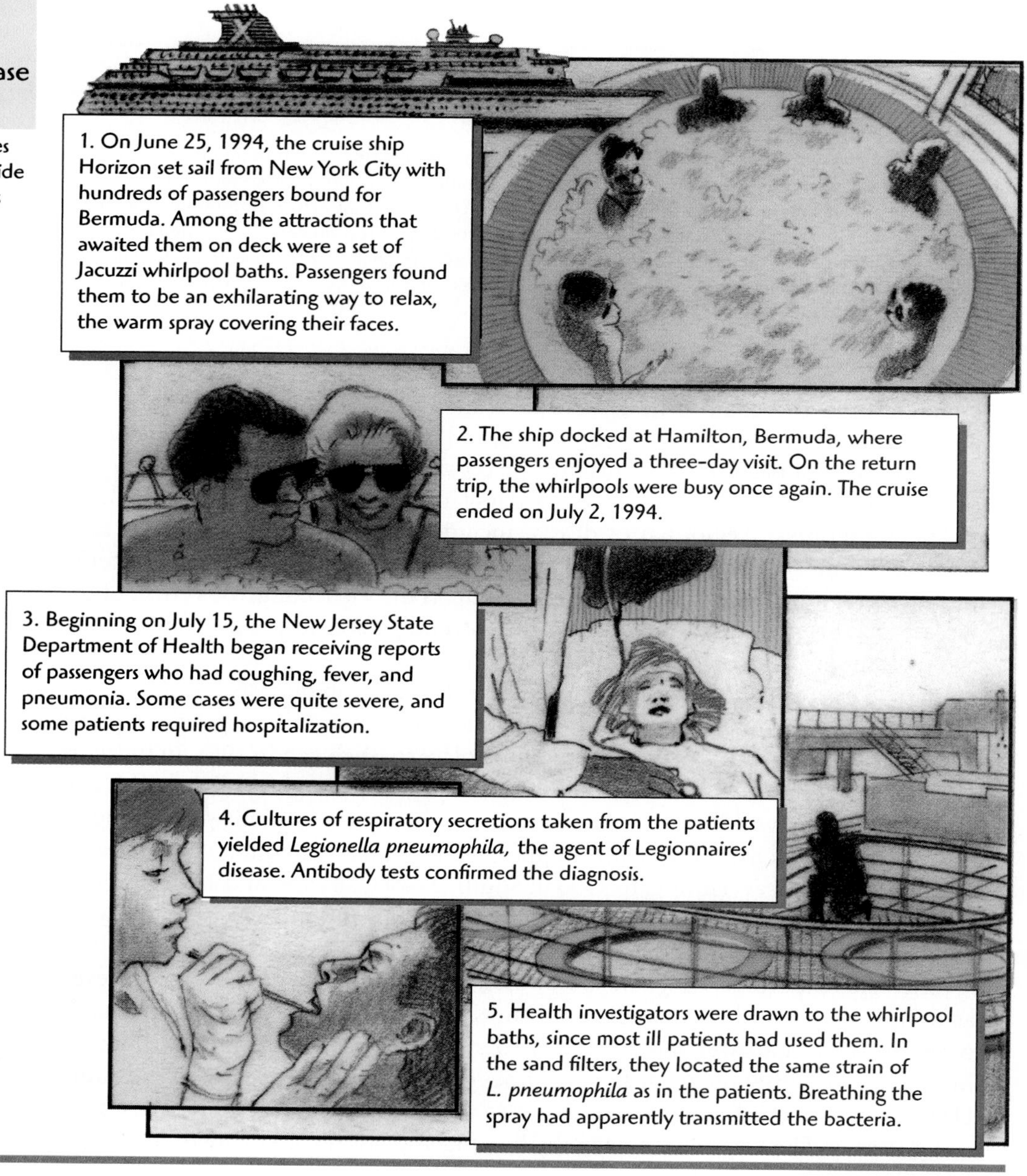

1. On June 25, 1994, the cruise ship Horizon set sail from New York City with hundreds of passengers bound for Bermuda. Among the attractions that awaited them on deck were a set of Jacuzzi whirlpool baths. Passengers found them to be an exhilarating way to relax, the warm spray covering their faces.

2. The ship docked at Hamilton, Bermuda, where passengers enjoyed a three-day visit. On the return trip, the whirlpools were busy once again. The cruise ended on July 2, 1994.

3. Beginning on July 15, the New Jersey State Department of Health began receiving reports of passengers who had coughing, fever, and pneumonia. Some cases were quite severe, and some patients required hospitalization.

4. Cultures of respiratory secretions taken from the patients yielded *Legionella pneumophila,* the agent of Legionnaires' disease. Antibody tests confirmed the diagnosis.

5. Health investigators were drawn to the whirlpool baths, since most ill patients had used them. In the sand filters, they located the same strain of *L. pneumophila* as in the patients. Breathing the spray had apparently transmitted the bacteria.

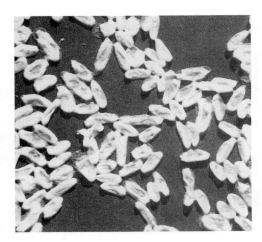

FIGURE 7.13

Coxiella burnetii

An electron micrograph of *Coxiella burnetii*, the agent of Q fever (×55,000). Note the coccobacillary form of the organism.

been derived either from "query," meaning unknown, or from Queensland, the province in which the disease occurred. The rickettsia that causes Q fever is named ***Coxiella burnetii*** (FIGURE 7.13), after H. R. Cox, who isolated it in Montana in 1935, and Frank Macfarlane Burnet, who studied its properties in the late 1930s.

kok'se-el'lah bur-net'e-e

Q fever is prevalent worldwide among livestock, especially in dairy cows, goats, and sheep, and outbreaks may occur wherever these animals are raised, housed, or transported. Transmission among livestock and to humans is accomplished primarily by airborne dust particles, as well as by respiratory droplets and by ticks. In addition, humans may acquire the disease by consuming unpasteurized milk infected with *C. burnetii* or milk that has been improperly pasteurized. Patients experience severe headache, high fever, a dry cough, and occasionally, lesions on the lung surface. The mortality rate is low, and treatment with tetracycline is effective.

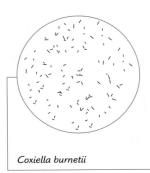

Coxiella burnetii

PSITTACOSIS AND CHLAMYDIAL PNEUMONIA

Psittacosis and chlamydial pneumonia are airborne diseases each caused by a different species of chlamydia (pl., chlamydiae). Chlamydiae are a subgroup of rickettsiae and are among the smallest bacteria (0.25 μm) related to disease in humans. They are cultivated only in living human cells and have a complex life cycle that includes a number of different forms. Three species of chlamydiae are recognized: *Chlamydia trachomatis*, the cause of trachoma and two sexually transmitted diseases (Chapter 10); ***Chlamydia psittaci***, the cause of psittacosis; and ***Chlamydia pneumoniae***, the cause of chlamydial pneumonia.

sit-ah-ko'sis
klah-mid'e-ah
(pl. klah-mid'e-e)

trah-ko'mah-tis
sit'ah-si

Psittacosis affects parrots, parakeets, canaries, and other members of the psittacine family of birds (*psittakos* is the Greek word for "parrot"). The disease also occurs in pigeons, chickens, turkeys, and seagulls, and some microbiologists prefer to call it **ornithosis** to reflect the more widespread occurrence (*orni-* is from the Greek for "bird"). Humans acquire *Chlamydia psittaci* by inhaling airborne dust or dried droppings of infected birds. Sometimes the disease is transmitted by a bite from a bird or via the respiratory droplets from another human. A notable series of cases occurred in 1992 after individuals came in contact with infected parakeets and cockatiels (FIGURE 7.14).

sit'ah-sin

The symptoms of psittacosis resemble those of primary atypical pneumonia or influenza. Fever is accompanied by headaches, dry cough, and scattered patches of lung infection. Tetracycline is commonly used in therapy. The incidence of psittacosis in the United States is currently very low (about 100 to 250 cases per year),

FIGURE 7.14

Two Outbreaks of Psittacosis

These outbreaks of psittacosis were traced to birds distributed by a single supplier. This incident occurred in 1992. Coincidence linked the disease to the distributor's birds, even though there was no evidence of widespread disease among his stock.

TEXTBOOK CASES

1. On February 13, a distributor in Mississippi shipped a supply of parakeets and cockatiels to retail pet stores in Massachusetts and Tennessee. The birds had been supplied to him by domestic breeders.

2. Four days later, on February 17, a man purchased one of the parakeets from the Massachusetts store. The man noted that the bird became very "tired-looking" some days after he brought it home.

3. On February 19, a family from Tennessee purchased a cockatiel sent by the distributor. The bird was taken home and kept in a bird cage where all family members could enjoy it. Some days later, family members observed that the bird was "irritable."

4. On March 1, the man from Massachusetts was hospitalized with fever, sore throat, and pneumonia. Two other members of his family were also sick.

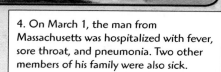

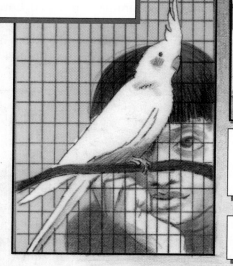

5. Also on March 1, six members of the Tennessee family were experiencing fever, cough, and sore throat.

6. In both families a diagnosis of psittacosis was made. All recovered.

partly because federal law requires a 30-day quarantine for imported psittacine birds. In addition, birds are given water treated with chlortetracycline hydrochloride (CTC) and CTC-impregnated feed. Psittacosis and other airborne bacterial diseases of the lower respiratory tract are summarized in TABLE 7.3.

Chlamydial pneumonia is caused by *Chlamydia pneumoniae* (FIGURE 7.15), an organism formerly called **TWAR** because two of the original isolates of the organism were specified TW-183 and AR-39. The chlamydia is transmitted by respiratory droplets and causes a mild walking pneumonia, principally in young

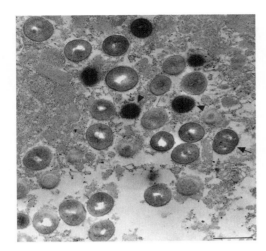

FIGURE 7.15

Chlamydia pneumoniae

An electron micrograph of *Chlamydia pneumoniae* in a glial cell from a patient suffering from Alzheimer's disease. Elementary bodies (a stage in the reproductive cycle of chlamydiae) are indicated by arrowheads, while reticulate bodies (another stage) are the less dense organisms. The arrow points to chlamydiae in binary fission. This photograph is among the first relating Alzheimer's disease to a microorganism. (Bar = 1 μm.)

adults and college students. The disease is clinically similar to psittacosis and primary atypical pneumonia and is characterized by fever, headache, nonproductive cough, and infection of the lower lobe of the lung. Treatment with tetracycline or erythromycin hastens recovery from the infection. The organism was first observed in Seattle, Washington, in 1983 and is now believed to infect many thousands annually in the United States. Its relationship to cardiovascular disease is explored in **MicroFocus 7.8**.

MicroFocus 7.8

THE (UN)USUAL SUSPECTS

Here's one to startle the senses: the "germ theory of cardiovascular diseases."

And why not, suggest researchers? New Age medications have not completely cleared away the fatty plaques lining the blood vessels. Nor have lasers, angioplasty, and other innovative devices. Why not try antibiotics?

But antibiotics for what? Why not start, they say, with *Chlamydiae pneumoniae*? As early as 1988, Pekka Saikku and his colleagues at the University of Helsinki in Finland located antibodies against *C. pneumoniae* in an unusually high number of heart attack patients (27 of 40 examined) and in numerous men with heart disease (15 of 30 examined). Their observations were later confirmed by eight research teams in five countries. Perhaps, researchers suggest,

the bacteria injure the blood vessels, triggering an inflammatory response in which immune system cells attack the vessel walls and induce large, fibrous lesions, or plaques, to form. When pieces of plaque break free, they start blood clots that clog the arteries and cause heart attacks (the condition is known as atherosclerosis).

A second suspect is cytomegalovirus (CMV), an invasive agent of the herpes virus family. Since 1997, scientists have known that people infected with CMV respond very poorly to arterial cleaning, the technique of angioplasty, and the arteries quickly close up. Another culprit may be *Streptococcus sanguis*, an agent of periodontal disease. Microbiologists believe that poor oral hygiene gives the bacterium access to the blood, where it produces blood-clotting proteins. It's no

coincidence, they maintain, that people with unhealthy teeth and gums tend to have more heart trouble. (Half jokingly, they suggest: "Floss or die.") The final suspect is *Helicobacter pylori*, the cause of most peptic ulcers. Italian scientists have linked a virulent strain with increased incidence of heart disease.

Whether *H. pylori* or *C. pneumoniae* or CMV or a streptococcus is ultimately found guilty remains uncertain. At the present time, experiments with antibiotics are underway with 3500 heart patients from medical centers in the United States, Canada, and Europe. It is conceivable that if the microbial connections hold up, antibiotics will become major weapons in the effort to stem heart disease.

TABLE 7.3

A Summary of Airborne Bacterial Diseases of the Lower Respiratory Tract

DISEASE	CAUSATIVE AGENT	DESCRIPTION OF AGENT	ORGANS AFFECTED	CHARACTERISTIC SIGNS
Tuberculosis	*Mycobacterium tuberculosis*	Acid-fast rod	Lungs, bones, other organs	Tubercle
Pneumococcal pneumonia	*Streptococcus pneumoniae*	Gram-positive encapsulated diplococcus in chains	Lungs	Rust-colored sputum
Primary atypical pneumonia	*Mycoplasma pneumoniae*	Mycoplasma No cell wall, 0.2 μm	Lungs	Dry cough
Klebsiella pneumonia	*Klebsiella pneumoniae*	Gram-negative encapsulated rod	Lungs	Pneumonia
Serratia pneumonia	*Serratia marcescens*	Gram-negative rod Red pigment at 25°C	Lungs	Pneumonia
Legionnaires' disease (legionellosis)	*Legionella pneumophila*	Gram-negative rod	Lungs	Pneumonia
Q fever	*Coxiella burnetii*	Rickettsia 0.45 μm	Lungs	Influenzalike symptoms
Psittacosis	*Chlamydia psittaci*	Chlamydia 0.25 μm	Lungs	Influenzalike symptoms
Chlamydial pneumonia	*Chlamydia pneumoniae*	Chlamydia	Lungs	Influenzalike symptoms

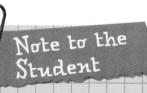

Note to the Student

In this text, we are surveying a broad group of diseases caused by an equally broad group of microorganisms. You will note, however, that other microorganisms generally do not induce the life-threatening situations posed by bacterial diseases. To be sure, there are nonbacterial diseases such as malaria, AIDS, and rabies that are deadly, but bacterial diseases are the ones that have ravaged humans for centuries. Tuberculosis, diphtheria, meningitis, and pneumonia are examples in this chapter. Typhoid fever, syphilis, cholera, and plague are examples encountered in other chapters.

Why do we not fear these bacterial diseases any more in the United States, and why can we blithely discuss them as if they were occurring on another planet? How often, for example, do newspaper headlines trumpet diphtheria or pertussis epidemics?

TOXIN INVOLVED	TREATMENT ADMINISTERED	IMMUNIZATION AVAILABLE	COMMENT
None	Isoniazid Rifampin Pyrazinamide Ethambutol	Bacille Calmette Guérin (BCG)	Extended treatment necessary Diagnosis by tuberculin test 25,000 new cases annually Related to AIDS
Not established	Penicillin Tetracycline Erythromycin	Polysaccharide vaccine to 23 strains	Over 80 strains identified Natural resistance high Deterioration of alveoli
Not established	Erythromycin	None	Called walking pneumonia Eaton agent involved Diagnosis by CAST
Not established	Various antibiotics	None	Common nosocomial disease Urinary tract infections, also
Not established	Various antibiotics	None	Common nosocomial disease Urinary tract infections, also
Not established	Erythromycin	None	Associated with airborne water droplets
Not established	Tetracycline	Vaccine for high-risk workers	Occurs in dairy cows Associated with raw milk
Not established	Tetracycline	None	Occurs in parrots and parrotlike birds
Not established	Tetracycline	None	Young adults affected

The fact of the matter is that serious bacterial diseases do break out occasionally, and some of us may be affected by them, but by and large we are insulated from widespread epidemics. This is because public health agencies understand bacterial diseases much better than in the past and can deal with them effectively by such means as sanitation measures, good hospital care, and a multitude of antibiotics. Perhaps this is a fitting place to pause and reflect on how much medical research has contributed to the quality of life. We might begin by trying to imagine what it might be like to fear infectious disease as our ancestors once did.

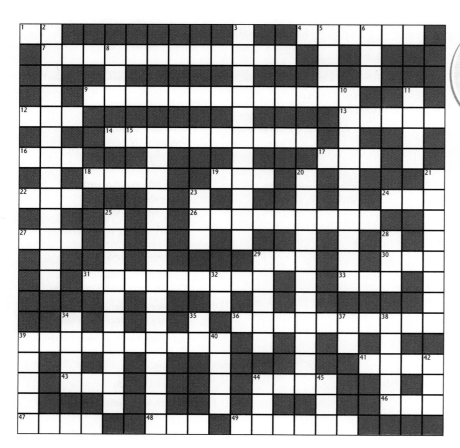

Review

The main subject of this chapter has been respiratory diseases caused by bacteria. To test your recall of these diseases, fill in the following crossword puzzle. The answers to the puzzle are in Appendix D.

■ ACROSS

1. Scarlet fever is caused by a species of streptococc_____
4. Respiratory secretions sometimes containing blood
7. Caused by a species of *Mycobacterium*
9. Genus of acid-fast rods
12. Used for immunization against two respiratory diseases
13. Bacteria can _____ the body by respiratory droplets
14. Not visible with the light microscope
16. Shape of *Legionella* bacterium
17. A valuable drug for treating meningitis is _____ -ampin

Summary

This chapter surveys a number of bacterial diseases of the respiratory tract, beginning with diseases of the upper tract and concluding with diseases of the lower tract and lungs. In many cases, the diseases are not confined to the respiratory organs, and a spread to distant organs takes place.

Among the diseases of the upper tract are streptococcal diseases, diphtheria, pertussis, and several forms of meningitis. Toxins contribute to the development of the first two diseases, and all the diseases are accompanied by fever, cough, and destruction of the local tissues. In strep throat, there is tissue erosion; in diphtheria, a pseudomembrane forms; and in pertussis, a narrowing of respiratory passages leads to the characteristic "whoop." Respiratory symptoms tend to be milder for *Neisseria*- and *Haemophilus*-induced meningitis, but serious problems arise after the bacteria pass through the blood and involve the meninges.

The lower tract infections include tuberculosis, various forms of pneumonia, Legionnaires' disease, Q fever, and psittacosis. In these instances, bacteria grow on the lung surface, and the destruction of lung tissue limits the body's ability to exchange gases. Oxygen starvation can develop in the more serious diseases such as tuberculosis and pneumococcal pneumonia, but the infection is usually milder in *Mycoplasma* pneumonia, Q fever, and psittacosis. In virtually all cases, antibiotics are available to control the diseases and help speed recovery.

18. Former name for *Chlamydia pneumoniae*
19. Incidence of diphtheria in the United States
22. Immunization to diphtheria is rendered using a _____-oid
24. The diphtheria toxin is a _____-tein
26. A species causes a form of meningitis
27. Used for immunization against tuberculosis
29. Global health group (abbr) concerned with infectious disease
30. In the CAST test, red blood cells agglutin_____
31. Species cause psittacosis and pneumonia
33. Streptococci can cause a blood disease called _____-ticemia
36. Transmitted by airborne droplets of water
39. Gram-negative rod that causes whooping cough
41. Certain strains of mycobacteria resist _____-biotics
43. Abbreviation for a mycobacterial disease
44. Accompanies meningococcal meningitis

46. The counterstain in the Gram stain technique is _____ranine
47. Abrasions of the _____ permit streptococci to enter
48. Spreading tuberculosis is said to be _____-iary
49. *Haemophilus* meningitis is not common in _____

■ **DOWN**

2. Alpha, beta, and gamma hemolytic forms
3. Disease of parrots, parakeets, and canaries, as well as humans
5. *S. pneumoniae* is often called the _____-mococcus
6. Psittacosis may be carried by exo_____ birds
8. Cases of legionellosis are treated with _____-thromycin
10. May be due to *Neisseria* or *Haemophilus*
11. *Mycoplasma* species have no _____ wall
15. Causes pseudomembranes to form
20. Small Gram-negative rod involved in meningitis in children

21. Rickettsia that causes Q fever
23. Drug (abbr) used to treat tuberculosis
25. Due to a species of *Corynebacterium*
28. A spinal _____ may be necessary to locate meningitis organisms
29. A symptom of meningitis may be the _____-house-Friderichsen syndrome
32. Q fever occurs in _____-mestic animals
34. The agent of pneumococcal pneumonia is _____-positive
35. Pneumonia may affect the termin_____ air sacs
37. Klebsiella may cause a _____-socomial infection
38. Organs affected by *Mycobacterium* species
39. Animals in which *C. psittaci* infects
40. An _____-fast rod is involved in cases of tuberculosis
42. A bout of _____-luenza may lead to streptococcal disease of the throat
44. Color of the pigment formed by *Serratia marcescens*
45. How a person feels when the fever is present in strep throat

Questions for Thought and Discussion

1. One of the remarkable public health stories of the 10-year period between 1986 and 1996 was the virtual elimination of *Haemophilus* meningitis as a concern to doctors and parents. Indeed, at the beginning of the period there were 18,000 cases annually in the United States, but in 1996, only 254 cases were reported. What factors probably contributed to the decline of the disease?

2. In 1997, in a widely publicized story, baseball pitcher Jason Isringhausen was diagnosed with tuberculosis. Doctors immediately put him on a regimen of four drugs. Which drugs do you suspect were prescribed? Why were four drugs needed? And why did the case generate so much press? (Postscript: Isringhausen was back in uniform for the 1999 season.)

3. A virus is apparently responsible for the ability of the diphtheria bacillus to produce the toxin that leads to disease. Do you believe that having the virus is advantageous to the bacterium? Why or why not?

4. In New York City, in lower Manhattan, stands a notable building between Water Street and Franklin D. Roosevelt Drive. The building has strange rounded edges that make it appear like a weird circular planter. Constructed in 1901, the building was a hospital for immigrants, especially those with tuberculosis. Can you guess what the shape of the building had to do with the disease?

5. At present there is no licensed vaccine for the prevention of any streptococcal diseases, even though these are among the most commonly experienced

bacterial diseases in the United States. Can you postulate why a vaccine, especially one composed of killed streptococci, might pose a threat to health?

6. It is a paradox of success that technology gives us appliances for better living but often provides breeding grounds for microorganisms. For example, *Legionella* probably lived undisturbed for millennia in ponds and lakes; but with the rise of air conditioning, powerful vents swept air over reservoirs of water and picked up droplets of *Legionella* to disperse to unsuspecting people who breathed the air. How many other examples of "technology" can you relate to the spreading problem of Legionnaires' disease?

7. Bacteria are generally designated Gram-positive or Gram-negative, but you may have noted that small bacteria such as rickettsiae and chlamydiae do not have this designation. Why do you think this is so? Also, why do you suppose the designation is lacking for members of the genus *Mycobacterium*?

8. It was February 1987. The patient was admitted to the hospital with high fever and a respiratory infection. Pneumococci and streptococci were eliminated as causes. Penicillin was ineffective. The most unusual sign was a continually dropping count of red blood cells. Can you guess the final diagnosis?

9. "Be sure to dress warmly when you go out or you'll catch pneumonia." This precaution, or something like it, is familiar to almost every child. In what respect is it wrong? Why is it right?

10. In a report appearing in 1997, epidemiologists noted in children a rising incidence of otitis media (middle ear infections). They attributed the increase, in part, to the larger numbers of children in day care. How are these factors related?

11. Each year, a group of "mushers" gathers in Nome, Alaska, for a 770-mile dogsled tour to Nenana, an inland city. The two-week expedition is called the Serum 25. It commemorates the 1925 run, during which life-saving serum was delivered by dogsled to quell a diphtheria epidemic. At that time there were no antibiotics, but "serum" was then widely used. What was in the serum that was so valuable?

12. Now that *Haemophilus influenzae* is no longer considered to be the agent of influenza, would you agree that a name change is in order? If so, what name might you suggest?

13. One of the major world health stories of 1995 was the outbreak of diphtheria in the new independent states of the former Soviet Union. What factors might have contributed to this international public health emergency, and what do you think was the plan to help quell the spread of the diphtheria?

14. In this chapter we have encountered organisms that are commonly named for their discoverers. Examples are Friedländer's bacillus, Pfeiffer's bacillus, and the Bordet-Gengou bacillus. However, certain organisms, such as *Legionella* and *Chlamydia* are not often referred to by the names of their discoverers. Can you postulate why?

15. How many professions can you name in which workers might be exposed to the organism of Q fever? Why is it likely that many more cases have occurred than have been diagnosed?

16. In 1997, the incidence of pneumonia was recorded in various states of the United States. Massachusetts had a very high rate, but so did Georgia. North Dakota had the third lowest rate, Florida the lowest. The highest rate was in California. Suppose you were an analyst of infectious diseases. What explanation(s) might you offer for these observations?

17. In 1996, meningococcal meningitis swept through Nigeria (on Africa's west coast). Over 150,000 cases were reported, and deaths were estimated at 15,000. The epidemic arrived with the arid season when the air in Nigeria becomes exceptionally dry and dusty. It left with the rainy season. How do you think the climate related to the epidemic?

18. A 1997 report from the CDC indicated that an estimated 40,000 people in the United States die annually from pneumonia due to *Streptococcus pneumoniae*. Despite this high figure, only 30 percent of older adults who could benefit from the pneumonia vaccine are vaccinated (compared to over 50 percent who receive an influenza vaccine yearly). Suppose you were the epidemiologist in charge of bringing the pneumonia vaccine to a greater percentage of Americans. How would you proceed?

19. Manitou Springs is a small town at the foot of Pike's Peak in Colorado. The town is about 7000 feet above sea level. Early in the twentieth century, people came to the town to drink from its mineral springs because the waters apparently helped cure tuberculosis. Many years later, scientists concluded there was no particular benefit to drinking the water. And yet, many patients had returned to good health after their visit to the town. How was this possible?

20. In 1998, Primary Children's Hospital in Salt Lake City reported a dramatic increase in the number of rheumatic fever cases. Doctors were alerted to start monitoring sore throats more carefully. Why do you suppose this prevention method was recommended?

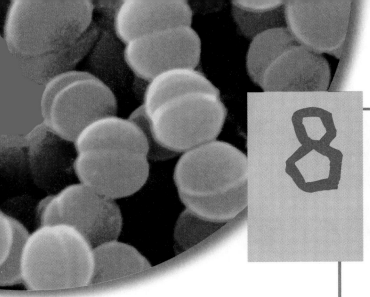

8 Foodborne and Waterborne Bacterial Diseases

Scramble or gamble.

—A CDC official succinctly advising consumers
how to avoid *Salmonella* infection from eggs

TWENTY-FIVE MILLION POUNDS? You want us to recall twenty-five *million* pounds of hamburger meat? Is this a joke?"

It was no joke, assured the inspectors from the United States Department of Agriculture (USDA). They were standing in the office of Hudson Foods, Inc. in Columbus, Nebraska. And they were demanding a recall of the company's total production between June 5 and August 12, 1998. That amounted to 25 million pounds of hamburger meat.

No one is quite sure exactly who the first patient was, but one of the first was a young supermarket worker who reported to the emergency room at the St. Mary Corwin Hospital in Pueblo, Colorado, on July 15. The young man had bloody diarrhea and painful abdominal cramps. The doctor took a stool sample, gave him some medication, and sent him home. Then she sent the stool sample to the laboratory for routine testing. A day later, the results were ready: The patient was infected with *E. coli* O157:H7 (FIGURE 8.1).

City and county health departments routinely employ a communicable disease specialist who tracks outbreaks and reports them to the Centers for Disease Control and Prevention (CDC). That day, the person on duty in Pueblo was Sandra Gallegos. Gallegos recognized the *E. coli* strain; it was associated with extensive blood infection, severe kidney damage, and, in some cases, death. She called the patient and learned that he had eaten grilled hamburger patties for dinner on July 9. It didn't take long to make the connection—hamburger meat contaminated with cattle feces is a prime method for *E. coli* transmission. On her way home

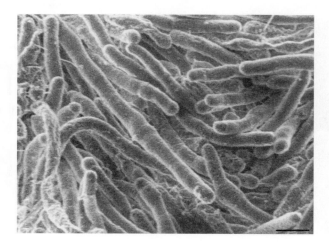

FIGURE 8.1

Escherichia coli

A scanning electron micrograph of the surface of a colony of *Escherichia coli*. A strain of this organism causes serious intestinal disease and was involved in a widespread outbreak in 1998. The strain was *E. coli* O157:H7. (Bar = 10 μm.)

from work, she stopped by the patient's house and picked up the leftover frozen hamburgers. The next day, they were off to the USDA testing lab in Athens, Georgia.

By this time, other public health officials were also awakening to the fact that something unusual was going on. In Denver, for example, the city epidemiologist Pam Shillam noted an upsurge in the incidence of *E. coli* cases, and she was investigating two cases, both associated with a July 4 barbecue. Both people had eaten hamburgers, and both had bloody diarrhea yielding *E. coli*.

Almost simultaneously, the USDA report confirming *E. coli* in the Pueblo hamburgers arrived on Shillam's desk. Shillam checked the *E. coli* "fingerprint" in the report with that of the two local cases and found a match. By August 11, there were 16 more cases in Colorado, and all of them were connected to hamburger meat bearing the Hudson Foods label. By August 12, USDA inspectors were pulling into the parking lot at Hudson. They had some bad news.

The recall that followed was the largest ever for meat or poultry in the United States. As the shell-shocked company complied with federal mandates, supermarkets and fast-food restaurants around the country adapted as best they could (some Burger King outlets were left without burgers). Meanwhile, inspectors tried to pinpoint the origin of the epidemic, even though it would probably be impossible because infected cattle generally show no symptoms. Hamburger contamination is particularly difficult to trace because grinding spreads the bacteria throughout the meat, so they grow in multiple places. Moreover, freezing does not kill *E. coli*, and many people still like their hamburgers medium or rare. At this writing, the origin of the epidemic remains unknown.

The outbreak in Colorado illustrates the extreme measures that public health departments take to safeguard the quality of our lives. Although health inspectors are constantly vigilant to prevent disease transmission, sometimes their strongest precautions are not good enough, and outbreaks occur. (We shall see numerous examples in this chapter.) But even when health officials cannot prevent an outbreak, it is comforting to know they react swiftly and strongly. In Colorado, many got sick—but no one died.

We shall categorize the foodborne and waterborne diseases as intoxications or infections. **Intoxications** are diseases in which bacterial toxins, or poisons, are ingested in food and water. Examples are botulism, staphylococcal food poisoning, and clostridial food poisoning. By contrast, **infections** refer to diseases in which live bacteria are ingested in food and water and subsequently grow in the body. These infections include typhoid fever, salmonellosis, shigellosis, cholera, and several other bacterial diseases.

8.1 Foodborne and Waterborne Intoxications

Intoxications are health problems in which a bacterial toxin is involved. Generally, there is a brief time between the entry of the toxin to the body and the appearance of symptoms (i.e., the incubation period), and the situation also resolves (for better or worse) in a relatively brief period. We shall observe this pattern in the diseases below.

BOTULISM

Of all the foodborne intoxications in humans, none is more dangerous than **botulism**. The causative agent, *Clostridium botulinum*, produces a toxin so powerful that one pint of the pure material could eliminate the entire population of the world; one ounce would kill all the people in the United States. The toxin is clearly a potent weapon for bioterrorism.

Clostridium botulinum is a Gram-positive anaerobic bacillus that forms spores. The spores exist in the intestines of humans as well as fish, birds, and barnyard animals. They reach the soil in manure, organic fertilizers, and sewage, and often, they cling to harvested products. When spores enter the anaerobic environment of cans or jars, they germinate to vegetative bacilli, and the bacilli produce the toxin. The toxin, a protein of high molecular weight (900,000 daltons), is called an **exotoxin** because the bacilli release it to the food environment as it is synthesized. The bacteria themselves are of little consequence, but the toxin is lethal once absorbed into the bloodstream.

The symptoms of botulism develop within hours. Patients suffer blurred vision, slurred speech, difficulty swallowing and chewing, and labored breathing. The limbs lose their tone and become flabby, a condition called **flaccid paralysis**. These symptoms result from a complex process in which the toxin penetrates the ends of nerve cells and inhibits the release of the neurotransmitter acetylcholine into the junctions between nerves and muscles. Without acetylcholine, nerve impulses cannot pass into the muscles, and the muscles do not contract. Failure of the diaphragm and rib muscles to function leads to respiratory paralysis and death within a day or two.

Because botulism is a type of foodborne intoxication (or poisoning), antibiotics are of no value as a treatment. Instead, large doses of specific antibodies called **antitoxins** must be administered to neutralize the toxins. Life-support systems such as respirators are also utilized. Frequently the nature of the problem is not recognized because the patient has done nothing extraordinary in the previous hours. Although the annual number of cases in the United States is low (about 75 to 100 per year), the percentage of deaths is considerable. A vaccine consisting of botulism toxoid is available for laboratory workers. Concern about the use of botulism toxin as a weapon of bioterrorism has stimulated additional vaccine research.

Botulism can be avoided by heating foods before eating them, because the toxin is destroyed on exposure to temperatures of 90°C for 10 minutes. However, experience shows that most outbreaks are related to food eaten cold. The largest episode recorded in the United States, for example, occurred in Michigan in 1977 when 58

klo-strid′e-um

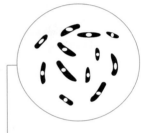

Clostridium botulinum

Exotoxin:
a poisonous protein chemical substance produced by bacteria and immediately excreted.

flak′sid

as′ĕ-til-ko′lēn
Acetylcholine:
the chemical substance that regulates impulse transfer at the junction of two nerves or a nerve and muscle.

Antitoxins:
antibody molecules that unite specifically with toxin molecules.

people became ill after eating home-canned peppers at a restaurant. Another notable outbreak is illustrated in FIGURE 8.2. Foods linked to botulism include mushrooms, olives, salami, and sausage. (Indeed, the word *botulism* is derived from the Latin *botulus,* for "sausage.")

Scientists have identified seven types of *Clostridium botulinum,* depending on the variant of toxin produced. Types A, B, and E cause most human disease. Knowing which type of *C. botulinum* caused the disease is important because antitoxin therapy must be type-specific. In animals, botulism is manifested as **fodder disease,** acquired when cattle ingest toxin from silage and feed; in fowl, it is called **limberneck.** Massive fish kills also occur periodically from the consumption of botulism toxin in water.

Silage:
animal food made by fermenting plants in tall silos.

FIGURE 8.2

An Outbreak of Botulism

This incident occurred during April 1994 in El Paso, Texas. It was the largest outbreak of botulism in 11 years.

TEXTBOOK CASES

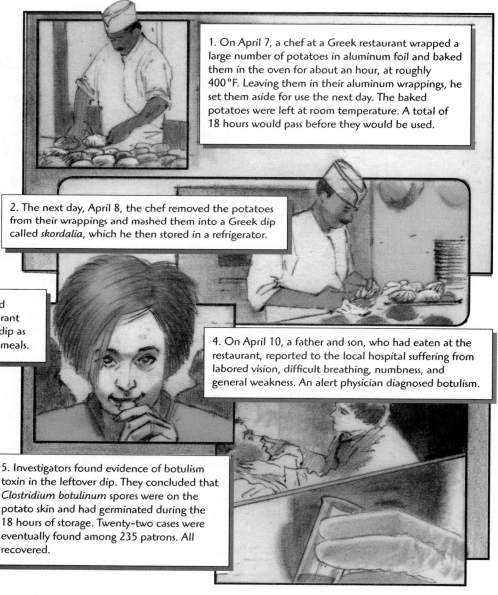

1. On April 7, a chef at a Greek restaurant wrapped a large number of potatoes in aluminum foil and baked them in the oven for about an hour, at roughly 400°F. Leaving them in their aluminum wrappings, he set them aside for use the next day. The baked potatoes were left at room temperature. A total of 18 hours would pass before they would be used.

2. The next day, April 8, the chef removed the potatoes from their wrappings and mashed them into a Greek dip called *skordalia,* which he then stored in a refrigerator.

3. That afternoon and evening, many restaurant patrons enjoyed the dip as an appetizer to their meals.

4. On April 10, a father and son, who had eaten at the restaurant, reported to the local hospital suffering from labored vision, difficult breathing, numbness, and general weakness. An alert physician diagnosed botulism.

5. Investigators found evidence of botulism toxin in the leftover dip. They concluded that *Clostridium botulinum* spores were on the potato skin and had germinated during the 18 hours of storage. Twenty-two cases were eventually found among 235 patrons. All recovered.

Studies in recent decades indicate that *Clostridium botulinum* can grow in the anaerobic tissue of a wound and cause **wound botulism**. Moreover, researchers have implicated the organisms in cases of **infant botulism** and have suggested that the disease may lead to sudden infant death syndrome (SIDS), which affects 8000 infants annually and is sometimes called crib death. Honey has been implicated as a possible source of the spores. Another species of *Clostridium, C. difficile,* may also be the cause.

We should note that in recent years, the botulism toxin has been put to practical use. Scientists have found that, in minute doses, the toxin can relieve a number of movement disorders (the so-called dystonias) caused by involuntary sustained muscle contractions. For example, **botox**, as the toxin is known, can be used to treat **strabismus**, or misalignment of the eyes, commonly known as cross-eye; it is also used against **blepharospasm**, or involuntarily clenched eyelids. Also, the toxin may be valuable in relieving stuttering, uncontrolled blinking, musician's cramp (the bane of the violinist), and spastic closure of the anal and urinary sphincter. In addition, the toxin could one day become an important treatment for cerebral palsy and multiple sclerosis.

stra-bis′mus

bleph′ă-ro-spasm

STAPHYLOCOCCAL FOOD POISONING

Years ago it was common for people to complain of **ptomaine poisoning** shortly after eating contaminated food. (Indeed, the recovery of ptomaines from the intestinal tract appeared to justify their reputation.) Modern microbiologists, however, have exonerated the ptomaines and placed the blame for most food poisonings on the Gram-positive bacterium *Staphylococcus aureus*. Today, **staphylococcal food poisoning** ranks as the second most reported of all types of foodborne disease (*Salmonella*-related illnesses are first). Because most staphylococcal outbreaks probably go unreported, staphylococcal food poisoning could be the most common type.

Like botulism, staphylococcal food poisoning is caused by an exotoxin excreted in foods. Since the symptoms are restricted to the intestinal tract, the toxin is called an **enterotoxin** (*entero* refers to the intestines). Patients experience abdominal cramps, nausea, vomiting, prostration, and diarrhea as the toxin encourages the release of water. (The word *diarrhea* is derived from the Greek stems *dia*, meaning "through," and *rhein*, meaning "to flow"; hence, water "flows through" the intestines). The symptoms last for several hours, and recovery is usually rapid and complete.

The **incubation period** for staphylococcal food poisoning is a brief 1 to 6 hours. Often the individual can think back and pinpoint the source. Examples are spoiled meats and fish, as well as contaminated dairy products, cream-filled pastries, and salads such as potato salad and coleslaw. Foods containing *S. aureus* lack an unusual taste, odor, or appearance, and the only clues to possible contamination are factors such as moisture content, low acidity, and improper heating previous to arrival at the table. The staphylococcal enterotoxin is among the most heat-resistant of all exotoxins.

A key reservoir of *S. aureus* in humans is the nose. Thus, an errant sneeze may be the source of staphylococci in foods. Studies indicate, however, that the most common **mode of transmission** is from boils or abscesses on the skin that shed staphylococci. The staphylococci grow over the broad temperature range of 8°C to 45°C, and since refrigerator temperatures are generally set at about 5°C, refrigeration is not

to-mān′

Ptomaines:
foul-smelling nitrogen compounds often recovered from the intestine.

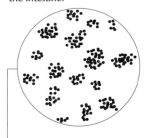

Staphylococcus aureus

Enterotoxin:
a toxin whose effects are experienced in the intestine.

Incubation period:
the time that elapses between entry of the disease agent to the host and the appearance of symptoms.

Boil:
a raised pus-filled lesion.

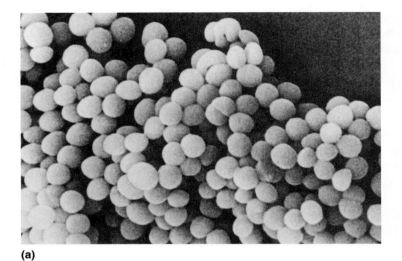

(a)

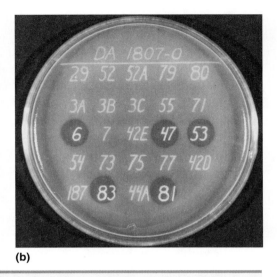

(b)

FIGURE 8.3

Staphylococcus aureus

(a) A scanning electron micrograph of *Staphylococcus aureus*, the most common cause of food poisoning in the United States. The typical grapelike cluster formation of the cocci can be seen (×15,000). (b) Typing of *S. aureus* with bacteriophages. The plate of nutrient medium was seeded with the unknown strain of staphylococci, and numbered bacteriophages were then placed into different areas. The clear areas indicate which of the phages interacted specifically with the bacteria. In this case, the strain of *S. aureus* is one that interacts with phages 6, 47, 53, 81, and 83. Tests like this are important in relating a specific strain of *Staphylococcus aureus* to an outbreak of food poisoning.

an absolute safeguard against contamination. Ham is particularly susceptible because staphylococci tolerate salt.

Staphylococcus aureus normally does not grow in human intestines because of competition by other organisms. Therefore, public health investigators are usually unable to locate the organisms in stool samples. Moreover, the contaminated food has often been consumed completely. Thus, case reports are often based on symptoms, patterns of outbreak, and type of food eaten. When investigators locate staphylococci, they can identify the organisms by growth on mannitol salt agar, Gram staining, and testing with bacteriophages to learn the strain involved, as FIGURE 8.3 illustrates.

Mannitol salt agar: a selective and differential medium in which staphylococci usually ferment the mannitol and produce yellow colonies.

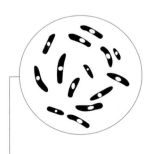

Clostridium perfringens

CLOSTRIDIAL FOOD POISONING

Since its recognition in the 1960s, **clostridial food poisoning** has risen to prominence as the second most common type of food poisoning, after staphylococcal food poisoning. The causative organism, ***Clostridium perfringens***, is also an agent of gas gangrene (Chapter 9). This Gram-positive anaerobic sporeformer contaminates protein-rich foods such as meat, poultry, and beans. If the spores survive the cooking process, they germinate to vegetative cells and produce an enterotoxin. Consumption of the toxin leads to illness. Large numbers of vegetative cells may also be consumed into anaerobic pockets in the large intestine, where the enterotoxin is produced.

The incubation period for clostridial food poisoning is a relatively long 8 to 14 hours, a factor that distinguishes it from staphylococcal food poisoning. Moderate to severe cramping, abdominal pain, and watery diarrhea are common symptoms, as the enterotoxin encourages the outward movement of water from epithelial cells lining the intestinal tract. Recovery is rapid, often within 24 hours, and therapy is generally unnecessary.

Epithelial cells:
cubelike cells that line the skin, blood vessels, and body cavities such as the respiratory and gastrointestinal tracts.

To this point . . .

We have surveyed three foodborne diseases in which toxins are responsible for the characteristic symptoms. In botulism, the toxin affects the transmission of nerve impulses and causes a life-threatening situation, while in staphylococcal food poisoning and clostridial food poisoning, the toxins affect the intestinal lining and induce a loss of water by diarrhea. This water loss is less severe on the body than the nerve interference in botulism, but the incidence of food poisoning is much higher than for botulism.

We shall now move on to a series of foodborne and waterborne diseases in which bacteria enter the body and grow profusely. These diseases are more correctly called food infections than food intoxications. We shall begin with a serious health problem, typhoid fever, then survey other Salmonella-related diseases, and next focus on shigellosis and cholera, in which patient dehydration is a prime concern. The discussion will conclude with a series of intestinal disturbances that generally are not life-threatening but have become widely recognized as detection methods continue to improve.

8.2

Foodborne and Waterborne Infections

Foodborne and waterborne infections have a longer incubation period than intoxications because bacteria must establish themselves in the body before symptoms develop. We shall see this pattern in the diseases that follow.

TYPHOID FEVER

Typhoid fever is among the classical diseases (the "slate-wipers") that have ravaged human populations for generations. The disease captured the attention of microbiologists a century ago and was studied by Karl Eberth and Georg Gaffky, both coworkers of Robert Koch. Eberth observed the causative organism, *Salmonella typhi*, in spleen tissue in 1880, and Gaffky isolated it in pure culture 4 years later.

Salmonella typhi, a Gram-negative rod, displays high resistance to environmental conditions outside the body. This factor enhances its ability to remain alive for long periods of time in water, sewage, and certain foods. *S. typhi* causes disease only in humans and is transmitted by the five Fs: flies, food, fingers, feces, and fomites.

Salmonella typhi is acid-resistant, and with the buffering effect of food and beverages, it survives passage through the stomach. In the small intestine it invades the tissues, causing deep ulcers and bloody stools. Blood invasion follows, and after a few days, the patient experiences mounting fever, lethargy, and delirium. (The word *typhoid* is derived from the Greek *typhos*, for "smoke" or "cloud," a reference to the delirium.) The abdomen becomes covered with **rose spots**, an indication that blood is hemorrhaging in the skin.

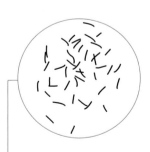

Salmonella typhi

Fomites:
lifeless objects that transmit the agents of disease.

Rose spots:
red-colored, blotchy skin spots reflecting hemorrhaged blood.

MicroFocus 8.1

TYPHOID MARY

By 1906, typhoid fever was claiming about 25,000 lives annually in the United States. During the summer of that year a puzzling outbreak occurred in the town of Oyster Bay on Long Island, New York. One girl died and five others contracted typhoid fever, but local officials ruled out contaminated food or water as sources. Eager to find the cause, they hired George Soper, a well-known sanitary engineer from the New York City Health Department.

Soper's suspicions centered on Mary Mallon, the seemingly healthy family cook. But she had disappeared 3 weeks after the disease surfaced. Soper was familiar with Robert Koch's theory that infections like typhoid fever could be spread by people who harbor the organisms. Quietly he began to search for the woman who would become known as Typhoid Mary.

Soper's investigations led him back over the 10 years' time during which Mary Mallon cooked for several households. Twenty-eight cases of typhoid fever occurred in those households, and each time, the cook left soon after the outbreak. One epidemic in 1903 in Ithaca, New York, claimed 1300 lives.

Ironically, Soper had gained his reputation during this episode.

Soper tracked Mary Mallon through a series of leads from domestic agencies and finally came face-to-face with her in March 1907. She had assumed a false name and was now working for a family in which typhoid had broken out. Soper explained his theory that she was a carrier, and pleaded that she be tested for typhoid bacilli. When she refused to cooperate, the police forcibly brought her to a city hospital on an island in the East River off the Bronx shore. Tests showed that her stools teemed with typhoid organisms, but fearing that her life was in danger, she adamantly refused the gall bladder operation that would eliminate them. As news of her imprisonment spread, Mary became a celebrity. Soon public sentiment led to a health department policy deploring the isolation of carriers. She was released in 1910.

But Mary's saga had not ended. In 1915, she turned up again at New York City's Sloane Hospital working as a cook under a new name. Eight people had recently died of typhoid fever, most of them doctors and nurses. Mary was taken back to the island, this time in

handcuffs. Still she refused the operation and vowed never to change her profession. Doctors placed her in isolation in a hospital room while trying to decide what to do. The weeks wore on.

Eventually Mary became less incorrigible and assumed a permanent residence in a cottage on the island. She gradually accepted her lot and began to help out with routine hospital work. However, she was forced to eat in solitude and was allowed few visitors. Mary Mallon died in 1938 at the age of 70 from the effects of a stroke. She was buried without fanfare in a local cemetery.

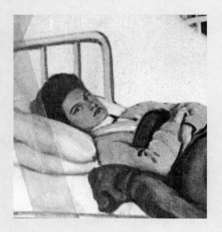

About 400 cases of typhoid fever are reported annually to the CDC, as FIGURE 8.4 indicates. Treatment is generally successful with the antibiotic chloramphenicol, except when antibiotic resistance due to R factors is noted (Chapter 6). About 5 percent of recoverers become **carriers** and continue to harbor and shed the organisms for a year or more. Because they are possible sources of disease to others, the public health department usually monitors the activities of carriers. The experiences of one of history's most famous carriers, Typhoid Mary, are recounted in MicroFocus 8.1.

Traditional vaccines for typhoid fever have consisted of dead *S. typhi* cells, but adverse reactions have introduced an element of risk. The newer TY21a vaccine is composed of weakened (attenuated) viruses genetically altered to carry *Salmonella* antigens. A vaccine currently under development (Typhin Vi) consists of capsular polysaccharides from *S. typhi*. Its supporters point to a stronger response than that rendered by the viral vaccine. MicroFocus 8.2 describes an interesting relationship between *S. typhi* and cystic fibrosis.

MicroFocus 8.2

THE DOWN SIDE, THE UP SIDE

Cystic fibrosis is a gruesome disease. Abnormal amounts of thick, sticky mucus build up in the respiratory tracts of children and clog the air passageways. Parents have to slap children on the back repeatedly to help clear the clogging. Life-threatening respiratory infections often accompany the disease.

Scientists now know that cystic fibrosis is a genetic disease that develops when two mutant genes are inherited from the parents. With the mutation in place, a regulatory protein is not produced, and the sticky mucus accumulates. About 30,000 individuals in the United States suffer the misery of cystic fibrosis each year.

But there is a strange twist to this story. Harvard researchers have discovered that the regulatory protein is an attachment site for the typhoid bacillus *Salmonella typhi*. Apparently the regulatory protein protrudes from cells and binds to *S. typhi* at the start of the disease process. Now the bacilli are free to invade and destroy the tissues. However, if there is no protein, then there is no binding, and no disease.

Occasionally, Mother Nature does things that seem to defy explanation. Evidence suggests that the cystic fibrosis patient is immune to typhoid fever. Before the age of antibiotics, that would have been a worthwhile trade-off, since typhoid fever was a major killer. Indeed, in developing countries, typhoid fever is still a serious health problem. Is it possible that cystic fibrosis is another of those "diseases of civilization"? What do you think?

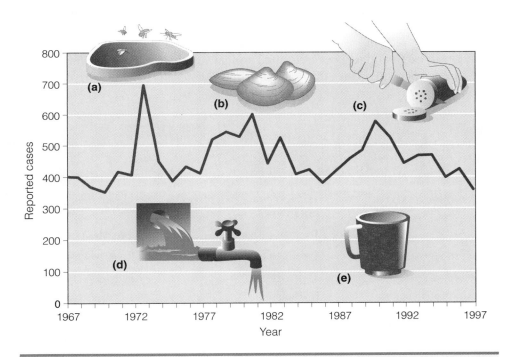

FIGURE 8.4

The Incidence of Typhoid Fever

Reported cases of typhoid fever in the United States by year, 1967 to 1997. For 1997, 365 cases were reported. In about half the cases, the disease was acquired during foreign travel. Portrayed on the graph are the five Fs important in the transmission of typhoid fever: (a) flies, (b) food, (c) fingers, (d) feces, and (e) fomites.

SALMONELLOSIS

sal'mo-nel-lo'sis

Serotypes:
variants of organisms that differ according to the antibodies they elicit from the immune system.

Dehydration:
excessive loss of body fluids.

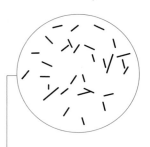

Salmonella typhimurium

Salmonellosis currently ranks as the most reported of all foodborne diseases in the United States, with almost 40,000 cases occurring annually (TABLE 8.1 compares the disease to staphyloccal food poisoning.) It is caused by hundreds of serotypes (serological types) of **Salmonella**. Serotypes are used for *Salmonella* instead of species because of the uncertain relationships existing among the organisms. The most common causes of salmonellosis include *S. typhimurium* (FIGURE 8.5), *S. heidelberg, S. enteritidis,* and *S. newport.* All are Gram-negative rods.

After an incubation period of 1 to 3 days, the patient with salmonellosis experiences fever, nausea, vomiting, diarrhea, and abdominal cramps. Intestinal ulceration is usually less severe than in typhoid fever, and blood invasion is uncommon. The symptoms may last a week or more, and dehydration may occur in some patients; fluid replacement may be necessary. Diagnosis usually consists of isolating the *Salmonella* serotype from stool specimens or rectal swabs, using differential media. Often the infection is called **gastroenteritis,** or simply **enteritis.** A notable outbreak occurred in 1991, as MicroFocus 8.3 describes.

With increased awareness and modern methods of detection, salmonellosis has been linked to a broad variety of foods. **Pasteurized milk** was linked to 5770 cases in the midwestern United States in 1985 (Chapter 24), and frozen pasta products were the source of dozens of cases in the northeastern states in 1986. **Poultry products** are particularly notorious because *Salmonella* serotypes commonly infect chickens and turkeys when the normal gut bacteria are absent (MicroFocus 8.4 explores a possible method for replacement). The organisms may be consumed directly from the poultry or in pot pies, processed chicken roll, turkey roll, or chicken salads. With over 4 billion chickens and turkeys consumed annually in the United States (an average of 75 pounds per American), the possibilities for *Salmonella* passage are plentiful.

TABLE 8.1

A Comparison of Staphylococcal Food Poisoning and Salmonellosis

CHARACTERISTIC	STAPHYLOCOCCAL FOOD POISONING	SALMONELLOSIS
Agent	*Staphylococcus aureus*	*Salmonella* serotypes
Description	Gram-positive cluster of cocci	Gram-negative rod
Toxin involved	Yes (enterotoxin)	No
Incubation period	Few hours	1–3 days
Incidence in U.S.	Possible millions annually	40,000 reported annually
Symptoms	Cramps, nausea, diarrhea; no ulceration; no fever	Cramps, nausea, diarrhea; some ulceration; fever
Duration of symptoms	Few hours	Few days
Foods involved	All	All, especially poultry/eggs
Animals involved	No	Yes (especially reptiles)
Treatment	None	Antibiotics possible
Source of bacteria	Skin infection, nose	Fecal contamination
Diagnosis	Isolate bacteria from food	Isolate bacteria from feces

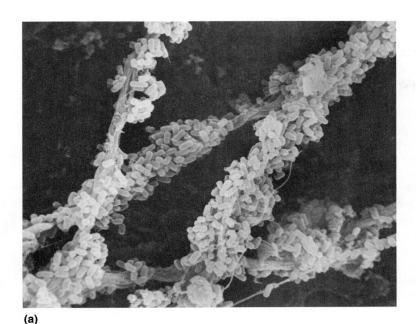

(a)

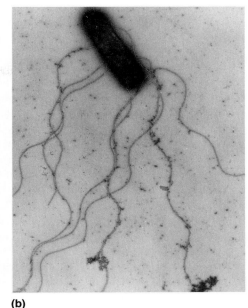

(b)

FIGURE 8.5

Salmonella Species

Two views of *Salmonella* involved in salmonellosis. (a) *S. typhimurium* observed on the collagen fibers of muscle tissue from an infected chicken ($\times$12,000). (b) A transmission electron micrograph of a *Salmonella* serotype showing peritrichous flagella ($\times$40,000). Note the long length of the flagella relative to the cell.

MicroFocus 8.3

YOU MAKE THE CALL

Poultry products and eggs are well known for their connections to *Salmonella* diseases, but the signs that summer did not point to the poultry and eggs; they pointed to the fruit salad.

There were 75 people at the party in New Jersey that June night in 1991. By the next week, 17 were ill with nausea, vomiting, diarrhea, abdominal cramps, and fever. Soon, investigators were visiting each one, asking questions and requesting stool samples. All 17 had eaten the fruit salad—the watermelon, cantaloupe, honeydew melon, strawberries, and grapes. The investigators scratched their heads because fruit salad and *Salmonella* just don't go together. Or do they? And if they do, which was the responsible fruit? They waited for additional cases to surface.

They did not have to wait long. In July, 20 cases of salmonellosis were reported in Minnesota, and several more occurred in Illinois, Pennsylvania, North Dakota, Missouri, and Michigan. Even Canada contributed 72 cases. All tolled, there were 400-plus cases of salmonellosis in 23 states and Canada during that June-July period. And the culprit seemed to be the cantaloupe.

At least the laboratory researchers suspected it was the cantaloupe, even though they could not isolate *Salmonella* from the fruit. But they recovered *Salmonella* from enough patients who had eaten cantaloupe; and they were able to pinpoint *Salmonella poona* as the epidemic's cause. In addition, they traced all the cantaloupes to a farm in south Texas where the soil was heavily

contaminated by *Salmonella* and where *S. poona* had probably infected the rinds. But people do not eat cantaloupe rinds; they eat the fruit. So how did the *Salmonella* get from the rind to the fruit? Any guesses?

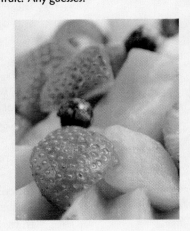

MicroFocus 8.4

"SORRY, NO VACANCY"

In the old days, chicks hatched from their eggs, scrambled to their feet, and nestled under their mother's wing until it was safe to come out. By staying close to their mother hen, the chicks received protection, caring, and bacteria. Bacteria? Yes, bacteria—hundreds of strains of harmless organisms that filled the chicks' guts and prevented *Salmonella* serotypes from causing infection. With all the enterococci, fusobacteria, lactobacilli, and other strains, there simply was no room for *Salmonella*. The chicks remained healthy.

But mother hen is gone. The high-tech chicken farms of the modern era use machines to remove the eggs from the hen as they are produced. The chicks hatch and develop without ever seeing who made them. To be sure, that is sad. But microbiologically, the sadness is compounded by the absence of the harmless bacteria from the chick's gut (and the tendency of the chick to develop salmonellosis).

As of 1998, there was an answer. That year, the Food and Drug Administration approved a spray (called Preempt) that showers chicks with a mix of 29 species of harmless bacteria. The chicks pick the bacteria off their feathers and ingest them. As the harmless bacteria set up housekeeping in the gut, they compete with and exclude the dangerous ones. (Scientists call the process "competitive exclusion.") Numerous tests show that *Salmonella* serotypes are significantly reduced or completely eliminated. Once again, science has replaced mother hen.

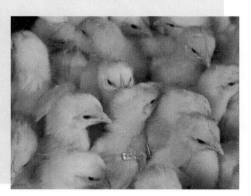

Eggs are another source of salmonellosis when used in foods such as custard pies, cream cakes, egg nog, ice cream, and mayonnaise (Chapter 24). In 1992, the CDC reported 38 cases associated with Caesar salad dressing made with raw eggs. In the past, salmonellosis was associated with cracked or contaminated egg shells, but researchers now believe that *Salmonella* serotypes infect the ovary of the hen and pass into the egg before the shell forms. If this is so, then even the highest-grade eggs may be contaminated. Consumers should store eggs in the main compartment of the refrigerator, refrigerate leftover egg dishes quickly in small containers (to accelerate cooling), and avoid "runny" or undercooked eggs. The current catchphrase at the CDC is "scramble or gamble." Indeed, in 1992, New Jersey outlawed "eggs over easy." (It later rescinded the ban.)

Live **animals** are also known to transmit salmonellosis, and many states now prohibit the sale of Easter chicks and ducklings for this reason. Moreover, some years ago, the FDA prohibited the distribution of pet turtles less than 4 inches long because a significant number of salmonellosis outbreaks were attributed to handling these animals. The sale of iguanas is also restricted, and a savannah monitor lizard was apparently the cause of an infant's disease in 1992, as MicroFocus 8.5 relates.

SHIGELLOSIS (BACTERIAL DYSENTERY)

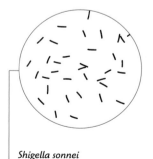

Shigella sonnei

shĭ′gel-lo′sis

Members of the genus *Shigella* were first described by the Japanese investigator Kiyoshi Shiga in 1898, and 2 years later by the European microbiologist Simon Flexner. *Shigella* species are small Gram-negative rods found mainly in humans and other primates. They cause digestive disturbances ranging from mild diarrhea to a severe and sometimes fatal dysentery. (Dysentery is a syndrome manifested by waves of intense abdominal cramps and frequent passage of small-volume, bloody mucoid stools.) For many years, *Shigella* diseases were known as **bacterial dysentery**. However, watery diarrhea without blood or mucus is a more common symptom than dysentery, and the name **shigellosis** is preferred. About 25,000 cases occur annually in the United States.

MicroFocus 8.5

"THANKS BUT NO THANKS"

I t just wasn't a nice pet at all," the parents told the health department people. "But the children really wanted a lizard, so we gave in." There was a pause, then they continued. "It had diarrhea all the time we had it, and the cage was so big we had to climb in to clean it. And oh, those heat rocks in the bottom of the cage—they all had to come out for cleaning. A month ago we got rid of it."

The "it" of the conversation was a 2-foot-long savannah monitor lizard. The lizard was the prime suspect in a case of salmonellosis affecting the 8-week-old infant of the family. A week previously,

the baby had been brought to the hospital clinic suffering from bloody diarrhea, severe flatulence, and a temperature of 101°F. The lab isolated *Salmonella poano* from its stools, and health investigators were now trying to track down the source of the *Salmonella*. It was June 1992 in suburban Salt Lake City, Utah.

"Mind if we take some samples?" the visitors asked. In the next few minutes they swabbed the cage, the rocks, the lizard's water dish, and the floor of the cage. Two days later, sure enough—*Salmonella poano* in almost every sample. But how could the infant have come in

contact with the animal? It was probably an error by the parents—cleaning the cage, handling the lizard, washing the rocks in the kitchen sink, forgetting to wash their hands or doing so poorly. Perhaps the bacteria made their way to the baby by feeding utensils.

No additional studies were performed, partly because the lizard could not be traced. Moreover, the family had already resolved that no more lizards would set foot in their house. They had traded the lizard back to the pet shop for another pet—a python.

Shigellosis may be caused by any of four species of **Shigella**, including *Sh. sonnei, Sh. dysenteriae, Sh. flexneri* (for Shiga and Flexner), and *Sh. boydii*. Humans ingest the organisms in contaminated water as well as in many foods, especially eggs, vegetables, shellfish, and dairy products. *Shigella* usually penetrates the epithelial cells lining the intestine and, after 2 to 3 days, it produces sufficient enterotoxins to encourage water release. Infection of the small intestine produces watery diarrhea, but infection of the large intestine results in bloody mucoid stools characteristic of dysentery. Indeed, the dysentery can be quite indisposing. It is said that at the Battle of Crécy in 1346, the English army was racked with dysentery. When the French attacked, they literally caught the English with their pants down.

sōn'e-i

Shigella species can be isolated from stools, and most cases of shigellosis subside within a week. Usually there are few complications, but patients who lose excessive fluids must be given salt tablets, oral solutions, or intravenous injections of salt solutions for **rehydration**. Antibiotics are sometimes effective, but many strains of *Shigella* are resistant because of R factors. Recoverers generally become carriers for a month or more and continue to shed the bacilli in their feces. Vaccines are not available, but 586 passengers aboard the cruise ship *Viking Serenade* wished they were. They were the unfortunate victims of a shigellosis outbreak in 1994 traced to bacteria in the water supply. Trapped hopelessly aboard ship, they could only wait for landfall and dream of a more pleasant "serenade" the next time.

Intravenous: injection directly into the vein.

CHOLERA

No diarrhea can compare with the extensive diarrhea associated with **cholera**. In the most severe cases, a patient may lose up to 1 liter of fluid every hour for several hours. The fluid is colorless and watery, with characteristic **rice-water stools** reflecting the conversion of the intestinal contents to a thin liquid like barley soup. The patient's eyes become gray and sink into their orbits. The skin is wrinkled, dry, and

kol'er-ah

Rice-water stools: thin, souplike intestinal contents characteristic of cholera.

FIGURE 8.6

The Bacilli of Cholera

Two views of *Vibrio cholerae*, the cholera bacillus. (a) A view of the edge of a colony of *Vibrio cholerae* on a solid culture medium (×5400). Many cells are seen in various stages of division, and the irregular arrangement of the vibrios is visible. (b) Two free cells, one of which is dividing (×20,000). Note the commalike shape of the cells.

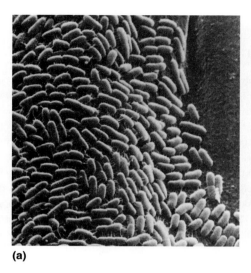 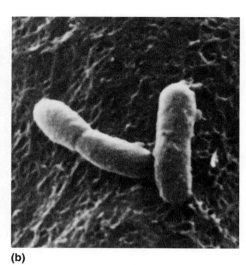

(a)   (b)

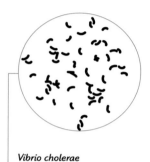

Vibrio cholerae

Tetracycline:
an antibiotic that interferes with protein synthesis, especially in Gram-negative bacteria.

cold, and muscular cramps occur in the arms and legs. Despite continuous thirst, sufferers cannot hold fluids. The blood thickens, urine production ceases, and the sluggish blood flow to the brain leads to shock and coma. In untreated cases, the mortality rate may reach 70 percent.

Cholera is caused by **Vibrio cholerae**, a curved Gram-negative rod (FIGURE 8.6) first isolated by Robert Koch in 1883. The bacilli enter the intestinal tract in contaminated water or food, such as raw oysters. *Vibrio cholerae* is extremely susceptible to stomach acid. However, if high numbers are ingested, enough remain to colonize the intestines. As the bacilli move along the intestinal epithelium, they secrete an enterotoxin that stimulates the unrelenting loss of fluid (MicroFocus 8.6). Antibiotics such as tetracycline may be used to kill the bacteria, but the key treatment is restoration of the body's water balance. Often, this entails **intravenous injections** of salt solutions. More commonly, patients can be treated with **oral rehydration solution (ORS)**, a solution of electrolytes and glucose that will restore the normal balances in the body.

MicroFocus 8.6

MEMORIES

It was supposed to be a simple evening together at a quiet, local restaurant—six women, dinner, some interesting scuttlebutt, and a pleasant memory or two. The August night was hot that summer in Maryland in 1991. All would go as planned, except for the memory. It would not be pleasant.

Two days later, one of the women developed vomiting and water diarrhea so severe she had to be hospitalized. Then two others had acute diarrhea requiring medical attention. When blood samples from the three were analyzed for antibodies, the results raised the eyebrows of health officials—it was cholera.

The first thing that came to mind were the crabs served that night. But Marylanders are proud of their crabs, and health investigators were relieved to learn that crabs had been served to others at the restaurant with no apparent effect. What about the Thai-style rice pudding? It came with a topping made from imported coconut milk, and several unopened packages of the milk were still in the freezer. Did the sick women have the rice pudding with the topping? Yes. How about the other restaurant patrons that night? They had ordered rice pudding but without the topping. Aha! Could the health officials

please have the unopened milk packages for testing?

During the next several days, emergency rooms were checked for additional cases of cholera, but none surfaced. Sewage collection points were tested for cholera bacilli, but samples turned up negative. Secondary contacts of the women were reached to see if they had any unusual symptoms; none reported any. By now the laboratory results on the coconut milk were ready. The milk was positive for *Vibrio cholerae* and a number of other bacteria. A voluntary product recall was issued by the distributor. Case closed.

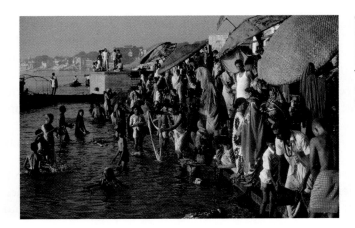

FIGURE 8.7

How Cholera Spreads

The Ganges River in India is considered sacred, and people wash in the river and drink from it. Cholera bacilli frequently inhabit the river and pass easily among unsuspecting bathers.

Cholera has been observed for centuries in human populations, and seven pandemics have been documented. The current pandemic began in 1961 in Indonesia and now involves about 35 countries (FIGURE 8.7). A major outbreak occurred in Peru and Ecuador early in 1991 and from there spread throughout the region, accounting for 731,000 cases by the end of 1992 and 6300 deaths in 21 countries in the Western Hemisphere. By 1998, the epidemic was spreading throughout Africa at what the World Health Organization called a "catastrophic rate." MicroFocus 8.7 describes how the responsible strain may have emerged.

Pandemic: a worldwide epidemic.

MicroFocus 8.7

HOW THE SHEEP GOT THE WOLF'S CLOTHES

The seventh pandemic of cholera began in Sulawesi, Indonesia, in 1961. Soon it spread to India, the Soviet Union, and the Middle East. By 1991, it had reached Latin America and affected all countries of South America, except Argentina. By 1995, over 5000 people had died of cholera, and many hundreds of thousands had been terribly sick.

The pandemic was apparently due to a toxin-producing strain of *Vibrio cholerae* known as O1. The toxin binds to intestinal cells, setting off a cascade of reactions, and water pours out of the cells—up to 5 gallons of water per day. Where did the toxin come from? Microbiologists from Harvard think they have the answer: a virus.

Matthew Waldor and John Mekalanos had been studying cholera for many years. They were impressed by the toxicity of the O1 strain and wondered why other strains were far less

lethal. Their interest centered on the toxin gene in *V. cholerae*, and they speculated that the gene might have been delivered by a virus through the process of transduction (Chapter 6). To test their theory, they removed the entire toxin gene by sophisticated genetic engineering techniques, then they replaced it with an antibiotic-resistance gene. Now they cultured the new antibiotic-resistant cholera cells with normal cholera cells susceptible to antibiotics. Bingo! The susceptible cells became antibiotic-resistant. Something (a virus?) seemed to be leaving the antibiotic-resistant cells and ferrying the resistance gene to the susceptible cells.

But maybe the bacteria were conjugating and exchanging their genes directly. To test this theory, Waldor and Mekalanos passed the genetically engineered (antibiotic-resistant) cells through a filter that would trap everything except viruses. They took the clear,

cell-free liquid and added it to a fresh batch of normal cells. Double bingo! The cells became resistant to antibiotics. The virus theory strengthened.

Still another test: They treated the clear, cell-free fluid with enzymes that destroy free-floating nucleic acids but have no effect on viruses. (This would eliminate any molecular DNA or RNA that might transform cells.) Then they combined the fluid with normal cells. Once again, the cells became antibiotic-resistant. And the coup de grace: Electron micrographs revealed long, stringy viruses in the cell-free fluid.

To be sure, the cholera bacterium is not the first to have its toxicity associated with a virus (the diphtheria and botulism organisms are others), but the finding helps explain how an organism can suddenly become lethal. The sheep had acquired the wolf's clothing.

At present, travelers to cholera regions of the world are immunized with preparations of dead *V. cholerae,* thereby obtaining protection for about 6 months. But this approach may change, because public health officials anticipate a genetically engineered cholera vaccine that will give longer-lasting protection without the risk of using dead pathogenic cells. In 1992, researchers at the University of Maryland identified the genes for enterotoxin production and successfully removed them from experimental *V. cholerae* cells. So treated, the vibrios became nonpathogenic but still alive (i.e., attenuated), and they could be used in a vaccine to stimulate an antibody response. Field trials for the new vaccine are ongoing at this writing.

For generations, scientists believed the cholera bacillus exists only within a human host. That principle was refuted by University of Maryland researchers led by Rita Colwell (current Director of the National Science Foundation). Colwell and her colleagues found *V. cholerae* in waters from the Chesapeake Bay, even though no cholera outbreaks were remotely close to the site. They postulated that the organisms enter a sporelike dormant state that cannot be cultivated. (Highly sensitive antibody tests detected the organism when more traditional tests failed.) Apparently, in the cold, nutrient-poor water, the organism's metabolic rate diminishes, and it stops reproducing. This state, says Colwell, allows the cholera bacillus to survive in habitats and environments ranging from seawater to the human intestinal tract. In the sea, moreover, the bacillus appears to be a regular gut inhabitant of a tiny crustacean known as a copepod. The findings are novel, and they may signal a new outlook for cholera in the decades ahead.

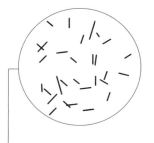

Escherichia coli

E. COLI DIARRHEAS

One of the major causes of **infantile diarrhea** is the Gram-negative rod ***Escherichia coli*** (FIGURE 8.8). This organism may induce diarrhea by either of two mechanisms: Certain *enterotoxic* strains produce an enterotoxin similar to that in cholera, while other *enteroinvasive* strains penetrate the intestinal epithelium, as in shigellosis. The toxin causes fluid loss in the small intestine, while penetration occurs primarily in the large intestine. Both mechanisms lead to dehydration and salt imbalance substantial enough to be life-threatening in

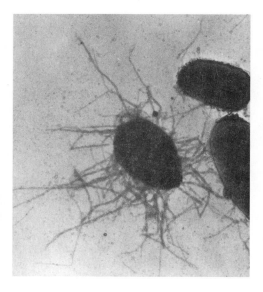

FIGURE 8.8

Escherichia coli

A transmission electron micrograph of *Escherichia coli,* the cause of many forms of traveler's and domestic diarrheas. The hairy fibers extending from the cell surface are pili, short appendages of protein the bacterium uses to adhere to the infected tissue (×40,000).

infants. Antibiotic therapy and fluid replacement are usually effective. Often the infection is nosocomial.

Traveler's diarrhea is a term usually applied to a disease in which the victim experiences diarrhea within 2 weeks of traveling to a tropical location; the diarrhea lasts 1 to 10 days. Sometimes this disease is called **Montezuma's revenge**, a reference to the leader of the Aztec nation decimated by smallpox and other diseases brought from Europe in the 1500s. A number of organisms including several types of bacteria, viruses, and protozoa may cause traveler's diarrhea, but recent studies point to *E. coli* as the principal agent. The bacilli adhere to the intestinal lining with pili (Figure 8.8) and produce enterotoxins, which induce water loss. The volume lost is usually low, but occasionally it may be considerable, and dysentery may occur. The possibility of traveler's diarrhea may be reduced by careful hygiene and attention to the food and water consumed during visits to other countries.

As described in the introduction to this chapter, it is possible to contract a rather serious *E. coli* diarrhea without traveling. In 1993, for example, *E. coli* **O157:H7**, an enterotoxic strain, was the cause of over 500 cases of serious illness in patrons of the Jack-in-the-Box fast-food chain (Chapter 3). Also that year, mayonnaise contaminated with *E. coli* was implicated in numerous cases of bloody diarrhea contracted at The Sizzler restaurants in Oregon; and some years ago, the McDonald's chain faced an outbreak of *E. coli* infection traced to its hamburgers. Despite their acidity, orange juice, apple juice, and apple cider also have been connected to outbreaks, as FIGURE 8.9 illustrates. When confined to the large intestine with grossly bloody diarrhea, the disease can lead to the complication known as **hemorrhagic colitis**. When the disease involves the kidney and leads to kidney failure, it is called **hemolytic uremic syndrome (HUS)**; seizures, coma, colonic perforation, liver disorder, and cardiomyopathy have been associated with HUS.

Epidemiologists at the CDC now estimate that approximately 20,000 cases of *E. coli* O157:H7 infection occur annually in the United States, with about 250 deaths. Forty-six clusters of infections were recognized in 1994. As of 1995, 32 states required that *E. coli* O157:H7 isolates be reported to the state health department, and physicians were alerted to watch for cases of bloody diarrhea. A toxin similar to that produced by *Shigella* species has been identified in *E. coli* isolates (it is called the "shigalike toxin"). Fresh-picked carrots in a garden salad were implicated in two incidents in 1993, and dry-cured salami was implicated in two 1994 outbreaks.

The prevailing wisdom is that *E. coli* O157:H7 exists in the intestines of **cattle** but causes no disease in these animals. (Researchers are considering an adjustment in cattle feeds to prevent the organism's proliferation.) Slaughtering brings *E. coli* to beef products, and excretion to the soil accounts for transfer to plants and fruits. The organism is particularly pathogenic because it has a low infectious dose (about 100 bacilli are enough to establish infection); it produces toxins at an unusually high rate; and, since it colonizes the intestines, it can deliver toxins to this area efficiently. The organism ferments the alcoholic carbohydrate **sorbitol** very slowly, and this factor is useful in a diagnostic test: In MacConkey agar, the lactose is replaced by sorbitol, and *E. coli* O157:H7 produces white colonies, while other *E. coli* strains produce red or pink colonies.

In recent years, ***E. coli* O111:NM** and ***E. coli* O104:H21** have also been identified as causes of intestinal illness. All told, over 100 serological types of *E. coli* have been implicated in hemolytic uremic syndrome and hemorrhagic colitis. Treatment regimens are not established, and in uncomplicated cases, the symptoms resolve within 5 to 10 days. Research continues on a vaccine for all *E. coli* diarrheas.

Nosocomial:
hospital-acquired.

Pili:
short hairlike appendages that anchor bacteria to surfaces.

car'di-o-my-op'a-the
Cardiomyopathy:
infection of the heart muscle.

FIGURE 8.9

An Outbreak of *E. coli* O157:H7 Infection

This outbreak occurred in New Haven County, Connecticut, during October 1996.

TEXTBOOK CASES

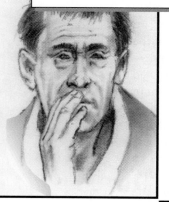

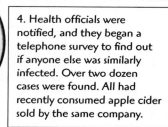

1. On October 6, 1996, a family from a large city in Connecticut decided to take a drive in the country. Along the way they stopped at a general store for a bite of lunch. The father and two children had apple cider; the mother had a soda instead.

2. Three days later, the father and children began to experience serious abdominal pains and vomitting. Moreover, there was blood in their stools. But the mother had no symptoms.

3. One of the children became worse. She had to be admitted to the hospital. The doctor said that the blood was infected and that the kidneys might be suffering. He advised dialysis to assist the kidney function.

4. Health officials were notified, and they began a telephone survey to find out if anyone else was similarly infected. Over two dozen cases were found. All had recently consumed apple cider sold by the same company.

5. Inspectors visited the cider plant. The cider was unpasteurized. It was made from apples picked directly from the tree as well as apples picked from the ground, where contamination with cow manure might have occurred. They recommended pasteurization.

PEPTIC ULCER DISEASE

One of the more remarkable discoveries of the modern era is that many cases of **peptic (stomach) ulcers** are caused by a bacterium. In past decades, scientists believed that all ulcers resulted from "excess acid" due to factors such as nervous stress, smoking, alcohol consumption, diet, and physiological dysfunction. However, the work of Barry Marshall and his coworkers has made it clear that the bacterium ***Helicobacter pylori*** is involved (MicroFocus 8.8). This Gram-negative micro-aerophilic curved rod is similar to *Campylobacter* species, and it is apparently transmitted by contaminated food and water, although a 1997 report indicates that it

he′li-co-bak′ter py-lor′e

MicroFocus 8.8

ULCERS ARE TRANSMISSIBLE?

The old claim "You're giving me an ulcer!" may be truer than anyone believed, if the latest laboratory evidence holds up. Why? The evidence indicates that ulcers are a transmissible disease.

The story began in 1982 when two Australian gastroenterologists, Barry J. Marshall and J. Robin Warren, identified bacteria living in the stomach lining of over 100 patients who had ulcers. The initial discovery was serendipitous because Marshall and Warren could not cultivate the bacterium under normal conditions. Only when they were swamped with work did they leave their culture plates in the incubator too long. And only then did the colonies of bacteria appear. Marshall (Figure a) and Warren identified the organism as the Gram-negative curved rod *Campylobacter pyloridis*. Since then, the organism's name has been changed to *Helicobacter pylori* (Figure b).

Marshall's initial speculation that *H. pylori* causes ulcers aroused widespread skepticism and intensified research. It took 10 years, but research has appeared to confirm Marshall's contention. In 1993, a study published in the *New England Journal of Medicine* indicated that 48 of 52 peptic ulcer patients could be cured of their ulcers in 6 weeks if treated with two antibiotics over a 12-day period. Another 52 patients received a placebo and 39 seemed to be cured, but a year later, the ulcers had returned in all 39 patients. By comparison, only 4 of the patients receiving antibiotics experienced a recurrence.

Marshall now conducts research at the University of Virginia Medical School and supervises an ongoing program to further elucidate the cause of ulcers. The bacterial cause of ulcers conflicts with the conventional wisdom, which says that stress, diet, or other factors trigger excess acid secretion and ulcer formation. (Indeed, two of the top-selling drugs in the United States are the antacids cimetidine [Tagamet] and ranitidine [Zantac], both used to control acid secretion.) Nevertheless, the evidence continues to mount that *H. pylori* is a major factor. In another study at Baylor University, researchers obtained results similar to Marshall's. The data have compelled some researchers to begin thinking of ulcers as a transmissible disease, thereby encouraging doctors to prescribe tetracycline together with Pepto-Bismol. Two biotechnology firms are even attempting to develop a vaccine against *H. pylori*.

And what of Marshall? It is said that once he drank a culture of *H. pylori* to prove his thesis that it causes peptic ulcers. Nowadays, he has adopted a more conservative approach to research, leaving the thesis-proving to his graduate students.

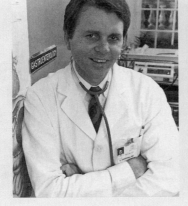 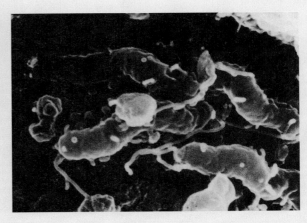

■ *(a) Barry J. Marshall and (b)* Helicobacter pylori, *the bacterium believed to be involved in most cases of peptic ulcers.*

survives in the gut of a housefly as well. Doctors have revolutionized the treatment of ulcers by prescribing antibiotics such as tetracycline clarithromycin (Biaxin), and omeprazole (Prilosec). They have achieved cure rates of up to 90 percent; relapses are uncommon.

How *H. pylori* manages to survive in the intense acidity of the stomach is interesting. Apparently, the bacterium twists its way through the mucus coating of the stomach lining and attaches to the stomach wall. There it secretes the enzyme **urease**. Urease digests urea in the area and produces ammonia as an end-product, as

cla-rith'ro-my'cin

om-e-pra'zōl

Urease:
a bacterial enzyme that digests urea to ammonia, an alkaline substance.

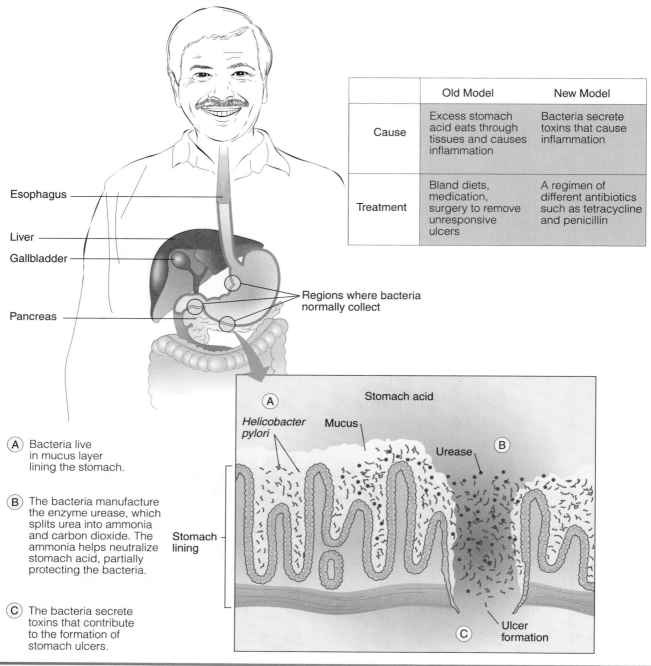

	Old Model	New Model
Cause	Excess stomach acid eats through tissues and causes inflammation	Bacteria secrete toxins that cause inflammation
Treatment	Bland diets, medication, surgery to remove unresponsive ulcers	A regimen of different antibiotics such as tetracycline and penicillin

Esophagus

Liver

Gallbladder

Pancreas

Regions where bacteria normally collect

Stomach acid

Ⓐ

Helicobacter pylori   Mucus

Urease   Ⓑ

Stomach lining

Ⓒ   Ulcer formation

Ⓐ Bacteria live in mucus layer lining the stomach.

Ⓑ The bacteria manufacture the enzyme urease, which splits urea into ammonia and carbon dioxide. The ammonia helps neutralize stomach acid, partially protecting the bacteria.

Ⓒ The bacteria secrete toxins that contribute to the formation of stomach ulcers.

FIGURE 8.10

The Progression of Peptic Ulcers

Scientists now believe that the majority of peptic ulcers are caused by the bacterium *Helicobacter pylori*. This figure illustrates how they cause an ulcer and highlights the old and new approaches to an ulcer.

FIGURE 8.10 shows. The ammonia neutralizes acid in the stomach, and the organism begins its destruction of the tissue, supplemented by digestive enzymes normally found in the stomach tissue. In the stomach lining, a sore 0.25 to 0.5 inch in diameter appears (although some ulcers may be up to 1 inch in diameter). The pain is severe and is not relieved by food or an antacid (as is a duodenal ulcer).

In the past, physician biopsies of a patient's stomach tissue were used to detect *H. pylori*, but in 1996, a new and relatively simple noninvasive **breath test** was approved by the FDA. The patient drinks a urea solution fortified with harmless carbon-13 isotopes. Because *H. pylori* breaks down urea rapidly, the carbon-13 is quickly expelled, and it can be detected easily if the organism is present. If no isotope is detected, the organism is probably not present. The test can be used to document eradication of the organism after therapy, but recent antibiotic use would also yield a negative result.

The treatment of peptic ulcers with antibiotics has brought permanent relief to thousands of sufferers worldwide. But research is ongoing, because the modes of transmission must be studied, the treatments await refining, and the organism's relationship to stomach cancer is not yet clear. Still, these are historic times for patients and physicians alike.

CAMPYLOBACTERIOSIS

kam'pi-lo-bak'te-re-o'sis

kam'pĭ-lo-bak'ter je-jun'ee

Since the early 1970s, **campylobacteriosis** has emerged from an obscure disease in animals to recognition as a widespread intestinal disease in humans. The pathogen is ***Campylobacter jejuni***, a curved (*campylo-* means "curved"), Gram-negative rod that moves by means of a single polar flagellum (FIGURE 8.11). Reservoirs for the organism include the intestinal tracts of many animals, including dairy cattle, chickens, and turkeys. Contaminated water is also a source of infection.

The clinical symptoms of campylobacteriosis range from mild diarrhea to severe gastrointestinal distress, with fever, abdominal pains, and bloody stools. *Campylobacter jejuni* colonizes the small or large intestine, causing inflammation and occasional mild ulceration. However, the signs and symptoms of campylobacteriosis are not unique. Most patients recover in less than a week without treatment, but some have high fevers and bloody stools for prolonged periods. Erythromycin therapy hastens recovery.

Raw milk was identified as a source of *Campylobacter* in 18 outbreaks between 1981 and 1990, most of which involved school field trips to local dairy farms. A notable incident in New Zealand in 1990 occurred at a camp where contaminated water was apparently the source of the *Campylobacter* (MicroFocus 8.9). Other species, including *C. coli* and *C. upsaliensis*, have also been identified as human pathogens, and as methods of detection improve, the number of reported cases of campylobacteriosis will probably continue to rise.

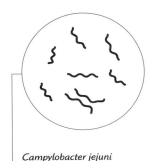

Campylobacter jejuni

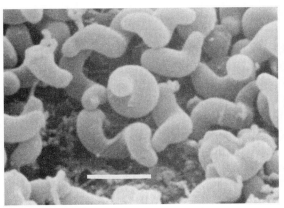

(a)

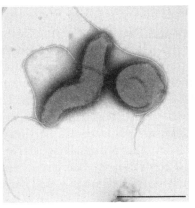

(b)

FIGURE 8.11

Campylobacter jejuni

Two views of *Campylobacter jejuni*, the cause of campylobacteriosis. (a) A scanning electron micrograph of *C. jejuni* taken from a colony of cells. (Bar = 1 μm.) Note the curved shape of most organisms and the coccus shape of several. (b) A transmission electron micrograph of negatively stained cells, showing the flagellar arrangement of both types of cells. (Bar = 0.5 μm.)

MicroFocus 8.9

HOLIDAY BLUES

The August rains had been torrential, but now the long winter was coming to an end and there was a touch of spring in the air. It was a grand time to take a break, and what better way to relax than to visit the camp and convention center at Christ Church—Christ Church, New Zealand, that is.

The weather was ideal, and the scenery was a touch of heaven. On all sides there were farms and pastures, and one could walk along the country lanes and greet the sheep and cattle grazing nearby. The housing was lovely, there was plenty to do, and the holiday was great. Great, that is, until one-by-one, the visitors fell ill. During early September, 44 people complained of nausea, diarrhea, and vomiting. Some had headaches; practically all had abdominal pains; and the disease did not discriminate—the age range was 3 to 51 years.

On September 4, the Canterbury Area Health Board began its investigation. Two people were already hospitalized with *Campylobacter jejuni* infection, and this curved bacterium appeared to be at fault. But where did it come from? Investigators found that three springs supplied water to the camp grounds; they noted that the water was neither chlorinated nor filtered. They also discovered bacteria-rich pasture lands bordering two of the three springs. The only missing link was a method for bringing contaminated soil into the springs. What do you think was the answer?

LISTERIOSIS

lis-ter'i-o-sis
mon'o-cy-toj'en-ēz

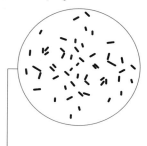

Listeria monocytogenes

Monocyte:
a type of large white blood cell that functions in phagocytosis.

Listeriosis is caused by *Listeria monocytogenes*, a small Gram-positive rod. At one time, this organism was dubbed the "Cinderella" of pathogenic bacteria because its ability to cause disease was not widely recognized. The bacillus is commonly found in the soil and in the intestines of many animals, including birds, fish, barnyard animals, dairy cattle, and household pets. It is transmitted to humans by food contaminated with fecal matter, as well as by the consumption of animal foods. Delicatessen cold cuts, as well as soft cheeses (e.g., Brie, Camembert, feta, and blue-veined cheeses), have been associated with a significant number of cases. Indeed, an outbreak of listeriosis associated with duck liver (used for *fois gras*) was among the first epidemics reported by the CDC in the twenty-first century.

Listeriosis occurs in many forms. One form, called **listeric meningitis**, is characterized by headaches, stiff neck, delirium, and coma. Another form is a blood disease accompanied by high numbers of white blood cells called **monocytes** (hence the organism's name) (FIGURE 8.12). A third form is characterized by infection of the uterus, with vague flulike symptoms. If contracted during pregnancy, the disease may result in miscarriage of the fetus or mental damage in the newborn. Other individuals suffer respiratory distress, diarrhea, back pain, skin itching, and other nonspecific symptoms that make diagnosing the disease difficult. Penicillin, tetracycline, and other antibiotics are effective treatments.

Listeriosis does not appear to be transmissible among humans. Although the prompt and prolonged use of antibiotics is an effective treatment, relapses are common. CDC epidemiologists estimate that 2000 cases of listeriosis occur in the United States annually and that 25 percent result in death. The causative organism has been isolated from vegetables, milk, poultry, sausages, and dairy products. The bacterium is considered psychotropic, meaning it is able to grow at refrigerator temperatures.

A notable outbreak of listeriosis occurred in late 1998 and early 1999. Close to 100 cases of illness were reported in 22 states, all linked to hot dogs and deli meats distributed by Sara Lee, Ball Park, Hygrade, and other companies. Although health

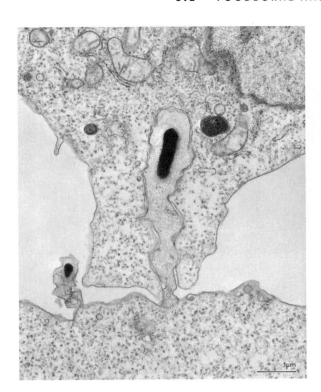

FIGURE 8.12

The Transmission of *Listeria monocytogenes*

An electron micrograph of *Listeria monocytogenes* spreading from one monocyte to another. A *Listeria* cell within one pseudopod (bottom) has been engulfed by a pseudopod from the second cell (top). On pinching off, the bacterium will be inside the cytoplasm of the second cell.

officials never found the bacterial source for certain, they postulated that dust from construction work on air-conditioning units at the production plant may have been involved. Fourteen adults died during the outbreak, and six pregnant women suffered miscarriages.

BRUCELLOSIS

Brucellosis (also known as Malta fever or Bang's disease) is an occupational hazard of farmers, veterinarians, dairy and meat plant workers, and others who work with large animals. Transmission can occur by splashing milk into the eye, by the accidental passage of fluids through skin abrasions, by contact with animals, and by the consumption of milk and other dairy products. In one example of food transmission, the CDC reported 29 cases in Mexican emigrants living in Houston, Texas. All had eaten goat cheese made from unpasteurized goat's milk. Human-to-human transmission is virtually unknown.

Among the organisms responsible for brucellosis are ***Brucella abortus*** from cattle, ***B. suis*** from swine, and ***B. mellitensis*** from goats and sheep. Another species, ***B. canis***, is associated with dogs and may be acquired by contact with pets. All are small Gram-negative rods. In animals, brucellosis manifests itself in several organs, especially the reproductive organs because the bacterium multiplies in the tissues of the uterus. Sterility is a common complication, and pregnant animals are known to abort their young. In veterinary literature, the disease is often referred to as **contagious abortion**.

The major focus of brucellosis in humans is the blood-rich organs, such as the spleen and lymph glands. Patients experience flulike weakness, as well as backache, joint pain, and a high fever (with drenching sweats) in the daytime and low fever

broo'sel-lo'sis

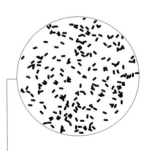

Brucella abortus

FIGURE 8.13

Brucellosis in Bison

Brucellosis poses a threat to bison in Yellowstone National Park, as well as to cattle they encounter outside the confines of the park. A vaccine has not yet been developed for wildlife like these, and resolution of the epidemic remains elusive.

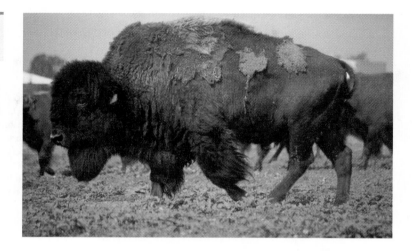

Undulant fever:
another name for brucellosis, based on alternating periods of fever and chills.

(with chills) in the evening. This fever pattern gives the disease its alternate name, **undulant fever** (*undulat-* is Latin for "vary"). The disease seldom causes death in humans, and tetracycline speeds recovery. The pasteurization of milk, and livestock immunization, have reduced the incidence of brucellosis in humans from 6300 cases in 1947 to about 100 cases annually. However, a major outbreak of the disease has been taking place since 1997 among bison and elk herds in Yellowstone National Park in Wyoming, Montana, and Colorado (FIGURE 8.13).

OTHER FOODBORNE AND WATERBORNE DISEASES

A number of other bacterial organisms transmitted by food and water merit brief consideration in this chapter. Some have been recognized as pathogens only in recent years; others have been known for decades.

par'a-he'mo-lit'ik-us

Among the recent concerns is ***Vibrio parahaemolyticus*** (FIGURE 8.14). This Gram-negative rod is a major cause of foodborne infections in Japan and other areas of the world where seafood is the main staple of the diet. Patients experience acute abdominal pain, vomiting, diarrhea, and watery stools. Some years ago, an outbreak aboard an American cruise ship was linked to seafood salad, and another incident in Louisiana was traced to unrefrigerated cooked shrimp.

vul-nif'i-cus

Another species of *Vibrio* has also caused recent concern. In 1996, the CDC reported on an outbreak of intestinal illness due to ***Vibrio vulnificus***. This organism occurs naturally in brackish and seawaters, where oysters and clams live. People who consume

FIGURE 8.14

Vibrio parahaemolyticus

A scanning electron micrograph of *Vibrio parahaemolyticus*, a Gram-negative rod associated with seafood. This marine bacterium is widely distributed in natural aquatic environments around the world and is a well-known foodborne pathogen of the gastrointestinal tract. (Bar = 1 μm.)

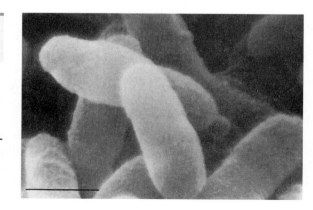

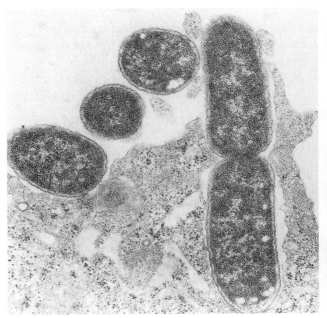

(a)

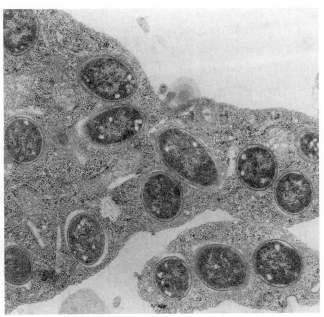

(b)

FIGURE 8.15

Yersinia enterocolitica

Transmission electron micrographs of invasive *Yersinia enterocolitica*. (a) A number of bacteria attached to the plasma membrane of infected cells. One bacterium appears to be undergoing cell division and entering the cell at the same time. (b) Several *Y. enterocolitica* cells observed within the cytoplasm of an infected cell. The bacteria are in membrane-enclosed vacuoles. Researchers postulate that a single gene is responsible for the invasive capacity displayed by this organism.

these molluscs raw are at risk, especially those with a compromised immune system and those who suffer from liver disease or low stomach acid. (Indeed, taking an antacid after a meal of any contaminated food may neutralize helpful stomach acid and facilitate the passage of the bacteria to the bloodstream.) The gastrointestinal infection involves fever, nausea, and severe abdominal cramps. Often it is accompanied by septicemia, necrotic skin lesions, and cellulitis (a diffuse inflammation of connective tissues of the skin). The mortality rate for the disease is over 50 percent. A notable outbreak related to eating raw seafood occurred in 1999 on New York's Long Island.

Bacillus cereus is a Gram-positive sporeforming bacillus that causes food poisoning in two distinct forms, both due to enterotoxins. The first form, *diarrheal*, is accompanied by diarrhea and abdominal pain, while the second form, *emetic*, is characterized by substantial vomiting, frequently experienced after consuming cooked rice. Neither form involves fever, and most patients recover within 2 days without treatment. In the 1980s, investigators traced a notable outbreak to a college cafeteria where a macaroni and cheese dish harbored a million bacilli per gram. Heat-resistant spores had apparently survived the cooking process. Fried rice prepared at a local restaurant was the cause of a 1993 outbreak in Virginia.

Another emerging cause of foodborne illness is ***Yersinia enterocolitica*** (FIGURE 8.15). This Gram-negative rod is widely distributed in animals and in river and lake waters. The largest episode of disease thus far recorded in the United States occurred in 1982 and involved 172 patients in Arkansas, Tennessee, and Mississippi. Patients experienced fever, diarrhea, and abdominal pain, and most required hospitalization. Investigators believed that contaminated milk was the source. A 1990 outbreak in Georgia involved raw chitterlings (pork intestines). In this case, *Y. enterocolitica* was apparently transferred to a group of children by hand-to-hand contact with the individual preparing the food.

Still another cause of intestinal illness is ***Plesiomonas shigelloides***, a Gram-negative, facultatively anaerobic rod. *P. shigelloides* is normally limited to the tropical and subtropical climates of Asia and Africa, and it is commonly found in the gut

yer-sin'i-a en'ter-o-co-lit'ĭ-ka

ples-e-o-mo'nas shig-el-oi'des

of tropical fish. It can cause intestinal illness in people who eat raw seafood or who travel in the tropics and consume contaminated water or eat contaminated food. A 1990 case, however, appeared to fit neither description. The case occurred in a year-old child who had apparently been infected by water in the bathroom tub. Her parents previously had poured water from their aquarium into the tub. The aquarium was home to a collection of piranhas, a type of tropical fish the family kept as pets.

TABLE 8.2

A Summary of Foodborne and Waterborne Bacterial Diseases

DISEASE	CAUSATIVE AGENT	DESCRIPTION OF AGENT	ORGANS AFFECTED	CHARACTERISTIC SIGNS
Botulism	Clostridium botulinum	Gram-positive sporeforming rod	Neuromuscular junction	Paralysis
Staphylococcal food poisoning	Staphylococcus aureus	Gram-positive staphylococcus	Intestine	Diarrhea Nausea Vomiting
Clostridial food poisoning	Clostridium perfringens	Gram-positive sporeforming rod	Intestine	Diarrhea Cramping
Typhoid fever	Salmonella typhi	Gram-negative rod	Intestine Blood Gall bladder	Ulcers Fever Rose spots
Salmonellosis	Salmonella serotypes	Gram-negative rods	Intestine	Fever Diarrhea Vomiting
Shigellosis	Shigella serotypes	Gram-negative rods	Intestine	Diarrhea Dysentery
Cholera	Vibrio cholerae	Gram-negative curved rod	Intestine	Rice-water stools Extreme diarrhea Shock
E. coli diarrheas	Escherichia coli	Gram-negative rod	Intestine	Diarrhea
Campylobacteriosis	Campylobacter jejuni	Gram-negative curved rod	Intestine	Diarrhea Fever
Listeriosis	Listeria monocytogenes	Gram-positive small rod	Intestine Meninges Monocytes	Diarrhea Meningitis
Brucellosis	Brucella species	Gram-negative rods	Spleen Lymph glands	Undulating fever Joint pain
Other foodborne and waterborne diseases	Vibrio parahaemolyticus	Gram-negative rod	Intestine	Diarrhea
	Vibrio vulnificus	Gram-negative rod	Intestine	Diarrhea
	Bacillus cereus	Gram-positive sporeforming rod	Intestine	Diarrhea
	Yersinia enterocolitica	Gram-negative rod	Intestine	Diarrhea
	Pleisomonas shigelloides	Gram-negative rod	Intestine	Diarrhea
	Aeromonas hydrophila	Gram-negative rod	Intestine	Diarrhea

Clinical reports in the 1980s documented that *Aeromonas* species, especially **Aeromonas hydrophila**, cause human gastrointestinal disease. The organisms are Gram-negative rods commonly found in soil and water. They appear to be transmitted by food. Both choleralike and dysenterylike diarrheas, ranging from mild to severe, have been reported in patients. An enterotoxin may be responsible for the symptoms.

a'er-o-mo'nas hi-drof'ĭ-lah

The foodborne and waterborne bacterial diseases discussed in this chapter are summarized in TABLE 8.2.

TOXIN INVOLVED	TREATMENT ADMINISTERED	IMMUNIZATION AVAILABLE	COMMENT
Yes	Antitoxin	None	Most powerful toxin known Infant and wound botulism possible
Yes	None	None	Affects millions of Americans annually Due to an enterotoxin Brief incubation period
Yes	None	None	Common in protein-rich foods Spores survive cooking
Not established	Chloramphenicol	Vaccine of dead bacteria	Spread from carriers About 400 cases annually in U.S.
Not established	Not recommended	None	Associated with poultry products Most reported foodborne disease in U.S. About 40,000 cases annually
Not established	Rehydration Antibiotics	None	May be accompanied by dysentery R factors limit antibiotic use
Yes	Rehydration	Vaccine of dead bacteria	Danger from dehydration Rare in U.S. Raw seafood involved
Yes	Antibiotics Rehydration	None	Symptoms due to enterotoxin Enteroinvasive strains observed Possible hemolytic uremic syndrome
Not established	Erythromycin	None	Associated with raw milk Symptoms mild to serious
Not established	Antibiotics	None	Dangerous in pregnancy Associated with animals Soft cheeses implicated
Not established	Tetracycline	None	Induces abortion in barnyard animals Hazardous to animal workers
Not established	Various antibiotics	None	Associated with seafood
Not established	Various antibiotics	None	Associated with shellfish
Yes	None	None	Spores survive in cooked foods
Not established	Various antibiotics	None	Widely found in animals
Not established	Various antibiotics	None	Occurs in tropical climates
Yes	Various antibiotics	None	Common in soil and water

Note to the Student

For over a half-century, *Escherichia coli* has been the tireless workhouse of biological research. In the 1940s, it was used as a host organism to determine the life cycle of viruses. Many of the important metabolic pathways, including the renowned Krebs cycle, were worked out first in this organism. In the 1950s, biochemists used *E. coli* to discover the three forms of microbial recombination. In the 1960s, it was the major research organism for deciphering the genetic code and learning how genes work. In the 1970s, *E. coli* became the guardian of public health as a valuable indicator of water pollution. It also emerged as an industrial giant for producing enzymes, growth factors, and vitamins. Since the 1980s, biochemists have used it as a living factory to produce an array of genetically engineered pharmaceuticals. And in the 1990s, *E. coli* continued to illustrate how bacteria can be put to work in the interest of science and for the betterment of humanity.

Then came *E. coli* O157:H7. To be sure, this strain has caused much human misery and pain because of its propensity to invade the intestinal tissues, pass to the blood, and cause serious injury to the kidneys. It has made us more careful of what we eat and has caused us to think twice about having a rare hamburger. Along the way it has become the "germ of the week" on "Dateline," "20-20," and other television news programs, where it has been portrayed as the chief villain among a world of villains. Unfortunately, it has also made us forget all the good things that *E. coli* has done for us. And what a shame that is! Perhaps one bad apple can, indeed, spoil the whole barrel.

Summary

A recurring theme of this chapter is that foodborne and waterborne bacterial diseases primarily affect the intestinal tract and are of two types: intoxications and infections.

Foodborne intoxications are exemplified by botulism, staphylococcal food poisoning, and clostridial food poisoning. In all three instances, the growing and multiplying bacteria deposit toxins in contaminated food, and the toxins bring on the illness after the food is consumed. In botulism, the toxins interfere with nerve transmission and induce paralysis, while in the remaining two diseases, the toxins induce a mild to moderate bout of diarrhea. The incubation periods tend to be short, since bacterial growth in the body is not a prerequisite to disease.

In contrast to intoxications, foodborne and waterborne infections have longer incubation periods because bacterial growth must occur before symptoms are experienced. In typhoid fever, there is tissue invasion and severe intestinal ulceration, followed by a life-threatening invasion of the blood. Cases of salmonellosis are less dangerous, most of them characterized by several days of fever, cramps, and diarrhea. In *Shigella*-related infections, some erosion of the intestinal tissue occurs, and small-volume, bloody stools may occur, a condition called dysentery. Massive often-fatal diarrhea is the key characteristic of cholera, and fluid-electrolyte imbalances are usually severe. Other infections, including *E. coli* diarrhea, listeriosis, and campylobacteriosis, are accompanied by varying intestinal symptoms, but in brucellosis the characteristic sign is a high-low fever pattern called undulating fever. This occurs because, although acquired by contaminated food, brucellosis is a blood disease with little evidence of intestinal infection.

Questions for Thought and Discussion

1. The story is told of an early nineteenth-century doctor in New York City who was an expert at diagnosing typhoid fever even before the symptoms of disease appeared. The doctor's forte was the tongue. He would go up and down the rows of hospital beds, feeling the tongues of patients and announcing that the patient was in the early stages of typhoid. Sure enough, a few days later the symptoms would surface. What do you think was the secret to his success?

2. In 1997, researchers in Boston reported that *Helicobacter pylori* accumulates in the gut of houseflies after the flies feed on food containing the bacteria. What are the implications of this research?

3. You have volunteered to do the supermarket shopping for the upcoming class barbecue. What are some precautions you can take to ensure that the event is remembered for all the right reasons?

4. In 1997, Swedish researchers provided evidence that *Salmonella* serotypes are infecting penguins on Bird Island, a remote island in the distant South Atlantic. The organisms, not normally found in the birds, are presumably of human origin. Assuming humans had not visited the island in the previous decades, how might the bacteria have reached the birds?

5. "Finding the source of an outbreak is like trying to go back to a forest fire to find a spark." So said an exasperated University of Saskatchewan researcher explaining the difficulty of tracing the origin of a 1997 botulism outbreak in water fowl in which millions of birds died. The risk of botulism appears to rise when wetlands have a neutral pH and are relatively salt-free. Also, it is known that water birds often acquire botulism by eating insect larvae that have concentrated the disease-related neurotoxin. With these facts in mind, develop a possible scenario in which such things as temperature, pH, salinity, pesticide use, and other wetland factors may contribute to a botulism epidemic.

6. Some years ago, the CDC noticed a puzzling trend: Reported cases of salmonellosis seemed to soar in the summer months, then drop radically in September. Can you venture a guess why this is so?

7. A popular contemporary gift is a bottle of olive oil infused with fresh herbs and/or garlic. Many people like to leave the gifts out on the kitchen counter as a display. What microbiological hazard exists here? What advice might you give the owner of such a bottle of oil?

8. A laboratory instructor proposes to demonstrate the growth of soilborne organisms in canned food in the following way: A can is to be punctured with an ice pick and a small pinch of rich soil introduced to the can; the hole will then be sealed with candle wax and the can incubated. A fellow laboratory instructor hears of the experiment, reacts with concern, and advises the first instructor not to perform it. Why?

9. Between February 18 and 22, 1987, botulism was diagnosed in 11 patrons of a restaurant in Vancouver, B.C. The disease was subsequently traced to mushrooms bottled and preserved in the restaurant. What special cultivation practice enhances the possibility that mushrooms will be infected with the spores of the organism of botulism?

10. It has been reported that some individuals have used botulinum toxin to ease facial wrinkles by relaxing the muscles. This practice has been denounced by the FDA. Why?

11. In preparation for a summer barbecue, a man cuts up chickens on a wooden carving board. After running the board under water for a few seconds, he uses it to cut up tomatoes, lettuce, peppers, and other salad ingredients. What sort of trouble is he asking for?

12. When a woman died of botulism in 1980, a public official was quoted in an interview as saying: "This death might have been prevented if any of the doctors involved had recognized and acted early on the symptoms of the disease they were dealing with." Do you believe the doctors were at fault? What might be your reply to the official?

13. During 1992, the North Carolina Department of Health received reports of illness in 18 workers at a local pork processing plant. All the affected employees worked on the "kill floor" of the plant. All had Gram-negative rods in their blood. Their symptoms included fever, chills, fatigue, sweats, and weight loss. Which disease was pinpointed in the workers?

14. Three days ago, two hamburgers were purchased at the local market. One was frozen, the other remained chilled in the refrigerator section. Both are now placed on the grill. All other things being equal (size of hamburger, cooking time, source of meat, use of condiments, and so on), which hamburger might be safer to eat if you wish to avoid food poisoning?

15. Most physicians agree that the illness called "stomach flu" is not influenza at all. They maintain that the cramps, diarrhea, and vomiting can be due to a variety of bacteria and viruses. Which organisms in this chapter might be good candidates?

16. "You don't have to travel anymore to get traveler's diarrhea." So announced a state epidemiologist to thousands of attendees at a recent convention on emerging diseases. He was referring to the unusually high incidence of foodborne and waterborne diseases in the United States. What conditions in modern society would lead him to make this announcement?

17. In 1986, a New Rochelle, New York, frozen-food manufacturer recalled thousands of packages of jumbo stuffed shells and cheese lasagna after a local outbreak of salmonellosis. Which parts of the pasta products would attract the attention of inspectors as possible sources of *Salmonella*? Why?

18. Studies have shown that bismuth subsalicylate (Pepto-Bismol) can be used to prevent traveler's diarrhea, but the treatment is not easy to follow: 2 ounces or 2 tablets four times a day for 3 weeks before travel begins. Short of turning pink, what other measures can you use to prevent traveler's diarrhea while visiting other countries?

19. An estimated 25 million Americans will have an ulcer at some time of their lives, yet a recent study indicates that two-thirds still don't know that *Helicobacter pylori* causes 90 percent of ulcers. Suppose you were a public health official. What would you do to get the word out?

20. The CDC estimates that each year, 20,000 individuals suffer diarrhea from *E. coli* O157:H7, and that over 200 people die as a result of infection. Despite this prevalence, relatively few cases are diagnosed. What factors may contribute to misdiagnoses or nondiagnoses?

Review

The preceding pages have summarized some of the major bacterial diseases transmitted by food and water. To test your knowledge of the chapter's contents, rearrange the scrambled letters and insert the correct word in each of the missing spaces. The answers are listed in Appendix D.

1. To treat patients who have botulism, large doses of _____ must be administered.

[I] [I] [T] [A] [X] [N] [N] [T] [O]

2. One of the most excessive diarrheas observed in an intestinal disease is associated with _____.

[R] [L] [H] [E] [A] [C] [O]

3. The fever pattern in brucellosis gives the disease its alternate name of _____ fever.

[A] [U] [U] [T] [L] [N] [N] [D]

4. Disease associated with *Shigella* species is usually accompanied by a syndrome of cramps and bloody stools called _____.

[N] [S] [D] [E] [E] [Y] [Y] [T] [R]

5. In cases of typhoid fever, the abdomen is often covered with a series of _____ spots.

[E] [S] [R] [O]

6. _____ food poisoning has a relatively short incubation period and is caused by a toxin deposited in food during aerobic bacterial growth.

[O] [H] [L] [A] [Y] [S] [P] [C] [C] [T] [L] [O] [C] [A]

7. Because *Salmonella* serotypes commonly infect _____, any products derived from these animals are potentially infected.

[H] [C] [N] [K] [I] [E] [S] [C]

8. A small percentage of those who recover from typhoid fever remain _____ and can spread the organism in their feces.

[A] [C] [R] [E] [I] [R] [S] [R]

9. *Escherichia coli* is a common Gram-_____ rod that can be a cause of infantile and traveler's diarrhea.

[G] [N] [V] [I] [A] [E] [T] [E]

10. A sporeforming aerobic rod that can cause food-borne illness is *Bacillus* _____.

R C E S U E

11. A curved rod belonging to the genus _____ is known to cause mild to severe diarrhea in humans.

Y E A P O C C L A T R M B

12. In an animal such as a cow, infection with *Brucella* may result in the _____ of the fetus.

O T O A R I N B

13. A major symptom in patients experiencing botulism is _____ of the limbs and respiratory muscles.

A L S P A Y S R I

14. Many instances of staphylococcal food poisoning originate with staphylococci found in the _____.

O S E N

15. *Salmonella typhi* is able to reach the human intestinal tract because it is highly resistant to _____.

C I A D

16. One of the dangers of shigellosis is excessive _____ loss in the patient.

L I D U F

17. Outbreaks of cholera in the United States can best be described as _____.

A E R R

18. Consumers of seafood are particularly vulnerable to intestinal infection due to a species of _____.

O I B R V I

19. The most reported foodborne infection in the United States is that caused by types of _____.

A M E A S O L L L N

20. To avoid staphylococcal food poisoning, consumers should be sure to _____ all left-over foods before eating them.

E H T A

21. The organism *Clostridium perfringens* multiplies in foods only under _____ conditions.

E O I N R C A A B

22. Diagnosis of many of the intestinal diseases is assisted by the isolation of bacteria from _____ specimens.

O O T S L

23. Diseases such as shigellosis, typhoid fever, and cholera may be contracted by consuming contaminated _____.

O E F O D S A

24. In recent years, raw _____ has been implicated in many outbreaks of campylobacteriosis.

L K M I

25. Those who work with large _____ may be exposed to the bacterium that causes brucellosis.

M N L A A I S

https://microbiology.jbpub.com

The site features **eLearning,** an on-line review area that provides quizzes and other tools to help you study for your class. You can also follow useful links for in-depth information, read more MicroFocus stories, or just find out the latest microbiology news.

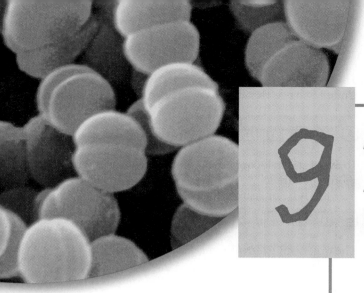

9 Soilborne and Arthropodborne Bacterial Diseases

This scourge had implanted so great a terror in the hearts of men and women that . . . fathers and mothers refused to nurse and assist their own children, as though they did not belong to them.

—Italian novelist Giovanni Boccaccio writing about the Black Death in the 1500s

BUBONIC PLAGUE, COMMONLY KNOWN as "the Black Death," was probably the greatest catastrophe ever to strike Europe. It swept back and forth across the continent for almost a decade, each year increasing in ferocity. By 1348, two-thirds of the European population were stricken and half of the sick had died. Houses were empty, towns were abandoned, and a dreadful solitude hung over the land. The sick died too quickly for the living to bury them, and at one point, the Rhône River was consecrated as a graveyard for plague victims. Contemporary historians wrote that posterity would not believe such things could happen, because those who saw them were themselves appalled. The horror was almost impossible to imagine; to many people, it was the end of the world.

Before the century concluded, the Black Death visited Europe at least five more times in periodic reigns of terror. During one epidemic in Paris, an estimated 800 people died each day; in Siena, the population dropped from 42,000 to 15,000; and in Florence, almost 75 percent of the citizenry perished. Flight was the chief recourse for people who could afford it, but ironically, the escaping travelers spread the disease. Those who remained in the cities were locked in their homes until they succumbed or recovered.

The immediate effect of the plague was a general paralysis in Europe. Trade ceased and wars stopped. Bewildered peasants who survived encountered unexpected prosperity because landowners had to pay higher wages to obtain help. Land values declined and class relationships were upset, as the system of feudalism gradually crumbled. The authority of the clergy, already in decline, deteriorated further because the Church was helpless in the face of the disaster. With many priests and monks dead, a new order of reformers arose to found Protestantism. Medical practices became increasingly sophisticated, with new standards of sanitation and a 40-day period of detention (a "quarantine") imposed on vessels docking at ports. Indeed, the mechanical clock came into widespread use, reflecting the urgency of life.

The graveyard of plague left fertile ground for the renewal of Europe during the Renaissance. To many historians, the Black Death remains a major turning point in Western civilization.

Nor did it end there. European populations were also devastated by typhus and relapsing fever. Both of these diseases, like the plague, are transmitted by arthropods, and both can be interrupted by arthropod control. Neither is a major problem in our society, but other arthropodborne diseases—such as Lyme disease, tularemia, and Rocky Mountain spotted fever—occasionally are reported in the news media. We shall study each of these diseases in this chapter.

Arthropods: insects and other animals with jointed appendages, segmented bodies, and outer skeletons of chitin.

To begin, we shall examine a number of soilborne diseases where organisms enter the body through a cut, wound, or abrasion, or by inhalation. Among these are anthrax, a feared disease in bioterrorism, and tetanus, a concern to anyone who has stepped on a nail or piece of glass. We shall also study other diseases receiving wider recognition as detection methods improve. These soilborne diseases, as well as the arthropodborne diseases, are primarily problems of the blood.

9.1
Soilborne Bacterial Diseases

Soilborne bacterial diseases are those whose agents are transferred from the soil to the unsuspecting individual. To remain alive in the soil, the bacteria must resist environmental extremes, and often the bacteria form spores, as the first three diseases illustrate.

ANTHRAX

Anthrax is primarily a disease of large animals such as cattle, sheep, and goats. It is caused by ***Bacillus anthracis,*** a Gram-positive sporeforming rod (pictured in FIGURE 9.1). Animals ingest the spores from the soil during grazing, and soon they are overwhelmed with bacteria as their organs fill with bloody black fluid (*anthrac* is the Greek word for "coal"; the disease name is thus a reference to the blackening of the blood). About 80 percent of untreated animals die, and since the bacteria remain in the dead body as spores, it is often necessary to cremate the carcass or bury it deeply in lime to prevent soil contamination. Burning the field may also be required.

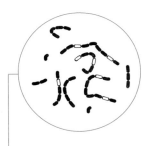

Bacillus anthracis

Humans acquire anthrax in a number of ways. Workers who tan hides, shear sheep, or process wool may inhale the spores and contract pulmonary anthrax, often called **woolsorter's disease**. Consumption of contaminated meat may lead to gastrointestinal anthrax. Contact with spores may lead to anthrax of the skin. Animal products related to past outbreaks of anthrax have included violin bows, shaving bristles, goatskin drums, and leather jackets.

Anthrax spores germinate rapidly on contact with human tissues. The thick capsule of the cells impedes phagocytosis, and the organisms produce a number of toxins.

FIGURE 9.1

Bacillus anthracis

Bacillus anthracis is the cause of anthrax. (a) Free spores and vegetative cells of *B. anthracis* visualized with the scanning electron microscope (×5400). Note the oval shape of the spores and the typical rod shape of the vegetative cells. (b) Anthrax spores in the process of germinating (×50,000). The spore coat of the spore in the center of the photograph has divided and is beginning to separate. A vegetative cell may be seen emerging from the spore at the bottom.

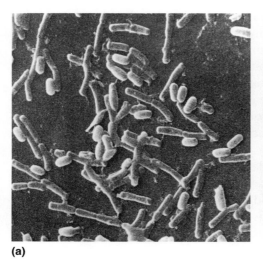
(a)

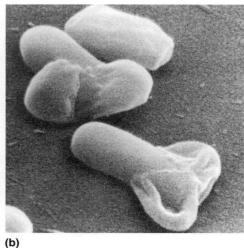
(b)

Pulmonary anthrax develops into a severe blood infection with extensive hemorrhaging. Skin and intestinal anthrax are accompanied by boil-like lesions covered with black crusts (FIGURE 9.2). Blood invasion follows, and violent dysentery with bloody stools accompanies the intestinal form. Penicillin is used for therapy. In untreated cases, the mortality rate is more than 80 percent.

In the 1990s, the total number of anthrax cases in the United States was less than a dozen, primarily because of the testing of imported animal products. A vaccine prepared with an attenuated strain of *B. anthracis* has been successful in reducing outbreaks in domestic herds. A variant of the vaccine is available to veterinarians and others who work with livestock. Six inoculations over an 18-month period are required for immunity.

Anthrax is also considered a threat in bioterrorism and in **biological warfare** (**MicroFocus 9.1**). This is because the spores can be aerosolized in microscopic droplets for widespread distribution to large areas and spread to substantial numbers of people. Moreover, the bacillus can be grown fairly easily and in large quantities, and the spores are extraordinarily resistant to destruction. An aerosol of spores could be released unobtrusively and could drift through a large city without being detected. At present, there is no vaccine for civilian use, but since 1998, all military personnel receive the vaccine containing attenuated *B. anthracis*, as noted above. The seriousness of bioterrorism has been underscored by a public health official who called anthrax "the poor man's atomic bomb."

FIGURE 9.2

An Anthrax Lesion

This cutaneous lesion is a result of infection with anthrax bacilli. Lesions like this one develop when anthrax spores contact the skin, germinate to vegetative cells, and multiply.

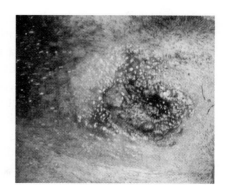

MicroFocus 9.1

THE LEGACY OF GRUINARD ISLAND

In 1941, the specter of airborne biological warfare hung over Europe. Fearing that the Germans might launch an attack against civilian populations, British authorities performed a series of experiments to test their own biological weapons. The spot chosen was Gruinard Island, a mile-long patch of land off the coast of Scotland. Investigators placed 60 sheep on the island and exploded a bomb containing anthrax spores overhead. Within days, all the sheep were dead.

Warfare with biological weapons never came to reality in World War II, but the contamination of Gruinard Island remained. A series of tests in 1971 showed that anthrax spores were still alive at and below the upper crust of the soil, and that they could be spread by earthworms. Officials posted signs

warning people not to set foot on the island, but did little else.

Then a strange protest occurred in 1981. Activists demanded that the British government decontaminate the island. They backed their demands with packages of soil taken from the island. Notes led government officials to two 10-pound packages of spore-laden soil, and the writers threatened that 280 pounds were hidden elsewhere.

Partly because of the protests, the British government instituted a decontamination of the island in 1986. Technicians used a powerful brushwood killer, combined with burning and treatment with formalin in seawater. Finally, they managed to rid the soil of anthrax spores. By April 1987, sheep were once again grazing on the island. However, people were somewhat reluctant to return.

Gruinard Island remains a monument of sorts to the effects of biological warfare.

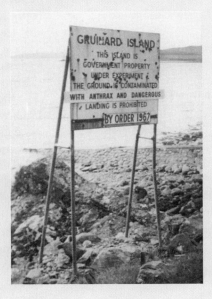

TETANUS

Tetanus is one of the most dangerous human diseases. *Clostridium tetani*, the bacillus that causes it, occurs everywhere in the environment, especially the soil. Spores enter a wound in very small numbers and revert to vegetative bacilli that produce the second most powerful toxin known to science (after the botulism toxin). The toxin provokes sustained and uncontrolled contractions of the muscles, and spasms occur throughout the body. Patients often experience violent deaths.

Clostridium tetani was first isolated in 1889 by the Japanese bacteriologist Shibasaburo Kitasato. It is a Gram-positive, anaerobic, sporeforming bacillus found in the intestines of many animals and humans. The bacillus possesses few invasive tendencies and does not cause intestinal disease. However, the spores are excreted in the feces to the soil, and later they enter the dead, oxygen-free tissue of a wound. The wound may result from a fracture, gunshot, animal bite, or puncture by a piece of glass, a thorn, or a needle. Rusty nails pose a threat because spores cling to the rough edges of the nail and the nail may cause extensive tissue damage as it penetrates. (The rust itself is of no consequence.)

Once inside the tissue, the spores germinate to vegetative cells that produce several toxins. The most important of these toxins appears to be **tetanospasmin**, an exotoxin of high molecular weight. At the synapse, this toxin is believed to block the relaxation pathway that follows muscle contraction. The toxin unites with glycine (an amino acid) and other neurotransmitters to inhibit muscle relaxation. Without any inhibiting influence, volleys of spontaneous impulses arise in the nerves and

Tetanus:
a physiological term meaning sustained, uncontrolled muscular contractions.

klo-strid'e-um

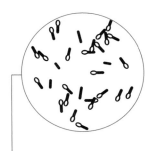

Clostridium tetani

crash into the muscles, causing the muscles to contract continuously and without control (FIGURE 9.3).

Symptoms of tetanus develop rapidly, often within hours. A patient experiences generalized muscle stiffness, especially in the facial and swallowing muscles. Spasms of the jaw muscles cause the teeth to clench and bring on a condition called **trismus,** or **lockjaw.** Severe cases are characterized by a "fixed smile," arching of the back (**opisthotonus**), spasmodic inhalation, and seizures in the diaphragm and rib muscles, leading to reduced ventilation and death. Patients are treated with sedatives and muscle relaxants, and are placed in quiet, dark rooms. Physicians prescribe penicillin to destroy the organisms and tetanus **antitoxin** to neutralize the toxin.

Immunization to tetanus may be rendered by injections of tetanus **toxoid** in the diphtheria-tetanus-acellular pertussis (DTaP) vaccine. The toxoid, developed in 1933 by Gaston Ramon, is prepared by treating the toxin with formaldehyde to eliminate its toxic quality. Children usually receive the first of several injections at the age of 2 months. Booster injections of tetanus toxoid in the **Td vaccine** (a "tetanus shot") are recommended every 10 years to keep the level of immunity high.

The United States has had a steady decline in the incidence of tetanus, with approximately 100 cases confirmed annually. Most cases occur in the young, who are more likely to have contact with soil, and in the elderly, in whom antibody levels have dropped or vaccination never took place. In other parts of the world, tetanus remains a major health problem and is often related to traditional customs. In some countries, for example, unsanitary ear-piercing is common, tattooing is widespread, and the umbilical stump of newborns is dressed with soil. In other cases, a simple splinter of wood may be the source of entry (as MicroFocus 9.2 illustrates).

GAS GANGRENE

To understand gas gangrene as an infectious disease, it is important to understand the physiological term *gangrene*. Gangrene is a condition that develops when the blood flow ceases to a part of the body, usually as a result of blockage by dead tissue. The body part, generally an extremity, becomes dry and shrunken, and the skin color changes to purplish or black. The gangrene may spread as enzymes from broken cells destroy other cells, and the tissue may have to be excised (debrided) or the body part amputated. This form of gangrene is called dry gangrene (FIGURE 9.4).

Gas gangrene, or moist gangrene, occurs when soilborne bacteria invade the dead, anaerobic tissue. The organisms responsible are ***Clostridium perfringens*** (formerly called *Clostridium welchii*), as well as several other species of *Clostridium* normally found in the large intestine and obtained from the soil when a wound is sustained. These anaerobic, sporeforming, Gram-positive rods multiply rapidly,

o-pis'tō-tō'nus

Toxoid:
a preparation of altered toxin molecules used for immunization purposes.

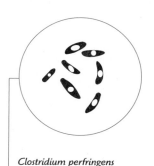

Clostridium perfringens

FIGURE 9.3

Tetanus

A photograph of a painting by Scottish surgeon Charles Bell showing a soldier dying of tetanus. The soldier was wounded at the battle of Corunna in 1809. Note that the muscles are fully contracting in virtually all parts of the body from head to toes. The soldier's face shows the clenched jaw and fixed ("sardonic") smile characteristic of lockjaw. The artist, Bell, was also the first to describe the paralysis and drooping of the facial muscles known as Bell's palsy.

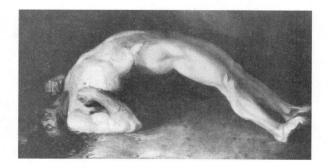

MicroFocus 9.2

SHOELACES

The untied shoelaces told the story—that and the difficult swallowing and distorted facial features. She had left the hospital the day before, but the symptoms were not gone—not yet, at least.

It began on Sunday, July 5, 1992. The 4th of July weekend was hot in Rutland, Vermont, and most of her friends were recovering from the previous day's celebrations. But she decided to catch up on her gardening. The ground was warm, and she took off her shoes to walk about the garden—nothing like good fertile soil, she must have been thinking.

Then it happened. "Ouch!" A splinter entered the base of her right big toe. No

matter. Take out the splinter and get on with the gardening. Gone and forgotten.

But it was not forgotten. Three days later, the pain on the left side of her face necessitated a visit to her family doctor. Probably a facial infection, she was told. Take the amoxicillin, and it should resolve.

It did not resolve—it worsened. Now it was July 12, and her jaw was so tight that she had not eaten for three days. The muscle spasms in her face were intense, and her friends nervously suggested that it looked like lockjaw. When she arrived at the hospital's emergency room, an alert doctor recognized the classic risus sardonicus (the grinning

expression caused by spasms of the facial muscles) and the trismus (the lockjaw caused by spasms of the chewing muscles). No question—she had tetanus.

Treatment was swift and aggressive—3250 units of tetanus antitoxin, intravenous penicillin, and a tetanus booster, plus removing the traces of wood still in the wound. She was placed in a quiet room and given muscle relaxants. Fifteen days would pass before she was discharged. She was well on her way to recovery . . . except she still could not tie those darn shoelaces.

while fermenting the muscle carbohydrates and putrefying the muscle proteins. Large amounts of gas result from this metabolism and tear the tissue apart. The gas also presses against blood vessels, thereby blocking the flow and forcing cells away from their blood supply. In addition, the organisms secrete **lecithinase**, an enzyme that dissolves cell membranes and releases toxic cellular enzymes. Two other bacterial enzymes, **hyaluronidase** and **hemolysin**, facilitate the passage of bacteria among the cells and destroy red blood cells, respectively. Neurotoxins are also released.

The symptoms of gas gangrene include intense pain and swelling at the wound site, as well as a foul odor. Initially the site turns dull red, then green, and finally blue-black. Anemia is common, and bacterial toxins may damage the heart and nervous system. Treatment consists of antibiotic therapy as well as debridement, amputation, or exposure in a hyperbaric oxygen chamber. The disease spreads rapidly, and death frequently results. Some microbiologists prefer the name **clostridial myonecrosis** ("muscle cell death") because gas is not always present in the early stages of disease.

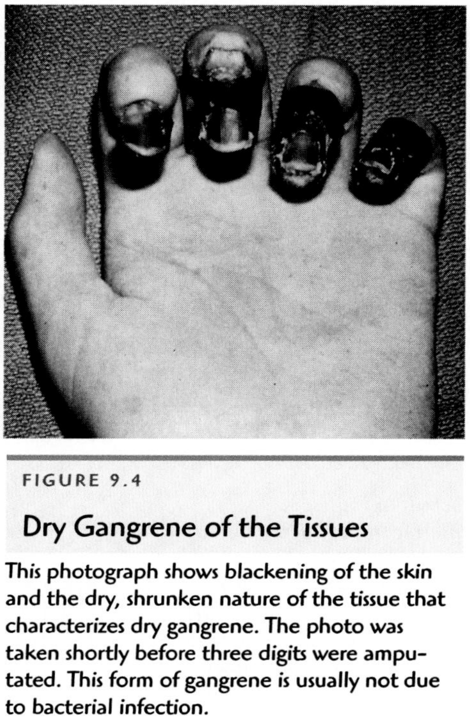

hi'ah-lu-ron'ĭ-das
he-mol'ĭ-sĭn

FIGURE 9.4

Dry Gangrene of the Tissues

This photograph shows blackening of the skin and the dry, shrunken nature of the tissue that characterizes dry gangrene. The photo was taken shortly before three digits were amputated. This form of gangrene is usually not due to bacterial infection.

LEPTOSPIROSIS

Leptospirosis is a typical **zoonosis**—that is, a disease of animals that can spread to humans. The disease affects household pets such as dogs and cats, as well as rats, mice, and barnyard animals. Humans acquire it by contact with these animals or from soil or water contaminated with their urine. Increasing rat populations in inner cities increase the risk for this disease through contact with standing water in parks.

lep'to-spi-ro'sis
spi'ro-kēt

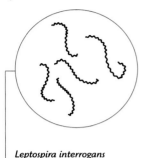

Leptospira interrogans

The agent of leptospirosis is ***Leptospira interrogans***, a small, delicate spirochete usually with a hook at one end that resembles a question mark, hence the name *interrogans* (FIGURE 9.5). The undulating movements of these organisms result from contractions of submicroscopic fibers called **axial filaments**. In animals, the spirochetes colonize the kidney tubules and are excreted in the urine to the soil. They enter the human body through the skin, especially through abrasions and the soft parts of the feet. Patients experience flulike symptoms, such as fever, aches, and muscle weakness. The systemic form of leptospirosis is **Weil's disease**. Here the spirochetes infect various organs, including the kidneys, liver, and meninges. Considerable jaundice may be present as bile seeps from the liver, and the patient may vomit blood from gastric hemorrhages. Despite the numerous tissues involved, the mortality rate from leptospirosis is low, and penicillin is generally used with success.

Leptospirosis occurs throughout the United States, and recognizing its symptoms, together with modern methods of diagnosis, have led to increased reports of its occurrence. In 1997, for example, a number of cases occurred in white water rafters in Costa Rica, and in 1997, the disease broke out in triathletes in Wisconsin (MicroFocus 9.3). The disease is considered an occupational hazard of veterinarians, as well as tunnel diggers, sugarcane cutters, dock workers, miners, and others who work in wet areas where rodents are present. Dogs may be immunized with a leptospirosis vaccine, usually combined with rabies, parvovirus, and distemper vaccines.

MELIOIDOSIS

me'le-oi-do'sis
soo'do-mo'nas soo'do-mal-la'e

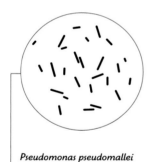

Pseudomonas pseudomallei

Melioidosis is a disease that, until recently, has been rare in the United States. It is caused by a Gram-negative rod named ***Pseudomonas pseudomallei***. This organism is common in soil and water, especially in Southeast Asia. Humans contract melioidosis by absorbing bacteria through soil-contaminated wounds, by inhalation, or by consuming contaminated food or water. The disease also affects horses, rodents, dogs, and cats.

Melioidosis has been called a "medical time bomb" because of its propensity to lie dormant in the body for years. Abscesses may eventually occur in the heart, lungs, liver, or spleen, and symptoms may vary widely, depending on which organs

FIGURE 9.5

Leptospira interrogans

Details of *Leptospira interrogans*, the agent of leptospirosis. (a) A scanning electron micrograph (×6000). Note the tightly coiling spirals and the absence of flagella in this spirochete. (b) A closer view of the terminal hook of one spirochete (×15,000).

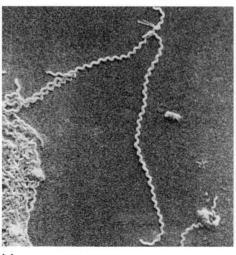

(a)

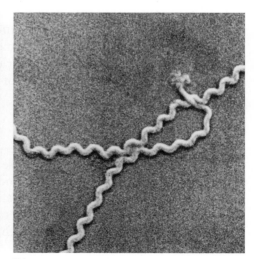

(b)

MicroFocus 9.3

BAD DAY AT LAKE SPRINGFIELD

They swam a brisk mile-and-a-half through Lake Springfield. They rode their bikes a long 45 miles over the Illinois hills. And to top it off, they ran a tough and painful 10 miles. It was the 1997 Springfield Ironhorse Triathlon. They fully expected to be tired. They didn't expect to get sick.

But they got sick in record numbers. Of about 1000 athletes, close to 100 were ill. Most had high fever, nausea, and headaches; some had red eyes. Seventy-two sought medical attention, and 23 were hospitalized. Two suffered

kidney failure and were on dialysis. And one had undergone an abdominal operation to find "an intestinal blockage." If it had happened to one or two people, doctors might have passed it off as influenza, but dozens of athletes were sick. And athletes don't get sick like this—especially triathletes!

By now, Illinois public health officials had publicized the outbreak, and many more people were coming forward to report their illness. No, they hadn't all been to the same restaurant. Nor were they all bitten by mosquitoes, or been

on a trip abroad together. Yes, they were all at Lake Springfield that fateful June day. Some were enjoying the beaches at the lake and swimming in the water; some were fishing; some were boating. And yes, they remembered watching the triathlon.

Eventually it all made sense: the symptoms, the bacterial isolations from the water, contact with the water, the blood tests. They all pointed to one disease—leptospirosis. In the end, no one died that summer, but Lake Springfield would never be the same.

are affected. Tropical experts have known of melioidosis since the early 1900s, but Americans did not appear to be involved until the Vietnam War, when several cases surfaced. This and other soilborne diseases are summarized in TABLE 9.1.

To this point . . .

We have surveyed several bacterial diseases commonly transmitted from the soil. Diseases such as tetanus and gas gangrene involve the contamination of wounds with bacteria in the form of spores. As the bacilli multiply in the dead anaerobic tissue of the wound, the symptoms of disease surface. Tetanus bacilli produce powerful toxins that lead to sustained muscle contractions, while gas gangrene bacilli ferment and putrefy the organic compounds in muscle to produce large amounts of gas that lead to gangrene.

Anthrax, leptospirosis, and melioidosis may also be contracted from the soil, as well as by other means, such as contact with animals or consuming contaminated food or water. Anthrax occurs in a number of forms, including pulmonary, gastrointestinal, and skin forms, all of which may be fatal. Leptospirosis, often spread by domestic animals and household pets, affects many abdominal organs. Melioidosis has contemporary significance because many cases in Americans were contracted from the soil in Southeast Asia during the Vietnam War. You may note that in many of the soilborne diseases there is substantial involvement of the blood, since bacteria spread through this tissue from the initial site of invasion.

We shall now turn to a series of bacterial diseases transmitted by arthropods. In these diseases, infected arthropods introduce bacteria into the circulation, and the symptoms of disease commonly occur in the bloodstream. High fever is usually associated with the disease, and a general feeling of illness is common. Our survey will include bubonic plague, one of the most historically important diseases, as well as two diseases that were observed for the first time in the United States.

TABLE 9.1

A Summary of Soilborne Bacterial Diseases

DISEASE	CAUSATIVE AGENT	DESCRIPTION OF AGENT	ORGANS AFFECTED	CHARACTERISTIC SIGNS
Anthrax	*Bacillus anthracis*	Gram-positive sporeforming rod	Blood Lungs Skin	Hemorrhaged blood Boil-like lesions
Tetanus	*Clostridium tetani*	Gram-positive sporeforming anaerobic rod	Nerves at synapse	Spasms Tetanus
Gas gangrene	*Clostridium perfringens*	Gram-positive sporeforming anaerobic rod	Muscles Nerves Blood cells	Gangrene Swollen tissue
Leptospirosis	*Leptospira interrogans*	Spirochete	Kidney Liver Spleen	Jaundice Vomiting
Melioidosis	*Pseudomonas pseudomallei*	Gram-negative rod	Heart Lung	Abscesses

9.2

Arthropodborne Bacterial Diseases

Arthropods transmit diseases to humans usually by taking a blood meal and themselves becoming infected. Then they pass the organisms to another individual during the next blood meal. Arthropodborne diseases occur primarily in the bloodstream, and they are often characterized by a high fever and a body rash.

BUBONIC PLAGUE

Few diseases have had the rich and terrifying history of **bubonic plague**, nor can any match the array of social, economic, and religious changes wrought by this disease.

Pandemic: a worldwide epidemic.

The first documented pandemic of plague probably began in Africa during the reign of the Roman emperor Justinian in A.D. 542. It lasted 60 years, killed millions, and contributed to the downfall of Rome. The second pandemic was known as the **Black Death** because of the purplish-black splotches on victims and the terror it evoked in the 1300s (MicroFocus 9.4). The Black Death decimated the world and, by some accounts, killed an estimated 40 million people in Europe, almost one-third of the population of that continent, as the chapter introduction relates. A deadly epidemic also occurred in London in 1665, where 70,000 people succumbed to the disease. Daniel Defoe's *Journal of the Plague Year* recounts how people reacted (FIGURE 9.6).

TOXIN INVOLVED	TREATMENT ADMINISTERED	IMMUNIZATION AVAILABLE	COMMENT
Yes	Penicillin	For animals	High mortality rate Affects many organs Rare disease in humans
Yes	Penicillin Antitoxin	Toxoid in DTaP	Second most powerful toxin Inhibits cholinesterase activity
Yes	Penicillin	None	Gas blocks flow of blood Called clostridial myonecrosis
Not established	Penicillin	For animals	Common in animals Typical zoonosis
Not established	Tetracycline	None	Symptoms develop slowly Occurs in Southeast Asia

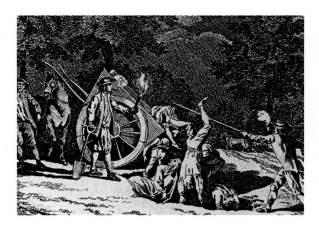

FIGURE 9.6

Bubonic Plague

An engraving drawn during the London plague of 1665. Bodies heaped on "dead carts" are being pulled into huge pits by men dragging the corpses off the carts with a hook attached to a ten-foot pole. This practice is probably the origin of the saying, "I wouldn't touch it with a ten-foot pole." The pipes the men are smoking give off noxious fumes to ward off the disease.

MicroFocus 9.4

A VOYAGE OF DEATH

In 1343, a group of Italian merchants from Genoa found themselves trapped behind the walls of the far-distant city of Caffa in the Crimea in Asia. The dreaded Tartars had laid siege to the city, and things looked bleak.

Three years later, the city was still under siege. Then one day, the Tartars began catapulting corpses over the walls. The corpses were their own men dead from the plague. Soon plague was sweeping through Caffa. The townspeople were terrified: Either the plague would kill them inside the walls, or the Tartars would kill them outside the walls. But the Tartars were equally terrified of the plague, and they were withdrawing.

Sensing an opportunity to escape, the merchants ran for their ships and sailed off. Unfortunately, their voyage home would be a voyage of death. Many died of the plague on board, and the survivors spread the disease wherever they stopped to replenish their supply of food and water. When the remaining few reached Genoa, they doomed their city. By this time, people throughout Europe were caught in the fangs of the Black Death. It was 1346. Western civilization was about to change forever.

In the late 1800s, Asian warfare facilitated the spread of a Burmese focus of plague, and migrations brought infected individuals to China and Hong Kong. During this epidemic in 1894, the causative organism was isolated by Alexandre Yersin and, independently, by Shibasaburo Kitasato. Plague first appeared in the United States in San Francisco in 1900, carried by rats on ships from the Orient. The disease spread to ground squirrels, prairie dogs, and other wild rodents, and it is now endemic in the southwestern states, where it is commonly called **sylvatic plague**. MicroFocus 9.5 recounts a case associated with wildlife.

Bubonic plague is caused by *Yersinia pestis* (formerly *Pasteurella pestis*). This Gram-negative rod stains heavily at the poles of the cell, giving it a safety-pin appearance and a characteristic called **bipolar staining**. As first demonstrated by Masaki Ogata in 1897, the bacillus is transmitted by the **rat flea *Xenopsylla cheopis***. A living organism such as a flea that transmits disease agents is called a **vector**, from the Latin *vehere*, meaning "to carry." Normally, the fleas infest only rats, but as the rats die, the fleas jump to humans and feed in the skin, thus transferring the bacilli into the bloodstream.

Bubonic plague is a blood disease. The bacteria multiply in the bloodstream and localize in the lymph nodes, especially those of the armpits, neck, and groin. Hemorrhaging in the lymph nodes causes substantial swellings called **buboes** (hence the name, bubonic plague). Dark, purplish splotches from hemorrhages can also be seen through the skin (the "rosies" in "Ring-a-ring of rosies"). From the buboes, the bacilli spread to the bloodstream, where they cause **septicemic plague**. Over 50 percent of untreated cases of bubonic or septicemic plague are fatal.

Human-to-human transmission of plague during epidemics has little to do with fleas. Instead, it is dependent upon respiratory droplets because *Y. pestis* localizes in

Sylvatic:
occurring in nature; wild.

zen'op-sil'ah ke-op'is

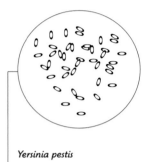

Yersinia pestis

Bubo:
a swelling, usually in the lymph nodes.

MicroFocus 9.5

"WHAT A SHAME!"

"Just an incredible day," he must have been thinking, as he trudged along. It was great to be out in the desert. Great to get away from the books for a while. Final exams were only a few weeks away, then summer, then college, then who knows? Maybe a career in physical education? Maybe a coaching job? Three miles completed, 5 miles to go. He had to keep moving to make it back home for dinner.

He didn't mind the solitude of the Arizona desert. It was cool up here in Flagstaff, just right for hiking. And there were plenty of animals to see and interesting plants to watch for. He would stop now and then for some water or to watch the horizon or feed a colony of prairie dogs as they bustled about the terrain. Then he continued on to home.

He enjoyed wrestling as well, and he was the team captain. Two days after the hike, he sustained a groin injury while wrestling. When the ache remained, he went to the doctor. The doctor noted the groin swelling and wondered whether it had anything to do with the fever the young man was experiencing. Was it just a coincidence—the ache, the swelling, the fever? This was no ordinary groin injury. "We'll watch it for a couple of days," the doctor said as he gave the young man a pain reliever.

Tragedy struck the next morning. All his mother remembered was a loud thud from the bathroom. She didn't remember her terrified shriek or dialing the emergency number. The emergency medical technicians were there in a flash, but it was too late. He was dead.

The investigation that followed took public health officials down many dead-ends. It wasn't the wrestling injury, they concluded. Still, the groin swelling made them suspicious. "That hiking trail," they asked his mother, "where is it?"

They set out in search of an elusive answer. About 3½ miles out, they came upon a colony of prairie dogs. The animals didn't look well. In fact, some were dead nearby. Carefully, they trapped a sick animal and carried it back to the lab. Two days later, the lab report was ready—the animal was sick with plague. Then the young man's tissues were tested—again, plague. The investigators shook their heads. "What a shame!"

the lungs of many of the first victims. In this form, the disease is called **pneumonic plague** and is highly contagious. Lung symptoms are similar to those in pneumonia, with extensive coughing and sneezing. Hemorrhaging and fluid accumulation are common. Many suffer cardiovascular collapse, and death is common within 48 hours of the onset of symptoms. Mortality rates for pneumonic plague approach 100 percent. One 1992 death was linked to a cat and rodents (FIGURE 9.7), and a notable outbreak appears to have occurred in India in 1994.

FIGURE 9.7

An Episode of Plague

This incident demonstrates that plague occurs in modern times in the United States.

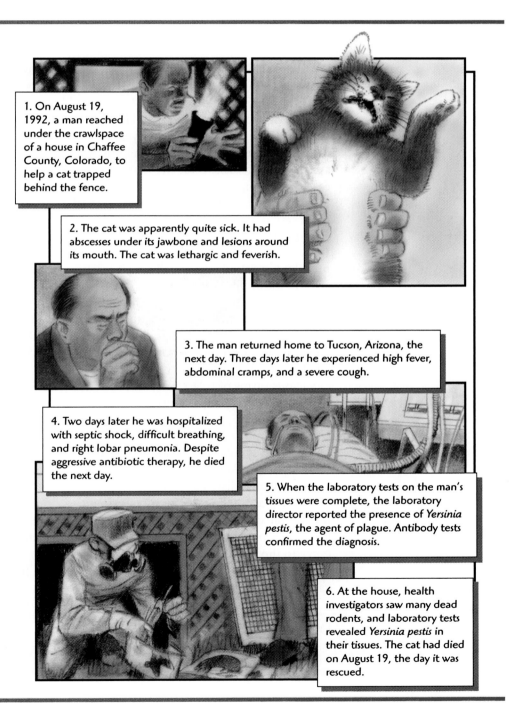

1. On August 19, 1992, a man reached under the crawlspace of a house in Chaffee County, Colorado, to help a cat trapped behind the fence.

2. The cat was apparently quite sick. It had abscesses under its jawbone and lesions around its mouth. The cat was lethargic and feverish.

3. The man returned home to Tucson, Arizona, the next day. Three days later he experienced high fever, abdominal cramps, and a severe cough.

4. Two days later he was hospitalized with septic shock, difficult breathing, and right lobar pneumonia. Despite aggressive antibiotic therapy, he died the next day.

5. When the laboratory tests on the man's tissues were complete, the laboratory director reported the presence of *Yersinia pestis*, the agent of plague. Antibody tests confirmed the diagnosis.

6. At the house, health investigators saw many dead rodents, and laboratory tests revealed *Yersinia pestis* in their tissues. The cat had died on August 19, the day it was rescued.

TEXTBOOK CASES

Tetracycline:
a broad-spectrum antibiotic that inhibits protein synthesis in bacteria.

Plague may be treated with tetracycline or streptomycin when detected early. Diagnosis consists of the laboratory isolation of *Y. pestis,* together with tests for plague antibodies and typing with bacteriophages. The disease occurs sporadically in Native American populations and in travelers through the Southwest. Small-game hunters, taxidermists, veterinarians, zoologists, and others who handle small rodents must be aware of the possibility of contracting plague. About two dozen cases are reported to the CDC annually. A vaccine consisting of dead *Y. pestis* cells is available for high-risk groups. Vaccine research has been stimulated by the possible use of plague bacilli in bioterrorism.

TULAREMIA

Tularemia is one of several microbial diseases first recorded in the United States (others include St. Louis encephalitis, Rocky Mountain spotted fever, Lyme disease, and Legionnaires' disease). In 1911, a U.S. Public Health Service investigator named George W. McCoy reported the plaguelike disease in ground squirrels from Tulare County, California, and within a year he isolated the responsible bacillus. By 1920, researchers identified tularemia in humans, and Edward Francis assumed a detailed study of the disease. Over the next 25 years, Francis amassed data on over 10,000 cases, including his own. In the 1960s, when a name was coined for the causative organism, *Francisella tularensis* was selected to honor him and the county of first observation.

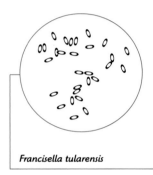

Francisella tularensis

Vector:
a living organism that transmits disease agents.

Francisella tularensis is a small Gram-negative rod that displays bipolar staining. It occurs in a broad variety of wild animals, especially rodents, and it is particularly prevalent in rabbits (in which case it is known as rabbit fever). Cats and dogs may acquire the bacillus during romps in the woods, and humans are infected by arthropods from the fur of animals. **Ticks** are important vectors in this regard, as evidenced by an outbreak of 20 tickborne cases in South Dakota in the 1980s. Other methods of transmission include contact with an infected animal (such as skinning an animal), consumption of rabbit meat, splashing bacilli into the eye, and inhaling bacilli, even from laboratory specimens.

Various forms of tularemia exist, depending on where the bacilli enter the body. An arthropod bite, for example, may lead to a skin ulcer (FIGURE 9.8) and swollen salivary glands. Splashing into the eye may cause an eye lesion, and inhalation may lead to pulmonary symptoms. In all forms, the disease is difficult to recognize because the symptoms are mild and nonspecific. Various patients with tularemia have been mistakenly treated for strep throat, rickettsial disease, lymphoid cancer, and cat-scratch disease.

Cat-scratch disease:
a bacterial disease acquired by a cat bite or scratch and accompanied by swollen lymph nodes, usually on one side of the body.

Tularemia usually resolves on treatment with tetracycline or streptomycin, and few people die of the disease. Epidemics are unknown, and evidence suggests that tularemia may not be communicable among humans despite the many modes of entry to the body. Physicians report about 200 cases annually in the United States, most from the Midwest. MicroFocus 9.6 describes how the disease unexpectedly came to Massachusetts.

LYME DISEASE

One of the major emerging problems of the contemporary era is Lyme disease, currently the most common tickborne (indeed, arthropodborne) illness in the

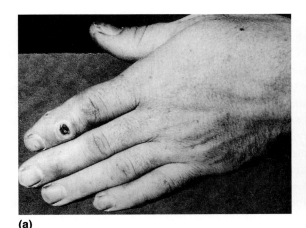

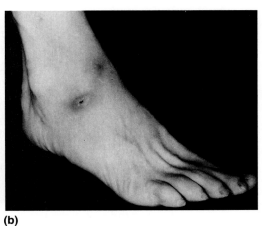

(a)   (b)

FIGURE 9.8

The Lesions of Tularemia

The lesions of tularemia occur where the bacilli enter the body. In (a), the patient acquired the disease by handling infected rabbit meat. In (b), infection was preceded by the bite of an infected arthropod. The craterlike form of the lesion can be seen in both cases.

MicroFocus 9.6

"BUT WE'VE NEVER HAD TULAREMIA ON CAPE COD!"

An epidemiologist is one who studies the pattern of disease in a community and attempts to locate its source and predict its spread. In the 1930s, the surprise observation of tularemia on Cape Cod, Massachusetts, tested the best epidemiologists of the day.

The story began when a young girl from Cape Cod was hospitalized with a fever lasting about 3 weeks. She had few other symptoms of illness, and physicians soon exhausted their list of diagnostic tests. When the girl's symptoms abated, her parents suggested that she be allowed to return home, and her doctors agreed. However, before she left, another round of tests was ordered. A week later, the results of one test were positive: The girl apparently had tularemia.

The physicians were perplexed. Cape Cod had plenty of rabbits and ticks, but

no case of tularemia had ever been reported. The girl could not recall a tick bite, but she did mention that her puppy had been ill with fever and was eating poorly some weeks before. Doctors tested the puppy and found that, indeed, it had been suffering from tularemia. The pieces of the puzzle were starting to fit together, but investigators still had no clue about how the disease might have entered the area.

After many weeks of judicious questions and possible leads, one was especially promising. Epidemiologists established that Cape Cod had experienced a short supply of rabbits that year. Rabbits were a favorite target of sportsmen, and a number of wealthy hunters had pooled their funds to import two freight cars full of rabbits from Kansas. Kansas, coincidentally, was a "homeland" of tularemia, and the ticks from

Kansas proved identical to their Cape Cod relatives.

Now the puzzle was solved: the girl with the mysterious fever, the positive test for tularemia, the puppy also sick with tularemia, the imported rabbits, and the tick carriers. It seemed logical that infected rabbits had brought the disease to Cape Cod, and that the puppy was bitten by a rabbit tick during one of its romps in the woods. An affectionate slurp had probably transmitted the disease to the girl.

The story has a bittersweet ending. The young girl recovered without complications, the puppy grew into a healthy dog, and hunters had plenty of game. But tularemia had come to Cape Cod to stay.

United States. Lyme disease has been reported in 46 states, and in 1997, it accounted for over 12,000 U.S. cases of infectious disease, as FIGURE 9.9 illustrates.

Lyme disease is named for Old Lyme, Connecticut, the suburban community where a cluster of cases was observed in 1975. That year, researchers led by Allan C. Steere of nearby Yale University traced the disease to **ticks** of the genus *Ixodes*. However, they were unable to locate a causative agent. Several years would pass until 1982, when a spirochete was observed in diseased tissue by investigators at the State University of New York at Stony Brook. Still another 2 years passed before the spirochete was isolated and cultivated (FIGURE 9.10). Researchers named it *Borrelia burgdorferi* for Willy Burgdorfer, the microbiologist who studied the spirochete in the gut of an infected tick.

Lyme disease has a variable incubation period that can be as long as 6 to 8 weeks. One of the first signs is a slowly expanding red rash at the site of the tick bite. The rash is called **erythema** (red) **chronicum** (persistent) **migrans** (expanding), or **ECM**. Beginning as a small flat or raised lesion, the rash increases in diameter in a circular pattern over a period of weeks, sometimes reaching a diameter of 10 to 15 inches, as FIGURE 9.11 shows. It has an intense red border and a red center, and it resembles a bull's eye (the **bull's eye rash**). It can vary in shape and is usually hot to the touch, but it need not be present in all cases of disease. Indeed, about one-third of patients do not develop ECM. The tick bite can be distinguished from a mosquito

iks-o'dēz

bŏ-rel'e-ah burg-dorf'er-e

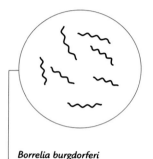

Borrelia burgdorferi

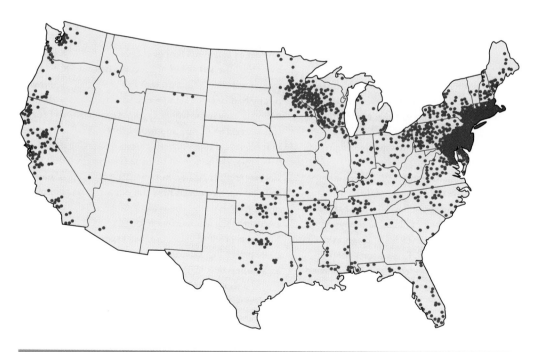

FIGURE 9.9

Lyme Disease in the United States, 1997

This map shows the location of the 12,801 cases of Lyme disease occurring in 1997. Forty-six states and the District of Columbia are involved in the epidemic. Ten northeastern states accounted for 92 percent of the reported cases.

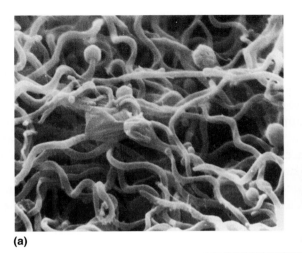
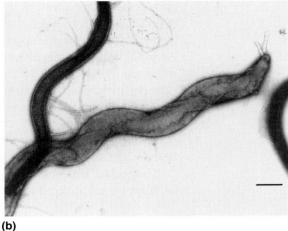

(a) (b)

FIGURE 9.10

Borrelia burgdorferi

Two views of *Borrelia burgdorferi*, the agent of Lyme disease. (a) A scanning electron micrograph showing an abundance of spirochetes. (b) A transmission electron micrograph in which the plasma membranes of two spirochetes have been disrupted, thereby releasing the endoflagella. These endoflagella run the length of the spirochete under the membrane and contribute to motility. (Bar = 0.5 μm.)

bite because the latter itches, while a tick bite does not. Fever, aches and pains, and flulike symptoms usually accompany the rash.

In the rash (or **early localized**) stage of Lyme disease, effective treatment can be rendered with penicillin and tetracycline. Left untreated, some cases resolve spontaneously, but others enter a second stage (**early disseminated**), when the disease spreads. Weeks to months later, the patient may experience pain, swelling, and **arthritis** in the large joints, especially the knee, shoulder, ankle, and elbow joints. Multiple rash sites may also be present at this stage, reflecting the spread of the spirochete. Vigorous treatment may effectively eliminate the spirochete, but the joint damage may be irreversible.

In the third stage (**late chronic**), the arthritis may be complicated by damage to the cardiovascular and nervous systems. Patients often experience irregular heartbeats, migraine headaches, hearing and vision abnormalities, and loss of muscle tone, especially in the facial muscles (Bell's palsy). Although Lyme disease is not known to have a high mortality rate, the overall damage to the body can be substantial.

The tick that transmits most cases of Lyme disease in the Northeast and Midwest is the deer tick *Ixodes scapularis* (formerly *I. dammini*); in the West, the major vector is the western black-legged tick *I. pacificus*. In its adult form, the tick is about the size of a pinhead or the period at the end of this sentence. It is smaller than the American dog tick, and it lives and mates in the fur of the white-tailed deer. Eventually it falls into the tall grass, where it waits for an unsuspecting dog, rodent, or human to pass by. The tick then attaches to its new host and penetrates into the skin. During the next 24 to 48 hours, it takes a blood meal and swells to the size of a small pea. While sucking the blood, it also defecates into the wound, and, if the tick is infected, spirochetes will be transmitted (as the life cycle

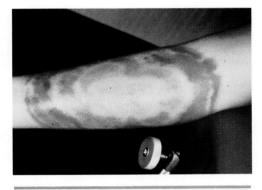

FIGURE 9.11

Erythema Chronicum Migrans (ECM)

Erythema chronicum migrans (ECM) is the rash that accompanies two-thirds of cases of Lyme disease. Note that the rash consists of a large patch with an intense red border. It is usually hot to the touch, and it expands with time.

ix-o′des scap-u-lar′is
dam-in′e
pa-cif′i-cus

in FIGURE 9.12 indicates). If the tick is observed on the skin, it should be removed with a forceps or tweezers, and the area should be thoroughly cleansed with soap and water and an antiseptic applied.

A diagnosis of Lyme disease is usually based on symptoms, and the physician will often use a pen to mark off the border of the skin rash to see if it expands with time. The patient's recent activities are noted (hiking in the woods, living in a tick-infested area, camping), and a blood sample may also be taken for a test for spirochetal antibodies. The test, however, may not be accurate because a number of weeks are required for the body to produce enough antibodies to show up in the test. A newer test designed to detect spirochetal DNA is now being developed.

Congenital transfers of *B. burgdorferi* have been documented, and pregnant women are encouraged to seek early diagnosis and treatment for the disease if they

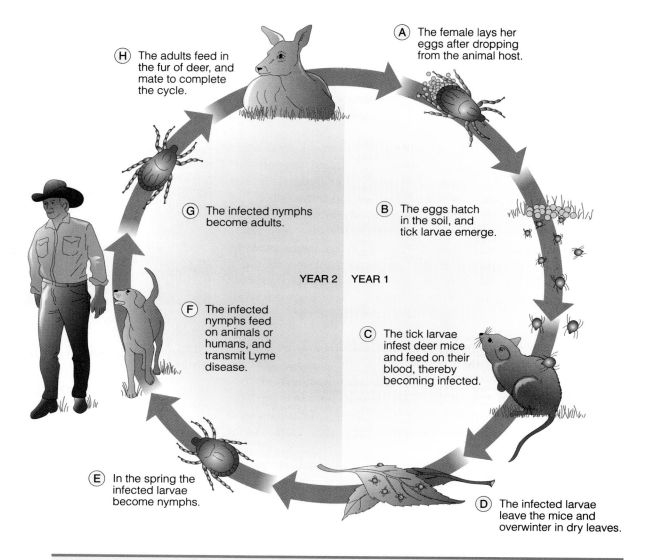

(A) The female lays her eggs after dropping from the animal host.

(H) The adults feed in the fur of deer, and mate to complete the cycle.

(G) The infected nymphs become adults.

(B) The eggs hatch in the soil, and tick larvae emerge.

YEAR 2   YEAR 1

(F) The infected nymphs feed on animals or humans, and transmit Lyme disease.

(C) The tick larvae infest deer mice and feed on their blood, thereby becoming infected.

(E) In the spring the infected larvae become nymphs.

(D) The infected larvae leave the mice and overwinter in dry leaves.

FIGURE 9.12

Life Cycle of the Tick

The life cycle of *Ixodes scapularis* and *Ixodes pacificus*, the ticks that transmit Lyme disease.

suspect they have been infected. At this writing, a vaccine for dogs has been licensed and is in routine use. A **vaccine** for humans (LYMErix) was approved by the U.S. Food and Drug Administration (FDA) in January 1999. The FDA approved the vaccine for people 15 to 70 years old, since experimental trials did not involve children. It is intended for those who live or work in grassy or wooded areas where infected ticks are probably present, and for those traveling to these areas. However, vaccination may be difficult for those with immediate travel plans because for full immunity, the FDA recommends an initial injection of vaccine, followed by a second injection after a month, and a third after a year. The vaccine is composed of a genetically engineered lipoprotein normally located on the outer surface of *B. burgdorferi*. (The lipoprotein is known as OspA, for outer surface protein A). Antibodies against the protein provide surveillance in the human body and are taken into the tick's gut when it takes a blood meal. There, the antibodies neutralize the bacteria in the arthropod as well. This action blocks transmission at the skin level.

Although Lyme disease is considered a "new" disease, there is evidence that it has existed for some decades, even though it has escaped recognition (**MicroFocus 9.7**). The disease is also called **Lyme borreliosis**.

RELAPSING FEVER

Relapsing fever is caused by a long spirochete currently referred to as ***Borrelia recurrentis***. Depending on the arthropod vector involved, various names have been given to strains of this spirochete. The CDC, for example, refers to two tickborne *Borrelia* species as *B. hermsii* and *B. turicatae*. However, we shall use the traditional name *B. recurrentis*, pending the outcome of DNA studies to determine the relationships among different strains.

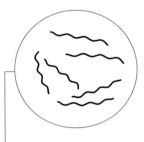

Borrelia recurrentis

MicroFocus 9.7

NOT SO NEW AFTER ALL

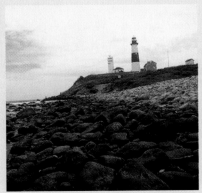

Is Lyme disease a totally new disease, or has it been present but unrecognized in human populations for some time?

One of the hotspots for Lyme disease is Long Island, a 120-mile-long island off the coast of New York City and the home of a certain author. At the easternmost tip of Long Island is the town of Montauk, an old fishing village and a resort community. It seems that for decades local doctors have spoken of "Montauk knee," a disease accompanied by swollen and inflamed knee joints and a skin rash. Was Montauk knee what we now call Lyme disease?

Pathologist David Pershing of the Mayo Clinic attempted to find out. He and several colleagues sought out 140 specimens of ticks collected between 1924 and 1951, many from natural history collections. Then they dissected the ticks and removed the intestines. They amplified the DNA in the intestinal matter by a technique called the polymerase chain reaction. Next they set out to identify any DNA that might belong to *Borrelia burgdorferi*, the cause of Lyme disease. The theory was simple: If the DNA of *B. burgdorferi* was present, then the spirochete must also have been present; if *B. burgdorferi* was present, Lyme disease would predate 1975. And present it was. Pershing's group identified the DNA of *B. burgdorferi* in 13 ticks. All 13 had been collected near Montauk.

bor-rel'e-ā

or'ni-tho-dor'us

The borreliae that cause relapsing fever are transmitted by **lice** and **ticks**. Lice are natural parasites of humans, and they thrive where personal hygiene is poor. Ticks of the genus *Ornithodorus* transmit the borreliae from rodent hosts. The ticks normally inhabit rodent burrows and nests, where the natural infection cycle proceeds without apparent disease in the rodents. Humans are incidental hosts, often bitten briefly and without notice by the ticks at night. Cabins in wilderness areas are favorable nesting sites for infected rodents and their ticks, especially when food is made available by occupants of the cabin (as FIGURE 9.13 illustrates).

FIGURE **9.13**

An Outbreak of Tickborne Relapsing Fever

Although relapsing fever is not a well-known disease, outbreaks can occur, as this episode demonstrates.

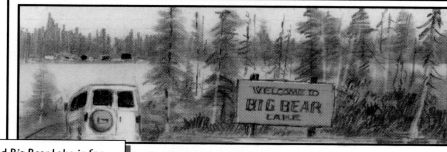

1. In August 1989, a family visited Big Bear Lake in San Bernardino County, California, for a week's vacation. They arrived early on a Saturday morning, and booked into cabin #4. They looked forward to a peaceful week in the country, free from the city's hustle and bustle.

2. The next week, a second group visited the lake and stayed in the same cabin. Several children were in the group. A good time was had by all.

3. After they left, cabin #4 was occupied by a third family. As before, the vacationers anticipated that nothing unusual would happen during their stay at the lake. It was a pleasure being in the woods.

4. By September, six people who had occupied cabin #4 were suffering from relapsing fever. Each of them had recurring bouts of high fever, severe headache, and extreme prostration.

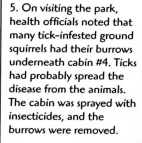

5. On visiting the park, health officials noted that many tick-infested ground squirrels had their burrows underneath cabin #4. Ticks had probably spread the disease from the animals. The cabin was sprayed with insecticides, and the burrows were removed.

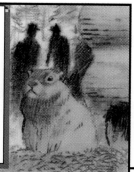

TEXTBOOK CASES

Cases of relapsing fever are characterized by substantial fever, shaking chills, headache, prostration, and drenching sweats. The symptoms last for a couple of days, then disappear, then reappear up to ten times during the following weeks. Microbiologists believe that different serotypes of *B. recurrentis* emerge from the organs after each attack. Treatment with tetracycline hastens recovery.

When lice are present, relapsing fever can occur in epidemics. One such epidemic descended upon Napoleon's lice-infested soldiers during the Russian campaign. Together with serious losses from another louseborne disease, typhus (discussed below), this disease so decimated the French army that the balance tipped in favor of the Russians. Peter Ilyich Tchaikovsky wrote the *1812 Overture* to celebrate the great Russian victory, one that might not have been possible without the intervention of microorganisms.

To this point . . .

We have studied four arthropodborne diseases of varying significance. Bubonic plague has had substantial impact on the course of history because it is among the most prolific killers of humans. Plague is still present in today's world. Tularemia, by contrast, is a plaguelike disease that has been recognized only in this century. Its symptoms are much milder than plague, and it often remains undiagnosed. Lyme disease has a history that is even more recent than tularemia's, having first been recorded in 1975. A distinctive lesion at the site of spirochete entry, and developing arthritis, are characteristic signs of the disease. In relapsing fever, disease is accompanied by recurring periods of fever.

In all these cases, the key element in control is the elimination of the arthropod vector. If the chain of transmission can be broken, the disease will not spread to the body. This is where the pest control operator plays a significant role in our system of public health. It is also where sanitation and personal hygiene contribute to good health.

In the final section of this chapter, we shall continue to examine arthropodborne diseases, emphasizing those diseases caused by rickettsiae, a group of small bacteria. Once again we shall encounter ticks, lice, and other arthropods as vectors, and we shall focus on their place in the disease process. Antibiotics are helpful in treatment of the diseases, but vector control is of prime importance.

9·3

Rickettsial Arthropodborne Diseases

In 1909, **Howard Taylor Ricketts**, a University of Chicago pathologist, described a new organism in the blood of patients with Rocky Mountain spotted fever and showed that ticks transmit the disease. A year later, he located a similar organism in the blood of animals infected with Mexican typhus, and discovered that fleas were the important vectors in this disease. Unfortunately, in the course of his work, Ricketts fell victim to the disease and died. When later research indicated that Ricketts had described a unique group of microorganisms, the name *rickettsiae* was coined to honor him. Originally, the rickettsiae were set apart from the bacteria, but microbiologists now consider them to be "small bacteria."

rik-et′se-e

ROCKY MOUNTAIN SPOTTED FEVER

am'ble-o'mah
der'mah-cent'or

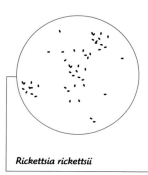

Rickettsia rickettsii

vīl fe'liks

Antigens:
substances that stimulate the immune system, often resulting in antibody production.

The agent of Rocky Mountain spotted fever is ***Rickettsia rickettsii.*** This organism is transmitted by **ticks**, especially those of the genera ***Amblyomma*** and ***Dermacentor*** (shown with other vectors in FIGURE 9.14). The hallmarks of Rocky Mountain spotted fever are a high fever lasting for many days and a skin rash reflecting damage to the small blood vessels. The rash begins as pink spots called **macules**, and progresses to pink-red pimplelike spots known as **papules**. Where the spots fuse, they form a **maculopapular rash**, which becomes dark red and then fades without evidence of scarring. The rash generally begins on the palms of the hands and soles of the feet and progressively spreads to the body trunk. Mortality rates of untreated cases are variable, with some outbreaks in Montana recording a rate as high as 75 percent. Treatment with tetracycline or chloramphenicol reduces this rate significantly.

Accurate and rapid diagnosis is essential in treating Rocky Mountain spotted fever. Evidence of a tick bite, progress of the rash, and the recent activities of the patient (camping, backpacking, and other outdoor activity) are taken into account. Traditionally, a procedure called the **Weil-Felix test** has been used as well. It is performed by mixing a sample of the patient's serum with the bacterium *Proteus OX19*. The bacteria clump together if the serum contains rickettsial antibodies. The test works because rickettsiae possess antigens also located in *Proteus* cells. However, the test is nonspecific and relatively insensitive, so antibody-detection tests are advised.

Rocky Mountain spotted fever was first observed in early settlers to the American Northwest. About a thousand cases were reported annually in the United States in the early 1980s, but public education about the disease, along with improved methods of diagnosis and treatment, caused a drop to about 400 cases by 1997 (FIGURE 9.15). Contrary to its name, Rocky Mountain spotted fever is not commonly reported in western states any longer, but it remains a problem in many southeastern and Atlantic Coast states. Children are its primary victims because of their contact with ticks.

EPIDEMIC TYPHUS

Epidemic typhus (also called **typhus fever**) is one of the most notorious of all bacterial diseases. It is considered a prolific killer of humans, and on several occasions it

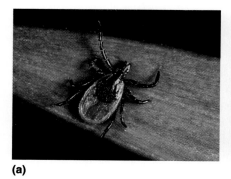

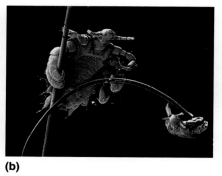

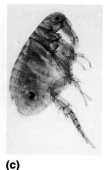

(a)   (b)   (c)

FIGURE 9.14

Three Arthropods That Transmit Bacterial Disease

(a) The tick (*Ixodes*). (b) The body louse (*Pediculus*). (c) The flea (*Xenopsylla*).

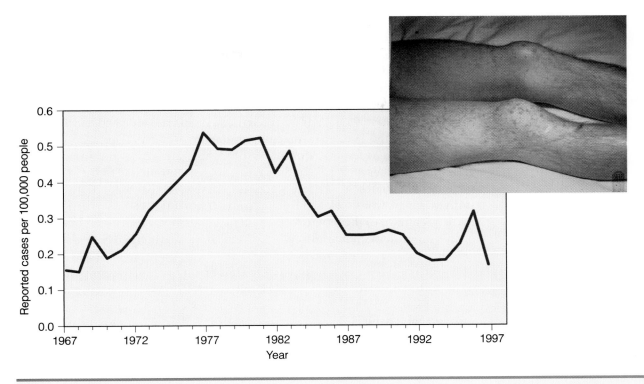

FIGURE 9.15

The Incidence and Symptoms of Rocky Mountain Spotted Fever

The incidence of Rocky Mountain spotted fever in the United States over the 30-year period preceding 1997. During the 1970s, this was the most prevalent tickborne disease, but insect control methods and antibiotic therapy have reduced the rate of incidence. Lyme disease is currently the most reported tickborne illness. Superimposed on the graph is a patient displaying the maculopapular rash associated with the disease.

has altered the course of history, as when it helped decimate the Aztec population in the 1500s. Historians report that Napoleon marched into Russia in 1812 with over 200,000 French soldiers but his forces were hit hard by typhus. Hans Zinsser's classic book *Rats, Lice, and History* describes events such as these and provides an engaging look at the effects of several infectious diseases on civilization (MicroFocus 9.8).

MicroFocus 9.8

RATS, LICE, AND HISTORY

The title of this box repeats the title of a book written by Hans Zinsser. Zinsser was born in New York City in 1878. He achieved fame for isolating the bacterium of epidemic typhus, but he is equally well known for his prose. Zinsser wrote some of the most uniquely personal, wise, and witty books of the twentieth century. Indeed, the unabridged title of his most famous book is (with tongue in cheek) *Rats,*

Lice, and History: Being a Study in Biography, Which, After Twelve Preliminary Chapters Indispensable for the Preparation of the Lay Reader, Deals with the Life History of Typhus Fever.

On a more serious note, here is a sample of Zinsser's writing from his 1935 book: "Soldiers have rarely won wars. They often mop up after the barrage of epidemics. And typhus, with its brothers and sisters—plague, cholera, typhoid,

dysentery—has decided more campaigns than Caesar, Hannibal, Napoleon, and all the other generals of history. The epidemics get the blame for defeat, the generals the credit for victory. It ought to be the other way 'round . . . ."

If you think you'd enjoy learning more about disease and its effect on civilization, Zinsser's book would be a worthwhile investment of your time.

pro'vaht-zek'e

pe-dik'u-lus

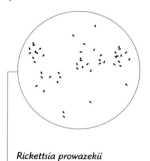

Rickettsia prowazekii

Serum:
the straw–colored fluid remaining after blood cells have been removed from blood.

Epidemic typhus is caused by ***Rickettsia prowazekii***. The bacteria are transmitted to humans by head and body **lice** of the genus ***Pediculus***. This was first noted by Charles Nicolle, winner of the 1928 Nobel Prize in Physiology or Medicine. Lice are natural parasites of humans. They flourish where sanitation measures are lacking and hygiene is poor. Often these conditions are associated with war, famine, poverty, and a generally poor quality of life.

The characteristic fever and rash of rickettsial disease are particularly evident in epidemic typhus. There is a **maculopapular rash**, but unlike the rash of Rocky Mountain spotted fever, it appears first on the body trunk and progresses to the extremities. Intense fever, sometimes reaching 104°F, remains for many days as the patient hallucinates and becomes delirious. (Typhus, like typhoid, takes its name from the Greek word *typhos*, meaning "smoke" or "cloud.") Some patients suffer permanent damage to the blood vessels and heart, and over 75 percent of sufferers die in epidemics. Tetracycline and chloramphenicol reduce this percentage substantially, and the disease is rare in the United States.

The diagnosis of epidemic typhus depends on observation of symptoms, evidence of lice infestation, and a number of tests using serum (Chapter 19), including the Weil-Felix test. Control of the disease requires destruction of lice populations through good hygiene. The use of insecticide powders on the clothes and body surface are also helpful. The fear generated by typhus was used to create the deception described in MicroFocus 9.9.

ENDEMIC TYPHUS

zen'op-sil'ah ke-op'is

Endemic typhus is a second form of typhus. This disease occurs sporadically in human populations because the **flea** that transmits it, ***Xenopsylla cheopis***, is not a natural parasite of humans. However, the disease is prevalent in rodent populations where fleas abound (such as rats and squirrels), and thus it is called **murine typhus**, from the Latin *murine*, referring to "mouse." Cats and their fleas are also involved, and lice may harbor the bacilli.

MicroFocus 9.9

THE COUNTERFEIT EPIDEMIC

Since first described in 1916 by Austrian physicians Edmund Weil and Arthur Felix, the Weil-Felix test has been an important diagnostic tool for the detection of typhus. The test is based on the principle that antibodies produced against the typhus bacteria also cause *Proteus OX19* cells to clump together. But what if a person were inoculated with *Proteus OX19* cells? Would the body produce the same antibodies? And if a diagnosis were based solely on the Weil-Felix test, could that person be mistaken to have typhus?

These questions occurred to two Polish physicians during World War II. Hundreds from their district had already been sent to German labor camps, and hundreds more were threatened with the same fate. However, the Germans were deathly afraid of typhus, and since Poland had experienced an outbreak decades before, Polish doctors were required to certify that the workers were typhus-free. Also, they were obligated to send blood samples to German laboratories for Weil-Felix testing to confirm the certification.

The two physicians decided to concoct a bogus epidemic of typhus. They injected anyone who came to them with *Proteus OX19* cells, explaining that the injection was a "serum therapy" for the patient's symptoms. When blood samples were later sent to Germany, the Weil-Felix test proved positive and the Germans became alarmed at the "typhus" epidemic. Eventually 12 villages in the district were declared epidemic zones, and the residents were not conscripted.

The doctors, Eugene S. Lazowski and Stanislaw Matulewicz, told their story in 1977. Through guile and imagination, their private immunological war had spared hundreds, perhaps thousands, of Polish people the atrocities of war. Their counterfeit epidemic had been a success.

The agent of endemic typhus is *Rickettsia typhi.* Both rodent and flea may harbor it for weeks without displaying any effects, but when an infected flea feeds in the human skin, it deposits the organism into the wound. Endemic typhus is usually characterized by a mild fever, persistent headache, and a maculopapular rash. Often the recovery is spontaneous, without the need of drug therapy. However, lice may transport the rickettsiae to other individuals and initiate an epidemic.

In the Southwest, endemic typhus is known as **Mexican typhus,** the disease from which Ricketts died. Since first described in 1570, it has also been called **tabardillo,** from *tabardo,* meaning "colored cloak," a reference to the mantlelike rash that covers the body.

tab'ar-dēl'yo

OTHER RICKETTSIAL DISEASES

Several other rickettsial diseases have microbiological significance because of their sporadic occurrence. These diseases are transmitted to humans by arthropod vectors, and most are characterized by fever and rash. The mortality rates are generally low.

Scrub typhus is so named because it occurs in scrubland, where the soil is sandy or marshy and vegetation is poor. *Trombicula,* the **mite** that transmits the disease, lives in areas such as these. Scrub typhus is also called **tsutsugamushi,** from the Japanese words *tsutsuga* for "disease" and *mushi* for "mite." The causative agent, *Rickettsia tsutsugamushi,* enters the skin during mite infestations and soon causes fever and a rash, together with other typhuslike symptoms. Outbreaks may be significant, as evidenced by the 7000 U.S. servicemen affected in the Pacific during World War II.

trom-bik'u-lah
soot'soo-gah-moosh'e

Rickettsialpox was first recognized in 1946 in an apartment complex in New York City. Investigators traced the disease to **mites** in the fur of local mice, and named the disease rickettsialpox because the skin rash was similar to that of chickenpox. Rickettsialpox is now considered a benign disease. It is caused by *Rickettsia akari* (*acari* is Greek for "mite"). Fever and rash are typical symptoms, and fatalities are rare.

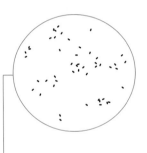

Rickettsia akari

Except for the great influenza pandemic of 1918 to 1919 (Chapter 12), **trench fever** was the most widespread disease encountered during World War I. An estimated 1 million soldiers are thought to have been infected. The disease is caused by *Rochalimaea quintana,* one of the few rickettsiae cultivated outside of living cells. Transmission takes place by head and body **lice** (MicroFocus 9.10). Symptoms include a maculopapular rash and a fever occurring at irregular intervals. Trench fever is prevalent where lice abound, and trench warfare provided a near-ideal setting. The disease is sometimes called **His-Werner disease** for the two investigators who studied it in the early 1900s.

ro'kah-li-me'ah

In various regions of the world, *Rickettsia conorii* causes a series of **tickborne fevers.** These diseases are known as boutonneuse fever, Marseilles fever, Nigerian typhus, and South African tick bite fever. All appear to be mild versions of Rocky Mountain spotted fever, and all are accompanied by a fever and rash. In addition, a **black spot** (*la tache noire*) develops where the tick has fed in the skin. Wild rodents harbor the disease in nature.

boo-ton-ez'

tahsh nwahr

In textbooks from the early 1900s, an illness called **Brill-Zinsser disease** was described as a mild form of typhus. The high fever was a distinguishing characteristic, and it was recognized that if a patient was infested with **lice,** an epidemic of typhus might ensue. Today microbiologists believe that Brill-Zinsser disease is a recurrence of an earlier case of typhus in which *Rickettsia prowazekii* lay dormant in the patient for many years.

er-lik'e-o'sis

mon-o-sit'ik
er-lik'e-ah chaf-e-en'sis
gran-u-lo-sit'ik

fag'o-si-to-phil'ah

Ehrlichiosis, the final disease we shall consider, was first described in humans in 1986. Formerly believed to be confined to dogs, ehrlichiosis has been recognized in two forms in the United States: **human monocytic ehrlichiosis (HME),** which is caused by the rickettsia *Ehrlichia chaffeensis* (because the first case was observed at Fort Chaffee, Arkansas); and **human granulocytic ehrlichiosis (HGE).** The current thinking is that ehrlichiosis is identical with HME, and that HGE is a separate disease. Indeed, in 1996 the causative agent of HGE was first identified (FIGURE 9.16). It was found to be almost identical to *Ehrlichia phago-cytophila* and to *Ehrlichia equi*, which causes ehrlichiosis in horses. As of this writing, the new organism has not been named.

Patients with either ehrlichiosis (HME) or HGE suffer from headache, malaise, and fever, with some liver disease and, infrequently, a maculopapular rash. Ehrlichiosis (HME) is transmitted by the **Lone Star tick** (prevalent in the South), while HGE is transmitted by the **dog tick** and the **deer tick**, the same one that transmits Lyme disease (prevalent in the Northeast). Indeed, both HGE and HME are quite

TABLE 9.2

A Summary of Arthropodborne Bacterial Diseases

DISEASE	CAUSATIVE AGENT	DESCRIPTION OF AGENT	ORGANS AFFECTED	CHARACTERISTIC SIGNS
Bubonic plague	*Yersinia pestis*	Gram-negative bipolar staining rod	Lymph nodes Blood Lungs	Buboes Pneumonia Septicemia
Tularemia	*Francisella tularensis*	Gram-negative bipolar staining rod	Eyes Skin Blood	Eye lesion Skin ulcer Pneumonia
Lyme disease	*Borrelia burgdorferi*	Spirochete	Skin Joints Heart	Erythema chronicum migrans Arthritis
Relapsing fever	*Borrelia recurrentis*	Spirochete	Blood Liver	Fever Jaundice
Rocky Mountain spotted fever	*Rickettsia rickettsii*	Rickettsia	Blood Skin	Fever Rash
Epidemic typhus	*Rickettsia prowazekii*	Rickettsia Skin	Blood Rash	Fever
Endemic typhus	*Rickettsia typhi*	Rickettsia	Blood Skin	Fever Rash
Scrub typhus	*Rickettsia tsutsugamushi*	Rickettsia	Blood Skin	Fever Rash
Rickettsialpox	*Rickettsia akari*	Rickettsia	Blood Skin	Fever Rash
Trench fever	*Rochalimaea quintana*	Rickettsia	Blood Skin	Fever Rash
Tickborne fevers	*Rickettsia conorii*	Rickettsia	Blood Skin	Fever Rash
Ehrlichiosis (HME) (HGE)	*Ehrlichia chaffeensis* *E. equi* (?)	Rickettsia	Blood	Fever

similar to Lyme disease, except that the symptoms come on faster in HGE and HME, they clear more quickly, and the rash is infrequent. HME affects the body's monocytes (hence "monocytic"), while HGE affects the neutrophils (a type of granulocyte, hence "granulocytic"). Thus, a lowering of the white blood cell count (leukopenia) occurs in both diseases. A notable outbreak of HGE affected 68 patients in New York City in 1994.

The arthropodborne diseases covered in this chapter are summarized in TABLE 9.2.

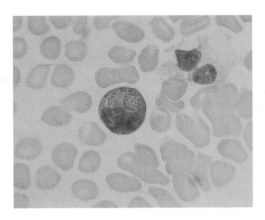

FIGURE 9.16

An *Ehrlichia* Species

The species of *Ehrlichia* that causes human granulocytic ehrlichiosis (HGE). This tick-borne organism is seen multiplying within a cell culture of human white blood cells called granulocytes. The granulocytes are neutrophils.

VECTOR	TOXIN INVOLVED	TREATMENT ADMINISTERED	IMMUNIZATION AVAILABLE	COMMENT
Rat flea	Yes	Tetracycline Streptomycin	Killed bacteria for high risk	Great historic significance Septicemic and pneumonic forms Rodents infected
Flea Tick	Yes	Tetracycline Streptomycin	None	Resembles many other diseases Many modes of transmission No epidemics
Tick	Not established	Penicillin Tetracycline	Genetically engineered lipoprotein	Recognized since 1975 Most prevalent tickborne disease Three possible stages
Louse	Not established	Tetracycline	None	Relapses common Rose spots develop on skin
Tick	Not established	Tetracycline	Killed bacteria for high risk	Most common rickettsial disease Rash first on extremities
Louse	Not established	Tetracycline	None	High mortality rate Rash first on body trunk
Flea	Not established	Tetracycline	None	Mild typhuslike disease Prevalent in rodents
Mite	Not established	Tetracycline	None	Occurs in scrubland Prevalent in Far East
Mite	Not established	Tetracycline	None	Rare disease Resembles chickenpox
Louse	Not established	Tetracycline	None	Common in World War I Cultivation in artificial medium
Tick	Not established	Tetracycline	None	Different forms
Tick	Not established	Tetracycline	None	Recognized since 1986

MicroFocus 9.10

A LOUSY PROBLEM

Because head lice transmit a number of infectious diseases, public health officers are somewhat concerned when outbreaks of these arthropods occur in children. Therefore, they were interested when a number of parents in Virginia reported lice in the hair of their children.

Subsequent investigation revealed that the outbreak began shortly after the children had their class pictures taken. Their teacher, a fastidious person, wanted to be sure the children looked their best, so she combed each one's hair with the same comb—a comb that was contaminated with lice.

Note to the Student

Several diseases discussed in this chapter have occurred in broad-scale epidemics in past centuries and have accounted for widespread death. Bubonic plague, relapsing fever, and epidemic typhus are three examples. In today's world, microbiologists can quell the spread of these diseases by controlling arthropod populations.

But there is one disease in this chapter that may be spread by airborne spores. In the human body, its effects are so devastating that whole populations may be wiped out. The disease is anthrax. Its causative agent, *Bacillus anthracis,* is a potent weapon in biological warfare.

Consider how easily biological warfare can be carried on with *B. anthracis* spores. Spores released into the atmosphere may settle onto food and into water for human consumption. They may also be inhaled into the lungs or enter the blood through an abrasion in the skin. The terrifying symptoms of anthrax quickly follow any of these exposures.

Can warfare of this type come to pass? Apparently so, because for many years, several countries have explored its possibilities. To preclude biological warfare, over 100 nations signed an international treaty in 1972 banning the development of biological weapons. Under one of its terms, all stockpiles of anthrax spores were to be destroyed, and all such weapons research was to cease. However, in 1979, observers reported an epidemic of anthrax in the city of Sverdlovsk in the Siberian region of Russia. The epidemic came only a few days after an explosion at a nearby military installation. Soviet officials denied that the two events were related but failed to provide a satisfactory explanation to critics. Then, in 1993, after the breakup of the Soviet Union, examination of autopsy notes and pathological specimens from victims confirmed that lesions in the lungs were characteristic of anthrax.

Many scientists believe that the threat of biological warfare still looms large, and the concern for the enemy's use of bacteriological weapons surfaced during the Persian Gulf War of 1992 (especially when stocks of biological weapons were discovered in 1995). The possibilities of genetically engineered biological weapons have added a new dimension to the issue and compounded the threat.

Summary

The common themes underlying this chapter are soil and arthropods and their ability to transmit bacterial disease. Soil is the source of sporeforming bacilli that cause anthrax, tetanus, and gas gangrene, and it can also harbor the organisms of leptospirosis and melioidosis. For all these diseases, there is some level of blood involvement. Anthrax is accompanied by severe blood hemorrhaging, and the toxins of tetanus and gas gangrene are transmitted by the blood. In a similar manner, the agent of leptospirosis uses the blood to distribute itself throughout the body.

Arthropods are the important modes of transmission for plague, tularemia, Lyme disease, Rocky Mountain spotted fever, typhus, and a number of other diseases, many due to rickettsiae. Since arthropods inject bacteria into the blood or deposit them into a wound, the involvement of blood is substantial. In plague, there is intense septicemia; tularemia is characterized by malaise and mild fever; and Lyme disease is accompanied by a red skin rash, with fever and headaches that reflect blood involvement. The pattern of skin rash and fever continues for the rickettsial diseases, as the blood remains the focus of infection.

Because of the involvement of soil and/or arthropods, the diseases in this chapter are more difficult to transmit than airborne, foodborne, or waterborne diseases. Soilborne diseases do not occur in epidemics, and incidence rates tend to be low. Moreover, arthropodborne diseases require that the tick, louse, flea, mite, or other arthropod be present in the environment for epidemics to occur. When the arthropod is available, however, epidemics can be substantial, as the descriptions of plague, Lyme disease, Rocky Mountain spotted fever, and epidemic typhus in this chapter illustrate.

Questions for Thought and Discussion

1. In February 1980, a patient was admitted to a Texas hospital complaining of fever, headache, and chills. He also had greatly enlarged lymph nodes in the left armpit. A sample of blood was taken and Gram stained, whereupon Gram-positive diplococci were observed. The patient was treated with cefoxitin, a drug for Gram-positive organisms, but soon thereafter he died. On autopsy, *Yersinia pestis* was found in his blood and tissues. Why was this organism mistakenly thought to be diplococci, and what error was made in the laboratory? Why were the symptoms of plague missed?

2. There is a town outside of London known as Gravesend. The town apparently acquired its name during the 1660s in connection with a great medical upheaval. What was the name of that upheaval, and how do you suppose the name came about?

3. Although the tetanus toxin is second in potency to the toxin of botulism, many physicians consider tetanus to be a more serious threat than botulism. Would you agree? Why?

4. Some estimates place epidemic typhus among the all-time killers of humans; one listing even has it in third place behind malaria and plague. In 1997, during a civil war, an outbreak of epidemic typhus occurred in the African country of Burundi. The outbreak was estimated to be the worst since World War II. What conditions may have led to this epidemic?

5. On February 13, 1976, a newspaper article requested purchasers of a certain brand of Pakistani wool yarn to check with their local health departments because the wool was thought to be contaminated with anthrax spores. The article read as follows: "Spores of anthrax, which is a livestock disease, have been found on the yarn. The disease affects people as a skin ailment and is usually not fatal." Does the article minimize a potential medical emergency? If yes, write a letter to the editor in reply. If not, explain why not.

6. In 1993, a 57-year-old man died of tetanus in a Kansas hospital. His experience had begun on August 14 with a puncture wound to the foot and ended on September 16. Family members reported that the man had never received a vaccination with tetanus toxoid. Hospital costs for his therapy totaled $145,329. The administration of a dose of tetanus vaccine, by comparison, costs $3.30. Setting aside the value of a human life for the moment, what does this disparity of costs tell you?

7. At various times, local governments are inclined to curtail deer hunting. How might this lead to an increase in the incidence of Lyme disease?

8. In 1982, endemic typhus was observed in five members of a Texas household. On investigation, epidemiologists learned that family members had heard rodents in the attic, and two weeks previously they had used rat poison on the premises. Investigators concluded that both the rodents and the rat poison were related to the outbreak. Why?

9. Leptospirosis has been contracted by individuals working in such diverse locales as subway tunnels, gold mines, rice paddies, and sewage-treatment plants. What precautions might be taken by such workers to protect themselves against the disease?

10. A young woman was hospitalized with excruciating headache, fever, chills, nausea, muscle pains in her back and legs, and a sore throat. Laboratory tests ruled out meningitis, pneumonia, mononucleosis, toxic shock syndrome, and other diseases. On the third day of her hospital stay, a faint pink rash appeared on her arms and ankles. By the next day, the rash had become darker red and began moving from her hands and feet to her arms and legs. Can you guess what the diagnosis eventually was?

11. In Chapter 9 of the Bible, in the Book of Exodus, the sixth plague of Egypt is described in this way: "Then the Lord said to Moses and Aaron, 'Take a double handful of soot from a furnace, and in the presence of Pharaoh, let Moses scatter it toward the sky. It will then turn into a fine dust over the whole land of Egypt and cause festering boils on man and cattle throughout the land.'" Which disease in this chapter is probably being described?

12. During the Civil War, some 92,000 soldiers died of battle wounds but 190,000 died of battle-related diseases. Which diseases in this chapter probably contributed to the enormous mortality rate? What conditions encouraged each disease cited?

13. In autumn, it is customary for homeowners in certain communities to pile leaves at the curbside for pickup. How might this practice increase the incidence of tularemia, Lyme disease, and Rocky Mountain spotted fever in the community?

14. At various times in past centuries, it was believed that cats were the medium through which witches spoke. Fearing cats, people would try to eliminate these animals from their neighborhood. Bubonic plague would occasionally break out shortly thereafter. Why?

15. Centuries ago, the habit of shaving one's head and wearing a wig probably originated in part as an attempt to reduce lice infestations in the hair. Why would this practice also reduce the possibilities of certain diseases? Which diseases?

16. An article in *Health* magazine (1996) opens with the following statement: "As pierce-o-mania sweeps the nation, it's bringing more ugly infections along with it." What are some possible infections that ear, nose, tongue, and other body piercings can lead to?

17. People from various government and civilian agencies continue to be concerned about a terrorist attack using anthrax spores. In various scenarios, try to paint a picture of how such an attack might happen. Then, using your knowledge of microbiology, present your vision of how agencies might deal with such an attack.

http://microbiology.jbpub.com

The site features **eLearning,** an on-line review area that provides quizzes and other tools to help you study for your class. You can also follow useful links for in-depth information, read more MicroFocus stories, or just find out the latest microbiology news.

Review

The bacterial diseases transmitted by soil and arthropods are the main focus of this chapter. To test your understanding of the chapter contents, match the statement on the left with the disease on the right by placing the correct letter in the available space. A letter may be used once, more than once, or not at all. Appendix D contains the answers.

_____ 1. Accompanied by erythema chronicum migrans.

_____ 2. Transmitted by lice; caused by *R. prowazekii*.

_____ 3. Affects neutrophils in the body; transmitted by ticks.

_____ 4. May be transmitted by contact with dogs.

_____ 5. Caused by a sporeforming rod that produces hemolysis and lecithinase.

_____ 6. Tickborne disease; caused by *R. rickettsii*.

_____ 7. Blood hemorrhaging in large animals such as cattle, sheep, and goats.

_____ 8. Also known as tabardillo and Mexican typhus.

_____ 9. Treated with antitoxins; caused by an anaerobic sporeformer.

_____ 10. Caused by *Borrelia burgdorferi*; transmitted by a tick.

_____ 11. Bubonic, septicemic, and pneumonic stages.

_____ 12. Maculopapular rash beginning on extremities and progressing to body trunk.

_____ 13. Caused by a spirochete that infects kidney tissues in pets and humans.

_____ 14. Occurs in small game animals, especially rabbits.

_____ 15. Transmitted by mites; also known as scrub typhus.

_____ 16. Caused by a Gram-negative rod with bipolar staining; transmitted by rat flea.

_____ 17. Long-range complications include arthritis in large joints.

_____ 18. Up to ten attacks of substantial fever, joint pains, and skin spots; *Borrelia* involved.

_____ 19. Immunization rendered by the DTaP vaccine.

_____ 20. Pulmonary, intestinal, and skin forms possible; due to a *Bacillus* species.

_____ 21. A typical zoonosis; caused by a spiral bacterium.

_____ 22. Caused by a *Francisella* species; has multiple modes of transmission.

_____ 23. Epidemics where sanitation is poor; louseborne rickettsial disease.

_____ 24. Sustained and uncontrolled contractions of the body's muscles.

_____ 25. Most commonly reported tickborne disease in the United States.

A. Plague

B. Epidemic typhus

C. Anthrax

D. Melioidosis

E. Relapsing fever

F. Tularemia

G. Lyme disease

H. Rickettsialpox

I. Tsutsugamushi

J. Endemic typhus

K. Ehrlichiosis

L. Leptospirosis

M. Tetanus

N. Rocky Mountain spotted fever

O. Gas gangrene

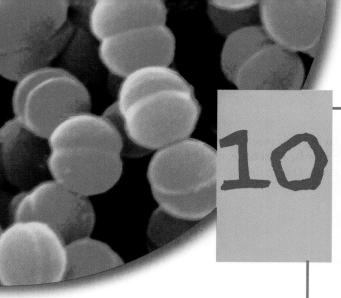

10 Sexually Transmitted, Contact, and Miscellaneous Bacterial Diseases

I just froze. Then I closed the door, and went in my room and cried.

—A soft-spoken, 38 year old woman recalling her reaction when she was visited by a health official and told she had syphilis

THE VICTORIAN ERA OF THE 1800s was notorious for its prudish attitude toward sex. Bulls were called "he-cows," and the legs of a piano were modestly covered with pantaloons. Women did not disrobe when visiting a physician; instead, they pointed to a chart to show where they hurt. An 1863 etiquette book stipulated that the works of male and female authors should be separated on bookshelves unless the authors were married. Even the biology books of that era mirrored the taboo on sex by carefully avoiding mention of the human reproductive system. It was as if the human species did not provide for the next generation.

Our era, by contrast, has been marked by broad sexual freedom, but it has also seen an alarming rise in diseases of the reproductive organs. Formerly, these diseases were called venereal diseases (VDs) from Venus, the Roman goddess of love. However, health departments now call them sexually transmitted diseases (STDs), a name that indicates the mode of transmission and avoids the "love" connotation. The STDs discussed in this chapter are of bacterial origin and include familiar names such as syphilis and gonorrhea, as well as emerging problems such as chlamydia. To underscore the seriousness of the STD problem, the Centers for Disease Control and Prevention (CDC) estimates that for each day in 1999, over 40,000 Americans contracted a sexually transmitted disease.

The increase in sexually transmitted diseases is but one example of how changing social patterns can affect the incidence of disease. Several other examples are evident in the diseases discussed in this chapter. For instance, the incidence of leprosy in the United States has risen because in the last decades, immigrant groups have brought the disease with them. Toxic shock syndrome was first recognized widely in 1980 when a new brand of high-absorbency tampon appeared on the commercial market. Finally, the mortality rate from nocardiosis rose when this disease was found to complicate cases of acquired immune deficiency syndrome (AIDS).

10.1

Sexually Transmitted Diseases

The sexually transmitted diseases of bacterial origin belong to a broad category of diseases that are transmitted by contact. The contact in this case is with the reproductive organs. This type of person-to-person transmission is necessary for bacterial survival because the bacteria usually cannot remain alive outside the body tissues. The list of sexually transmitted diseases is diverse, as the following examples will demonstrate. Other STDs are discussed in Chapters 13, 14, and 15.

SYPHILIS

Over the centuries, Europeans have had to contend with four pox diseases: chickenpox, cowpox, smallpox, and the Great Pox, a disease now known as syphilis. The first European epidemic was recorded in the late 1400s, shortly after the conquest of Naples by the French army (MicroFocus 10.1). For decades the disease had various names, but by the 1700s, it had come to be called syphilis.

Syphilis is caused by *Treponema pallidum*, literally the "pale spirochete." This spiral bacterium moves by means of axial filaments and spreads by human-to-human contact, usually during sexual intercourse. It penetrates the skin surface through the mucous membranes or via a wound, abrasion, or hair follicle. Then it causes a disease that progresses in three stages, described below. The variety of clinical symptoms that accompany the stages, and their similarity to other diseases, have led some physicians to call syphilis the "great imitator."

trep'o-ne'mah

The incubation period for syphilis varies greatly, but it averages about 3 weeks. **Primary syphilis** is the first stage to appear. This stage is characterized by the **chancre**, a painless circular, purplish ulcer with a raised margin and hard edges described as being like cartilage (FIGURE 10.1a). The chancre develops at the site of entry of the spirochetes, often the genital organs. However, any area of the skin may be affected, including the pharynx, rectum, or lips. (Centuries ago, people discovered that kissing could transmit syphilis, and even though they did not know what was causing the dreaded disease, they began to substitute hand-shaking and gentle kisses on the cheek for kissing on the lips.) The chancre teems with spirochetes. It persists for 2 to 6 weeks, and then it disappears spontaneously.

shang'ker

Pharynx:
the throat region.

Several weeks later, the patient experiences **secondary syphilis**. Symptoms include fever and a constitutional flulike illness, as well as swollen lymph nodes reminiscent of infectious mononucleosis. The skin rash that appears may be mistaken for measles, rubella, or chickenpox (FIGURE 10.1b). Loss of the eyebrows often occurs, and a patchy loss of hair results in "moth-eaten" areas commonly seen on the head. Involvement of the liver may lead to jaundice and suspicion of hepatitis. In untreated patients, the symptoms last several weeks, and death may result. Most patients

Infectious mononucleosis:
a viral disease accompanied by swollen lymph nodes, sore throat, and mild fever.

Jaundice:
yellow tinting of the eyes and skin due to seepage of bile into the bloodstream.

MicroFocus 10.1

THE ORIGIN OF A DISEASE

Among the more intriguing questions in medical history are how and why syphilis suddenly emerged in Europe in the late 1400s. Writers of that period tell of an awesome new disease that swept over Europe and on to India, China, and Japan. But where did the disease come from?

One oft-told story is that syphilis existed in the New World, and that members of Columbus' crew acquired it during stopovers in the Caribbean islands. Columbus returned to Palos in northern Italy in 1493, and some of his crew reportedly joined the army of Charles VII of France. In 1494, Charles' army attacked Naples in Italy, but mounting losses from the strange new sickness forced him to withdraw. His army of 30,000 French, German, Swiss, English, Polish, Spanish, and Hungarian troops returned to their native lands, and apparently brought the disease home with them.

A second theory holds that the disease first came to Spain and Portugal with slaves imported from Africa in the

mid-1400s. An African disease called yaws is very similar to syphilis in causative organism, transmission, and stages of development. Certain historians believe that some unknown factor caused yaws to flare up in the form of syphilis in the late 1400s. They speculate that the army of Charles VII provided a highly susceptible population of diverse men who spread the disease wherever they traveled. Indeed, recent studies of Native American burial grounds show no traces of syphilis before the arrival of Columbus. By contrast, remains of those dying after Columbus' arrival show signs that the disease was present in the community.

With its devastating effects, syphilis inspired a variety of epithets. The Italians called it the French disease (*morbus Gallicus*), while the French called it the Italian disease (*la maladie Italienne*); to the Japanese, it was the Chinese disease. The English impartially termed it the Great Pox. The name "syphilis" derives from the works of Girolamo Fracostoro, a sixteenth-century poet-scientist of

Verona. In 1530, Fracostoro wrote a long poem about a shepherd named Syphilus who momentarily left his pastoral responsibilities to commit a sexual indiscretion. The angered gods punished him with the horrible sores of the disease. In a later work on disease transmission, Fracostoro suggested that the illness be called syphilis after the mythical shepherd.

Syphilis was as international in effect as in name, and proved to be no respector of rank. Henry VIII of England, Napoleon of France, and Peter the Great of Russia all contracted the disease. Poets such as Keats, musicians such as Beethoven, and artists such as Gauguin also succumbed, as did millions of common people. For many generations, epidemics of syphilis swept back and forth across the world. As Lord Byron wrote in one of his poems:

The smallpox has gone out of late;
Perhaps it may be follow'd by the
Great.

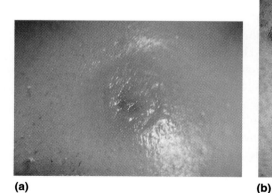 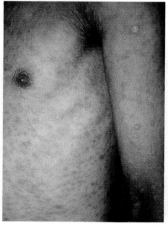 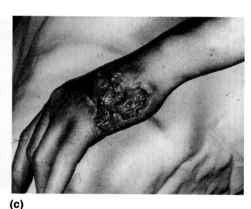

(a)   (b)   (c)

FIGURE 10.1

The Stages of Syphilis

Views of the skin lesion in the three stages of syphilis. (a) The chancre of primary syphilis as it occurs on the body surface. The chancre is circular with raised margins and is usually painless. It occurs where penetration of syphilis spirochetes has taken place. (b) The flat, wartlike lesions characteristic of secondary syphilis. (c) The gumma that forms in tertiary syphilis. Note the granular, diffuse nature of this lesion compared with the primary chancre shown in (a).

recover, but they bear pitted scars from the lesions and remain "pockmarked." These individuals now enter a latent stage, during which they continue to be infectious.

About one-third of untreated patients eventually develop **tertiary syphilis**. This stage occurs in many forms, but most commonly it involves the skin, cardiovascular system, and nervous system. The hallmark of tertiary syphilis is the **gumma**, a soft, gummy granular lesion (FIGURE 10.1c). In the cardiovascular system, gummas weaken the major blood vessels, causing them to bulge and burst. In the spinal cord and meninges, gummas lead to degeneration of the tissues and paralysis. In the brain, they alter the patient's personality and judgment and cause insanity so intense that for many generations, people with tertiary syphilis were confined to mental institutions. It is conceivable that our ancestors failed to equate the chancre of primary syphilis with the horrible symptoms of tertiary syphilis because the stages were so distantly separated in time.

gum'ah

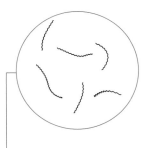

Treponema pallidum

Syphilis is a serious problem in pregnant women because the spirochetes penetrate the placental barrier after the fourth month of pregnancy, causing **congenital syphilis** in the fetus. Syphilitic skin lesions and open sores may be apparent in the newborn, or symptoms may develop weeks after birth. Affected children often suffer poor bone formation, meningitis, or **Hutchinson's triad**, a combination of deafness, impaired vision, and notched, peg-shaped teeth.

The cornerstone of syphilis control is the identification and treatment of the sexual contacts of patients. Penicillin is the drug of choice for the primary, secondary, and latent stages of the disease, but antibiotics are ineffective in tertiary syphilis because gummas appear to be an immunological response to the spirochetes. *T. pallidum* multiplies very slowly in the tissues, partly because of its 33-hour generation time. This factor encourages successful therapy.

Generation time: the time period that elapses between divisions in bacteria.

Since *T. pallidum* (FIGURE 10.2) was first observed in 1905 by Fritz R. Schaudinn and P. Erich Hoffman, exhaustive attempts have been made to cultivate it on laboratory media, but none have been successful. Diagnosis in the primary stage therefore depends on the observation of spirochetes from the chancre using the dark-field microscope. As the disease progresses, a number of tests to detect syphilis antibodies become useful, including the rapid plasma reagin test, the

Dark-field microscope: an instrument that displays live, unstained bacteria on a dark background.

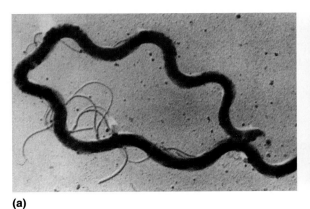

(a)

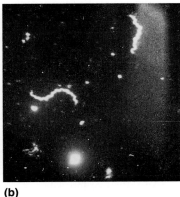

(b)

FIGURE 10.2

Treponema pallidum

Two views of *Treponema pallidum*, the agent of syphilis. (a) A scanning electron micrograph taken at 13,500 power magnification. The thin threads are axial filaments extending along the periphery of the spirochete. (b) A dark-field microscope view of the spirochetes seen in a sample taken from the chancre of a patient.

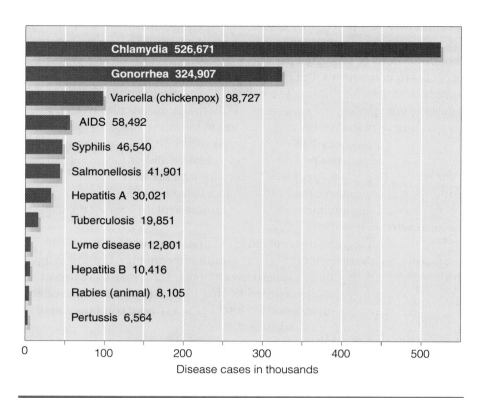

Disease	Cases
Chlamydia	526,671
Gonorrhea	324,907
Varicella (chickenpox)	98,727
AIDS	58,492
Syphilis	46,540
Salmonellosis	41,901
Hepatitis A	30,021
Tuberculosis	19,851
Lyme disease	12,801
Hepatitis B	10,416
Rabies (animal)	8,105
Pertussis	6,564

Disease cases in thousands

FIGURE 10.3

Reported Cases of Microbial Diseases in the United States, 1997

For the year, chlamydia was considerably more prevalent than the next most common reportable disease, gonorrhea. Chickenpox was the third most common.

Venereal Disease Research Laboratory (VDRL) test, and others (Chapter 19). The complement-fixation test devised by Wassermann is rarely used anymore.

Syphilis is currently among the most reported microbial diseases in the United States (FIGURE 10.3). Statistics indicate that about 45,000 people are afflicted with the disease annually, of whom about 9000 are in the primary or secondary stage. Taken alone, these figures suggest the magnitude of the syphilis epidemic, but some public health microbiologists believe that for every case reported, as many as nine cases go unreported.

GONORRHEA

Gonorrhea is the second most frequently reported microbial disease in the United States, after chlamydia (Figure 10.3). During the 1960s, the incidence of gonorrhea rose dramatically; since 1975, several hundred thousand cases have been reported annually. Epidemiologists suggest that 3 to 4 million cases go undetected or unreported each year. Despite effective antibiotic therapy and national attempts at close surveillance, gonorrhea remains an epidemic.

The agent of gonorrhea is *Neisseria gonorrhoeae*, a small Gram-negative diplococcus named for Albert L. S. Neisser, who isolated it in 1879. The organism, commonly known as the **gonococcus**, has a characteristic double-bean shape exhibited by neisseriae (FIGURE 10.4). *N. gonorrhoeae* is a very fragile organism susceptible to

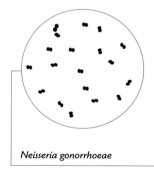

Neisseria gonorrhoeae

ni-se're-ah gon'o-re'a

most antiseptics and disinfectants. It survives only a brief period outside the body and is rarely contracted from a dry surface such as a toilet seat. The great majority of cases of gonorrhea are therefore transmitted in person-to-person contact during sexual intercourse. (Gonorrhea is sometimes called "the clap," from the French *clappoir* for "brothel.")

The incubation period for gonorrhea ranges from 2 to 6 days. In females, the gonococci invade the epithelial surfaces of the cervix and the urethra. The cervix may be reddened, and a discharge may be expressed by pressure against the pubic area. Patients often report abdominal pain and a burning sensation on urination, and the normal menstrual cycle may be interrupted.

In some females, gonorrhea also spreads to the Fallopian tubes, which extend from the uterus to the ovaries. As these thin passageways become riddled with pouches and adhesions, the passage of egg cells becomes difficult. Complete blockage, or **salpingitis**, may take place. A condition of the pelvic organs such as this is called **pelvic inflammatory disease (PID)**. Sterility may result from scar tissue remaining after the disease has been treated, or a woman may experience an ectopic pregnancy. It should be noted that symptoms are not universally observed in females, and that an estimated 50 percent of affected women exhibit no symptoms. Such asymptomatic women may spread the disease unknowingly.

In males, gonorrhea occurs primarily in the urethra, the tube from the bladder that passes through the penis to the exterior. Onset usually is accompanied by a tingling sensation in the penis, followed in a few days by pain when urinating. There is also a thin, watery discharge at first, and later a more obvious whitened, thick fluid that resembles semen. Frequent urination and an urge to urinate develop as the disease spreads further into the urethra. The lymph nodes of the groin may also swell, and sharp pain may be felt in the testicles. Unchecked infection of the epididymis may lead to sterility. Symptoms tend to be more acute in males than in females, and males thus tend to seek diagnosis and treatment more readily.

Gonorrhea does not restrict itself to the urogenital organs. **Gonococcal pharyngitis**, for example, may develop in the pharynx if bacteria are transmitted by

Cervix:
the opening to the uterus.

Urethra:
the tube that leads from the bladder to the exterior.

sal'pin-ji'tis
Salpingitis:
blockage of the Fallopian tubes.

Ectopic pregnancy:
a pregnancy taking place in the Fallopian tube.

Epididymis:
the thin tube leading from the testicle.

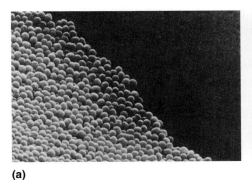 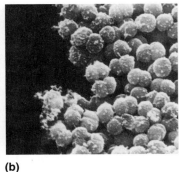 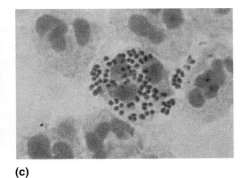

(a) **(b)** **(c)**

FIGURE 10.4

Neisseria gonorrhoeae

Three views of *Neisseria gonorrhoeae*, the agent of gonorrhea. (a) A scanning electron micrograph of the edge of a colony of *Neisseria gonorrhoeae* (×5400). (b) An enlarged view of the cocci (×10,000). Note the typical pairing of the cells and the dustlike granules on the cell surfaces. The significance of these granules is not clear. (c) A stained smear of discharge from the male urethra showing the diplococci of gonorrhea. Some of the diplococci have been taken into the cytoplasm of phagocytes (×1000).

Keratitis:
a disease of the cornea of
the eye.

of-thal'me-ah
Ophthalmia:
severe inflammation of the eyes.

cef-tri-ax'ōn
cef-ix'ēm

oral-genital contact; patients complain of sore throat or difficulty in swallowing. Infection of the rectum, or **gonococcal proctitis**, is also observed, especially in individuals performing anal intercourse. Transmission to the eyes may occur by fingertips or towels, and **keratitis** may develop.

Gonorrhea is particularly dangerous to infants born to infected women. The infant may contract gonococci during passage through the birth canal and develop a disease of the eyes called **gonococcal ophthalmia**. To preclude the blindness that may ensue, most states have laws requiring that the eyes of newborns be treated with drops of 1 percent silver nitrate or antibiotics such as erythromycin or tetracycline.

Traditionally, gonorrhea has been treated with a single large dose of penicillin. In 1976, however, a strain of *N. gonorrhoeae* appeared that resists the drug. In succeeding years, therapy shifted to spectinomycin and then to tetracycline. The latter is still recommended together with ceftriaxone and cefixime. An attack of gonorrhea does not immunize one to future attacks, apparently because the immune system does not respond strongly enough to the first attack. No vaccine is available at this writing, but an antipili vaccine is in the experimental stage.

Gonorrhea can be detected by observing Gram-negative diplococci in the discharge from the urogenital tract, as well as in colonies from swab samples cultivated on Thayer-Martin medium. For an immunological test, physicians take a swab sample and dip the swab into an antibody solution. An immunoassay reaction takes place (Chapter 19), and within a few hours, a color reaction indicates the presence or absence of gonococci. The test allows doctors to detect gonorrhea early so that treatment can start immediately. A test to detect the DNA of gonococci is also available.

CHLAMYDIA

Chlamydia, also known as chlamydial urethritis, is one of several diseases collectively known as **nongonococcal urethritis**, or **NGU**. Nongonococcal urethritis is a general term for a condition in which people without gonorrhea have a demonstrable infection of the urethra usually characterized by inflammation, and often accompanied by a discharge. Evidence is convincing that over 50 percent of cases of NGU are actually chlamydia (chlamydial urethritis). Another 25 percent of cases are believed to be ureaplasmal urethritis, and the remaining 25 percent are of unknown cause.

Chlamydia is a gonorrhealike disease transmitted by sexual contact. The causative agent is ***Chlamydia trachomatis***, a species of chlamydiae. *Chlamydia trachomatis* is an exceptionally small organism, measuring about 0.25 μm in diameter. It grows only in living tissue, such as fertilized chicken eggs and tissue cultures, and it has a complex reproductive cycle, as illustrated in FIGURE 10.5. The organism appears to be a specific parasite of humans.

As of 1999, over 500,000 cases of chlamydia were occurring in Americans annually. The disease has an incubation period of about 1 to 3 weeks, and the symptoms are remarkably similar to those of gonorrhea, although somewhat milder. Females often note a slight vaginal discharge, as well as inflammation of the cervix. Burning pain is also experienced on urination, reflecting disease in the urethra. In complicated cases, the disease may spread to the Fallopian tubes, causing adhesions that block the passageways (salpingitis). Certain researchers report that **pelvic inflammatory disease (PID)** is a more likely consequence of chlamydia than of gonorrhea. (PID from gonorrhea and chlamydia is believed to affect about 50,000 women in the

klah-mid'e-ah tra-ko'mah-tis

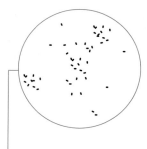

Chlamydia trachomatis

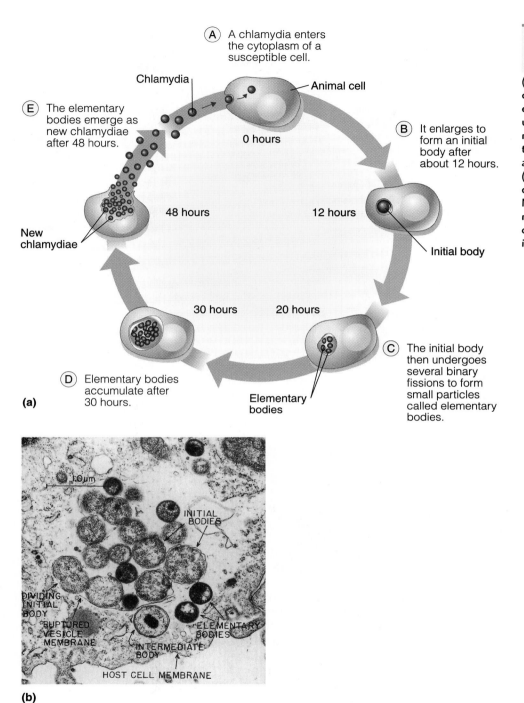

(A) A chlamydia enters the cytoplasm of a susceptible cell.

Chlamydia

Animal cell

(E) The elementary bodies emerge as new chlamydiae after 48 hours.

0 hours

(B) It enlarges to form an initial body after about 12 hours.

48 hours

12 hours

New chlamydiae

Initial body

30 hours

20 hours

(D) Elementary bodies accumulate after 30 hours.

(a)

Elementary bodies

(C) The initial body then undergoes several binary fissions to form small particles called elementary bodies.

FIGURE 10.5

The Chlamydiae

(a) The reproductive cycle of the chlamydiae. (b) An electron micrograph of an ultrathin section through a microcolony of *Chlamydia* in the cytoplasm of a tissue cell after 48 hours of incubation (×34,000). The various developmental forms are labeled. Note where the vesicular membrane has ruptured and chlamydiae are being released into the cytoplasm.

1.0 µm

INITIAL BODIES

DIVIDING INITIAL BODY

RUPTURED VESICLE MEMBRANE

ELEMENTARY BODIES

INTERMEDIATE BODY

HOST CELL MEMBRANE

(b)

United States annually.) Often, however, there are few symptoms of disease before the salpingitis manifests itself, thus adding to the danger (FIGURE 10.6).

In males, chlamydia is characterized by painful urination and a discharge that is more watery and less copious than in gonorrhea. The discharge is often observed after urinating for the first time in the morning. Tingling sensations in the penis are generally evident. Inflammation of the epididymis may result in sterility, but this complication is uncommon. Chlamydial pharyngitis and proctitis are also possible.

FIGURE **10.6**

A Case of Chlamydia

This case occurred in a 32 year old professional woman. Tragic complications of the disease resulted because she and her doctor neglected to consider that she could be suffering from a sexually transmitted disease.

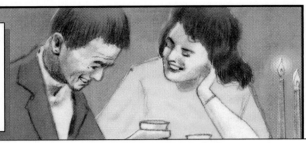

1. An educated, professional woman met a gentleman at a friend's house one evening. She was director of a New York law firm. The man was equally successful in his professional career.

2. The couple hit it off immediately. There were many evenings of quiet candlelit dinners, and soon, they became sexually intimate. Neither one used condoms or other means of protection.

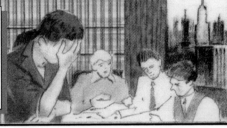
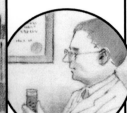

3. Three days after having intercourse, the woman began experiencing fever, vomiting, and severe abdominal pains. She immediately made an appointment to see her doctor.

4. Assuming the illness was an intestinal upset, the physician prescribed appropriate medication. The woman was actually suffering from chlamydia, but the fact that she was sexually active did not come up during the examination.

5. Feeling better, the woman continued her normal routine. But 6 months later, with no apparent warning, she collapsed on a New York City sidewalk.

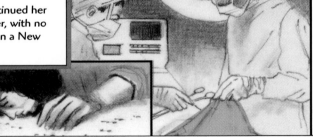

6. The woman was rushed to a local hospital, where doctors diagnosed a chlamydial infection of the peritoneum. They performed emergency surgery: her uterus and Fallopian tubes were badly scarred. She recovered, however, the scarring left her unable to have children.

TEXTBOOK CASES

Newborns may contract *C. trachomatis* from an infected mother and develop a disease of the eyes known as **chlamydial ophthalmia**. The silver nitrate used to prevent gonococcal ophthalmia is not effective as a preventative, so erythromycin therapy is required. Studies in the 1980s also revealed that **chlamydial pneumonia** may develop in newborns from an exposure to *C. trachomatis* during birth. Health officials estimate that each year, over 75,000 newborns suffer chlamydial ophthalmia and 30,000 newborns experience chlamydial pneumonia.

Chlamydia may be successfully treated with tetracycline. (If a woman is pregnant, erythromycin is substituted because tetracycline affects bone formation in newborns.) Since 1983, two relatively fast and simple laboratory tests have been available to detect *C. trachomatis*. In the first test, a physician takes a swab sample from the penis or the cervix (as in a Pap smear) and places the swab in a vial of fluid for transport to a local laboratory. A fluorescent antibody test using monoclonal antibodies (Chapter 19) is then performed, and within 30 minutes the results are available. The second test is an immunoassay test, also performed with a swab sample. It is completed in the doctor's office and is similar to the test for gonorrhea. A test to detect the DNA of *C. trachomatis* is available as well. It uses a urine sample and is said to detect as few as five cells in a sample.

Monoclonal antibodies: antibodies experimentally produced against a single type of cell or substance.

The big news of 1998 was the deciphering of the genome of *C. trachomatis*. (One researcher exclaimed: "It's like we were working in a room with the lights turned off, and now someone has turned on the lights.") The successful mapping of the 900 genes was achieved by Richard Stephens and his colleagues at the University of California at Berkeley. One interesting observation was a set of genes for synthesizing peptidoglycan. The organism was not thought to use this organic substance, but the presence of the genes indicates that it is employed somewhere in the cell, though no one is sure where. Also, the organism has genes for synthesizing ATP, another surprise since researchers believed that chlamydiae use host cell ATP for their energy needs. And the organism has about 20 genes it apparently "borrowed" from a host cell sometime during its evolution millennia ago.

UREAPLASMAL URETHRITIS

Ureaplasmal urethritis is another type of nongonococcal urethritis. It is caused by ***Ureaplasma urealyticum***, a mycoplasma, so-named because of its ability to digest urea in culture media. The organism is often referred to as a **T-mycoplasma** because "tiny" colonies of the organisms develop on laboratory media. At about 0.15 μm in size, *U. urealyticum* is one of the smallest known bacteria that cause human disease.

u-re'ah-plaz'ma
u-re'ah-lit'ī-kum

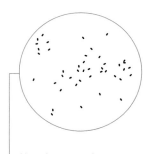

Ureaplasma urealyticum

The symptoms of ureaplasmal urethritis are similar to those of gonorrhea and chlamydia. A distinction can be made between the diseases because in ureaplasmal urethritis, the discharge is variable in quantity, and the urethral pain is usually aggravated during urination. Symptoms are often very mild. Transmission is generally by sexual contact.

Penicillin cannot be used to treat ureaplasmal urethritis because *U. urealyticum* has no cell wall. Tetracycline is currently the drug of choice. Diagnosis often depends on eliminating gonorrhea or other types of NGU as possibilities, and for this reason, cases are not often recognized.

Infertility is one consequence of ureaplasmal urethritis because low sperm counts and poor movement of sperm cells have been observed in males. Salpingitis in females has also been described. Moreover, *Ureaplasma* is capable of colonizing the placenta during pregnancy, and reports have linked it to spontaneous abortions and premature births. As previously noted, 25 percent of NGU cases may be ureaplasmal urethritis.

CHANCROID

Chancroid is a sexually transmitted disease believed to be more prevalent worldwide than gonorrhea or syphilis. The disease is endemic in many undeveloped nations, and it is common in tropical climates and where public health standards are low. Immigrants account for a large percentage of the approximately 3500 cases detected in the United States annually.

shang'kroid

he-mof'i-lus doo-krāy'e

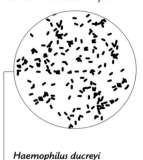

Haemophilus ducreyi

The causative agent of chancroid is *Haemophilus ducreyi*, a small Gram-negative rod named for Augusto Ducrey, who observed it in skin lesions in 1889. The earliest sign of chancroid is a tender papule surrounded by a narrow zone of redness (erythema). The papule quickly becomes pus-filled and then breaks down, leaving a shallow, saucer-shaped ulcer that bleeds easily and is painful. The ulcer has ragged edges and soft borders, a characteristic that distinguishes it from the primary lesion of syphilis. For this reason, the disease is often called **soft chancre**.

The lesions in chancroid most often occur on the penis in males and the labia or clitoris in females. Substantial swelling of the inguinal lymph nodes may be observed. However, the disease generally goes no further. The clinical picture in chancroid makes the disease recognizable, but definitive diagnosis depends on isolating *H. ducreyi* from the lesions.

The transmission of chancroid depends on contact with the lesion. Tetracycline, erythromycin, and sulfonamide drugs are useful for therapy, but the disease often disappears without treatment.

OTHER SEXUALLY TRANSMITTED DISEASES

A number of other sexually transmitted diseases merit brief attention in this chapter. None of these diseases normally presents a life-threatening situation to humans.

lim'fo-gran'u-lo'mah ven-e're-um

kla-mid'e-ah tra-ko'mah-tis

Inguinal lymph nodes: lymph nodes of the groin.

Lymphogranuloma venereum (LGV) is caused by a variant of *Chlamydia trachomatis*, slightly different from the variant that causes chlamydial urethritis. LGV is more common in males than females, and is accompanied by fever, malaise, and swelling and tenderness in the inguinal lymph nodes. Females may experience infection of the rectum (proctitis), if the chlamydiae pass from the genital opening to the nearby intestinal opening. Approximately 500 cases are detected annually in the U.S. Lymphogranuloma venereum is prevalent in Southeast Asia and Central and South America. Sexually active individuals returning from these areas may show symptoms of the disease, but treatment with tetracycline leads to rapid resolution.

kah-lim'mah-to-bak-te're-um gran-u-lo'mah-tis

Granuloma inguinale is a rare disease in Europe and North America, but it remains an endemic problem in tropical and subtropical areas of the world, such as Caribbean countries and Africa. It is caused by *Calymmatobacterium granulomatis*, a small Gram-negative encapsulated bacillus. The disease begins with a primary lesion starting as a nodule and progressing to a granular ulcer that bleeds easily. In most cases, this ulcer forms in the external genital organs but it may spread to other regions by contaminated fingers. The inguinal lymph nodes may swell, but fever and other body symptoms are usually absent, a factor that distinguishes the disease from LGV. Tissue samples reveal masses of bacteria called **Donovan bodies** within phagocytes in the lesion. The disease responds to various antibiotics, especially tetracycline.

Vaginitis is a general term for various mild infections of the vagina and sometimes the vulva. One cause of vaginitis is *Gardnerella vaginalis*, formerly called *Haemophilus vaginalis*. This small Gram-negative rod usually lives uneventfully in the vagina, but flare-ups of disease may take place and transmission by sexual contact may occur during these times. A foul-smelling discharge is the most prominent symptom, and tetracycline therapy generally provides relief.

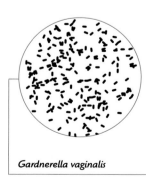

Gardnerella vaginalis

The final organism that we shall consider is *Mycoplasma hominis* (FIGURE 10.7). This mycoplasma causes **mycoplasmal urethritis**, a disease similar to ureaplasmal urethritis. In addition, the organism can colonize the placenta and cause spontaneous

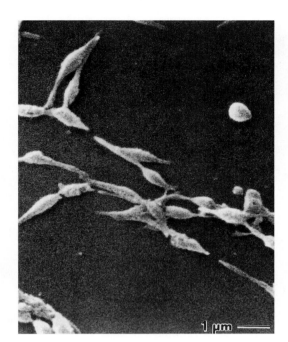

FIGURE 10.7

A Species of *Mycoplasma*

A species of *Mycoplasma* seen with the scanning electron microscope. A closely related species called *M. hominis* causes mycoplasmal urethritis, an STD that is similar to chlamydia. The pleomorphic (multishape) appearance of the organism is due to the absence of a cell wall. (Bar = 1 μm.)

abortion or premature birth. *M. hominis* is distinguished from *Ureaplasma* by its inability to digest urea, its larger colony growth on agar, and its preference for anaerobic conditions during laboratory cultivation. Tetracycline is prescribed for active cases of mycoplasmal urethritis. The disease can also be caused by ***Mycoplasma genitalium***, as reported first in 1993 by a joint American-British research team. *M. genitalium* has another distinction in microbiology—it was the second organism of any kind (the first was *Haemophilus influenzae*) to have its entire genome deciphered, an achievement completed in 1995 by Craig Venter and his associates.

TABLE 10.1 summarizes the sexually transmitted bacterial diseases.

To this point . . .

We have studied a series of sexually transmitted diseases and have noted their prevalence in modern society. Syphilis is the only disease in the group that regularly spreads to other organs of the body. The remaining diseases are largely restricted to the urogenital organs. In addition, syphilis is the only STD that is life-threatening. The other diseases generally are mild and may resolve even without treatment. However, with gonorrhea and chlamydia, there may be long-range complications, such as sterility or spontaneous abortion.

We also pointed out some sexually transmitted diseases that are less publicized, but which may occur widely in the United States. Chancroid and ureaplasmal urethritis are examples. It is conceivable that the incidence of lymphogranuloma venereum, granuloma inguinale, and Mycoplasma and Gardnerella infections may be equally high, but detection methods are currently lacking. The true extent of STDs may never be known.

We shall now turn our attention to a group of bacterial diseases usually acquired by contact, though generally not sexual contact. Some of these diseases have been long known and, left untreated, they may persist for years. Others were unknown a generation ago and are of short duration. Few are fatal, but all have contributed to our knowledge of the broad spectrum of bacterial diseases.

TABLE 10.1

A Summary of Sexually Transmitted Bacterial Diseases

DISEASE	CAUSATIVE AGENT	DESCRIPTION OF AGENT	ORGANS AFFECTED	CHARACTERISTIC SIGNS
Syphilis	*Treponema pallidum*	Spirochete	Skin Cardiovascular organs Nervous system	Chancre Skin lesions Gumma
Gonorrhea	*Neisseria gonorrhoeae*	Gram-negative diplococcus	Urethra, cervix Fallopian tubes Epididymis Eyes, pharynx	Pain on urination Discharge Salpingitis
Chlamydia (Chlamydial urethritis)	*Chlamydia trachomatis*	Chlamydia	Urethra, cervix Fallopian tubes Epididymis Eyes, pharynx	Pain on urination Watery discharge Salpingitis
Ureaplasma urethritis	*Ureaplasma urealyticum*	Mycoplasma	Urethra Fallopian tubes Epididymis	Pain on urination Variable discharge Salpingitis
Chancroid (Soft chancre)	*Haemophilus ducreyi*	Gram-negative rod	External genital organs Inguinal lymph nodes	Soft chancre Erythema Swollen inguinal lymph nodes
Lymphogranuloma venereum	*Chlamydia trachomatis*	Chlamydia	Inguinal lymph nodes Rectum	Swollen inguinal lymph nodes Proctitis
Granuloma inguinale	*Calymmatobacterium granulomatis*	Gram-negative rod	External genital organs	Bleeding ulcer Swollen inguinal lymph nodes
Vaginitis	*Gardnerella vaginalis*	Gram-negative rod	Vagina	Foul-smelling discharge
Mycoplasmal urethritis	*Mycoplasma hominis* *M. genitalium*	Mycoplasma	Urethra Fallopian tubes Epididymis	Pain on urination Variable discharge Salpingitis

10.2

Contact Bacterial Diseases

Numerous bacterial diseases are transmitted by contact other than sexual contact. Usually, some form of skin contact is required, as these diseases will illustrate.

LEPROSY (HANSEN'S DISEASE)

For many centuries, **leprosy** was considered a curse of the damned. It did not kill, but neither did it seem to end. Instead, it lingered for years, causing the tissues to degenerate and deforming the body. In biblical times, the afflicted were required to call out "Unclean! Unclean!" and usually they were ostracized from the community. Among the more heroic stories of medicine is the work of Father Damien de Veuster, the Belgian priest who in 1870 established a hospital for leprosy patients on the

TOXIN INVOLVED	TREATMENT ADMINISTERED	IMMUNIZATION AVAILABLE	COMMENT
Not established	Penicillin	None	Primary, secondary, and tertiary stages The "Great Imitator" Congenital transmission
Not established	Penicillin Spectinomycin Tetracycline Ceftriaxone	None	One of the most reported U.S. microbial diseases Complicated by pelvic inflammatory disease Eye infection in newborns
Not established	Tetracycline Erythromycin	None	Leads to infertility Antibody test for diagnosis Estimated 3–5 million cases annually in U.S.
Not established	Tetracycline	None	Leads to infertility Linked to spontaneous abortion
Not established	Tetracycline Erythromycin Sulfonamides	None	Few complications Many immigrant cases
Not established	Tetracycline	None	Prevalent in Central and South America
Not established	Tetracycline	None	Donovan bodies seen in lesions
Not established	Tetracycline	None	Organism commonly found in the vagina
Not established	Tetracycline	None	Similar to ureaplasmal urethritis

island of Molokai in Hawaii. An equally heroic story was written more recently (MicroFocus 10.2).

The agent of leprosy is **Mycobacterium leprae**, an acid-fast rod related to the tubercle bacillus. This organism was first observed in 1874 by the Norwegian physician Gerhard Armauer Hansen. It is referred to as Hansen's bacillus, and leprosy is commonly called **Hansen's disease**. Ironically, *M. leprae* has not yet been cultivated in artificial laboratory medium, and thus, Koch's postulates (Chapter 1) have not been fulfilled. In 1960, researchers at the CDC succeeded in cultivating the bacillus in the footpads of mice, and in 1969, scientists found that it would grow in the tissues of armadillos. Growth in apes was reported in 1982.

Leprosy is spread by multiple skin contacts, as well as by droplets from the upper respiratory tract. The disease has an unusually long incubation period of 3 to 6 years, a factor that makes diagnosis very difficult. Because the organisms are heat-sensitive, the symptoms occur in the skin and peripheral nerves in the cooler parts of the body, such as the hands, feet, face, and earlobes. Severe cases also involve the eyes and the respiratory tract.

Patients with leprosy experience disfiguring of the skin and bones, twisting of the limbs, and curling of the fingers to form the characteristic **claw hand**. Loss of facial

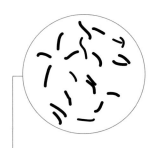

Mycobacterium leprae

Koch's postulates:
a series of procedures for relating a specific organism to a specific disease.

Peripheral nerves:
nerves that extend from the brain and spinal cord to the body tissues.

MicroFocus 10.2

THE "STAR" OF CARVILLE

On December 1, 1894, seven leprosy patients arrived at an old plantation on a crook in the Mississippi River. Soon thereafter, four nuns of the Order of St. Vincent de Paul joined them. Together this small band formed the nucleus of what was to become the National Hansen's Disease Center at Carville, Louisiana.

Change came slowly. In 1921, the federal government acquired the institution, but it remained essentially a prison, patrolled by guards and surrounded by a cyclone fence with barbed wire. Then, in 1931, a leprosy patient named Stanley Stein arrived. Stanley Stein was not his real name—he had forsaken that for fear of bringing shame to his family. Soon, Stein instituted a weekly paper to bring a sense of community to the patients. Originally named *The Sixty-Six Star* (Carville was

Marine Hospital Number 66), the name was eventually shortened to *The Star*.

As the circulation of *The Star* increased, Stein and others launched a campaign for change. In 1936, the patients acquired a telephone so they could hear the voices of their families. Three years later, the swamps were drained to reduce the incidence of malaria. Soon there came a better infirmary, a new recreation hall, and removal of the barbed wire. In 1946, the State of Louisiana allowed the patients to vote in local and national elections.

Through all these years, Stein's leprosy worsened. Originally he had tuberculoid leprosy, the form in which the nerves are damaged. Afterward, however, he developed lepromatous leprosy, which causes lesions to form on the face, ears, and eyes. Soon he was totally blind.

Without feeling in his fingers, he could not even learn Braille.

But Stein was not finished. He and his newspaper tirelessly fought for a new post office and weekend passes for patients. In 1961, President Kennedy paid tribute to *The Star* on its thirtieth anniversary and singled out its indomitable editor for praise. Stanley Stein died in 1968. By that time, *The Star* had a circulation of 80,500 in all 50 states and 118 foreign countries.

■ *Stanley Stein stands next to the printing press as copies of* The Star *are printed.*

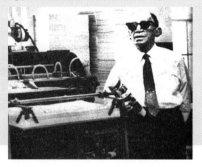

Lepromas:
tumorlike growths accompanying leprosy in the tissues.

clo-faz'i-mēn

of-laks'a-cin

BCG:
a preparation of modified tubercle bacilli used for immunization against tuberculosis.

features accompanies thickening of the outer ear and collapse of the nose. Tumor-like growths called **lepromas** form on the skin and in the respiratory tract (lepromatous leprosy). However, the largest number of deformities develop from the loss of pain sensation due to nerve damage (tuberculoid leprosy). Inattentive patients can pick up a pot of boiling water without flinching, and they accidentally let cigarettes burn down and sear their fingers.

For many years, the principal drug for the treatment of leprosy was a sulfur compound known commercially as **Dapsone** ("Zap it with dap"). In many cases, such as the one shown in FIGURE 10.8, the results were dramatic. However, studies indicate that *M. leprae* is becoming increasingly resistant to this drug, and alternative antibiotics, such as rifampin and clofazimine, are being used. In 1992, the WHO began a campaign to treat the disease with oflaxacin, and in 1998, thalidomide was approved as a therapy (MicroFocus 10.3). Some attempts have been made to immunize populations with BCG, the vaccine used for tuberculosis. Early diagnosis relies on a procedure called the lepromin test, performed in basically the same way as the tuberculin test (Chapter 7).

The World Health Organization estimates that there are over 10 million people with leprosy in the world today. Cases in the United States have risen during the last generation, in large measure because of infected immigrants. Approximately 7000 patients are currently being treated in American hospitals. About 300 come each year to the National Hansen's Disease Center in Carville, Louisiana, for 2 to 6 weeks of initial diagnosis and treatment, followed by subsequent care at any of ten specially designated medical facilities around the country.

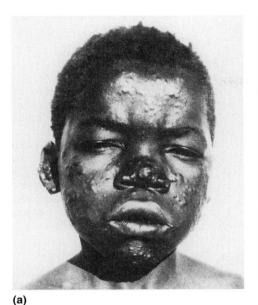

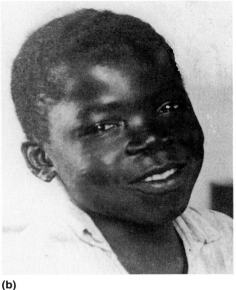

(a)   **(b)**

FIGURE 10.8

Treating Leprosy

The young boy with leprosy is pictured (a) before treatment with Dapsone and (b) some months later, after treatment. Note that the lesions of the ear and face and the swellings of the lips and nose have largely disappeared.

MicroFocus 10.3

BACK BY POPULAR DEMAND

In 1998, the infamous drug thalidomide (tha-lid'o-mid) continued its long road back to respectability, when the Food and Drug Administration (FDA) approved its use for treating a form of leprosy.

In the 1950s, thalidomide was administered to pregnant women as a treatment for morning sickness. But by 1961, investigators realized, to their horror, that the drug was causing facial disfiguring in newborns and crippling birth defects. Over 12,000 children were born with limbs that were either missing or malformed. Many of those individuals live in our neighborhoods today.

Things began to change in 1996, when Celgene, a biotechnology company, filed an application with the FDA to use thalidomide to treat a form of leprosy called erythema nodosum leprosum. This skin condition is accompanied by inflamed skin nodules. Extensive tests yielded positive results, and the approval process was completed in 1998.

But approval was not rendered without restrictions. At the outset, the American Academy of Pediatrics lobbied strongly against the drug. Celgene was encouraged to provide a multistep education campaign and a program for safety. For example, doctors wishing to use the drug must register with Celgene; a doctor must confirm that a woman is not pregnant before a prescription is filled; women using the drug must be tested for pregnancy weekly; and male partners must be educated about contraceptive measures, including condom use.

Health officials estimate that worldwide, over 2 million people with leprosy can benefit from the therapeutic effects of thalidomide (including about 7000 Americans). However, the drug must be used with strong precautions. Then the benefits will outweigh the risks.

STAPHYLOCOCCAL SKIN DISEASES

Staphylococci are normal inhabitants of the human skin, mouth, nose, and throat. Although they generally live in these areas without causing harm, they can initiate disease when they penetrate the skin barrier or the mucous membranes. Penetration is assisted by open wounds, damaged hair follicles, ear-piercing, dental extractions, or irritation of the skin by scratching. **Staphylococcus aureus**, the grapelike cluster of Gram-positive cocci, is the species usually involved in disease.

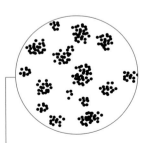

Staphylococcus aureus

FIGURE 10.9

Staphylococci and Skin Abscesses

(a) Staphylococci at the base of a hair follicle during the development of a skin lesion. Phagocytes (white blood cells that engulf bacteria) have begun to collect at the site as pus accumulates, and the skin has started to swell. (b) A severe abscess on the head of a young boy. Abscesses often begin as trivial skin pimples and boils, but they can become serious as staphylococci penetrate to the deeper tissues.

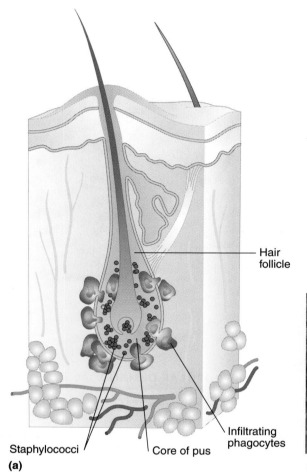

Hair follicle

Staphylococci
Core of pus
Infiltrating phagocytes

(a)

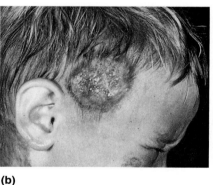

(b)

Abscess:
a circumscribed pus–filled lesion, often caused by staphylococci.

The hallmark of staphylococcal skin disease is the **abscess**, a circumscribed pus-filled lesion (**FIGURE 10.9**). A **boil** is a skin abscess, which often begins as a pimple. Deeper skin abscesses, called **carbuncles**, develop when the staphylococci work their way down to the tissues below the skin. Skin contact with other people spreads the disease. Food handlers should be aware that staphylococci from boils and carbuncles can be transmitted to food, where they can cause food poisoning (Chapter 8).

Another skin disease caused by *S. aureus* is the **scalded skin syndrome**, or **Ritter's disease**, which is occasionally seen in infants. The skin becomes red, wrinkled, and tender to the touch, with a sandpaper appearance. It may then peel off. Toxins produced by the staphylococci living at a point distant from the skin appear to be responsible for this condition. Mortality rates may be high in untreated cases.

im-pē-tī'go con-ta'je-o'sum

A more widespread staphylococcal skin disease is **impetigo contagiosum**. Here the infection is more superficial and involves patches of epidermis just below the outer skin layer. Impetigo first appears as thin-walled blisters that ooze a yellowish fluid and form yellowish-brown crusts. Usually the blisters occur on the exposed parts of the body, but they may also occur around the nose and upper lip after a child has had a cold with a runny nose, since the constant irritation provides a mechanism for penetration by the staphylococci. *Streptococcus pyogenes* (Chapter 7) may also cause impetigo.

pi-oj'ĕ-nez

Staphylococcal skin diseases and bloodborne infections are commonly treated with penicillin, but resistant strains of *S. aureus* are well known, and physicians may need to test a series of alternatives before an effective antibiotic is located. This problem was brought to public awareness during the 1990s, when reports of antibiotic resistance in staphylococci became widespread. Resistances to numerous antibiotics were reported, and **multidrug-resistant *Staphylococcus aureus* (MRSA)** soon appeared in many hospitals. The last-resort antibiotic for the bacteria was vancomycin, a very expensive and somewhat toxic drug. However, by 1997, **vancomycin-resistant *S. aureus* (VRSA)** was detected in clinical settings. New drugs and new treatment approaches are being made available to the medical community to help stem the tide of MRSA and VRSA. Chapter 23 discusses the issue of antibiotic resistance in more detail.

A staphylococcal skin disease can also be treated by vigorously scrubbing the lesions with Betadine applied with 2-by-2-inch gauze pads under the direction of a physician. The disease should be treated with caution because staphylococci commonly invade the blood and penetrate to other organs. For example, staphylococcal blood poisoning (septicemia) may develop, as well as staphylococcal pneumonia, endocarditis, meningitis, or nephritis. A trivial skin boil is often the source.

Betadine:
an iodine-based antiseptic that kills many bacterial species.

Nephritis:
disease of the kidney.

TOXIC SHOCK SYNDROME

In 1978, James Todd of Children's Hospital in Denver, Colorado, coined the name **toxic shock syndrome (TSS)** for a blood disorder characterized by sudden fever and circulatory collapse. The name remained in relative obscurity until the fall of 1980, when a major outbreak occurred in menstruating women who used a particular brand of highly absorbent tampons. News of TSS dominated the media for about 6 months and led to a recall of the tampons. With that episode, toxic shock syndrome assumed a position of significance in modern medicine. Incidence rates are shown in FIGURE 10.10.

Toxic shock syndrome is caused by a toxin-producing strain of *Staphylococcus aureus*. The earliest symptoms of disease include a rapidly rising fever, accompanied by vomiting and watery diarrhea. Patients then experience a sore throat, severe muscle aches, and a sunburnlike rash with peeling of the skin, especially on the

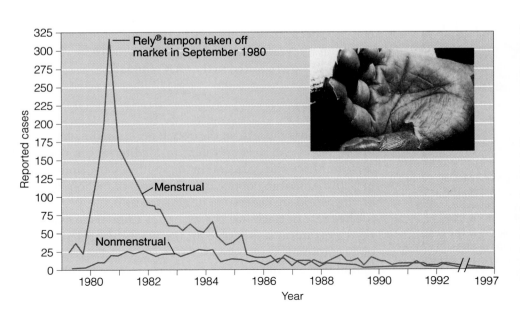

FIGURE 10.10

Reported U.S. Cases of Toxic Shock Syndrome, 1979 to 1997
The total number of cases per year is the sum of the numbers of monthly cases. The disease reached a peak in the fall of 1980; then, the incidence rates dropped with the recall of the highly absorbent tampons. Nonmenstrual episodes currently account for a significant number of cases. The photograph shows the peeling skin often associated with TSS.

MicroFocus 10.4

"IT SEEMED LIKE A GOOD IDEA!"

The idea of a tattoo seemed okay. All her friends had them, and a tattoo would add a sense of uniqueness to her personality. After all, she was already 22. It took some pushing from her friends, but she finally made it into the tattoo parlor that day in Fort Worth, Texas.

Two weeks later the pains started—first in her stomach, then all over. Her fever was high, and now a rash was breaking out; it looked like her skin was burned and was peeling away. One visit to the doctor, then immediately to the emergency room of the local hospital. The gynecologist guessed it was an

inflammation of the pelvic organs (pelvic inflammatory disease, they called it), so he gave her an antibiotic and sent her home.

But it got worse—the fever, the rash, the peeling, the pains. Back she went to the emergency room. This time they would admit her to the hospital, give her intravenous blood transfusions and antibiotics, keep her for 11 days, and discover a severe blood infection due to *Staphylococcus aureus*. And there was an unusual diagnosis: toxic shock syndrome. Don't women get that from tampons? Most do, she was told, but a few get it from staph entering a skin wound—a

wound that can be made by a contaminated tattooing needle.

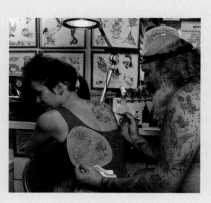

palms of the hands and soles of the feet. A sudden drop in blood pressure also occurs, possibly leading to shock and heart failure. Antibiotics may be used to control the growth of bacteria, but measures such as blood transfusions must be taken to control the shock.

Although the staphylococci involved in TSS exist in various places in the body, the ones inhabiting the vagina have received the most attention. During the 1980 outbreak, scientists speculated that lacerations or abrasions of the tissue by tampon inserters gave the staphylococci access to the tissues. Others suggested that staphylococci grow in the warm, stagnant fluid during the long period that the tampon is in place. It appears certain that multiple factors play a role in toxic shock syndrome, because males, prepubertal girls, and postmenopausal women also have been stricken. Indeed, in 1994 one woman contracted TSS from a contaminated needle (MicroFocus 10.4). About 500 cases of TSS are reported to the CDC annually.

TRACHOMA

Trachoma is a disease of the eyes. It occurs in hot, dry regions of the world and it is prevalent in Mediterranean countries, parts of Africa and Asia, and in the southwestern United States in Native American populations. Hundreds of millions throughout the world are believed to be afflicted by it.

The cause of trachoma is a variant of *Chlamydia trachomatis*, the organism responsible for the STDs chlamydia and lymphogranuloma venereum (FIGURE 10.11). Fingers, towels, optical instruments, and face-to-face contact are possible modes of transmission. The chlamydiae multiply in the **conjunctiva**,

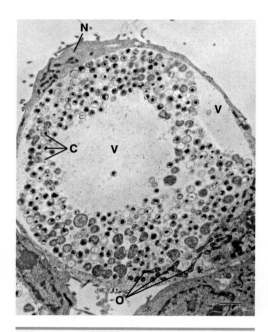

FIGURE 10.11

Chlamydia trachomatis Within a Host Cell

A transmission electron micrograph of a McCoy cell infected with *Chlamydia trachomatis*, the agent of trachoma. In this view, innumerable chlamydiae (C) can be seen within the cell cytoplasm, but not in the large vacuole (V) in the center and right of the cell. The cellular nucleus (N) has been compressed at the periphery, and many organelles (O) are also forced to the edge of the cell. (Bar = 1 μm.)

the thin membrane that covers the cornea and forms the inner eyelid. A series of tiny, pale **nodules** forms on this membrane, giving it a rough appearance. (The word *trachoma* is derived from the Greek *trachi-*, meaning "rough.") In serious cases, the upper eyelid turns in, causing abrasion of the cornea by the eyelashes. Blindness develops from corneal abrasions and lesions.

Tetracycline and erythromycin help reduce the symptoms of trachoma, but in many patients, the relief is only temporary because chlamydiae reinfect the tissues. The World Health Organization maintains squads of trachoma nurses who travel from village to village, identifying trachoma cases in their early stages and treating them before they become serious. Trachoma is believed to be the world's leading cause of preventable blindness.

Conjunctiva: the thin membrane that covers the cornea and forms the inner eyelid.

BACTERIAL CONJUNCTIVITIS (PINKEYE)

Several microorganisms cause conjunctivitis, among them the bacterium ***Haemophilus aegyptius***, the Koch-Weeks bacillus. This organism is also known in the literature as *Haemophilus influenzae* biotype III because of its close relationship to *H. influenzae*. The organism is a small Gram-negative rod that grows in chocolate agar, a rich medium that contains disrupted red blood cells (*Haemophilus* means "blood-loving").

Conjunctivitis is a disease of the conjunctiva. When infected, the membrane becomes inflamed, a factor that imparts a brilliant pink color to the white of the eye (hence the name pinkeye). A copious discharge runs down the cheek in the waking hours and crusts the eyelids shut during sleep. The eyes are swollen and itch intensely, and vision in bright light is impaired (photophobia).

Conjunctivitis may be transmitted in a number of ways, including face-to-face contact and via airborne droplets. Contaminated optometric instruments, microscopes, and towels may also transmit the bacilli. The disease normally runs its course in about 2 weeks, and therapy is usually not required. Neomycin may be administered to hasten recovery. Conjunctivitis is extremely contagious, especially where people congregate.

In recent years, a variant of *H. aegyptius* has also been isolated from the blood of patients suffering from a disease called **Brazilian purpuric fever**. This life-threatening disease is accompanied by nausea, vomiting, fever, and hemorrhagic skin lesions. Many patients display conjunctivitis before the onset of more serious symptoms.

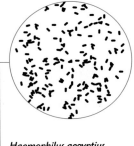

Haemophilus aegyptius

Photophobia: impaired vision in bright light.

Neomycin: an antibiotic that binds to ribosomes in many Gram-negative bacteria.

YAWS

Yaws commonly occurs in tropical countries of Africa, South America, and Southeast Asia. It is caused by ***Treponema pertenue***, a spirochete identical in appearance and similar in chemistry to the syphilis spirochete. Yaws is usually acquired by skin contact. A red, raised lesion called a **mother yaw** develops at the site of entry. Blood associated with the lesion gives it the appearance of a raspberry, and the disease is sometimes called **frambesia**, from *framboise*, the French word for "raspberry."

In time the lesion disappears, but months later the patient develops numerous other yaws. Left untreated, these also disappear, only to reappear as soft granular lesions. The similarities have led investigators to postulate that syphilis may have originated as yaws, or vice versa. **Bejel** and **pinta** are two other diseases very similar to yaws. TABLE 10.2 provides a summary of this and other contact bacterial diseases.

per-ten'u

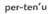

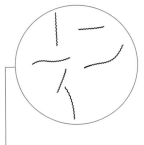

Treponema pertenue

TABLE 10.2

A Summary of Contact Bacterial Diseases

DISEASE	CAUSATIVE AGENT	DESCRIPTION OF AGENT	ORGANS AFFECTED	CHARACTERISTIC SIGNS
Leprosy (Hansen's disease)	*Mycobacterium leprae*	Acid-fast rod	Skin, bones Peripheral nerves	Tumorlike growths Skin disfigurement "Claw hand"
Staphylococcal skin diseases	*Staphylococcus aureus*	Gram-positive cluster of cocci	Skin	Abscess, boil Scalded-skin syndrome Impetigo contagiosum
Toxic shock syndrome	*Staphylococcus aureus*	Gram-positive cluster of cocci	Blood	Fever Watery diarrhea Sore throat Sunburnlike rash
Trachoma	*Chlamydia trachomatis*	Chlamydia	Eyes	Nodules on conjunctiva Scarring in eye
Bacterial conjunctivitis	*Haemophilus aegyptius*	Gram-negative rod	Eyes	Pinkeye Photophobia
Yaws	*Treponema pertenue*	Spirochete	Skin	Red, raised lesion

To this point . . .

We have discussed several bacterial diseases spread by contact by focusing on six examples. In leprosy, multiple contacts may be necessary for the transmission of the bacteria. Staphylococcal skin diseases are also spread by contact, although many episodes of infection begin by simply irritating the skin and allowing staphylococci to penetrate. Tissue irritation may also be the source of the staphylococci involved in toxic shock syndrome. Indeed, researchers who studied the tampon problem of 1980 concluded that the bacteria were already present in the body. Contact spreads the staphylococci to others.

In trachoma, conjunctivitis, and yaws, we discussed three other diseases spread by contact. Trachoma and yaws are prevalent in warm countries where less clothing is worn than in temperate climates. This yields a greater area of skin surface for contact with an infected individual. Bacterial conjunctivitis spreads where people congregate. You might note that the symptoms of the six diseases studied are largely restricted to the skin, where penetration has occurred. Except for the staphylococcal diseases, deeper organs seldom become involved, and life-threatening situations are uncommon. Also, we see the broad range of bacterial organisms that can cause disease including two rods, a staphylococcus, a chlamydia, and a spirochete.

In the final section of this chapter, we shall consider a number of miscellaneous bacterial diseases grouped into discrete categories. Certain of these diseases (the endogenous diseases) are caused by bacteria already in the body; other diseases (the animal bite diseases) are associated with bite wounds; still other diseases (oral diseases) occur in the mouth. A final group (nosocomial diseases) are contracted during a stay in the hospital. We shall also make brief mention of urinary tract and burn infections as we complete our survey.

TOXIN INVOLVED	TREATMENT ADMINISTERED	IMMUNIZATION AVAILABLE	COMMENT
None	Dapsone Rifampin Clofazimine	BCG	Lepromin test for diagnosis Long incubation period
Probable	Penicillin Vancomycin	None	Antibiotic resistance in staphylococci Food handlers involved
Yes	Penicillin Blood transfusions	None	Occurs in all groups, especially menstruating women 500 cases annually
Not established	Tetracycline Erythromycin	None	Leading cause of preventable blindness
Not established	Neomycin	None	Extremely contagious Copious discharge
Not established	Penicillin	None	Found in tropical countries Related to bejel and pinta

Miscellaneous Bacterial Diseases

The miscellaneous bacterial diseases include a diverse mix of diseases related to animal bites, poor oral hygiene, and hospital stays. Also in this group are diseases related to organisms already in the body, the so-called endogenous diseases. We shall discuss them first.

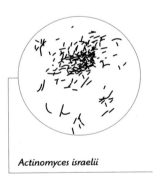

Actinomyces israelii

ENDOGENOUS BACTERIAL DISEASES

Endogenous bacterial diseases are caused by organisms that normally inhabit the body. Natural host resistance generally prevents proliferation of the causative organisms, but when the resistance is suppressed, disease may follow.

An example of an endogenous disease is **actinomycosis**. This disease is caused by *Actinomyces israelii*, named for James A. Israel, who described the bacillus in 1878. It is a Gram-positive, anaerobic, funguslike rod often found in the gastrointestinal and respiratory tracts. On entering the gum tissues during a dental extraction, *A. israelii* multiplies and grows toward the facial surface, causing a red swelling that is lumpy and hard as wood. The condition, known as **lumpy jaw**, may develop into a skin problem with draining sinuses. Another form of actinomycosis involves **draining sinuses** of the chest wall, while a third form is characterized by **abdominal sinuses**, often as a complication of ulcers.

ak'ti-no-mi-ko'sis

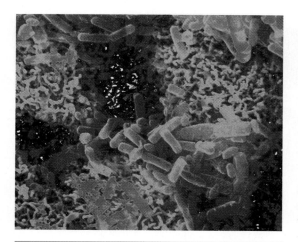

FIGURE 10.12

Endogenous Microorganisms

A scanning electron micrograph of the lining of the human large intestine. Endogenous disease may develop when bacteria like these invade the tissue during periods of suppressed host resistance.

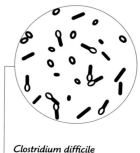

Clostridium difficile

mul-toc'i-da

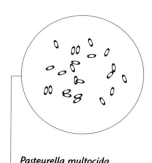

Pasteurella multocida

hens'e-la

Nocardiosis, another example of an endogenous disease, is due to an acid-fast, funguslike rod called ***Nocardia asteroides***. The disease strikes the lungs, where multiple abscesses form. Fever, coughing, and bloody sputum develop, and the symptoms may be mistaken for tuberculosis. Reports of death from nocardiosis have been linked to AIDS (Chapter 13). *N. asteroides* may also cause abscesses and swelling of the foot, a condition called **Madura foot**. This condition follows penetration from the soil via a wound.

Species of ***Bacteroides*** are Gram-negative anaerobic rods that inhabit the large intestine and the feces of most individuals (as FIGURE 10.12 displays). These organisms enter the bloodstream when a person sustains an intestinal injury and cause blood clots that clog the vessels, causing oxygen depletion and possible gangrene in the tissues. ***Bacteroides fragilis*** is the most common pathogenic species of the group.

One of the side effects of excessive antibiotic use is the elimination of many species of intestinal bacteria that normally keep other species in check. Under the circumstances, an endogenous disease may develop from infection by ***Clostridium difficile***, a Gram-positive anaerobic rod. As other organisms disappear, the clostridia multiply and produce a series of toxins that induce a condition called **pseudomembranous colitis**. Yellowish-green membranous lesions cover the intestinal lining, and patients experience diarrhea with watery stools. Infants appear to be particularly susceptible to this condition, especially if a normal population of bacteria has not yet been established. Research in the 1980s also linked *Clostridium difficile* and its toxins to sudden infant death syndrome (SIDS).

ANIMAL BITE DISEASES

Public health officials estimate that each year in the United States, about 3.5 million people are bitten by animals. Most of these wounds heal without complications, but in certain cases, bacterial disease may develop.

An important cause of bite infections is ***Pasteurella multocida***, a Gram-negative rod. This organism is a common inhabitant of the pharynx of cats and dogs, where it causes a local disease called **pasteurellosis**. In humans, the symptoms of pasteurellosis develop rapidly, with local redness, warmth, swelling, and tenderness at the site of the bite wound. Abscesses frequently form, especially if the wound has been sutured. Some patients may experience arthritis. The disease responds slowly to antibiotic therapy.

Although cats transmit few diseases to humans, a notable problem is **cat-scratch disease** (also known as **cat-scratch fever**). The disease affects an estimated 20,000 Americans each year, primarily children, and it is transmitted by a scratch, bite, or lick from a cat (or, in some cases, a dog). Symptoms include a papular or pustular lesion at the site of entry, followed by headache, malaise, and low-grade fever. Swollen lymph glands, generally on the side of the body near the bite, accompany the disease, as shown in FIGURE 10.13. In rare cases, the brain and central nervous system may be involved. Most episodes of disease end after several days or weeks, and antibiotics such as rifampin hasten recovery.

The causative agent of cat-scratch disease has not yet been isolated with certainty, but a leading candidate is ***Bartonella henselae***, a rickettsia. Antibodies against

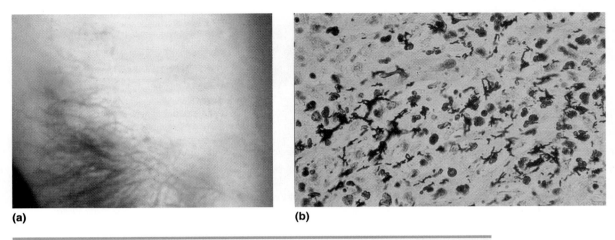

(a) **(b)**

FIGURE 10.13

Cat-Scratch Disease

(a) A patient displaying in the armpit the considerable lymph node swelling that accompanies cat-scratch disease. (b) A photomicrograph of *Bartonella henselae*, considered by many researchers to be the causative agent of cat-scratch disease.

this organism are usually present in people with cat-scratch disease, and the rickettsia is usually isolated from cats whose scratch has led to disease. *B. henselae* also appears to cause **bacillary angiomatosis**, a disease characterized by tumors whose cells organize themselves to form blood vessels. Occurring in the body's cardiovascular system, bacillary angiomatosis resembles Kaposi's sarcoma (Chapter 13) and may be a late manifestation of cat-scratch disease. Another possible cause of cat-scratch disease is *Afipia felis*, a Gram-negative rod.

an'ge-o-mah-to'sis

a-fip'e-ah

Two different species of bacteria can cause **rat-bite fever**. One is *Streptobacillus moniliformis*, a Gram-negative rod that occurs in long chains. It is found in the pharynx of rats and other rodents. Patients experience a lesion at the site of the bite, then a typical triad of fever, arthritislike pain in the large joints, and skin rash. The second organism is *Spirillum minor*, a rigid spiral bacterium with polar flagella. A lesion occurs at the wound site, and a maculopapular rash spreads out from this point. In Japan and other parts of Asia, *Spirillum*-related rat-bite fever is known as **sodoku**. Antibiotic therapy is generally recommended for both forms of rat-bite fever.

TABLE 10.3 summarizes the endogenous and animal bite bacterial diseases.

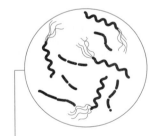

Streptobacillus moniliformis and *Spirillum minor*

ORAL DISEASES

The oral cavity is a type of ecosystem, with complex interrelationships among the members of the resident population of microorganisms and the oral environment. The cavity has various ecological niches, each with a different physical property and nutrient supply dictating the number and type of microorganism that can survive. At least 20 different species of bacteria have been isolated from the normal oral environment, among them a variety of streptococci, diphtherialike bacilli, lactobacilli, spirochetes, and filamentous bacteria. Scientists estimate that there are between 50 billion and 100 billion bacteria in the adult mouth at any one time. (To put the number in perspective, consider that about 78 billion people have lived on Earth since the beginning of time.)

TABLE 10.3

A Summary of Miscellaneous Bacterial Diseases

DISEASE	CAUSATIVE AGENT	DESCRIPTION OF AGENT	ORGANS AFFECTED	CHARACTERISTIC SIGNS
Endogenous Diseases				
Actinomycosis	*Actinomyces israelii*	Gram-positive anaerobic funguslike rod	Gum tissues Chest wall Abdominal organs	Draining sinus
Nocardiosis	*Nocardia asteroides*	Acid-fast funguslike rod	Lungs	Abscesses Rusty sputum Madura foot
Bacteroides infection	*Bacteroides fragilis*	Gram-negative anaerobic rod	Intestine Blood	Blood clots
Pseudomembranous colitis	*Clostridium difficile*	Gram-positive sporeforming rod	Intestine	Intestinal lesions Diarrhea
Animal Bite Diseases				
Pasteurellosis	*Pasteurella multocida*	Gram-negative rod	Skin	Abscess at site of bite Arthritis
Cat-scratch disease	*Bartonella henselae* (?) *Afipia felis* (?)	Rickettsia Gram-negative rod	Skin	Lesion at site of bite Swollen lymph glands
Rat-bite fever	*Streptobacillus moniliformis*	Gram-negative streptobacillus	Skin	Lesion at site of bite Rash, fever
	Spirillum minor	Spirochete	Skin	Lesion at site of bite Rash, fever

Dental plaque:
an oral deposit of dense gelatinous material consisting of organic compounds and bacteria.

a-cid-o-gen'ik

hi'drox-y-ap'a-tite

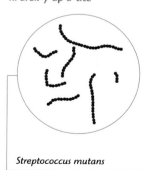

Streptococcus mutans

The material that accumulates on the tooth surface is known by many terms, the most common of which is **dental plaque**. Plaque is essentially a deposit of dense gelatinous material consisting of protein, polysaccharide, and an enormous mass of bacteria. By some accounts there are more than a billion bacteria per gram of net weight of plaque. Most bacterial species have been cultivated in the laboratory, and two-thirds are either anaerobic or facultative species.

Dental caries, or tooth decay, takes its name from the Latin *cariosus*, meaning "rotten." In order for dental caries to develop, three elements must be present: a caries-susceptible tooth with a buildup of plaque; dietary carbohydrate, usually in the form of sucrose (sugar); and acidogenic (acid-producing) plaque bacteria (**FIGURE 10.14**). The bacteria produce acid that breaks down the calcium phosphate salts in hydroxyapatite, the major compound in the enamel and underlying dentin.

One of the primary bacterial causes of caries is acidogenic ***Streptococcus mutans***. This Gram-positive coccus has a high affinity for the smooth surfaces, pits, and fissures of a tooth. Its enzymes react with the glucose and fructose in sucrose and convert them to long-chain carbohydrates called glucans and levans. These materials give *S. mutans* its special adherence qualities. The bacilli then ferment dietary carbohydrates to lactic acid, with smaller amounts of acetic acid, formic acid, and butyric acid. The acids dissolve hydroxyapatite, after which protein-digesting enzymes break down any remaining organic materials. Other streptococcal species involved in caries include ***S. sanguis***, ***S. mitis***, and ***S. salivarius***.

TOXIN INVOLVED	TREATMENT ADMINISTERED	IMMUNIZATION AVAILABLE	COMMENT
Not established	Various antibiotics	None	Lumpy jaw possible Associated with IUD use Normal lung inhabitant
Not established	Various antibiotics	None	Associated with AIDS Endogenous disease Soil transmission via wound
Not established	Various antibiotics	None	May lead to gangrene Normal intestinal inhabitant
Possible	Various antibiotics	None	Accompanies excessive antibiotic use
Not established	Various antibiotics	None	Common in cats and dogs
Not established	Various antibiotics	None	Treatment not always necessary
Not established	Various antibiotics	None	Typical fever, arthritis, and rash
Not established	Various antibiotics	None	Common in Japan

MicroFocus 10.5

AND NOW FOR SOMETHING DIFFERENT

In the war against tooth decay, people have armed themselves with floss, toothpaste, toothbrushes, and many innovative variations of these. Still the bacteria seem to win, especially *Streptococcus mutans*. Modifying the diet helps, adding fluoride to the water tips the balance still further, and using a vaccine may be a future answer. But as of now, the bacteria still seem to win.

British researchers have a different approach: Stop *Streptococcus mutans* at its point of attachment. Charles G. Kelly is leading a research team that has produced a peptide for coating the teeth. The peptide binds to the teeth

surfaces where *S. mutans* attaches, and prevents bacterial attachment. No attachment means no bacteria, which means no acid, which means no tooth decay. Voila!

Kelly's group began with *S. mutans* and its adhesin protein. This large molecule at the bacterial surface binds to receptors on the teeth, like a key fits into a lock. The researchers located a critical 20 amino acid chain in the adhesin protein that does the actual binding (i.e., the "teeth" of the key). Next they found a way to synthesize large amounts of the amino acid chain. They smeared their synthetic preparation on the teeth of volunteers whose

mouths were cleansed of bacteria, thereby muddying up the attachment sites. Control volunteers were treated with a placebo. Those receiving the synthetic preparation remained free of *S. mutans* for over 3 months. By contrast, the bacteria appeared in the mouths of control volunteers after only 3 weeks.

For the present, the dental wars go on. It is comforting to know, however, that scientists have imaginative solutions that extend beyond a new flavor of toothpaste. Dental caries is the most widespread infectious disease in today's world. Putting it to an end would be a considerable feather in the scientific cap.

FIGURE 10.14

Dental Caries

(a) Overlapping circles depicting the interrelationships of the three factors that lead to caries activity. (b) *Streptococcus mutans*, a major cause of dental caries, as visualized by the scanning electron microscope (×10,000).

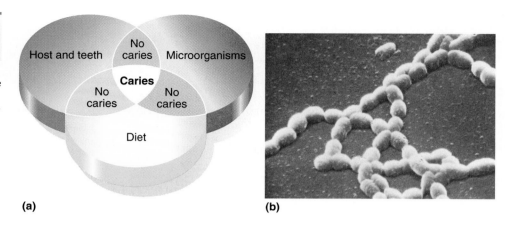

(a)   **(b)**

Fluorides:
derivative compounds of the chemical halogen fluorine.

The prevention of dental caries relates to three principal areas: protecting the tooth, modifying the diet, and combatting cariogenic bacteria (Figure 10.14). Tooth protection may be accomplished by the ingestion and topical application of **fluorides**. These compounds displace hydroxyl ions in hydroxyapatite, thus reducing the solubility of the enamel. Teeth can also be protected by applying polymers to cover pits and fissures in the teeth, thereby preventing bacterial adhesion. Diet modification requires minimizing sucrose in foods. Some success has been observed by substituting **xylitol**, an alcoholic derivative of xylose, for the sugar in candy. Efforts to eliminate cariogenic bacteria focus on preventing the synthesis of dextrans and levans by streptococci, as well as stimulating antibody production against the bacteria. A novel approach is explored in MicroFocus 10.5.

Some dental researchers even foresee a **vaccine** against tooth decay. Such a vaccine would be a polar opposite in sophistication to a toothbrush. With recognition of *S. mutans* as the dominant cariogenic organism and advances in immunology, the vaccine has come closer to reality. British researchers have concentrated on an injectable vaccine using a cell wall constituent of *S. mutans*, while American investigators have been developing oral vaccines to stimulate immune factors at the oral surface. (Oral vaccines are considered safer because streptococcal antigens in the blood could bring on heart problems, as Chapter 7 indicates.) In recent years, researchers have successfully used synthetic *S. mutans* peptides to stimulate antibody responses, and they have employed *S. mutans* antigens coupled to such carriers as harmless *Salmonella* cells and cholera subunits. High-tech laboratories have isolated and cloned the genes from *S. mutans* and attached them to fat droplets called liposomes for use as a vaccine. Indeed, the inventiveness of vaccine developers underscores an optimism that an anticaries vaccine is a real possibility.

Caries is not the only form of dental disease. The teeth are surrounded by tissues that provide the support essential to tooth function. These tissues, called the periodontal tissues, may be the site of a **periodontal disease** called **acute necrotizing ulcerative gingivitis (ANUG)**. Microbiologists believe that ANUG is the result of the invasion of the tissues by several bacteria, among which are *Porphyromonas gingivalis*, a Gram-negative rod; *Leptotrichia buccalis*, a long, thin Gram-negative rod; *Treponema vincentii*, a spirochete; and species of *Eikenella*, another Gram-negative rod. Indeed, in 1990 researchers at Mount Sinai Hospital in New York reported that *E. corrodens* can cause severe cellulitis and arthritis of the knee after entering the blood through trauma of the gingival tissues.

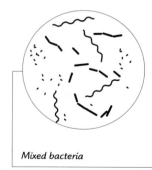

Mixed bacteria

por-fir'o-mon'as

lep'to-trik'e-ah

i'ken-el'ah

ANUG is characterized by punched-out ulcers that appear first along the gingival margin and interdental papillae, and then spread to the soft palate and tonsil areas. Infections in the latter area are sometimes called **Vincent's angina** after Jean Hyacinthe Vincent, who described the spirochete in 1892. A foul odor and bad taste come from gases produced by anaerobic bacteria. As the periodontal tissues decay, the teeth may become loosened and eventually dislodged completely. Diagnosis depends on the observation of rods and spirochetes from the ulcers. The disease is sometimes called **fusospirochetal disease** because the rods have a long, thin fusiform shape and are mixed with spirochetes (FIGURE 10.15). Antibiotic washes may be used in therapy, and some physicians suggest painting the area with a traditional remedy of gentian violet.

ANUG has long been associated with conditions such as malnutrition, viral infection, excessive smoking, poor oral hygiene, and mental stress. The disease was common among soldiers in World War I and was known at that time as **trench mouth**. It is not considered a transmissible disease, but one that develops from bacteria already in the mouth.

Studies in the 1990s highlighted the hazards associated with dental equipment as a transfer mode for bacteria. Interest centered around **biofilms**, the populations of waterborne and airborne microorganisms that adhere to macromolecules on a solid surface. Among the pathogens found in biofilms are *Pseudomonas* species, *Legionella pneumophila*, and *Mycobacterium* species. At risk are dental patients with diminished resistance to infection, including elderly people, transplant recipients, and AIDS and cancer patients.

Of particular concerns are the **waterlines** in hand pieces, air-water syringes, and ultrasonic scalers. Biofilms build up as microorganisms (most originating from the public water supply) colonize the narrow, smooth-walled waterlines. Counts as high as 1 million microorganisms per milliliter of water have been reported.

Although there is no established risk from biofilms in waterlines, the American Dental Association has issued several recommendations to ensure safety. They recommend that independent water reservoirs be used, rather than the public supply; that chemical treatment regimens be put in place; that daily draining and air purging regimens be established; and that point-of-use filters be employed. Through a proactive program, biofilms can be controlled and disease transmission can be interrupted.

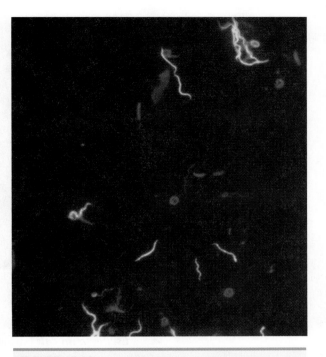

FIGURE 10.15

Bacteria of the Oral Plaque

A photomicrograph of treponemes found in the subgingival plaque of a patient with periodontal disease. These spirochetes have been stained by fluorescence microscopic methods. The organisms cannot be cultivated in laboratory media and must be studied directly as they come from the patient.

URINARY TRACT INFECTIONS

According to a study reported in 1996 in the *New England Journal of Medicine*, about 7 million episodes of **urinary tract infections** occur annually in the United States. Urinary tract infections are the second most frequent cause of visits to the doctor's office (after respiratory tract infections). Sufferers report abdominal discomfort, burning pain on urination, and frequent urges to urinate. Most infections develop in the urinary bladder, where urine is stored before it leaves the body

FIGURE 10.16

Pathogens of the Urinary Tract

(a) An unusual electron micrograph of a colony of *Escherichia coli* in which the cells appear as long, filamentous forms following treatment to cause a genetic mutation. The mutation has resulted in loss of the ability to undergo cell division. In its normal form, *E. coli* is a major cause of urinary tract infections.
(b) A scanning electron micrograph of *Proteus mirabilis*. This large cell contains hundreds of flagella that permit motion among the tissue cells of the urinary tract. (Bar = 5 µm.)

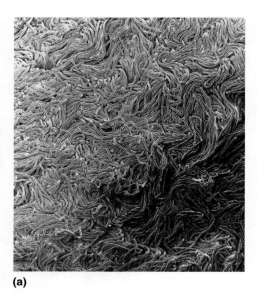

(a)

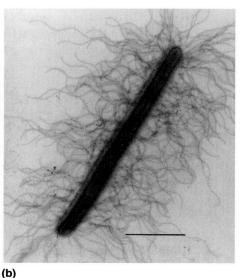

(b)

through the urethra. Among the major causes of infection are **Proteus mirabilis** and **Escherichia coli** (shown in FIGURE 10.16).

Women are apparently infected more often than men, most likely because of anatomical differences: The male urethra is about 9 inches long, and infecting organisms must travel this lengthy distance from the environment before reaching the bladder; the female urethra, by comparison, is only about 1 inch long. Furthermore, the female urethra opens in front of the vagina, and various microorganisms reside normally in the vaginal tract. In addition, the proximity of the urethra to the anus permits intestinal organisms to pass from the gastrointestinal tract to the urinary tract. Sexual intercourse increases the possibility of urinary tract infection because bacteria can enter the urethra during organ contact.

Most urinary tract infections are successfully treated with sulfur-related compounds such as Bactrim or Septra, or antibiotics such as ciprofloxacin (Cipro) or ofloxacin. Such practices as avoiding tight-fitting clothes and urinating soon after sexual intercourse can also reduce the possibility of infection. Studies have shown that cranberry juice and vitamin C may inhibit the bacteria by increasing the acidity of the urinary tract. Left untreated, the infection can involve the entire bladder or spread to the kidneys. Various cultivation methods are used in diagnosis, including one in which different bacteria give different color reactions, as FIGURE 10.17 shows.

Researchers have investigated the possibility of a vaccine against *E. coli* as a way of preventing urinary tract infections. In 1997, a research group tested a genetically engineered, injectable vaccine in mice. The vaccine consists of proteins that trigger the immune system to produce antibodies against the bacterium's adhesion molecules of the pili. When coated with antibodies, the bacterium cannot adhere to the urinary tract tissues. A second group was experimenting with a different vaccine composed of killed bacteria delivered to the vaginal tract by suppository. Local delivery of the vaccine would ensure a local immune response and avoid inflammation caused by injection at distant sites. At this writing, both studies remain preliminary.

Mounting evidence has shown that **biofilms** can be a key factor in urinary tract infections. Bacteria sequestered in these slimy conglomerates are shielded from attack by the body's immune system, and they are difficult to kill with antibiotics. Biofilms in urinary catheters often provide starting points for bladder infections, as bacteria creep up the catheters. In males, biofilms have also been implicated in infections of

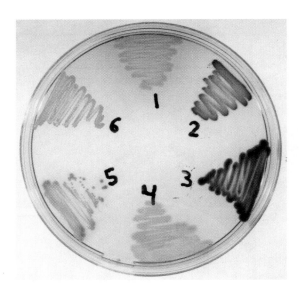

FIGURE 10.17

Detecting Urinary Tract Pathogens

Various urinary tract pathogens are cultivated on a laboratory medium called CHROMagar. The different bacteria display different color reactions, which aid identification. 1: *Proteus mirabilis.* 2: *Enterobacter faecalis.* 3: *Klebsiella pneumoniae.* 4: *Pseudomonas aeruginosa.* 5: *Escherichia coli.* 6: *Staphylococcus aureus.*

the prostate gland, which are accompanied by chronic pain and sexual dysfunction. Researchers have demonstrated that biofilms are highly organized clumps of bacteria bound together by a carbohydrate matrix and surrounded by water channels for nutrient delivery and waste disposal. The carbohydrate shields the bacteria from defensive mechanisms, including antibodies and antibiotics. Finding ways to penetrate this barrier is important to stemming the tide of urinary tract infections.

NOSOCOMIAL DISEASES

Nosocomial diseases are those acquired during hospitalization. The CDC has estimated that up to 10 percent of all hospital patients may develop a nosocomial disease during their stay, with surgical patients particularly susceptible. Certain types of operations such as amputations and intestinal surgery are accompanied by an infection rate approaching 30 percent. Over 1 million patients may be involved annually, and an estimated $6 billion in hospital costs is spent to treat the nosocomial diseases.

A hospital's patient population is a high-density community composed of unusually susceptible individuals. A variety of pathogenic bacteria abound, and new ones are continually being introduced as new patients arrive (**FIGURE 10.18**). In addition, the extensive use of antimicrobial agents contributes to the development of resistant strains of microorganisms, and staff members become carriers of these strains. Many of the patients have already experienced some interference with their normal immune defenses, such as a breach of the skin barrier in surgery, radiation therapy for cancer, immunosuppressive medication, or indwelling apparatus such as catheters and intravenous tubes. When all these factors meet, nosocomial diseases break out.

The organisms that cause nosocomial diseases are generally **opportunistic**—that is, they do not cause disease in normal humans, but they are dangerous in compromised individuals. Among the most common opportunistic bacteria are Gram-negative rods such as *Escherichia coli, Serratia marcescens, Enterobacter aerogenes, Enterobacter cloacae, Klebsiella pneumoniae,* and *Proteus* species. Often these bacteria are the cause of urinary tract infections. *Staphylococcus aureus* is another important cause of nosocomial diseases, as are various types of streptococci.

Opportunistic:
referring to microorganisms that invade the tissues of an immuno-compromised individual.

sĕ-ra'she-ah mar-ses'ens

FIGURE 10.18

A Hospital Epidemic of *Burkholderia* Infection

This epidemic occurred over an extended period—from August 31, 1996, to June 1, 1998—when the causative organism was finally identified at its source.

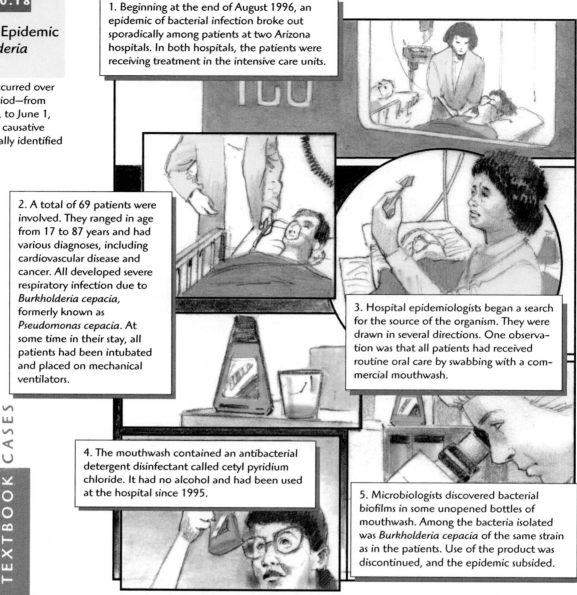

1. Beginning at the end of August 1996, an epidemic of bacterial infection broke out sporadically among patients at two Arizona hospitals. In both hospitals, the patients were receiving treatment in the intensive care units.

2. A total of 69 patients were involved. They ranged in age from 17 to 87 years and had various diagnoses, including cardiovascular disease and cancer. All developed severe respiratory infection due to *Burkholderia cepacia,* formerly known as *Pseudomonas cepacia.* At some time in their stay, all patients had been intubated and placed on mechanical ventilators.

3. Hospital epidemiologists began a search for the source of the organism. They were drawn in several directions. One observation was that all patients had received routine oral care by swabbing with a commercial mouthwash.

4. The mouthwash contained an antibacterial detergent disinfectant called cetyl pyridium chloride. It had no alcohol and had been used at the hospital since 1995.

5. Microbiologists discovered bacterial biofilms in some unopened bottles of mouthwash. Among the bacteria isolated was *Burkholderia cepacia* of the same strain as in the patients. Use of the product was discontinued, and the epidemic subsided.

soo-do-mon'as a'er-jin-o'sa

Pseudomonas aeruginosa, a Gram-negative rod, is a particular problem in burn victims (FIGURE 10.19). The organism grows rapidly and produces a sickly sweet odor, as well as a green fluorescent pigment that causes the tissue to glow under ultraviolet light. It is also a cause of serious disease in patients with **cystic fibrosis**. The respiratory cells of these individuals cannot produce a regulatory protein. The protein normally reacts with *Pseudomonas aeruginosa* and helps the cells take the bacteria inside, where they are destroyed (FIGURE 10.20). Without the regulatory protein, the *P. aeruginosa* remains in a **biofilm** in the air passageways, where it grows and causes inflammation, leading to an insidious decline in respiratory function. An estimated 80 to 90 percent of cystic fibrosis patients suffer from infection with *P. aeruginosa;* indeed, the organism is a primary cause of respiratory failure. The regulatory protein also has a relationship to the typhoid bacillus (Chapter 8).

To deal with nosocomial diseases, hospitals designate a specialist, usually a **nurse epidemiologist**, whose primary responsibility is to locate problem areas and report them to an infection-control committee. The local committee consists of nurses, doctors, dieticians, engineers, and housekeeping and laboratory workers who monitor equipment and procedures to interrupt the disease cycle. All authorities agree that frequent and conscientious hand-washing is the all-important first step.

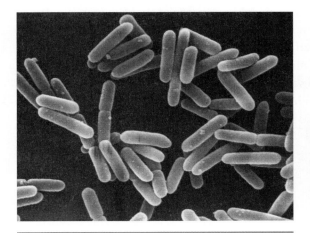

FIGURE 10.19

Pseudomonas aeruginosa

A scanning electron micrograph of *Pseudomonas aeruginosa*, an important cause of nosocomial diseases, especially in patients who have suffered burns.

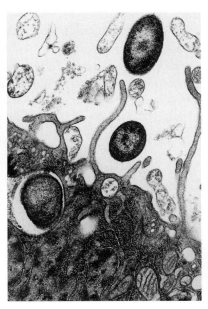

FIGURE 10.20

Cystic Fibrosis and *Pseudomonas aeruginosa*

An electron micrograph of *Pseudomonas aeruginosa* cells being internalized by an epithelial cell of the human respiratory tract. *P. aeruginosa* infection is normally held in check by this action, but in cystic fibrosis patients, an essential protein is not produced, and the cells cannot internalize the bacterial cells and destroy them. Patients therefore suffer from respiratory infections caused by *P. aeruginosa.*

Note to the Student

We have surveyed numerous diseases in this chapter, but one group stands out and merits additional comment. I am referring to the sexually transmitted diseases.

Prior to World War II, doctors had to contend with five classical diseases transmitted by sexual contact. These were syphilis, gonorrhea, chancroid, lymphogranuloma venereum, and, rarely, granuloma inguinale. With the widespread use of antibiotics after the war, the annual incidence of syphilis and gonorrhea declined, and the other three diseases virtually disappeared.

Then came the 1960s and the sexual revolution. It was a time of affluence and defiance of traditional values. Birth control pills, vasectomies, and contraceptive devices offered sexual liberation to go along with social and economic freedoms. Not surprisingly, the incidence rates of STDs soared, and today, the United States is in the grip of an STD epidemic of unprecedented proportions.

The statistics are awesome: Public health officials estimate that one out of every four Americans between the ages of 15 and 55 will acquire an STD at some point in his or her life; 15 million Americans visit clinics and doctors' offices annually for treatment; and over $2 billion is spent each year in health-care costs related to STDs. Moreover, the list of sexually transmitted diseases continues to expand, and at least 25 diseases are now involved, including the ones noted in this chapter, as well as genital warts, hepatitis B, shigellosis, genital herpes, candidiasis, AIDS, and numerous diseases discussed in other chapters.

Is the epidemic likely to end? Some sociologists contend that the fear of getting an STD may be a motivating factor in limiting promiscuous sex. However, a more realistic view is that there has been a shift in attitude toward such things as pre-marital sex and sex in books and films. Condom use can do much to interrupt the transmission of an STD, but while values continue to be sorted out, it appears that the incidence of STDs will remain high, and that an end to the epidemic is still beyond expectation.

Summary

Two general categories of bacterial diseases are discussed in this chapter: contact diseases and miscellaneous diseases. The contact diseases are spread among individuals by sexual contact and by skin contact. Diseases transmitted by sexual contact are some of the most numerous in society today. They range from the life-threatening disease syphilis to the milder diseases gonorrhea and chlamydia. Untreated, syphilis occurs in three stages, the last stage involving mental and cardiovascular deterioration. Although gonorrhea and chlamydia result in less damage to the body, an important effect of both is the possibility of sterility owing to blockage of the reproductive tubules. Other sexually transmitted diseases, such as ureaplasmal urethritis, chancroid, lymphogranuloma, vaginitis, and mycoplasmal urethritis, are also relatively mild.

Skin contact diseases discussed in this chapter include leprosy, staphylococcal skin diseases, trachoma, conjunctivitis, and yaws. Staphylococcal infections can be complicated by blood involvement, but the other diseases rarely go further than the skin, and they can be controlled by drug therapy.

The miscellaneous bacterial diseases fall into identifiable groups: endogenous diseases and animal bite diseases. Endogenous diseases result from bacteria that normally reside in the body but cause infection when body defenses diminish, such as in an immunocompromised host. Animal bite diseases include pasteurellosis from dogs and cats, cat-scratch disease, and rat-bite fever. Oral diseases, urinary tract infections, and nosocomial diseases are also discussed briefly to provide an overview of their importance.

Questions for Thought and Discussion

1. In 1995, the Rockefeller Foundation offered a $1 million prize to anyone who could successfully develop a simple and rapid test to detect chlamydia and/or gonorrhea. The test had to use urine as a test sample and be performed and interpreted by someone with a high school education. To date, no one has claimed the prize. Can you guess why?

2. One of the major problems of the current worldwide epidemic of AIDS is the possibility of transferring the human immunodeficiency virus (HIV) among those who have a sexually transmitted disease. Which diseases in this chapter would make a person particularly susceptible to penetration of HIV into the bloodstream? What explanation can you give for each example?

3. Studies indicate that most cases of *Staphylococcus*-related impetigo occur during the summer months. Why do you think this is the case?

4. Suppose a high incidence of leprosy existed in a particular part of the world. Why is it conceivable that there might be a correspondingly low level of tuberculosis?

5. It has been suggested that women should avoid vaginal douching because the practice can encourage the development of pelvic inflammatory disease (PID) if there is an underlying STD. How can you explain the connection to an inquisitive friend?

6. One day in the late 1980s, a Senegalese patient reported to a New York hospital with an upper lip swollen to about three times its normal size. Probing with a safety pin at facial points where major nerve endings terminate showed that the area to the left of the nose and above the lip was without feeling. When a biopsy of the tissue was examined, it revealed round reservoirs of immune system cells called granulomas within the nerves. On bacteriological analysis, acid-fast rods were observed in the tissue. What disease do all these data suggest?

7. On January 9, 1984, an undergraduate psychology student was bitten by a laboratory rat on the left index finger. Within 12 hours, her finger was swollen and throbbing. Soon thereafter she was hospitalized with swollen lymph nodes, a skin rash, fever, and exquisite sensitivity of the finger. Gram-negative branching rods were found in the tissue. What disease was she suffering from?

8. Researchers at the University of Maryland have suggested a "dip and brush" method of controlling oral diseases. The idea is to dip a toothbrush into an antiseptic several times while brushing to reduce the level of plaque bacteria. Do you think this method will reduce dental problems?

9. In some African villages, blindness from trachoma is so common that ropes are strung to help people locate the village well, and bamboo poles are laid to guide farmers planting in the fields. What measures can be taken to relieve such widespread epidemics as this?

10. Certain microscopes have the added feature of a small hollow tube that fits over the eyepiece or eyepieces. Viewers are encouraged to rest their eyes against the tube and thereby block out light from the room. Why is this feature hazardous to health?

11. A quote from the Book of Leviticus reads: "And the leper . . . shall be defiled; he is unclean; he shall dwell alone; without the camp shall his habitation be." Short of editing the Bible, how can this attitude toward leprosy be changed?

12. After a young man suffers an abrasion on the right arm, his affectionate cat licks the wound. Several days later, a pustular lesion appears at the site and a low-grade fever develops. He also experiences "swollen glands" on the right side of his neck. What disease has he acquired?

13. A woman suffers two miscarriages, each after the fourth month of pregnancy. She then gives birth to a child, but impaired hearing and vision become apparent as it develops. Also, the baby's teeth are shaped like pegs and have notches. What medical problem existed in the mother?

14. In the early 1990s, the CDC was reporting approximately 100,000 instances of ectopic pregnancy in the United States annually, a fivefold increase over the rate in 1970. What could account for this significant increase?

15. One of the diseases discussed in this chapter is probably the most widespread disease in all the world. Students go to special schools and earn a special degree to learn how to deal with it. Then they spend years developing their skill in treating it. What is the disease?

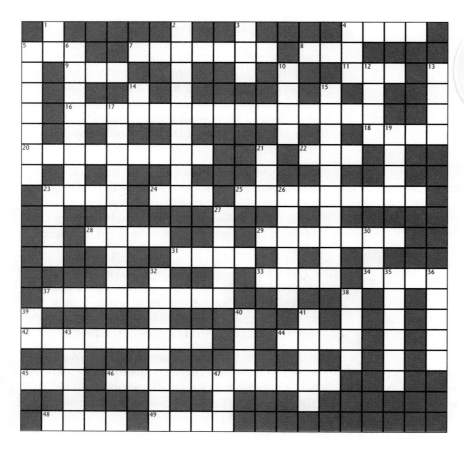

Review

A major topic of this chapter has been sexually transmitted diseases. To test your recall of these diseases, fill in the following crossword puzzle. The answers to the puzzle are in Appendix D.

■ ACROSS

4. The _____ of transmission for STDs is contact.
5. Health organization that charts epidemics of STDs.
7. Occurs during primary syphilis.
8. Number of exposures necessary to establish STD infection.
9. Living tissue for chlamydia cultivation.
11. Ureaplasmal urethritis is a type of _____.
16. Accompanied by swelling of inguinal lymph nodes.
18. Gender in which gonorrhea symptoms are more apparent.
20. Caused by *Haemophilus ducreyi.*

16. A 1998 report indicated that levels of syphilis in the United States were, until then, the lowest in history (about 70,000 new cases per year). The report suggested that the prospects for elimination may be emerging. Why do you think the incidence of syphilis has reached these low levels, and what can be done to hasten its elimination?

17. A recent column by Ann Landers carried the following letter: "I am a 34-year-old married woman who is trying to get pregnant, but it doesn't look promising. . . . When I was in college, I became sexually active. I slept with more men than I care to admit. . . . Somewhere in my wild days, I picked up an infection that left me infertile. . . . The doctor told me I have quite a lot of scar tissue inside my Fallopian tubes." The young woman, who signed herself "Suffering in St. Louis," went on to implore readers to be careful in their sexual activities. What advice do you think the woman gave to readers?

18. At a specified hospital in New York City, hundreds of patients pay a regular visit to the "neurology ward." Some sign in with numbers; others invent fictitious names. All receive treatment for leprosy. Why do you think this disease still carries such a stigma?

19. While on their honeymoons, women are sometimes confronted with "honeymoon cystitis," a type of urinary tract infection. They have pain on urination, a frequent urge to urinate, and burning and abdominal discomfort. Why is this condition often related to one's honeymoon?

20. Cosmetic counters often have a number of eye makeup testers for consumers to sample. A recent survey of these testers revealed that over 50 percent were contaminated with bacteria involved in eye infections. What can consumers do to avoid exposure to the bacteria, and what should producers do to limit the danger to consumers?

22. STD (abbr) caused by *Chlamydia trachomatis*.
23. Colloquial expression for gonorrhea.
24. Number of exposures necessary to establish STD infection.
25. Syphilis stage with skin rash, loss of hair, and flulike symptoms.
28. Occurs during urination in gonorrhea patient.
29. Urine tube infected by *Neisseria gonorrhoeae*.
31. Syphilis stages are separated by substantial amounts of _____.
33. Container for sample transported to lab.
34. The _____ of choice for syphilis is penicillin.
37. Gonorrhealike disease transmitted by sexual contact.
42. Caused by a Gram-_____ diplococcus discovered by Neisser.
44. Digested by T-mycoplasma in laboratory culture.
45. Possible complication of gonorrhea (abbr).
46. Blockage of Fallopian tube as a result of gonorrhea.
48. Continent where lymphogranuloma is prevalent.
49. Can display symptoms of syphilis.

■ **DOWN**

1. Older name (initials) for a sexually transmitted disease.
2. Tubes invaded by gonococci during time of infection.
3. Gonorrhea is rarely contracted by exposure to a _____ surface.
4. Often display a discharge when gonorrhea is present.
5. Sexual _____ is generally required for transmission of syphilis spirochetes.
6. Absent in *Mycoplasma* species.
10. Odor of discharge from vaginitis patient.
12. Stain technique to identify gonococci.
13. Possibly 3 to _____ million chlamydia cases in U.S. annually.
14. Bacterium (initials) that causes syphilis.
15. Syphilis that passes from mother to child.
17. One species can cause a form of urethritis.
19. Chlamydiae do not grow on nutrient _____ media.
21. Organ that can be infected by gonococci and chlamydiae.
23. The organism that causes chlamydia is a very tiny _____.

26. Opening to uterus infected by gonococci.
27. Soft, granular lesion in tertiary syphilis.
30. Shape of *Haemophilus ducreyi*.
32. Caused by *Treponema pallidum*.
35. Organ infected by gonococci leading to proctitis.
36. Syphilis sometimes called the _____ imitator.
38. Object used to obtain sample from gonorrhea patient.
39. Bacterium (initials) that causes gonorrhea.
40. Gonococci that are resistant to penicillin (abbr).
41. Body region affected during cases of gonorrhea.
43. Swollen _____ nodes accompany LGU and are a major symptom.
47. STDs can also be transmitted by _____-sexual methods.

http://microbiology.jbpub.com

The site features **eLearning,** an on-line review area that provides quizzes and other tools to help you study for your class. You can also follow useful links for in-depth information, read more MicroFocus stories, or just find out the latest microbiology news.

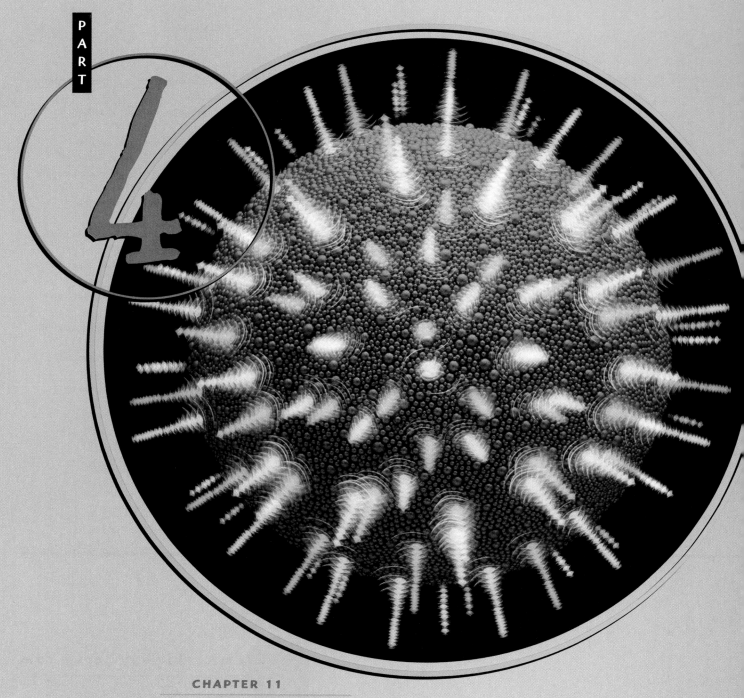

PART 4

Other Microorganisms

Bacteria are but one of several groups of microorganisms interwoven with the lives of humans. Other prominent groups are the viruses, fungi, protozoa, and multicellular parasites. Knowledge of these microorganisms developed slowly during the early 1900s, partly because they were generally more difficult to isolate and cultivate than bacteria. (Indeed, viruses remained unseen and unphotographed until the late 1930s.) Another reason is that methods for research into bacteria were more advanced than for other microorganisms, and investigators often chose to build on established knowledge rather than pursue uncharted courses of study. Moreover, the urgency to learn about other microorganisms was not great because they did not appear to cause such great epidemics.

Much of that changed in the second half of the 1900s. Many bacterial diseases came under control with the advent of vaccines and antibiotics, and the increased funding for biological research allowed attention to shift to other infectious agents. The viruses finally were identified and cultivated, and microbiologists laid the foundations for their study. Fungi gained prominence as tools in biological research, and scientists soon recognized their significance in ecology and industrial product manufacturing. As remote parts of the world opened to trade and travel, public health microbiologists realized the global impact of protozoal disease. Moreover, as concern for the health of the world's peoples increased, observers expressed revulsion at the thought that hundreds of millions of human beings were infected by multicellular parasites.

In Part 4, we shall study four groups of microorganisms over the course of six chapters. Chapter 11 is devoted to a study of the viruses, and Chapters 12 and 13 outline the multiple diseases caused by these infectious particles. In Chapter 14, the discussion moves to fungi, while in Chapter 15, the area of interest is the protozoa, and in Chapter 16, we discuss the multicellular parasites. Throughout these chapters, the emphasis is on human disease. You will note some familiar terms, such as malaria, hepatitis, and chickenpox; as well as some less familiar terms, such as toxoplasmosis, giardiasis, and dengue fever. The spectrum of diseases continues to unfold as scientists develop new methods for the detection, isolation, and cultivation of microorganisms.

VIROLOGY

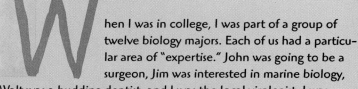

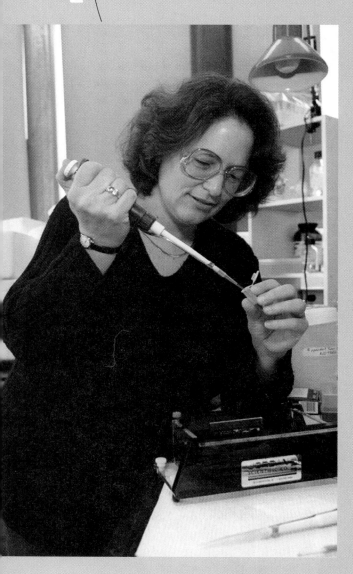

When I was in college, I was part of a group of twelve biology majors. Each of us had a particular area of "expertise." John was going to be a surgeon, Jim was interested in marine biology, Walt was a budding dentist, and I was the local virologist. I was fascinated with viruses, the ultramicroscopic bits of matter, and at one time I wrote a term paper summarizing arguments for the living or nonliving nature of viruses. (At the time, neither side was persuasive, and even my professor gracefully declined to place himself in either camp.)

I never quite made it to being a virologist, but if your fascination with these infectious particles is as keen as mine was (and continues to be), you might like to consider a career in virology. Virologists investigate dread diseases such as AIDS, polio, and rabies. They also study the beautiful variegations found in certain types of tulips. Some virologists concern themselves with many types of cancer, and others study the chemical interactions of viruses with various tissue culture systems and animal models. Virologists are working to replace agricultural pesticides with viruses that will destroy mosquitoes and other pests. Some virologists are inserting viral genes into plants and are hoping the plants will produce viral proteins to lend resistance to disease. One particularly innovative group is trying to insert genes from hepatitis B viruses into bananas. They hope that one day we can vaccinate ourselves against hepatitis B by having a banana for lunch.

If you wish to consider the study of viruses, there is one very important proviso you should know–virologists are chemists. I realize that to a biologist, "chemistry" ranks with "root canal," but the fact of the matter is that to do virology, you must be able to do chemistry. You must have general, organic, and, if possible, physical chemistry in your undergraduate program. Then, prepare for lots more chemistry in your graduate program as you pursue the dream I was never quite able to attain. (Actually, it all worked out very well, because I am extremely happy doing what I do.)

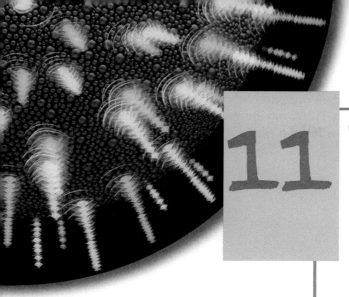

11 The Viruses

It's just bad news wrapped in protein.

—Nobel laureate Peter Medawar describing a virus

OVER THE SPAN OF SEVERAL GENERATIONS, the word *virus* has had two meanings. More than a century ago at the time of Pasteur and Koch, "virus" referred to a vague poison associated with disease and death. Physicians would suggest that the air was filled with virus, or that a virus was in the blood. Louis Pasteur and his contemporaries wrote freely about the "cholera virus" and the "rabies virus"; and in the vernacular of Koch's times, a bacterium was the virus of tuberculosis (which makes reading the reports of the 1890s very confusing).

The modern notion of a virus is dramatically different. In today's world, viruses are recognized as particles of nucleic acid and protein, often with a covering membrane. They replicate in living cells and cause a number of important diseases, such as genital herpes, influenza, hepatitis, and infectious mononucleosis. Viruses vary considerably in size, shape, and chemical composition, and the methods used in their cultivation and detection are completely different than for other microorganisms. The term *rabies virus* is still a common expression in microbiology, but with a vastly different meaning than in Pasteur's time.

In this chapter, we shall study the properties of viruses and focus on their unique mechanism for replication. We shall also see how they are classified, how they are eliminated outside the body, and how the body deals with them during a period of disease. You will note a simplicity in viruses that has led many microbiologists to question whether they are living organisms or fragments of genetic material leading an independent existence. Most of the information in this chapter has only been known since the 1950s, and the current era might be called the Golden Age of Virology. Our survey will begin with a review of some of the events that led to this period.

Foundations of Virology

No single person discovered viruses. Instead, an understanding of the viruses evolved in the late 1800s with the general understanding of the germ theory of disease. Different diseases had recognizable patterns, and although a bacterium, protozoan, fungus, or other agent could be isolated for most diseases, some diseases had no identifiable agent. Many of these diseases would turn out to be viral diseases.

THE EARLY YEARS

A mechanical device, the **filter**, led to early interest in viruses. In 1884, Charles Chamberland, an associate of Pasteur, devised a porcelain filter to trap the smallest known bacteria, and in 1892, the Russian pathologist **Dimitri A. Iwanowski** used Chamberland's filter in his studies on tobacco mosaic disease. In **tobacco mosaic disease**, the tobacco leaves shrivel and assume a mosaic (patchwork) appearance before dying (as FIGURE 11.1 shows). Iwanowski filtered the crushed leaves of a diseased plant and found that the clear sap dripping from the filter (rather than the crushed leaves on the filter) contained the infectious agent. Unable to see any microorganism, Iwanowski reported that a **filterable virus** was the agent of disease. This implied that the unseen agent, whatever its nature, would pass through a bacterial filter. At the time it was a remarkable discovery, because scientists could scarcely comprehend anything smaller than bacteria as disease agents.

Six years later, in 1898, **Martinus Beijerinck** repeated Iwanowski's work and added considerably to the knowledge of viruses. Beijerinck found that the tobacco mosaic virus remains active in dried leaves and soil. By testing the activity of many dilutions of viral fluid, he was able to demonstrate the fluid's potency, and he showed that it was inactivated by boiling. Beijerinck concluded that the disease agent was a "contagious living fluid" (*contagium vivum fluidum*) rather than a discrete object.

Before the excitement of these discoveries subsided, **Paul Frosch** and **Friederich Löeffler** reported in 1898 that foot-and-mouth disease is caused by a filterable virus. This finding implied that "virus" could be transmitted among animals as well as plants. Three years later, in 1901, **Walter Reed** and his group in Cuba wrote that yellow fever is also due to a filterable virus, and with this report, they established human involvement. For a while, the criterion of filterability remained significant, but scientists soon found that some viruses, such as those of rabies and cowpox, did not easily pass through filters. Hence, the agents came to be described simply as "viruses," using the word in a more limited and specific sense.

A unique virus was discovered in 1915 by the English bacteriologist **Frederick Twort**, and independently in 1917 by the French scientist **Felix d'Herrelle**. The virus of Twort and d'Herrelle came to be called the **bacteriophage** ("bacteria-eater") for its ability to destroy bacteria (MicroFocus 11. 1). When a drop of virus was placed in

Tobacco mosaic disease:
a viral disease that causes tobacco leaves to shrivel and assume a mosaic appearance.

bi'jer-ink

lef'ler

Yellow fever:
a mosquitoborne viral disease of the liver and blood.

de-rel'

bak-te're-o-faj'

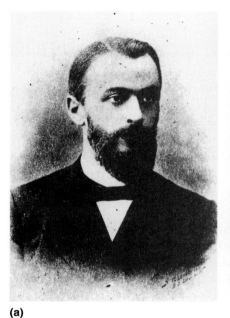
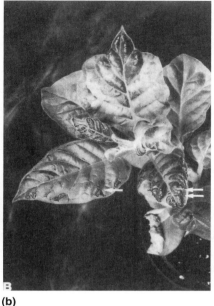
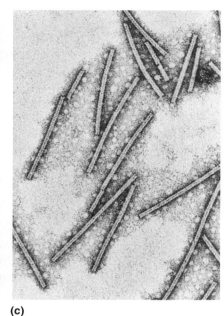

(a)   (b)   (c)

FIGURE 11.1

The Investigator, the Disease, and the Virus

In 1892, the Russian pathologist Dmitri Iwanowski (a) used an ultramicroscopic filter to separate the clear juice from crushed leaves of tobacco plants suffering from tobacco mosaic disease. He placed the juice on healthy leaves and reproduced the disease as the leaves (b) became shriveled (arrow) with a mosaic appearance. Iwanowski had no idea what was causing the disease, since his microscope revealed no particles of any sort. He wrote that tobacco mosaic disease is caused by a "filterable virus," meaning some unknown poison that passes through a filter. Fifty years would pass before microbiologists finally saw (c) the particles that cause the disease. The particles are tobacco mosaic viruses.

MicroFocus 11.1

WHY NOT TRY?

When bacteriophages were identified in 1915, some scientists came to believe they might be useful for curing the dreaded bacterial diseases then raging throughout the world. After all, bacteriophages could destroy bacteria in test tubes, so why not try them in the human body? Unfortunately, the bacteriophages turned out to be highly specific viruses, attacking only certain strains of bacteria. Moreover, no one knew much about them or had the means to work with them effectively.

Fast-forward to the modern era of electron microscopes, sophisticated laboratory analyses, and genetic engineer-ing. Technology had advanced substantially, and in the 1980s, the Polish microbiologist Stefan Slopek decided to try again. He identified a bacterium in the blood of an ill patient, then searched out and isolated a bacteriophage specific for that bacterium. He injected a solution of the phages into the patient and waited to see what would happen. Over a period of days, the infection gradually resolved. Slopek tried again—this time with 137 patients. Each patient benefited from the treatment, and several seemed completely cured.

Could bacteriophages be the answer to the growing problem of antibiotic resistance in bacteria? Perhaps so, but there is the potential problem that phages could convert benign or avirulent bacteria to toxin-producing strains (as for diphtheria or botulism), or that phages could alter the expression of host genes and promote the transfer of virulence genes. Still, some novel approaches to treating infectious disease must be found, and bacteriophages may be a candidate.

Here's a postscript: Martin Arrowsmith, the idealistic young physician of Sinclair Lewis' *Arrowsmith*, traveled to the West Indies to treat bubonic plague—with phage therapy.

MicroFocus 11.2

"BIG FLEAS HAVE LITTLE FLEAS"

For the person suffering the miseries of bacterial disease, there is some consolation in knowing that bacteria get sick too. It is a small consolation, perhaps, but that's apparently what happens. Numerous bacterial species have viruses that prey upon them and use them for replication purposes. Without the host bacterium, the virus remains as inert as a grain of sand. Possibly this is the ultimate test of the eternal predator-prey relationship first enunciated by the English mathematician Augustus DeMorgan:

Big fleas have little fleas upon their backs to bite 'em.

And little fleas have lesser fleas, and so on ad infinitum.

a broth culture of bacteria, the bacteria disintegrated within minutes. D'Herrelle believed that bacteriophage (or, simply, phage) could be used to kill bacteria in the body, but investigators later found that the viruses are easily eliminated from the body and are highly specific for the bacterial strain they attack (MicroFocus 11.2). Bacteriophages have since become important tools in transduction research (Chapter 6) and in bacterial identification (Chapters 7 and 8).

THE TRANSITION PERIOD

By the 1930s, it was generally assumed that viruses were some sort of invisible microorganism below the resolving power of available microscopes. As the years passed, a long list of viral diseases had developed, and work with plant viruses had been productive because of the ease of viral cultivation. For example, virologists learned that tobacco mosaic viruses were composed exclusively of nucleic acid and protein.

Work with animal viruses, however, was less productive because cultivation in live animals was a difficult procedure. A breakthrough finally came when a living analog of Koch's nutrient agar was discovered for viruses. In 1931, **Alice M. Woodruff** and **Ernest W. Goodpasture** published a paper describing the use of **fertilized chicken eggs** as a nutrient for cultivating some viruses (FIGURE 11.2). The shell of the egg was a natural Petri dish for the nutrient medium, and viruses multiplied within the chick embryo tissues.

Resolving power:
the ability of a lens system to transmit light without variation and permit nearby objects to be clearly distinguished.

FIGURE 11.2

Viral Cultivation

(a) Inoculation of fertilized eggs by a technician in the virology laboratory. Techniques such as these are standard practice in virology research. (b) Inoculations to various sites of the fertilized egg for various viruses.

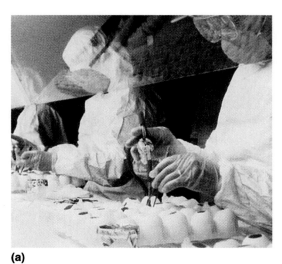

(a)

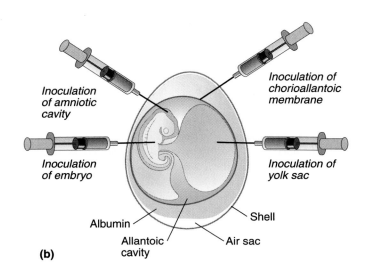

Inoculation of amniotic cavity

Inoculation of chorioallantoic membrane

Inoculation of embryo

Inoculation of yolk sac

Albumin

Allantoic cavity

Shell

Air sac

(b)

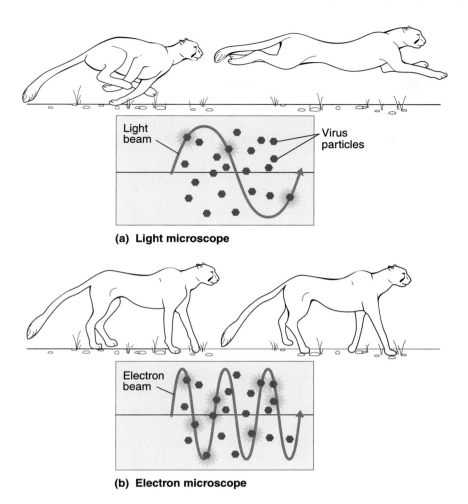

FIGURE 11.3

Wavelength and the Electron Microscope

How the wavelength of the electron beam contributes to the visualization of viruses. (a) When a light microscope is used, the relatively long wavelength of the visible light causes most of the energy to miss the viruses. A running cheetah misses most small rocks in similar fashion. (b) Since the electron beam has a short wavelength, the energy strikes many more viruses, bouncing away and creating an image. Similarly, a walking cheetah steps on more rocks.

The assumption had been that viruses, though incredibly small, were living things, but a discovery by **Wendel M. Stanley** of Rockefeller Institute raised doubts. In the early 1930s, three protein enzymes were crystallized by biochemists, and in 1935, Stanley made the startling announcement that tobacco mosaic viruses could also be crystallized. Crystals are composed of identical molecules, and many scientists now suggested that viruses were as lifeless as any crystalline chemical molecules. Virologists pointed out, however, that the viruses replicate, cause fevers, and elicit antibody responses, properties not associated with chemical molecules. Stanley received the 1946 Nobel Prize in Chemistry. His work opened a debate on the living or nonliving nature of viruses that remains unresolved, and it cut across preconceived ideas that only living things could cause disease.

Just as one technological device, the filter, led to the early notion of viruses, another technological device, the **electron microscope**, revealed the nature of the viruses. The innovative feature of the electron microscope is the incredibly short wavelength of the electron beam, which dramatically increases the instrument's resolving power. To understand the principle involved, consider the difference between a cheetah running and walking on the arid African plain (FIGURE 11.3). With a running stride, the cheetah misses most small rocks, just as visible light with its long wavelength passes over the viruses without striking them. When his stride is shortened, as in walking, more rocks are contacted, just as the electron

Antibody:
a protein produced by immune system cells in response to a specific chemical substance.

Electron microscope:
a magnifying device that uses an electron beam to increase the resolving power.

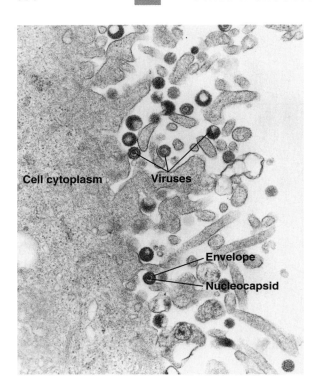

Cell cytoplasm

Viruses

Envelope

Nucleocapsid

FIGURE 11.4

Cells and Viruses

A transmission electron micrograph of tissue cells and associated viruses. In this view at the margin of the cell, the viruses are the dark, round objects in the space outside the cell. The envelope of the virus is seen as a ring at the viral surface, and the nucleocapsid of the virus is the darker center. These viruses are herpesviruses ($\times$48,000).

beam with its short wavelength contacts more viruses. By 1941, virologists were beginning to visualize the tobacco mosaic virus and other viruses, as FIGURE 11.4 shows.

The second key development of the 1940s was sparked by the national epidemic of poliomyelitis (or, simply, polio). Polio attacks people indiscriminately and often leads to permanent paralysis. Attempts at vaccine production were stymied by the inability to cultivate polio viruses outside the body, but **John Enders**, **Thomas Weller**, and **Frederick Robbins** of Children's Hospital in Boston solved that problem. Meticulously, they developed a **test tube medium** of nutrients, salts, and pH buffers in which living cells would remain alive. In the living cells, polio viruses replicated to huge numbers, and by the late 1950s, Jonas Salk and Albert Sabin had adapted the technique to produce massive quantities of virus for use in polio vaccines (Chapter 13). Enders, Weller, and Robbins did not invent tissue cultivation of viruses, but their work showed it had a practical value for vaccine production. In 1954 they shared the Nobel Prize in Physiology or Medicine.

The electron microscope and the test tube cultivation of viruses paved the way for the discoveries in virology that have followed during our era. We shall explore these discoveries in the following pages.

To this point . . .

We have outlined some of the major events in the development of virology, beginning with the early concept of viruses in the late 1800s and continuing through to the 1940s. Iwanowski was one of the first to note that something smaller than any known bacterium could cause disease. His work was further developed by Beijerinck, and expanded by the discoveries of Löeffler, Frosch, and Reed. In time, viruses were found to affect plants, animals, humans, and bacteria. Viruses were also related to cancer.

A surprising announcement of the 1930s was that viruses could be crystallized. This gave an insight into their simplicity and suggested that they might be nothing more than large chemical molecules. When the electron microscope was used to study viruses in the 1940s, scientists observed that viruses had structural details unlike anything seen in chemical compounds. An understanding of viral functions soon developed, as we shall see presently. Also, great strides were made toward the production of viral vaccines, the advances sparked by the tissue cultivation of polio viruses by Enders, Weller, and Robbins. Vaccines opened the way to the prevention of certain viral diseases.

In the next section we shall discuss the characteristics of viruses, beginning with their structure and continuing with their method of replication. You will note a level of structural simplicity matched by few other disease agents and a replication process not encountered elsewhere in the biological world. These attributes lend uniqueness to viruses.

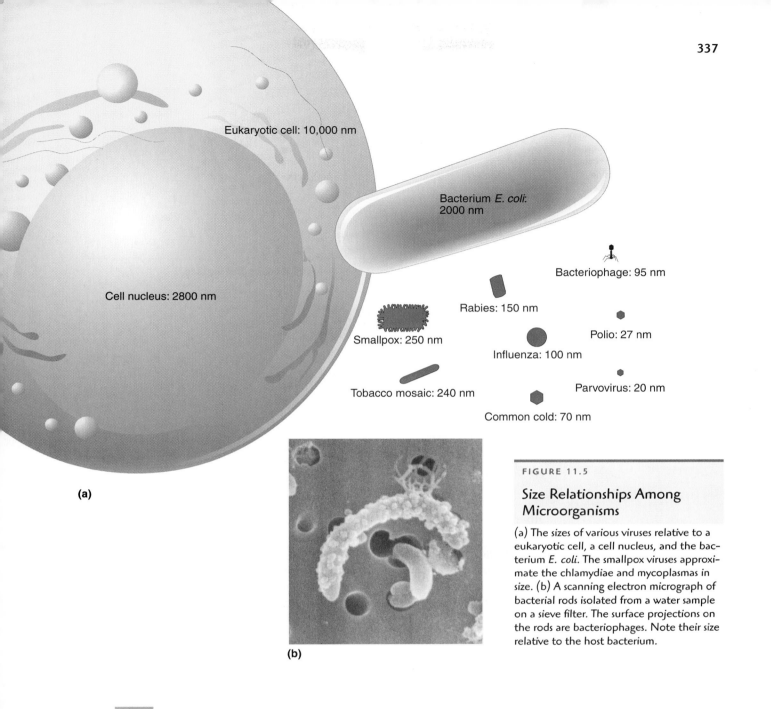

(a)

(b)

FIGURE 11.5

Size Relationships Among Microorganisms

(a) The sizes of various viruses relative to a eukaryotic cell, a cell nucleus, and the bacterium *E. coli*. The smallpox viruses approximate the chlamydiae and mycoplasmas in size. (b) A scanning electron micrograph of bacterial rods isolated from a water sample on a sieve filter. The surface projections on the rods are bacteriophages. Note their size relative to the host bacterium.

11.2

The Structure and Replication of Viruses

Viruses are among the smallest agents able to cause disease in living things. They range in size from the large 250 nanometers (nm) of poxviruses to the 20 nm of parvoviruses (FIGURE 11.5). At the upper end of the spectrum, viruses approximate the size of the smallest bacterial cells, such as the chlamydiae and mycoplasmas; at the lower end, they have about the same diameter as a DNA molecule.

Viruses occur in various shapes, as shown in FIGURE 11.6. Certain viruses, such as rabies and tobacco mosaic viruses, exist in the form of a **helix** and are said to have helical symmetry. The helix is a tightly wound coil resembling a corkscrew or spring.

Nanometer:
a billionth of a meter.

kla-mid'e-e

Helix:
a tightly wound coil.

FIGURE 11.6

Various Viral Shapes

Viruses exhibit numerous variations in symmetry. (a) The nucleocapsid has helical symmetry in the tobacco mosaic, measles, and rabies viruses. The helix resembles a tightly coiled spiral. (b) Certain viruses, such as herpesviruses, polio viruses, and parvoviruses, exhibit icosahedral symmetry in their nucleocapsids. The icosahedron is a polyhedron having 20 triangular faces and 12 points. (c) In other viruses, neither helical nor icosahedral symmetry exists exclusively. The bacteriophage, for example, has an extended icosahedral "head" and a helical tail with extended fibers. The smallpox virus has a series of rodlike filaments embedded within the membranous envelope at its surface. And the influenza virus consists of a series of helical segments enclosed by an envelope.

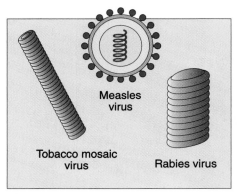

(a) Helical viruses

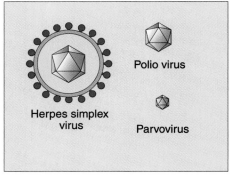

(b) Icosahedral viruses

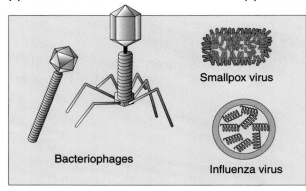

(c) Complex viruses

i-kos'ah-hēd'ron

je'nōm

Subunit:
a chemical substance derived from a microorganism.

Capsomeres:
protein subunits in the capsid of a virus.

Other viruses, such as herpes simplex and polio viruses, have the shape of an **icosahedron** and hence, icosahedral symmetry. The icosahedron is a polyhedron with 20 triangular faces and 12 corners. Certain viruses have a combination of helical and icosahedral symmetry, a construction described as **complex**. Some bacteriophages, for example, have complex symmetry, with an icosahedral head and a collar and tail assembly in the shape of a helical sheath. Poxviruses, by contrast, are brick-shaped, with submicroscopic filaments occurring in a swirling pattern at the periphery of the virus.

All viruses consist of two basic components: a core of nucleic acid called the **genome**, and a surrounding coat of protein known as the **capsid**. The genome contains either DNA or RNA, but not both; and the nucleic acid occurs in double-stranded or single-stranded form. Usually the nucleic acid is unbroken, but in some instances (as in influenza viruses) it exists in segments. The genome is usually folded and condensed in icosahedral viruses, and coiled in helical fashion in helical viruses. FIGURE 11.7 shows the components of a virus.

The capsid protects the genome. It also gives shape to the virus and is responsible for the helical, icosahedral, or complex symmetry. Generally, the capsid is subdivided into individual protein subunits called **capsomeres** (the organization of capsomeres yields the viral symmetry). The number of capsomeres is characteristic for a particular virus. For example, 162 capsomeres make up the capsid in herpesviruses, and 252 capsomeres compose the capsid in adenoviruses, one of the causes of the common cold.

The capsid provides a protective covering for the genome because the construction of its amino acids resists temperature, pH, and other environmental fluctuations. In some viruses, the capsid contains enzymes to assist cell penetration during

Naked forms

Enveloped forms

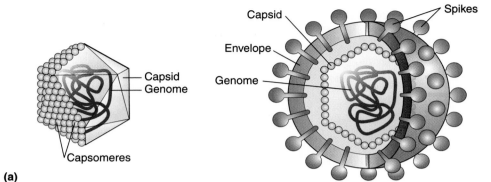

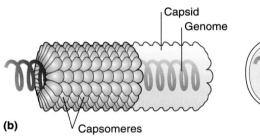

(a)

(b)

FIGURE 11.7

The Components of Viruses

(a) An icosahedral virus in both naked and enveloped forms. Capsomere units are shown on one face of the capsid. The genome consists of either DNA or RNA and is folded and condensed. (b) A helical virus in both naked and enveloped forms. The genome winds in a helical fashion. The capsomeres are protein subunits that form the capsid cover.

replication. Also, the capsid is the structure that stimulates an immune response during periods of disease. The capsid plus the genome is called the **nucleocapsid** (though a better term is probably *genocapsid*, to maintain the structure-to-structure consistency). FIGURE 11.8 shows an icosahedral nucleocapsid.

Many viruses are surrounded by a flexible membrane known as an **envelope**. The envelope is composed of lipids and protein and is similar to the host cell membrane, except that it includes viral-specified components. It is acquired from the cell during replication and is unique to each type of virus. In some viruses, such as influenza and measles viruses, the envelope contains functional projections known as

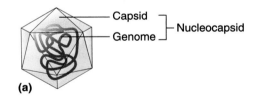

(a)

FIGURE 11.8

An Icosahedral Virus

(a) A schematic view of an icosahedral virus showing the genome and capsid. (b) A transmission electron micrograph of an iridovirus displaying icosahedral symmetry. The points of the icosahedron can be seen clearly since this virus has no envelope. The virus causes African swine fever (×295,000).

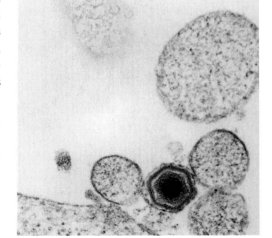

(b)

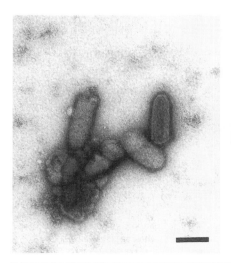 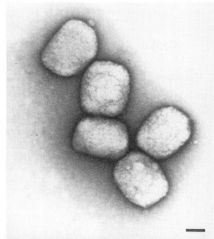 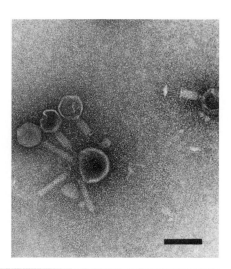

FIGURE 11.9

Viral Symmetry

Transmission electron micrographs of viruses displaying various forms of nucleocapsid symmetry. (a) The vesicular stomatitis virus, which causes skin sores in bovine animals. This virus has a helical nucleocapsid and appears in the shape of a bullet. It is related to the rabies virus. (Bar = 100 nm.) (b) The vaccinia virus, which causes cowpox. This viral nucleocapsid is rectangular with a series of rodlike fibers at its surface. The symmetry is described as complex. (Bar = 100 nm.) (c) A bacteriophage with an icosahedral head and an extended tail. This symmetry is also designated complex. (Bar = 100 nm.)

Spike:
a projection of the viral envelope that helps in attachment to the host cell.

Virion:
a complete virus outside its host cell.

esh'er-ik'e-ah

spikes. The spikes often contain enzymes to assist viral attachment to host cells. Indeed, enveloped viruses lose their infectivity when the envelope is destroyed. Also, when the envelope is present, the symmetry of the capsid may not be apparent since the envelope is generally a loose-fitting structure. Some authors refer to viruses as spherical or cubical because the envelope gives the virus this appearance.

A completely assembled and infectious virus outside its host cell is known as a **virion.** (We shall use the terms *virus* and *virion* interchangeably.) Compared to a prokaryote such as a bacterium, a virion is extraordinarily simple. As we have seen, it consists essentially of a segment of nucleic acid, a protein coat, and in some cases, an envelope. (Three variations are pictured in FIGURE 11.9.) Virions lack the chemical machinery for generating energy and synthesizing large molecules. Therefore, they must rely upon the structures and chemical components of their host cells to replicate. We shall examine how this takes place next.

THE REPLICATION OF BACTERIOPHAGES

The process of viral replication is one of the most remarkable events in nature. A virion invades a living cell a thousand or more times its size, utilizes the metabolism of the cell, and produces copies of itself, often destroying the cell. The virion cannot replicate independently, but within the cell, the replication takes place with high efficiency.

Replication has been studied in a wide range of virions and their host cells. Among the best known processes of replication is that carried on by **bacteriophages** of the T-even group (T for "type"). Bacteriophages T2, T4, and T6 are in this group. They are large, complex DNA virions with the characteristic head and tail of bacteriophages but without an envelope. We shall use their replication cycle in *Escherichia coli* as a model for the viruses. An overview of the process is presented in FIGURE 11.10.

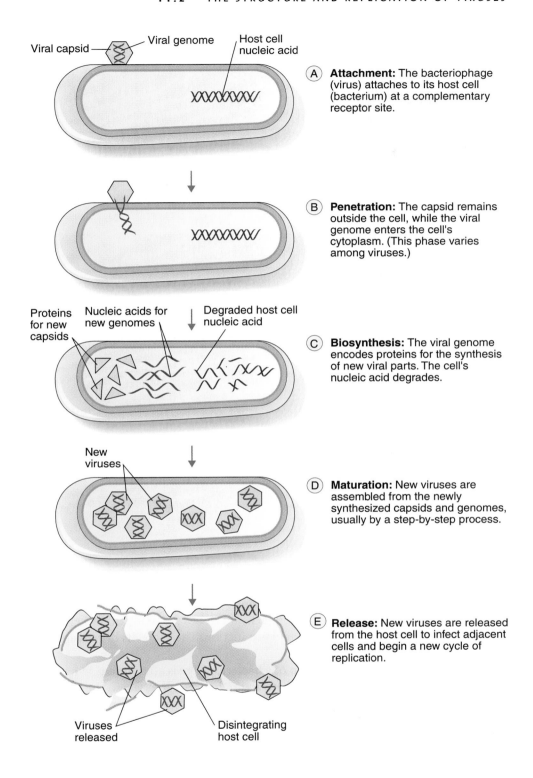

Viral capsid — Viral genome   Host cell nucleic acid

(A) **Attachment:** The bacteriophage (virus) attaches to its host cell (bacterium) at a complementary receptor site.

(B) **Penetration:** The capsid remains outside the cell, while the viral genome enters the cell's cytoplasm. (This phase varies among viruses.)

Proteins for new capsids   Nucleic acids for new genomes   Degraded host cell nucleic acid

(C) **Biosynthesis:** The viral genome encodes proteins for the synthesis of new viral parts. The cell's nucleic acid degrades.

New viruses

(D) **Maturation:** New viruses are assembled from the newly synthesized capsids and genomes, usually by a step-by-step process.

(E) **Release:** New viruses are released from the host cell to infect adjacent cells and begin a new cycle of replication.

Viruses released   Disintegrating host cell

FIGURE 11.10

Bacteriophage Replication

The pattern of replication in bacteriophages (bacterial viruses) has been studied for many generations. It serves as a model for the replication of other viruses.

FIGURE 11.11

Viral Attachment

Scanning electron microscope views of the attachment of bacteriophages to their host cells. (a) Numerous bacteriophages are attached to the surface of the cells. The arrow indicates the tail fibers (×70,000). (b) A remarkable close-up view of the point of attachment showing the tail assembly (arrow). The magnification is ×200,000.

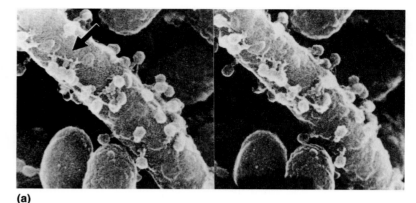

(a)

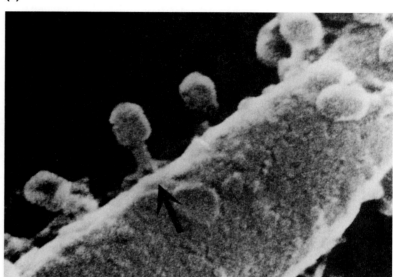

(b)

It is important to note that the nucleic acid in a virion contains only a few of the many genes needed for viral synthesis and replication. It contains, for example, genes for synthesizing viral structural components, such as capsid proteins, and for a few enzymes used in the synthesis; but it lacks the genes for many other key enzymes, such as those used during nucleic acid production. Therefore, its dependence on the host cell is substantial.

The first phase in the replication of a bacteriophage is **attachment** to its host cell. There is no long-distance chemical attraction between the two, so the collision is a chance event. For attachment to occur, a site on the phage must match with a complementary **receptor site** on the cell wall of the bacterium. The actual attachment consists of a weak chemical union between virion and receptor site. (In some cases, the bacterial flagellum or pilus contains the receptor site.) FIGURE 11.11 depicts the attachment phase.

In the next phase, **penetration**, the tail of the phage releases the enzyme lysozyme to dissolve a portion of the bacterial cell wall. Then the tail sheath contracts, and the tail core drives through the cell wall. As the tip of the core reaches the cell membrane below, the DNA passes through the tail core and on through the cell membrane into the bacterial cytoplasm. For most bacteriophages, the capsid remains outside (MicroFocus 11.3).

Receptor site:
the chemical group on a host cell where a virus attaches.

MicroFocus 11.3

EMPTY BOXES

What do you do after you've opened the box and removed the gift? You probably admire the gift, thank the giver, and think about how you'll use it. Perhaps you try it on or otherwise begin weaving it into your life. The poor box gets shunted aside until someone thinks to put it in the garbage pail (or the recycle bin).

It's not much different with viruses: The DNA or RNA genome enters the cell's cytoplasm and encodes new viruses, while the capsid gets broken down, or, in the case of bacteriophages, is left outside the cell. But things may be different in the future. Researchers are investigating viral capsids as miniature reaction chambers for designing ultramicroscopic wires or synthesizing crystals for microelectronic components. Because of a capsid's uniform size and shape, scientists see it as the ultimate small test tube.

Investigators at Montana State University have put the theory to work. Mark Young and his colleagues cultivated masses of viruses, separated the capsids from the genomes, then reassembled the capsid. They combined the protein shells with tungsten salts and found that tungsten molecules penetrate when the acidity level is varied to control the pore size. Soon they were dreaming of constructing computer chips inside a viral capsid—and perhaps a new meaning for the phrase "computer virus."

Next comes the period of **biosynthesis**. First the phage DNA uses bacterial nucleotides and enzymes to synthesize multiple copies of itself. Then the DNA is used to encode viral proteins. Messenger RNA molecules transcribed from phage DNA appear in the cytoplasm, and the biosynthesis of phage enzymes and capsid proteins begins. Bacterial ribosomes, amino acids, and enzymes are all enlisted for the biosynthesis. Because viral capsids are repeating units of capsomeres, a relatively simple genetic code can be used over and over. For a number of minutes, called the **eclipse period**, no viral parts are present. Then they begin to appear.

Ribosomes: ultramicroscopic particles of RNA and protein important in protein synthesis.

The next phase is known as **maturation**. Now the segments of bacteriophage DNA and the capsids are assembled into complete virions. The enzymes encoded by viral genes guide the assembly in step-by-step fashion. In one area, phage heads and tails are assembled from protein subunits; in another, the heads are packaged with DNA; and in a third, the tails are attached to the heads.

The final stage of viral replication is the **release** phase. For bacteriophages, this is also called the **lysis stage** because the cell membrane lyses, or breaks open. For some phages, the important enzyme in this process is **lysozyme**, encoded by the bacteriophage genes late in the sequence of events. The enzyme degrades the bacterial cell wall, and the newly released bacteriophages are set free to infect other bacteria. The progressive disintegration of bacteria by lysis inspired Twort and d'Herrelle to name the viruses bacteriophages, or "bacteria-eaters."

Lysozyme: an enzyme that degrades bacterial cell walls, especially those of Gram-positive species.

The time that passes from phage attachment to the release of new viruses is commonly referred to as the **burst time**. For bacteriophages, the burst time averages from 20 to 40 minutes. At the conclusion of the process, 50 to 200 new phages emerge from the host cell. This number is commonly called the **burst size**.

THE REPLICATION OF ANIMAL VIRUSES

The method of replication displayed by T-even phages is similar to that in animal viruses, but with some notable exceptions. One example is the attachment phase. Like bacteriophages, animal viruses have attachment sites, but the receptor sites exist on the host cell membrane rather than the cell wall. Furthermore, animal viruses have no tails, so the attachment sites are distributed over the entire surface of the capsid. And the sites themselves vary. For example, adenoviruses have small fibers at

Adenoviruses: a collection of icosahedral DNA viruses that cause diseases of the upper respiratory tract.

TABLE 11.1

The Replication of Bacteriophages and Animal Viruses Compared

	BACTERIOPHAGE	ANIMAL VIRUS
Attachment	Precise attachment of special tail fibers to cell wall	Attachment of spikes, capsid, or envelope to cell surface receptors
Penetration	Phage tail dissolves cell wall; nucleic acid passes through	Whole virus enters cell, or viral envelope fuses with cell membrane; nucleic acid is released
Biosynthesis and maturation	Occurs in cytoplasm Host cell activity ceases Viral DNA replicates and begins to function Viral components synthesized	Occurs in cytoplasm and nucleus Host cell activity ceases Viral DNA or RNA replicates and begins to function Viral components synthesized
Release from host cell	Cell lyses when viral enzymes weaken it	Some cells lyse; enveloped viruses bud through host cell membrane
Cell destruction	Immediate	Immediate; some delayed

the corners of the icosahedron, while influenza viruses have spikes on the envelope surface. TABLE 11.1 summarizes some differences we shall discuss.

An understanding of the attachment phase can have practical consequences because the host's receptor sites are inherited characteristics. The sites vary from person to person, which may account for the susceptibility of different individuals to a particular virus. In addition, a drug aimed at an attachment site could conceivably bring an infection to an end. Many pharmaceutical scientists are investigating this approach to antiviral therapy. Indeed, a drug that prevents the attachment of influenza viruses to their host cells is now available (Chapter 12).

Penetration is also different. Phages inject their DNA into the host cell cytoplasm, but animal viruses are usually taken *in toto* into the cytoplasm. In some cases, the viral envelope fuses with the cell membrane and releases the nucleocapsid into the cytoplasm. In other cases, the virion attaches to a small outfolding of the cell membrane, and the cell then enfolds the virion within a vesicle and brings it into the cytoplasm like a piece of food during phagocytosis. FIGURE 11.12 illustrates this process.

Uncoating takes place after the nucleocapsid has entered the cytoplasm. In this process, the protein coat is separated from the nucleic acid, probably by the activity of lysosomal enzymes derived from **lysosomes**, which are enzyme-containing organelles found in most eukaryotic cells. In a DNA virus, a specific enzyme encoded by the viral DNA contributes to uncoating.

Now the process diverges once again because some animal viruses contain DNA, while some contain RNA. The DNA of a DNA virus supplies the genetic codes for enzymes that synthesize viral parts from available building blocks. A number of DNA viruses, such as poxviruses, replicate entirely in the host cell cytoplasm. Other DNA viruses employ a division of labor: DNA genomes are synthesized in the host cell nucleus, and protein capsids are produced in the cytoplasm (FIGURE 11.13). The proteins then migrate to the nucleus and join with the nucleic acid molecules for assembly. Adenoviruses and herpesviruses follow this pattern.

RNA viruses follow a slightly different pattern. The RNA can act as a messenger RNA molecule (Chapter 5) and immediately begin supplying the codes for protein

Lysosomal enzymes:
enzymes from the lysosome, a saclike organelle of eukaryotic cells.

Herpesviruses:
a group of icosahedral DNA viruses involved in herpes simplex, chickenpox, and infectious mononucleosis.

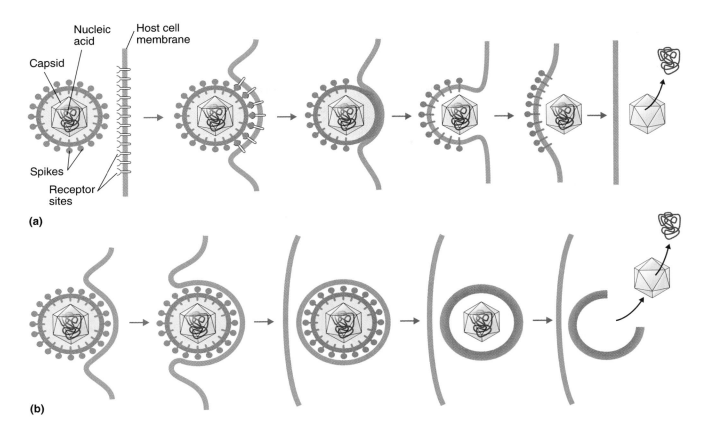

FIGURE 11.12

The Entry of Animal Viruses into Their Host Cells

Animal viruses enter their host cells by two major methods. (a) In the first method, an enveloped virus contacts the cell (plasma) membrane, and the spikes interact with receptor sites on the membrane surface. This action is highly specific for the viral spikes and receptor sites. The envelope lipids "blend" with lipids of the membrane, and the nucleocapsid passes into the host cell's cytoplasm. Then the nucleic acid is released. (b) In the second method, a specific interaction between spikes and receptor sites takes place, and a vesicle forms around the virus. The vesicle pinches off into the cytoplasm, then the envelope "blends" with the vesicle membrane. This liberates the nucleocapsid into the cytoplasm, and the nucleic acid is released.

synthesis. Such a virus is said to have "sense"; it is called a **positive-stranded RNA virus,** or **sense virus.** In other RNA viruses, however, the RNA is used as a template to synthesize a complementary strand of RNA. The latter is then used as a messenger RNA molecule for protein synthesis. The original RNA strand is said to have "antisense," and the virus is therefore an **antisense virus.** It is also called a **negative-stranded RNA virus.** Usually the enzyme RNA polymerase is present in the virus to synthesize the complementary strand. Measles viruses are antisense (negative-stranded) viruses, whereas polio viruses are sense (positive-stranded) viruses.

One RNA virus called the **retrovirus** has a particularly interesting method of replication. Retroviruses carry their own enzyme, called **reverse transcriptase.** The enzyme uses the viral RNA as a template to synthesize single-stranded DNA (the terms *reverse transcriptase* and *retrovirus* are derived from this reversal of the usual

Reverse transcriptase:
an enzyme that synthesizes DNA using the genetic message contained in RNA.

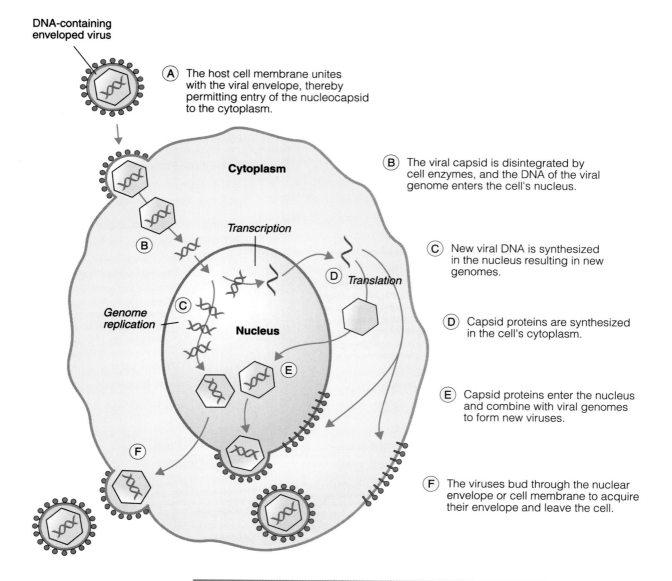

DNA-containing enveloped virus

(A) The host cell membrane unites with the viral envelope, thereby permitting entry of the nucleocapsid to the cytoplasm.

Cytoplasm

(B) The viral capsid is disintegrated by cell enzymes, and the DNA of the viral genome enters the cell's nucleus.

Transcription

(C) New viral DNA is synthesized in the nucleus resulting in new genomes.

(D) Translation

Genome replication

Nucleus

(D) Capsid proteins are synthesized in the cell's cytoplasm.

(E) Capsid proteins enter the nucleus and combine with viral genomes to form new viruses.

(F) The viruses bud through the nuclear envelope or cell membrane to acquire their envelope and leave the cell.

FIGURE 11.13

Replication of a DNA Animal Virus

The virus illustrated here is a herpesvirus (such as one that might cause genital herpes), and the host cell is from human skin.

biochemistry). Once formed, the DNA serves as a template to form a complementary DNA strand. The viral RNA is then destroyed, and the two DNA strands twist around each other to form a double helix. The DNA now migrates to the cell nucleus and integrates into one of the host cell's chromosomes, where it is known as a **provirus**, as shown in FIGURE 11.14. From this position, the DNA encodes new retroviruses. The process we have described here applies to certain leukemia viruses and to the human immunodeficiency virus (HIV) that causes AIDS (Chapter 13).

The final steps of viral replication may include the acquisition of an envelope. In this step, envelope proteins are synthesized and incorporated into a membrane within the cytoplasm or at the surface of the cell. Then the virus pushes through the

Retrovirus:
a virus whose reverse transcriptase uses RNA as a template to synthesize DNA for incorporation into a cell's nucleic acid.

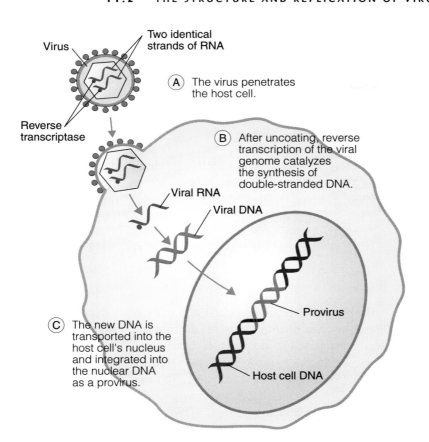

FIGURE 11.14

The Formation of a Provirus

Virus

Two identical strands of RNA

(A) The virus penetrates the host cell.

Reverse transcriptase

(B) After uncoating, reverse transcription of the viral genome catalyzes the synthesis of double-stranded DNA.

Viral RNA

Viral DNA

(C) The new DNA is transported into the host cell's nucleus and integrated into the nuclear DNA as a provirus.

Provirus

Host cell DNA

membrane, forcing a portion of the membrane ahead of it and around it, resulting in an envelope. This process, called **budding**, need not necessarily kill the cell during the virus' exit. The same cannot be said for unenveloped viruses, however. They leave the cell when the cell membrane ruptures, a process that generally leads to cell death.

Before we leave viral replication, we should note that living cells may not be an absolute necessity for the process to occur. Recent research indicates that cell debris may provide enough essentials to ensure viral replication (MicroFocus 11.4).

LYSOGENY

In the replication cycles, infection need not result in new viral particles or cell lysis. Rather, the virus may integrate its DNA or its RNA (via DNA) into a chromosome of the cell (as described in the previous paragraphs) and achieve a state called **lysogeny**. When bacteriophages are involved, the phage DNA in the lysogenic state is called a **prophage**; when an animal virus (such as a retrovirus) is involved, the viral DNA is known as a **provirus**. In both cases, it appears that the viral genome is encoding a repressor protein that prevents activation of the genes necessary for replication.

Lysogeny may have several implications. Viruses in the lysogenic state, for example, are immune to body defenses since the body's antibodies cannot reach them (antibodies do not penetrate into cells). Moreover, the virus is propagated each time the cell's chromosome is reproduced, such as during mitosis in animal cells. And the prophage or provirus can confer new properties on the infected cell, such as when a toxin-encoding prophage infects a bacterium. A case in point is *Clostridium botulinum*, a bacterium whose lethal toxin is encoded by an indwelling prophage (Chapter 8).

li-soj'ih-ne
Lysogeny:
the condition in which viruses and bacteria coexist without damage to each other.

MicroFocus 11.4

OUT TO DINNER

A fundamental tenet of microbiology is that viruses replicate only in living cells. This principle was challenged during the winter of 1992, when researchers at the State University of New York at Stony Brook managed to cultivate viruses outside of intact cells.

A research group, led by Eckard Wimmer, had been trying for years to replicate polio viruses in the right combination of crushed human cell debris, plus salts, ATP, nucleotides, and amino acids. Dozens of their combinations had been unsuccessful, but they persisted in the research. On that fateful January afternoon, they added fragments of RNA from polio viruses to their latest test tube concoction and set up the myriad controls necessary for a successful experiment. Then they went to dinner.

By the time they returned, history had been made. There in the mixture were whole, intact polio viruses—viruses produced without the benefit of living cells. The scientists gasped in disbelief, congratulated one another, and began to ponder the implications of their discovery. The research implications would be enormous, as would the philosophical implications. At the very least, the definition of a virus would have to change forever.

T-lymphocyte:
an immune system cell that functions in cell-mediated immunity.

Another is the bacterium of diphtheria (Chapter 7). A third is the situation where the body's T-lymphocytes harbor the human immunodeficiency virus (HIV) in its provirus form. Such an individual has **HIV infection**.

A phenomenon traced to lysogeny is **specialized transduction**. In this process, a fragment of DNA from one cell is transferred to a second cell in combination with bacteriophage DNA (Chapter 6). A final implication involves cancer. As we shall see later in this chapter, cancer may develop when a virus enters a cell and assumes a lysogenic relationship with that cell. The proteins encoded by the virus often bring about the profound changes associated with this dreaded condition.

To this point . . .

We have begun a study of viruses by discussing their size, shape, and method of replication. We noted that some viruses have icosahedral symmetry, while others have helical symmetry, and others have a complex symmetry with a variety of shapes. However, all viruses consist of a genome of RNA or DNA, and a protein capsid. Some viruses are surrounded by a flexible membranous envelope. The complete virus is a virion.

We then studied the replication of viruses using the bacteriophage and its bacterial host as a model. The process begins with a union between phage and bacterium, followed by penetration of the viral DNA to the bacterial cytoplasm. Synthesis and release of new virions are the final two stages. Using the model as a basis, we noted how animal viruses differ in their replication mode, especially with respect to adsorption and penetration. Differences are also observed in DNA and RNA viruses. The discussion concluded with the concept of lysogeny, where viruses remain in their host cells for long time periods as proviruses or prophages.

Our survey of viral characteristics will continue in the final section. We shall see how viruses are classified and how viral diseases are detected. Inhibition of viruses using drugs inside the body will be surveyed, and we shall mention the types of viral vaccines. We shall also see how viruses can be inactivated outside the body. There will be an extensive treatment of the role of viruses in cancer, and the chapter will conclude with discussions of viroids and prions, two types of infectious subviral particles.

11.3

Other Characteristics of Viruses

Like all other microorganisms, viruses have characteristics that set them apart and help virologists understand their activities and deal with them effectively. In this section, we shall examine some of these characteristics.

NOMENCLATURE AND CLASSIFICATION

A widely accepted classification system for viruses has not yet been devised, in part because sufficient data are not yet available to determine how different viruses relate to one another. Viruses therefore lack formal names (a fact that does not seem to bother students). Instead, they have acquired their names from several sources. Examples are the measles virus (after the disease); the adenovirus (after the adenoids, where it is commonly located); the Coxsackie virus (after Coxsackie, New York, where it was originally isolated); and the Epstein-Barr virus (after researchers who studied it). The situation is reminiscent of the late 1800s, when different bacteria were called the "tubercle bacillus," or the "diphtheria bacillus," or the "cholera bacillus."

cook-sak'e

This is not to say, however, that no classification system exists for viruses. Indeed, one classification scheme is loosely based on the body tissues affected by the virus. Though inexact, this scheme places viruses into four convenient groups, depending on whether they replicate in the respiratory, skin, visceral, or nervous tissue (TABLE 11.2). We shall use this scheme in Chapters 12 and 13.

Visceral: pertaining to the organs in the large cavities of the body, especially the abdominal cavity.

A second classification system is in the process of evolving. At periodic meetings of the International Committee on Taxonomy of Viruses, a revised and updated viral classification scheme is presented. At this writing, no orders, divisions, or kingdom have been established for viruses, but virologists have prepared a working document in which a viral species is defined as a group of viruses sharing the same genetic information and ecological niche. Names have not yet been established for species, but the viruses have been categorized into genera; each genus name ends with the

TABLE 11.2

Classification of Human Viral Diseases by Tissue Affected

GROUP	TISSUES AFFECTED	IMPORTANT DISEASES
Pneumotropic	Respiratory system	Influenza, respiratory syncytial disease, adenovirus diseases, rhinovirus infection
Dermotropic	Skin and subcutaneous tissues	Chickenpox, herpes simplex, measles, mumps, smallpox, molluscum contagiosum, rubella
Viscerotropic	Blood and visceral organs	Yellow fever, dengue fever, infectious mononucleosis, cytomegalovirus disease, viral fevers, viral gastroenteritis, hepatitis A, hepatitis B, AIDS
Neurotropic	Central nervous system	Rabies, polio, bovine spongiform encephalopathy, arboviral encephalitis

TABLE 11.3

Major Families of Animal Viruses and Their Characteristics

FAMILY	STRAND TYPE	CAPSID SYMMETRY	ENVELOPE	DIAMETER (NM)	COMMON NAME OF IMPORTANT MEMBERS
DNA Viruses					
Poxviridae	Double	None	+	130–300	Smallpox virus, cowpox virus
Herpesviridae	Double	Icosahedral	+	150–200	Herpes simplex virus, varicella zoster virus, Epstein–Barr virus, cytomegalovirus
Adenoviridae	Double	Icosahedral	−	70–90	Human adenoviruses
Papovaviridae	Double	Icosahedral	−	45–55	Human papillomavirus
Hepadnaviridae	Single or double	Icosahedral	+	42	Hepatitis B virus
Parvoviridae	Single	Icosahedral	−	18–26	Parvovirus B19
RNA Viruses					
Picornaviridae	Single	Icosahedral	−	20–30	Hepatitis A virus, polio virus, Coxsackie viruses, rhinoviruses
Calciviridae	Single	Icosahedral	−	35–40	Norwalk virus
Togaviridae	Single	Icosahedral	+	45–70	Rubella virus, equine encephalitis viruses
Flaviviridae	Single	Icosahedral	+	40–70	Yellow fever virus, Japanese encephalitis virus, dengue fever virus, hepatitis C virus
Filoviridae	Single	Helical	+	80–10,000	Ebola and Marburg viruses
Bunyaviridae	Single	Helical	+	90–100	Bunyamwera virus, hantavirus
Reoviridae	Double	Icosahedral	−	60–80	Human rotavirus, Colorado tick fever virus
Orthomyxoviridae	Single	Helical	+	80–120	Influenza viruses
Paramyxoviridae	Single	Helical	+	125–250	Parainfluenza virus, mumps virus, measles virus
Rhabdoviridae	Single	Helical	+	60–175	Rabies virus, animal viruses
Retroviridae	Single	Icosahedral	+	100	Human immunodeficiency virus (HIV), tumor viruses
Arenaviridae	Single	?	+	50–300	Lassa virus, lymphocytic choriomeningitis virus
Coronaviridae	Single	Helical	+	80–130	Coronaviruses

suffix -*virus* (e.g., *Herpesvirus*). The genera have then been organized into 73 families, each ending with -*viridae* (e.g., Herpesviridae). A selection of viral families and genera affecting humans, together with some of their characteristics, is presented in TABLE 11.3. Note that due to the rapid changes taking place in viral taxonomy, some new names may be in use by the time you read this.

THE DETECTION OF VIRUSES

The methods used to detect viruses are more involved and considerably more time-consuming than for bacteria and other microorganisms. Plant and animal tissues are difficult and expensive to maintain, and pathogenic viruses often replicate only in human host cells, which causes additional complications. By contrast, bacteriophages are easily cultivated in bacterial cultures, and bacteriophages have been used as models for studying viral characteristics.

One common method of cultivating viruses is to inoculate them into fertilized chicken eggs. A hole is drilled in the shell of the egg, and a suspension of viral material is introduced. Because different viruses replicate in different membranes or parts of the chick embryo, virologists must anticipate which virus is present. Viral replication is detected by either the death of the embryo, cell damage to the embryo or its membranes, or the formation of characteristic lesions at the site of inoculation.

Another method of detecting viruses is to inoculate suspensions of material to **tissue cultures**. To prepare the culture, cells are separated from a tissue with enzymes and suspended in a solution of nutrients, growth factors, pH buffers, and salts. The cells adhere to the wall of the container and reproduce to form a single layer, or monolayer. When viruses replicate in these cells, a noticeable deterioration occurs. This is called a **cytopathic effect (CPE)**.

An indirect method for detecting viruses is to search for viral antibodies in a patient's serum. This can be done by combining serum (the blood's fluid portion) with known viruses. In some serological tests, the viruses are attached to carrier particles, and the reaction results in a visible clumping. Certain viruses—such as those of influenza, measles, and mumps—have the ability to agglutinate (clump) red blood cells. This phenomenon, called **hemagglutination (HA)**, can be used for detection purposes. In addition, it is possible to detect antibodies against certain viruses because antibodies react with viruses and tie up the reaction sites, thereby inhibiting hemagglutination. Thus, a laboratory test for antibodies can be performed by combining the patient's serum with known viruses and red blood cells. Hemagglutination indicates that antibodies are absent from the serum, but the **hemagglutination-inhibition (HAI) test** points to the presence of serum antibodies (FIGURE 11.15). Such a finding implies that the patient has been exposed to the viruses. Chapter 19 explores gene probes and other contemporary approaches to viral detection.

In certain instances, viruses leave signs of their presence in infected tissue. For example, the brain cells of a rabid animal contain cytoplasmic granules called **Negri bodies**, and cells from herpes simplex patients have nuclear granules known as

Cytopathic effect:
deterioration and destruction of host cells by viruses.

Serological test:
a test that detects the presence of antibodies or antigens.

heme'ag-glu-tin-a'shun
Hemagglutination:
the clumping of red blood cells.

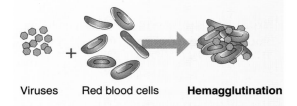

Viruses   Red blood cells   Hemagglutination

(a)

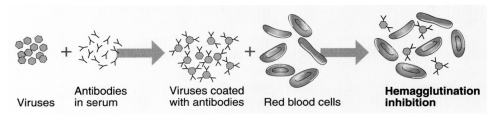

Viruses   Antibodies in serum   Viruses coated with antibodies   Red blood cells   Hemagglutination inhibition

(b)

FIGURE 11.15

The Hemagglutination-Inhibition Test

(a) Viruses of certain diseases, such as measles and mumps, are able to agglutinate (clump) red blood cells. (b) In the hemagglutination-inhibition (HAI) test, known viruses are combined with serum from a patient. If the serum contains antibodies for that virus, the antibodies coat the virus, and when the viruses are then combined with red blood cells, no agglutination will take place. Since the nature of the virus is known, the type of antibody present can be determined.

MicroFocus 11.5

ESCAPE

European rabbits had been a scourge in Australia ever since English settlers released a dozen of them in 1840. True to their reputation, the new arrivals bred prolifically, and by 1995, over 300 million rabbits dotted the Australian landscape.

But Australian scientists had a plan: They quarantined several thousand rabbits on Wardang Island off Australia's southern coast and infected them with calciviruses. (Calciviruses are a group of RNA viruses with cuplike projections on their surfaces. They quickly kill rabbits by causing blood clots in vital organs.) To reduce the spread of either viruses or rabbits, the scientists inspected the fences daily and tested the blood of wild rabbits outside the pens for evidence of calciviruses. If the experiment was successful on the island, they would consider releasing viruses on the Australian mainland.

Unfortunately, the viruses escaped. By September 1995, scientists were finding dead rabbits outside the pens and then on the mainland. The dead rabbits had evidence of calcivirus disease. There was no question: The virus was out of quarantine.(Research conducted in 1997 indicates that various insects carry the virus; in retrospect, that may have been the escape route.)

Now the scientists had some difficult days ahead. They would have to wait to learn whether the virus interrupts the breeding success of survivors; also, they would have to go without knowing how long the virus lasts in the environment. The escape was final and irrevocable. The genie was out of the bottle. They would have to go ahead with the general release.

Virologists and veterinarians acted swiftly. With government approval, they released infected rabbits at hundreds of sites on the mainland and hoped for the best. Soon, dead rabbits were everywhere. Within 2 years, the rabbit population was reduced by 95 percent in some areas; and many plant and animal species, preyed on by the rabbits, were rebounding after remaining unseen for generations. At this writing, the native wildlife remain unaffected, except that eagles and other predators of rabbits have declined in numbers. At first, scientists were discouraged at having to act in haste, but in this instance, the escape apparently had a beneficial twist. At least, so far.

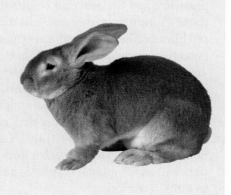

Lipschütz bodies:
granules in the nucleus of cells infected by herpes simplex viruses.

Lymphocyte:
a type of white blood cell important in specific immune system defenses.

Lipschütz bodies. Moreover, a series of cellular or tissue modifications may signal the presence of viruses. Infectious mononucleosis, for example, is characterized by large numbers of swollen lymphocytes with foamy, highly vacuolated cytoplasm. Physicians call these cells **Downey cells**. Measles is accompanied by **Koplik spots**, a series of bright red patches with white pimplelike centers on the lateral mouth surfaces. Swollen salivary glands and teardroplike skin lesions are associated with mumps and chickenpox, respectively. Blood clots are associated with certain viruses, as MicroFocus 11.5 indicates.

The most obvious method for detecting viruses is by direct observation with the electron microscope. In this procedure, tissue samples may be examined directly or after viral cultivation. Virologists are often able to identify unknown viruses by comparison to known viruses.

Plaque:
a clear area on a lawn of bacteria where bacteriophages have destroyed the cells.

Phage typing:
a method of identifying an unknown bacterium by its reaction with a known bacteriophage.

Bacterial viruses (bacteriophages) may be detected by the formation of plaques. A **plaque** is a clear "moth-eaten" area on a cloudy "lawn" of bacteria where bacteriophages have destroyed the cells. Technologists first cultivate the bacteria on an agar surface, then add the viruses by spraying or other methods (FIGURE 11.16). If the viruses are specific for that particular bacterium, they infect and replicate in the cells, thereby destroying them and forming plaques. This method can also be reversed, so that a known phage is used to detect an unknown bacterium. Epidemiological surveys of several bacterial diseases such as staphylococcal food poisoning are aided by this procedure, often called **phage typing** (FIGURE 11.17).

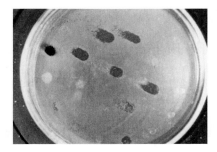

FIGURE 11.16

The Process of Plaque Formation

Susceptible bacteria are inoculated into plates of nutrient medium. Bacterial viruses are then sprayed onto the
surface, and the plate is incubated. As viruses replicate
in the bacteria, they destroy the cells and leave clear
"moth-eaten" areas containing no bacteria. These areas
are the plaques shown on the plate in the photograph.

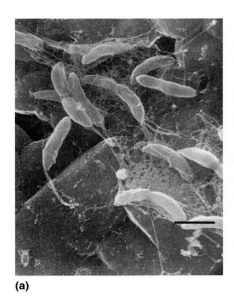

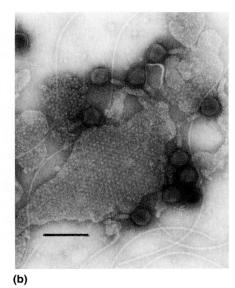

(a)   **(b)**

FIGURE 11.17

A Bacterium and Its Bacteriophage

(a) The bacterium *Caulobacter crescentus*, a Gram-negative rod typically found in freshwater environments. (Bar = 0.2 μm.) (b) The bacteriophage φCR30, the phage that replicates within *C. crescentus*.
The icosahedral head and the tail of the phages are visible. The long lines in the photograph are bacterial flagella amid the debris. (Bar = 5 μm.)

The difficulty in detecting viruses has a bearing on relating a particular virus to a
particular disease. In the classical sense, Koch's postulates cannot be applied to a viral
disease because the viruses cannot be cultivated in pure culture. To circumvent this
problem, **Thomas M. Rivers** in 1937 expanded Koch's postulates to include viruses
as follows: Filtrates of the infectious material shown not to contain bacteria or
other cultivatable organisms must produce the disease or its counterpart; or, the filtrates must produce specific antibodies in appropriate animals. This concept has
come to be known as **Rivers' postulate**.

THE INHIBITION OF VIRUSES

During periods of disease, the human body attempts to rid itself of viruses
mainly by phagocytosis, neutralization with antibodies, and interactions with T-
lymphocytes. **Antibodies** are immune system protein molecules that react with
viruses. Usually one antibody molecule unites specifically with a single virion,

Phagocytosis:
a defensive measure of the body
in which white blood cells engulf
and destroy microorganisms.

thereby preventing the virion from binding to its host cell. Antibodies also clump viruses into large masses efficiently removed by **phagocytosis**. In addition, viruses activate the complement system, a group of substances that encourage phagocytosis (Chapter 18). Finally, an important source of defense is the body's **T-lymphocytes** (also called T-cells). When activated by viruses, T-lymphocytes migrate to virus-infected cells and interact directly with the cells, destroying the cells and the viruses within the cells (Chapter 18).

Normal body defenses against viral disease cannot be supplemented by common antibiotics because viruses lack the structures and metabolic substances with which antibiotics interfere. For example, penicillin is useless for inhibiting viruses because viruses have no cell wall. However, several drugs have been proven effective against viruses. One drug, called **amantadine** (Symmetrel), prevents the attachment of influenza viruses to the host cell surface. Another drug, **vidarabine** (Vira-A), is used for treating herpes zoster (shingles) and encephalitis (brain disease) due to the herpes simplex virus. A third drug, **acyclovir** (Zovirax), has been available since 1985 as a topical ointment for genital herpes and more recently, for chickenpox.

ah-man'tah-dēn

vi-dar'ah-bēn

a-si'klo-vir

Acyclovir is typical of antimicrobial agents called **base analogs**. These substances resemble nitrogenous bases and are erroneously incorporated into viral DNA. Other base analogs called **idoxuridine (IDU)** and **trifluridine** are taken up by herpesviruses in place of thymine, and the resulting genome cannot replicate itself. The base analog **azidothymidine (AZT)** has been used since 1987 to treat HIV infection and AIDS, and two other analogs called **dideoxyinosine (ddI)** and **dideoxycytidine (ddC)** are approved, also for treating AIDS. Another drug called **foscarnet** is used in patients having retinal disease (retinitis) caused by the cytomegalovirus (CMV). **Ganciclovir** is also used against CMV infection.

i-doks-ur'ĭ-dēn
tri-floor'ĭ-dēn

a-zi'do-thi'-mi-dēn

fos-kar'net

gan-si'klo-vir

Another class of antiviral drug is called **reverse transcriptase inhibitors**. These drugs bind directly to reverse transcriptase and inhibit its activity, thereby preventing the synthesis of DNA in retroviruses. Used primarily against HIV, these medications include **nevirapine** and **delavirdine**. Still another class is **protease inhibitors**. These drugs react with protease, the enzyme that trims viral proteins down to working size for the construction of the capsid. Examples are **saquinavir** (Invirase), **indinavir** (Crixivan), and **ritonavir** (Norvir). They are used in patients with HIV infection and AIDS.

ne-vir'a-pin
de-la-vir'din
sa-quin'a-vir
in-din'a-vir
ri-ton'a-vir
Protease:
an enzyme that digests protein.

A final class of antiviral drug currently in the testing stage is called **neuraminidase inhibitors**. Neuraminidase is an enzyme in the spike of the influenza virus. It encourages attachment of the viruses to the respiratory cells in humans (Chapter 12). The new neuraminidase inhibitor drugs clog the site where neuraminidase attaches, thereby preventing attachment and encouraging resistance to the virus. One such drug, named **zanamivir**, was developed by biochemists based on their knowledge of the molecular structure of neuraminidase and its attachment site. Zanamivir and a similar drug named oseltamivir (Tamiflu) are products of human ingenuity. Indeed, medical science may one day provide an antiviral drug to deal with obesity (MicroFocus 11.6).

za-nam'i-vir

o-sel-tam'i-vir

Interferon represents one of the most optimistic approaches to inhibiting viruses. First identified in 1957 by Alick Isaacs and Jean Lindenmann, interferon is not a single substance but a group of over 20 substances designated alpha, beta, and gamma interferons. Each group has several members, and all appear to be proteins. Interferons are produced by various body cells on stimulation by viruses. (Dendritic cells of the immune system—Chapter 18—produce large amounts of alpha-interferon.) They trigger a nonspecific reaction that protects against the stimulating virus, as well

in'ter-fēr'on
Interferons:
a group of cellular proteins
that provide protection against
viruses.

MicroFocus 11.6

OVERWEIGHT? TAKE AN ANTIBIOTIC

It's far out, to be sure, but as of 1997, University of Wisconsin researchers have linked a virus to obesity. And, they maintain, it may be possible one day to eliminate the virus and slim down quickly by taking an antiviral antibiotic.

The road to this startling conclusion began in 1990 with a veterinarian's chance remark that chickens infected with adenoviruses gain considerable weight. The conversation took place in Bombay, India, and the second participant in was Nikhil V. Dhurandhar (du-ran'dar). Dhurandhar was a nutritionist on his way to Wisconsin to do research. The veterinarian's observation was intriguing, and Dhurandhar resolved to pursue it.

At the medical school in Wisconsin, the fledgling researcher obtained a flock of chickens and a culture of adenoviruses (respiratory viruses often involved in the common cold). He soon confirmed that in chickens, the viruses are pathogenic and bring on rapid mortality—but not before the chickens become unusually obese, just as the vet had said.

But did it work that way with people? Dhurandhar solicited volunteers and got responses from 45 lean individuals and 154 obese people, each weighing over 250 pounds. The investigator was working with adenovirus strain 36 (AD-36), and antibodies against this virus would prove that it was currently in the body or that it had once been there. Dhu-

randhar took blood samples and analyzed them: None of the lean individuals had AD-36 antibodies, but 15 percent of the obese people had the telltale antibodies.

Although the results pointed to a relationship between virus and obesity, the waters soon became muddy: Obese individuals usually have high blood levels of cholesterol and triglycerides; however, the 15 percent with AD-36 antibodies had normal levels. This observation remains perplexing.

In the early 1980s, few people were willing to believe that gastric ulcers are related to a bacterium (Chapter 8), but the relationship is now an accepted tenet of medicine. Linking obesity to a virus may seem like a stretch. Still . . .

---

as many other viruses. In addition, some interferons have anticancer properties. However, human interferon is the only one that will work in humans. Mouse, chicken, dog, or other animal interferons are ineffective.

Unlike antibodies, interferons do not interact directly with viruses, but with the cells they protect. For this reason, they have a broader inhibitory effect. Interferons are produced when a virion releases its genome into the cell. The viral material (probably a double strand of RNA) induces the cell to synthesize and secrete interferons. These bind to specific receptor sites on the surfaces of adjacent cells and trigger the production of several proteins within those cells. The proteins inhibit viral replication by methods not completely understood, although many virologists believe that at least one protein binds to messenger RNA molecules encoded by the virus (FIGURE 11.18). Interferons also appear to mobilize natural killer cells, which attack tumor cells (Chapter 20).

The inability to obtain sufficient funding stifled interferon research for many years. (One approach was to inoculate huge batches of white blood cells with harmless viruses.) However, a breakthrough came in 1980 when Swiss and Japanese scientists deciphered the genetic code for interferon, and spliced *E. coli* plasmids with the genes for interferon synthesis (Chapter 6). Experiments showed that interferon from bacterial factories would reduce hepatitis symptoms, diminish the spread of herpes zoster, and shrink certain cancers. In 1984, a Swiss biotechnology firm began marketing alpha-interferon using the trade name Intron. In 1986, the U.S. Food and Drug Administration approved the sale of alpha-interferon for use against a form of leukemia; in 1988, it approved its use against genital warts; and in 1992, against chronic hepatitis B.

Plasmid:
a closed-loop unit of bacterial DNA existing apart from the chromosome.

FIGURE 11.18

The Production and Activity of Interferon

Left: A host cell produces interferon following exposure to the RNA associated with a virus. Viruses replicate in the same cell. Right: The interferon reacts with receptors at the surface of a neighboring cell and induces the cell to produce antiviral proteins. The proteins interfere with viral replication in the cell, possibly by binding to messenger RNA molecules.

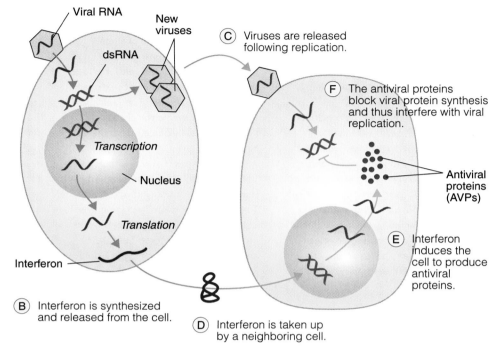

(A) Viral RNA stimulates the host to synthesize interferon while also directing replication of new viruses.

Viral RNA

New viruses

dsRNA

(C) Viruses are released following replication.

(F) The antiviral proteins block viral protein synthesis and thus interfere with viral replication.

Transcription

Nucleus

Antiviral proteins (AVPs)

Translation

(E) Interferon induces the cell to produce antiviral proteins.

Interferon

(B) Interferon is synthesized and released from the cell.

(D) Interferon is taken up by a neighboring cell.

VIRAL VACCINES

Despite the optimism inspired by the new drugs, the major approach to viral disease continues to be prevention through public education and the use of **vaccines**. Vaccines stimulate antibody production by the immune system and thereby induce specific defense (**MicroFocus 11.7**). They can also stimulate the production of killer T-cells (Chapter 18).

Several types of viral vaccines are currently in use. One type contains **inactivated viruses**, which are viruses treated with a physical agent (such as mild heat) or a chemical agent (such as formaldehyde). This treatment alters the genome of the virus, thereby preventing replication, but it does not severely affect the capsid, which remains intact and stimulates antibody production. Opponents of inactivated viral vaccines point out that treatment may not reach all viruses, and that untreated viruses may remain active and cause disease. They also note that the vaccine must be given by injection to ensure an immune response, and that the immune response is low relative to that elicited by the second type of vaccine.

The second type of vaccine contains **attenuated viruses**, which are viruses that continue replicating in body cells but at an extremely low rate. Attenuated viruses stimulate the immune system for a longer period of time than inactivated viruses, and thus the immune response is higher. They are obtained by transferring viruses from culture to culture for a period of months or years, until a variant emerges with a greatly reduced replication rate. Opponents of attenuated viral vaccines suggest that the viruses may revert to their original form and cause disease, and that the viruses

Inactivated viruses: viruses that cannot replicate due to alteration of the genome.

ah-ten'u-a'ted
Attenuated viruses: viruses that replicate at a very low rate.

MicroFocus 11.7

USEFUL INTERFERENCE

In order for a virus to infect a cell, it must first dock at the cell's receptor site. After this "marriage" of sorts has taken place, the viral genome enters the cell and replication proceeds. But suppose the cell receptors were hidden from the virus? Would that prevent viral replication from taking place? And would the cell be protected?

Apparently, the answer is yes on both counts. In a canyon near Lake Casitas, about 40 miles northwest of Los Angeles, lives a unique population of mice. Somewhere in the ancient past, the cells of these mice acquired the ability to produce proteins normally found in a virus. In an amazing twist of evolution, a virus probably entered the mouse cells, and viral genes that normally encode capsid production became part of the mouse cell chromosomes. So endowed, the mouse cells began producing capsid proteins, and the proteins adhered to viral receptors at the cell surface. With the receptors tied up, the mice became

immune to the virus, and, as natural selection proceeded, an entire colony of immune mice developed. The key piece of biochemical evidence was presented in the late 1980s when researchers from the University of California pinpointed the gene for capsid protein inside cells of the Lake Casitas mice.

Does this finding mean that cells can be protected by incorporating genes for viral proteins? Again, the answer is yes. For several years now, DNA technologists and genetic engineers have been splicing into plant cells the genes for viral proteins and have been developing disease-resistant plants. In 1993, for example, French biotechnologists protected champagne grapevines from disease by incorporating the capsid genes from grape fan-leaf viruses. Wine from these new transgenic plants is expected to reach market soon.

Can we protect humans the same way? Perhaps so, but with slight modifications. Researchers are currently

attempting to develop an AIDS vaccine by using envelope proteins from HIV. These proteins will elicit antibody production in the body. The antibodies would react with and neutralize envelope proteins on HIV, thereby preventing HIV's union with receptor sites on the body's cells. To be sure, this is not the same as the mouse-generated viral proteins, but the principle is similar: Interfere with attachment, and thereby prevent infection.

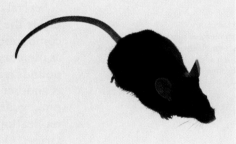

may infect cells other than the usual host cells or activate proviruses already in host cells. Moreover, attenuated viruses have been known to cause disease in rare cases.

Inactivated and attenuated viruses are sometimes called "dead" and "live" viruses, respectively, and the vaccines are therefore known by these terms (e.g., live measles vaccine). The words "dead" and "alive" are misleading, however, because they signify the life status of viruses, which remains uncertain. The **Salk vaccine** for polio typifies a vaccine made with inactivated viruses, while the **Sabin vaccine** for polio represents a vaccine made with attenuated viruses.

Another type of vaccine is composed of **viral subunits**. These are protein molecules, usually produced by genetic engineering methods. The vaccine for hepatitis B is typical. This vaccine (Chapter 13) contains capsid proteins synthesized by yeast cells genetically altered with the DNA from hepatitis B viruses. Researchers are currently pursuing a number of **DNA vaccines** for viral diseases such as AIDS. The spectrum of viral and other microbial vaccines is discussed in Chapter 19.

THE INACTIVATION OF VIRUSES

Viruses may be inactivated by many of the physical and chemical agents routinely used for other microorganisms. Among the **physical agents** are heat and ultraviolet light. **Heat** alters the structure of viral proteins and nucleic acids, causing them to unfold and denature. Sterilization temperatures reached in the autoclave (Chapter 21) will destroy all viruses, and boiling water for a few minutes will eliminate most

Autoclave:
a device that generates high-temperature steam under pressure for the destruction of microorganisms.

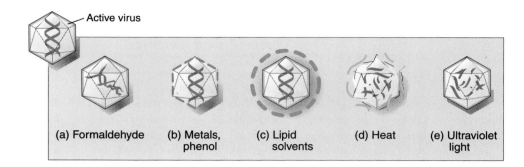

FIGURE 11.19

Six Methods of Inactivating Viruses

(a) Formaldehyde combines with free amino groups on nucleic acid bases. (b) Metals react with the protein of the viral capsid. (c) Lipid solvents dissolve the envelope in enveloped viruses. (d) Phenol reacts with proteins in the capsid. (e) Heat denatures proteins of the capsid. (f) Ultraviolet light binds together thymine molecules in the genome and distorts the nucleic acid.

Halogen:
an element whose atoms have seven electrons in the outer shell, such as chlorine, iodine, and bromine.

viruses (with the notable exception of the hepatitis A virus, which requires a longer time). **Ultraviolet (UV) light** inactivates viruses by stimulating adjacent thymine or cytosine bases on DNA molecules to bind together and form pairs called **dimers**. The dimers twist the molecule out of shape, and the distorted viral genome cannot replicate. Ultraviolet light is used in the preparation of some vaccines. **X rays** are another type of useful radiation. X rays cause breaks in the sugar-phosphate backbone of the nucleic acid.

Several **chemical agents** can be used outside the body to inactivate viruses, but not inside the body because of their toxic effects on the tissues. Examples are halogen compounds, such as chlorine and iodine derivatives; heavy metal compounds, such as mercury and silver derivatives; and phenol derivatives (Chapter 22). These compounds react strongly with protein, thereby altering the viral capsid. **Formaldehyde** is another useful chemical agent because it reacts with free amino groups on adenine, guanine, and cytosine molecules to modify the viral genome and prevent replication. The Salk polio vaccine is prepared with formaldehyde-inactivated viruses. Other valuable chemical agents are **lipid solvents**, such as ether, chloroform, and detergents, all of which dissolve the lipid in the envelope of viruses. Enzymes directed against viral proteins and nucleic acids are also useful. FIGURE 11.19 summarizes the activity of chemical and physical agents against viruses.

11.4

Viruses and Cancer

Cancer is indiscriminate. It affects humans and animals, young and old, male and female, rich and poor. In the United States, over 450,000 people die of cancer annually, making the disease the second most common cause of death after cardiovascular disease. Worldwide, over 2 million people die of cancer each year.

THE NATURE OF CANCER

Cancer results from the uncontrolled reproduction of cells through the process of mitosis: The frequency of mitosis is greater for cancer cells than for normal cells. The cells escape controlling factors and as they continue to multiply, a cluster of cells soon forms. Eventually, the cluster yields an abnormal, functionless mass of cells. This mass is called a **tumor**.

Normally, the body will respond to a tumor by surrounding it with a capsule of connective tissue. Such a tumor is designated **benign**. If, however, the cells multi-

Tumor:
an abnormal, functionless mass of cells.

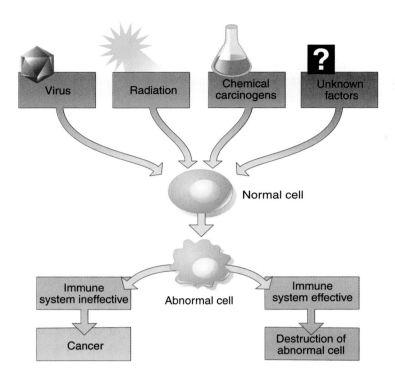

FIGURE 11.20

The Onset of Cancer

Viruses and other factors induce a normal cell to become abnormal. When the immune system is effective, it destroys the abnormal cell, and no cancer develops. However, when the abnormal cell evades the immune system, it develops first into a tumor and then into a spreading cancer.

ply too rapidly and break out of the capsule and spread, the tumor is described as **malignant**. The individual now has **cancer**, a reference to the radiating spread of cells that resemble a crab (the word is derived from the Greek *karkinos*, meaning "crab"). **Oncology**, the study of cancer, is derived from *onkos*, the Greek word for "tumor."

Cancer cells differ from normal cells in three major ways: They grow and undergo mitosis more frequently than normal cells, they stick together less firmly than normal cells, and they undergo dedifferentiation. **Dedifferentiation** means that normal cells revert to an early stage in their development. For example, when ciliated cells of the bronchi become cancer cells, they lose their cilia and dedifferentiate into formless cells that divide as rapidly as early embryonic cells. Moreover, the cells fail to exhibit **contact inhibition**; that is, they do not adhere tightly to one another, as normal cells do. Thus, they overgrow one another to form a tumor. Sometimes, they **metastasize**, or spread, to other body parts where new tumors begin. Also, they invade and grow in a broad variety of body tissues, since they do not stick to tissue cells. Through all this, the cells are evading or overcoming the natural body defenses centered in the immune system (**FIGURE 11.20**). There appears to be no boundary limiting the growth of a tumor.

How can such a mass of cells bring illness and misery to the body? By their sheer force of numbers, cancer cells invade and erode local tissues, thereby interrupting normal functions and choking organs to death. For example, a tumor in the kidney prevents kidney cells from performing their excretory function, a brain tumor cripples this organ by compressing the nerves and interfering with nerve impulse transmission, and a tumor in the bone marrow may block blood cell production.

In addition, tumor cells rob the body of vital nutrients to satisfy their own growth needs. Thus, the cancer patient will commonly experience weight loss even while maintaining a normal diet. Anemia and a general feeling of tiredness may develop when the tumor cells use up essential minerals for red blood cell

Oncology:
the study of cancer.

Metastasize:
to spread to distant locations.

Anemia:
a condition characterized by a below-normal level of red blood cells.

production. Moreover, some tumor cells are known to produce hormones identical to those normally produced by the body's endocrine glands, thereby overloading the body with chemical regulators. Some tumors block air passageways; others interfere with the immune system so that microbial diseases take hold. Tumor cells weaken the body until it fails.

THE INVOLVEMENT OF VIRUSES

Carcinogens:
cancer-causing substances.

Scientists are uncertain as to what triggers a normal cell to multiply without control. However, they know that certain chemicals are **carcinogens**, or cancer-causing substances. The World Health Organization (WHO) estimates that carcinogens may be associated with 60 to 90 percent of all human cancers. Among the known carcinogens are the hydrocarbons found in cigarette smoke, as well as asbestos, nickel, certain pesticides and dyes, and environmental pollutants in high amounts. Physical agents such as UV light and X rays are also believed to be carcinogens.

roos

There is considerable evidence that **viruses** are also carcinogens. Experiments with animals indicate that some viruses can induce tumor formation. Federal law, however, prohibits these experiments from being repeated with human volunteers, because of the serious consequences. Nevertheless, a number of viruses have been isolated from human cancers, and when these viruses are transferred to animals and tissue cultures, an observable transformation of normal cells to tumor cells takes place. Examples of such viruses are the herpesviruses associated with tumors of the human cervix and the Epstein-Barr virus, which is linked to Burkitt's lymphoma, a tumor of the jaw. As early as 1911, Peyton Rous postulated that a virus was involved in tumors in chickens.

One of the clearest virus-cancer links emerged in 1980 when a research team led by **Robert T. Gallo** of the National Cancer Institute isolated a virus that transforms normal T-lymphocytes into the malignant T-lymphocytes found in a rare cancer called **T-cell leukemia**. A year later, the same virus was found responsible for a relatively high rate of both T-cell leukemia and a form of lymphoma in Japan. Gallo identified the virus as an RNA-containing retrovirus and named it **HTLV** (**for human T-cell leukemia virus**). His expertise with retroviruses proved valuable in 1984 when his research group set out to isolate the AIDS virus, also an RNA-containing retrovirus. Instead of transforming T-lymphocytes, however, the AIDS virus destroyed them (Chapter 13).

In the 1990s, increasing evidence demonstrated that HTLV can cause leukemia, as well as neurological pain disorder and another condition marked by destruction of the sheaths that surround the nerve fibers. The virus appears to be bloodborne, and the primary mode of transport is through the use of illegal intravenous drugs. The growing incidence among patients also poses a threat to health-care workers who are exposed to patients' blood. A second virus, named **HTLV-II**, has also been located. Although the virus has not been definitely linked to any cancer, it is apparently common in patients suffering from a condition called **hairy-cell leukemia**, a type of leukemia in which the white blood cells develop long hairlike extensions to their cytoplasm at the surface.

HOW VIRUSES TRANSFORM CELLS

Oncogene:
a gene that can transform a normal cell to a cancer cell.

The mechanism by which viruses and other carcinogens transform normal cells into tumor cells remained obscure until the **oncogene theory** was developed in the 1970s. First postulated by **Robert Huebner** and **George Todaro** in 1969, this theory suggests that transforming genes, the so-called oncogenes, normally reside in the chromosomal DNA of a cell. In the late 1970s, researchers **J. Michael Bishop** and **Harold Varmus**, of the University of California at San Francisco, located oncogenes in a wide variety of creatures from fruit flies to humans. Bishop and Varmus also made the astonishing discovery that practically the same genes exist in certain viruses, and they hypothesized that the genes could have been captured by the viruses. It appeared that the oncogenes were not viral in origin but part of the genetic endowment of every living cell. Bishop and Varmus received the 1989 Nobel Prize in Physiology or Medicine for their work.

The discovery of oncogenes demonstrated that some forms of cancer have a genetic basis. As research continued, oncology researchers extracted DNA from tumors and used it to turn healthy cells into cancerous ones in the test tube. Moreover, they surmised that the transforming substance was in a small segment of the tumor cell DNA—probably a single gene. Finally, in 1981, three separate research groups isolated an oncogene residing in a human bladder cancer. At this writing, over 60 different oncogenes have been identified.

In recent years, the theory of oncogene activity has been revised slightly. Researchers now propose that normal genes, called **proto-oncogenes**, are the fore-runners of oncogenes (FIGURE 11.21). Proto-oncogenes may have important functions as regulators of growth and mitosis. Indeed, research reported in 1985 linked proto-oncogenes to the production of cyclic adenosine monophosphate (cAMP), an organic substance central to many physiological processes. That proto-oncogenes exist in diverse forms of life argues for their important role in cell metabolism, perhaps as growth regulators. (As one researcher notes, "They would not have survived through evolution just to make tumors.") It seems certain that proto-oncogenes can be converted to oncogenes by carcinogens, such as viruses, radiation, or chemicals, or by chromosomal breakage and rearrangement, after which tumor formation begins. Indeed, the bladder cancer oncogene differs from its counterpart proto-oncogene by only one nucleotide in 6000.

Proto-oncogenes: Human genes that can be transformed by carcinogens into oncogenes.

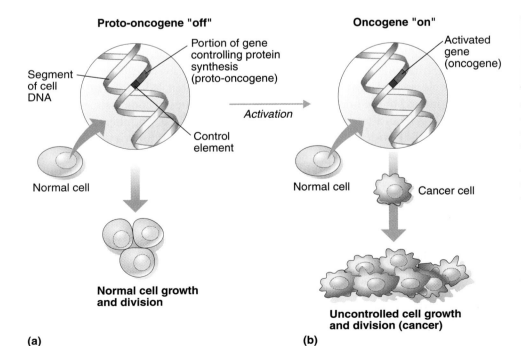

Proto-oncogene "off"

Segment of cell DNA

Portion of gene controlling protein synthesis (proto-oncogene)

Control element

Normal cell

Activation

Oncogene "on"

Activated gene (oncogene)

Normal cell

Cancer cell

Normal cell growth and division

Uncontrolled cell growth and division (cancer)

(a)

(b)

FIGURE 11.21

The Oncogene Theory

The oncogene theory helps explain the process of cancer development. (a) The normal cell grows and divides without complications. Within its DNA it contains proto-oncogenes that are "turned off." When the genes are activated by viruses or other factors, they revert to oncogenes, which "turn on." An abnormal cancer cell (b) results. The oncogenes encode proteins that regulate the transformation from a normal cell to a cancer cell and the development of a tumor.

But how do viruses convert proto-oncogenes to oncogenes? Virologists have observed that when a virus enters a cell, it may enter a lysogenic relationship with the cell and thereby transform it. If the viral genome is composed of DNA, for example, the DNA may integrate itself directly into the chromosome (like a prophage integrates into a bacterial chromosome) and become a provirus. If the viral genome is composed of RNA, the enzyme reverse transcriptase synthesizes DNA using RNA as a template. The double-stranded DNA then inserts into the cell chromosome as a provirus (see Figure 11.14). This system applies to the retroviruses studied by Gallo.

Another mechanism of transformation has been studied with the virus of **Burkitt's lymphoma**. In this cancer of the lymphoid connective tissues of the jaw, the viral genome appears to insert itself into a chromosome of B-lymphocytes, the white blood cells important in immunity. The insertion triggers proto-oncogenes involved in cell growth to move from chromosome 8 to chromosome 14, far from the influence of their control genes. A segment of DNA from chromosome 14 replaces the proto-oncogenes from chromosome 8. The proto-oncogenes, now oncogenes, appear to produce elevated amounts of their protein product.

Once the proto-oncogene becomes an oncogene, it can influence cellular growth and mitosis in several ways. Oncogenes, for example, may provide the genetic codes for growth factors that stimulate uncontrolled cell development and reproduction. Or the oncogenes may become incapable of encoding substances that turn off cell growth, a function the proto-oncogenes once had. During the 1980s in a particularly interesting series of studies at Cold Spring Harbor Laboratories, a team led by **Michael Wigler** isolated a protein whose production was directed by an oncogene. The protein was injected into normal cells, and within hours, the normal cells began to multiply rapidly and show unmistakable signs of conversion to cancer cells. In a later experiment, they injected antibodies to neutralize the protein in cancer cells and observed signs of reversion to normal cells. The experiments strengthened the evidence that abnormal products of oncogenes enhance cell transformation and that, in theory, countermeasures are possible.

One gene that has received considerable attention is a viral oncogene known as the *ras* gene, so named because it induces *ra*t *s*arcoma, a tumor of the rat connective tissue. When the *ras* gene is inserted in human bladder cells, it causes a human tumor to form. Normally, the proto-oncogene encodes a protein that, when activated, encourages other molecules to induce cell division. Following several cell divisions (enough, for example, to heal a wound), the protein is deactivated. When the *ras* proto-oncogene is mutated to the oncogene, however, *ras* continues to code for the protein, but the protein is in an altered form that cannot be deactivated. The altered protein keeps telling the cell "Divide, divide, divide!" In a short period of time, a tumor forms.

Technological advances in cancer research and detection have been remarkable in recent years (FIGURE 11.22). However, investigators are quick to point out that there will probably be no cures in the near future. Nevertheless, several innovative chemical substances loom on the horizon that can influence the course of certain types of cancer. Interferons are one such group of substances, interleukins another, and monoclonal antibodies still another (Chapter 20). Oncogene studies are significant because they may help in early cancer detection and assist the development of anticancer drugs. The oncogene theory provides an explanation of a unifying mechanism by which all carcinogens may act, regardless of whether they are chemical substances, physical agents, or viruses.

Burkitt's lymphoma: cancer in the lymphoid connective tissue of the jaw.

FIGURE 11.22

Cancer Detection

A patient is examined for cancer by a radioisotope scanner. An injected radioactive substance concentrates in certain "hot spots" where cancer cells concentrate. The scanner passes back and forth across the body, recording the patterns of radioactivity.

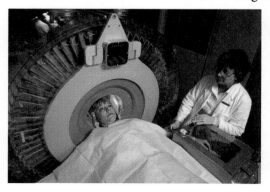

11.5

Subviral Particles

W hen viruses were discovered, scientists believed they were the ultimate infectious particles. It was difficult to conceive that anything smaller than ultramicroscopic viruses could cause disease in plants, animals, and humans. In recent years, however, that thinking has been revised, as scientists have researched a new class of disease agents—the subviral particles. We shall examine three types of subviral particles in this section.

VIROIDS

Viroids are tiny fragments of nucleic acid known to cause several diseases in plants and thought to be involved in human and animal diseases. Their discovery resulted from studies conducted in the 1960s at the U.S. Department of Agriculture's Beltsville, Maryland, research center near Washington, D.C. A team of scientists led by Theodore O. Diener were investigating a suspected viral disease, **potato spindle tuber (PST)**, which results in long, pointed potatoes shaped like spindles. Nothing would destroy the disease agent except an RNA-dissolving enzyme, and in 1971, the group postulated that a fragment of single-stranded RNA was involved. Diener called the agent a **viroid**, meaning "viruslike." The next year, a team led by Joseph Semancik at the University of California found a similar agent in a disease of citrus trees.

Currently, at least a dozen plant diseases have been related to viroids. The largest of these particles is about one-twentieth of the size of the smallest virus (FIGURE 11.23). The RNA chain of the PST viroid has a known molecular sequence (359 nucleotides), but it contains so few genetic codes that the replication cycle is not understood. Diener speculates that the viroids originated as introns, the sections of RNA spliced out of messenger RNA molecules before the messengers are able to function (Chapter 5). The similarity in size between introns and viroids, and the ring shape for both, have fueled the speculation. Semancik theorizes that viroids may be regulatory genes interacting with the host genome, because viroid diseases are characterized by interference with plant growth.

An interesting twist in viroid research occurred in 1981 when studies showed that viroids could infect animals. Researchers from Knoxville, Tennessee, reported DNA viroids in hamster colonies afflicted with lymphatic cancer. Currently, some microbiologists believe that viroids may cause the mysterious slow virus diseases of humans (Chapter 13).

PRIONS

Prions are described as **pro**teinaceous **in**fectious particles thought to cause a number of diseases, including kuru and mad cow disease (Chapter 13). Prions were named in 1982 by **Stanley B. Prusiner**, a leading researcher in prion study and winner of the 1997 Nobel Prize in Physiology or Medicine (FIGURE 11.24). Tests indicate that prions can survive the heat, radiation, and chemical treatment that normally inactivate viruses. Moreover, prions appear to be composed only of protein because they are susceptible to some protein-digesting enzymes but not nucleases. These factors indicate that prions are not viruses and raise the question of how prions replicate,

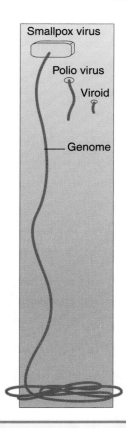

FIGURE 11.23

Viral Relationships

The size relationships of a smallpox virus, polio virus, and viroid. If the viroid were magnified 60,000 times, it would measure only one-eighth of an inch. By contrast, the genome of the smallpox virus would extend almost 14 feet and the genome of the polio virus 4.5 inches. The genome of the potato spindle tuber viroid has 359 nucleotides, while that of the smallpox virus has almost 500,000.

pre'onz

Pru'sin-er

Prions:
infectious particles of protein possibly involved in human disease.

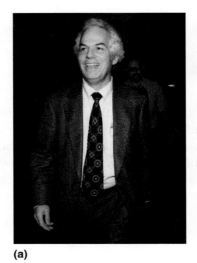

(a)

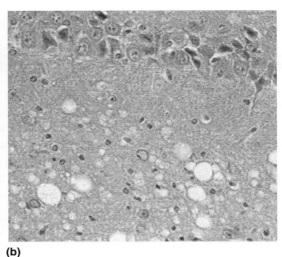

(b)

FIGURE 11.24

Prion Research and Disease

(a) Stanley Prusiner, winner of the 1997 Nobel Prize in Physiology or Medicine for his work on prions as agents of infectious disease. The award surprised the scientific community because the Nobel Prize is generally awarded to two or more individuals in each category, and because the work on prions remains somewhat speculative and incomplete. (b) A photomicrograph showing the vacuolar degeneration of gray matter characteristic of human and animal prion diseases. Mad cow disease in animal species is believed to be a spongiform encephalopathy (Chapter 13).

because one of the central dogmas in biology is that inheritance operates through DNA and RNA.

Research in the 1990s shed light on the mystery of prions. Investigators discovered that prions apparently are deviant versions of a harmless protein found on the membrane surfaces of most mammalian cells, particularly brain cells. The harmless protein is called **prion protein (PrP)**. In 1997, researchers reported that the role of PrP is to bind copper ions and thereby help the cell resist the toxic effects of highly reactive oxygen radicals. Their evidence shows that after exposure to copper, the brain cells of mice lacking PrP die more readily than do normal brain cells. Apparently, the enzyme that protects cells from oxygen radicals (superoxide dismutase) requires copper for its activity. Thus, without PrP, no copper is bound, and the enzyme is inactive, thereby leading to toxicity and cell death.

In the normal state, the PrP protects its cell. Then a transformation occurs, and the PrP folds into a different form. Now it is a **prion**. In the normal form, PrP is soluble in some detergents and can be digested by the enzyme protease; but in the abnormal form, the prion is insoluble in those detergents and resistant to the action of protease. Prusiner designated the normal protein PrP^C and the abnormal protein PrP^{Sc}. The abnormal form (prion) consists primarily of pleated sheets of misshapen protein that tend to clump together. In doing so, they may block the molecular traffic of cells by the sheer force of large size and eventually kill the cells. The symptoms of disease soon follow, and brain tissues develop a spongelike appearance with empty areas of dead tissue. These are the so-called **spongiform encephalopathies** discussed in Chapter 13. Mad cow disease is one example.

sponj'i-form
en'ceph-a-lop'a-thies

At this writing, many questions remain: For example, researchers have not yet shown how the transformation from normal to abnormal PrP takes place; the question of normal PrP's function waits to be confirmed; how prions transfer from host to host and how they bring about disease symptoms has not been established; and absolutely pure, synthetic prions (free of any possible contaminating substance) have not yet been shown to be capable of causing disease. Moreover, some scientists believe that prions are shrouds of protein enclosing ultrasmall viruses (termed *virinos*). Presumably, further research will clarify these issues.

NANOBES

Though still rudimentary, research evidence indicates the existence of microorganisms below the size of the smallest bacteria and more complex than viruses. The organisms have been named **nanobes** because their size ranges from about 20 to about 100 nanometers (the mycoplasmas are the smallest bacteria, with a size of about 150 nanometers). Recovered in sandstone deposits by Australian researchers, the organisms were first reported in 1999. They apparently form colonies, contain DNA, and have chemical and biological structures consistent with those of other living things. Researchers have found evidence of their presence in patients with large cysts in their kidneys. Amid speculation concerning their existence, nanobes, like prions and viroids, represent new frontiers for research.

nan'obes

Note to the Student

Every science has its borderland where known and visible things merge with the unknown and invisible. Startling discoveries often come from this hazy, uncharted realm of speculation, and certain objects manage to loom large. In the borderland of microbiology, one curious and puzzling object is the virus.

Are viruses alive? At present, the tendency of many biologists is to sidestep the question. However, I shall make a suggestion. Although we have referred to viruses as microorganisms for the sake of convenience, I have avoided references to "live" or "dead" viruses. Instead, I have used the words "active" for replicating viruses and "inactive" for viruses unable to replicate. I suggest, therefore, that we consider viruses to be inert chemical molecules with at least one property of living things—the ability to replicate. Thus, viruses are neither totally inert nor totally alive, but somewhere in the threshold between. Perhaps viruses are transitional forms between inert molecules and living organisms. Indeed, a prominent virologist has suggested calling them "organules" or "molechisms," depending on one's preference.

Summary

The fundamental principles of this chapter are the structure and replication of viruses. Studying viruses was extremely difficult until the 1940s, when the electron microscope enabled scientists to see viruses and innovative methods allowed researchers to cultivate them. In the decades that followed, it became clear that viruses are extraordinarily small particles composed of nucleic acid surrounded by a protein coat and, in some cases, a membranelike envelope. The nucleic acid core known as the genome can be either DNA or RNA in either a single-stranded or double-stranded form. The protein coat, known as the capsid, is usually subdivided into smaller units called capsomeres. Capsids can have icosahedral, helical, or complex symmetry. The envelope, when present, is obtained from the host cell during replication and contains viral-specified proteins.

Viral replication occurs only in living cells. The process involves attachment, penetration, biosynthesis, maturation, and release phases, and it varies according to the virus. For example, penetration can occur by a number of different methods, and the biochemistry of synthesis varies among DNA and RNA viruses. Viruses have no binomial names, but instead are named according to their disease (e.g., measles virus), their discoverer (e.g., Epstein-Barr virus), or another method. Classification schemes are based on physiological and biochemical characteristics, or on the tissue where replication takes place.

Various detection methods for viruses are based on such things as characteristic changes in tissue cultures, antibody responses, or pathological signs in diseased tissue. Certain drugs such as AZT can be used to inhibit viral replication, but the primary public health response to viral disease is through the use of vaccines. Vaccines consisting of inactivated viruses are available for polio and rabies, and vaccines containing weakened (attenuated) viruses are used to treat measles, mumps, and rubella. Many of the physical and chemical methods routinely used on microorganisms can be employed to inactivate and destroy viruses.

Cancer is a complex condition in which cells multiply without control. Among the many cancer-inducing agents are viruses, and although the mechanisms of cancer induction are still unclear, viruses may bring about cancers by converting preliminary genes into cancer-causing oncogenes. Their relationship to cancers and to infectious diseases has secured an important place for viruses in the study of microbiology.

Questions for Thought and Discussion

1. If you were to stop 1000 people on the street and ask if they recognize the term *virus*, all would probably respond in the affirmative. If you were then to ask the people to *describe* a virus, you might hear answers like "It's very small" or "It's a germ," or a host of other colorful but not very descriptive terms. As a student of microbiology, how would you describe a virus?

2. A textbook author referring to viruses once wrote: "Certain organisms seem to live only to reproduce, and much of their activity and behavior is directed toward the goal of successful reproduction." Would you agree with this concept? Can you think of any creatures other than viruses that fit the description?

3. Oncogenes have been described in the recent literature as "Jekyll and Hyde genes." What factors may have led to this label, and what does it imply? In your view, is the name justified?

4. Suppose the viroid turned out to be an infectious particle able to cause disease in humans. What difficulties might occur when dealing with this protein-free nucleic acid fragment both inside and outside the body?

5. Stanley's 1935 announcement that viruses could be crystallized stirred considerable debate about the living nature of viruses. Imagine that one day, a virus was discovered to contain both DNA and RNA. Might this stir an equal amount of controversy on the nature of viruses? Why?

6. Why was the cultivation of viruses in test tubes by Enders' group as significant as the cultivation of bacteria in test tubes by Koch? Why was each achievement critically important to the times? What type of follow-up experiment came after each foundation was established?

7. Researchers studying the bacteria that live in the oceans have long been troubled by the question of why bacteria have not saturated the oceanic environments. What might be a reason?

8. In broad terms, the public health approach to dealing with bacterial diseases is treatment. Can you guess the nature of the general public health approach to viral diseases? What evidence do you have to support your answer?

9. Bacteria can cause disease by using their toxins to interfere with important body processes; by overcoming body defenses, such as phagocytosis; by using their enzymes to digest tissue cells; or other similar mechanisms. Viruses, by contrast, have no toxins, cannot overcome body defenses, and produce no digestive enzymes. How, then, do viruses cause disease?

10. When Ebola fever broke out in Africa in 1994, the death toll was high, but the epidemic was short-lived. By comparison, when influenza breaks out at the start of winter, the toll is low, but the epidemic lasts for 6 or more months. From the standpoint of the virus, what dynamics do you see in these two types of epidemics?

11. Some virologists believe that the agent of kuru, scrapie, and other diseases is a prion. The term *prion* is derived from the words *pro*teinaceous *in*fectious particle. You will note that if these word parts are put together, the word is *proin*, not *prion*. How do you suppose the word got to be *prion*?

12. The eminent researcher Peter Medawar once described a virus using the derogatory words on the opening page of this chapter. How did the virus gain this questionable reputation? Explain whether it will ever change, and if so, how.

13. Many textbooks attempt to simplify biological concepts, and in doing so, they often oversimplify a particular thought. For example, it is not unusual to read that "viruses were discovered by Dimitri Iwanowski." How would you react to this statement?

14. How have revelations from studies on viruses, viroids, and prions complicated some of the traditional views about the principles of biology?

15. When discussing the multiplication of viruses, virologists prefer to call the process replication, rather than reproduction. Why do you think this is so? Would you agree with virologists that *replication* is the better term?

http://microbiology.jbpub.com

The site features **eLearning**, an on-line review area that provides quizzes and other tools to help you study for your class. You can also follow useful links for in-depth information, read more MicroFocus stories, or just find out the latest microbiology news.

Review

Use the following syllables to compose the term that answers each clue from virology. The number of letters in the term is indicated by the dashes, and the number of syllables in the term is shown by the number in parentheses. Each syllable is used only once. The answers are listed in Appendix D.

A A A AC AL AN AT AT BAC BO CAP CAP CEP CLO CO CO CY DE DERS DIES DINE DRON ED EN EN FER FORM GE GEN GENE HE HE HYDE I I I IN IN LET LEY LIX LY MAN MERES MOR NEG NOME O O OID ON ON ON ONS OPE PHAGE PRI RE RI SA SID SO SO STAN TA TED TEN TER TER TI TIV TOR TRA TU U UL VEL VI VIR VIR VIR Y

1. Viral protein coat (2) __ __ __ __ __ __

2. Viral shape (2) __ __ __ __ __

3. Bacterial virus (5) __ __ __ __ __ __ __ __ __ __

4. Neutralize viruses (4) __ __ __ __ __ __ __ __ __

5. Rabies granules (2) __ __ __ __ __

6. Herpes drug (4) __ __ __ __ __ __ __ __ __

7. Natural antiviral (4) __ __ __ __ __ __ __ __ __

8. Weakened virus (5) __ __ __ __ __ __ __ __ __ __

9. Disease RNA fragment (2) __ __ __ __ __ __

10. Functionless cell mass (2) __ __ __ __ __

11. Virus-inactivating light (5) __ __ __ __ __ __ __ __ __ __

12. Cancer gene (3) __ __ __ __ __ __

13. Site where virus attaches (3) __ __ __ __ __ __ __

14. Shape of polio virus (5) __ __ __ __ __ __ __ __ __

15. Viral core (2) __ __ __ __ __ __

16. Cultivated polio virus (2) __ __ __ __ __ __

17. Completely assembled virus (3) __ __ __ __ __

18. Virus incorporated to cell (4) __ __ __ __ __ __ __

19. Drug for influenza (4) __ __ __ __ __ __ __ __ __

20. Surrounds the nucleocapsid (3) __ __ __ __ __ __ __ __

21. Crystallized viruses (2) __ __ __ __ __

22. Modifies viral genome (4) __ __ __ __ __ __ __ __ __ __

23. Protein particles (2) __ __ __ __ __ __

24. Capsid subunits (3) __ __ __ __ __ __ __ __

25. Vaccine virus (5) __ __ __ __ __ __ __ __ __

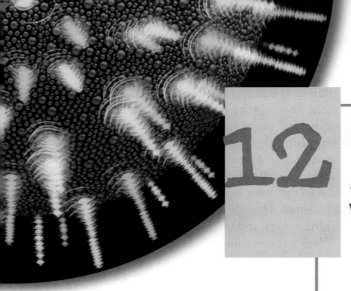

12

Pneumotropic and Dermotropic Viral Diseases

Medicine has never before produced any single improvement of such utility.

—Thomas Jefferson congratulating Edward Jenner on his development of a smallpox vaccine

HOW DOES ONE GO ABOUT eradicating a disease from the face of the Earth? How, indeed, when the disease at one time was killing one-third of English newborns; when the disease helped topple the highly civilized Aztec nation to a few hundred Spanish invaders; and when the ferocious disease was the major epidemic of the fledgling American colonies? How does one mount a global campaign against **smallpox**?

Apparently, the World Health Organization (WHO) was determined to try, and in 1966, it received $2.5 million to begin its campaign. The goal was to stamp out smallpox in 10 years using global vaccination programs. Under the direction of Donald A. Henderson, vaccine-producing laboratories were established in countries where epidemics were raging. Wyeth Laboratories developed and donated a two-tined needle for administering the vaccine in 15 rapid jabs to the arm. By 1971, vaccination programs had been begun in 44 countries.

Next came surveillance containment. The WHO set up teams to improve the reporting and discovery of outbreaks, and every known contact of victims was vaccinated to break the chain of transmission. Vaccinators used persuasion and, in some cases, coercion to learn the whereabouts of people suffering from the disease. A favorite tool was the threat to withhold food ration cards. Rewards were offered for information, and people gradually came forward. By 1970, the number of smallpox countries had dropped to 17, and by 1973, only 6 countries were left.

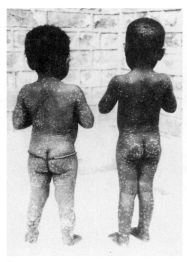

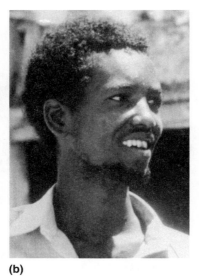

(a)   **(b)**

FIGURE 12.1

Smallpox

(a) Two young boys infected with smallpox. This photograph was taken during the Bangladesh epidemic in 1973. (b) Ali Maow Maalin, the Somali cook who had the last case of smallpox.

But these countries included India, Pakistan, and Bangladesh, and 700 million people lived there (FIGURE 12.1). Now the WHO employed more rigorous techniques, including posting guards to prevent patients from leaving their homes, and vaccinating everyone within 5 miles of an infected village. By 1976, the job in Asia was done, and only Ethiopia remained. Despite a civil war, famine, several kidnappings, and torrential summer rains, the WHO pressed on. When victory seemed in sight, however, smallpox broke out in neighboring Somalia. Now, all efforts were directed at this African country, and a campaign involving 200,000 public health officials, 700 advisors, 55 countries, and untold millions of dollars eventually focused on a hospital cook named Ali Maow Maalin. Maalin developed smallpox on October 26, 1977. He was placed under guard, and vaccination was administered to 161 people previously in contact with him. None developed smallpox. In fact, no one has developed smallpox since that epic date.

In the minds of many scientists, the eradication of smallpox was the major medical event of the twentieth century. No claim of eradication had ever before been made for a disease, and nowhere have the potential benefits of applied public health been manifested better. Indeed, the eradication of smallpox has probably been public health's finest hour.

So, one might say, that's one less disease to worry about (and one less to learn for the test). Unfortunately not, because students need to know about the classical diseases of history in order to understand the contemporary ones. This is one reason why we study smallpox and numerous other diseases we probably will not encounter in our lifetimes. We also study viral diseases because, with the control of many bacterial diseases, viral diseases have become an important focus of attention in the medical community: For example, influenza continues to be an ongoing problem in the twenty-first century, and chickenpox is still among the most commonly reported diseases of childhood years. Another viral disease, genital herpes, has become so rampant that, by some estimates, 10 to 20 million Americans are currently infected. Indeed, the virus causing this disease may even be involved in clogged arteries (**MicroFocus 12.1**).

But scientists are learning to control many viral diseases even as we study them. For example, mumps and rubella were part of the fabric of life only a generation ago, but the annual case reports have dropped from hundreds of thousands to mere hundreds (and some officials are bold enough even to whisper the word "eradication").

In this chapter we shall focus on the pneumotropic viral diseases, which affect the respiratory system, and the dermotropic viral diseases, whose symptoms are found in the skin. As in Chapter 13, each disease is presented as an independent essay, so you can establish an order that best suits your needs. The pneumotropic and dermotropic divisions are an artificial classification simply for grouping convenience. Therefore, you may note that the symptoms go beyond the respiratory system or skin, respectively.

nu'mo-trōp'ik
der'mo-trōp'ik

MicroFocus 12.1

THE MISSING LINK?

During the late 1970s, Catherine Fabricant of Cornell University made the interesting observation that chickens infected with fowl herpesvirus develop a condition that looks suspiciously like atherosclerosis (fat accumulation on the inner walls of the coronary arteries, often resulting in heart disease). Her observation was intriguing, but there was more: The chickens were on a cholesterol-free diet. And more: Chickens whose diet included cholesterol suffered even greater fat accumulation. And still more: Chickens vaccinated against infection by fowl herpesvirus suffered no fat buildup. The link between herpesvirus and atherosclerosis appeared unmistakable.

Fabricant's work opened a set of inquiries that continues today. In 1993, for example, David Hajjar, also of Cornell, reported evidence that herpes-infected cells encourage blood clot formation while trapping fat deposits and accelerating fat buildup. These factors would speed up atherosclerosis and lead to heart attack. Hajjar's theory is that infected artery cells produce a glycoprotein that accumulates at the cell surface. The glycoprotein unites with a clotting protein and sets the clotting mechanism into motion. Allied to clot formation is the arrival of white blood cells called monocytes. The monocytes collect fat and begin the process that will eventually lead to fat buildup and atherosclerosis.

Hajjar's theory is compelling not only because he has the evidence in molecular biology to support it, but because it could also explain why atherosclerosis occurs even though there are low cholesterol levels in certain patents. Although the link between herpesviruses and heart disease is still speculative, some futurists are already thinking about immunizing against heart disease by using a herpes vaccine. It may seem unusual, but that is what futurists are for.

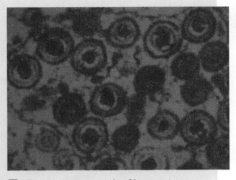

■ *Electron micrograph of herpesvirus.*

12.1

Pneumotropic Viral Diseases

The pneumotropic viral diseases occur within the human respiratory tract. Certain ones, such as influenza, primarily affect the upper regions of the tract, while others, such as respiratory syncytial disease, involve the lungs and lead to viral pneumonia. Also included in this group are the ubiquitous common colds and head colds that affect millions of Americans annually.

INFLUENZA

Influenza is an acute, contagious disease of the upper respiratory tract transmitted by droplets. The disease is believed to take its name from the Italian word for "influence," a reference either to the influence of heavenly bodies, or to the *influenza de freddo*, "influence of the cold." Since the first recorded epidemic in 1510, scientists have described 31 pandemics. The most notable pandemic of the twentieth century occurred in 1918 (**MicroFocus 12.2**); others took place in 1957 (the Asian flu) and in 1968 (the Hong Kong flu).

The influenza virion belongs to the Orthomyxoviridae family of viruses. It is composed of eight single-stranded segments of RNA, each wound helically and associated with protein to form a nucleocapsid. Additional protein surrounds the core of

influenza virus

Droplets:
tiny particles of mucus and saliva expelled from the respiratory tract.

Pandemic:
a worldwide epidemic.

or'tho-mik'so-vir'ĭ-da

MicroFocus 12.2

THE EPIDEMIC OF THE CENTURY

One theory suggests that it began when soldiers at Fort Riley, Kansas, were exposed to dust from burning manure piles during a March storm. Another theory implies that the source was an outbreak among hogs at an Iowa swine-breeders' show in September. Regardless of the origin, the epidemic that followed would be remembered as the most incredible of the twentieth century. The year was 1918; the disease was influenza.

At the time, influenza was called Spanish flu because it resembled an epidemic originating in Spain in 1893. American soldiers were the first to experience it, and as they traveled off to World War I in Europe, they carried the disease with them. Germany, France, and Great Britain soon were involved. Most of those affected were in their twenties and thirties—young, healthy, and vigorous.

The disease struck rich and poor alike, beginning with a cold. By the second day, victims were cyanotic (blue lips and face), and by the fourth or fifth day, they were dead from an overwhelming pneumonia as the lungs filled with fluid.

On October 6, 1918, the *Washington Post* recorded 658 fatalities from pneumonia, the most deaths from disease ever recorded in the United States in a single day. Indeed, October 1918 was the deadliest month in U.S. history.

People adapted as best they could. Some wore camphor balls or bulbs of garlic; others consumed hot peppers or bootleg whiskey as medicinal agents. Public health officials fumigated street cars and trains daily with phenol and prohibited standing on a public conveyance. The police arrested people for not wearing masks or for spitting in the streets. Schools were closed, but homework assignments were printed in local newspapers, and students were expected to mail them in. On the sidewalks, girls skipped rope to:

I had a little birdie
His name was enza
I opened the window
and in-flu-enza.

Medicinal remedies ranged from aspirin and laxatives to morphine and caffeine. Some people burned sulfur candles; others tried daily enemas. Many houses were trimmed with crepe to signify death—white for babies, purple for younger people, and black for the elderly. Survivors stacked coffins in cemeteries and behind funeral homes, and the army often had to be called in to bury the dead.

By late 1919, influenza had claimed 20 million lives throughout the world, a figure comparable to deaths from bubonic plague centuries before. Over 500,000 succumbed in the United States in a 10-month period. Some 24,000 American servicemen died of the disease (compared to a total of 34,000 World War I casualties). The notion of the Spanish flu remained until 1936 when Patrick Laidlaw, a British microbiologist, related the human disease to swine influenza. Memories of the great epidemic of 1918 to 1919 were vividly recalled when swine influenza was identified in 500 U.S. Army recruits at Fort Dix, New Jersey, in the summer of 1976. The vaccination program that followed was the most ambitious ever mounted in the United States.

hem′ah-gloo′tin-in
nūr-ah-min′ĭ-dās

Antigen:
a chemical substance that stimulates a response by the immune system.

segments, and an envelope lies outside the protein. The envelope contains a series of projections called **spikes** (FIGURE 12.2). One type of spike contains the enzyme **hemagglutinin (H)**, a substance that facilitates the attachment of influenza viruses to host cells. The second type contains another enzyme, **neuraminidase (N)**, a compound that assists the entry of the virion into the host cell for replication and out of the host cell when replication is complete. Both enzymes are antigens.

Three types of influenza virus are recognized: type A, which causes most pandemics; type B, which is less widespread than type A; and type C, which is rare. Each type is known for its **antigenic variation**, a process in which chemical changes occur periodically in hemagglutinin and neuraminidase, thereby yielding new strains of virus. The process is also called **genetic drift** if it involves a tiny mutation, or **genetic shift** if it involves a major change. These changes have practical consequences because as a result of genetic drift, the antibodies produced during a previous attack of influenza fail to recognize the new strain, and a person may suffer another reasonably mild attack of disease. In addition, genetic shift may give rise to such new strains that everyone is defenseless, and pandemics ensue. Also, antigenic variation precludes the development of a universally effective vaccine, although several have been developed over the years for particular strains. Moreover, the nomenclature for influenza viruses is based on the variant of antigen present. It is not uncommon to see references to strains such as A(H3N2), which predominated in the U.S. in 1999.

The onset of influenza is abrupt, with sudden chills, fatigue, headache, and pain most pronounced in the chest, back, and legs. Over a 24-hour period, body temperature can rise to 104°F, and a severe cough develops. Patients experience nasal congestion, dry throat, and tight chest, the latter a probable reflection of viral invasion of tissues of the trachea and bronchi. Despite these severe symptoms, influenza is normally short-lived and has a favorable prognosis. The disease is self-limiting and usually resolves in 1 week to 10 days, although certain outbreaks raise public health concerns (MicroFocus 12.3). Secondary complications may occur if bacteria such as staphylococci or *Haemophilus influenzae* (Pfeiffer's bacillus) invade the damaged respiratory tissue.

A diagnosis of influenza is based on several factors, including the pattern of spread in the community, observation of disease symptoms, laboratory isolation of viruses, and agglutination of human type O red blood cells. Active cases of type A influenza may be treated with **amantadine** (Symmetrel), a drug believed to interfere with uncoating in the replication cycle. An alternate drug is **rimantadine**. High-risk individuals, such as the elderly and very young, may be immunized with inactivated

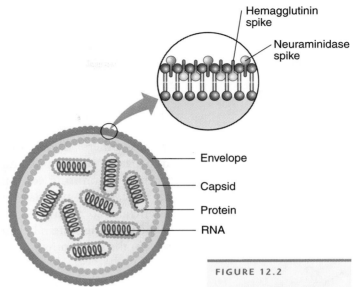

FIGURE 12.2

The Influenza Virus

This diagram of the influenza virus shows its eight segments of RNA and its envelope with two types of spikes.

ah-man'tah-dēn
ri-man'tah-dēn

MicroFocus 12.3

CARNAGE

In May 1997, worried parents brought their 3-year-old son to a Hong Kong doctor for treatment for influenza. The doctor gave the boy aspirin and an antibiotic and sent them home. But soon he was at Queen Elizabeth Hospital with a massive lung infection. Then his lungs collapsed, his liver shut down, and his kidneys failed. The boy died soon thereafter.

Baffled by his illness, doctors sent samples of the boy's tissues to experts in The Netherlands and the United States. Three months later, the diagnosis was complete: The boy's death was due to influenza virus A (H5N1), a virus fiercely pathogenic in chickens, but until then, unknown in humans.

An air of tension quickly developed among public health officials around the world. They recalled the 20 million dead of influenza in 1918 and 1919, the 100,000 dead of Asian flu in 1957, and the 36,000 who died of Hong Kong flu in 1968. They watched for other cases of the avian virus in humans (as a nervous Hong Kong community filled hospital emergency rooms with people having symptoms of routine colds). And they monitored the epidemic as it spread among the population of chickens: One moment a chicken stood contentedly in its cage; the next moment it leaned over and fell dead, blood oozing from its orifices. By November, 4 more human cases were confirmed; by Christmas, another 13.

On December 28, 1997, Hong Kong's Chief Executive decided to act swiftly: "No chicken will be allowed to walk free in the territory," he declared. Knives flashed, blood splattered, and the carnage began, as a million-and-a-half chickens were slaughtered. Thousands of workers were mobilized to stuff dead chickens into garbage bags and haul them to landfills. Carcasses rotted and rats picked apart bags left by the roadside. A thousand tons of chickens disappeared from the Hong Kong landscape.

In January 1998, the Chinese New Year came and went without the traditional poultry dishes. There were no live chickens or chicken dishes to offer to the gods or to honor Chinese ancestors. To be sure, it was a strange holiday. But there were no more deaths from influenza. It had been a close call.

influenza viruses of the type and strain predicted for the impending flu season. A new drug directed at neuraminidase is also being tested, as MicroFocus 12.4 explains.

Two serious complications of influenza have surfaced during recent decades. One complication is **Guillain-Barré syndrome (GBS)**. This condition is characterized by nerve damage, poliolike paralysis, and coma. Some nonparalytic cases are characterized by numbness in the arms and legs, and general weakness and shakiness. The second complication is **Reye syndrome**, named for Ramon D. K. Reye, who reported it in 1963. Reye syndrome (pronounced "ray" by some and "rye" by others) usually makes its appearance when a child is recovering from influenza or chickenpox and has received aspirin. The fever rises, and repeated, protracted vomiting continues for a period of hours. The child may become lethargic, sleepy, and glassy-eyed (or "starry-eyed"), as well as disoriented, incoherent, and combative. Reye syndrome, like GBS, is believed to be due to activity of the immune system because viruses cannot be found in sufficient numbers to explain the symptoms.

ge-yan' bar-rā'

Lethargic:
drowsy or indifferent.

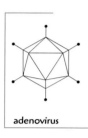

adenovirus

Inclusions:
bodies composed of numerous virions in a crystalline pattern.
Adenoids:
patches of lymphoid tissue in the human pharynx.

ADENOVIRUS INFECTIONS

Adenoviruses are a group of over 30 types of icosahedral virions having double-stranded DNA and belonging to the family Adenoviridae (FIGURE 12.3). They multiply in the nuclei of host cells and induce the formation of **inclusions**, a series of bodies composed of numerous virions arranged in a crystalline pattern. The viruses take their name from the adenoid tissue from which they were first isolated in 1953.

Adenoviruses are among the most frequent causes of upper respiratory diseases collectively called the **common cold**. Adenoviral colds are distinctive because the fever is substantial, the throat is very sore, and the cough is usually severe. In addition, the lymph nodes of the neck swell and a whitish-gray material appears over the throat

MicroFocus 12.4

THE ACHILLES HEEL

Students of ancient history know that the Greek warrior Achilles was cloaked in armor except at one vulnerable spot near his heel. An arrow directed at his heel in battle would eventually kill Achilles (and signify a tendon connecting three lower leg muscles to the bone).

In their search for antimicrobial agents, scientists are continually on the lookout for an organism's Achilles heel. And for influenza, such a spot may exist at the enzyme neuraminidase (nur-ah-min'i-dase). This enzyme is found in the spike of the virus. It destroys the scialic acid present in the viral envelope at the conclusion of the replication cycle. This function is important because if left in

place, scialic acid would clump influenza viruses together on the cell surface, and they could not enter the cell to replicate. But neuraminidase efficiently breaks down the scialic acid, and without this organic "glue," the viruses are free to enter the respiratory cells and begin the disease process.

Enter the scientists. Graeme Laver and his colleagues at the Australian National Laboratory found that neuraminidase exists in crystals whose proteins consist of four units extending out from the envelope like four ultramicroscopic balloons. The chains of amino acids in the units are similar among influenza viruses, so a drug that would react with one influenza virus would react with all.

The group set to work to synthesize a drug to "plug" the neuraminidase site where it binds to scialic acid. They hunted for the key amino acids reacting in the site (amino acids where a drug could anchor itself) and features for tight binding to the drug. It was molecular biology at its best, plus a bit of logic and a helping of luck. Fifteen long years passed as the group slogged on. Finally, the new drug was ready: Its name is zanamivir (Relenza). A second drug called oseltamivir (Tamiflu) is also available at this writing. Both portend a new generation of antiviral drugs.

surface. Another common cold virus is the **coronavirus**, an RNA virus enclosed in a crownlike series of projections.

One strain of adenovirus causes **keratoconjunctivitis**, an inflammation of the cornea (*kerato-*) and conjunctiva of the eye. Patients experience reduced vision for several weeks, but recovery is usually spontaneous and complete. Transmission may be by respiratory droplets, contact, or ophthalmic instruments. Contaminated water may also transmit the viruses, as illustrated in an early 1970s outbreak where the chlorinator in a swimming pool malfunctioned, resulting in 44 cases of eye infection ("swimming pool conjunctivitis").

Another strain of adenovirus causes **viral meningitis**, an inflammation of the meninges. Viral meningitis is often called **aseptic meningitis** because no visible agent (such as a bacterium or fungus) can be located. Still another type of adenovirus causes tumors in animals.

In recent years, adenoviruses have developed a more positive image as vectors (carriers) for genes during **gene therapy experiments**. In the 1990s, for example, researchers rendered adenoviruses incapable of replication, then reengineered them with a collection of genes to help control cystic fibrosis (CF). The genetically altered viruses ferried the helpful genes into the respiratory cells of CF patients, where they encoded proteins to help clear away the mucus and sticky material accumulating in the airways. The experiments continue as of this writing.

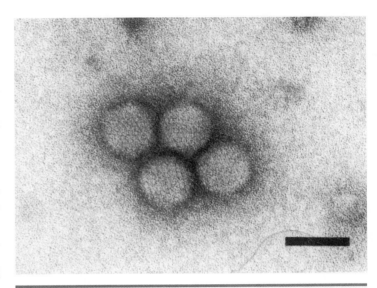

FIGURE 12.3

A Transmission Electron Micrograph of Adenoviruses

These viruses have no envelope, and the icosahedral symmetry of the nucleocapsid can be observed. The rough surface of the viruses is due to the presence of capsomeres. Adenoviruses are agents of common colds. (Bar = 100 nm.)

RESPIRATORY SYNCYTIAL DISEASE

Since 1985, **respiratory syncytial (RS) disease** has been the most common lower respiratory tract disease affecting infants and children under 2 years of age. Infection takes place in the bronchioles and air sacs of the lungs, and the disease is often described as **viral pneumonia**. Maternal antibodies passed from mother to child probably provide protection during the first few months of life, but the risk of infection increases as these antibodies disappear. Indeed, researchers have successfully used preparations of antibodies (called immune globulin) to lessen the severity of established cases of RS disease. Ribavirin has also been used with success.

The respiratory syncytial virus is an enveloped RNA helical virion of the Paramyxoviridae family. When the virus infects tissue cells, the latter tend to fuse (**FIGURE 12.4**) and form giant cells called **syncytia** (sing., syncytium).

RS disease can also occur in adults, usually as an upper respiratory disease with influenzalike symptoms. Outbreaks occur yearly throughout the United States, but most cases are misdiagnosed or unreported. Some virologists believe that up to 95 percent of all children have been exposed to the disease by the age of 5, and CDC epidemiologists estimate that 90,000 hospitalizations and 4500 deaths occur in infants and children each year in the United States as a result of RS disease. A 1999 study linked the disease to a major proportion of middle ear infections in children.

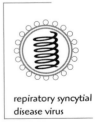

repiratory syncytial disease virus

par'ah-mik'so-vir'ĭ-da

sin-sish'ah
sin-sish'e-um

FIGURE 12.4

Syncytium Formation by Respiratory Syncytial Viruses

A syncytium is a giant cell formed from the union of several smaller cells. The syncytium results in a formless mass of tissue that functions abnormally and leads to disease symptoms. It also provides a mechanism by which viruses can spread from one cell to many cells, as shown here for RS viruses.

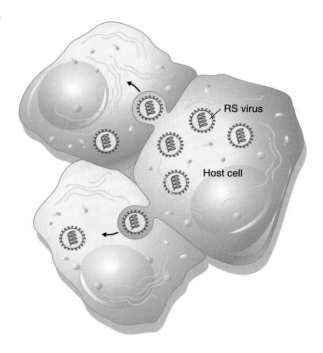

RS virus

Host cell

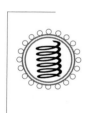

parainfluenza virus

PARAINFLUENZA

Parainfluenza is caused by an RNA helical virion of the Paramyxoviridae family of viruses (the RS and measles viruses are included in this family). Although as widespread as influenza, parainfluenza is a much milder disease. It is characterized by minor upper respiratory illness, often referred to as a cold. Bronchitis and croup may accompany the disease, which is most often seen in children under the age of 6. The disease predominates in the late fall and early spring, and is seasonal, as FIGURE 12.5 indicates.

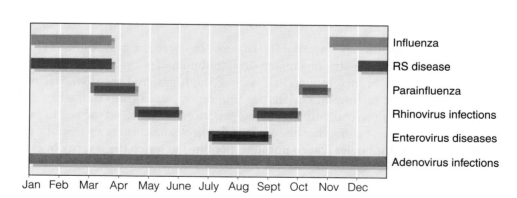

Influenza

RS disease

Parainfluenza

Rhinovirus infections

Enterovirus diseases

Adenovirus infections

Jan Feb Mar Apr May June July Aug Sept Oct Nov Dec

FIGURE 12.5

The Seasonal Variation of Viral Respiratory Diseases

This chart shows the seasons associated with various viral diseases of the respiratory tract. Note that the influenza and RS disease seasons overlap and are the primary diseases of the winter season. Enteroviruses (Chapter 13) cause diseases of the gastrointestinal tract as well as respiratory disorders and are usually acquired from the environment.

MicroFocus 12.5

BLAMING THE MESSENGER

Why do we feel so miserable when we develop a cold or the flu? Scientists think they may have an answer. The key, they suggest, is a protein called interleukin-6. Interleukin-6 is produced by white blood cells of the immune system (its T-lymphocytes). Acting like a hormone, the protein travels to other white blood cells (the phagocytes), where it encourages an immune response to disease. When too much interleukin-6 is produced, however, tissue inflammation develops, and fever, achiness, and extreme exhaustion follow.

That's where the flu and common cold viruses come in. Working with student volunteers, scientists from various institutions have found that respiratory viruses stimulate the production of excessive amounts of interleukin-6 during infection. Their studies, reported in 1998, confirm that the amount of interleukin-6 in nasal washings is directly proportional to the amount of virus present and the severity of respiratory symptoms. Essentially, they point out, the body's response helps fight the infection but makes us miserable as well. The trick, researchers say, is for the body to produce enough interleukin-6 to combat the virus, but not so much that we have to suffer the symptoms of illness. Apparently the body has not yet learned the trick.

RHINOVIRUS INFECTIONS

Rhinoviruses are a broad group of over 100 different RNA viruses with icosahedral symmetry. They belong to the family Picornaviridae (*pico-* means "small"; hence small-RNA-viruses). Rhinoviruses take their name from the Greek *rhinos*, meaning "nose," referring to their infection site. The viruses are among the major causes of **common colds**, also called head colds.

pi-kor'nah-vir'ĭ-da

A **head cold** involves a regular sequence of symptoms beginning with headache, chills, and a dry, scratchy throat. A "runny nose" and obstructed air passageways are the dominant symptoms, but the cough is variable and fever is often absent or slight. Some children suffer from **croup**. Antihistamines can sometimes be used to relieve the symptoms, which are often due to histamines released from damaged host cells. Another possible cause of symptoms is explored in MicroFocus 12.5.

Croup: hoarse coughing.

Rhinoviruses thrive in the human nose, where the temperature is a few degrees cooler than in the rest of the body. This may be one reason that the fumes from hot chicken soup appear to hasten recovery. Research on the use of **vitamin C** as a preventive has been promising. One study, for example, indicates that this vitamin induces the body to produce interferon, while another suggests that it encourages the formation of collagen to strengthen the "intercellular cement."

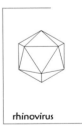

rhinovirus

Scientists have identified the receptor sites in nasal tissues where rhinoviruses attach. Furthermore, they have synthesized an antibody that binds to these sites and blocks viral attachment. Supposedly the antibody could be used as an anticold drug. Another group of researchers have used copies of the receptor sites as a drug to bind to the virus before it can find its host cell. And still another group conducted tests with a three-ply Kleenex tissue composed of two regular tissues sandwiched around a middle tissue impregnated with acidic compounds (the press dubbed them "killer Kleenexes").

Receptor site: an area of chemical activity on a cell surface where a virus can attach.

The prospects for developing a cold vaccine are not promising, partly because many different viruses are involved. In addition to the rhinoviruses, the common cold viruses include adenoviruses and respiratory syncytial viruses, as well as coronaviruses, Coxsackie viruses, echoviruses, and reoviruses. A new nasal spray

TABLE 12.1

A Summary of Pneumotropic Viral Diseases

DISEASE	CLASSIFICATION OF VIRUS	TRANSMISSION	ORGANS AFFECTED	VACCINE	SPECIAL FEATURES	COMPLICATIONS
Influenza	Orthomyxoviridae	Droplets	Respiratory tract	Available	Antigenic variation Strains A, B, C	Reye syndrome Guillain-Barré syndrome
Adenovirus infections	Adenoviridae	Droplets Contact	Lungs, meninges Eyes	Not available	Common cold syndrome	Pneumonia Aseptic meningitis
Respiratory syncytial disease	Paramyxoviridae	Droplets	Respiratory tract	Not available	Syncytia of respiratory cells	Pneumonia
Parainfluenza	Paramyxoviridae	Droplets Contact	Upper respiratory tract	Not available	Common cold syndrome	None
Rhinovirus infections	Picornaviridae	Droplets Contact	Upper respiratory tract	Not available	Head-cold syndrome	None

in'ter-fēr'on

containing interferon has stimulated interest, but the side effects of this compound need to be understood before commercial products appear on the pharmacy shelf. The pneumotropic viral diseases are summarized in TABLE 12.1.

To this point . . .

We have surveyed a number of pneumotropic viral diseases that affect the respiratory tract. Our initial emphasis was on influenza, one of the most common diseases in our society. The influenza virus has a unique composition among viruses, with eight segments of RNA in its nucleocapsid. Antigenic variation in the virus accounts for the myriad strains that appear from year to year and that make resistance and vaccine development very difficult. Secondary infection, as well as Reye and Guillain-Barré syndromes, can complicate cases of influenza.

We then concentrated on respiratory viruses that cause the familiar common cold. The adenoviruses were discussed as cold agents, and their role in keratoconjunctivitis, meningitis, and tumors was briefly mentioned. We then turned to the respiratory syncytial (RS) virus, one of the most common causes of lower respiratory diseases in children. Finally, we focused on rhinoviruses, a group of RNA viruses that cause the widely encountered head cold, and parainfluenza viruses, also the cause of colds. Throughout the discussions, the broad variety of viral strains and types that cause respiratory diseases were noted. This variety will probably preclude the development of a vaccine for many years.

We shall now turn our attention to the dermotropic viral diseases. These are viral diseases of the skin. In this group we shall discuss herpes simplex and chickenpox, two of the most widespread diseases in humans; measles and rubella, two viral diseases whose incidences are declining; and smallpox, a viral disease that is apparently extinct. In this diversity, we see the spectrum of viral diseases in the modern era.

Dermotropic Viral Diseases

The dermotropic viral diseases are a diverse collection of human maladies. Certain ones, such as herpes simplex, remain epidemic in contemporary times; while others, such as measles, mumps, and chickenpox, are being brought under control through effective vaccination programs. Indeed, there are relatively few antiviral drugs, and prevention programs remain a major course of action in dealing with these diseases.

HERPES SIMPLEX

Herpes simplex is an array of viral diseases caused by a large DNA virion having icosahedral symmetry and an envelope with spikes. A member of the family Herpesviridae, it is one of the most common viruses in the environment. Indeed, some virologists contend that over 90 percent of Americans have been exposed to it by age 18. The virus passes among cells by intercellular bridges and remains in the nerve cells until something triggers it to multiply. Granules called **Lipschütz bodies** are seen in the cell nucleus.

Physicians recognize many manifestations of herpes simplex infection, including **cold sores** (fever blisters), the unsightly lesions that form around the lips or nose (FIGURE 12.6); **herpes encephalitis**, a rare but potentially fatal brain disease; **neonatal herpes**, a life-threatening disease transmitted by mothers to newborns during childbirth; **gingivostomatitis**, a series of cold sores of the throat usually occurring in children; **herpes keratitis**, a disease of the eye and an important cause of blindness in young adults; and genital herpes, a troublesome sexually transmitted disease. The

herpes simplex virus

Lipschütz bodies: granules in the nucleus of cells infected with herpes simplex or other herpesviruses.

jin'jĭ-vo-sto'mah-ti'tis

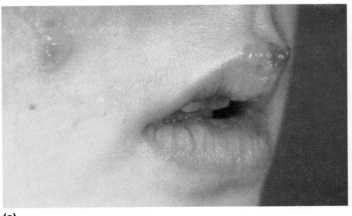

(a)

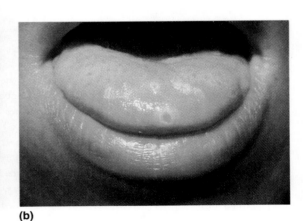

(b)

FIGURE 12.6

Two Manifestations of Herpes Simplex

(a) The cold sores (fever blisters) of herpes simplex erupting as tender, itchy papules and progressing to vesicles that burst, drain, and form scabs. Contact with the sores accounts for spread of the virus.
(b) Gingivostomatitis involving the oral mucosa, tongue, and cheeks with sores and blisters.

word *herpes* is Greek for "creeping," a reference to the spreading nature of herpes infections through the body after contact has been made (MicroFocus 12.6).

The sores and blisters of herpes simplex have been known for centuries. In ancient Rome, an epidemic was so bad that the Emperor Tiberius banned kissing; Shakespeare, in *Romeo and Juliet*, writes of "blisters o'er ladies lips"; and in the 1700s, genital herpes was so common that French prostitutes considered it a vocational disease. In current times, **genital herpes** is estimated to affect between 10 and 20 million Americans yearly, of whom about 500,000 are new cases. (The figures are inexact because genital herpes is not a reportable disease.) Signs generally appear within a few days of sexual contact, often as itching or throbbing in the genital area. This is followed by reddening and swelling of a small area where painful blisters erupt. The blisters crust over and the sores disappear, usually within about 3 weeks. In the majority of cases, however, the symptoms reappear, often in response to stressful triggers, such as sunburn, fever, menstruation, or emotional disturbance. FIGURE 12.7 shows the effect of ultraviolet light on the outbreak of infection. People with active herpes lesions pass the viruses to others during sexual contact.

In the 1960s, scientists learned that the herpes simplex virus has two different forms: type I and type II. For reasons that remain unclear, **type I virus** often inhabits areas above the waist and is the cause of herpes keratitis and most cold sores, while **type II virus** appears prevalent below the waist. This principle does not always hold true, however. Type II herpes simplex virus is especially worrisome because it is associated with **cervical cancer**, a disease that strikes over 15,000 American women annually. Though evidence is inconclusive, studies show that women who have suffered from genital herpes are several times more likely to develop cervical cancer than those who have not had herpes. Regular checkups, including Pap smears at frequent intervals, are recommended for women in this high-risk group.

Genital:
referring to the organs of sexual reproduction.

Keratitis:
infection of the cornea of the eye.
Cold sores:
herpes-induced blisters occurring on the lips, gums, nose, and adjacent areas.

MicroFocus 12.6

GLADIATORS

The situation appeared normal: a camp for high school wrestlers in Minnesota from July 2 to July 28, 1989. The camp attracted 175 wrestlers from all over the United States. As they gathered that first day, they looked forward to daily sessions of grunting and wrestling their way to excellence. Three groups would participate: lightweights, middleweights, and heavyweights.

But this would be no ordinary experience. During the final week of camp, the first case of herpes simplex was observed. Then there was another, and another. Soon, there were too many infected participants for the camp to

continue and, with 2 days remaining on the schedule, the camp was suspended and the wrestlers sent home.

Subsequent contacts by the federal Centers for Disease Control and Prevention (CDC) revealed that 60 of the 175 participants had contracted herpes simplex during that 2-week period. All experienced symptoms during the camp session or within 1 week of leaving. Lesions developed on the head or neck (73 percent of cases), the extremities (42 percent of cases), and the trunk (28 percent of cases). Five individuals experienced infection of the eye, and wrestlers in the heavyweight division were most frequently involved.

Herpes simplex in wrestlers and rugby players is called herpes gladiatorum ("herpes-of-the-gladiators," probably a whimsical term at first, but now technically acceptable). First described in the mid-1960s, herpes gladiatorum has broken out several times since then. Transmission occurs primarily by skin contact, and transmission on the fingertips can account for infection at several body sites. The disease illustrates another possible manifestation of herpes-related illness, and its swift passage by contact through a group of susceptible individuals demonstrates the ease of transfer.

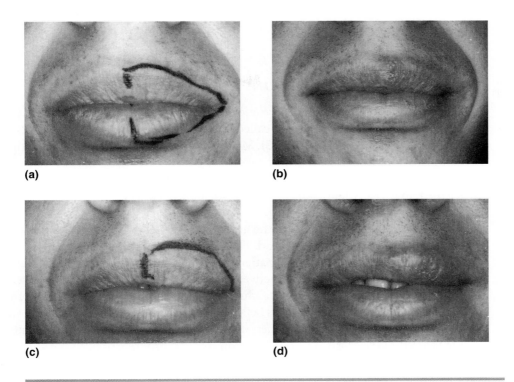

(a)   (b)

(c)   (d)

FIGURE 12.7

Ultraviolet Light and Herpes

An experiment showing the effects of ultraviolet (UV) light on the formation of herpes simplex sores of the lips. This patient usually experienced sores on the left upper lip. (a) The patient was exposed to UV light from a retail cosmetic sunlamp on the left upper and lower lips in the area designated by the line. The remainder of the face was protected by a sunscreen. (b) Sores formed on the left upper lip. (c) The patient was later exposed a second time to the sunlamp, but only on the left upper lip. (d) Sores formed and were larger than the previous ones. The results indicate that herpes sores can be experimentally stimulated by UV light, such as in sunlamps and sunlight.

Herpes encephalitis is a brain disease often accompanied by blindness, convulsions, or a range of neurological disorders, including mental impairment, and it may lead to death. The herpesviruses may be acquired by contact with an infected individual and may possibly reach the brain by the olfactory nerves after breathing into the nose. Herpes encephalitis can also occur in a newborn, where it is called **neonatal herpes**. In this case, the viruses infect the infant during passage through the birth canal. Indeed, if a woman has active genital herpes, her obstetrician may recommend birth by cesarean section. The passage of viruses across the placenta may also lead to neonatal herpes. In recent years, the acronym **TORCH** has been coined to focus attention on diseases with congenital significance: T for toxoplasmosis, R for rubella, C for cytomegalovirus, and H for herpes. O is for other diseases, such as syphilis.

Certain drugs have been approved by the Food and Drug Administration for the treatment of the various forms of herpes simplex. For example, **idoxuridine (IDU)** and **trifluridine** are used against herpes keratitis, and **vidarabine** is used to treat eye infections and herpes encephalitis, especially in newborns. Currently, the only drug approved for use against genital herpes is **acyclovir** (Zovirax). Acyclovir is a guanine

Olfactory nerves:
nerves used in the sense of smell.

i-doks-ur'ĭ-dēn

tri-floor'ĭ-dēn
vi-dār'ah-bēn

a-si'klo-vir

derivative and a base analog that interferes with viral replication (FIGURE 12.8). Eye infections also respond to this drug.

OTHER HERPESVIRUS INFECTIONS

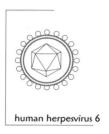

human herpesvirus 6

rose-e-o'-lah

kap-o'si
Angiogenic:
having many blood vessels.

Although a direct cause-and-effect relationship has not been established, scientists have found that a type of herpesvirus called **human herpesvirus 6 (HHV-6)** bears a relationship to **multiple sclerosis (MS)**. Multiple sclerosis is a disease in which cells of the body's immune system attack myelin, the sleeve of tissue that surrounds nerve cells; the attack leads to the formation of numerous lesions called scleroses (hence the name). Muscle weakness, visual disturbances, and an array of other neurological impairments follow.

In 1998, researchers reported that the great majority of MS patients tested have antibodies against HHV-6 in their blood. These signatures of the virus, together with the finding of herpesviral DNA in patients and HHV-6 in myelin lesions, have helped strengthen the relationship between the virus and the disease. Moreover, HHV-6 is also known to be a cause of childhood **roseola**, a condition marked by fever and a red body rash. Researchers believe that HHV-6 may remain dormant in the body from the childhood years, then resurface to be part of the chain of events leading to multiple sclerosis. The relapsing, on-and-off progress of multiple sclerosis is reminiscent of the recurrent attacks that characterize herpesvirus infections. As many as 350,000 Americans suffer from multiple sclerosis.

Another herpesvirus called **human herpesvirus 8 (HHV-8)** is now regarded as the most probable cause of **Kaposi's sarcoma (KS)**, a highly angiogenic tumor most commonly seen in immunocompromised individuals, such as those with AIDS.

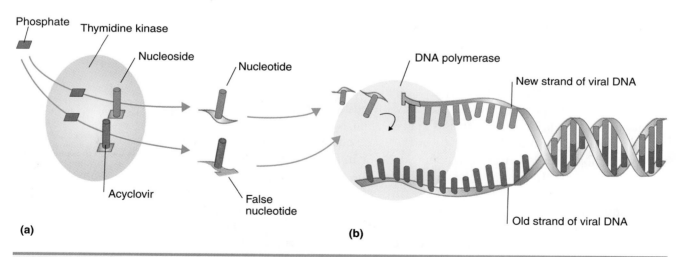

(a)   (b)

FIGURE 12.8

The Mode of Action of Acyclovir

Acyclovir interferes with the replication of herpesviruses. (a) The enzyme thymidine kinase (circle, left) functions by combining phosphate groups with sugar-base combinations (nucleosides) to form nucleotides. Acyclovir resembles nucleosides, and the enzyme mistakenly adds phosphate groups to the acyclovir to form a false nucleotide. (b) During viral replication, another enzyme, DNA polymerase (circle, right) attaches the false nucleotide onto a developing DNA molecule. However, the false nucleotide lacks an attachment point for the next nucleotide. The elongation of DNA thus comes to a halt, and viral replication stops.

Indeed, KS, which is marked by purple skin tumors, has become one of the most common tumors in parts of Africa where AIDS is endemic. The DNA of HHV-8 is present in most biopsies of tissue from KS patients, and antibodies against the virus are invariably detected in those with the disease or at risk of developing it. In 1997, two HHV-8 proteins were found to be instrumental in promoting blood vessel formation associated with the tumor.

Before leaving herpesviruses, we shall briefly mention a herpeslike illness called **B virus infection**. B virus infection is a relatively benign and common disease of Old World monkeys. Caused by a herpesvirus related to that of herpes simplex, human B virus infection is accompanied by serious neurological symptoms such as pain and numbness, with dizziness, local paralyses, and possible respiratory arrest. The disease is relatively rare in humans, but laboratory researchers who work with monkeys are at risk.

CHICKENPOX (VARICELLA)

In the centuries when pox diseases regularly swept across Europe, people had to contend with the Great Pox (syphilis), the smallpox, the cowpox, and the chickenpox, a benign disease that made the skin resemble that of a freshly plucked chicken. As of 1998, **chickenpox** remained the third most reported disease in the United States, with about 82,500 cases reported annually (chlamydia was first and gonorrhea second). The causative agent is a double-stranded DNA virion with icosahedral symmetry and an envelope. It is a herpesvirus of the family Herpesviridae.

Chickenpox is a highly communicable disease. It is transmitted by respiratory droplets and skin contact, and it has an incubation period of 2 weeks. The disease begins in the respiratory tract, with fever, headache, and malaise. Viruses then pass into the bloodstream and localize in the peripheral nerves and skin. As they multiply in the cutaneous tissues, they trigger the formation of up to 500 small, teardrop-shaped, fluid-filled vesicles (FIGURE 12.9). **Varicella**, the alternate name for chickenpox, is the Latin word for "little vessel."

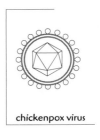

chickenpox virus

Malaise:
a general feeling of illness.

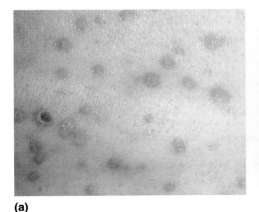
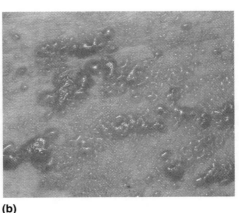

(a)   **(b)**

FIGURE 12.9

The Lesions of Chickenpox and Shingles

(a) A typical case of chickenpox. The lesions may be seen in various stages, with some in the early stage of development and others in the crust stage. (b) Dermal distribution of shingles lesions on the skin of the body trunk. The lesions contain less fluid than in chickenpox and occur in patches as red, raised blotches.

Pox:
pitted scars remaining in recoverers from smallpox.

The **vesicles** in chickenpox develop over 3 or 4 days in a succession of **crops**. They itch intensely and eventually break open to yield highly infectious virus-laden fluid. Although many refer to the vesicles as pox, the latter term is more correctly reserved for the pitted scars of smallpox. In chickenpox, the vesicles form crusts that fall off without leaving a scar. **Acyclovir** has been shown to lessen the symptoms of chickenpox and hasten recovery. Development of this drug is described in MicroFocus 12.7. Varicella immune globulin has also been used.

The mortality rate from chickenpox is low, and the disease is considered benign. However, **Reye syndrome** may occur during the recovery period, and public health officials have issued warnings against using aspirin to reduce fever. Other complications of chickenpox include pneumonia, encephalitis (brain inflammation), and bacterial infection of the skin. In pregnant women, the virus has been known to cross the placenta and cause damage in the fetus.

In 1995, the FDA licensed a vaccine for chickenpox. Known as Varivax, the vaccine consists of attenuated viruses administered subcutaneously and is recommended for all individuals over 1 year of age. One dose is given to children between ages 1 and 12, and two doses are given to adolescents and adults. It is hoped that use of the vaccine

ah-ten'u-a'ted
Attenuated virus:
a virus that replicates at a very low rate.

MicroFocus 12.7

THE PREFERRED WAY

Gertrude Belle Elion was getting dressed at 6:30 on the morning of October 17, 1988. Then the telephone rang. A moment later, Elion was speechless. She had won the Nobel Prize in Physiology or Medicine.

Only a few times in the century-long history of the Nobel Prize has the award been granted to researchers who developed drugs or worked for drug companies. This was one of those years. Gertrude B. Elion shared the award with George H. Hitchings, her former coworker at Burroughs Wellcome Research Laboratories in North Carolina, and with Sir James Black of King's College Medical School in London. The Nobel Committee named the three scientists for "their discovery of important principles of drug treatment" and for developing an intelligent method for designing new compounds based on an understanding of basic biochemical processes.

For Gertrude Elion, the award culminated a research career that almost did not happen. Even though she had a Bachelor of Science degree in biochemistry, Elion had difficulty obtaining a laboratory position because of her gender. She therefore accepted a job as a chemistry teacher. After World War II,

she went to Wellcome Laboratories, then to New York as an assistant to Hitchings. Although she never attained an advanced degree, Elion's technique and expertise were so respected that she soon came to be accepted as a colleague at the laboratory.

In 1944 Elion and Hitchings set out to learn how normal cell growth differs from that of abnormal cells, such as cancer cells. They hoped to find a way to destroy abnormal cells. The pair focused on differences in how various species metabo-

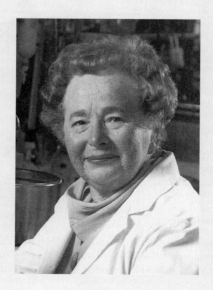

lize nucleic acid components, confining their studies mainly to nitrogenous bases of nucleic acids. In the 1950s, they developed antileukemia drugs called thioguanine and 6-mercaptopurine. Then the biochemical clues led them to a series of other drugs including azathioprine (Imuran), which stalls the rejection mechanism in transplants; allopurinol, which is used to treat gout; and pyrimethamine and trimethoprim, for malaria and other diseases. In 1977, they developed acyclovir, now used widely against herpes simplex and more recently against chickenpox. Other colleagues, applying the basic ideas of Elion and Hitchings, synthesized AZT for AIDS patients.

Elion and Hitchings were part of the so-called "fundamentalist" world of chemotherapy. By concentrating on the fundamental physiology and biochemistry of cells, they came to understand essential cellular metabolic pathways and how to interfere with them. Other researchers, dubbed "screeners," preferred to bypass the cellular biochemistry and devote their efforts to screening a number of compounds, trusting their intuition and luck. It was the more rational approach that the Nobel Committee cited in its award.

will reduce the 9000 hospitalizations and 100 deaths related to chickenpox annually. Pregnant women should not be immunized.

Herpes zoster, or **shingles,** is an adult disease caused by the same virus that causes chickenpox. For this reason, the virus is often referred to as the **varicella-zoster (VZ) virus.** The viruses multiply in ganglia (knots of nerve tissue) along the spinal cord, and travel down the nerves to the skin of the body trunk. Here they cause blisters with blotchy patches of red that appear to encircle the trunk (*herpes* is Greek for "creeping," and *zoster* is Greek for "girdle"). Many sufferers also experience a series of headaches, as well as facial paralysis and sharp "ice-pick" pains described as among the most debilitating known. The condition can occur repeatedly and is linked to emotional and physical stress (such as radiation therapy), as well as to a suppressed immune system or aging.

There is substantial evidence that herpes zoster is caused by the same virus that caused chickenpox decades before in the individual. Most cases occur in people over age 50, and a person with an active case of herpes zoster can induce chickenpox (but not herpes zoster) in another susceptible person. AIDS patients may be susceptible to the disease because of their compromised immune systems (FIGURE 12.10). For herpes zoster, acyclovir therapy lessens the symptoms, but the immune globulin used to treat varicella has limited value.

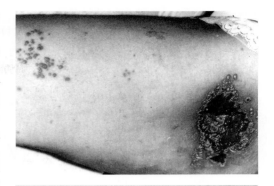

FIGURE 12.10

Herpes Lesions on a Patient's Leg

This patient suffered from disseminated herpes zoster associated with an immune deficiency due to HIV. The large lesion is a necrotic skin ulcer; the smaller lesions are herpetic pustules. The patient was treated intravenously with acyclovir, and the lesions healed. However, she later succumbed to the effects of HIV infection.

MEASLES (RUBEOLA)

Measles is a highly contagious disease caused by an RNA helical virion first isolated in tissue culture by John Enders and Thomas Peebles in 1954. The virion is enveloped, with hemagglutinin spikes, and is closely related to the mumps and RS viruses in the Paramyxoviridae family. Transmission usually occurs by respiratory droplets during the early stages of disease.

par'ah-mik'so-vir'ĭ-da

Measles symptoms commonly include a hacking cough, sneezing, nasal discharge, eye redness, sensitivity to light, and a high fever. Red patches with white grainlike centers appear along the gumline in the mouth 2 to 4 days after the onset of symptoms. These diagnostic patches are the **Koplik spots** first described in 1896 by Henry Koplik, a New York pediatrician.

The characteristic **red rash** of measles appears about 2 days after the first evidence of Koplik spots. Beginning as pink-red pimplelike spots (maculopapules), the rash breaks out at the hairline, then covers the face and spreads to the trunk and extremities (FIGURE 12.11). **Rubeola,** the alternative name for measles, is derived from the Latin *rube* for "red." Rashes resemble those in scarlet fever, but the severe sore throat of scarlet fever generally does not develop. Within a week, the rash turns brown and fades.

mac'u-lo-pap'ules

Measles is usually characterized by complete recovery. In some cases, however, bacterial disease may develop in the damaged respiratory tissue. Another possible problem is subacute sclerosing panencephalitis (SSPE), a rare brain disease characterized by a decrease in cognitive skills and loss of nervous function. There is also some evidence that the measles virus may be linked to multiple sclerosis and diabetes.

In 1978, the U.S. Public Health Service launched a campaign to eliminate measles in the United States. The cornerstone of the campaign was immunization of all school-age children with attenuated measles viruses in the **measles-mumps-rubella (MMR)** vaccine. Measles viruses have no known hosts other than humans, a factor

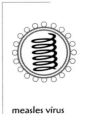

measles virus

FIGURE 12.11

The Rashes of Measles and Scarlet Fever

A comparison of the rashes accompanying cases of measles and scarlet fever. Note the progression of the respective rashes and the unique characteristics of each disease.

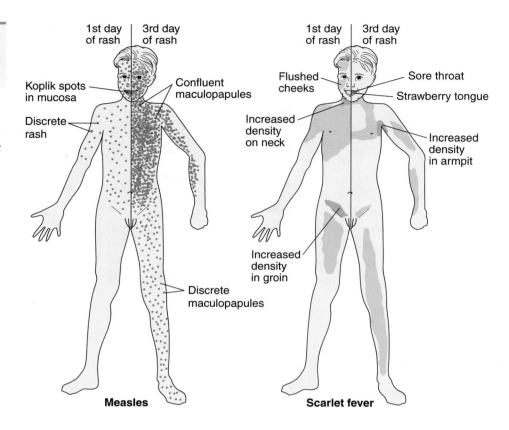

Measles   **Scarlet fever**

that is helpful in containing the disease. By 1983, the total number of reported cases was 1463, a reduction of 99.7 percent from the prevaccine era (FIGURE 12.12). However, the number skyrocketed to over 27,000 cases in 1990, reflecting outbreaks of measles in unimmunized children and college-age students inoculated with ineffective vaccines. Immunization of children entering grade school is now mandatory in all 50 states. By 1991, the number of cases had dropped to about 9500, and by 1999, there were only 60 cases; the epidemic was over.

RUBELLA (GERMAN MEASLES)

For generations, **rubella** was thought to be a mild form of measles. The distinction was not made until 1829 when Rudolph Wagner, a German physician, noted the differences in symptoms and suggested the two diseases were different. Thereafter, the new disease was known as German measles (from Wagner's homeland) to distinguish it from measles. ("German" may also have been derived from the Latin *germanus*, meaning "akin"—in this case, akin to measles.) The name *rubella* ("small red") was suggested in the 1860s because the disease is accompanied by a slightly red rash.

Rubella is caused by an RNA virus of the Togaviridae family. The virion is icosahedral with an envelope and spikes containing hemagglutinin. Viral transmission generally occurs by contact or respiratory droplets, and the disease is usually mild. It is accompanied by occasional fever with a variable, pale-pink maculopapular rash beginning on the face and spreading to the body trunk and extremities. The rash develops rapidly, often within a day, and fades after another 2 days. Recovery is usually prompt, but relapses appear to be more common than with other diseases, possibly because the viruses remain active within body cells.

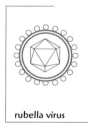

rubella virus

Maculopapular:
referring to pink-red pimplelike spots that spread.

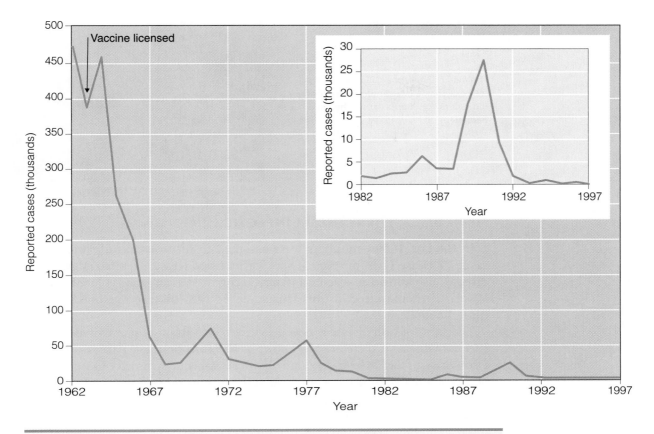

FIGURE 12.12

Reported U.S. Cases of Measles (Rubeola), 1962–1997

Note the sharp dropoff in cases after licensing of the vaccine in the mid-1960s. Unfortunately, the immunity from this vaccine was not long-lasting, and a new epidemic of measles broke out in the late 1980s. The inset shows the rise from a low of 1400 cases in 1983 to over 27,000 cases in 1990. The recent reduction in cases is partly due to renewed efforts to revaccinate susceptible individuals.

Rubella is dangerous to the developing fetus in a pregnant woman. This condition, called **congenital rubella syndrome**, occurs about 50 times each year in the United States. Destruction of the fetal capillaries takes place, and blood insufficiency follows. The organs most often affected are the eyes, ears, and cardiovascular organs, and children may be born with cataracts, glaucoma, deafness, or heart defects. If rubella is contracted during the first month of pregnancy, the probability of damage to the fetus is about 50 percent. The probability declines sharply thereafter. In the 1965 to 1966 epidemic of rubella in the United States, over 50,000 instances of stillbirth and fetal deformity were recorded. The R in the TORCH group of diseases stands for rubella.

Since its introduction in 1969, the **rubella vaccine** has had a dramatic effect on the rate of incidence of the disease. That year, physicians reported 58,000 cases of rubella, but by 1999, the number was down to 238. The vaccine consists of attenuated viruses cultivated in human tissue cultures. It is combined with the measles and mumps vaccines (MMR) for subcutaneous inoculation of children. More than 95 percent of children entering grade school now provide evidence of rubella vaccination. Adult females are advised to avoid pregnancy for 3 months after immunization as a precaution against contracting rubella from viruses in the vaccine.

Cataract:
clouding of the lens of the eye.
Glaucoma:
visual defects due to high pressures exerted by eye fluids.

MMR:
a three-component vaccine providing immunity to measles, mumps, and rubella.

FIGURE 12.13

Fifth Disease

The fiery red rash of a child with fifth disease (erythema infectiosum). The confluent red rash makes it appear as if the child has been slapped.

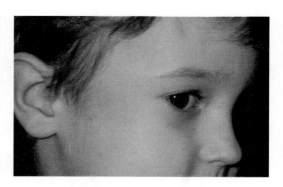

FIFTH DISEASE (ERYTHEMA INFECTIOSUM)

In the late 1800s, numbers were assigned to diseases accompanied by skin rashes. Disease I was measles, II was scarlet fever, III was rubella, IV was Duke's disease (also known as **roseola** and now recognized as any rose-colored rash), and V was **erythema infectiosum**. This so-called **fifth disease** remained a mystery until the modern era.

The agent of fifth disease is now believed to be a strain of **parvovirus** designated **B19**; fifth disease is therefore also known as **B19 infection**. The parvovirus is a small DNA virion of the Parvoviridae family, having icosahedral symmetry. Community outbreaks of fifth disease occur worldwide, and transmission appears to be by respiratory droplets. Rubella is often suspected, especially if the child has not been immunized.

Fifth disease primarily affects children. The outstanding characteristic is a fiery red rash on the cheeks and ears, making it appear as if the child has been slapped, as FIGURE 12.13 shows. (The disease is sometimes called **slapped-cheek disease**.) The rash may spread to the trunk and extremities, but it fades within several days, leaving a "lacy" rash on the skin. Recurrences during ensuing days or weeks are related to bathing, sunlight, exercise, or stress. This characteristic, and the "slapped-cheek" appearance, are important to diagnosis.

Fifth disease is not limited to children. Adults suffer from painful joints similar to the symptoms of rheumatoid arthritis, especially in the fingers, wrists, knees, and ankles. Infection of the bone marrow may also lead to anemia, and pregnant women may suffer miscarriage (but birth defects generally do not occur). Although antibody preparations (immune globulin) are available for treatment, the symptoms usually resolve spontaneously.

MUMPS

Mumps takes its name from the English "to mump," meaning to be sullen or to sulk. The characteristic sign of the disease is enlarged jaw tissues arising from swollen salivary glands, especially the parotid glands. **Epidemic parotitis** is an alternate name for the disease.

The mumps virus is an RNA helical virion of the Paramyxoviridae family. Spikes with hemagglutinin are present in its envelope. The virus was among the first human viruses cultivated in fertilized chicken eggs, an achievement of Claud D. Johnson and Ernest Goodpasture in 1934.

Mumps is generally transmitted by droplets, contact, and fomites; it is considered less contagious than measles or chickenpox. The virus is found in human blood, urine, and cerebrospinal fluid, even though its effects are observed primarily in the **parotid glands**. Obstruction of the ducts leading from the glands retards the flow

---

er'i-thē'mah
Erythema:
reddening.

fifth disease virus

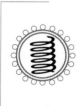

mumps virus

pah-rot'id
pa-ro-ti'tis

Fomites:
lifeless objects that transmit the agents of disease.
Parotid gland:
the large salivary gland below the ear where the upper and lower jawbones come together.

of saliva, which causes the characteristic swelling. The skin overlying the glands is usually taut and shiny, and patients experience pain when the glands are touched.

In male patients, the mumps virus may pose a threat to the **reproductive organs**. As long ago as 1790, the Scottish physician Robert Hamilton observed swelling and damage to the testes and named the condition **orchitis**, from the Greek *orchi-*, referring to the testicles. The sperm count may be reduced, but sterility is not common. An estimated 25 percent of mumps cases in postadolescent males develop into orchitis.

The **mumps vaccine**, developed in 1967, consists of attenuated viruses and is usually combined with the measles and rubella vaccines (MMR). Although the campaign against mumps never attained the fame of the campaigns against measles or rubella, the reduction of mumps cases has been equally notable. Almost 200,000 cases were recorded in 1967 but only 352 cases occurred in 1999, the lowest number ever recorded. Humans are the only hosts for the virus.

or-ki′tis
Orchitis:
an infection of the male genital organs, a complication of mumps.

To this point . . .

We have surveyed a number of viral diseases whose symptoms occur largely on the skin surface. Herpes simplex infections are manifested as blisterlike lesions in cold sores, genital herpes, and herpes keratitis. With chickenpox, the lesions are more like fluid-filled teardrops. Measles is not accompanied by lesions but rather a blushlike rash that begins on the head and then spreads to the extremities. The rubella rash is similar, but it develops and fades rapidly and often does not occur at all. A fiery red rash on the cheeks and ears is a sign of fifth disease, and swollen parotid glands typify mumps.

None of the dermotropic diseases that we have studied is known to be life-threatening, but the long-ranging effects may be consequential. For example, we have seen how SSPE is associated with measles, how orchitis may complicate mumps, how herpes zoster is an adult form of chickenpox, and how genital herpes recurs in a patient for many years. Also, a severe congenital problem is associated with rubella. Thus, many of the diseases formerly considered benign are currently viewed in a new light.

In the concluding section of this chapter, we shall study other dermotropic diseases, including smallpox, a viral disease that has been known to be potentially fatal for centuries. The remarkable feature of smallpox is that it has not been observed in humans for over 25 years. This claim cannot be made for any other disease. We shall also give brief mention to the skin warts caused by different viruses, and to Kawasaki disease, a malady not yet related to a virus with certainty.

12.3

Other Dermotropic Viral Diseases

Though dermotropic viral diseases tend to be benign, certain ones, such as smallpox, have exacted heavy tolls of human misery. Smallpox and other skin diseases are discussed in the final section of this chapter.

SMALLPOX (VARIOLA)

Smallpox has ravaged people around the world since prebiblical times. It moved swiftly across Europe and Asia, often doubling back on its path, and it was apparently brought to the New World in the 1500s by Cortez' troops. There it killed 3.5 million Native Americans and contributed to the collapse of the Inca and Aztec civilizations.

smallpox virus

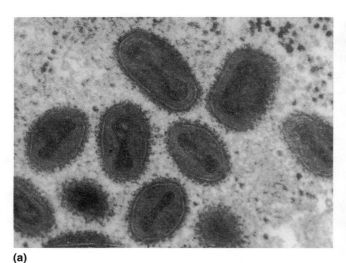

(a)

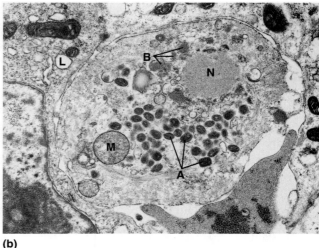

(b)

FIGURE 12.14

The Smallpox Virus

(a) A colored electron micrograph of the smallpox virus cultivated in cell culture. Note the brick-like shape of the virus and the characteristic rods at its surface. Smallpox viruses have no envelope. (b) A transmission electron micrograph of a cell infected with smallpox viruses (×30,000). Rectangular mature virions can be observed (A) as well as immature virions (B). Also visible are the cell nucleus (N), mitochondrion (M), and lysosome (L).

Nucleocapsid:
the nucleic acid core and protein coat of a virus.

Pustules:
deep pus–containing lesions that extend to the lower skin layers.

Cowpox:
a pox disease in animals that may also occur in humans.

Few people escaped the pitted scars that accompanied the disease, and children were not considered part of the family until they had survived smallpox.

Smallpox is caused by a brick-shaped DNA particle of the Poxviridae family (FIGURE 12.14). It is one of the largest virions, approximately the size of chlamydiae. The nucleocapsid is surrounded by a series of fiberlike rods with an envelope. Transmission is by contact.

The earliest signs of smallpox are high fever and general body weakness. Pink-red spots, called **macules**, soon follow, first on the face and then on the body trunk. (In chickenpox, the spots appear randomly in crops.) The spots become pink pimples, or **papules**, then fluid-filled **vesicles** so large and obvious that the disease is also called **variola**, from the Latin *varus* meaning "vessel" (FIGURE 12.15). The vesicles become deep **pustules**, which break open and emit pus. If the person survives, the pustules leave pitted scars, or **pocks**. These are generally smaller than the lesions of syphilis (the Great Pox) or varicella (chickenpox).

Centuries ago, people discovered that they could survive smallpox if they were fortunate enough to experience the disease during a mild year. The custom thus arose of "buying the pox": One would approach a person who had a mild form and offer money to rub skin together. An Oriental custom of injecting oneself with pox fluid eventually spread to Europe, and later to North America. In 1721, a hospital was established in Boston for anyone interested in **variolation**, as the process was called.

In 1798, the English physician Edward Jenner noted that milkmaids contracted a mild form of smallpox named **cowpox**, or **vaccinia** (*vacca* is Latin for "cow"). Anyone who experienced cowpox apparently did not contract smallpox. Jenner therefore utilized material from a cowpox lesion for variolation and established the process of **vaccination** (FIGURE 12.16). His method was so successful that Napoleon ordered his entire army vaccinated in 1806. The effort to vaccinate the American population was led by President Thomas Jefferson.

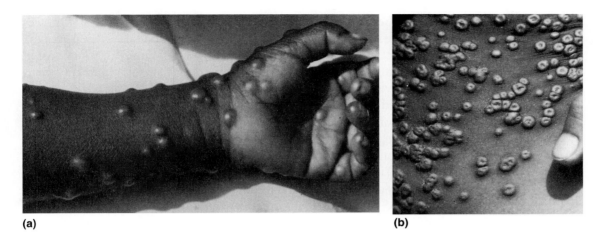

(a)

(b)

FIGURE 12.15

The Lesions of Smallpox

(a) The lesions are raised, fluid-filled vesicles similar to those in chickenpox. For this reason, cases of chickenpox have been misdiagnosed as smallpox. Later, the lesions will become pustules (b), and then form pitted scars, the pocks.

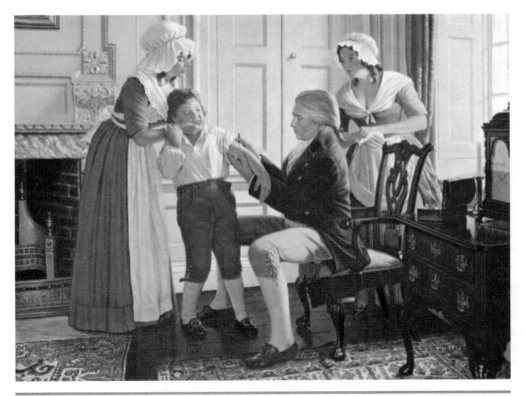

FIGURE 12.16

The First Vaccination

A painting by Robert Thom showing Edward Jenner vaccinating a young boy. The woman at the right is holding her wrist at the spot from which cowpox material was taken.

Vaccination has been hailed as one of the greatest medical and social advances because it was the first attempt to control disease on a national scale. It was also the first effort to protect the community rather than the individual. A century passed before it was understood that the antibodies produced against the mild cowpox virus were equally effective in neutralizing the smallpox virus.

In 1966, the World Health Organization (WHO) received funding to attempt the global eradication of smallpox. **Surveillance containment** methods were used to isolate every known pox victim, and all contacts were vaccinated (as noted in the chapter introduction). The eradication was aided by the fact that smallpox viruses apparently do not exist anywhere in nature except in humans. On October 26, 1977, health-care workers reported isolation of the last case, and the WHO instituted a 2-year waiting period to see if any new cases would appear. Finally, in 1979, the WHO announced worldwide smallpox eradication, the first such claim made for any disease.

As of this writing, no naturally occurring cases of smallpox have been reported. Smallpox viruses still remain in two laboratories (one at the CDC, the other in Moscow), and the 1978 smallpox death of a laboratory worker in England points up their hazard. The WHO has recommended that stocks of smallpox viruses be destroyed, especially since scientists have deciphered the base sequence of the smallpox virus genome. Not all scientists agree, however, and by the time you read this, the questions should have been resolved and the important decisions made (MicroFocus 12.8). For safety's sake, the World Health Organization maintains stocks of smallpox vaccine at depots throughout the world to immunize 300 million people.

MicroFocus 12.8

"SHOULD WE OR SHOULDN'T WE?"

One of the liveliest debates in microbiology is whether the last remaining stocks of smallpox viruses should be destroyed. Here are some of the arguments.

For Destruction:

■ People are no longer vaccinated, so if the virus should escape the laboratory, a deadly epidemic could ensue.

■ The DNA of the virus has been sequenced, and many clones of fragments are available for performing research experiments; therefore, the whole virus is no longer necessary.

■ Eradicating the disease means eradicating the remaining stocks of laboratory virus, and the stocks must be destroyed to complete the project.

■ If the United States and Russia destroy their smallpox stocks, it will send a message that biological warfare cannot be tolerated.

Against Destruction:

■ Future studies of the virus are impossible without the whole virus. Indeed, certain sequences of the viral genome defy deciphering by current laboratory means.

■ Studying the genome of the virus without the whole virus will not provide insights into how the virus causes disease.

■ Mutated viruses could cause smallpoxlike diseases, so continued research on smallpox is necessary in order to be prepared.

■ Smallpox viruses may be secretly retained in other labs in the world, so destroying the stocks may create a vulnerability. Smallpox viruses may also remain active in buried corpses.

■ Destroying the virus impairs the scientist's right to perform research, and the motivation for destruction is political, not scientific.

Now we turn to you. Can you add any insights to either list? Which argument do you prefer? Please let us know when you can.

P.S. June 1999 was originally set as the date to "throw the switch," and destroy the last stocks, but 3 months before, President Bill Clinton revoked the plan. At this writing, no new date has been set.

MOLLUSCUM CONTAGIOSUM

Molluscum contagiosum is a viral disease accompanied by **wartlike skin lesions**. The lesions are firm, waxy, and elevated with a depressed center. When pressed, they yield a milky, curdlike substance. Although usually flesh-toned, the lesions may appear white or pink. Possible areas involved include the facial skin and eyelids in children, and the external genitals in adults. The lesions may be removed by excising them (cutting them out).

The virus of molluscum contagiosum is an enveloped DNA virion of the Poxviridae family (FIGURE 12.17). Transmission is generally by contact, such as by sexual contact. A characteristic feature of the disease is the presence of large cytoplasmic bodies called **molluscum bodies** in infected cells from the base of the lesion.

mol-lus'kum
kon-ta'je-o'sum

molluscum
contagiosum virus

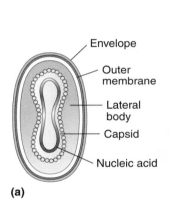

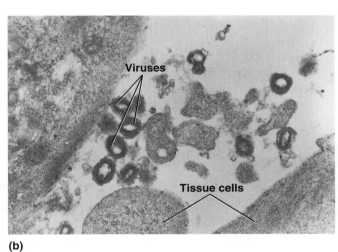

(a)   (b)

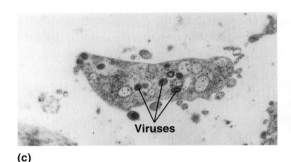

(c)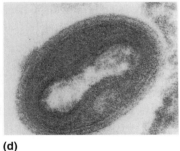

(d)

FIGURE 12.17

Poxviruses

(a) A drawing of a poxvirus, showing its complex features. Fiberlike rods (not shown) are embedded in the outer membrane and envelope of the virus. In (b) and (c), poxviruses can be seen within diseased tissue (×27,500). (d) A closeup view of a poxvirus with a transmission electron microscope (×280,000).

WARTS

Warts are small, usually benign skin growths that are commonly due to viruses. **Plantar warts** occur on the soles of the feet. **Genital warts** are often transmitted in sexual contact. These warts are sometimes called **condylomata**, from the Greek *kondyloma*, meaning "knob," a reference to the figlike appearance of the warts. They are usually moist and pink.

One of the primary causes of warts are the **human papilloma viruses**, a collection of over two dozen types of icosahedral DNA virions of the Papovaviridae family. In most cases, the skin warts they cause are a minor problem. However, evidence suggests that certain papilloma viruses may be associated with **cervical cancer**. Indeed, in 1994 researchers reported the identification of DNA from 25 types of papilloma viruses in the tumor cells of 95 percent of patients having cervical cancer.

Genital warts caused by papilloma viruses may be transferred during sexual intercourse, and some virologists suggest that this condition may be more prevalent than genital herpes. An estimated 4 million Americans are believed to be infected, and many harbor and transmit the virus without experiencing symptoms. Malignancies of the cervix, vagina, penis, and anus have also yielded papilloma viruses. Moreover, a pregnant woman with genital warts may transmit the viruses during the birth process, and studies show that in the newborn the viruses may lodge in the larynx, trachea, and the lungs. A controversial study reported in 1999 has linked the viruses to prostate cancer.

TABLE 12.2 presents a summary of the dermotropic viral diseases covered in this chapter.

con'di-lo-mah'tah

pap-i-lo'mah

human papilloma virus

KAWASAKI DISEASE

Although Kawasaki disease has not yet been identified as a viral disorder, the course of the disease suggests that an infectious agent is involved. We shall therefore consider it here.

Kawasaki disease takes its name from the Japanese pediatrician Tomisaku Kawasaki, who described its symptoms in 1967. Children 1 to 2 years old account for most patients. The illness is characterized by a high fever and sore throat; then, **red spots** appear, first on the extremities and next the body trunk. As the disease progresses, there is a characteristic peeling of the skin about the fingers, a phenomenon called **desquamation**. Complications of Kawasaki disease usually involve the cardiovascular system, and internal bleeding may occur. Treatment is generally directed at minimizing these possibilities.

Kawasaki disease was first detected in the United States in 1971. Since then, it has been reported with increasing frequency, and about 2500 cases were reported through the 1980s. A notable outbreak in 1985 in the Denver, Colorado, area involved 61 people.

There is some laboratory evidence that a staphylococcus or a streptococcus may be involved in Kawasaki disease. The possibility also exists that the disease is an immune-related syndrome complicating some unknown viral disease in the same manner that Reye syndrome follows influenza and chickenpox. Some physicians therefore refer to the illness as **Kawasaki syndrome**. Indeed, the CDC has made no mention of the disease in its reports since 1989, and most other microbiology textbooks do not discuss it. Perhaps Kawasaki disease will also disappear from this textbook one day, but for the time being, it is important to be aware of its existence.

des'kwa-ma'shun

Syndrome:
a collection of symptoms.

TABLE 12.2

A Summary of Dermotropic Viral Diseases

DISEASE	CLASSIFICATION OF VIRUS	TRANSMISSION	ORGANS AFFECTED	VACCINE	SPECIAL FEATURES	COMPLICATIONS
Herpes simplex	Herpesviridae	Contact	Skin Pharynx Genital organs	Not available	Characteristic lesions Lipschütz bodies Acyclovir treatment	Encephalitis Congenital infections Neonatal herpes
Chickenpox (varicella)	Herpesviridae	Droplets Contact	Skin Nervous system	Attenuated viruses	Characteristic lesions Crops Acyclovir treatment	Herpes zoster (shingles) Reye syndrome Pneumonia
Measles (rubeola)	Paramyxoviridae	Droplets Contact	Respiratory tract Skin, blood	Attenuated viruses	Koplik spots Progress of rash Hemagglutination inhibition	SSPE Pneumonia Encephalitis
Rubella (German measles)	Togaviridae	Droplets Contact	Skin, blood	Attenuated viruses	Skin rash Mild cold symptoms	Congenital rubella syndrome
Fifth disease (Erythema infectiosum)	Parvoviridae	Droplets(?)	Skin, blood	Not available	"Slapped-cheek" appearance Lacy skin patterns	None established
Mumps (epidemic parotitis)	Paramyxoviridae	Droplets	Salivary glands Blood	Attenuated viruses	Swollen glands Hemagglutination inhibition	Orchitis Encephalitis Meningitis
Smallpox (variola)	Poxviridae	Contact Droplets Fomites	Skin Blood	Cowpox viruses	Characteristic lesions Macules, papules, vesicles, pox	Permanent scarring
Molluscum contagiosum	Poxviridae	Contact	Skin	Not available	Characteristic lesions	None
Warts	Papovaviridae	Contact	Skin	Not available	Characteristic lesions	None
Kawasaki disease	(Unknown)	(Unknown)	Skin, blood	Not available	Skin rash Desquamation	Heart involvement

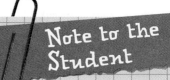

Note to the Student

In this chapter, we have had an opportunity to note the changing complexion of microbiology. We have seen, for example, how measles viruses are increasingly associated with neurological problems, how Reye syndrome has become linked to influenza and chickenpox, how an association is growing between cervical tumors and herpes simplex viruses, and how chickenpox and herpes zoster, once thought to be separate diseases, are now linked to the same virus. Moreover, we note that despite modern detection devices, there is still no identifiable agent for Kawasaki disease.

The point is that microbiology is a dynamic and ever-changing science. This dynamism implies that microbiologists and physicians must continually adjust to new truths as they emerge. A friend once told me that if you dip a tennis ball into the ocean, the water dripping from the ball represents all that is known; the ocean represents all that is waiting to be discovered.

Summary

Within broad limits, viral diseases usually occur in specific parts of the body. Accordingly, the diseases can be classified into four categories, two of which are pneumotropic viral diseases and dermotropic viral diseases. Pneumotropic diseases occur in the respiratory tract, while dermotropic diseases display their symptoms on the skin or close to the skin surface.

Among the important pneumotropic diseases are influenza, adenovirus infections, respiratory syncytial (RS) disease, and rhinovirus infections. Varying degrees of fever and respiratory distress accompany all these diseases, and life-threatening situations are rare except if secondary infection takes place, as is possible with influenza. Various sites of infection within the respiratory tract are seen, ranging from the air sacs for RS disease to the nose for rhinoviral infec-tion. Adenovirus infections can occur outside the respiratory tract as well.

The dermotropic viral diseases include mild infections such as chickenpox and serious infections such as smallpox. Infection can begin with skin contact, such as in herpes simplex, smallpox, or warts, or it may be initiated by airborne viruses. In the latter case, the viruses infect the respiratory tract causing mild respiratory symptoms, then invade the blood and localize near the skin where they induce manifestations of disease. The skin rashes of measles, rubella, and fifth disease are typical. Mumps also follows this pattern but a skin rash is not present; rather, there is salivary gland swelling and a painfully tight skin. Kawasaki disease is included in this chapter because of its skin symptoms, even though a viral agent has not yet been identified.

Questions for Thought and Discussion

1. In the mid-1980s, the nation's colleges for the deaf reported an unprecedented demand for admission. For example, at the National Technical Institute for the Deaf at Rochester Institute of Technology, the student body swelled from 750 students to 1250 students. How was this related to the events of a previous generation involving rubella?

2. In February 1992, the CDC reported an outbreak of measles at an international gymnastics competition in Indianapolis, Indiana. A total of 700 athletes and numerous coaches and managers from 51 countries were involved. Although the potential for a disastrous international epidemic was high, it never materialized. What steps do you think the local health agencies took to quell the spread of the disease?

3. A little girl experiences frequent and severe vomiting for a period of hours. She soon becomes sleepy and glassy-eyed. When disturbed, she quickly becomes irritated and combative. One week before, she had recovered from chickenpox. What is she experiencing, and what course of action must be taken?

4. Thomas Sydenham, the "English Hippocrates," was a London physician in the seventeenth century. In 1661, he differentiated measles from scarlet fever, smallpox, and other fevers, and set down the foundations for studying these diseases. How would a modern Thomas Sydenham go about distinguishing the variety of look-alike skin diseases discussed in this chapter?

5. In the United Kingdom, the approach to rubella control is to concentrate vaccination programs on young girls just before they enter the childbearing years. In the United States, the approach is to immunize all children at the age of 15 months. Which approach do you believe is preferable? Why?

6. One way of avoiding the viruses that cause common colds is to adopt the motto, "Let us spray." This motto refers to using a disinfectant spray to destroy viruses on environmental surfaces. How many *other* ways can you name for avoiding cold viruses?

7. In 1994, the fitness file of a local newspaper carried a story on "The New Herpes." The reference was to human papilloma viruses and genital warts as the herpes simplex of the 1990s. How many similarities can you find between these two diseases? Would you agree with the comparison?

8. Despite its availability and effectiveness, many physicians do not recommend the chickenpox vaccine to parents and their children. Indeed, the CDC reported that fewer than 20 percent of candidate

children were immunized during 1995 and 1996. Why do you think some physicians are reluctant to use the vaccine? Do you believe their skepticism is warranted? What might you recommend to justify or to overcome the reluctance to use the vaccine?

9. Most physicians agree that there would be great demand for a genital herpes vaccine. However, there is much opposition to marketing a vaccine that contains attenuated herpes simplex viruses. Why is this so? What alternatives are there for a useful vaccine against genital herpes?

10. It is not uncommon for a person with respiratory disease to visit the doctor and be told: "Don't worry about it. It's just a touch of the flu. I'll give you a shot of penicillin before you leave." Suppose the person wanted to know if it really was influenza. What diagnostic tests would have to be performed? Also, why is the doctor inclined to give a penicillin injection?

11. A child experiences "red bumps" on her face, scalp, and back. Within 24 hours, they have turned to tiny blisters and become cloudy, some developing into sores. Finally, all become brown scabs. New "bumps" keep appearing for several days, and her fever reaches 102°F by the fourth day. Then the blisters stop coming and the fever drops. What disease has she had?

12. The great seventeenth-century physician William Harvey, who discovered how blood circulates, was a great fan of garlic therapy to treat disease. In one of his writings, Harvey recommended putting a clove of garlic inside your shoe when you have a respiratory illness. What do you think of Harvey's recommendation?

13. One day in March 1977, a Boeing 737 bound for Kodiak, Alaska, developed engine trouble and was forced to land. While the company rounded up another aircraft, the passengers sat waiting for 4 hours in the unventilated cabin. One passenger, it seemed, was in the early stages of influenza and was coughing heavily. By the week's end, 38 of the 54 passengers on the plane had developed influenza. What lessons does this incident teach?

14. Although smallpox viruses are considered to be gone from the environment, there remains a closely related virus that causes monkeypox in nature. By what genetic mechanisms could this virus conceivably become a smallpox virus?

15. A man experiences an attack of shingles and is warned by his doctor to stay away from children as much as possible. Why is this advice given? Is it justified?

Review

On completing your study of pneumotropic and dermotropic viral diseases, test your comprehension of the chapter contents by circling the choices that best complete each of the following statements. The answers are listed in Appendix D.

1. Rhinoviruses are a collection of (RNA, DNA) viruses having (helical, icosahedral) symmetry and the ability to infect the (air sacs, nose), causing (mild, serious) respiratory symptoms.

2. Herpes simplex is a viral disease that can be transmitted by (breathing contaminated air, contact) and is characterized by thin-walled (blisters, ulcers) that often appear during periods of (emotional stress, exercising), but can be treated with a drug called (deoxycyclovir, acyclovir).

3. In children, the skin lesions of chickenpox occur (all at once, in crops) and resemble (teardrops, pitted scars), but in adults the lesions are known as (shingles, erythemas) and resemble blotchy patches of (blue, red) that are very (itchy, painful).

4. For generations, rubella was thought to be a mild form of (chickenpox, measles) because it was also accompanied by (a skin rash, brain lesions) and was transmitted by (contaminated water, airborne droplets).

5. The complications of influenza include (Reye, Koplik) syndrome; for mumps, the complication is a disease of the (testes, pancreas) called (colitis, orchitis), and for measles, it is a disease of the (brain, liver) known as (SSPE, GBS).

6. One of the early signs of (smallpox, measles) is a series of (Koplik spots, Lipschütz bodies) occurring in the (lungs, mouth) and signaling that a (red rash, blue-green rash) is forthcoming.

7. Although the agent of (fifth, sixth) disease has not been identified with certainty, the leading candidate is the (B29, B19) strain of (picornavirus, parvovirus), a small (DNA, RNA) virus.

8. After transmission by (mosquitoes, airborne droplets), the virus of (mumps, Kawasaki disease) spreads by the blood to the (salivary, sweat) glands, where it interferes with fluid secretion.

9. Although now eradicated, (mumps, smallpox) can be prevented by immunizations with (fowlpox, cowpox) virus in a method first devised in 1798 by Edward (Jennings, Jenner).

10. Antigenic variation among (mumps, influenza) viruses seriously hampers the development of a highly effective (vaccine, treatment), and a life-threatening situation can occur if secondary infection due to (fungi, bacteria) complicates the primary infection.

11. Respiratory syncytial disease is caused by a (DNA, RNA) virus that infects the (lungs, intestines) of (adults, children) and induces cells to (clump together, move apart) and form giant cells called (syncytia, tumors).

12. Warts are small, benign skin growths caused by human (parvoviruses, papilloma viruses), transmitted by (sexual contact, contaminated milk), and somewhat similar to the growths associated with (chickenpox, molluscum contagiosum).

13. Adenoviruses include a collection of (DNA, RNA) viruses that induce the formation of (granules, inclusions) and are responsible for (yellow fever, common colds), as well as infections of the (eye, ear) and (kidneys, meninges).

14. Genital herpes is caused by a (helical, icosahedral) virus that is believed to affect 10 to 20 (thousand, million) Americans each year, causing blisters with (thick, thin) walls that disappear in about 3 (days, weeks), only to reappear when (stress, physical injury) occurs.

15. The TORCH diseases are a set of (infectious, physiological) diseases transmitted by (airborne droplets, transplacental passage), occurring in (the elderly, newborns), and including (rubeola, rubella) and (herpes simplex, humoral disease).

16. The MMR vaccine contains (inactivated, attenuated) viruses and is used primarily in (children, older adults) to provide (long-term, short-term) immunity to such diseases as (measles, molluscum contagiosum), (mononucleosis, mumps), and (German measles, influenza).

http://microbiology.jbpub.com

The site features **eLearning,** an on-line review area that provides quizzes and other tools to help you study for your class. You can also follow useful links for in-depth information, read more MicroFocus stories, or just find out the latest microbiology news.

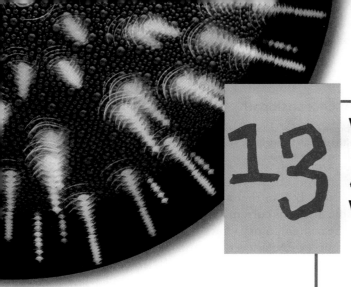

13

Viscerotropic and Neurotropic Viral Diseases

Gone are hamburgers, beef stew, beef sausages, and even Yorkshire pudding, that drippings-soaked symbol of British culinary aplomb.

—From an article in *Discover* magazine describing the 1997 British response to mad cow disease

I T APPEARED IN ENGLAND IN 1986. First one cow showed the symptoms, then another and another. All of them were apprehensive and twitchy, overreacting to a sound or touch. Soon the whole herd developed a peculiar, high-stepping, swaying gait with an unsteady lurch. Some cows became overly aggressive, and soon the local residents were talking about the day the cows went mad.

By 1990, cows were becoming ill at the rate of hundreds per week, and cartoon writers were having a field day, with mad cows descending on farmhouses and milk factories. To health officials, however, the situation was more foreboding than mirthful (FIGURE 13.1). Were the milk and meat supplies contaminated, and would humans be next? Indeed, there were reports of mad cats, and speculation arose that cat food made from bovine parts was to blame.

Through all the months, virologists had been drawing a parallel between the unknown disease and **scrapie**, the disease in which sheep develop neurological symptoms. Under the microscope, scrapie-infected tissue looks spongy, with tiny fluid-filled holes, exactly like the cows' brain tissue. But how was the agent transferred to cows? Then, veterinary researchers discovered that young calves are often fed a protein-rich feed made from the carcasses of sheep.

Today, the term "**mad cow disease**" is used primarily by journalists. The proper name for the disease is **bovine spongiform encephalopathy,** or **BSE**. (The parts of the name refer to cow, spongy appearance, and brain disease.)

bo'vine sponj'i-form
en-cef-a-lop'a-thē

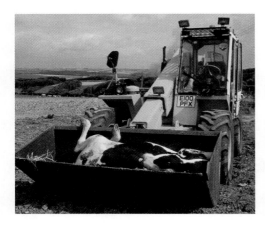

FIGURE 13.1

Bovine Spongiform Encephalopathy

During the 1990s, an outbreak of BSE—"mad cow disease"—brought a strong response from public health officials in England. The epidemic subsided after extreme measures were taken to destroy all animals that might possibly be infected.

Most investigators consider BSE in the same terms as scrapie, and a human equivalent of the disease is currently being researched.

BSE will be one of the contemporary viral diseases we study in this chapter. We shall also survey Ebola fever, hepatitis, polio, and other diseases that are discussed in the news media regularly. In addition, a major focus of the chapter will be on acquired immune deficiency syndrome, better known as AIDS. This disease was probably the longest-lived and most notorious epidemic of the late twentieth century.

vis'er-o-trōp'ik

The diseases we shall study in this chapter fall into two general categories. Some illnesses, such as yellow fever and mononucleosis, are regarded as viscerotropic diseases because they affect the blood and visceral organs. The second category of illnesses are the neurotropic diseases, such as BSE, polio, and rabies, which affect the central nervous system. As in Chapter 12, each disease is presented as a separate essay, and you may select the order of study most suitable to your needs.

nur'o-trōp'ik
Visceral organs:
the internal organs of the chest, abdominal, and pelvic regions.

13.1

Viscerotropic Viral Diseases

he viscerotropic viral diseases affect such organs as the blood, liver, spleen, and the small and large intestines. To reach these organs, the viruses are generally introduced to the body tissues by arthropods or by contaminated food and drink, as we shall see in the discussions that follow.

YELLOW FEVER

The earliest known outbreak of **yellow fever** in the Western Hemisphere took place in Central America in 1596. The disease spread rapidly, and it soon rendered large regions of the Caribbean and tropical Americas almost uninhabitable. In time, natives developed immunity or suffered only mild cases, but the mortality rate in outsiders remained high. Finally, in 1901, a group led by Walter Reed identified **mosquitoes** as the agents of transmission (MicroFocus 13.1). With widespread vector control, the incidence rate of the disease gradually declined.

yellow fever virus

Yellow fever was the first human disease associated with a virus. The causative agent is an RNA virion of the Flaviviridae family with icosahedral symmetry and an envelope. It is one of the smallest known viruses and is often referred to as an **arbovirus** because it is *ar*thropod-*bo*rne.

Yellow fever occurs in nature in monkeys and other jungle animals, where the virus is transmitted by various mosquitoes, including species of *Haemogogus*. In the cities, a different mosquito, *Aedes aegypti*, transmits the virus among humans. (The tiger mosquito *Aedes albopictus* has also been implicated in transmission.) *Aedes aegypti* is common in the Caribbean region and in the southern and eastern United

hem'ah-go'gus
a-e'dez a-gip'ti
al-bo-pic'tus

MicroFocus 13.1

"FOR THE CAUSE OF HUMANITY . . ."

During the Spanish American War, the U.S. government became disease-conscious because more soldiers were dying from disease than from bullet wounds. Yellow fever was particularly bad in Cuba, where it exacted a heavy toll. When the war was over, Cuba remained under U.S. control, and the Surgeon General sent a commission of four men to study the disease. Led by Major Walter Reed, the group included three assistant surgeons: James Carroll, Jesse W. Lazear, and Aristides Agaramonte. On June 25, 1900, the four men assembled in Cuba and began their work.

At first the commission devoted its energy to isolating a bacterium, but none could be found. As the weeks wore on, the investigators were impressed with the peculiar way the disease jumped from house to house, even when there was no contact with infected persons or contaminated objects. They also visited Carlos J. Finlay, a physician from Havana who insisted that mosquitoes were involved in transmission. If his theory was true, then the disease could be interrupted by simply killing the mosquitoes.

By now it was August, and Reed had been called back to Washington. Carroll, Lazear, and Agaramonte pushed forward and bred mosquitoes from eggs given them by Finlay. They allowed the mosquitoes to feed on patients with established cases of yellow fever, and then they applied the insects to the skin of volunteers, including themselves. The results were inconclusive: Some volunteers got yellow fever, but others did not. Two accidents then saved the research. One was fortunate, the other tragic.

One day in late August, Carroll decided to feed an "old" mosquito some of his own blood, lest it die. Three days later, Carroll was ill with the fever.

Lazear's notebook recorded that the insect had fed "*twelve days* before on a yellow fever patient, who was then in his *second day* of the disease." This, they discovered, was the proper combination of two factors necessary for a successful transmission. The disease could be reproduced over and over again, if this procedure was followed.

Then came tragedy. Lazear was working at the bedside of a yellow fever patient when a stray mosquito settled on his wrist. For reasons not clear, Lazear let the insect drink its fill. Five days later, he developed yellow fever; on the seventh day of his illness, he died. Lazear had been bitten previously, but apparently by uninfected mosquitoes. This time, the mosquito was infected.

Reed returned to Cuba in October, and a new set of experiments was planned to prove once and for all that clothing and other objects could not transmit yellow fever. The experiments were gruesome: Some volunteers slept in blood-soaked and vomit-stained garments of disease victims; others allowed themselves to be mercilessly bitten by mosquitoes; still others came forward to be injected with blood from yellow fever victims. By late 1900, there was no doubt that mosquitoes were the carriers of yellow fever.

It has been said that the experiments performed in Cuba are among the noblest in the history of medicine. Two volunteers, Private John R. Kissinger and clerk John J. Moran, were asked why they were agreeing to such life-threatening experiments. "We volunteer," they replied, "solely for the cause of humanity and in the interest of science."

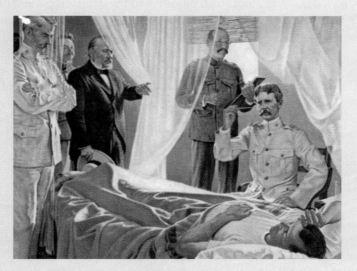

■ A painting by Robert Thom depicting members of the yellow fever commission at the bedside of Private John Kissinger, after he was bitten by infected mosquitoes. Left to right: Major W. C. Gorgas (Havana sanitation officer), Aristides Agaramonte, Carlos J. Finlay, James Carroll, and Walter Reed. The experiments were conducted at Camp Lazear, named for Jesse Lazear, who had died of yellow fever the previous summer.

MicroFocus 13.2

MOVING DAY

Bank Street is a well-known thoroughfare in New York City, but in 1798, it did not even exist. That year, yellow fever struck the city, and a clerk at the Bank of New York, then on downtown Wall Street, developed the disease. Both he and the bank were quarantined for a spell, and the

bank suffered a considerable loss of business. Determined to avoid a recurrence, the bank directors purchased eight lots on a nameless lane in Greenwich Village, a suburban area north of the city. There they erected an outpost of the bank "for emergencies," as they put it.

Sure enough, yellow fever returned

in 1822. People were fleeing the city for the peace and solitude of Greenwich Village, and the bank directors figured now was the time to move. And move they did—lock, stock, and barrel—to their new neighborhood, and to their new street, which they eventually named (you guessed it) Bank Street.

States, and yellow fever was a problem in these areas for many generations (**Micro-Focus 13.2**). In 1803, for example, emperor Napoleon of France sent troops to quell an uprising in Haiti, but yellow fever killed thousands of his men. Soon thereafter, Napoleon came to think of the Americas as a fever-ridden land, and when President Thomas Jefferson sent emissaries to negotiate the purchase of the French New Orleans region, Napoleon offered the entire Louisiana territory at a bargain price.

Yellow fever can be a fatal disease. Mosquitoes inject the viruses into the bloodstream, and fever mounts within days. Infection of the liver causes an overflow of bile pigments into the blood, a condition called **jaundice**, and the complexion becomes yellow (the disease is often called "yellow jack"). The gums bleed, the stools turn bloody, and the delirious patient often vomits blood. Patients die of internal bleeding, and mortality rates are very high, as in a notable Philadelphia epidemic of 1793 (**MicroFocus 13.3**).

Except for supportive therapy, no treatment exists for yellow fever. However, the disease can be prevented by immunization with either of two **vaccines**. The more widely used vaccine contains the 17D strain of yellow fever virus cultivated in chicken eggs. Max Theiler, a South African physician, won the 1951 Nobel Prize in Physiology or Medicine for the development of this vaccine.

Bile:
a yellow-brown mixture of acids, salts, pigments, and other substances produced by the liver and stored in the gall bladder; assists fat digestion.

ti'ler

MicroFocus 13.3

THE PHILADELPHIA STORY

Yellow fever was one of the most dramatic diseases ever to strike the United States. During the 1700s, historians chronicled 35 separate outbreaks as the disease ravaged the country. Nowhere did yellow fever strike harder than in Philadelphia.

In 1793, Philadelphia was the capital of the United States, and its largest city, with a population of 40,000. When yellow fever broke out, the panic rivaled that in Europe during the plague years. In patients, the eyes glazed, the flesh

yellowed, and delirium developed. People died, not here and there, but in clusters and in alarming patterns. Friends recoiled from one another. If they met by chance, they did not shake hands but nodded distantly and hurried on. The air felt diseased, and people dodged to the windward of those they passed. The deaths went on, great ugly scythings of humanity.

At the height of the epidemic, thousands fled Philadelphia, and officials posted warning notices on all homes

where people were infected. Those who could not get away, including most of the city's poor, sought protection by breathing through cloth masks soaked in garlic juice, vinegar, or camphor. Benjamin Rush, a noted American physician (and signer of the Declaration of Independence), prescribed a frightening course of purges, blood lettings, vomiting, and immersion in icewater to reduce fever. Nearly all the 24,000 people who remained in Philadelphia were afflicted. Almost 5000 died.

DENGUE FEVER

Dengue fever has been known since David Bylon, a physician in the Dutch East Indies, described an outbreak in 1779. The disease takes its name from the Swahili word *dinga*, meaning "cramplike attack," a reference to the symptoms. Dengue fever is caused by an RNA icosahedral virion of the Flaviviridae family that multiplies in white blood cells and platelets. The virus is closely related to the yellow fever virus, except that four strains of dengue fever virus are known to exist. Transmission is by the ***Aedes aegypti* mosquito** and by the tiger mosquito ***Aedes albopictus*** (FIGURE 13.2).

High fever and prostration are early signs of dengue fever. These are followed by sharp pain in the muscles and joints, and patients often report sensations that their bones are breaking. The disease is therefore also called **breakbone fever**. Another name, **saddleback fever**, is used because of temperature fluctuations. After about a week, the symptoms fade. Death is uncommon, but if one of the other strains of dengue virus later enters the body, a condition called **dengue hemorrhagic fever** may occur. In this condition, a rash from skin hemorrhages appears on the face and extremities, and severe vomiting and shock ensue as the blood pressure decreases dramatically.

Dengue fever has traditionally been confined to Southeast Asia. However, in 1963, the disease broke out in Central America, and it has occurred sporadically in the Americas since then.

deng'e

dengue fever virus

Breakbone fever:
an alternate name for dengue fever, accompanied by bone-breaking sensations.

INFECTIOUS MONONUCLEOSIS

The name **infectious mononucleosis** (or "mono" in the vernacular) is familiar to young adults because the disease is common in this age group. It is sometimes called the "kissing disease" because it is spread by contact with saliva. Droplets and fomites, such as table utensils and drinking glasses, may also carry the virus.

Infectious mononucleosis is a blood disease, especially of antibody-producing **B-lymphocytes** of the lymph nodes and spleen. Enlargement of the lymph nodes ("swollen glands") is accompanied by a sore throat, fever, and a high count of damaged **B-lymphocytes**, a type of mononuclear white blood cell (hence the disease's name, mononucleosis). Mononucleosis usually runs its course in 3 to 4 weeks. Among the most dangerous complications are defects of the heart, paralysis of the face, and rupture of the spleen. The liver may be involved and jaundice may occur,

infectious
mononucleosis virus

B-lymphocyte:
a type of mononuclear white blood cell that functions in the immune system.

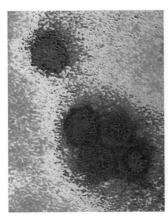

(a)

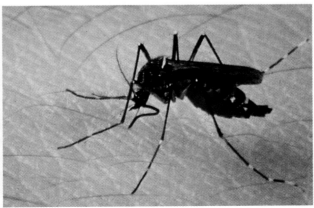

(b)

FIGURE 13.2

The Dengue Fever Virus and Its Vector

(a) A colored transmission electron micrograph of dengue fever viruses (red clusters) in the cytoplasm of host tissue cells (×210,000). (b) The *Aedes aegypti* mosquito, which transmits dengue fever as well as yellow fever.

a condition some physicians refer to as hepatitis. Those who recover usually become carriers for several months and shed the viruses into their saliva.

The diagnostic procedures for mononucleosis include detection of an elevated lymphocyte count and the observation of **Downey cells**, the damaged B-lymphocytes with vacuolated and granulated cytoplasm. The patient also experiences an elevation of **heterophile antibodies** (antibodies reacting with antigens from unrelated species). Such antibodies can be detected by the **Paul-Bunnell test**, performed by mixing samples of the patient's serum with sheep or horse erythrocytes and observing the cells for agglutination. FIGURE 13.3 describes an adaptation of this test. The disease strikes an estimated 100,000 people annually in the United States.

The virus of infectious mononucleosis is a DNA herpesvirus having icosahedral symmetry and an envelope. Some virologists suggest that the virus enters the body when the person is very young, then replicates and remains inside the lymphocytes before emerging in the young adult. A substantial body of evidence indicates that it is identical to the **Epstein-Barr (EB) virus**. This virus has been detected in patients

het'er-o-fil'
Antigens:
substances that stimulate the immune system, often resulting in antibodies.

FIGURE 13.3

The Monospot Slide Test for Infectious Mononucleosis

This test is based on an agglutination reaction between horse erythrocytes and infectious mononucleosis antibodies. Suitable controls not shown in the figure must also be included.

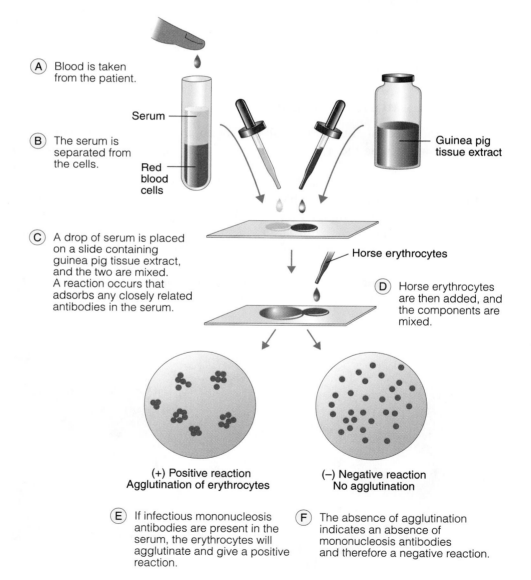

(A) Blood is taken from the patient.

Serum

(B) The serum is separated from the cells.

Red blood cells

Guinea pig tissue extract

(C) A drop of serum is placed on a slide containing guinea pig tissue extract, and the two are mixed. A reaction occurs that adsorbs any closely related antibodies in the serum.

Horse erythrocytes

(D) Horse erythrocytes are then added, and the components are mixed.

(+) Positive reaction
Agglutination of erythrocytes

(−) Negative reaction
No agglutination

(E) If infectious mononucleosis antibodies are present in the serum, the erythrocytes will agglutinate and give a positive reaction.

(F) The absence of agglutination indicates an absence of mononucleosis antibodies and therefore a negative reaction.

who have **Burkitt's lymphoma**, a tumor of the connective tissues of the jaw that is prevalent in areas of Africa. First isolated in the early 1960s by British virologists M. Anthony Epstein and Yvonne M. Barr, the Epstein-Barr virus was a surprising revelation and an important breakthrough in medicine because it demonstrated the link between viruses and cancer. **Epstein-Barr virus disease** is assumed to be a precursor to mononucleosis.

Contemporary virologists continue to search for reasons why the EB virus is associated with tumors on one continent and infectious mononucleosis on another. Some cancer specialists theorize that the malaria parasite, common in Africa, acts as an irritant of the lymph gland tissue, thereby stimulating tumor development. Another possibility is that there are really two viruses, a mononucleosis virus and an Epstein-Barr virus, and that one triggers the other to function.

The EB virus has also been linked to **chronic fatigue syndrome**. The symptoms include sore throat, aching muscles, sleep disturbances, swollen lymph nodes, and prolonged, overwhelming fatigue (patients say they feel as limp as Raggedy Ann dolls). Evidence of EB virus involvement is based on the presence of these viruses and their antibodies in some affected individuals. The relationship is not conclusive, however, and some investigators remain skeptical of any microbial involvement. In 1996, for instance, a high-ranking CDC official wrote: "The current body of scientific evidence argues against the possibility that chronic fatigue syndrome is caused by an infectious agent." That same year, scientists found that some cases were related to poor regulation of blood pressure by autonomic nerves; adjusting the body's salt levels via the diet resolved the syndrome. The tendency at present is to diagnose chronic fatigue syndrome by excluding other potential causes of prolonged fatigue.

Burkitt's lymphoma:
a type of cancer occurring in connective tissues of the jaw.

Malaria:
a serious protozoal disease of the red blood cells, transmitted by mosquitoes.

HEPATITIS A

Some years ago, the members of a university football team paused during practice and drank water taken from a local well. But this was no ordinary water. During the previous week, the water had been contaminated by viruses seeping into the well from a cesspool high above. Within days, all the players began to feel ill, and soon the unmistakable signs of hepatitis appeared. MicroFocus 13.4 recounts another such incident.

MicroFocus 13.4

THIRTY-TWO AND COUNTING

For some, the number 13 is unlucky, but for the town of Peter's Creek, Alaska, the unlucky number was 32. It was late spring 1988, and the weather was unusually hot for that time of year. Between May 23 and June 10, 32 unfortunate people contracted hepatitis A, and things went downhill fast.

The outbreak of hepatitis was traced to a local convenience market, and the culprit was the ice slush that so many people enjoy on a hot day. The slush was contaminated, possibly by a certain store employee. Although the employee refused to be tested, his sister had had hepatitis A recently, and he had looked somewhat jaundiced at the time. He was one of two store employees responsible for preparing the slush each day. (Later, it was learned that he used water from the bathroom sink to make the slush.)

For the unlucky patients, there were many days of abdominal pain, fever, jaundice, and a serious liver disease. They would have to avoid fats and oils (no fried foods, mayonnaise, or oily salad dressings), and they could not have alcohol of any type. For many, there was the added burden of knowing they had infected others, because 23 additional cases soon developed. It was not a summer to remember fondly.

FIGURE 13.4

Hepatitis A Viruses

An electron micrograph of hepatitis A viruses (×241,000). The particles were coated with antibodies to assist staining. The coating accounts for the halo around the viruses.

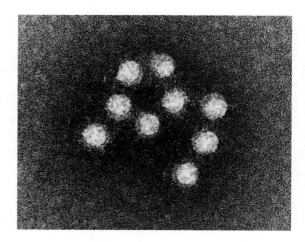

hepatitis A virus

pi-kor'nah-vir'ĭ-da

Incubation period:
the time that elapses between entry of the microorganism to the host and the appearance of symptoms.
Anorexia:
a prolonged loss of appetite.
Jaundice:
a yellowing of the complexion and eyes caused by an overflow of bile pigments to the bloodstream.

Immune globulin:
an antibody preparation used as a preventative or treatment for disease.

Hepatitis is an acute inflammatory disease of the liver caused by several viruses. **Hepatitis A (infectious hepatitis)** is the form most commonly transmitted by food or water contaminated by the feces of an infected individual. An infected food handler is often involved, and outbreaks have also been traced to day-care centers where workers contact contaminated feces. In addition, the disease may be transmitted by raw shellfish such as clams and oysters, since these animals filter and concentrate the viruses from contaminated seawater.

Hepatitis A is caused by a small RNA virion considered by most virologists to belong to the Picornaviridae family and referred to as a **heparnavirus** (*hepatitis-RNA-virus*). The virion lacks an envelope and appears to have cubic symmetry (resembling a cube), but this factor is not fully documented (**FIGURE 13.4**). Hepatitis A viruses are very resistant to chemical and physical agents, and several minutes of exposure to boiling water may be necessary to inactivate them.

The incubation period for hepatitis A is usually between 2 and 4 weeks. Therefore, hepatitis A is sometimes called **short-incubation hepatitis** (relative to hepatitis B, or long-incubation hepatitis). Initial symptoms include anorexia, nausea, vomiting, and low-grade fever. Discomfort in the upper-right quadrant of the abdomen follows as the liver enlarges. Considerable jaundice usually follows the onset of symptoms by 1 or 2 weeks (the urine darkens, as well), but many cases are without jaundice. The symptoms may last for several weeks, and relapses are common. A long period of convalescence is generally required, during which alcohol and other liver irritants are excluded from the diet.

Diagnostic procedures for hepatitis A are based on liver function tests, observation of characteristic symptoms, and the demonstration of hepatitis A antibodies in the serum. The virus is excreted in large numbers in the stools about 2 weeks before symptoms appear. In one recent incident, for example, a restaurant worker in New Jersey became infected on May 9 but showed no symptoms, even though he was shedding hepatitis viruses. Hepatitis symptoms developed at the end of May, and during the first 3 weeks of June, 56 cases of hepatitis broke out among patrons of the restaurant.

There is no treatment for hepatitis A except for prolonged rest and relieving symptoms. In those exposed to the virus, it is possible to prevent development of the disease by administering **hepatitis A immune globulin** within 2 weeks of infection. This preparation consists of antiviral antibodies obtained from blood donors. Blood is routinely screened for hepatitis antibodies, and if large amounts are found, the blood serum is used for immune globulin. In the New Jersey outbreak cited previously, 1430 people were given injections during a 2-day clinic held on June 19 and 20. And over 30,000 individuals received injections during a 1997 outbreak related to strawberries (**MicroFocus 13.5**).

Maintaining high standards of personal and environmental hygiene, and removing the source of contamination, are essential to interrupting the spread of hepatitis A. Moreover, in 1995, the Food and Drug Administration (FDA) licensed a **vaccine** composed of formalin-inactivated viruses. Known commercially as Havrix, the vaccine is administered into the deltoid muscle in two doses to those between ages 2 and 18 (pediatric formulation) and in three doses to those over age 18 (adult formulation). A second vaccine (Vaqta) requiring only one dose was licensed in 1996. Over 20,000 Americans contract hepatitis A each year.

Deltoid muscle: the shoulder muscle.

TABLE 13.1 compares hepatitis A with hepatitis B and hepatitis C, the other major types of hepatitis.

HEPATITIS B

Hepatitis B (serum hepatitis) is the second major type of hepatitis. It is caused by a DNA virus known as a **hepadnavirus** (*hepa*titis-*DNA*-*virus*) of the family Hepadnaviridae. The hepadnavirus can appear in three forms. In its most frequently observed form, the virus is seen as spherical particles measuring about 22 nm in diameter. These small particles appear to be composed exclusively of an antigenic protein substance called **hepatitis B surface antigen**, or **HBsAg**. A second

hep-ad'na-virus

TABLE 13.1

A Comparison of Three Types of Hepatitis

CHARACTERISTIC	HEPATITIS A	HEPATITIS B	HEPATITIS C
Alternate names	Infectious hepatitis	Serum hepatitis	Posttransfusion hepatitis NANB hepatitis
Virus	RNA virus Picornaviridae	DNA virus Dane particle Hepadnaviridae	RNA virus Flaviviridae
Incubation period	2–4 weeks	4 weeks to 6 months	2 weeks to 6 months
Major transmission	Food and water Saliva contact Sexual contact	Body fluids Blood Sexual contact	Blood
Symptoms	Jaundice Abdominal pain	Jaundice Abdominal pain	Jaundice Abdominal pain
Illness severity	Moderate	High	High
Diagnosis	Liver function tests Symptoms Antibodies in serum	Liver function tests Symptoms HBsAg in serum	Liver function tests Symptoms Antibodies in serum
Carrier state	Rarely develops	Develops	Develops
Nosocomial problem	No	Yes	Yes
Prevention	Vaccine	Vaccine	None
Liver cancer	Not likely	Possible	Not established

OUTFLOW

During March 1997, a fourth-grade student at Madison Elementary School in Michigan became violently ill with fever, vomiting, terrible abdominal pains, and urine the color of dark tea. When her parents took her to the hospital emergency room in Marshall, they learned that other children from her school were equally ill. An outbreak of hepatitis A had begun.

By the end of March, over 100 children and staff members had hepatitis A, and three school districts from two separate counties were involved. Investigators began a hunt for the epidemic's source and narrowed the list of suspected foods to frozen sliced strawberries. By mid-April, 264 children, parents, staff members, and visitors to the three schools were sick with hepatitis A. The outbreak was one of the largest in public health history.

The search for the source of the contaminated strawberries was exhaustive but fruitless. By June 1997, CDC officials confirmed their failure to locate an origin. In the interim period, however, much had happened. For example, the strawberries were traced to farms in northern Mexico, and relations between the United States and Mexico became strained as diplomats traded insinuations and insults. Moreover, the strawberry industry, already reeling from a 1996 erroneous involvement with *Cyclospora*, was crashing further.

In San Diego, the company supplying the strawberries was also in trouble. Federal law requires that U.S. farmers supply all produce for federally supported school lunch programs (as in Madison); the company had purchased its strawberries in Mexico. A federal indictment of the company followed.

There was also a rush on immune globulin, the antibody preparation used to prevent the development of hepatitis A. Because strawberries from the implicated batch were traced to California school freezers, 9000 children from Los Angeles received injections of immune globulin; in Georgia, 10,000 children lined up for shots; and in Tennessee, 8600 children rolled up their sleeves. Fortunately, no cases developed outside of Michigan.

A final effect of the epidemic was a review of questionable sanitary conditions associated with strawberry picking, preparation, freezing, and distribution. New laws and regulations were in the offing, as public health agencies sought some benefit amid the wrongful suffering of the Michigan children. Next time, they assured, things would be different.

---

form are elongated particles also composed of HBsAg in tubular or filamentous rods up to 200 nm long. The third form is the more traditional virus, a virion containing HBsAg as an outer envelope surrounding an inner nucleocapsid of double-stranded DNA enclosed in a core antigen called **hepatitis B core antigen**, or **HBcAg**. This third form has been called the **Dane particle** since it was first reported by D. S. Dane in 1970. Apparently, the overproduction of the surface HBsAg during viral replication yields this protein in large amounts. The antigen was previously known as the **Australia antigen**; it has remained an important diagnostic sign for hepatitis B since first reported by Nobel laureate Baruch Blumberg in the early 1970s.

Transmission of hepatitis B usually involves direct or indirect contact with an infected body fluid such as blood or semen. For example, transmission may occur by contact with blood-contaminated needles used in hypodermic syringes or for tattooing, acupuncture, or ear-piercing. Blood-contaminated objects such as fiber optic endoscopes, instruments, and renal dialysis tubing are also implicated. Moreover, transmission may take place by contact with saliva, including contact made in the dental office (FIGURE 13.5). Hepatitis B is also an important **sexually transmitted disease**, particularly when anal intercourse takes place. This is because bleeding often occurs during anal intercourse, and viruses are able to enter the bloodstream of the receptive partner from the semen of the infected individual. (A similar situation holds for AIDS.)

The clinical course of hepatitis B is basically the same as for hepatitis A, but more severe illness is generally associated with hepatitis B. The disease has an incubation

Australia antigen:
an antigen located on the surface of the hepatitis B virus.

Fiber optic endoscope:
an instrument consisting of a fiberlike strand that is inserted into tissue to observe it.
Renal dialysis:
the process of cleansing the blood in an artificial kidney machine.

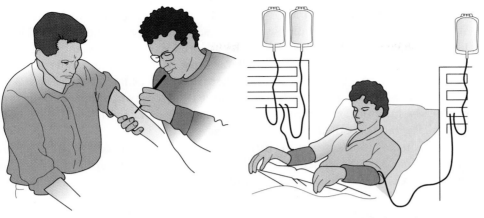

(a) Nonsterile tatooing needles   **(b)** Contaminated dialysis equipment

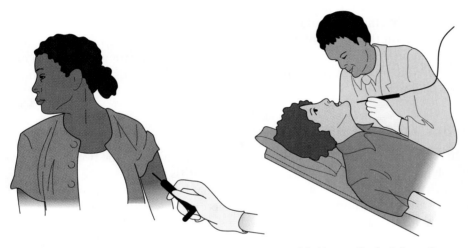

(c) Contaminated vaccination equipment   **(d)** Nonsterile dental practices

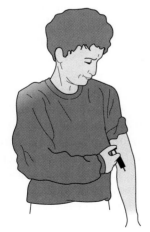
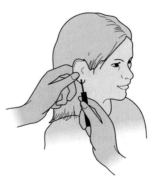

(e) Contaminated drug needles   **(f)** Nonsterile body piercing equipment

FIGURE 13.5

Some Methods for the Transmission of Hepatitis B

period of 4 weeks to 6 months and is therefore known as **long-incubation hepatitis** (relative to hepatitis A). Among adults, the common findings during the early stage are fatigue, anorexia, and taste changes. (Smokers experience a notable distaste for cigarettes.) Dark urine and clay-colored stools are present several days before jaundice appears. An uncomfortable sense of fullness and tenderness is felt in the upper-right quadrant of the abdomen. Recovery usually occurs about 3 to 4 months after the onset of jaundice, and about 10 percent of patients remain carriers for several months. In rare cases, extensive liver damage may occur, including cancer. The latter is called **hepatocarcinoma**.

hep-at'o-car-sin-o'ma

Injections of alpha-interferon (Intron A) can influence the course of hepatitis B. Lamivudine (3TC, Epivir), a base analog, has also been FDA-approved as a treatment. Moreover, prophylactic therapy may be rendered by injections of **hepatitis B immune globulin**. This preparation consists of antibodies concentrated from the serum of blood donors. In addition, the disease can be prevented by immunization with the hepatitis B vaccine. Since 1987, this **vaccine** has consisted of hepatitis B surface antigens (HBsAg) produced by genetically engineered yeast cells. The vaccine is known commercially as Recombivax HB or Engerix-B (depending on the company that produces it). Recommended for all age groups (including infants), it is particularly valuable for health-care workers who might be exposed to blood from patients. For infant use, it is combined with the Hib vaccine as Comvax.

Prophylactic: protective.

OTHER TYPES OF HEPATITIS

In recent years, other types of hepatitis have been added to the two that were previously recognized. Among the new ones is **hepatitis C**. This disease is caused by an RNA virus of the Flaviviridae family, a virus that has not yet been cultivated in laboratory animals or human cell cultures. There are few early symptoms associated with hepatitis C, and liver damage develops slowly, but insidiously. Often, the liver cirrhosis is beyond repair when the disease is finally recognized. Indeed, damage from hepatitis C is the primary reason for liver transplants in the United States.

Cirrhosis: progressive deterioration.

Hepatitis C was formerly a serious problem in **blood transfusion recipients**, but a laboratory screening test for the virus has reduced the risk to 1 in 100,000 units of blood transfused. (A home screening test called Hepatitis C Check has also received FDA approval.) The disease is most often observed in injection drug users and is sometimes diagnosed in individuals who use cocaine or have tattoos or body piercings. Alpha-interferon and riboflavin are approved therapies for the disease.

The screening test for hepatitis C followed identification of the virus by Michael Houghton of the biotechnology company Chiron. In addition to its diagnostic purpose, the test has been used to hunt for antibodies against hepatitis C in preserved blood. One such search in 1999 uncovered antiviral antibodies in frozen blood samples taken from servicemen in 1948 during a serious epidemic of strep infection. The finding confirmed that hepatitis C has been in the United States at least 50 years and is not a new disease, as some epidemiologists suspected. Indeed, the late blooming of hepatitis C suggests that this disease may be a major factor during the twenty-first century.

Delta hepatitis appears to be caused by two viruses: the hepatitis B virus and the delta virus (delta is the fourth letter of the Greek alphabet, equivalent to D). Delta viruses were discovered by Italian investigators in 1977. They consist of a protein fragment called the **delta antigen** and a segment of RNA. Apparently, the viruses can only cause liver damage when hepatitis B virus is also present (the press labeled them the "piggyback viruses"). Injection drug users were a major focus of an outbreak in Massachusetts in 1984.

Hepatitis E appears to be caused by at least three strains of an RNA virus not yet identified. Also found in pigs, the virus is apparently transmitted to humans via drinking water. Pregnant women seem to be particularly susceptible to illness, especially in the later stages of pregnancy. Hepatitis F has not been confirmed as a separate clinical entity, but **hepatitis G** appears to involve chronic liver illness. In 1996, investigators from Abbott Laboratories identified a 9400-base RNA virus as the cause of hepatitis G. Other forms of hepatitis await identification. At present they are simply termed **non-A non-B (NANB) hepatitis**.

To this point . . .

We have begun a study of the viscerotropic viral diseases by focusing on several diseases of the blood and visceral organs. The first two diseases, yellow fever and dengue fever, are caused by viruses injected directly into the bloodstream by mosquitoes. Yellow fever has great historical interest because epidemics were widespread during past generations, but vaccines and arthropod control now limit its spread in many parts of the world. Dengue fever remains a threat in many countries. High fever reflects viral invasion of the blood in both cases.

We then turned to infectious mononucleosis and hepatitis. Ongoing research into these diseases reveals new information, while questions continue to surface. For example, the role of the Epstein-Barr virus in infectious mononucleosis is still uncertain, and the relationship of the disease to Burkitt's lymphoma is a debatable issue. In hepatitis, we saw how numerous different forms have emerged since the 1970s, each caused by a different virus. Infection of the liver is the common element in all types of hepatitis, and convalescence is generally long because damage to the liver is not easily repaired. Liver disease is also a consequence of yellow fever, and often it occurs in infectious mononucleosis.

We shall now focus attention on a series of viral diseases of the gastrointestinal tract as we study viral gastroenteritis, and we shall study a number of viral fevers in which the pathogens affect the bloodstream. In addition, we will consider acquired immune deficiency syndrome (AIDS). Many of the viscerotropic diseases in this section occur sporadically and are not well understood. However, the potential for epidemics is great.

13.2

Other Viscerotropic Viral Diseases

We continue with the viscerotropic diseases by examining additional diseases of the gastrointestinal tract and blood. Many emerging viral diseases are in this section, and we include a discussion of acquired immune deficiency syndrome (AIDS). Recall that our classification system is arbitrary, and that many of the diseases also affect organs other than the visceral organs. An example is seen in some of the agents of viral gastroenteritis that we examine first.

VIRAL GASTROENTERITIS

gas'tro-en-ter-i'tis

Viral gastroenteritis is a general name for a common illness occurring in both epidemic and endemic forms. It affects all age groups worldwide and may include some of the frequently encountered traveler's diarrheas. Public health officials believe that the disease is second in frequency to the common cold, among infectious illnesses affecting people in the United States. (In developing nations, gastroenteritis is estimated to be the second leading killer of children under the age of 5, accounting for 23 percent of all deaths in this age group.) Clinically the disease varies, but usually it has an explosive onset with varying combinations of diarrhea, nausea, vomiting, low-grade fever, cramps, headache, and malaise. It can be severe in infants, the elderly, and patients whose immune systems are compromised by other illnesses. Some people mistakenly call it "stomach flu."

One cause of viral gastroenteritis is the human **rotavirus**, a virus first described in 1973 in Australia. The virion contains segmented, double-stranded RNA as well as inner and outer capsids, but no envelope. A member of the Reoviridae family, it is named for its circular appearance (*rota* is Latin for "wheel"). FIGURE 13.6a shows this virus. A possible mechanism for its action on the body is summarized in **MicroFocus 13.6**. The CDC considers rotaviruses the single most important cause of diarrhea in infants and young children admitted to hospitals. Many cases involve severe dehydration and death.

Rotavirus:
A circular RNA virus that can cause gastroenteritis.

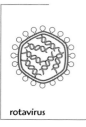

rotavirus

In 1999, officials at the U.S. Food and Drug Administration (FDA) approved RotoShield, a **vaccine** to protect against rotavirus infection. Administered orally, the vaccine consists of the four most common strains of rotavirus (it is a "tetravalent" vaccine). To formulate the vaccine, molecular biologists at Wyeth-Ayerst Laboratories inserted a protein-encoding gene from a human rotavirus into the genome of a monkey rotavirus. Thus, every part of the virus in the vaccine is monkey virus, except for a capsid protein on the outer surface encoded by the new gene. The immune system responds to this protein and produces protective antibodies. The main target populations for the vaccine are children who reside in developing countries. In the early weeks of vaccine use, cases of bowel obstruction were observed, and the vaccine was withdrawn for further study.

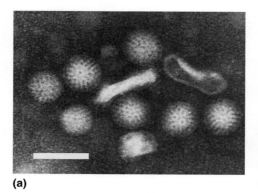
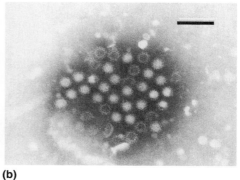

(a)   (b)

FIGURE 13.6

Two Viruses That Cause Gastroenteritis

(a) Rotaviruses observed in the diarrheal stool of an infant with gastroenteritis. (Bar = 100 nm.) Note the wheel-like circular appearance from which the rotavirus takes its name. (b) Norwalk viruses from stool specimens of a patient with gastroenteritis. (Bar = 100 nm.) The viruses appear to have icosahedral symmetry.

MicroFocus 13.6

SMELLY INSIGHTS

The cage was not supposed to smell of diarrhea. Mouse number 3 had received the control protein, not the intact rotavirus. The protein should have been harmless. Where did all this mess come from?

Then it hit—could the protein be causing the diarrhea? And if so, how? Is this one of those moments every researcher dreams about? Quick, check the data. Who do I tell? Can I repeat the experiment? Where do we go from here? Wow!

It happened to Judith M. Ball, virus researcher at Baylor College of Medicine. She and her colleague Mary Estes were studying rotaviruses, a cause of

often-fatal diarrhea in millions of children. They had isolated a protein called nonstructural glycoprotein number 4 (NSP4), so named because it was not involved in the structure of the rotaviral capsid (*nonstructural*), it was a *protein*, and it was number 4 in the series of proteins studied. Now they were testing NSP4 to confirm that it was simply another viral protein of little pathological consequence. It was not supposed to cause diarrhea.

But it did. And Bell's insight opened the door to a new biochemical process and a novel concept of viral pathology: Experiments showed that biochemically, NSP4 protrudes through the capsid and

frees the virus from surrounding cellular membranes so it can replicate. For the viral pathologist, further studies indicated that in the body, the protein induces diarrhea by mobilizing intracellular calcium; this leads to increased calcium secretion and an outpouring of water characteristic of diarrhea. The protein is a toxin, the first digestive tract toxin of viral origin ever detected.

As she prepared her research paper for *Science* magazine in 1996, Ball recalled how it began with a messy cage and a glorious moment in time. Ball contends she was lucky. Her colleagues prefer to point to the dictum of Louis Pasteur: "Chance favors the prepared mind."

A second cause of viral gastroenteritis is the **Norwalk virus** (FIGURE 13.6b), named for Norwalk, Ohio, where it caused a notable outbreak of intestinal disease in 1968. The virion is transmitted by contaminated water and food, especially seafood (FIGURE 13.7). The virus is more common than rotavirus in older children and adults. Outbreaks of disease can be detected by the symptoms and by a rise in antibodies to the virus. In 1987, over 300 participants at a South Dakota outing were infected by Norwalk virus from well water. The well was adjacent to a septic dump station.

The Norwalk virus belongs to the family Calciviridae, a group called **calciviruses**. These viruses contain RNA and have capsids with icosahedral symmetry. With an electron microscope, the viruses appear as six-pointed stars ("star of David") and have an abundance of calcium in their capsids. Another calcivirus known as a **Norwalklike virus** was implicated in 1996 and 1997 as causing outbreaks of viral gastroenteritis associated with the consumption of raw oysters.

Viral gastroenteritis can also be caused by either of two **enteroviruses**. Enteroviruses are small, icosahedral RNA virions of the Picornaviridae family. They are currently considered a less frequent cause of gastroenteritis than other viruses and are notable for the variety of infections they may cause. An antiviral drug called **pleconaril** appears to limit their replication.

One enterovirus is the **Coxsackie virus**, first isolated in 1948 by Gilbert Dalldorf and Grace Mary Sickles from the stool of a patient residing in Coxsackie, New York. The viruses occur in many strains within two groups, A and B. Strains B4 and B5 Coxsackie viruses are most commonly associated with gastroenteritis. Group B viruses are also implicated in **pleurodynia** (or Bornholm's disease), a painful disease of the rib muscles; and **myocarditis**, a serious disease of the heart muscle and valves, sometimes resulting in a heart attack or the need for a heart transplant. In addition, group B Coxsackie viruses are among the most frequent causes of **aseptic meningitis**. Group A viruses have been isolated from cases of respiratory infections, conjunctivitis, and **herpangina**, a disease of children with abrupt fever onset and

Norwalk virus

cal'-ci-vir'i-dā

Coxsackie virus

cook-sak'e

ploor'o-din'e-ah

Aseptic meningitis:
a type of meningitis in which no microbial agent is observed.

FIGURE 13.7

A Case of Norwalk Virus Gastroenteritis

This outbreak occurred in New Jersey during December 1979. It was one of the first reports of Norwalk virus gastroenteritis linked to any food other than shellfish.

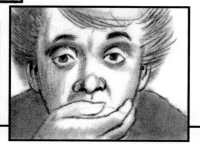

1. In early December 1979, a New Jersey restaurant and catering facility received a shipment of lettuce from a produce market in Philadelphia.

2. A worker who had just finished washing some shrimp then washed some of the lettuce in the same sink. The shrimp and the lettuce were prepared on the same table.

3. On December 6, 1979, a group of businesspeople attended a luncheon banquet at the restaurant. The restaurant served green salad made with the lettuce. A second group of businessmen and women received cole slaw instead of salad.

4. About 30 hours later, 63 of the 87 people who ate green salad developed gastroenteritis. None of those who had cole slaw became ill. Health department microbiologists identified Norwalk virus as the agent and theorized that it had entered the lettuce from contaminated shrimp.

TEXTBOOK CASES

punched-out vesicles on the soft palate, tongue, tonsils, and hands ("hand, foot, and mouth disease"). Enterovirus 71 is involved.

Some virologists believe that Coxsackie viruses are the so-called **24-hour viruses** responsible for brief bouts of diarrhea. And an intriguing 1994 report in the *New England Journal of Medicine* indicated that Coxsackie viruses might trigger the development of insulin-dependent **diabetes** in genetically susceptible individuals. According to the report, the viruses stimulate the immune system to produce antibodies that attack the pancreatic cells responsible for producing insulin.

The second enterovirus that causes viral gastroenteritis is the **echovirus**. Echoviruses were discovered in the early 1950s. They take their name from the

Diabetes:
a disease in which the passage of glucose into body cells is interrupted.

acronym ECHO, for enteric (intestinal), cytopathogenic (pathogenic to cells), human (human host), and orphan (a virus without a famous disease). Echoviruses occur in many strains and cause gastroenteritis as well as aseptic meningitis. The meningitis, however, is usually less severe than bacterial meningitis. Echoviruses are also a cause of respiratory infections and maculopapular skin rashes called **exanthems**. A Massachusetts outbreak called the Boston exanthem attracted attention in 1954.

eg-zan'them
Exanthem:
a skin rash that develops rapidly.

VIRAL FEVERS

A series of viruses may cause human illnesses characterized by high fever. These diseases occur sporadically and are usually rare in the United States.

An example of a viral fever is **Colorado tick fever**. This disease is caused by an RNA virus of the Reoviridae family. It is transmitted by the tick ***Dermacentor andersonii*** and accounts for about 200 cases of disease per year, chiefly in the state of Colorado. Characteristic symptoms include alternating periods of fever and relief (saddleback fever), with pain in the muscles, joints, and eyes. Leukopenia, and the presence of viruses inside the red blood cells, are other factors that mark the disease.

der-ma-cen'tor

Leukopenia:
a reduced number of white blood cells.

Sandfly fever is another example of a viral fever. The disease is prevalent where sandflies of the genus ***Phlebotomus*** abound. It occasionally breaks out in Mediterranean regions, Southeast Asia, and parts of Central America. Patients suffer recurrent high fever and joint and bone pains resembling those in dengue fever. The responsible virus is an RNA virion of the Bunyaviridae family.

flĕ-bot'o-mus

Rift Valley fever is named for a region in eastern Africa called the Rift Valley. This is an immense earthquake-prone area. In addition to affecting humans, the disease affects animals and causes extensive losses of sheep and cattle. Indeed, the virus is so dangerous to animals that federal law prohibits its transport to the mainland of the United States. Transmission is by several genera of mosquitoes, and denguelike pain in the bones and joints accompanies the fever, which lasts for about a week. The virion is an RNA virus of the Bunyaviridae family.

bun'ya-vir'i-dā
Hemorrhagic:
referring to bleeding and accumulating blood.

Certain viral fevers are accompanied by severe hemorrhagic lesions of the tissues. These diseases are classified as **viral hemorrhagic fevers**. One example, **Lassa fever**, is so named because it was first reported in the town of Lassa, Nigeria, in 1969 (FIGURE 13.8). The disease is caused by an RNA virus of the Arenaviridae family (an arenavirus). Infection is accompanied by severe fever, prostration, and patchy blood-filled hemorrhagic lesions of the throat. The fever persists for weeks, the pharyngeal lesions bleed freely, and profuse internal hemorrhaging is common. At least four epidemics have been identified in Africa since 1969, and the disease is occasionally seen in the United States. John G. Fuller has written a lucid and vivid account of the discovery of Lassa fever in his book *Fever! The Hunt for a New Killer Virus*. The book should be read by anyone who believes there are no remaining frontiers in medicine.

a-re'na-vir'i-dā

Another viral hemorrhagic fever is **Marburg disease**, named for Marburg, West Germany, where an outbreak occurred in 1967. Virologists identified the virus in tissues of green vervet monkeys imported from Africa. Saddleback fever, bleeding from the gums and throat, and gastrointestinal hemorrhaging are characteristic features; mortality rates during epidemics tend to be high. The viral agent is a **filovirus**, a long threadlike virus (*filum* is Latin for "thread") that often takes the shape of a fishhook or U. Its genome is composed of RNA.

Saddleback fever:
alternating periods of fever and relief.

Another filovirus, the **Ebola virus**, captured headlines in 1995. During that summer, an outbreak of **Ebola hemorrhagic fever** occurred in Zaire and Sudan, and an astonished world watched as newspaper reports spoke of blood spouting from

e-bol'ah

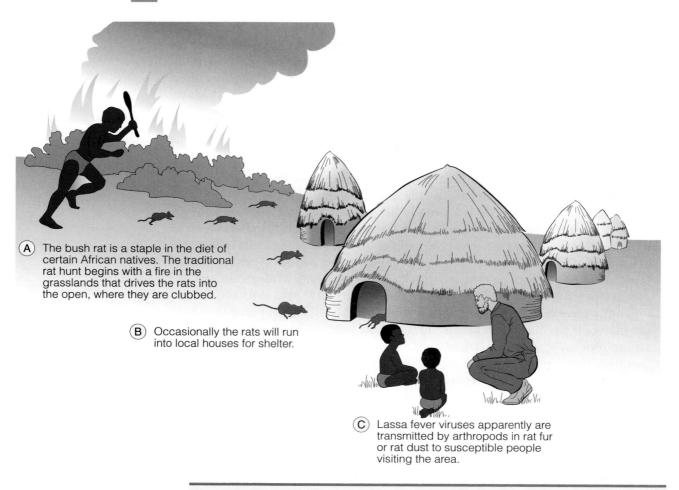

(A) The bush rat is a staple in the diet of certain African natives. The traditional rat hunt begins with a fire in the grasslands that drives the rats into the open, where they are clubbed.

(B) Occasionally the rats will run into local houses for shelter.

(C) Lassa fever viruses apparently are transmitted by arthropods in rat fur or rat dust to susceptible people visiting the area.

FIGURE 13.8

An Emerging Virus

A suggested method for the emergence of Lassa fever from nature.

patients' eyes, nose, ears, and gums; organs turning to liquid; and a horror story similar to the one recounted in *The Hot Zone* by Richard Preston. (The salient difference was that the Ebola viruses in Preston's book were loose near Washington, D.C.) To make matters worse, theaters had recently screened *Outbreak,* and a nervous public watched as Dustin Hoffman and Rene Russo battled an Ebolalike epidemic in Africa. Now the real thing was happening. When it was over, hundreds of Africans had died and the media were alerting readers to an unknown microbial world lurking in the wilderness. The phrase "emerging viruses" was being mentioned with increased frequency on the late news.

How Ebola virus causes massive internal bleeding and hemorrhaging was a subject of speculation until 1998, when researchers at the University of Michigan discovered that the virus encodes at least two glycoproteins. One attaches to endothelial cells lining the veins and arteries, where it encourages viral entry. Viral replication and damage to the cells weaken the blood vessels, causing them to leak; catastrophic bleeding follows. The second glycoprotein apparently attaches to neutrophils (types of white blood cells) and thereby limits phagocytosis and the immune response.

Thus, the patient bleeds to death internally before a reasonable defense can be mounted. The Ebola virus is shown in FIGURE 13.9a.

Other viral hemorrhagic fevers, all caused by Bunyaviridae or Arenaviridae are Congo-Crimea hemorrhagic fever, which occurs worldwide; Oropouche fever, which affects regions of Brazil; and Junin and Machupo, the hemorrhagic fevers of Argentina and Bolivia, respectively. An arenavirus called the **Sabia virus** has caused hemorrhagic illnesses in Brazil, and in 1994, it caused disease in a Yale University researcher, who survived the ordeal. A virus called the **Guanarito virus** is associated with Venezuelan hemorrhagic fever.

Still another hemorrhagic fever is **Korean hemorrhagic fever**, caused by the RNA-containing **Hantaan virus (Hantavirus)**, named for the Hantaan River in Korea. American servicemen experienced the bunyaviral disease during the Korean War, and an outbreak occurred among Marines in Korea in 1986. Then, in the summer of 1993, a brief epidemic occurred among Native Americans living in the southwestern United States. It was named the "four corners disease" for the place where four states come together; its diagnosis is described in MicroFocus 13.7. Symptoms of the disease included a rapidly developing flulike illness, with blood hemorrhaging and acute renal and respiratory failure. The disease was given the technical name **hantavirus pulmonary syndrome**, and the strain of virus was named Sin Nombre virus (Spanish for "no name"); another strain isolated later was called Muerto Canyon virus (FIGURE 13.9b). CDC investigators identified airborne viral particles from the dried urine and feces of rodents (especially deer mice) as the vector for the virus. By the end of 1993, 91 cases were confirmed in 20 states. Forty-eight patients died.

Hantavirus pulmonary syndrome has now became a "regular" in the lexicon of medicine. During the first 5 months of 1999, for example, the disease was identified in 30 states. NATO peacekeeping troops in Bosnia experienced the disease in 1996, and an epidemic occurred in Argentina in 1997. Human-to-human spread was postulated in Argentina because individuals were infected at a far distance from the

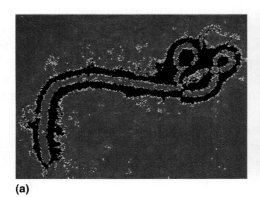

(a)

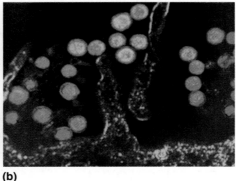

(b)

FIGURE 13.9

The Ebola Virus and the Hantavirus

(a) A colored transmission electron micrograph of the Ebola virus, the agent of Ebola hemorrhagic fever. This lethal virus is possibly transmitted in the dust of rodents and/or by contact with human tissues. Note that the virus is a long threadlike filovirus. (b) A colored transmission electron micrograph of the hantavirus, the cause of hantavirus pulmonary syndrome. This enveloped virus with a helical nucleocapsid was first isolated in 1993 following an outbreak of hantavirus disease at the Four Corners region in the southwestern United States.

MicroFocus 13.7

"WE CAN'T FIND IT BUT WE KNOW IT'S THERE!"

A microbial identification of an unusual sort was made in 1994. That year, a strange epidemic of viral disease broke out in the southwestern United States at the border area of four states (Arizona, Colorado, New Mexico, and Utah). The disease came to be known as the "four corners disease." It spread quickly among Native Americans, causing severe hemorrhaging, pneumonia, and kidney disease, and it resulted in 35 deaths among 52 patients. Scientists performed a battery of tests, hunting for myriad viruses and their antibodies, but they came up empty each time.

Then they hit on a novel idea. Instead of looking for the virus, why not look for the viral genome—the DNA of the virus.

Scientists obtained DNA from numerous different viruses in culture collections and replicated the DNA fragments to produce a variety of "gene probes." A gene probe is a small, single-stranded molecule of DNA that will hunt down and unite with its complementary single-stranded DNA molecule. Acting like a right hand searching for a left hand, the gene probe emits a radioactive signal when the union has taken place (if the complementary strand cannot be found, no signal is sent).

Now the scientists were ready to give their theory a try. They began by extracting DNA from the tissues of disease patients. Then they combined the DNA with gene probes from a constellation of

viruses and held their breath to see which would send a signal. Their answer came a few short minutes later when a sooty band of radioactivity appeared on their instruments; the DNA from the patient was uniting with the gene probe from the hantavirus, a very rare virus named for the Hantaan River in Korea. The infecting virus must be a hantavirus.

Not only was the mystery solved, but scientists now had a useful tool for diagnosing and tracking the disease. And they could work to interrupt its spread because they knew how to locate the disease and what was causing it. They could also point out the face of the enemy—well, not really, because they had not seen the virus, only its footprint.

outbreak's epicenter, and no rodents were found in many areas where patients developed the disease. Researchers are attempting to produce a hantavirus vaccine by inserting hantaviral genes into a cowpox (vaccinia) virus. This type of genetically engineered vaccine has been produced for other diseases as well.

In the 1960s and 1970s, public health officials believed they had triumphed over infectious disease. Smallpox was on the way to extinction; polio was under control; and, thanks to antibiotics, sanitation, and pesticides, such maladies as tuberculosis, cholera, and malaria were disappearing. But then in one wave after another, nature counterattacked with Marburg disease, Lassa fever, Ebola fever, and hantavirus disease, as well as Legionnaires' disease, hepatitis C, *E. coli* O157:H7, Lyme disease, and AIDS. In all, at least 30 newly identified pathogens emerged. By the end of the century, health officials were concluding that new pathogens will continue to threaten human existence for all time. The trick, researchers suggest, is to adopt a guerrilla strategy in which reliable intelligence and rapid reaction are the keys to survival. The viral fevers taught science a valuable lesson for the new century.

CYTOMEGALOVIRUS DISEASE

si'to-meg'ah-lo-vi'rus

Epithelium:
the tissue that lines blood vessels and numerous body cavities.

The **cytomegalovirus (CMV)** is an icosahedral DNA virion of the herpesvirus group. The virus takes its name from the enlarged cells ("cyto-megalo") found in infected tissues. Usually, these are cells of the salivary glands, epithelium, or liver.

Cytomegalovirus disease may be among the most common diseases in American communities. Fever, malaise, and, in some cases, an enlarged spleen, develop, but few other signs of disease are observed. Most patients recover uneventfully. However, if a woman is pregnant, a serious congenital disease may ensue as the viruses pass into the fetal bloodstream and damage the fetal tissues. Mental impairment is sometimes observed in young patients. The C in the **TORCH** group of diseases refers to cytomegalovirus disease. The other letters stand for toxoplasmosis (T), rubella (R), and herpes simplex (H). The O is for other diseases, such as syphilis.

The cytomegalovirus has also demonstrated its invasive tendency in patients who have acquired immune deficiency syndrome (AIDS). Up to one-third of AIDS patients experience **CMV-induced retinitis**, a serious infection of the retina that can lead to blindness. **Ganciclovir** is often used to treat the disease, with **foscarnet** as an alternative drug. In immunocompromised individuals, cytomegaloviruses can also infect the lungs, liver, brain, and kidneys and cause death. Patients undergoing cancer therapy or receiving organ transplants may be susceptible to CMV disease because immunosuppressive drugs are often administered to these patients. The virus has also been implicated in cardiovascular disease (Chapter 7).

HIV INFECTION AND AIDS

In 1981, physicians described a syndrome involving a deficiency of the immune system. This clinical entity included the development of certain opportunistic infections, as well as an unusual type of skin cancer called Kaposi's sarcoma. The most plausible factor was a virus, but a definitive agent was not identified until 1984, when a French group led by **Luc Montagnier** isolated the infectious agent. In 1986, the virus was given its current name of **human immunodeficiency virus (HIV)**. By that time, the disease was well known as **acquired immune deficiency syndrome (AIDS)**.

The human immunodeficiency virus (HIV) is an RNA-containing icosahedral virus with an envelope that contains spikes, as FIGURE 13.10 illustrates. Within its genome it contains molecules of an enzyme called **reverse transcriptase**. When the RNA is released in the cytoplasm of a host cell, the enzyme synthesizes a molecule of DNA utilizing the genetic message in the RNA as a template. (This reversal of the usual mode of genetic information transfer [transcription] gives the virus its name, retrovirus, and the enzyme its name, reverse transcriptase.) The DNA molecule, now termed a **provirus**, integrates into the host's DNA, and from that location, it transcribes its genetic message into new particles of HIV. The whole viruses then

TORCH:
an acronym for diseases transmitted from a pregnant woman to her unborn child.

gan-ci'klo-vir
fos-car'net

kap'o-sē sar-ko'mah

mon'tan-yā

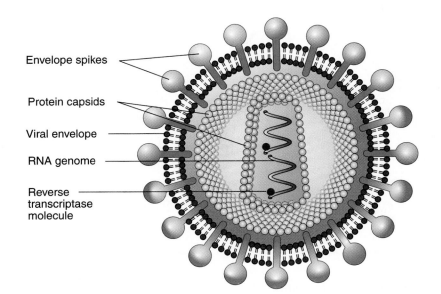

Envelope spikes

Protein capsids

Viral envelope

RNA genome

Reverse transcriptase molecule

FIGURE 13.10

A Diagram of the Human Immunodeficiency Virus (HIV)

The virus consists of two molecules of RNA and molecules of reverse transcriptase. A protein capsid surrounds the genome, and an envelope with spikes of protein lies outside the capsid.

"bud" from the host cell to infect other cells, as FIGURE 13.11 indicates. This individual now has **HIV infection**.

The normal host cell of HIV is a cell of the immune system called a **T-lymphocyte**. These cells participate in cell-mediated immunity. In this process, the cells mature and proliferate to form a colony of cytotoxic T-lymphocytes that respond to the presence of protozoa, fungi, and infected cells. (These processes are explored in more detail in Chapter 18.) Infection by HIV leads to the failure of this immune

Cell-mediated immunity: immunity derived from the activity of T-lymphocytes that encompasses an interaction between stimulated T-lymphocytes and antigen-bearing cells.

(A) **Attachment, entry, and uncoating:**
The virus enters the host cell and is uncoated in the cytoplasm.

(B) **Reverse transcription and integration:**
Reverse transcriptase uses the viral RNA as a template to synthesize a strand of DNA, and then uses the DNA strand as a template to complete a DNA double helix (the original viral RNA is degraded.) The DNA then enters the nucleus and integrates into the chromosomal DNA of the host, becoming a provirus.

(C) **Synthesis of viral parts:**
The proviral DNA is transcribed into viral RNA fragments and translated into viral proteins.

(D) **Assembly and release:**
New capsids assemble around viral RNA fragments and reverse transcriptase molecules, and the nucleocapsids "bud" from the cell membrane as complete viruses.

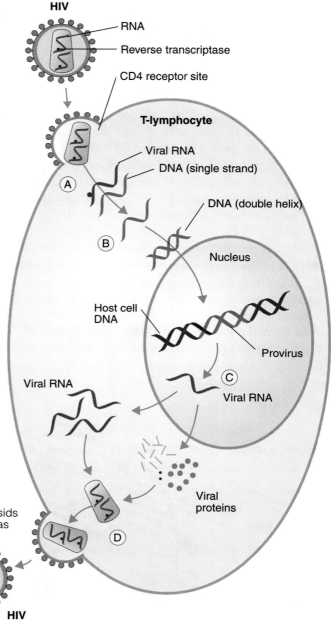

FIGURE 13.11

The Replication Cycle of the Human Immunodeficiency Virus (HIV)

response and places the host at risk for opportunistic pathogens and cancers, similar to those in patients with other immunodeficiencies.

The major T-lymphocyte infected by HIV is the helper T-lymphocyte that bears the **CD4 receptor site**. (The helper T-lymphocyte is also called a CD4 cell because of the site.) A second coreceptor site is also involved. Other cells infected may include those of the central nervous system and macrophages in the blood and tissue. For a period of time, the body keeps up with the virus and replaces T-lymphocytes as they are destroyed. Eventually, however, the infected individual suffers a decline from the normal 1000 T-lymphocytes per microliter of blood to less than 100 per microliter. Infections and neoplasms follow. Scientists have also discovered a simian immunodeficiency virus (SIV) in rhesus monkeys.

As of January 2000, a total of over 750,000 cases of AIDS were reported to the CDC since the epidemic's beginning. Close to 500,000 deaths have occurred from complications such as opportunistic illnesses. It is important to note that AIDS is the end result of HIV infection. Approximately 1.0 to 1.5 million Americans are believed to have HIV infection. Worldwide, scientists estimate that about 20 million people are infected with HIV.

A person with HIV infection manifests generalized symptoms and an ever-weakening condition. Fever, diarrhea, rash, swelling of the lymph nodes, night sweats, malaise, and fatigue may be present. These symptoms occur sporadically and last several weeks at a time. There is also severe depression from the never-ending series of illnesses. Antibody evidence for HIV at this point is substantial, and it is now recognized that an ongoing production of HIV is taking place. This stage was previously known as **AIDS-related complex**.

AIDS develops when the individual experiences **neurological disease**, including dementia, memory loss, mood swings, and other nerve-related pathologies. AIDS also is present when the individual develops a **wasting syndrome** with excessive diarrhea and loss of muscle mass. The most widespread evidence of AIDS is the presence of **opportunistic illnesses** such as Kaposi's sarcoma, *Pneumocystis carinii* pneumonia, cytomegalovirus infection, cryptosporidiosis, *Candida albicans* infection, and cryptococcosis. These illnesses are explored in Chapters 14 and 15 and are summarized in FIGURE 13.12. Tuberculosis and other mycobacterial diseases may also be significant problems.

Transmission of HIV occurs primarily by contamination with infected blood or semen. Intimate sexual contact, including anal intercourse, is a common method of transmission. Rectal tissues bleed and give access to the virus. Unprotected vaginal intercourse is also a high-risk sexual activity, especially if lesions, cuts, or abrasions of the vaginal tract exist. The use of condoms has been shown to decrease the transmission of HIV significantly. The sharing of blood-contaminated needles by injection drug users also transmits HIV. Needle-exchange programs are now being used as a way of interrupting this transmission method. Moreover, transplacental transfer from mother to child is an acknowledged method of HIV transmission.

Viral transmission can also occur through blood products used for medical purposes. Packed red blood cells and blood factor concentrates may contain the virus, but extensive tests are now performed to preclude their presence. Health-care workers are at risk of acquiring HIV during their professional activities, such as through an accidental needle stick. Health-care workers should always practice established infection-control procedures (universal precautions).

A number of **diagnostic tests** can be used to determine whether an exposed person is HIV infected. HIV antibodies are detected by the ELISA test (discussed in Chapter 19). The Western blot analysis is also used to confirm the diagnosis. A newer test called

Lymph nodes:
pockets of white blood cells located in the neck, armpits, groin, and other body regions; site of the cells of the immune system.

krip'to-spoor-id'e-o'sis
krip'-to-kok-o'-sis

Needle stick:
an injury to the skin tissues from an unintentional injection with a needle.

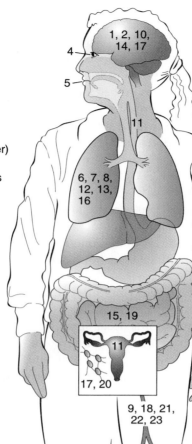

Viral diseases
1. HIV encephalopathy
2. Progressive multifocal leukoencephalopathy
3. Shingles, recurrent (herpes zoster)
4. Cytomegalovirus retinitis
5. Recurrent herpes simplex lesions

Bacterial diseases
6. Persistent pneumonia
7. Tuberculosis
8. *Mycobacterium avium* complex
9. *Salmonella* septicemia

Fungal diseases
10. Cryptococcosis
11. Candidiasis
12. Histoplasmosis
13. Coccidioidomycosis

Protozoal diseases
14. Toxoplasmosis
15. Chronic *Cryptosporidium* diarrhea
16. *Pneumocystis* pneumonia

Cancers
17. Lymphomas of brain, lymphatic tissue
18. Kaposi's sarcoma

Miscellaneous conditions
19. Persistent diarrhea
20. Persistent generalized lymphadenopathy
21. Wasting syndrome
22. Night sweats
23. Persistent fever

FIGURE 13.12

Opportunistic Illnesses in AIDS Patients

This figure illustrates the variety of opportunistic illnesses that affect the body when its immune system has been compromised as a result of infection with HIV. Note the various systems that are affected and the myriad organisms involved.

Gene probe:
a segment of radioactive DNA used in diagnostic tests to seek out and combine with a complementary segment of DNA.

a-zi′do-thi′-mi-dēn

di′de-ox′e-in′o-sēn
di′de-ox′e-si′ti-dēn

the **viral load test** detects the RNA of HIV and is also available to assess the extent of infection. Using this test, almost 100 percent of infected individuals can be detected. Gene probes and PCR amplification methods can also be used, as Chapter 19 explains.

Treatment protocols for HIV infection and AIDS have been researched for many years. The drug used since 1987 is **azidothymidine**, commonly known as **AZT**. AZT interferes with reverse transcriptase activity and acts as a chain terminator as it inhibits DNA synthesis (**FIGURE 13.13**). The drug decreases the viral load in patients, and increases the survival of patients with HIV infection. Other anti-HIV agents approved for use include **dideoxyinosine (ddI)** and **dideoxycytidine (ddC)**. Both are similar to AZT, but have fewer side effects. Another agent is **3TC**, also known as **lamivudine**. Like AZT, the mechanism of 3TC is inhibiting DNA synthesis.

Still another group of anti-HIV agents are the **protease inhibitors**. These drugs interfere with the processing step of capsid production in the synthesis of HIV particles. The drugs inhibit the enzyme protease, which is responsible for sectioning molecules of large protein for use in the capsid. Several protease inhibitors are now in use, including **saquinavir (Invirase), indinavir (Crixivan)**, and **ritonavir (Norvir)**. They are used with AZT and 3TC in **highly reactive antiretroviral therapy (HAART)**.

As of this writing, a **vaccine** for HIV infection and AIDS is being sought with great anticipation, but it is not yet available. Evidence indicates that inactivated whole viruses may protect susceptible individuals, but there is reluctance to use such vaccines because of the possibility that active viruses may be present. Other vaccines use synthetic viral fragments, such as the gp41 and gp120 proteins found in the envelope of HIV. More information about a possible AIDS vaccine is presented in Chapter 19. While the vaccine is being developed, emphasis continues to be placed on preventing the infection, because vaccine development will probably require several more years. TABLE 13.2 summarizes AIDS and other diseases in this section.

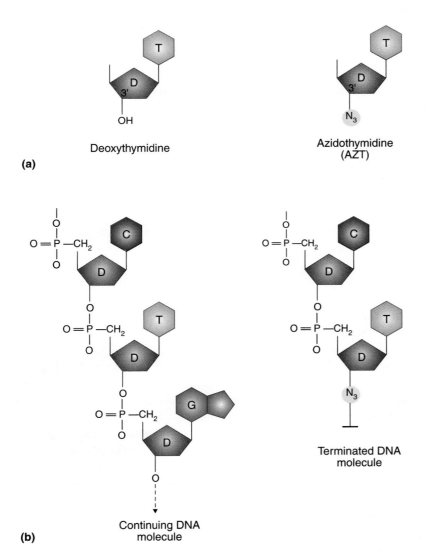

(a)

(b)

Deoxythymidine

Azidothymidine
(AZT)

Terminated DNA
molecule

Continuing DNA
molecule

FIGURE 13.13

How AZT Works

(a) Azidothymidine (AZT) is similar to the nucleotide deoxythymidine, except at the 3' position, where deoxythymidine has an $-OH$ group and AZT has an $-N_3$ group. The $-OH$ is used to hook onto the next nucleotide in the growing DNA chain, but the $-N_3$ cannot perform this function, and nothing will attach to it. (b) When AZT is present, the DNA molecule sometimes picks it up instead of deoxythymidine because of the structural similarity between the two molecules. After the AZT molecule is placed in the chain, however, another nucleotide cannot attach, and the DNA chain stops growing. With DNA synthesis halted, the virus cannot be constructed. AZT is said to be a chain terminator.

TABLE 13.2

A Summary of Viscerotropic Viral Diseases

DISEASE	CLASSIFICATION OF VIRUS	TRANSMISSION	ORGANS AFFECTED	VACCINE	SPECIAL FEATURES	COMPLICATIONS
Yellow fever	Flaviviridae	*Aedes aegypti* (mosquito)	Liver Blood	Inactivated viruses	Jaundice	Hemorrhaging
Dengue fever	Flaviviridae	*Aedes aegypti* (mosquito)	Blood Muscles	Not available	Breakbone fever	Hemorrhagic fever
Infectious mononucleosis	Herpesviridae	Saliva Contact Droplets	Blood Lymph nodes Spleen	Not available	Downey cells Paul-Bunnell test	Splenic rupture Jaundice
Hepatitis A	Picornaviridae	Food Water Contact	Liver	Inactivated virus	Jaundice	Liver damage
Hepatitis B	Hepadnaviridae	Contact with body fluids	Liver	Synthetic proteins	Jaundice	Liver cancer
Hepatitis C	Flaviviridae	Contact with body fluids	Liver	Not available	Jaundice	Liver damage
Viral gastroenteritis	Many viruses	Food Water	Intestine	Not available	Diarrhea	Dehydration Meningitis
Viral fevers	Many viruses	Contact Arthropods Animals	Blood	Not available	Fever Joint pain	Hemorrhaging
Cytomegalo-virus disease	Herpesviridae	Contact Congenital transfer	Blood Lung	Not available	Enlarged cells	Fetal damage
Acquired immune deficiency syndrome	Retroviridae	Contact with body fluids and blood products	T-lymphocytes Brain	Not available	Immune deficiency	Opportunistic illnesses

To this point . . .

We have discussed additional viscerotropic viral diseases, beginning with a series of diseases of the gastrointestinal tract. Many viruses are involved in this disorder, including the rotavirus, the Norwalk virus, and two types of enteroviruses. We noted that infections are accompanied by varying combinations of diarrhea and malaise, and that the diseases can be severe in certain individuals.

We then surveyed a number of viral fevers, three of which are transmitted by arthropods. The viral fevers are rare in the United States, but they commonly occur in other parts of the world, such as South America and Africa, and represent a potential source of epidemics if they break out in susceptible populations. We also saw how cytomegalovirus is widespread in Americans but of little consequence except in pregnant women and those with suppressed immune systems, such as people infected with HIV.

The section closed with a discussion of HIV infection and AIDS, a disease that is currently considered a major health problem in the United States. The disease is caused by human immunodeficiency virus (HIV). It involves the immune system and paves the way for opportunistic illnesses.

In the final section of this chapter, we shall survey several neurotropic viral diseases. These diseases have substantial importance because they affect the nervous system and *often result in death or permanent paralysis. Two of the diseases, rabies and polio, can be prevented with immunization. Another neurotropic disease, called slow virus (prion) disease, represents an area of intensive investigation in microbiology because of its contemporary nature.*

13-3

Neurotropic Viral Diseases

Neurotropic viral diseases affect the human nervous system. This fragile system suffers substantial damage when viruses replicate in the tissue. Rabies, a highly fatal and well known disease, is symbolic, as we shall see in the paragraphs ahead. Other diseases and their viruses are less well-known. For example, in 1999, an episode of brain illness was linked to a newly recognized paramyxovirus called the **Nipah virus**. Over 250 cases of illness occurred in Malaysia and Singapore, and exposure to pigs seemed to be the primary mode of transmission.

RABIES

Rabies is notable for having the highest mortality rate of any human disease, once the symptoms have fully materialized. Few people in history have survived rabies, and in those who did, it is uncertain whether the symptoms were due to the disease or the therapy.

Rabies can occur in most warm-blooded animals, including dogs and cats, horses and rats, and skunks and bats. The disease has been identified in Alaskan caribou, Russian wolves, and American prairie dogs. Public health microbiologists have also voiced concerns for the raccoon epizootic that is currently working its way up the eastern seaboard into New England (**MicroFocus 13.8**). **Raccoons** are well adapted to urban dwelling (one writer calls them "garbage can gourmets"), and the symbiotic relationship with humans may encourage the spread of rabies. Of equal concern is an emerging epizootic in coyotes.

Epizootic: an epidemic in animals. rab'do-vir'ĭ-da

The rabies virus is an RNA virion of the Rhabdoviridae family with a meager five genes in its genome. It is rounded on one end, flattened on the other, and looks like a bullet (**FIGURE 13.14**). The virus enters the tissue through a skin wound contaminated with the saliva, urine, blood, or other fluid from an infected animal. The air in a cave inhabited by diseased bats can also transmit the virus. Indeed, rabid bats are a primary source of human infection in the United States.

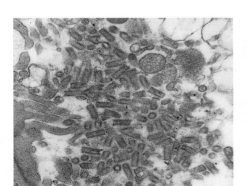

FIGURE 13.14

The Rabies Virus

An accumulation of rabies viruses in the salivary gland tissue of a canine (×58,000). The viruses are elongated particles, some having the tapered shape of bullets. This configuration is characteristic of the rhabdoviruses.

MicroFocus 13.8

BEWARE THE GARBAGE CAN GOURMET

Human cases of rabies are very rare (10 confirmed cases in the 1980 to 1992 period), but animal rabies continues to be common. In 1998, for instance, almost 7000 cases of rabies among animals were reported to the CDC. Almost half the cases were reported in raccoons.

Rabid raccoons were probably introduced to the mid-Atlantic region of the United States in the mid-1970s, when hunters brought them up from the Southeast to replenish hunting stocks. While raccoons remained in their original territories, rabies was reasonably under control, but in a new rabies-free area, the disease spread rapidly among the raccoon population. The first cases occurred in West Virginia (1977). Then the disease was detected in raccoons from Virginia (1978), Maryland (1981), Pennsylvania (1982), New Jersey (1989), New York (1990), Connecticut (1991), and New Hampshire (1992)—and on from there, as the figure shows. The disease also spread east to North Carolina (1991) and north to Ohio (1992).

Given that raccoons live in close proximity with humans in urban, suburban, and rural areas, the possibility of contracting rabies from a raccoon is real. Pet immunizations may interrupt the

chain of transmission to humans, but stray raccoons remain a threat for direct transmission to humans via a bite. And should that occur, it is somewhat sobering to know that death is a virtual certainty once rabies symptoms have developed. Indeed, a CDC writer stated: "There is no evidence that any pharmocologic intervention is effective for the treatment of human rabies" (*MMWR*, 1992, 41:663).

To interrupt the animal epidemic, researchers are testing oral rabies vaccines distributed by means of raccoon baits. On Parramore Island, a barrier island off the coast of Virginia, thousands of doses of a new vaccine have been distributed inside baited tubes to attract the raccoons living on the strip of land. The island must be used because the vaccine has been genetically engineered by grafting genes from the rabies virus to the harmless vaccinia (cowpox) virus formerly used against smallpox. Such genetically engineered vaccines cannot be released without careful supervision, and the island provides the opportunity to control the spread of the virus. Over the months, raccoons will be trapped to deter-

mine whether the vaccine is eliciting an immune response. The hope is that one day the vaccine can be routinely used to interrupt the raccoon epidemic.

While the vaccine work is continuing, public education has remained the chief method for intervention. Health departments provide these warnings: Minimize exposures to wild raccoons; keep pet immunizations current; if bitten by or exposed to an animal seek prompt medical attention; and consider preexposure immunization if you must work where there is an animal population.

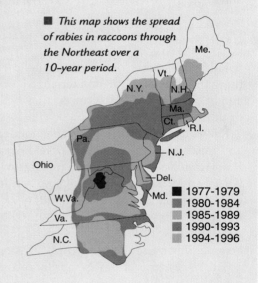

■ *This map shows the spread of rabies in raccoons through the Northeast over a 10-year period.*

■ 1977-1979
■ 1980-1984
■ 1985-1989
■ 1990-1993
■ 1994-1996

The incubation period for rabies varies according to the amount of virus entering the tissue and the wound's proximity to the central nervous system. As few as 6 days or as long as a year may elapse before symptoms appear. A bite from a rabid animal does not ensure transmission, however, because experience shows that only 5 to 15 percent of inoculated individuals develop the disease.

Early signs of rabies are abnormal sensations such as tingling, burning, or coldness at the site of the bite. Fever, headache, and increased muscle tension develop, and the patient becomes alert and aggressive. Soon there is paralysis, especially in the swallowing muscles of the pharynx, and saliva drips from the mouth. Brain degeneration, together with an inability to swallow, increases the violent reaction to the sight, sound, or thought of water (the word "rabies" comes from the Latin *rabere* for "rage"). The disease has therefore been called **hydrophobia**—literally, the fear of water. Death usually comes within days from respiratory paralysis.

A person who is bitten by an animal, particularly a wild carnivore, should be treated as if the animal were rabid. Before 1980, this meant up to two-dozen injec-

Hydrophobia:
an alternate name for rabies based on extreme sensitivity to water.

Carnivore:
a meat-eating animal with canine teeth.

tions of duck embryo **vaccine** given at a 45-degree angle in the abdominal fat. Since 1980, however, physicians have used a vaccine composed of inactivated viruses cultivated in human embryonic lung cells. (A less expensive vaccine prepared in chick embryo cells is now being tested.) Because human tissue is used, allergic responses are much reduced. For people suffering from animal bites, five injections are given in the deltoid muscle of the arm. These injections are preceded by thorough cleansing and one dose of rabies immune globulin to provide immediate antibodies at the site of the bite. This **postexposure immunization** is usually accompanied by a tetanus booster, but the latter is omitted if exposure is not certain, as occurred in the incident described in FIGURE 13.15. For high-risk individuals such as veterinarians, trappers,

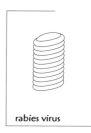

rabies virus

FIGURE 13.15

An Unusual Case of Rabies

This case was unusual because rabies is not usually associated with calves. Transmission had probably occurred during contact with a wild animal.

TEXTBOOK CASES

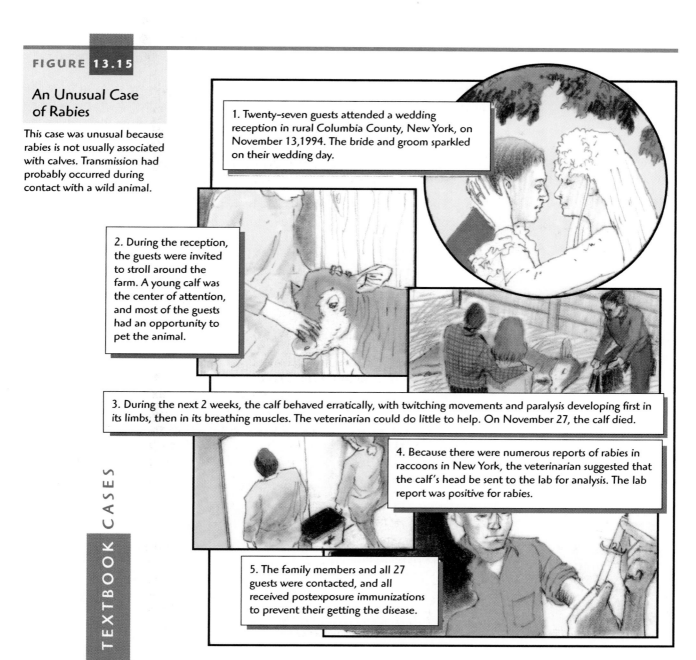

1. Twenty-seven guests attended a wedding reception in rural Columbia County, New York, on November 13, 1994. The bride and groom sparkled on their wedding day.

2. During the reception, the guests were invited to stroll around the farm. A young calf was the center of attention, and most of the guests had an opportunity to pet the animal.

3. During the next 2 weeks, the calf behaved erratically, with twitching movements and paralysis developing first in its limbs, then in its breathing muscles. The veterinarian could do little to help. On November 27, the calf died.

4. Because there were numerous reports of rabies in raccoons in New York, the veterinarian suggested that the calf's head be sent to the lab for analysis. The lab report was positive for rabies.

5. The family members and all 27 guests were contacted, and all received postexposure immunizations to prevent their getting the disease.

and zoo workers, a preventive immunization of three injections may be given. This **preexposure immunization** currently costs about $125.

Rabies has historically been a major threat to animals. One form, called **furious rabies**, is accompanied by violent symptoms as the animal becomes wide-eyed, drools, and attacks anything in sight. In the second form, **dumb rabies**, the animal is docile and lethargic, with few other symptoms. In 1998, almost 7000 wildlife cases were reported throughout the United States (half in raccoons). However, the number of human cases is usually less than 5 per year, due in part to postexposure immunizations, of which over 25,000 are given annually. (However, over 50,000 die of rabies worldwide.) Health departments are now conducting a novel campaign to immunize wild animals using vaccine air-dropped within biscuit-sized baits of dog-food and fishmeal.

POLIO

The name **polio** is a shortened form of **poliomyelitis**, a word derived from the Greek *polios* for "gray" and *myelon* for "matter." The "gray matter" is the nerve tissue of the spinal cord and brain, which are affected in the disease. Viruses that cause polio are among the smallest virions, measuring 27 nm in diameter. They are composed of RNA and are icosahedral virions of the Picornaviridae family (FIGURE 13.16).

Polio viruses usually enter the body by contaminated water and food. They multiply first in the tonsils and then in lymphoid tissues of the gastrointestinal tract, causing nausea, vomiting, and cramps. In many cases, this is the extent of the problem. Sometimes, however, the viruses pass through the bloodstream and localize on the meninges, where they cause **meningitis**. Paralysis of the arms, legs, and body trunk may result. In the most severe form of polio, the viruses infect the medulla of the brain, causing **bulbar polio** (the medulla is bulblike). Nerves serving the upper body torso are affected. Swallowing is difficult, and paralysis develops in the tongue, facial muscles, and neck. Paralysis of the diaphragm muscle causes labored breathing and may lead to death.

Virologists have identified three types of polio virus: type I, the **Brunhilde** strain, causes a major number of epidemics and is sometimes a cause of paralysis; type II, the **Lansing** strain, occurs sporadically but invariably causes paralysis; and type III, the

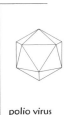

polio virus

Tonsils:
patches of lymphoid tissue in the pharynx of humans.

FIGURE 13.16

Polio Viruses

An electron micrograph of the viruses that cause polio (×286,000). Although the particles appear to be circular, their symmetry has been found to be icosahedral. With a diameter of about 27 nm, these are among the smallest viruses that cause human disease.

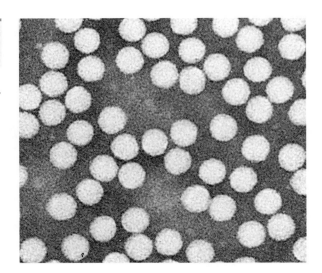

Leon strain, usually remains in the intestinal tract. Once the method of laboratory cultivation of polio viruses was established by Enders, Weller, and Robbins, a team led by Jonas Salk grew large quantities of the viruses and inactivated them with formaldehyde to produce the first polio vaccine in 1955. Albert Sabin's group subsequently developed a vaccine containing attenuated (weakened) polio viruses. This vaccine was in widespread use by 1961 and could be taken orally as compared with Salk's vaccine, which had to be injected. Both vaccines are referred to as **trivalent** because they contain all three strains of virus. The vaccines have contributed substantially to the reduction of polio, as FIGURE 13.17 shows. Chapter 19 details their use.

Although the gradual disappearance of polio from media headlines has brought some complacency regarding the need for immunization, the disease still breaks out

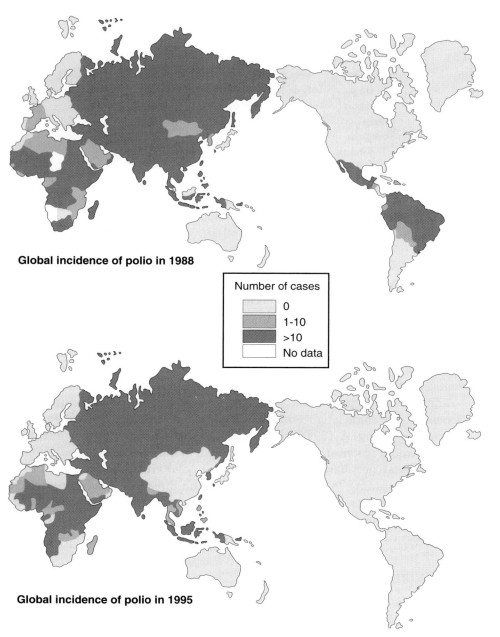

Global incidence of polio in 1988

Number of cases

- 0
- 1-10
- >10
- No data

Global incidence of polio in 1995

FIGURE 13.17

The Race to Eradicate Polio

The World Health Organization and other health agencies are attempting to eradicate polio from the face of the Earth by early in the twenty-first century. Progress of the campaign is illustrated by the global incidence rate of polio in 1988 compared to that in 1995.

MicroFocus 13.9

BLITZ

One ordinary morning at the end of December 1997, two million people set out to eradicate polio in India. Coming from every conceivable corner of a vast country, they arrived at 650,000 Indian villages, where they set up immunization posts. Children came to them by the thousands, then the hundreds of thousands, then the millions. By the end of the day, 127 million children had received polio immunizations.

This was the National Immunization Day for India, one in a series of such events across the world. The campaigns are coordinated by the World Health Organization, with help from UNICEF (which provides the oral polio vaccine) and Rotary International (which helps recruit volunteers). Their success is illustrated by the 1996 achievement—over

420 million children under age 5 vaccinated, nearly two-thirds of the world's population of children in that age group.

Then, there are the Days of Tranquility. These are pauses in wars and civil strife to allow children to be immunized. In El Salvador, a day is designated each year, and health-care workers cross enemy lines to vaccinate the local children. In Sri Lanka, polio vaccine was passed across front lines during Days of Tranquility in 1995 and 1996. And cease-fires have been called in the Sudan to pass out polio vaccine (the days also give warring armies a glimpse of peace).

Polio is a particularly desirable target for eradication because, like smallpox, the disease occurs only in humans. Moreover, the virus exists in the body for only a short period of time, and the

vaccine provides effective intervention for the disease. These reasons, plus the involvement of the world's nations, have generated high optimism that one day, polio may be nothing more than a memory.

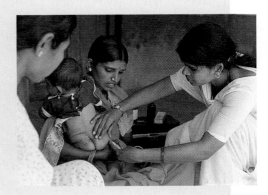

occasionally. For example, a 1993 epidemic affected close to 100 individuals in The Netherlands who had chosen to refuse immunization. Recent events in the Americas have been more positive, however. The attempt at polio eradication by the Pan American Health Organization has apparently been successful, and no case of polio due to a "wild" environmental virus has occurred since August 23, 1991 (MicroFocus 13.9 details the effort to eradicate polio in other parts of the world). This does not necessarily mean that polio viruses have been eradicated from individuals. Indeed, when CDC researchers undertook a screening of Canadian residents related to the affected individuals from The Netherlands (in the episode related above), they isolated the identical polio virus that had affected their European relatives.

A discouraging legacy of the polio epidemics is **postpolio syndrome**, a series of ailments that include fatigue, muscle weakness and atrophy, and some instances of difficult breathing. A 1994 report indicated that these symptoms affect about 500,000 Americans, nearly one-third of the 1.6 million survivors of past polio epidemics. Researchers have found fragments of polio viruses in the tissues of these individuals, leading to the suggestion that the infection is reemerging. Other researchers, however, offer that viral fragments do not indicate reinfection. As of this writing, no whole viruses have been found. Another suggestion is that Coxsackie B viruses may be involved.

SLOW VIRUS (PRION) DISEASES

Certain viruses appear to cause slow-developing degenerative diseases in which many years elapse between the infection and any detectable symptoms. The viruses, known as **slow viruses,** have not yet been visualized with the electron microscope.

Moreover, no nucleic acid has been detected in material that transmits the disease. Many scientists believe that viruses will eventually be isolated and that nucleic acid will be identified; nevertheless, many investigators support the theory that slow viruses are really **prions** (discussed at length in Chapter 11). Thus, we refer to the agents as slow viruses (prions).

pre'onz

Virologists have related three diseases to slow viruses (prions). The first such disease to be identified was **kuru**, a fatal disorder found in villages of the Fore people who live in the remote highlands of New Guinea. Villagers suffer a gradual loss of limb control and eventually all bodily control because of the destruction of their brain cells. Kuru was considered a genetic disease until D. Carleton Gajdusek of the National Institutes of Health researched it and helped prove that it was due to an infectious agent. For his work, Gajdusek shared the 1976 Nobel Prize. The time between injection of the infectious material and the first signs of disease is measured in months or years.

koo'roo

gad'u-sek

The second disease in this group is **scrapie**, a disease of sheep and goats. Known for centuries, scrapie interferes with nervous coordination in animals so they cannot walk or stand. Tortured by itching, the animals scrape constantly against rocks and tree trunks, hence the disease's name. In the late 1930s, over 1500 sheep in Scotland died from a scrapie-contaminated vaccine.

Scrapie:
a disease of sheep and goats
thought to be due to a slow virus.

A somewhat similar disease in cattle has recently emerged, as discussed in the chapter opening. The disease is **bovine spongiform encephalopathy (BSE)**, also called **mad cow disease**. BSE has an incubation period of 8 to 12 years. It affects the brain tissue in cattle, causing their brains to develop a "spongy" appearance with large numbers of empty spaces called **plaques** (FIGURE 13.18). The animals become apprehensive and unable to stand on their feet; they behave erratically and soon die.

In 1996, British researchers announced a possible link between BSE and a human malady called **Creutzfeldt-Jakob disease (CJD)**. This disease has been recognized for decades in humans and is much like kuru in effects. Patients suffer from nervousness, bizarre behavior, memory loss, wobbly walk, lethargy, and hunched posture, and, eventually, death. In the past, researchers have been unsure of the cause of CJD or how the disease is transmitted, but cases were linked to corneal transplant as well as transplanted dura mater (one of the meninges, the membranes that cover the brain and spinal cord). Another possible mode of transmission is by contaminated needle electrodes inserted to the brain for diagnostic purposes. In 1996, the disease was related to BSE, and the $6.5 billion British cattle industry was under a cloud of suspicion. The British government reacted by reluctantly destroying 4 million cattle from a national herd of about 11 million. It also imposed a ban on adding tissues from sheep, goats, and other animals to livestock feed. (The United States did likewise.)

kroits'felt yak'ob

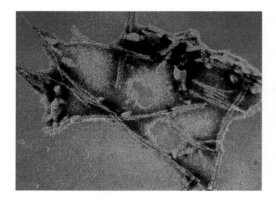

FIGURE 13.18

The Signs of BSE

A colored transmission electron micrograph of prion fibrils (green) from the brain of a cow that died of bovine spongiform encephalopathy (BSE), also called mad cow disease. Fibrils and spongy lesions in the brain tissue are typical of the disease and are similar to those in the brains of patients with new variant Creutzfeldt-Jakob disease.

The link between BSE and Creutzfeldt-Jakob disease was strengthened in 1997 when two research groups reported that a new variant of CJD had infected 19 young British patients over a 3-year period (the traditional CJD affects older individuals). One group reported that new variant CJD could be reproduced in animals by inoculations of brain material from infected cows. The second group focused on **prions**, the nucleic-acid-free protein particles researched by Stanley Prusiner (Chapter 11). This group reengineered mice so they possessed the human version of prion protein (PrP) on their brain cells. When the mice were injected with either brain material from BSE cows or CJD victims, they developed similar neurological symptoms. And they harbored the same abnormal and misshapen prion protein (the prion) found in patients with prion diseases.

The research does not prove conclusively that the young CJD patients were infected by contaminated beef, but the research draws a strong parallel between bovine spongiform encephalopathy and Creutzfeldt-Jakob disease. The definitive proof will come from the isolation of the disease agent (slow virus or prion) from infected animals and the demonstration that it—and it alone—can cause the disease. The current thinking is that a prion is involved and that a misshapen prion may be ingested in food, travel to the brain, and subvert the patient's normal PrP, prompting it to become misshapen and thereby encourage the disease to develop. Through 1999, no case of BSE had been reported in the United States, although PrP has been found in numerous mammals and salmon, and BSE has been observed in mice, cats, and some zoo animals fed ruminant tissues. A protein-antibody test is now available to detect evidence of BSE in spinal fluid.

alz'hi-mer

a-mi'o-trof'ik

Continuing research on slow viruses (prions) has substantial importance with respect to other diseases. For example, evidence indicates that the agents may be involved in Alzheimer's disease, a condition that involves dementia and the deterioration of physical health. Other possibilities are that the agents may cause Parkinson's disease and amyotrophic lateral sclerosis (Lou Gehrig's disease), as well as Gerstmann-Straussler-Scheinker (GSS) syndrome, a spongiform encephalopathy that affects humans like BSE affects cows. In addition, research may shed light on the relationship between childhood diseases and the slow-developing mental-deterioration illnesses that afflict the elderly.

ARBOVIRAL ENCEPHALITIS

en-cef'a-li'tis
Encephalitis:
acute inflammation of the brain.

The term **encephalitis** means acute inflammation of the brain. Used in the general sense, encephalitis may refer to any brain disorder, much as pneumonia refers to a lung disorder. In this section, we shall use encephalitis to mean a number of viral disorders that are *ar*thropod*bo*rne (hence arboviral).

Arboviral encephalitis may be caused by a series of RNA viruses, usually of the Togaviridae or Bunyaviridae families. In humans, viral encephalitis is characterized by sudden, very high fever and a severe headache. Normally, the patient experiences pain and stiffness in the neck, with general disorientation. Patients become drowsy and stuporous, and may experience a number of convulsions before lapsing into a coma. Paralysis and mental disorders may afflict those who recover. Mortality rates are generally high.

equine encephalitis virus

There are many forms of arboviral encephalitis and various vectors of the disease. One form is **St. Louis encephalitis (SLE)**, named for the city where it was first identified in 1933. This disease, transmitted by mosquitoes, resurfaced in 1975 with 1300 cases nationwide. Other forms are California encephalitis, La Crosse encephalitis, Japanese B encephalitis, and West Nile encephalitis, all transmitted by mosquitoes. Russian encephalitis and Louping ill encephalitis are forms transmitted by ticks. A notable outbreak of mosquitoborne West Nile encephalitis occurred in New York City in 1999.

Arboviral encephalitis is also a serious problem in **horses**, causing erratic behavior, loss of coordination, and fever (FIGURE 13.19). In addition to the economic loss sustained by the death of the horse, the disease is transmissible from horses to humans by ticks, mosquitoes, and other arthropods (FIGURE 13.20). Important forms are Eastern equine encephalitis (EEE), Western equine encephalitis (WEE), and Venezuelan Eastern equine encephalitis (VEEE). The diseases occur in many

TEXTBOOK CASES

FIGURE 13.19

An Outbreak of Eastern Equine Encephalitis

This outbreak occurred in Florida during 1991. Horses in transit or flocks of birds may have been responsible for transporting the viruses from central to northern Florida.

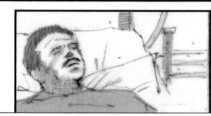

1. During the summer of 1991, a group of horses at a northern Florida stable were observed displaying erratic behaviors. Many horses were unsteady on their feet, and some walked in circles.

2. As the days passed, the symptoms worsened. Many of the horses held their heads low, as if asleep. Worried veterinarians suspected Eastern equine encephalitis (EEE).

3. Shortly thereafter, a number of the stable's trainers, jockeys, and stable hands developed piercing headaches, occasional numbness in the arms and legs, and stiff necks.

4. Some of them were hospitalized. Blood tests confirmed that they harbored the EEE virus. To interrupt the epidemic, investigators began a search for the agent of transmission.

5. Heavy mosquito swarms were reported at a tire depot in central Florida. Suspecting arthropod involvement, researchers collected *Aedes albopictus* mosquitoes from pools of water in the tires.

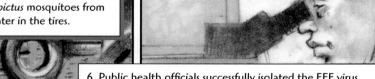

6. Public health officials successfully isolated the EEE virus from the mosquitoes and concluded they were the epidemic's source. This was the first isolation of the EEE virus from *A. albopictus*.

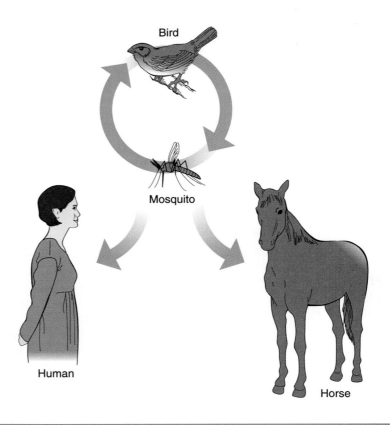

FIGURE 13.20

The Transmission of Viral Encephalitis

The generalized pattern of viral encephalitis transmission among various animals, including humans. Epidemics of viral encephalitis are difficult to interrupt because numerous animals are involved. Polio, by comparison, infects only humans.

animals in nature and are a particular problem in birds because birds are natural reservoirs of the viruses and spread them during annual migrations.

LYMPHOCYTIC CHORIOMENINGITIS

lim′fo-sit′ĭk ko′re-o-men′in-ji′tis

Lymphocytic choriomeningitis (LCM) is usually found in mice, hamsters, and other **rodents**, where it is transmitted by feces and dustborne viruses from urine. Several outbreaks in humans have been recorded since 1960, most related to pet hamsters or hamster colonies in laboratories. In 1984, a case was traced to mice in the patient's home.

LCM is a mild disorder, often with influenzalike symptoms. Fever and malaise precede headache, drowsiness, and stupor, and the meninges of the brain are infiltrated with large numbers of lymphocytes (hence the disease's name). The symptoms subside within a week, and the mortality rate is very low. An RNA virus of the Arenaviridae family appears to be the cause. Aseptic meningitis may be the only symptom of disease.

TABLE 13.3 summarizes the neurotropic viral diseases.

TABLE 13.3

A Summary of Neurotropic Viral Diseases

DISEASE	CLASSIFICATION OF VIRUS	TRANSMISSION	ORGANS AFFECTED	VACCINE	SPECIAL FEATURES	COMPLICATIONS
Rabies	Rhabdoviridae	Contact with body fluids	Brain Spinal cord	Inactivated viruses	Paralysis Hydrophobia	Death
Polio	Picornaviridae	Food Water Contact with human feces	Intestine Spinal cord Brain	Inactivated viruses Attenuated viruses	Infection of medulla	Permanent paralysis
Slow virus (prion) disease	(Unknown)	Not established	Brain	Not available	Brain degeneration	Paralysis Mental deterioration
Arboviral encephalitis	Many viruses	Arthropods	Brain	Not available	Encephalitis	Coma Seizures
Lymphocytic choriomeningitis	Arenaviridae	Dust Contact	Brain Meninges	Not available	Lymphocytes in brain	Paralysis

Note to the Student

In the remote tropics of South America and Africa there lurks a coterie of viruses that infect animals, but seldom bother humans. Occasionally, however, humans stumble into their paths, with results horrifying enough to mark the annals of medicine. The hemorrhagic fever viruses, for example, make the internal organs bleed and rot, and patients ooze contagious, virus-laden blood from their eyes, ears, nose, and other orifices. Marburg viruses appeared in 1967, then Lassa fever viruses in the 1970s, followed by Ebola viruses and hantaviruses in the years thereafter. In 1994, another hemorrhagic fever virus, the Sabia virus, escaped from a high-security laboratory at Yale University and roamed the streets of New Haven and Boston before felling its human host with symptoms (the patient recovered, and none of his 80 contacts developed the disease).

Where have these viruses come from and what do they portend? The strange new pathogens erupting on American soil are believed to be ancient organisms that lacked the opportunity to attack until humans blundered into their habitat. Lassa virus, Marburg virus, Ebola virus, hantavirus—all were probably confined for millennia to isolated human groups or animals; then civilization's encroachment on the forest let them broaden their range. Now it was up to nature to trigger an expansion of the host organism. Previous to the 1993 hantavirus epidemic, for instance, heavy rains had disturbed the desert and mountain ecology of the southwestern United States, leading to an abundance of piñon nuts and grasshoppers. Suddenly, the deer mouse population exploded, and hantaviruses had a ready mode of transport. In other cases, humans luck out before the viruses can find an alternate host: Ebola virus kills its victims so quickly that it does not have time to spread. And it does not have an animal host—not yet, at least.

As the world shrinks to a global village, a great biological soup is emerging. It is a soup into which dangerous microorganisms of long-isolated ecologies are being mixed. Air travel provides an excellent opportunity for an ill person to carry viruses across the ocean in a matter of hours. Military bases in far corners of the globe, and increased trade with new nations, promote the exposure of foreigners to exotic viruses. Europeans once encountered dangerous new microorganisms in the New World. Now their descendants are confronting novel pathogens in their own new worlds.

To many scientists, these are exciting times because their search for disease agents is reminiscent of searches made by Pasteur and Koch over 100 years ago. To others, the times are foreboding because they must deal with immediate threats to life. And, they ask, what else is out there? What, for instance, is the agent of Kawasaki disease? Or kuru? Or bovine spongiform encephalopathy?

Contrary to what some people believe, science does not have an answer for everything. If you find yourself becoming complacent about disease and its control, I urge you to read Fuller's book about Lassa fever (*Fever*) or Preston's book about Ebola fever (*The Hot Zone*). Better yet, read Laurie Garrett's *The Coming Plague*. It will help you realize that the wave of emerging diseases is far from spent.

Summary

The major focal points of this chapter are the viscerotropic and neurotropic viral diseases. Viscerotropic diseases are those that affect the visceral organs, while neurotropic diseases affect the spinal cord and brain.

Two important viscerotropic diseases are yellow fever and dengue fever, both of which occur in the tropics where the agent of transmission, the mosquito, is common. Viral invasion of the blood characterizes both diseases, and high fever is a notable symptom. Several forms of hepatitis, including hepatitis A, B, and C, are also considered viscerotropic diseases because the major organ affected is the liver. Hepatitis A is caused by a resistant RNA virus that can remain active outside the body and be transmitted by a fecal-oral route. Hepatitis B, by comparison, is caused by a fragile DNA virus that must be trans-ferred directly from person to person by blood or semen to remain active. Infectious mononucleosis, another viral disease in this category, is also transferred from person to person, often by saliva.

The viscerotropic diseases also include several forms of viral gastroenteritis that occur in the intestinal tract and are accompanied by diarrhea. A number of serious viral fevers including Lassa fever, Ebola fever, and sandfly and Colorado tick fevers are in the group, as are cytomegalovirus disease and AIDS. AIDS is caused by an RNA retrovirus called the human immunodeficiency virus (HIV). The virus attacks and destroys the body's lymphocytes, thus weakening the immune system and encouraging disease by opportunistic organisms. HIV is transmitted by blood-to-blood contact, or semen to blood, and HIV infection is the first of several syndromes culminating in AIDS.

Among the neurotropic viral diseases, rabies is notable for its high mortality rate. The disease affects the brain tissue of most species of warm-blooded animals in nature and is generally transmitted by inoculation with their saliva. Another neurotropic disease, polio, is currently under control due in large measure to mass immunization programs using Salk and Sabin polio vaccines. Also in the group are a collection of slow-developing brain diseases such as kuru, scrapie, and Creutzfeldt-Jakob disease. Several arthropodborne central nervous system diseases collectively called encephalitis are also considered neurotropic diseases.

Questions for Thought and Discussion

1. In 1995, the New York newspaper *Newsday* reported that during the previous year, 1700 cases of rabies had occurred in New York State. Public health officials report, to the contrary, that rabies cases in the entire United States rarely exceed single digits. What might have been the source of *Newsday*'s error?

2. In 1996, a medical school student at the University of Maryland was assigned a case for a seminar on undetermined diagnoses in difficult cases. His subject was identified only as E.P., a gentleman who lived in the mid-1800s and was a well-known poet and animal lover. The man was taken to a hospital with delirium and tremors. He was confused and combative, and he refused to drink any water or other liquid. He died on October 7, 1849. The traditional diagnosis had been alcoholism, but the student made a different diagnosis. What do you think it was? When told the man's name, the student thought "Nevermore!" Who was the man?

3. A *New York Times* crossword puzzle once contained a space in the Across column for a term containing 14 letters. The only clue given was "dengue." By using the Down column, you could see that the second-to-last letter was an e and that the fifth-to-last letter was an f. What was the answer?

4. In 1996, the CDC's Advisory Committee on Immunization Practices (ACIP) recommended that the polio vaccine be used on a sequential schedule: two doses of injectable, inactivated (Salk) vaccine at 2 and 4 months of age, followed by two doses of oral, attenuated (Sabin) vaccine at 12 to 18 months and 4 to 6 years. This was a departure from a policy established in 1987, when the ACIP first recommended exclusive use of the oral Sabin vaccine. Why do you believe it changed its recommendations? And how well do you think the public and medical community will react to this change? (Chapter 19 details still more modifications to the policy.)

5. Health authorities shifted into adrenaline overdrive when an outbreak of Ebola hemorrhagic disease occurred in Reston, Virginia, in 1989. What sparks such a dramatic response when a disease like Ebola fever breaks out?

6. Walt Disney World uses a series of sentinel chickens strategically placed on the grounds to detect any signs of viral encephalitis. Why do you suppose they use chickens? Why is Disney World particularly susceptible to outbreaks of viral encephalitis? And what recommendations might be offered to tourists if the disease broke out?

7. During 1997, El Niño brought abundant rain and a mild winter to the southwestern United States. The conditions encouraged a burgeoning rodent population. (For example, deer mice that usually reproduce twice a year were able to turn out three litters.) Which viral disease did public health officials anticipate for 1998? What precautions did epidemiologists give residents?

8. Written on some blood donor cards is the notation "CMV(+)." What do you think the letters mean, and why are they placed there?

9. A student in a biology laboratory uses a sterile lancet from a package to pierce the skin and obtain blood for a blood-typing exercise. The student places the lancet down on the desktop, whereupon a nearby student picks it up and uses it again to pierce the skin. What is the danger?

10. Sometimes the use of acronyms becomes absurd. A recent headline in the medical section of a newspaper blared: "CDC blames HPS on MCV." Would you care to take a stab at what this gibberish means?

11. At a college campus some years ago, a group of students were passing around a wine bottle. Several days later, one member of the group developed hepatitis A and the others requested that the college

infirmary distribute immune globulin shots. When the infirmary refused, the students demonstrated, causing a stir. A reporter from a local newspaper wrote about the incident and recounted it accurately except for the last line of the article, which read: "Hepatitis A is normally transmitted by contaminated syringes." What is microbiologically wrong with this statement, and what are its implications?

12. Since 1990, the makers of one of the recombinant hepatitis B vaccines (Engerix-B) have offered free immunizations to emergency medical technicians (EMTs) throughout the United States. If you were an EMT, would you accept the offer?

13. The control of yellow fever in Central America was a principal factor in the construction of the Panama Canal. The work began in 1904 and was completed in 1914. It is said that during construction, a group of workers made up the following phrase: A MAN A PLAN A CANAL—PANAMA. What two things are unique about this phrase?

14. Sicilian barbers are renowned for their skill and dexterity with razors (and sometimes their singing voices). In 1995, French researchers studied a group of 37 Sicilian barbers and found that 14 had antibodies against hepatitis C, despite never having been sick with the disease. By comparison, when a random group of 50 blood donors was studied, none had the antibodies. What might account for the high incidence of exposure to hepatitis C among the barbers?

15. In many diseases, the immune system overcomes the infectious agent, and the person recovers. In certain diseases, the infectious agent overcomes the immune system, and death follows. Compare this broad overview of disease and resistance to what is taking place with AIDS, and explain why AIDS is probably unlike any other disease encountered in medicine.

16. The restaurant industry is currently weighing a requirement that all restaurant workers be immunized with hepatitis A vaccine. Would you favor or oppose this requirement?

17. A diagnostic test has been developed to detect hepatitis C in blood intended for transfusion purposes. Obviously, if the test is positive, the blood is not used. However, there is a lively controversy as to whether the blood donor should be informed of the positive result. What is your opinion? Why?

18. An epidemiologist notes that India has a high rate of dengue fever but a very low rate of yellow fever. What might be the cause of this anomaly?

Review

On completing your study of these pages, test your understanding of their contents by deciding whether the following statements are true or false. If the statement is true, write "True" in the space. If false, substitute a word for the underlined word to make the statement true. The answers are listed in Appendix D.

_____ 1. Both yellow fever and dengue fever are caused by a <u>DNA</u> virus transmitted by the mosquito.

_____ 2. One of the most common causes of death in AIDS patients is pneumonia due to <u>*Toxoplasma gondii*</u>.

_____ 3. The Coxsackie virus is a well-known cause of <u>gastroenteritis</u> in humans.

_____ 4. Downey cells are a characteristic sign of the viral disease <u>infectious mononucleosis</u>.

_____ 5. The echovirus is known to cause disease of the <u>spleen</u> in humans who acquire the virus.

_____ 6. Polio may be caused by any of <u>three</u> strains of polio virus.

_____ 7. The term *hydrophobia* means "fear of water," and it is commonly associated with patients who have <u>encephalitis</u>.

_____ 8. Hepatitis is primarily a disease of the <u>liver</u>.

_____ 9. The cell most often affected by HIV, the AIDS virus, is the human <u>monocyte</u>.

_____10. Because of the characteristic symptoms, dengue fever is sometimes called <u>breakbone fever</u>.

_____11. A small RNA virus is regarded as the cause of hepatitis <u>A</u>.

_____12. Norwalk virus and rotavirus are both considered to be agents of viral <u>encephalitis</u>.

_____13. The cytomegalovirus can cause serious disease of the <u>lungs</u> in AIDS patients.

_____14. The <u>Epstein-Barr</u> virus is most probably the cause of infectious mononucleosis.

_____15. A vaccine is available to prevent <u>yellow fever</u> but not to prevent AIDS.

_____16. Slow virus diseases include <u>kuru</u> and scrapie, but not encephalitis.

_____17. The Salk and Sabin vaccines are used for immunizations against <u>hepatitis</u>.

_____18. HIV is a <u>reovirus</u> in which the RNA of the genome is used as a template to synthesize DNA.

_____19. Pleurodynia and myocarditis are both related to infection by <u>Norwalk</u> virus.

_____20. Hepatitis B is most commonly transmitted by contact with infected semen or infected <u>blood</u>.

_____21. One of the organs that suffers damage during infections with yellow fever virus is the <u>kidney</u>.

_____22. The vaccine currently in use to protect against hepatitis A consists of <u>genetically engineered proteins</u>.

_____23. One of the most important causes of diarrhea in infants and young children admitted to hospitals is the <u>Epstein-Barr virus</u>.

_____24. Filoviruses are long, threadlike viruses that cause hemorrhagic fevers and include the <u>Marburg virus</u>.

_____25. Both *Aedes aegypti* and *Aedes albopictus* may be capable of transmitting the virus of <u>dengue fever</u>.

_____26. Enlargement of the lymph nodes, sore throat, mild fever, and a high count of B-lymphocytes are characteristic symptoms in people who have <u>polio</u>.

_____27. The resistance of hepatitis A viruses to chemical and physical changes in the environment is generally considered to be <u>low</u>.

_____28. The "four corners disease" that broke out in the United States in 1993 was eventually related to <u>Lassa fever viruses</u>, which were possibly transmitted among individuals by the deer mouse.

_____29. The C in the TORCH group of diseases stands for the <u>cephalovirus</u>, which can be transmitted from a pregnant woman to her unborn child.

_____30. The current protocol for rabies immunizations is to give the injections into the <u>stomach</u>.

http://microbiology.jbpub.com

The site features **eLearning,** an on-line review area that provides quizzes and other tools to help you study for your class. You can also follow useful links for in-depth information, read more MicroFocus stories, or just find out the latest microbiology news.

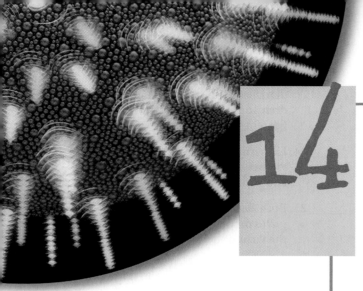

14 The Fungi

Mushrooms always grow in damp places, which is why they look like umbrellas.

—A midwestern eighth-grader sharing his insightful observation of a typical fungus

RELAND OF THE 1840s was an impoverished country of 8 million people. Most were tenant farmers paying rent to landlords who were responsible, in turn, to the English property owners. The sole crop of Irish farmers was potatoes, grown season after season on small tracts of land. What little corn was available was usually fed to the cows and pigs.

Early in the 1840s, heavy rains and dampness portended calamity. Then, on August 23, 1845, *The Gardener's Chronicle and Agricultural Gazette* reported: "A fatal malady has broken out amongst the potato crop. On all sides we hear of the destruction. In Belgium, the fields are said to have been completely desolated."

The potatoes had suffered before. There had been scab, drought, "curl," and too much rain, but nothing was quite like this new disease. It struck down the plants like frost in the summer. Beginning as black spots, it decayed the leaves and stems, and left the potatoes a rotten, mushy mass with a peculiar and offensive odor. Even the harvested potatoes rotted.

The winter of 1845 to 1846 was a disaster for Ireland. Farmers left the rotten potatoes in the fields, and the disease spread. The farmers first ate the animal feed and then the animals. They also devoured the seed potatoes, leaving nothing for spring planting. As starvation spread, the English government attempted to help by importing corn and establishing relief centers. In England, the potato disease had few repercussions because English agriculture included various grains. In Ireland, however, famine spread quickly.

After 2 years, the potato rot seemed to slacken, but in 1847 ("Black '47") it returned with a vengeance. Despite relief efforts by the English, over 2 million Irish died from starvation. Eventually, about 900,000 survivors set off for Canada and the United States. Those who stayed had to deal with economic and political upheaval as well as misery and death.

The potato blight faded in 1848, but it did not vanish. Instead, it emerged again during wet seasons and blossomed anew. In the end, hundreds of thousands of Irish left the land and moved to cities or foreign countries. During the 1860s, great waves of Irish immigrants came to the United States. Many Americans are descended from those starving, demoralized farmers.

Such are the historic, political, economic, and sociological effects of one species of fungus. Other fungal diseases of fruits, grains, and vegetables can be equally devastating, and we shall see numerous examples in this chapter as we survey the fungi. In addition, we shall take note of several widespread human and animal diseases caused by fungi, and we shall encounter many beneficial fungi such as those used to make antibiotics, breads, foods, and insecticides. Our study will begin with a focus on the structures, growth patterns, and life cycles of fungi.

fun'ji

Characteristics of Fungi

The fungi (sing., fungus) are a diverse group of eukaryotic microorganisms, with over 80,000 identifiable species. For many decades, fungi were classified as plants, but laboratory studies have revealed at least four properties that distinguish fungi from plants: Fungi lack chlorophyll, while plants have this pigment; the cell walls of fungal cells contain a carbohydrate called **chitin**, not found in plant cell walls; though generally filamentous, fungi are not truly multicellular like plants, because the cytoplasm of one fungal cell mingles through pores with the cytoplasm of adjacent cells; and fungi are heterotrophic eukaryotes, while plants are autotrophic eukaryotes. Mainly for these reasons, fungi are placed in their own kingdom **Fungi**, in the Whittaker classification of organisms.

Fungi generally are saprobes with complex life cycles usually involving spore formation. A major group of fungi, the **molds**, grow as long, tangled strands of cells that give rise to visible colonies (FIGURE 14.1). Another group, the **yeasts**, are unicellular organisms whose colonies resemble bacterial colonies.

STRUCTURE OF THE FUNGI

With the notable exception of yeasts, fungi consist of masses of intertwined filaments of cells called **hyphae**. Each cell of a single hypha is eukaryotic, with one or more nuclei, as well as other organelles. The cell wall is composed of small amounts of cellulose (but only in a small group of fungi) and large amounts of chitin. **Chitin** is a polymer of acetylglucosamine units, that is, glucose molecules containing amino

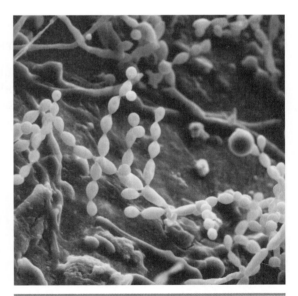

FIGURE 14.1

A Typical Fungus

A scanning electron micrograph of *Cladosporium cladosporioides*, one of the most common fungi isolated from air samples. Outdoors, this fungus is commonly found on decaying vegetation. Indoors, it may be isolated from refrigerator moldings, tile grout in showers, and vinyl shower curtains. The conidiophores and conidia of the fungus can be seen (×2970).

ki'tin

Saprobes:
organisms that feed on dead
organic matter.

sē–no–sit'ik
ri–zo'pus

hi'fah
hi'fā

mi–se'le–um

Mycology:
the study of fungi.

and acetyl groups. Chitin gives the cell wall rigidity and strength, a function it also performs in the exoskeletons of arthropods.

Fungal cells lack chlorophyll, and photosynthesis is therefore impossible. Since they consume preformed organic matter, fungi are described as **heterotrophic** organisms. They are **saprobic**, except for the parasitic fungi, which cause disease. Together with the bacteria, fungi decompose vast quantities of dead organic matter that would otherwise accumulate and make the Earth uninhabitable (MicroFocus 14.1). In industrial settings, these decompositions can be profitable. The fungus *Trichoderma*, for example, produces enzymes that degrade cellulose and give jeans a "stone-washed" appearance.

In many species of fungi, individual cells are separated by cross-walls, or **septa** (sing., septum). Such fungi are described as **septate**. The septa are incomplete, however, and pores allow adjacent cytoplasms to mix. In other fungal species, the cells have no septa, and the cytoplasms and organelles of neighboring cells mingle freely. These fungi are said to be **coenocytic**. The common bread mold *Rhizopus stolonifer* is coenocytic, while the blue-green mold that produces penicillin, *Penicillium notatum*, is septate.

The hypha is the morphological unit of the fungus and is visible only with the aid of a microscope (FIGURE 14.2). Hyphae have a broad diversity of forms (as photographs in this chapter illustrate), and many hyphae are highly branched with reproductive structures. A thick mass of hyphae is called a **mycelium** (pl., mycelia). This mass is usually large enough to be seen with the unaided eye, and generally it has a rough, cottony texture. The study of fungi is called **mycology**, and a person who studies fungi is a mycologist. Invariably, the prefix *myco-* will be part of a word referring to fungi, since *mycote* is Greek for "fungus."

GROWTH OF THE FUNGI

In nature, the fungi are important links in ecological cycles because they rapidly digest animal and vegetable matter. Working in immense numbers (MicroFocus 14.2), they release carbon and minerals back to the environment and make them available for recycling in plants. However, fungi may be a liability for industries

MicroFocus 14.1

WHEN FUNGI RULED THE EARTH

About 250 million years ago, at the close of the Permian period, a catastrophe of epic proportions visited the Earth. Apparently, over 90 percent of animal species in the seas vanished. The great Permian extinction, as it is called, also wreaked havoc on land animals and cleared the way for dinosaurs to inherit the planet.

But land plants managed to survive, and before the dinosaurs came, they spread and enveloped the world. At least, that is what paleobiologists tradi-

tionally believed. Now, however, they are revising their outlook and finding a significant place for the fungi. In 1996, Dutch scientists from Utrecht University presented evidence that land plants were decimated by the extinction and that for a brief geologic span, dead wood covered the planet. During this period, they suggest, the fungi emerged, and wood-rotting species experienced a powerful spike in their populations. Support for their theory is offered by numerous findings of fossil fungi from the

post-Permian period. The fossils are bountiful, and they come from all corners of the globe. Significantly, they contain fungal hyphae, the active feeding forms rather than the dormant spores.

And so it was that fungi proliferated wildly and entered a period of feeding frenzy where they were the dominant form of life on Earth. It's something worth considering next time you turn up your nose at a lowly fungus contaminating a cup of yogurt.

because they also contaminate leather, hair products, lumber, wax, cork, and polyvinyl plastics.

Many fungi live in a mutually beneficial relationship with other species in nature, an association called **mutualism**. In the southwestern Rocky Mountains, for instance, a fungus of the genus *Acremonium* thrives on the blades of a species of grass called *Stipa robusta* ("robust grass"). The fungus produces a powerful poison that can put horses and other animals to sleep for about a week (the grass is called "sleepy grass" by the locals). Thus the grass survives where others are nibbled to the ground, reflecting the mutually beneficial interaction between plant and fungus.

Other fungi called **mycorrhizal fungi** also live harmoniously with plants. The hyphae of these fungi invade the roots of plants (and sometimes their stems) and plunge into their cells. Though poised to suck the plants dry, the fungi are gentle neighbors. Mycorrhizal fungi consume some of the carbohydrates produced by the plants, but in return they contribute minerals and fluids to the plant's metabolism. Mycorrhizal fungi have been found in plants from salt marshes, deserts, and pine forests. Indeed, in 1995, researchers from the University of Dayton reported that over 50 percent of the plants growing in the large watershed area of southwestern Ohio contain mycorrhizal fungi.

Most fungi grow best at about 25°C, a temperature close to normal room temperature (about 75°F). Notable exceptions are the pathogenic fungi, which thrive at 37°C, body temperature. Usually these fungi also grow on nutrient media at 25°C. Such fungi are described as **biphasic** (two phases) or **dimorphic** (two forms). Many have a yeastlike phase at 37°C and a moldlike phase at 25°C. Certain fungi grow at still lower temperatures, such as the 5°C found in a normal refrigerator.

Many fungi thrive under acidic conditions at a pH from 5 to 6. Acidic soil may therefore favor fungal turf diseases, in which case lime should be used to neutralize the soil. Mold contamination is also common in acidic foods such as sour cream,

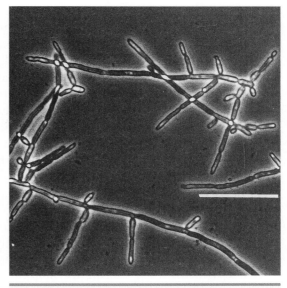

FIGURE 14.2

The Hypha

A phase-contrast photomicrograph of *Candida albicans* in its hyphal form. In the human body, phagocytes have a difficult time coping with these filamentous structures, a factor that may contribute to the pathogenicity of the fungus. (Bar = 40 μm.)

mi-co-rī z'al
Mycorrhizal fungi:
fungi living in a harmonious relationship with plant roots.
bi-fāz'ik

dī -mor'fik

Lime:
calcium carbonate.

MicroFocus 14.2

BIG AS THE BLUE WHALE

The most obvious thing to call it is a "humongous fungus," for indeed, it is gigantic. The fungus weighs over 100 tons, occupies 37 acres of forest ground, and is about 1500 years old. Located in the Upper Peninsula of Michigan, it was found in 1992 by James B. Anderson, Myron Smith, and their colleagues from the University of Toronto.

The enormous underground fungus is called *Armillaria bulbosa*. It consists of colossal numbers of hyphae that intertwine to unimagined lengths and push their fruiting bodies up to the surface as edible mushrooms. To prove their case that the massive structure is a single fungus, Anderson and Smith gathered 20 samples of the fungus and performed DNA analyses on 16 fragments from each sample. The genetic material was identical in every specimen.

Can the behemoth stand with the redwood trees and other domineering giants of our times? Possibly so. But then again, is a field of grass with all its blades coming from a single root system a single organism? It depends on how you interpret the rules. Nevertheless, it is becoming clear that a fungus is certainly not a lesser organism in the scheme of things—certainly not in terms of size.

applesauce, citrus fruits, yogurt, and most vegetables. Moreover, the acidity in breads and cheese encourages fungal growth. Blue cheese, for example, consists of milk curds in which the mold *Penicillium roqueforti* is growing.

Fungi are aerobic organisms, with the notable exception of the fermentation facultative yeasts that multiply in the presence or absence of oxygen. Normally, a high concentration of sugar is conducive to growth, and laboratory media for fungi usually contain extra glucose in addition to an acidic environment. Examples of such media are **Sabouraud dextrose agar** and **potato dextrose agar**. It should be noted that the nature of the medium may influence the appearance of the fungus, as FIGURE 14.3 shows.

sab'oo-rō

REPRODUCTION IN FUNGI

Reproduction in fungi may take place by **asexual processes** as well as by a sexual process. The principal structure of asexual reproduction is the **fruiting body**. In the asexual process, hyphae usually contain thousands of **spores**, all resulting from the mitotic divisions of a single cell and all genetically identical. Each spore has the capability of germinating to reproduce a new hypha that will become a mycelium (FIGURE 14.4).

Certain asexual spores develop within a sac called a **sporangium**. Appropriately, these spores are called **sporangiospores**. Other spores develop on supportive structures called **conidiophores**. These spores are known as **conidia** (sing., conidium), from the Greek *conidios*, meaning "dust." The bread mold *Rhizopus* produces sporangiospores, while the blue-green mold *Penicillium* produces conidia. Fungal spores are extremely light and are blown about in huge numbers by wind currents. Many people have an allergic reaction when they inhale spores, and local radio stations may report the daily mold spore count to alert sufferers.

Conidia:
unprotected asexually produced fungal spores formed on a supportive structure.

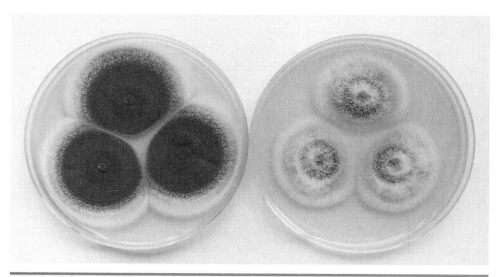

FIGURE 14.3

Variations in a Mold

The mold *Metarrhizium* growing on two different types of fungal medium and displaying two different growth patterns. In microbiology, the nature of the growth environment often influences the appearance of the microorganism.

Some asexual modes of reproduction do not involve a spore-containing structure. For example, spores may form by fragmentation of the hypha. This process yields **arthrospores**, from the Greek *arthro-* for "joint." The fungi that cause athlete's foot multiply in this manner. Another asexual process is called **budding**. In budding, the cell becomes swollen at one edge, and a new cell called a **blastospore**, or **bud**, develops from the parent cell and breaks free to live independently. Yeasts multiply in this way. **Chlamydospores** and **oidia** are other forms of asexual spores. Chlamydospores are thick-walled spores formed along the margin of the hypha, while oidia develop at the tip of the hypha. FIGURE 14.5 shows the asexual spores of *Aspergillus niger*.

Many fungi also produce spores by a **sexual process** of reproduction. In this process, the cells of opposite mating types of fungi come together and fuse. A fusion of nuclei follows, and the mixing of chromosomes temporarily forms a double set of chromosomes, a condition known as **diploid** (from the Greek *diploos*, meaning "twofold"). Eventually the chromosome number is halved, and the cell returns to having a single set of chromosomes, the so-called **haploid** condition (from the Greek *haploos* for "single"). Spores develop

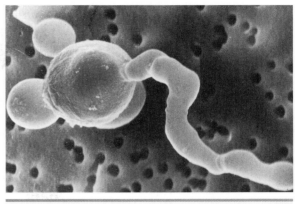

FIGURE 14.4

A Germinating Spore

A scanning electron micrograph of a spore of the fungus *Cephalosporium* germinating to form a hypha (×6000). Note the septa between cells of the hypha.

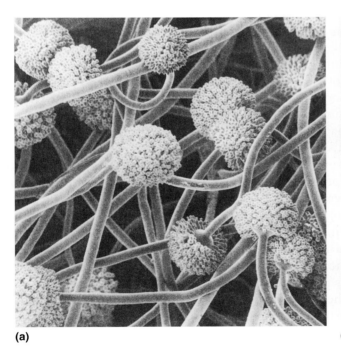

(a)

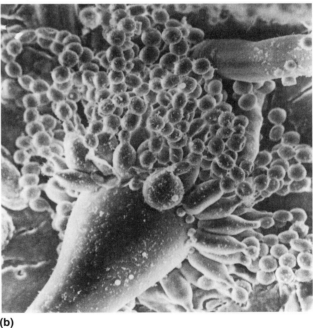

(b)

FIGURE 14.5

The Fungus *Aspergillus niger*

(a) A scanning electron micrograph showing the moldlike phase of *Aspergillus niger* (×600). Many conidiophores are present within the mycelium. Conidiophores contain conidia, the unprotected spores of certain fungi. This photograph demonstrates the three–dimensional image possible with the scanning electron microscope. (b) A close-up view of one conidiophore with a mass of conidia (×4000).

from cells in the haploid condition. A visible **fruiting body** often results during sexual reproduction, and it is the location of the spores. A mushroom is a fruiting body.

Sexual reproduction is advantageous because it provides an opportunity for the **evolution** of new genetic forms better adapted to the environment than the parent forms. For example, a fungus may become resistant to fungicides as a result of chromosomal changes during sexual reproduction. Separate mycelia of the same fungus may be involved in sexual reproduction, or the process may take place between separate hyphae of the same mycelium.

14.2

The Classification of Fungi

The classification of fungi is currently in a state of flux, owing in part to new biochemical analyses and DNA studies. Originally, fungi were considered part of the plant kingdom (they are still discussed in many botany courses). Then in 1968, they received their own kingdom status with Whittaker's classification scheme. Currently, they are still considered a kingdom, but under the domain Eukarya in Woese's three-domain system. Therefore, we continue to speak of the kingdom Fungi. Within the kingdom, the subcategories have traditionally been called divisions, as they are in botany. However, mycologists are gradually accepting the term *phylum* (pl., phyla) to further distance the fungi from the plants. In this time of transition, we shall retain the traditional term, division, while incorporating the newer term, phylum, in parentheses.

The fungi we discuss in this chapter are classified in three divisions (phyla) in the kingdom Fungi, and we shall examine them momentarily. However, other organisms are erroneously called fungi, and they merit brief attention. For example, biologists place in the kingdom Protista a series of organisms called **water molds** (Oomycota). Water molds have coenocytic hyphae, but their cell walls are composed predominantly of cellulose (versus chitin in true fungi); also, the diploid condition prevails in most species (versus haploid in true fungi); and finally, flagellated zoospores occur in the life cycle (no true fungi produce motile cells).

Most water molds are important saprobic decomposers in freshwater ecosystems. Some species, however, are parasitic, such as those that infect fish in aquaria. Also included in the parasite group are the organisms that cause downy mildew in grapes, white rust disease in cabbages, and the infamous late blight in potatoes. The effects of this disease, caused by *Phytophthora infestans*, are discussed in the chapter opening.

The kingdom Protista also includes the **plasmodial slime molds** (Myxomycota) and the **cellular slime molds** (Acrasiomycota). Although these organisms resemble amoebas and slugs, they produce a type of highly resistant spore during their life cycle. These spores are the basis for the "mold" connotation in the term slime mold. Another marginal group of fungi are the **chytrids**. These organisms are discussed in *MicroFocus 14.3*.

Within the kingdom Fungi, mycologists recognize three divisions (phyla) based on the format of sexual reproduction, and they delineate one division (phylum) where sexual stages have not yet been identified for the members. Generally, fungal distinctions are made on the basis of structural differences or physiological or biochemical patterns. However, DNA analyses are becoming an important tool for drawing relationships among various fungi. Indeed, the first-place winner of the

woes

fi'lum

o-o-my-ko'tah

zoo'o-spores

fi-tof'tho-rah in-fes'tans
mix'o-my-ko'tah
a-cras'i-o-my-ko'tah

kitch'rids

MicroFocus 14.3

THE DAY THE FROGS DIED

As taxonomists continue to sort out the differences between fungi, protists, and other eukaryotes, one group of organisms stand out for special consideration. They are the chytrids (kitch-rids), a group of aquatic fungi that produce flagellated spores. Normally, the presence of flagellated cells would exclude an organism from the kingdom Fungi, but molecular systematists have discovered that chytrids have cell walls of chitin and coenocytic hyphae, as well as proteins and nucleic acids more like the fungi than any other group. (In some taxonomic schemes, the name [phylum] Chytridiomycota has been established for these organisms.)

And now the zoological world is also turning to study the chytrid fungi. Researchers in Queensland, Australia, have reported the deaths of tens of thousands of frogs from lethal infection with a parasitic chytrid fungus. Massive die-offs occurred in nineteen species of frogs. Already, four species of frogs have become extinct, and scientists fear that other species may succumb as well. Once filled with frog song, the forests are now quiet. "They're just gone," said one researcher.

The fungus is apparently able to move long distances. In Australia, for example, it leapt across the 6000-kilometer-wide Nullarbor Desert and infected frogs in western Australia. It also crossed the oceans to cause a catastrophic disappearance of frogs in Panama and Costa Rica. (Researchers considered the horrible scenario of a fungus traveling on their boots.) And it made headlines in 1998 when it turned up wild in Arizona. To many epidemiologists, it was like watching the first cases of cholera and knowing it would turn up again. The question was, and continues to be: Where? And when?

1993 Westinghouse Science Talent Search was an Illinois student, named Elizabeth M. Pine, who showed that two structurally related mushrooms should probably be reclassified on the basis of their DNA content. We shall briefly examine each of the four groups next.

ZYGOMYCOTA

The first division (phylum) of fungi is **Zygomycota**, a group of zygomycetes that inhabit terrestrial environments. The zygomycetes have coenocytic hyphae, with septa where the reproductive cells are formed. During sexual reproduction, sexually opposite hyphae fuse, and a highly resistant **zygosporangium** forms at the site of fusion. This structure breaks down to yield one or more sexually produced spores, often referred to as **zygospores** (FIGURE 14.6). Elsewhere in the mycelium, thousands of asexually produced sporangiospores are being produced within sporangia. Both sexually produced and asexually produced spores are dispersed on wind currents.

zi′go-my-ko′tah
zi′go-my′cetes
Coenocytic: lacking cross-walls between adjacent cells.
zi′go-spor-an′ji-um
zi′go-spores

The well-known member of the Zygomycota is the common bread mold, ***Rhizopus stolonifer***. The hyphae of this fungus form a white or gray mycelium, with upright sporangiophores each bearing globular sporangia. Thousands of sporangiospores are formed in each sporangium. Occasional contamination of bread is compensated by the beneficial roles *Rhizopus* plays in industry. One species, for example, ferments rice to sake, the rice wine of Japan; another species is used in the production of cortisone, a drug that reduces inflammation in body tissues. These processes are explored further in Chapter 26.

ri-zo′pus

ASCOMYCOTA

Members of the **Ascomycota** are usually called ascomycetes. They are very diverse, varying from unicellular yeasts to powdery mildews, cottony molds, and large and

as′co-my-ko′tah
as′ko-mi-se′tēz

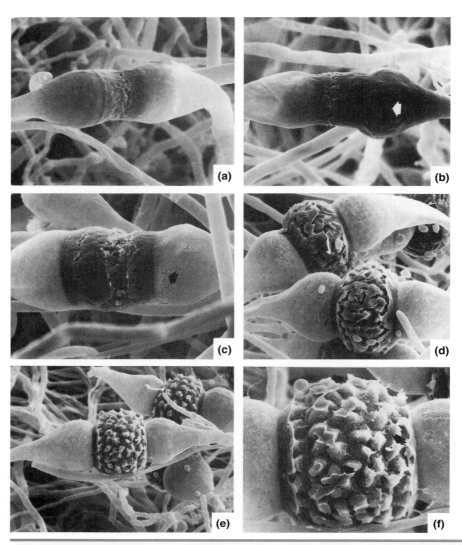

FIGURE 14.6

Reproduction in Fungi

A sequence of scanning electron micrographs showing zygosporangium formation in the mold *Rhizopus*. (a) Sexually opposite hyphae fuse and form a fusion septum. (b) Cells at the septum begin to swell and show early signs of a zygosporangium. (c) The outer primary wall begins to rupture. (d) The rupturing continues and (e) the zygosporangium is revealed. The zygosporangium continues to mature as the primary wall separates away. (f) A magnified view of the zygosporangium, showing its surface characteristics and the remnants of the primary wall. When the zygosporangium later breaks down, it will release sexually produced zygospores to propagate the fungus.

complex "cup fungi" (FIGURE 14.7). The latter form a **fruiting body**, a cup-shaped structure composed of hyphae tightly woven and packed together. The structure is called an **ascocarp**. The hyphae of an ascomycete are septate, with large pores allowing a continuous flow of cytoplasm.

Though their mycelia vary considerably, all ascomycetes form in the ascocarp a reproductive structure called an **ascus** during sexual reproduction. An ascus is a sac (ascomycetes are "sac fungi"), within which up to eight haploid **ascospores** form (FIGURE 14.8). Most of the ascomycetes also reproduce asexually by means of conidia, produced in chains at the end of a conidiophore.

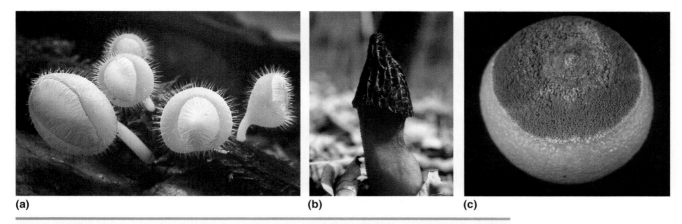

(a)   (b)   (c)

FIGURE 14.7

Three Common Ascomycetes

(a) The cup fungus *Cookeina tricholoma*, an ascomycete whose ascocarp resembles a cup. This fungus is often found on rotting wood. (b) The edible morel, an ascomycete prized for its delicate taste. (c) A *Penicillium* species growing on a piece of rotten citrus fruit. The waste products of this ascomycete contain the antibiotic penicillin.

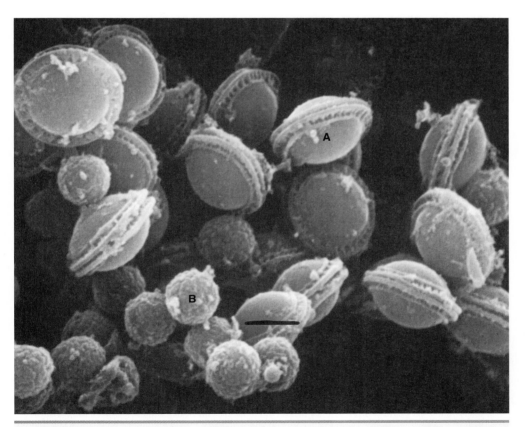

FIGURE 14.8

Two Types of Fungal Spores

Ascospores (A) and conidia (B) of the fungus *Aspergillus quadrilineatus*. This fungus was cultivated from the nasal sinuses of an ill patient who had recently received a bone marrow transplant. The sexually produced ascospores display a series of so-called equatorial crests at their midlines. The asexually produced conidia are rounder, with tightly folded ("rugous") surfaces. (Bar = 1 μm.)

sak'ah-ro-mi'sēz
as'per-jil'us

li'kens

cy'an-o-bac-ter'i-a

Certain members of the Ascomycetes are extremely beneficial. One example is the **yeast _Saccharomyces_**, used in brewing and baking (to be discussed shortly). Another example is **_Aspergillus_**, which produces such products as citric acid, soy sauce, and vinegar and is used in genetics research (**FIGURE 14.9**). A third is **_Penicillium_**, various species of which produce the antibiotic penicillin, as well as such cheeses as Roquefort and Camembert (Chapter 24). The edible morels and truffles are also classified in this group.

Ascomycetes are also the most frequent fungal partner in **lichens**. A lichen is a symbiotic association between a fungus and a photosynthetic organism such as a series of cyanobacteria or green algae or both. Most of the visible body of a lichen is the fungus. Its hyphae penetrate the cells of the photosynthetic partner and receive carbohydrate nutrients. The photosynthetic organism receives fluid from the water-husbanding fungus. Together, the organisms form a composite that readily grows in environments where neither organism could survive by itself (e.g., rock surfaces). Indeed, in some harsh environments, lichens support entire food chains. In the Arctic tundra, for example, reindeer graze on carpets of rein-

FIGURE 14.9

Normal and Mutant Fungi

Scanning electron micrographs of the conidiophores of _Aspergillus nidulans_. (a) The normal or "wild type" of the fungus is depicted. At the tip of the hypha, the conidiophore contains hundreds of asexually produced spores (conidia), any of which can germinate to reproduce the fungus. (b) A mutated form of _A. nidulans_. This organism was produced by mutating the regulatory genes of the fungus. As a result of the molecular manipulations, distinctive structural variations have occurred in the fungus, and the production of spores has been interrupted.

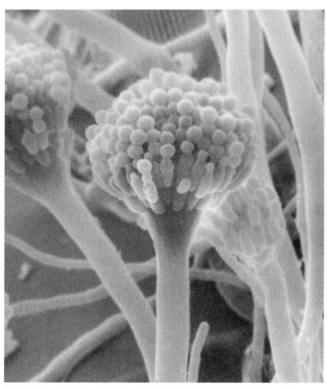

(a)

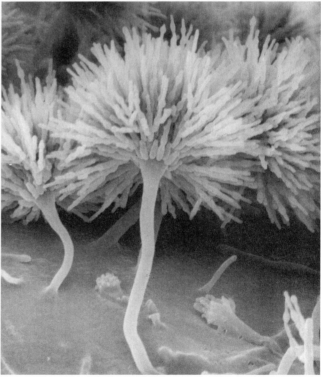

(b)

deer moss, actually a type of lichen. Lichens are often grouped by appearance into leafy lichens (foliose), shrubbery lichens (fruticose), and crusty lichens (crustose), as FIGURE 14.10 shows.

fo′li-ose
fru′ti-cose
crus′tose

On the deficit side, some ascomycetes attack valuable plants. For instance, one member of the group parasitizes crops and ornamental plants, causing powdery mildew. Another species has almost entirely eliminated the chestnut tree from the American landscape. Still another ascomycete is presently attacking elm trees in the United States (Dutch elm disease) and is threatening the extinction of this plant. Two other ascomycete pathogens are **Claviceps purpurea**, which causes ergot disease of rye plants, and **Aspergillus flavus**, which attacks a variety of foods and grains (Chapter 24).

klav′ĭ-seps pur-pur′e-a

BASIDIOMYCOTA

Members of the Basidiomycota, commonly known as basidiomycetes, are club fungi. They include the common mushroom (MicroFocus 14.4), as well as the shelf fungi, puffball, and other fleshy fungi, plus the parasitic rust and smut fungi. The name basidiomycete refers to the reproductive structure on which sexual spores are produced after hyphal fusion and meiosis have taken place. The structure, resembling a club, is called a **basidium** (pl., basidia), which is Latin for "small pedestal." Its sexually produced spores are known as **basidiospores**.

bah-sid′e-o-my-ko′tah
bah-sid′e-o-my′cetes

bah-sid′e-um

Perhaps the most familiar member of the class is the edible **mushroom.** Indeed, the Italian word *fungi* means "mushroom." Its mycelium forms below the ground, and after sexual fusion has taken place, the tightly compacted hyphae force their way to the surface and grow into a fruiting body called a **basidiocarp**, which is the

---

FIGURE 14.10

Lichens

(a) A cross section of a lichen, showing the upper and lower surfaces where tightly coiled fungal strands enclose photosynthetic algal cells. On the upper surface, a fruiting body, or ascocarp, has formed. Airborne clumps of algae and fungus called soredia are dispersed from the ascocarp to propagate the lichen. Loosely woven fungi at the center of the lichen permit the passage of nutrients, fluids, and gases. (b) A typical "crusty" lichen growing on the surface of a rock. Lichens are rugged organisms that can tolerate environments where there are few nutrients and extreme conditions. Their organic matter often forms the foundation of a local food chain.

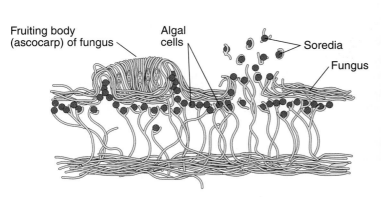

(a)

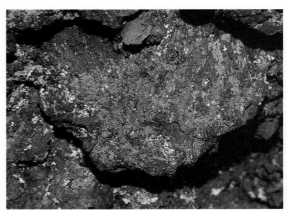

(b)

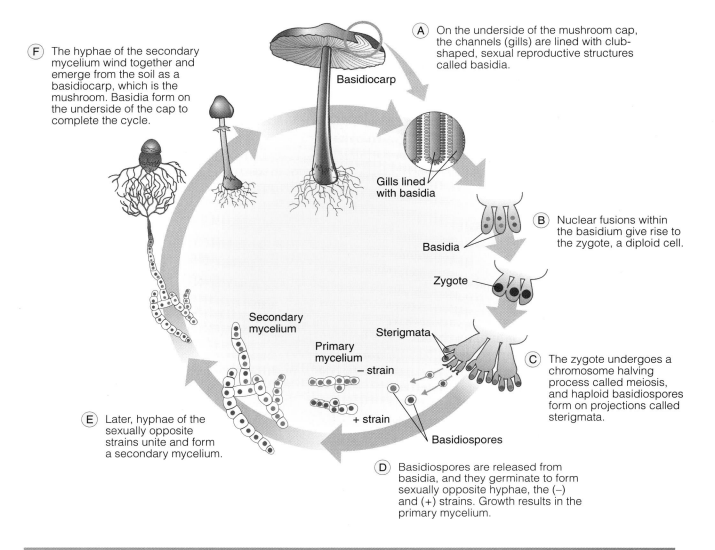

F The hyphae of the secondary mycelium wind together and emerge from the soil as a basidiocarp, which is the mushroom. Basidia form on the underside of the cap to complete the cycle.

Basidiocarp

A On the underside of the mushroom cap, the channels (gills) are lined with club-shaped, sexual reproductive structures called basidia.

Gills lined with basidia

Basidia

B Nuclear fusions within the basidium give rise to the zygote, a diploid cell.

Zygote

Secondary mycelium

Primary mycelium

Sterigmata

– strain

+ strain

Basidiospores

C The zygote undergoes a chromosome halving process called meiosis, and haploid basidiospores form on projections called sterigmata.

E Later, hyphae of the sexually opposite strains unite and form a secondary mycelium.

D Basidiospores are released from basidia, and they germinate to form sexually opposite hyphae, the (–) and (+) strains. Growth results in the primary mycelium.

FIGURE 14.11

The Life Cycle of a Typical Basidiomycete

a-gar′i-cus

am′ah-ni′tah

mushroom and its cap (FIGURE 14.11). Basidia develop on the underside of the cap along the gills, and each basidium may have up to eight basidiospores. Edible mushrooms belong to the genus *Agaricus*, but one of the most potent toxins known to science is produced by another species of a visually similar genus, *Amanita*. Sixteen outbreaks of mushroom poisoning, most related to this genus, were reported to the CDC in recent years, including the episode described in FIGURE 14.12. Another mushroom, the huge puffball, caused serious respiratory illness in eight people when the spores were inhaled in an incident in Wisconsin in 1994.

Agricultural losses due to the basidiomycetes of rust and smut diseases are considerable. **Rust diseases** are so named because of the orange-red color of the infected plant. The diseases strike wheat, oats, and rye, as well as trees used for lumber, such as white pines. Many rust fungi require alternate hosts to complete their life cycles, and local laws often prohibit the cultivation of certain crops near rust-

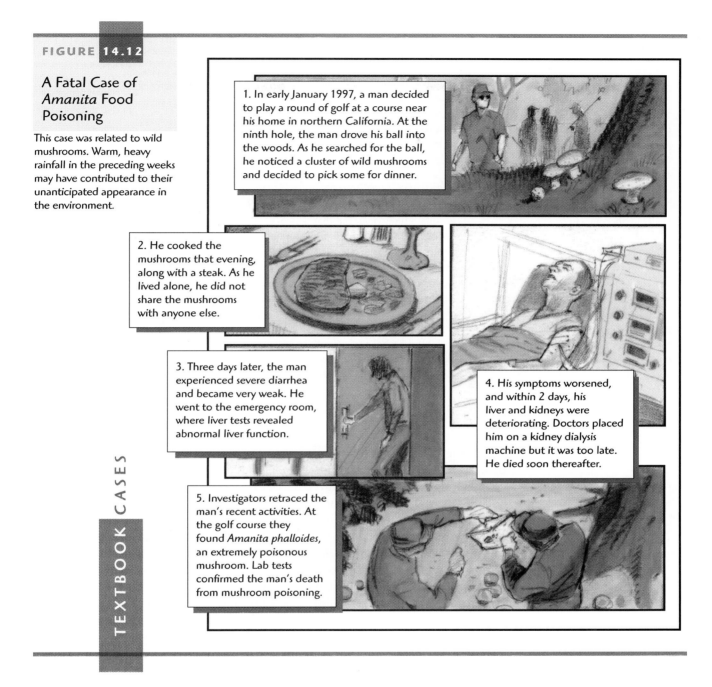

FIGURE 14.12

A Fatal Case of *Amanita* Food Poisoning

This case was related to wild mushrooms. Warm, heavy rainfall in the preceding weeks may have contributed to their unanticipated appearance in the environment.

TEXTBOOK CASES

1. In early January 1997, a man decided to play a round of golf at a course near his home in northern California. At the ninth hole, the man drove his ball into the woods. As he searched for the ball, he noticed a cluster of wild mushrooms and decided to pick some for dinner.

2. He cooked the mushrooms that evening, along with a steak. As he lived alone, he did not share the mushrooms with anyone else.

3. Three days later, the man experienced severe diarrhea and became very weak. He went to the emergency room, where liver tests revealed abnormal liver function.

4. His symptoms worsened, and within 2 days, his liver and kidneys were deteriorating. Doctors placed him on a kidney dialysis machine but it was too late. He died soon thereafter.

5. Investigators retraced the man's recent activities. At the golf course they found *Amanita phalloides*, an extremely poisonous mushroom. Lab tests confirmed the man's death from mushroom poisoning.

sensitive plants. For example, it may be illegal to raise gooseberries near white pine trees. **Smut diseases** give a black, sooty appearance to plants. They affect corn, blackberries, and a number of grains, and cause untold millions of dollars' worth of damage yearly.

DEUTEROMYCOTA

Certain fungi lack a known sexual cycle of reproduction and consequently are labeled with the botanical term "imperfect." These imperfect fungi are placed in the fourth division (phylum) **Deuteromycota**, where reproduction occurs only by an

doo'ter-o-my-ko'tah

MicroFocus 14.4

A GUIDE FOR THE MUSHROOM HUNTER

In ancient Rome, mushrooms were the food of the gods, and only the emperors were permitted to partake of their delights. Today, exotic mushrooms enjoy an equally high reputation among gourmets of the world. Some experts know how to spot them in the wild, but for amateurs, the key word is "caution," because in mushroom hunting, ignorance is disaster.

Mushrooms come in a huge variety of shapes, colors, and sizes. Among the interesting wild mushrooms are the Jack-O-Lantern fungus, known for its luminous gills; the Beefsteak fungus, whose cap resembles a piece of raw beef; and the Bird's Nest fungus, in which the fruiting body and its spores look like a bird's nest with eggs. On the debit side, about 100 of the 2000 known species can cause mushroom poisoning and death. High on the list of dangerous organisms are *Amanita verna*, the Destroying Angel, and *Amanita phalloides*, the Deathcap. Mortality rates of 50 percent have been observed in people who consume these mushrooms.

Botanists urge that mushrooms be hunted with a camera rather than a fork and plate. They point out that the colors and settings encourage prize-winning photography, and they urge that mushroom consumption be limited to those species cultivated for use as food. After all, they reason, birdwatchers do not eat birds, so why should mushroom-watchers eat mushrooms?

For those who insist on stalking wild mushrooms, mycologists recommend joining a society, reading extensively, and treading lightly into this hobby. As the sage writes:

There are old mushroom hunters,
And there are bold mushroom hunters,
But there are no old, bold mushroom hunters.

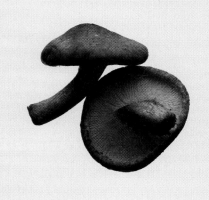

---

asexual method. It should be noted that a sexual cycle probably exists for these "deuteromycetes," but it has thus far eluded mycologists.

When the sexual cycle is discovered, the deuteromycete is reclassified into one of the other three divisions. A case in point is the fungus known as **Histoplasma capsulatum**. This fungus causes histoplasmosis, a disease of the human lungs and other internal organs. When the organism was found to produce ascospores, it was reclassified with the Ascomycetes and given the new name **Emmonsiella capsulata**. However, some traditions die slowly, and certain mycologists insisted on retaining the old name because it was familiar in clinical medicine. Thus, mycologists decided to use two names for the fungus: the new name, *Emmonsiella capsulata*, for the sexual stage; and the old name, *Histoplasma capsulatum*, for the asexual stage.

Many fungi pathogenic for humans are deuteromycetes. These fungi usually reproduce by budding or fragmentation, and segments of hyphae are commonly blown about by dust or deposited on environmental surfaces. For example, fragments of the athlete's foot fungus are sometimes left on towels and shower room floors. Nonpathogenic fungi are also classified here, as exemplified by species of *Pseudomassaria*. In 1999, this fungus was found to produce a compound that mimics insulin by assisting glucose passage into human cells; it could possibly be used by diabetics one day. (The compound has an advantage over insulin because it can be taken orally.) Recently discovered fungi are also placed in the Deuteromycota until more is known about them (MicroFocus 14.5).

The four divisons (phyla) of fungi are compared in TABLE 14.1.

doo'ter-o-mi'sēt

his'to-plaz'mah
cap-su-lat'um

ĕ'mon-si-el'ah

soo'do-mas-ar'i-ah

MicroFocus 14.5

NOT ALL FUNGI ARE BAD

In 1989, researchers at Johns Hopkins University discovered that taxol, a chemical derived from yew trees, could greatly reduce the size of tumors in women suffering from ovarian cancer. Two years later, in January 1993, the Food and Drug Administration approved taxol for ovarian cancer, while noting that the drug might be useful for breast, head, and neck tumors. Unfortunately, the exhilaration that accompanied approval of the new treatment was counterbalanced by the cost of the drug (about $1000 per treatment cycle) and the fear that the yew tree might be overfarmed to provide bark for the drug.

Then, in 1993, a new twist was added to the taxol story. In April, Montana researchers discovered growing within the bark of the yew a fungus that produces taxol on its own. Plant pathologist Gary Strobel and chemist Andrea Stierle, both from Montana State University, led the research. Under Strobel's intuitive direction, Stierle searched the Montana woods for local yews (*Taxus pacifica*) that would yield taxol. Finding one such yew, they went a step further and isolated a fungus from within the folds of the yew's bark. The fungus continued to produce taxol even after removal from its host

plant. They named the fungus *Taxomyces andreanae* (Andrea's taxus-fungus). Although *T. andreanae*'s yield of taxol is low, the potential for increasing the yield is great. For example, enormous fermentation tanks can be used to produce enormous amounts of the fungus and much larger amounts of the drug. Moreover, genetic engineering techniques can be used to pinpoint and clone the taxol

genes, then transfer them to high-yield vector organisms such as bacteria. Apparently the drug companies believe that these and other approaches can work. Months before their scientific paper appeared in print, the Montana researchers had secured a patent on the fungal production of taxol and were being courted by numerous drug companies. The fungus' future appears bright.

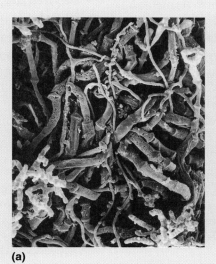

(a)

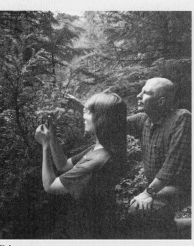

(b)

■ (a) The fungus *Taxomyces andreanae showing its hyphal strands and fruiting bodies with spores (×2300). (b) Strobel and Stierle with the yews from which the fungus was obtained.*

TABLE 14.1

Comparisons of the Divisions (Phyla) of Fungi

DIVISION (PHYLUM)	COMMON NAME	CROSS WALLS (SEPTA)	SEXUAL STRUCTURE	SEXUAL SPORE	ASEXUAL SPORE	REPRESENTATIVES
Zygomycota	Zygomycetes	No	Zygosporangium	Zygospore	Sporangiospore	*Rhizopus*
Ascomycota	Ascomycetes, sac fungi	Yes	Ascus	Ascospore	Conidia	*Saccharomyces Aspergillus Penicillium*
Basidiomycota	Basidiomycetes, club fungi	Yes	Basidium	Basidiospore	Conidia fragments	*Agaricus Amanita*
Deuteromycota	Deuteromycetes, imperfect fungi	Yes	Unknown	Unknown	Conidia fragments	*Candida Trichophyton*

14.3

The Yeasts

The word *yeast* refers to a large variety of unicellular fungi (as well as the single-cell stage of any fungus). Included in the group are nonspore-forming yeasts of the Deuteromycota, as well as certain yeasts that form basidiospores or ascospores and thus belong to the Basidiomycota or Ascomycota. The yeasts we shall consider here are the species of *Saccharomyces* used extensively in brewing, baking, and as a food supplement. Pathogenic yeasts will be discussed shortly.

Saccharomyces literally means "sugar-fungus," a reference to the ability of the organism to ferment sugars. The most commonly used species of *Saccharomyces* are **S. cerevisiae** and **S. ellipsoideus**, the former used for bread baking and alcohol production, the latter for alcohol production. Yeast cells are about 8 μm long and about 5 μm in diameter. They reproduce chiefly by budding (**FIGURE 14.13**), but a sexual cycle also exists in which cells fuse and form an enlarged cell (an ascus) containing smaller cells (ascospores). The organism is therefore an ascomycete.

The cytoplasm of *Saccharomyces* is rich in B vitamins, a factor that makes yeast tablets valuable **nutritional supplements**. One pharmaceutical company adds iron to the yeast and markets its product as Ironized Yeast, recommended for people with iron-poor blood.

The **baking** industry relies heavily upon *S. cerevisiae* to supply the texture in breads. Flour, sugar, and other ingredients are mixed with yeast, and the dough is set aside to rise. During this time, the yeasts break down glucose and other carbohydrates, and produce carbon dioxide through the chemistry of glycolysis and the Krebs cycle (Chapter 5). The carbon dioxide expands the dough, causing it to rise. Protein-digesting enzymes, also from the yeast, partially digest the gluten protein of the flour to give bread its spongy texture (**MicroFocus 14.6**). To make bagels, the

sak'ah-ro-mi'sēz

ser'e-vis'e-a
e-lip-soid'e-us

Budding:
an asexual reproductive process in which new cells form at the periphery of parent cells.

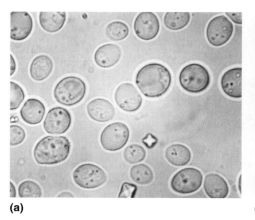
(a)

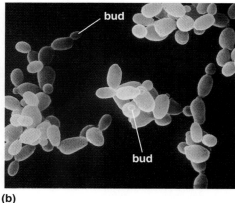
(b)

FIGURE 14.13

Yeasts

Two views of *Saccharomyces*, the common baking and brewing yeast. (a) A photomicrograph of yeast cells used in beer fermentation (×1000). (b) A colored scanning electron micrograph of *Saccharomyces cerevisiae*. Several cells are budding.

MicroFocus 14.6

THE DRIER THE BETTER

Need a quick microbiology laboratory? Simply go to the grocery store and purchase a package of "active dry yeast." Open the package, pour the contents into a bit of warm water, and you're on your way—instant microorganisms. You can study the yeasts with the microscope, investigate their physiology, and if you're really with it, rearrange their genes. All this from a package.

It wasn't always that way, though. Scientists could never figure out how to keep yeasts alive and in a dry state at the same time. If someone wanted to make bread, they had to get a starter from the "mother" dough where the yeast was growing; if the objective was wine fermentation, a trip to the culture supply or the old wine was necessary.

Then, during World War II, German prisoners were found in possession of a curious brown powder—it was the elusive dry yeast. They had the yeast for use as a nutritious food, or for bread when added to a bit of dough (or "Battlefield Red," if added to crushed grapes). Of course, the prisoners were not about to reveal the secret of the dried yeast, probably because they did not know what it was.

The postwar period was a different matter. In the euphoria of sharing, the Western world learned the secret of trehalose. Trehalose is a disaccharide, a simple two-molecule sugar. Added to yeast cells, it stabilizes the cell membrane, prevents cell damage due to drying, and keeps the yeast alive and active. Now everyone knew the answer, including an entrepreneur named Arthur Fleischmann—millionaire founder and owner of Fleischmann's Active Dry Yeast.

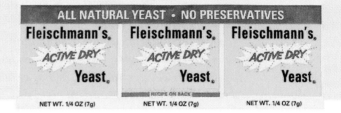

dough is boiled before baking; for sourdough bread, *Lactobacillus* species are added to give an acidic flavor to the bread; for rye bread, rye flour is substituted. In all these modifications, yeast remains an essential ingredient.

Yeasts are plentiful where there are orchards or fruits (the haze on an apple is a layer of yeasts). In natural alcohol **fermentations**, wild yeasts of various *Saccharomyces* species are crushed with the fruit; in controlled fermentations, *S. ellipsoideus* is added to the prepared fruit juice. Now the chemistry is identical with that in dough: The fruit juice bubbles profusely as carbon dioxide evolves through the reactions of glycolysis and the Krebs cycle. When the oxygen is depleted, the yeast metabolism shifts to fermentation, and the pyruvic acid from glycolysis changes to consumable ethyl alcohol (Chapter 5).

The products of yeast fermentation depend on the starting material. For example, when yeasts ferment barley grains, the product is **beer**; if grape juice is fermented, the product is **wine**. Sweet wines contain leftover sugar, but dry wines have little sugar. Sparkling wines such as champagne continue to ferment in thick bottles as yeast metabolism produces additional carbon dioxide. For **spirits** such as whiskey, rye, or scotch, some type of grain is fermented and the alcohol is distilled off. Liqueurs are made when yeasts ferment fruits such as oranges, cherries, or melons. Virtually anything that contains simple carbohydrates can be fermented by *Saccharomyces*. The huge share of the U.S. economy taken up by the wine and spirits industries is testament to the significance of the fermentation yeasts. A fuller discussion of fermentation processes is presented in Chapter 26.

Lactobacillus:
a genus of Gram-positive rods that ferment lactose to lactic acid.

Glycolysis:
the multistep enzyme process in which glucose *is* converted to pyruvic acid.

To this point . . .

We have discussed aspects of the structure, growth, and reproductive patterns in fungi. We began by exploring some details of the hypha and mycelium, and then we examined the temperature, pH, and oxygen requirements for growth. Most fungi grow at temperatures close to room temperature and under conditions that are acidic.

The discussion then turned to the two processes of reproduction that take place in the fungi. All fungi reproduce by an asexual process, and most species reproduce by a sexual process in which sexually opposite hyphae fuse to form sexual spores. Genetic variation is an advantage of such a process. The sexual cycle is also the basis for the classification of fungi into four divisions, also called phyla. Members of the Zygomycota form single free zygospores. In fungi of the Ascomycota, a sac forms containing up to eight ascospores. Members of the Basidiomycota form a clublike supportive structure, the basidium, on which basidiospores develop. Deuteromycota members have no known sexual cycle. The section closed with a discussion of the economically important baking and fermentation yeasts.

We shall now focus our attention on the fungal diseases of humans. Because these diseases generally do not occur in widespread epidemics, their names may be unfamiliar. However, some diseases may endanger human life, especially if the immune system has been compromised. For this reason, fungal diseases commonly occur as complications of other diseases, or in situations where a patient is undergoing treatment for an unrelated problem.

14.4

Fungal Diseases of Humans

In humans, the fungal diseases affect many body regions. For example, several diseases, including ringworm and athlete's foot, involve the skin areas, while others, such as cryptococcosis and histoplasmosis, occur in the lungs before spreading to other body areas. One disease, candidiasis, may take place in the oral cavity, intestinal tract, skin, vaginal tract, and other body locations depending on the conditions that stimulated its development. In a great many fungal diseases, a weakened immune system contributes substantially to the occurrence of the infection, as we shall often see in this section.

CRYPTOCOCCOSIS

krip'to-kok-o'sis

Cryptococcosis is among the most dangerous fungal diseases in humans. It affects the lungs and the meninges (the coverings of the brain and spinal cord) and is estimated to account for over 25 percent of all deaths from fungal disease.

krip'to-kok'us
nē-o-form'anz

Cryptococcosis is caused by a yeast known as ***Cryptococcus neoformans***. The organism is found in the soil of urban environments and grows actively in the droppings of pigeons, but not within the pigeon tissues. Cryptococci may become airborne with gusts of wind, and the organisms subsequently enter the respiratory

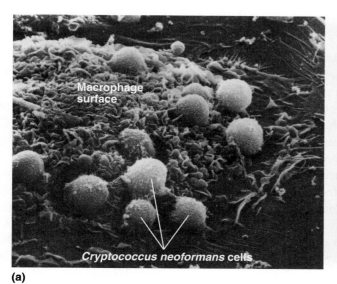

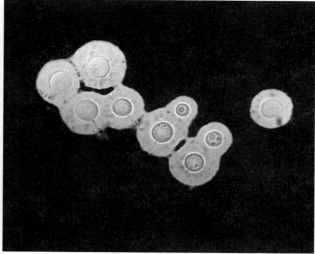

(a)   (b)

FIGURE 14.14

Cryptococcus neoformans

(a) A scanning electron micrograph of *Cryptococcus neoformans* clinging to the surface of a human macrophage (a type of phagocytic white blood cell). Internalization of the fungal cells is retarded by the capsules they possess. In this view, the cells have been attached to the macrophage surface for a long 30 minutes, and still they have not been internalized. (b) A negatively stained photomicrograph of *Cryptococcus neoformans*. A distinct capsule surrounds each oval, yeastlike cell. This capsule provides resistance to phagocytosis and enhances the pathogenic tendency of the fungus.

passageways of humans. Air conditioner filters are hazardous because they trap large numbers of cryptococci.

Cryptococcus neoformans cells, having a diameter of about 5 to 6 μm, are embedded in a gelatinous capsule that provides resistance to phagocytosis (FIGURE 14.14). The cells penetrate to the air sacs of the lungs, but symptoms of infection are generally rare. However, if the cryptococci pass into the bloodstream and localize in the meninges and brain, the patient experiences piercing headaches, stiffness in the neck, and paralysis. Diagnosis is aided by the observation of encapsulated yeasts in respiratory secretions or cerebrospinal fluid (CSF) obtained by a spinal tap.

Untreated cryptococcosis may be fatal. However, intravenous treatment with the antifungal drug **amphotericin B** is usually successful, even in severe cases. Because this drug has toxic side effects such as kidney damage and anemia, the patient should be continually monitored.

Resistance to cryptococcosis appears to depend upon the proper functioning of a branch of the immune system governed by T-lymphocytes (or T-cells). When these cells are absent in sufficient quantities, the immune system becomes severely compromised, and cryptococci can invade the tissues as opportunists. In patients with **acquired immune deficiency syndrome (AIDS)**, one of the causes of death is cryptococcosis.

During the early 1980s, mycologists identified a sexual stage for *C. neoformans*. The stage is related to the smut fungi of the Basidiomycota and is called *Filobasidiella neoformans*.

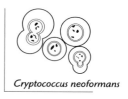

Cryptococcus neoformans

am′fo-ter′ĭ-sin

fi′lo-bah′sid-ē-el′ah

CANDIDIASIS

kan-di-di'ah-sis

Candida albicans is often present in the skin, mouth, vagina, and intestinal tract of healthy humans and other animals, where it lives without causing disease (FIGURE 14.15). The organism is a small yeast that forms filaments called pseudohyphae when cultivated in laboratory media. When immune system defenses are compromised, or when changes occur in the normal microbial population (i.e., the normal flora), *C. albicans* flourishes and causes numerous forms of **candidiasis**. (Older texts refer to the condition as **moniliasis** because the organism was once called *Monilia albicans*.)

One form of candidiasis occurs in the vagina and is often referred to as **vulvo-vaginitis**, or a **yeast infection**. Symptoms include itching sensations (pruritis), burning internal pain, and a white "cheesy" discharge. Reddening (erythema) and swelling of the vaginal tissues also occur. Diagnosis is performed by observing *C. albicans* in a sample of vaginal discharge or vaginal smear, and by cultivating the organisms on laboratory media. Treatment is usually successful with **nystatin** (Mycostatin) applied as a topical ointment or suppository. **Miconazole, clotrimazole**, and **ketoconazole** are useful alternatives.

nis'tah-tin
mǐ-kon'ah-zōl
kē'to-kon'ah-zōl

Vulvovaginitis is considered a sexually transmitted disease (but the disease is usually much milder in men than in women). Studies have shown that excessive antibiotic use may encourage loss of the rod-shaped lactobacilli that are normally present in the vaginal environment. Without lactobacilli as competitors, *C. albicans* flourishes. Other predisposing factors are the contraceptive intrauterine device (IUD), corticosteroid treatment, pregnancy, diabetes, and tight-fitting garments, which increase the local temperature and humidity.

Oral candidiasis is known as **thrush**. This disease is accompanied by small, white flecks that appear on the mucous membranes of the oral cavity and then grow together to form soft, crumbly, milklike curds. When scraped off, a red, inflamed base is revealed. Oral suspensions of gentian violet and nystatin ("swish and swallow") are effective for therapy. The disease is common in newborns, who acquire it during passage through the vagina (birth canal) of infected mothers. Children may also contract thrush from nursery utensils, toys, or the handles of shopping carts. Candidiasis may

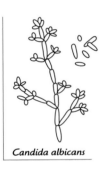

Candida albicans

FIGURE 14.15

The Agent of Candidiasis

A scanning electron micrograph of *Candida albicans* associated with the tissues of an animal. The oval structure of the cells and the tendency to form hyphae are apparent.

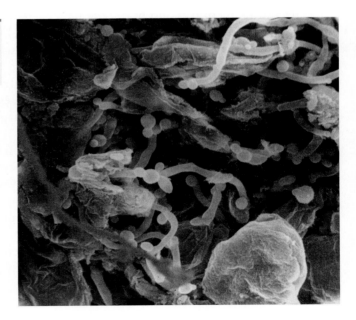

also be related to a suppressed immune system. Indeed, thrush may be an early sign of **AIDS** in a patient.

Candidiasis in the **intestinal tract** is closely tied to the use of antibiotics. Certain drugs destroy bacteria normally found here and allow *C. albicans* to flourish. In the 1950s, yogurt became popular as a way of replacing the bacteria. Today when intestinal surgery is anticipated, the physician often uses antifungal agents to curb *Candida* overgrowth. Moreover, people whose hands are in constant contact with water may develop a hardening, browning, and distortion of the fingernails called **onychia**, also caused by *C. albicans*.

o-nik'e-ah

DERMATOMYCOSIS

Dermatomycosis is a general name for a fungal disease of the hair, skin, and nails caused by a wide variety of fungi. The diseases are commonly known as **tinea infections**, from the Latin *tinea* for "worm," because in ancient times, worms were thought to be the cause. The tinea diseases include tinea pedis, **athlete's foot**; tinea capitis, **ringworm of the head**; tinea corporis, **ringworm of the body**; tinea cruris, ringworm of the groin, or "jock itch"; tinea unguium, ringworm of the nails; and tinea favosa, ringworm of the scalp, or **favus**.

der-mah'to-mi-ko'sis

The causes of dermatomycosis are a series of fungi called **dermatophytes**. One example is species of **Trichophyton**, an ascomycete whose sexual stage is named *Arthroderma*. Another example is certain species of **Microsporum**, also an ascomycete, whose sexual stage is named *Nannizzia*. A third cause is species of **Epidermophyton**, currently considered a deuteromycete.

tri-kof'ĭ-ton
ar'thro-derm'ah
na-niz'e-ah
ep'e-der-mof'ĭ-ton

Dermatomycosis is commonly accompanied by blisterlike lesions appearing on the skin, along the nail plate, or in the webs of the toes or fingers. Often a thin, fluid discharge exudes when the blisters are scratched or irritated. As the blisters dry, they leave a scaly ring (FIGURE 14.16). Centuries ago, people believed that worms inhabited the scaly ring, hence the name ringworm. The symptoms of dermatomycosis vary considerably and may include loss of hair, change of hair color, and local inflammatory reactions.

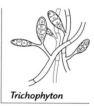

Trichophyton

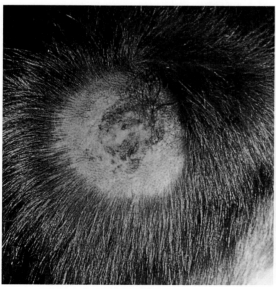

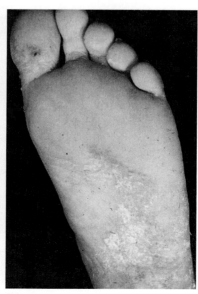

FIGURE 14.16

Two Views of Dermatomycosis

(a) Ringworm of the scalp, due to *Trichophyton mentagrophytes*. The lesions have crusted to form scaly blisters in this view. (b) Athlete's foot, caused by *Trichophyton rubrum*. The scaly blisters can be seen on the soles of the feet and in the webs between the toes.

(a)   (b)

The majority of dermatophytes grow readily on Sabouraud dextrose agar, and trained mycologists can usually diagnose the disease by observing the type of hypha and arthrospore present. Moreover, infected hairs and fungal cultures fluoresce in ultraviolet light. If protected from dryness, the dermatophytes live for weeks on wooden floors of shower rooms or on mats. People transmit the fungi by contact (FIGURE 14.17) and on towels, combs, hats, and numerous other types of fomites (inanimate objects). They also acquire the fungi by contact with **household pets**, because tinea diseases affect cats and dogs.

Treatment of dermatomycosis is often directed at changing the conditions of the skin environment. Commercial powders dry the diseased area, while ointments

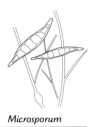

Microsporum

FIGURE 14.17

An Outbreak of Ringworm

This outbreak occurred among participants at an international wrestling meet. The incident happened in Schaumberg, Illinois, in 1992. It was believed to be one of the first epidemics of transmissible ringworm reported in the United States.

TEXTBOOK CASES

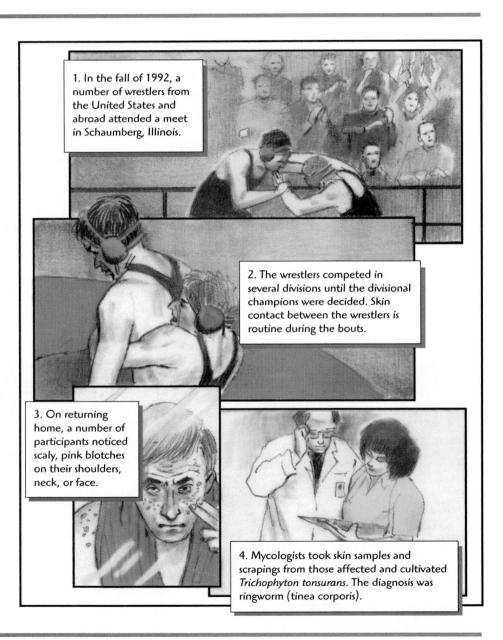

1. In the fall of 1992, a number of wrestlers from the United States and abroad attended a meet in Schaumberg, Illinois.

2. The wrestlers competed in several divisions until the divisional champions were decided. Skin contact between the wrestlers is routine during the bouts.

3. On returning home, a number of participants noticed scaly, pink blotches on their shoulders, neck, or face.

4. Mycologists took skin samples and scrapings from those affected and cultivated *Trichophyton tonsurans*. The diagnosis was ringworm (tinea corporis).

change the pH to make the area inhospitable for the organism. Certain acids such as undecylenic acid (Desenex) and mixtures of acetic acid and benzoic acid (Whitfield's ointment) are active against the fungi. Also, **tolnaftate** (Tinactin) and **miconazole** (Micatin) are useful as topical agents for infections not involving the nails and hair. **Griseofulvin**, administered orally, is a highly effective chemotherapeutic agent for severe dermatomycoses. This drug causes shriveling of the hyphae, possibly by interfering with nucleic acid synthesis. FIGURE 14.18 shows a case treated with **itraconazole**.

un'dec-ĕ-len'ik

tahl-naf'tate

gris'e-o-ful'vin

it'rah-kon'ah-zōl

HISTOPLASMOSIS

On January 4, 1988, a group of 17 students from an American university crawled into a cave in a national park in Costa Rica to observe the numerous bats whose droppings covered the floor. Within 3 weeks, 15 students developed fever, headache, cough, and severe chest pains. Twelve patients tested positive for *Histoplasma capsulatum*, and all were treated for histoplasmosis.

Histoplasmosis is a lung disease prevalent in the Ohio River valley and the Mississippi River valley. The causative agent is ***Histoplasma capsulatum***, an ascomycete whose sexual phase is named *Emmonsiella capsulata*. Infection usually occurs from the inhalation of spores in dry, dusty soil, and the disease is often called summer flu. Most people recover without treatment. However, a small percentage of people develop a disseminated form of histoplasmosis with tuberculosislike lesions of the lungs and other visceral organs. (The singer Bob Dylan suffered from lung and pericardial disease in 1997, as a result of histoplasmosis.) AIDS patients are vulnerable to this condition. Amphotericin B or ketoconazole may be used in treatment.

The fungus of histoplasmosis is often found in the air of **chicken coops** and **bat caves**. Although *Histoplasma* does not affect birds or bats, it grows in the droppings of these animals, as the outbreak in Costa Rica illustrates. Prolonged exposure to the

his'to-plaz-mo'sis
his'to-plaz'mah
cap-su-lat'um

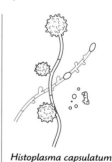

Histoplasma capsulatum

FIGURE 14.18

A Pathogen and the Disease

(a) A phase-contrast photomicrograph of *Microsporum racemosum*, an ascomycete and the cause of fungal disease of the nails. The long oval bodies are the conidia of the fungus (×389). (b) The nail of a 60-year-old female patient infected with *M. racemosum*. This incident began with a puncture wound by a fish bone. The fungus was identified by genetic analysis of its ribosomal RNA, and the disease was successfully resolved by treatment with itraconazole for 12 weeks.

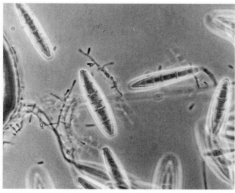

(a)

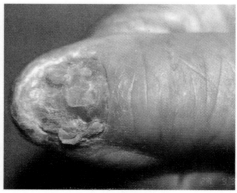

(b)

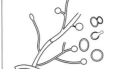

Blastomyces dermatitidis

ah'jĕ-lo-mi'sēz
derm'a-ti'ti-dis

air may therefore be hazardous. The disease is sometimes called **Darling's disease** after Samuel Darling, who described the cause in 1915.

BLASTOMYCOSIS

Blastomycosis occurs principally in Canada, the Great Lakes region, and areas of the United States from the Mississippi River to the Carolinas. The pathogen is ***Blastomyces dermatitidis***, an ascomycete whose sexual phase is named *Ajellomyces dermatitidis*. The fungus is dimorphic, appearing in the human as a yeast with a figure-8 appearance. Blastomycosis is also referred to as **Gilchrist's disease** for Thomas C. Gilchrist, the American dermatologist who first described it in 1896.

Blastomycosis is associated with dusty soil and **bird droppings**, particularly in and near barns and sheds. Entry to the body may occur through cuts and abrasions, and raised wartlike lesions are often observed on the face, hands, and legs. Inhalation leads to lung lesions with persistent cough and chest pains. Healing is generally spontaneous.

The progressive form of blastomycosis may involve many internal organs and may prove fatal. Amphotericin B used in therapy is thought to change the permeability of the fungal cell membrane and induce a leakage of cytoplasm.

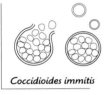

Coccidioides immitis

kok-sid'e-oi'do-mi-ko'sis
kok-sid'e-oi'dēz

COCCIDIOIDOMYCOSIS

Travelers to the San Joaquin Valley of California and dry regions of the southwestern United States may be exposed to a fungal disease known as **coccidioidomycosis**, or "valley fever." Its cause is ***Coccidioides immitis***, a protozoanlike fungus of the Deuteromycota. The organism produces arthrospores by a unique process of endospore and **spherule** formation, shown in FIGURE 14.19. When inhaled into the human lungs, *C. immitis* induces an influenzalike disease, with a dry, hacking cough, chest pains, and high fever. During most of the 1980s, about 450 annual cases of coccidioidomycosis were reported to the CDC. In 1991, however, that number jumped to over 1200 cases, and in 1992, the number of reports exceeded 4500, mostly from southern California.

Coccidioidomycosis is usually transmitted by dust particles laden with fungal spores. Cattle, sheep, and other animals deposit the spores in soil, and they become airborne with gusts of wind. Indeed, cases have been traced to standing on a railroad platform in the southwestern United States "to get a breath of fresh air." Many cases are self-limiting, but others are progressive and involve myriad internal organs and structures, including the meninges of the spinal cord. Spherules can be located in the sputum and biopsied

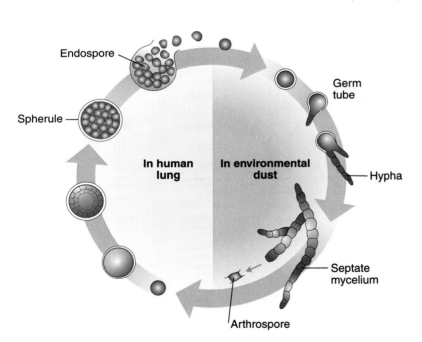

Endospore

Spherule

In human lung   **In environmental dust**

Germ tube

Hypha

Septate mycelium

Arthrospore

FIGURE 14.19

The Developmental Cycle of *Coccidioides immitis*

Outside the body, the organism exists as a septate mycelium. It segments to form airborne arthrospores, which are inhaled. In the respiratory tract, the arthrospores swell to yield a large body, the spherule, that segments and breaks down to release endospores. When released to the environment, the endospores form germ tubes and then the mycelium.

tissue of patients. Amphotericin B is prescribed for severe cases; most cases, however, resolve without treatment.

OTHER FUNGAL DISEASES

A number of other fungal diseases deserve brief mention because they are important in certain parts of the United States, or they affect individuals in certain professions. Generally the diseases are mild, although complications may lead to serious tissue damage.

Aspergillosis is a unique disease because the fungus enters the body as conidia, then grows as a mycelium. Disease usually occurs in a compromised host or where an overwhelming number of conidia has entered the tissue. The most common cause is *Aspergillus fumigatus*, an ascomycete. Infection of the lung may yield a round ball of mycelium called an **aspergilloma**, requiring surgery for removal. Conidia in the earwax lead to a painful ear disease known as **otomycosis**. Disseminated *Aspergillus* causes blockage of blood vessels, inflammation of the inner lining of the heart, or clots in the heart vessels. Amphotericin B therapy is usually necessary. It should be noted that one species of *Aspergillus* is very helpful, as **MicroFocus 14.7** discusses.

A closely related fungus, *Aspergillus flavus*, produces toxic compounds called **aflatoxins**. The mold is found primarily in warm, humid climates, where it contaminates agricultural products such as peanuts, grains, cereals, sweet potatoes, corn, rice, and animal feed. Aflatoxins are deposited in these foods and ingested by humans where they are thought to be carcinogenic, especially in the liver. Contaminated meat and dairy products are also sources of the toxins. Fungal toxins are called **mycotoxins**.

Another fungus that produces a powerful toxin is *Claviceps purpurea*. This member of the Ascomycetes class grows as hyphae on kernels of rye, wheat, and barley. As hyphae penetrate the plant, the fungal cells gradually consume the substance of the grain, and the dense tissue hardens into a purple body called a **sclerotium**. A group of peptide derivatives called alkaloids are produced by the sclerotium and deposited in the grain as a substance called **ergot**. Products such as bread made from rye grain may cause ergot rye disease, or **ergotism** (**MicroFocus 14.8**). Symptoms may include numbness, hot and cold sensations, convulsions with epileptic-type seizures, and paralysis of

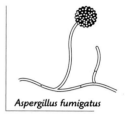
Aspergillus fumigatus

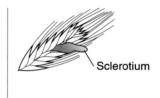
Sclerotium

clav′i-ceps pur-pur′e-a

skler-o′she-um

MicroFocus 14.7

"NOT WITHOUT MY BEANO!"

Some people would not dare sit down to a meal of corned beef and cabbage without a knife, fork, soda bread—and, of course, their Beano. Neither would they have Brussels sprouts with their steak, or broccoli with their fried chicken unless they were sure their Beano was nearby. Same for *pasta y fagiola* ("pasta fahzoole")—no Beano? No thanks!

To the scientist, there is really no mystery: Beano is the trade name for an enzyme preparation from the mold *Aspergillus niger*. The enzyme breaks down galactose, a disaccharide in beans,

cabbage, broccoli, Brussels sprouts, and other "strong vegetables" and high-fiber foods. Normally, galactose is broken down by the body's natural enzyme (alpha-galactosidase). But in the absence of the enzyme, bacteria in the large intestine will break down the galactose. Unfortunately, they do so at a heavy price: gas (flatulence), bloating, embarrassment—and an unwillingness to go back for seconds.

Enter Beano. All that's necessary is a couple of tablets or drops of liquid with the first bites of food (it tastes somewhat like soy sauce). Then the fungal enzyme

takes over and breaks down the galactose, leaving none for the bacteria. And leaving a happy memory of the meal—or so says the manufacturer.

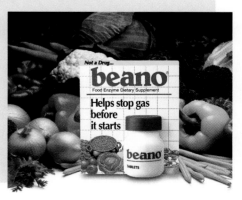

MicroFocus 14.8

A FUNGUS AND THE FRENCH REVOLUTION

In the early summer of 1789, a great wave of panic spread over France. Rumors circulated that brigands were everywhere, and many townsfolk fled to the woods to hide. Peasants stockpiled weapons, and soon turned their hostility on landowners, burning homes, and destroying records of their debts.

The incident came to be called the Great Fear (la Grand Peur). After it subsided, the rich remained apprehensive. They gradually realized that the peasants had enough power to seize property and commit acts of violence. The momentum for reform soon built to a fever pitch, and on the night of August 4, 1789, the French Assembly met and voted to abolish many ancient rights of the nobility. The French Revolution was under way.

Historians have often wondered what roused the peasants and precipitated the events of 1789. Essentially the fears were groundless: no more brigands than usual were about; and no evidence of a conspiracy existed among the peasants because the panic broke out in widely scattered communities, some separated by mountains. The episode seemed to be one of sheer wildness and not necessarily a manifestation of resentment. Nor

did the timing seem to fit any political, economic, or sociological pattern.

In 1984, Mary Kilbourne Matossian, from the University of Maryland, proposed a solution to the mystery of the Great Fear. She blamed the episode on ergot rye disease. Her studies of provincial records revealed a deterioration in public health in sections of France during mid-1789, and instances of nervous attacks and manic behavior. "Bad flour" was thought to be the cause, a factor that would tie in with the ergot rye theory. Another important clue had surfaced in 1974, when a historian reported that the rye crop of the late 1700s was "prodigiously" affected by ergot. He reported evidence of *Claviceps purpurea* in one-twelfth of all the rye. (By contrast, today if one three-hundredth of the rye is infected, it cannot be sold.)

But why would so many peasants eat bad bread in 1789? Apparently it was a bad year for rye, and the cold winter and wet spring contributed to widespread ergot disease. Coincidentally, the Great Fear broke out just after the rye harvest. Thus, the timing of the panic and behavior of the peasants appear to go hand-in-hand.

In retrospect, it is clear that the peasants resembled victims of ergot poisoning. Hallucinations are common and delirium often sets in. There are seizures, jaundice, numbness, and a belief that ants are crawling under the skin. Tremors, loss of speech, and a sense of suffocation occur. During the Middle Ages, the disease was called the "holy fire."

It would be simplistic to suggest that a fungus precipitated the French Revolution. Nevertheless, the evidence is substantial that ergot disease was a contributing cause. Certainly, the wild displays of the peasants must have been a terrifying sight to landowners. No doubt the fever pitch of the panic and the far-reaching consequences are better explained by the political and cultural climate of the times. Still, if the ergot disease had not happened. . . .

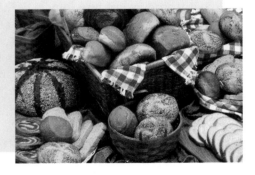

the nerve endings. Lysergic acid diethylamide (LSD) is a derivative of an alkaloid in ergot. Commercial derivatives of these alkaloids are used to cause contractions of the smooth muscles, such as to induce labor or relieve migraine headaches.

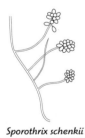

Sporothrix schenkii

Sporotrichosis is an occupational hazard of those who work with wood, wood products, or the soil. The disease can be contracted by handling sphagnum (peat) moss used to pack tree seedlings. It is also transmitted by punctures with rose thorns and is often referred to as **rose thorn disease**. The causative agent is ***Sporothrix schenkii*** (sometimes called *Sporotrichum schenkii*), which is a dimorphic fungus (FIGURE 14.20). Pus-filled purplish lesions form at the site of entry, and "knots" may be felt under the skin. Dissemination, though rare, may occur to the bloodstream, where blockages may cause swelling of the tissues (edema). In 1988, an outbreak of 84 cases of cutaneous sporotrichosis occurred in people who handled conifer seedlings packed with sphagnum moss from Pennsylvania (FIGURE 14.21). Cutaneous infections are controlled with potassium iodide, but systemic infections require amphotericin B therapy.

TABLE 14.2 summarizes the fungal diseases of humans.

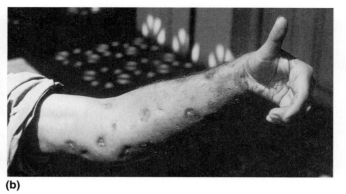

(a) **(b)**

FIGURE 14.20

Sporothrix schenkii

(a) A transmission electron micrograph of conidia of *Sporothrix schenkii* formed at the tip of a conidiophore. (Bar = 10 μm.) (b) A patient showing the lesions of sporotrichosis on an infected arm. Characteristic "knots" can be felt under the skin.

FIGURE **14.21**

An Outbreak of Sporotrichosis

In this outbreak, *Sporothrix schenkii* was isolated from the packing moss used at the Pennsylvania nursery, which supplied the trees and seedlings. Eighty-four cases of sporotrichosis in 15 states were identified in the outbreak.

TEXTBOOK CASES

1. In May 1988, a man visited an Illinois physician complaining of a swollen right hand and forearm. He had almond-sized "knots" under the skin of his right arm. The physician diagnosed sporotrichosis and placed the man on potassium iodide therapy.

2. On the next visit, the man brought along his neighbor, who had similar symptoms. Once again, the physician diagnosed sporotrichosis. The neighbor mentioned that the two men work together to raise and sell Christmas trees: to make a little money on the side.

3. In July, the physician examined a third patient. On questioning, the patient explained that he had recently participated in a sale of Colorado blue spruce seedlings to children. The source of the seedlings was the same Pennsylvania nursery that supplied Christmas tree seedlings to the first two men.

4. The physician reported his observations to the Illinois State Health Department. He learned that his patients were part of a growing list of cases of sporotrichosis being reported nationally. All the cases were related to fungus-contaminated moss used to pack trees and seedlings at the same nursery in Pennsylvania.

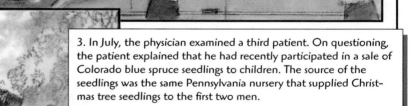

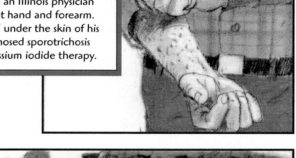

TABLE 14.2

A Summary of Fungal Diseases of Humans

ORGANISM	DIVISION (PHYLUM)	DISEASE	TRANSMISSION
Cryptococcus neoformans	Basidiomycota	Cryptococcosis	Airborne cells
Candida albicans	Deuteromycota	Candidiasis Vaginitis Thrush, onychia	Airborne Sexual contact Skin contact
Trichophyton species *Microsporum* species *Epidermophyton* species	Ascomycota Ascomycota Deuteromycota	Tinea pedis Tinea capitis Tinea corporis	Contact with hyphal fragments
Histoplasma capsulatum	Ascomycota	Histoplasmosis	Airborne spores
Blastomyces dermatitidis	Ascomycota	Blastomycosis	Airborne spores Open wound
Coccidioides immitis	Deuteromycota	Coccidioidomycosis	Airborne spores
Aspergillus fumigatus	Ascomycota	Aspergillosis Otomycosis	Airborne spores
Sporothrix schenkii	Deuteromycota	Sporotrichosis	Spores Puncture wound

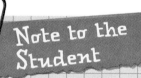

Note to the Student

During the 1980s, an epidemiologist at the University of Virginia initiated a study of infectious diseases acquired in the hospital, fully expecting most diseases to be caused by viruses and bacteria. To his surprise, almost 40 percent of the diseases were due to fungi.

The study was one of the first pieces of evidence pointing to an emerging threat of fungal disease. In most cases, an impaired immune system is involved—a system overwhelmed with human immunodeficiency virus, or a system depressed by cancer chemotherapy or antirejection drugs following a transplant. But there is also the problem of a meager arsenal of antifungal drugs, and the fungal pathogens are developing resistances to drugs of long-standing use. Moreover, clinical research in mycology has not kept up with that in clinical virology and bacteriology, in part due to the lack of established cultivation methods for fungal pathogens.

ORGAN AFFECTED	DIAGNOSIS	TREATMENT	COMMENT
Lungs Spinal cord Meninges	Examination of spinal fluid	Amphotericin B	Associated with pigeon droppings
Intestine Vagina Skin, mouth	Urine examination Vaginal smears Lab cultivation	Nystatin Miconazole Ketoconazole	Normally in human intestine
Skin	Lab cultivation Tissue examination	Undecylenic acid Griseofulvin Miconazole Itraconazole	Widely encountered skin diseases
Lungs Various organs	Lab cultivation Tissue examination	Amphotericin B	Associated with birds and bats
Lungs Various organs	Lab cultivation Tissue examination	Amphotericin B	Associated with bird droppings
Lungs	Lab cultivation Tissue examination	Amphotericin B	Common in southwestern U.S.
Lungs Ears	Lab cultivation Tissue examination	Amphotericin B	Hyphae grow in body
Skin Lymph vessels	Lab cultivation Tissue examination	Amphotericin B Potassium iodide	Associated with rotten wood

The list of fungal pathogens also appears to be expanding. In addition to the well-known pathogens (*Candida, Histoplasma, Cryptococcus,* and others), mycologists are proposing that up to 150 species of fungi may be pathogenic. *Aspergillus* species, for example, have increasingly been related to pneumonia; the plant pathogen *Fusarium* has been isolated from human blood disease; the mushroom *Coprinus* riddled a prosthetic heart valve in a recent case of endocarditis; and even the yeast *Saccharomyces* was found to cause infection in one person's burnt tissue.

At this writing, the CDC requests physicians to report 49 infectious diseases, but not one is of fungal origin. However, this policy may change in the years ahead because more and more fungi are being recognized for their pathogenic potential. Once considered a nuisance, fungi are now coming out of the shadows as serious threats to human health.

Summary

Fungi are a group of eukaryotic microorganisms distinguished from plants by their lack of chlorophyll, by differences in their cell walls, and by the fact that fungi are not truly multicellular. Moreover, fungi are heterotrophic (they utilize organic matter for food), while plants are autotrophic (they synthesize their own food).

Fungi generally consist of masses of intertwined filaments of cells called hyphae. Cross-walls separate the cells of hyphae in some fungal species but not in others. Reproductive structures generally occur at the tips of hyphae. Masses of asexually produced spores within or at the tip of the hypha provide the mechanisms for propagating the fungi. Spores can also be produced by a sexual mode, in which case the format of the reproductive process provides a basis for separating fungi into three divisions (phyla). In a fourth group, no sexual reproduction structure is formed, and reproduction occurs solely asexually. Most fungi grow best at room temperature and prefer conditions that are acidic.

Fungi are very diverse microorganisms capable of causing a broad variety of plant diseases. Many species have industrial significance as producers of valuable products. Yeasts, for example, are nonfilamentous fungi that ferment carbohydrates into alcohol; they also produce large amounts of carbon dioxide that encourages bread to rise, and they are useful vitamin supplements.

Among the many fungal diseases of humans are cryptococcosis and candidiasis. Both diseases often occur in immunosuppressed individuals, such as AIDS patients, and both are opportunistic diseases. Cryptococcosis affects the lungs and spinal cord, while candidiasis can occur in numerous organs such as the skin, intestines, vaginal tract, and oral cavity. Various antibiotics are available to alleviate the symptoms of these diseases.

Other important fungal diseases include ringworm infections of the skin, airborne lung diseases such as histoplasmosis and blastomycosis, and toxin-induced ergot disease of rye and other grains. A final disease, sporotrichosis, occurs on the skin and within blood vessels following a puncture wound.

Questions for Thought and Discussion

1. In the 1980s in a suburban community, a group of residents obtained a court order preventing another resident from feeding the flocks of pigeons that regularly visited the area. Microbiologically, was this action justified? Why?

2. A homemaker decides to make bread. She lets the dough rise overnight in a warm corner of the room. The next morning she notices a distinct beerlike aroma in the air. What is she smelling, and where did the aroma come from?

3. Fungi are extremely prevalent in the soil, yet we rarely contract fungal disease by consuming fruits and vegetables. Why do you think this is so?

4. In 1991, the U.S. Food and Drug Administration approved for over-the-counter sales a number of antifungal drugs such as clotrimazole and miconazole (Gyne-Lotrimin and Monistat, respectively). It thus became possible for a woman to diagnose and treat herself for a vaginal yeast infection. Should she do it?

5. Why is it a good idea to occasionally empty a package of yeast into the drain leading to a cesspool or a septic tank? Why are yeasts accused of having "metabolic schizophrenia"?

6. A woman has a continuing problem of ringworm, especially of the lower legs in the area around the shins. Questioning reveals that she has five very affectionate cats at home. Is there any connection between these facts?

7. A student of microbiology proposes a scheme to develop a strain of bacteria that could be used as a fungicide. Her idea is to collect the chitin-containing shells of lobsters and shrimp, grind them up, and add them to the soil. This, she suggests, will build up the level of chitin-digesting bacteria. The bacteria would then be isolated and used to kill fungi by digesting the chitin in fungal cell walls. Do you think her scheme will work? Why?

8. A certain restaurant advertises on its menu "Pizza con Funghi." Suppose you ordered this dish. What would you receive?

9. Mr. A and Mr. B live in an area of town where the soil is acidic. Oak trees are common, and azaleas and rhododendrons thrive in the soil. In the spring, Mr. A spreads lime on his lawn, but Mr. B prefers to save the money. Both use fertilizer, and both have magnificent lawns. Come June, however, Mr. B notices that mushrooms are popping up in his lawn and that brown spots are beginning to appear. By July, his lawn has virtually disappeared. What is happening in Mr. B's lawn, and what can Mr. B learn from Mr. A?

10. A mushroom walks into a bar and orders a beer. "Sorry," says the bartender, "we don't serve mushrooms." The mushroom thinks for a moment and replies, "But I'm a fun-guy." When you have recovered from this dreadful attempt at humor, you might like to try your hand at another "fun-guy" joke, or a "fun-gus" joke.

11. On June 27, 1995, a crew of five workers began a partial demolition of an abandoned city hall building in a Kentucky community. Three weeks later, all five required treatment for acute respiratory illness, and three were hospitalized. Cells obtained from the patients by lung biopsy revealed oval bodies. When the construction site was inspected, epidemiologists found an accumulation of bat droppings, and neighbors said they had seen bats in the area in recent weeks. From the information, can you surmise the nature of the disease in the demolition crew?

12. The baking or fermentation yeast *Saccharomyces* can be pronounced at least three ways: sa-kar´-o-myces, sak-a-ro-my´-ces, and sak-a-rom´-a-ces. Which pronunciation does your instructor prefer, and how do you suppose the three pronunciations evolved?

13. In 1992, residents of a New York community, unhappy about the smells from a nearby composting facility and concerned about the health hazard posed by such a facility, had the air at a local school tested for the presence of fungal spores. Investigators from the testing laboratory found abnormally high levels of *Aspergillus* spores on many inside building surfaces. Is there any connection between the high spore count and the composting facility? Is there any health hazard involved?

14. On January 17, 1994 a serious earthquake struck the Northridge section of Los Angeles County in California. From that date through March 15, 170 cases of coccidioidomycosis were identified in adjacent Ventura County. This number was almost four times the previous year's number of cases. Can you guess the connection between the two events?

15. In Arizona, during the 5-year period of 1990 to 1995, the incidence of cases of coccidioidomycosis increased 144 percent. How many reasons can you postulate for this extremely high increase?

http://microbiology.jbpub.com

The site features **eLearning**, an on-line review area that provides quizzes and other tools to help you study for your class. You can also follow useful links for in-depth information, read more MicroFocus stories, or just find out the latest microbiology news.

Review

The significance of the fungi is broad and diverse, as this chapter has demonstrated. To test your knowledge of the important fungi, match the statement on the left to the organism on the right by placing the correct letter in the available space. A letter may be used once, more than once, or not at all. Answers are listed in Appendix D.

_____ 1. Causes late blight of potatoes.

_____ 2. Produces a widely used antibiotic.

_____ 3. Converts carbohydrates to alcohol in beer.

_____ 4. Growth can be interrupted with griseofulvin.

_____ 5. Causes "valley fever" in the southwestern U.S.

_____ 6. Common white or gray bread mold.

_____ 7. Poisonous mushroom.

_____ 8. Sexual phase known as *Emmonsiella*.

_____ 9. Agent of rose thorn disease.

_____ 10. Edible mushroom.

_____ 11. Can overgrow the intestine when antibiotic consumed.

_____ 12. Known to cause Darling's disease.

_____ 13. A coenocytic mold.

_____ 14. Produces citric acid, soy sauce, and vinegar.

_____ 15. Associated with the droppings of pigeons.

_____ 16. Blue-green mold that has septa.

_____ 17. Agent of ergot disease in rye plants.

_____ 18. Cause of vaginal yeast infections in women.

_____ 19. Used to produce wine from grape juice.

_____ 20. One of the causes of athlete's foot.

_____ 21. Often found in chicken coops and bat caves.

_____ 22. Produces a toxic aflatoxin.

_____ 23. Agent of dermatomycosis.

_____ 24. Reproduction includes a spherule.

_____ 25. Nystatin and miconazole to inhibit.

A. *Amanita phalloides*

B. *Claviceps purpurea*

C. *Sporothrix schenkii*

D. *Blastomyces dermatitidis*

E. *Agaricus* species

F. *Mucor racemosus*

G. *Aspergillus* species

H. *Saccharomyces ellipsoideus*

I. *Phytophthora infestans*

J. *Myzeloblastanon krausi*

K. *Coccidioides immitis*

L. *Mucor mellitensis*

M. *Epidermophyton floccosum*

N. *Uncinocarpus reesii*

O. *Cryptococcus neoformans*

P. *Candida albicans*

Q. *Penicillium notatum*

R. *Acrotheca pedrosoi*

S. *Histoplasma capsulatum*

T. *Wangiella dermititidis*

U. *Rhizopus nigricans*

V. *Volutella graphii*

W. *Saccharomyces cerevisiae*

X. *Drechslera rostrata*

Y. *Streptothrix bovis*

Z. *Aspergillus flavus*

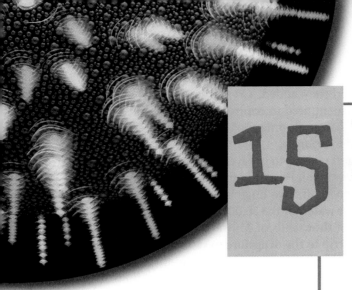

15 The Protozoa

It races through the bloodstream, hunkers down in the liver, then rampages through red blood cells before being sucked up by its flying, buzzing host to mate, mature, and ready itself for another wild ride through a two-legged motel.

—The editor of *Discover* magazine describing, in flowery terms, the life cycle of the protozoan that causes malaria

APRIL 12, 1993, SHOULD HAVE BEEN a festive day in Milwaukee, Wisconsin. The baseball home opener was scheduled, and fans were eager to see the Brewers play the California Angels. But the scoreboard contained an ominous message: "For your safety, no city of Milwaukee water is being used in any concession item." The city was in the throes of an epidemic, and a protozoan was to blame.

The protozoan was *Cryptosporidium coccidi*, an intestinal parasite that causes mild to serious diarrhea, especially in infants and the elderly. As the protozoa attach themselves to the intestinal lining, they mature, reproduce, and encourage the body to release large volumes of fluid. The infection is accompanied by abdominal cramps, extensive water loss, and in many cases, vomiting and fever.

krip′to-spor-id′e-um
kok-sid′e

Even as the first ball was being thrown out at the stadium, health inspectors were analyzing Milwaukee's water purification plants to see how a protozoan could have reached the city's water supply. *Cryptosporidium* is a waterborne parasite commonly found in the intestines of cows and other animals. Perhaps, they guessed, the heavy rain and spring thaw had washed the protozoan from farm pastures and barns into the Milwaukee River. The river might have brought *Cryptosporidium* into Lake Michigan from which the city drew its water. Indeed, the

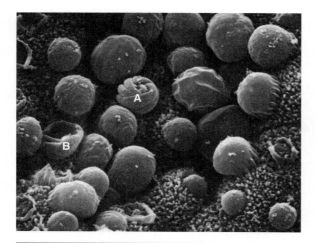

FIGURE 15.1

A Waterborne Protozoan

A scanning electron micrograph of *Cryptosporidium coccidi* at the surface of intestinal tissue. The parasites are globular saclike bodies 2 to 6 μm in diameter. Within the globes are numerous long, thin forms of the parasite called merozoites. After release from the globes, the merozoites will infect nearby cells. One parasite (A) has lost its membrane and the merozoites can be seen crowded together. The craterlike structures (B) are parasites from which the merozoites have already been released.

mouth of the river was very close to the intake pipe from the lake. Moreover, they added, *Cryptosporidium* can resist the chlorine treatment used to control bacteria in water; and the tests to detect bacterial contamination do not detect protozoa, such as *Cryptosporidium.*

As researchers worked to unravel the mystery, the game went on. Soda was available, but only from bottles. Drinking fountains were turned off. Two huge U.S. Army tanks stood by to provide reserve water for the 50,000 fans in attendance. And in the city, tens of thousands of Milwaukeeans made the mildly embarrassing trip to the drugstore to stock up on toilet paper and antidiarrheal medications. (A large window sign at a local Walgreen's proudly proclaimed: "We have Imodium A-D.") Back at the ballgame, things were not going much better—the Brewers lost to the Angels 12 to 5.

Cryptosporidium coccidi (**FIGURE 15.1**) will be one of the protozoa we study in this chapter. We shall encounter other protozoa that infect the human intestine, as well as several protozoa that live primarily in the blood and other organs of the body. Many of the diseases we encounter (for example, malaria) will have familiar names, but others, such as *Cryptosporidium* infections, are emerging diseases in our society (indeed, *Cryptosporidium* was not known to infect humans before 1976). Our study will begin with a focus on the characteristics of protozoa.

15.1 Characteristics of Protozoa

Protozoa are a group of about 30,000 species of single-celled organisms. They take their name from the Greek words *protos* and *zoon*, literally meaning "first animal." This name refers to the position many biologists formerly believed protozoa occupy in the evolution of living things. Though often studied by zoologists, protozoa also interest microbiologists because they are unicellular, have a microscopic size, and are involved in disease. The discipline of **parasitology** is generally concerned with the medically related protozoa and the multicellular parasites (Chapter 16).

Parasitology:
the discipline of biology concerned with pathogenic protozoa and multicellular parasites.

THE STRUCTURE OF PROTOZOA

Protozoa are among the largest organisms encountered in microbiology, some forms reaching the size of the period at the end of this sentence. With only a few exceptions, protozoa have no chlorophyll in their cytoplasm and thus cannot produce carbohydrates by photosynthesis. Although each protozoan is composed of a single cell, the functions of that cell bear a resemblance to the functions of multicellular animals rather than to those of an isolated cell from that animal.

Most protozoa are free-living and thrive where there is water. They may be located in damp soil and mud, in drainage ditches and puddles, and in ponds, rivers, and

Chlorophyll:
a green plant pigment essential to photosynthesis.

oceans. Some species of protozoa remain attached to aquatic plants or rocks, while other species swim about. The film of water on an ordinary dirt particle often contains protozoa. FIGURE 15.2 illustrates some of the diversity that exists within the protozoal groups.

Protozoal cells are surrounded only by a membrane. However, outside the membrane, some species of protozoa possess a rigid structure of protein called a **pellicle**. The cytoplasm contains eukaryotic features, each cell having a nucleus and nuclear membrane. In addition, freshwater protozoa continually take in water by the process of osmosis and eliminate it via organelles called **contractile vacuoles**. These vacuoles expand with water drawn from the cytoplasm and then appear to "contract" as they

Pellicle:
the thick, rigid structure outside the cell membrane of some protozoa.
Osmosis:
the movement of water through a membrane from a region of low concentration of a chemical substance to one of higher concentration.

FIGURE 15.2

Diversity Among Protozoa

The four groups are represented, with the organs of motion shown for members of each group.

I. Amoebas

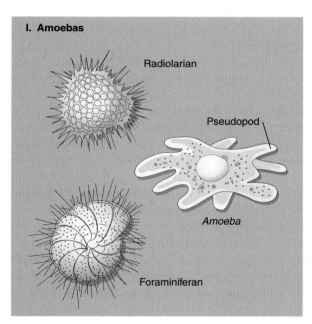

II. Flagellates

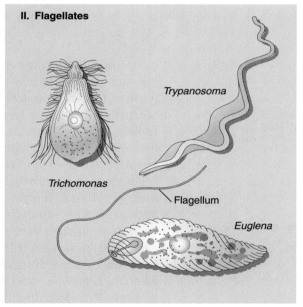

III. Ciliates

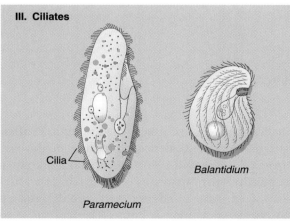

IV. Apicomplexans (Sporozoa)

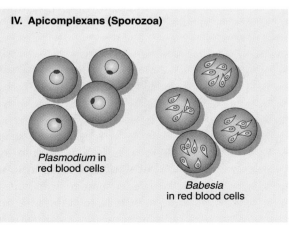

FIGURE 15.3

Feeding Behavior in Protozoa

This scanning electron photograph shows three amoebas attacking and devouring a fourth, presumably dead, amoeba. The amoebas are *Naegleria fowleri*, a cause of meningoencephalitis in humans. Each amoeba possesses a series of suckerlike structures that stick to the prey and serve as portals for ingestion. The researchers who first described the structures in 1984 recommend that they be called amoebastomes. (Bar = 10 μm.)

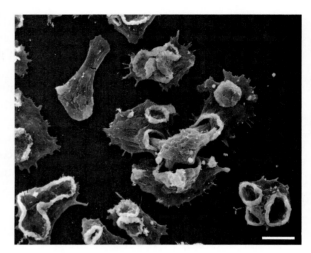

release water through a temporary opening in the cell membrane. Many protozoa also contain locomotor organelles, which permit independent motion.

THE GROWTH OF PROTOZOA

Protozoa obtain their nutrients by engulfing food particles by phagocytosis or through special organs of ingestion (FIGURE 15.3). A membrane then encloses the particles to form an organelle called a **food vacuole**. The vacuole joins with another organelle known as the **lysosome**, and digestive enzymes from the lysosome proceed to break down the particles. Nutrients are absorbed from the vacuole, and the remaining material is eliminated from the cell. Some protozoa have the ability to digest the cellulose in wood.

Nutrition in protozoa is primarily heterotrophic, since chlorophyll pigments are generally absent. Except for the parasitic organisms of disease and the species that feed on bacteria, protozoa are saprobic. Most protozoa are aerobic, obtaining their oxygen by diffusion through the cell membrane. The feeding form of a protozoan is commonly known as the **trophozoite** (*troph-* is the Greek stem for "food"). Another form, the **cyst**, is a dormant, highly resistant stage that develops in some protozoa when the organism secretes a thick case around itself during times of environmental stress. **Reproduction** in protozoa usually occurs by the asexual process of mitosis, although many protozoa also have a sexual stage.

Lysosome:
a vacuolelike cell organelle that contains digestive enzymes.

Saprobic:
living on dead organic matter.

trof'o-zo'ite

15.2

The Classification of Protozoa

When Robert Whittaker assigned protozoa to the **kingdom Protista** in 1969, he did so as a matter of convenience, rather than on the basis of evolutionary relationships. During the 1970s and 1980s, the kingdom's boundaries were extended to include some multicellular organisms (e.g., certain seaweeds), as well as some funguslike organisms (e.g., slime molds and water molds), and a potpourri of other organisms that needed a taxonomic home. The tendency was to

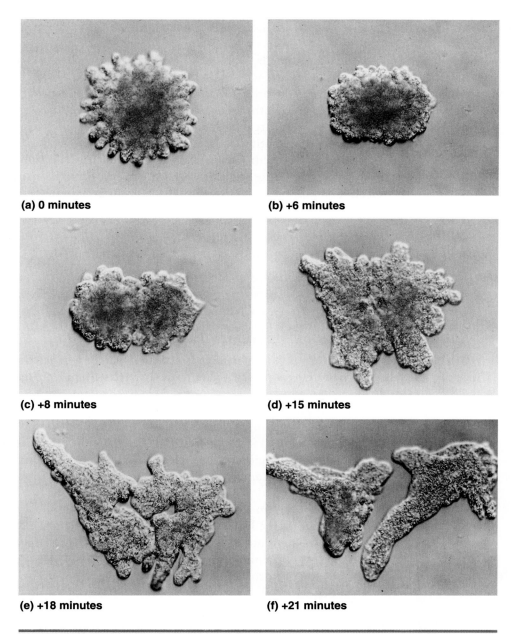

(a) 0 minutes

(b) +6 minutes

(c) +8 minutes

(d) +15 minutes

(e) +18 minutes

(f) +21 minutes

FIGURE 15.4

Binary Fission in *Amoeba proteus*

In this sequence of photomicrographs, the cytoplasm is seen separating to form two new individuals. Few visible changes are apparent for the first 15 minutes, but once cell division begins, separation takes place rapidly.

place in the Protista any eukaryotes that did not comfortably fit into the definitions of plants, fungi, or animals.

The kingdom Protista probably is a product of ignorance that reflects how many different types are related to one another. However, excellent new research in the area is shedding light on the taxonomic relationships, and in the years ahead, the kingdom Protista may be replaced by several new kingdoms. Molecular variations in ribosomal subunits, for example, are the basis for one new classification scheme, the three-domain system.

But that does not resolve the immediate problem of what to do with the protozoa. While the classification system is in a state of flux, we shall use type of motion as a criterion and discuss four groups of protozoa using the terms familiar to most students of biology: **amoebas** (protozoa that move by pseudopodia); **flagellates** (protozoa moving by flagella); **ciliates** (organisms with cilia); and **apicomplexans**, or **sporozoa** (protozoa exhibiting no motion in the adult form). This organization will give us considerable latitude when considering the protozoa of medical significance, while permitting us to introduce some protozoa of ecological and industrial importance. However, it should be remembered that the groupings are artificial, informal, and temporary.

AMOEBAS

sar'ko-di'nah

Pseudopodia:
temporary projections of an amoeba used for motion and phagocytosis.

Amoebas have been placed in the group **Sarcodina** (sarcodines) by many biologists and in the group **Rhizopoda** (rhizopods) by others. These organisms move as their cell contents flow into temporary formless projections called **pseudopodia** ("false-feet"). The amoeba is the classic example of the group, and thus the motion is called **amoeboid motion**. Pseudopodia also capture small algae and other protozoa in the process of phagocytosis. It is interesting to note that filaments of **actin** and **myosin**, the well-known proteins of muscle tissue, are associated with movement of the pseudopod.

An amoeba may be as large as 1 millimeter in diameter. It usually lives in freshwater and reproduces by binary fission, as shown in the sequence in FIGURE 15.4.

Amoebas may be found in home humidifiers, where they have been known to cause an allergic reaction called **humidifier fever**. Far more serious are the parasitic amoebas that cause amoebiasis and a form of encephalitis.

Two large groups of marine amoebas have ecological significance. The first group, the **radiolaria**, are abundant in the Indian and Pacific oceans. These amoebas have spherical shells with highly sculptured glassy skeletons, reminiscent of vintage Christmas ornaments. When the protozoa die, their skeletal remains litter the ocean floor with deposits called radiolarian ooze. The second group, the **foraminifera**, have chalky skeletons, often in the shape of snail shells with openings between sections (the name means "little window"). Foraminifera flourished during the Paleozoic era, about 225 million years ago. Their shells in ocean sediments therefore serve as depth markers for oil-drilling rigs and as estimates of the age of the rock. Geologic upthrust has brought the sediments to the surface in several places around the world, such as the White Cliffs of Dover (FIGURE 15.5).

Reports first published in 1987 indicated that amoebas in the genus *Acanthamoeba* (e.g., *A. castellani*) can cause corneal infection in people who wear contact lenses. They were reminded to adhere to recommended care and use procedures, and ophthalmologists and optometrists were advised to increase patient education. Recent research indicates that bacterial infection can be a cofactor in *Acanthamoeba* infection of the eye (FIGURE 15.6). Many cases are misdiagnosed as herpes simplex infections.

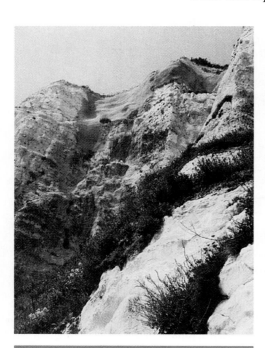

FIGURE 15.5

The White Cliffs of Dover, England

These cliffs are composed of the remains of foraminifera that thrived in the oceans millions of years ago.

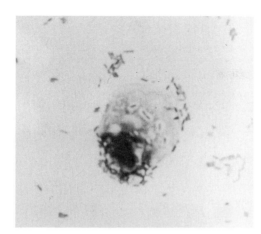

FIGURE 15.6

Acanthamoeba

A photomicrograph of an *Acanthamoeba* trophozoite in a field of bacteria of the genus *Xanthomonas*. Several bacteria are also contained within vesicles in the amoeba. It is postulated that contaminating bacteria in contact lens cleaning solutions support the growth of *Acanthamoeba* and thereby encourage it to multiply and adhere to the lens. Later, when the contact lens is inserted into the eye, the amoebas infect the cornea.

FLAGELLATES

Flagellates have traditionally been placed in the group **Mastigophora**. They often have the shape of a vase, and all move by means of one or more whiplike, undulating **flagella** (*mastig-* is Greek for "whip"). The flagellum can either push or pull the organism, depending on the species. Flagella occur singly, in pairs, or in large numbers. Each flagellum has the characteristic 9 + 2 arrangement of microtubules found in all eukaryotic flagella. Undulations sweep down the flagella to the tip, and the lashing motion forces water outward to provide locomotion. The movement resembles the activity of a fish sculling in water. (Flagella also occur in bacteria, but their structure, size, and type of movement differ.)

Almost half the known species of protozoa are flagellates. An example is the green flagellate *Euglena* often found in freshwater ponds. This organism is unique because it is one of the few genera of protozoa that contain chloroplasts with chlorophyll, and it is thus capable of photosynthesis. Some botanists claim it to be a plant, but zoologists point to its ability to move and suggest that it is more animal-like. Still other biologists point out that it may be the basic stock of evolution from which both animal and plant forms once arose.

Some species of flagellated protozoa are free-living, but most live together with plants or animals. Several species, for example, are found in the gut of the termite, where they participate in a symbiotic relationship. Other species are parasitic in humans and cause disease of the nervous, urogenital, or gastrointestinal systems. Still others include the dinoflagellates that cause the infamous **red tides**. Chapter 25 discusses these species in more detail. One dinoflagellate, *Pfiesteria piscicida*, has been linked to extensive fish kills in waters from Alabama to Delaware (**MicroFocus 15.1**).

CILIATES

Ciliates, which have been traditionally classified as **Ciliophora**, are among the most complex cells on Earth. They range in size from a microscopic 10 μm to a huge 3 mm (about the same relative difference between a football and a football field). All species are covered with hairlike **cilia** (sing., cilium) in longitudinal or spiral rows. The movement of the cilia is coordinated by a network of fibers running beneath the surface of the cell. Cilia beat in a synchronized pattern, much like a field of wheat bending in the breeze or the teeth on a comb bending if you pass your thumb across the row. The organized "rowing" action that results speeds the

mas'tĭ-gof'o-rah

Flagellum:
the whiplike organ of motion in certain species of protozoa.

Euglena:
a flagellated protozoan with plantlike properties.

Symbiotic relationship:
one in which two populations coexist.

sil'e-of'o-rah

MicroFocus 15.1

TOO SOON FOR A LABEL

In 1997, *Newsweek* magazine labeled it the "cell from hell." It was a protozoan known as *Pfiesteria piscicida* (fis-ter'er-i-ah pis-i-ci'dah), and apparently it was destroying the fish population along the southeastern coast of the United States. Silvery menhaden (a type of herring) were turning up with quarter-sized lesions on their bodies, and a *Pfiesteria*-hysteria was setting in. The seminal research had been done by scientists from North Carolina State University. Their research was pointing to one or more toxins produced by the protozoan. During August of that year, tens of thousands of fish died in a 4.5 mile stretch of Maryland's Pocomoke River.

But was the protozoan the real culprit? Possibly there were other organisms involved, said researchers from the Virginia Institute of Marine Sciences. They maintained that a fungal pathogen was infecting the fish, perhaps after the protozoal toxin had weakened them. Their research was based on the recovery of fungal threads from the lesions and the previous observations of fungi in the ulcers of menhaden. Another possibility was that the lesions were due to the fungus, but the massive fish kill was due to the protozoan. And this observation can be important because the lesions are used as a sign of *Pfiesteria* infection when public health officials consider closing waters to public use.

The answers are still waiting to be learned as the research continues with haste. For the time being, the more prudent course is to avoid labeling organisms with derogatory epithets until the scientists are sure. Darn sure.

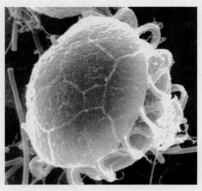

■ *Pfiesteria shumwayae, a member of the toxic* Pfiesteria *complex responsible for killing millions of fish.*

---

ciliate along in one direction. By contrast, flagellar motion tends to be jerky and much slower.

The complexity of ciliates is illustrated by the slipper-shaped ***Paramecium***. This organism has a primitive gullet, as well as a "mouth" into which food particles are swept, a single large macronucleus, and one or more micronuclei. During **sexual recombinations**, two cells make contact, and a cytoplasmic bridge forms between them. A micronucleus from each cell undergoes two divisions to form four micronuclei, of which one remains alive and undergoes division. Now a "swapping" of micronuclei takes place, followed by a union to re-form the normal micronucleus (**FIGURE 15.7**). This genetic recombination is somewhat analogous to what occurs in bacteria. It is observed during periods of environmental stress, a factor that suggests the formation of a genetically different and, perhaps, better adapted organism. Reproduction at other times is by mitotic cell division.

Another feature of *Paramecium* is the **kappa factors**. These nucleic acid particles are apparently responsible for the synthesis of toxins that destroy ciliates lacking the factors. *Paramecium* species also possess **trichocysts**, organelles that discharge filaments to trap prey. A third feature is the **contractile vacuole** used to "bail out" excess water from the cytoplasm. These organelles are present in freshwater ciliates but not in saltwater species because little excess water exists in the cells.

Ciliates have been the subject of biological investigation for many decades. They are readily found in almost any pond or gutter water; they have a variety of shapes; they exist in several colors, including light blue and pink; they exhibit elaborate and controlled behavior patterns; and they have simple nutritional requirements, which makes cultivation easy.

Micronucleus:
one of several smaller nuclei found in the cytoplasm of certain ciliates.

trik'o-sists

Contractile vacuole:
a clear, circular, cellular organelle used to remove water from the cytoplasm in certain protozoa.

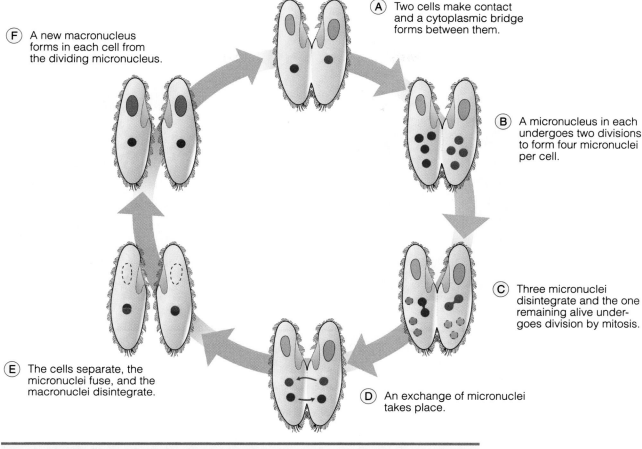

A new macronucleus forms in each cell from the dividing micronucleus.

(A) Two cells make contact and a cytoplasmic bridge forms between them.

(B) A micronucleus in each undergoes two divisions to form four micronuclei per cell.

(C) Three micronuclei disintegrate and the one remaining alive undergoes division by mitosis.

(D) An exchange of micronuclei takes place.

(E) The cells separate, the micronuclei fuse, and the macronuclei disintegrate.

(F) A new macronucleus forms in each cell from the dividing micronucleus.

FIGURE 15.7

Sexual Recombination in *Paramecium*

APICOMPLEXANS (SPOROZOA)

Apicomplexans are so named because one end of the cell (the apex) contains a *complex* of organelles used for penetrating host cells. The group name is **Apicomplexa**. Another name for the group is **Sporozoa**, because the organisms (sporozoa) were once believed to form spores. Another reason is because one stage in the life cycle is an infectious form known as the sporozoite.

a′pē-com-plex′ans

Apicomplexans (sporozoa) include a number of parasitic protozoa with complex life cycles that include alternating sexual and asexual reproductive phases. These life cycles include intermediary forms that resemble bacterial or fungal spores. However, the spores lack the resistance of other spores.

Protozoa in this group are notable for the absence of locomotor organelles in the adult form. Two species, the organisms of malaria and toxoplasmosis, are of special significance, the first because it is one of the most prolific killers of humans, the second because of its association with the disease AIDS. Other notable species include ***Isospora belli***, a cause of the human intestinal disease **coccidiosis**; ***Sarcocystis*** species, which live in the intestines as well as the muscle tissue of humans and animals; and ***Encephalitozoan*** species, which cause disseminated illness in AIDS patients (FIGURE 15.8).

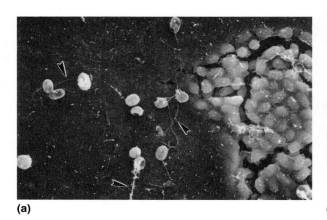

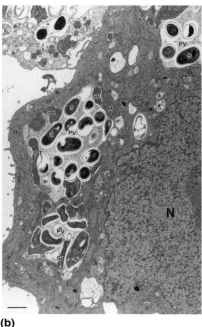

(a)   (b)

FIGURE 15.8

Encephalitozoon species

(a) A scanning electron micrograph of an *Encephalitozoon* species from cell culture. Note the delicate thread-like tubules extending from the ends of the cells (arrowheads). The significance of these tubules is unknown. (b) A transmission electron micrograph of a cell infected with *Encephalitozoon*. The parasite is multiplying within a vacuole termed the parasitophorus vacuole (PV). Within the vacuole, the *Encephalitozoon* cells have formed young, sporelike bodies called sporoblasts (SB), sporelike bodies (S), and developmental forms called the meront (M) and sporont (ST). The nucleus (N) of the cell can be observed. (Bar = 200 μm.)

To this point . . .

We have introduced the protozoa and have noted that they are a group of het-erotrophic, unicellular, microscopic organisms often involved in human disease. Most protozoa are found in aquatic environments, and the majority are free-living. Nutrients are commonly obtained by phagocytosis by the trophozoite form of the organism. A cyst may be formed under conditions of environmental stress.

We then outlined the salient features of the four groups of protozoa. Members of the first group, the amoebas, move by means of amoeboid motion using their pseudopodia. Radiolaria and foraminifera are important members of this group. The second group includes flagellated protozoa, and Euglena is an often-studied, photosynthetic member of the group. Ciliates are extremely complex, with many features of multicellular ani-mals. The genetic recombination mechanism exhibited by Paramecium illustrates the complexity. The final group, apicomplexans (sporozoa), contains protozoa whose life cycles are complex. Motion is not observed in the adult forms of these organisms.

We shall now examine several human diseases caused by protozoal parasites and studied by parasitologists. The survey will be organized according to the groups of pro-tozoa, beginning with amoebas and concluding with the most complex forms. Protozoal diseases occur worldwide, and public health agencies consider them to be a global health problem. The diseases are particularly prevalent in tropical and subtropical regions.

15·3

Protozoal Diseases Caused by Amoebas and Flagellates

Diseases from amoebas and flagellates occur in a variety of systems of the human body. For example, some diseases, such as amoebiasis and giardiasis, take place in the digestive system, while others, such as sleeping sickness and leishmaniasis, occur in the blood. Still others, such as trichomoniasis, develop in the urogenital tract. Associated with these diseases is an equally diverse series of modes of transmission, as we shall observe in the discussions ahead.

AMOEBIASIS

Amoebiasis occurs throughout all areas of the world, from tropical to subpolar regions. The disease primarily affects people who are undernourished and living in unsanitary conditions. Although an intestinal illness at first, it can spread to various organ systems.

am'e-bi'ah-sis

The causative agent of amoebiasis is ***Entamoeba histolytica***. In nature, the organism exists in the **cyst** form. It enters the body by food or water contaminated with human or animal feces, or by direct contact with feces. Contact with soiled diapers, such as in a day-care center, may thus be hazardous. The organisms pass through the stomach as cysts, and the **trophozoite** amoebas emerge in the distant portion of the small intestine and in the large intestine (FIGURE 15.9).

en'tah-me'bah his'to-lit'ĭ-ka

Trophozoite:
the feeding form of a protozoan.

Entamoeba histolytica has the ability to destroy tissue (*histolytica* means "tissue-breaking"). Using their protein-digesting enzymes, the amoebas penetrate the wall of the large intestine, causing lesions and deep ulcers. Patients experience sharp pain similar to that in appendicitis, but relatively little diarrhea or dysentery because the ulcers are separated and do not drastically affect water absorption (the older term **amoebic dysentery** has thus been replaced by amoebiasis). In severe cases, tissue invasion will extend to blood vessels of the intestinal wall, and bloody stools will follow. Ulcer perforation into the peritoneum is a possibility. The amoebas also invade the blood and may spread to the liver or lung, where fatal abscesses may develop.

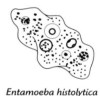

Entamoeba histolytica

Peritoneum:
the cavity outside the visceral organs.
me'tro-ni'dah-zŏl
par'o-mo-mi'sin

Metronidazole and paromomycin are commonly used to treat amoebiasis, but the drugs do not affect the cysts, and repeated attacks of amoebiasis may occur for months or years. The patient often continues to shed cysts in the feces to infect other people. Amoebiasis was originally a disease of the tropics, but soldiers returning after World War II brought it to the United States, and about 5 percent of Americans are believed to be infected. In recent years, waves of immigrants from Mexico and Caribbean nations have added to the incidence of the disease.

PRIMARY AMOEBIC MENINGOENCEPHALITIS

In the summer of 1980, the Centers for Disease Control and Prevention (CDC) noted an unusual cluster of seven cases of **primary amoebic meningoencephalitis (PAM)**. All the patients had been in contact with freshwater in a tropical setting. Since the first description of the disease in 1965, fewer than three dozen cases had been reported. In the 1980 cluster, all seven victims died.

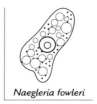

Naegleria fowleri

PAM may be caused by several species of amoeba in the genus *Naegleria*, especially ***Naegleria fowleri***. The amoebas appear to enter the body through the mucous

na-gle'rĭ-ah fow-ler'i

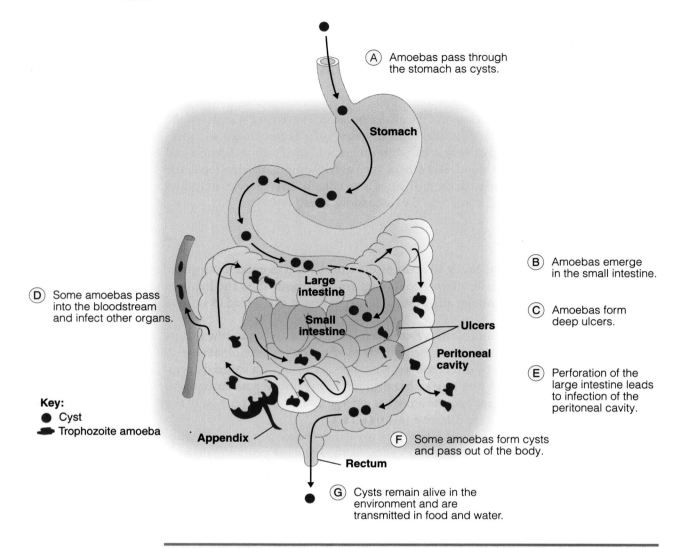

Ⓐ Amoebas pass through the stomach as cysts.

Stomach

Ⓑ Amoebas emerge in the small intestine.

Ⓓ Some amoebas pass into the bloodstream and infect other organs.

Ⓒ Amoebas form deep ulcers.

Large intestine

Small intestine

Ulcers

Peritoneal cavity

Ⓔ Perforation of the large intestine leads to infection of the peritoneal cavity.

Key:
● Cyst
🞄 Trophozoite amoeba

Appendix

Ⓕ Some amoebas form cysts and pass out of the body.

Rectum

Ⓖ Cysts remain alive in the environment and are transmitted in food and water.

FIGURE 15.9

The Course of Amoebiasis Due to *Entamoeba histolytica*

membranes of the nose and then follow the olfactory tracts to the brain. Nasal congestion precedes piercing headaches, fever, delirium, neck rigidity, and occasional seizures. The symptoms resemble those in other forms of encephalitis and meningitis. *Naegleria* in the spinal fluid is a sign of PAM.

GIARDIASIS

ji'ar-di'ah-sis

je-ar'de-ah

Since the 1970s, **giardiasis** has become the most commonly detected protozoal disease of the intestinal tract in the United States. Though not reportable to the CDC, the disease is estimated to occur in thousands of Americans annually. The causative agent is a flagellate named ***Giardia lamblia***. This organism is distinguished by four pairs of anterior flagella and two nuclei that stain darkly to give the appearance of eyes on a face. The protozoan can be divided equally along its longitudinal axis and is therefore said to display **bilateral symmetry**. Some microbiologists believe that *Giardia lamblia* was described as early as 1681 by Anton van Leeuwenhoek in samples of his stool.

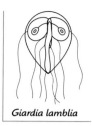

Giardia lamblia

Giardiasis is commonly transmitted by water that contains *Giardia* cysts stemming from cross-contamination of drinking water with sewage. In the 1970s, for example, 38 cases in Aspen, Colorado, broke out after a sewer line was obstructed and sewage leaked into the town's water supply. Recent years have also witnessed outbreaks in day-care centers and schools resulting from contact with feces (**Micro-Focus 15.2**). In addition, the disease has spread to wild animals (especially beavers), where it is now very common and from which it can be obtained via contaminated water. In 1989, a notable cluster of 22 cases in Albuquerque, New Mexico, was related to contamination of taco ingredients by water used to wash the lettuce.

Giardia lamblia passes through the stomach as cysts, and the trophozoites emerge as flagellates in the duodenum. They adhere to the intestinal lining using sucker devices and multiply rapidly. The patient feels nauseous, experiences gastric cramps and flatulence, and emits a foul-smelling watery **diarrhea** that may last for weeks. Some microbiologists maintain that the diarrhea arises from overgrowth of the intestinal wall with parasites, while others suggest injury to the tissue (**FIGURE 15.10**).

Flatulence: gas expelled from the intestinal tract through the anus.

Diagnosis of giardiasis depends on the microscopic identification of trophozoites or cysts in freshly passed fecal material. A reliable alternative to stool examination is the use of the **Enterotest capsule**. In this procedure, the patient swallows a weighted gelatin capsule attached to a string. The free end of the string is then taped to the mouth. After 4 hours the capsule is withdrawn, and the bile-stained mucus is scraped from the capsule and examined for trophozoites. The organisms exhibit an erratic turning motion, similar to a falling leaf.

MicroFocus 15.2

HAWAII TO MINNESOTA

On December 13, 1979, the Minnesota Department of Health learned that employees of a local school were being treated for *Giardia lamblia* infections, and that half the members of the staff were involved. Health officials subsequently distributed a questionnaire requesting information on symptoms, travel, type of water consumed, and contact with other sick people. Those with symptoms were asked for stool samples to test for *Salmonella, Shigella, Campylobacter,* and *Giardia lamblia.* Giardiasis was confirmed.

In the ensuing days, the Department of Health examined the eating, drinking, and plumbing facilities at the school and found that all of them were sanitary. Analysis of the questionnaire, however, provided a promising lead: Most of the affected individuals had eaten home-canned salmon. Officials narrowed their search in this direction.

Two months previously, an employee of the school had gone fishing on Lake Michigan and caught a bevy of salmon. He marinated the fish in vinegar and canned it. Wishing to share his bounty, the employee had recently brought several jars to school. Microbiologists were able to obtain four unopened jars of salmon and sample them for *Giardia.* To their dismay, all samples were negative.

Investigators now turned their attention to how the salmon was prepared for serving in the staff lunchroom. They established that several days before the outbreak, a female employee had opened the jars and tipped them over to drain the juice. In doing so, she held back the fish with her fingertips. When the woman was questioned, she admitted that before coming to work, she had changed her grandson's diaper and had soiled her hands with his loose stools. At the time the boy was visiting from Hawaii, but he had since gone home.

Health officials now contacted their counterparts in Hawaii and requested that the child be tested for *Giardia lamblia.* A few days later, a telephone call confirmed their suspicions: The test proved positive.

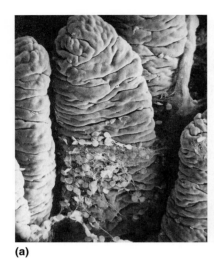
(a)

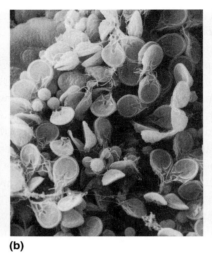
(b)

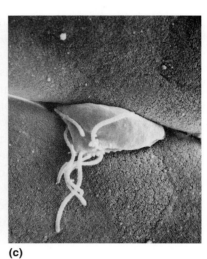
(c)

FIGURE 15.10

Giardia lamblia Infection of the Intestine

(a) A mass of trophozoites adhering to the base of a villus in the intestine of an animal (×1000). (b) A view of the *Giardia* population at the base (×2000). Note the flat shape of the cells with numerous flagella and a disklike sucker device for attaching to the tissue. (c) A single *Giardia* trophozoite wedged into the wall of the villus. Three pairs of flagella protrude posteriorly (×5200).

kwin'ah-krin
fu'rah-zol'ĭ-dēn
me'tro-ni'dah-zōl

Treatment of giardiasis may be administered with drugs such as quinacrine (Atabrine), furazolidine (Furoxone), and metronidazole. However, these drugs have side effects that the physician may wish to avoid by letting the disease run its course without treatment. Those who recover often become **carriers** and excrete the cysts for years. Giardiasis is sometimes mistaken for viral gastroenteritis and is considered a type of **traveler's diarrhea**. Latin America, Russia, and the Far East are prime areas for contracting the disease.

TRICHOMONIASIS

trik'o-mo-ni'ah-sis

Trichomoniasis is among the most common diseases in the United States, with an estimated 2.5 million people affected annually. The disease is transmitted primarily by sexual contact and is considered a **sexually transmitted disease**. Fomites (inanimate objects) such as towels and clothing have also been implicated in transmission.

trik'o-mo'nas

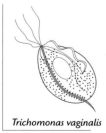
Trichomonas vaginalis

Trichomonas vaginalis, the causative agent, is a pear-shaped protozoan with two pairs of anterior flagella and one posterior flagellum. It thrives in the slightly acidic environment of the human vagina. Establishment may be encouraged by physical or chemical trauma, including poor hygiene, drug therapy, diabetes, or mechanical contraceptive devices such as the intrauterine device (IUD). The organism has no cyst stage.

In females, trichomoniasis is accompanied by intense itching (pruritis), and **burning pain** during urination. Usually, a creamy white, frothy **discharge** is also present. The symptoms are frequently worse during menstruation, and erosion of the cervix may occur. In males, the disease occurs primarily in the urethra, with pain on urination and a thin, mucoid discharge. The disease can occur concurrently with gonorrhea (FIGURE 15.11).

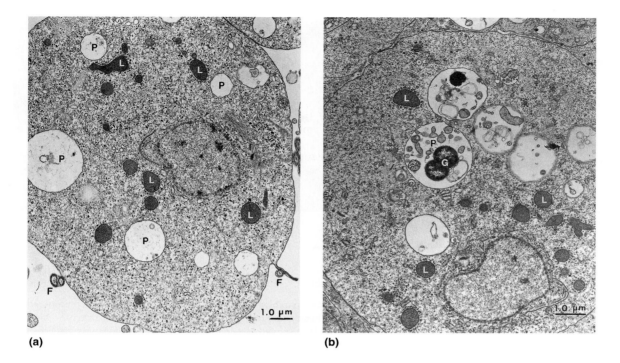

(a) (b)

FIGURE 15.11

Trichomoniasis and Gonorrhea

Electron micrographs illustrating that *Trichomonas* cells have the capacity to phagocytize *Neisseria gonorrhoeae*, the bacterial agent of gonorrhea, when the two organisms are incubated together. (a) Prior to experimental infection with *N. gonorrhoeae*, the protozoan contains many lysosomes (L) as well as relatively empty food vacuoles, or phagosomes (P). (b) After 5 minutes of incubation with *N. gonorrhoeae*, an intact diplococcus (G) is observed within a phagosome, and other phagosomes show evidence of bacterial debris. When trichomoniasis and gonorrhea occur simultaneously, the bacteria apparently serve as a food source for the protozoa.

Direct microscopic examination of clinical specimens is the most rapid and least expensive technique for identifying *T. vaginalis.* This is accomplished by making a wet mount preparation of the discharge and observing the quick, jerky motion of the protozoa. The drug of choice for treatment is orally administered metronidazole (Flagyl). Tinidazole and miconazole have also been used with success. Both the patient and the sexual partner should be treated concurrently to prevent transmission or reinfection.

ti-nid′ah-zōl
mĭ-kon′ah-zōl

TRYPANOSOMIASIS

Trypanosomiasis is a general name for two diseases caused by species of *Trypanosoma.* Protozoa in this genus are elongated flagellates having a characteristic undulating membrane that waves as the organism moves (FIGURE 15.12). The two diseases caused by trypanosomes are traditionally known as African sleeping sickness and South American sleeping sickness.

tri-pan′o-so-mi′ah-sis
tri′pan-o-so′mah

African sleeping sickness cycles between humans and the **tsetse fly** *Glossina palpalis.* The insect bites an infected patient, and the trypanosomes localize in the insect's salivary gland. Transmission occurs during the next bite. The point of entry

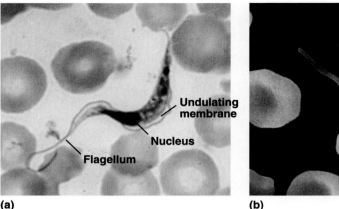
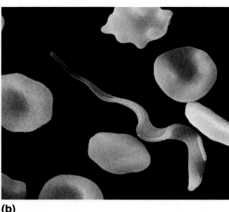

(a)   **(b)**

FIGURE 15.12

Two Views of Trypanosomes

(a) A photomicrograph of a species of *Trypanosoma*. The area about the trypanosome contains red blood cells. (b) A scanning electron micrograph of *T. brucei* among red blood cells. Internal details of the trypanosome are not visible, but the undulating membrane and short flagellum are clear.

bru'cē-i

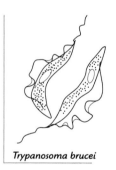

Trypanosoma brucei

mel-ar-so'prol
di'flu-ro-meth'il-or'ni-theen

cru'zi

tri-at'o-mah
rod'ne-us

becomes painful and swollen in several days, and a chancre similar to that in syphilis is observed. Invasion of the bloodstream follows soon thereafter.

Two types of African sleeping sickness exist. One form, common in Central Africa, is caused by ***Trypanosoma brucei* variety *gambiense***. It is accompanied by chronic bouts of fever, as well as severe headaches, changes in sleep patterns and behavior, and a general wasting away. As the trypanosomes invade the brain, the patient slips into a coma (hence the name, "sleeping sickness"). The second form, common in East Africa, is due to ***Trypanosoma brucei* variety *rhodesiense***. This disease is more acute, with higher fever and rapid coma and death.

African sleeping sickness exists wherever the tsetse fly is found, and Africa provides the right combination of temperature and moisture for this insect. In 1898, **David Bruce** identified the trypanosomes in tsetse flies and recommended insect control (MicroFocus 15.3). Bruce's discovery opened the door to the British colonization of Africa. Today the disease is checked by clearing brushlands and treating areas where the insects breed. Patients are treated with a drug known as pentamidine isethionate. Alternative drugs are arsenic-based melarsoprol and difluoromethylornithine, both of which are extremely expensive.

South American sleeping sickness is caused by ***Trypanosoma cruzi***, a trypanosome discovered by Carlos Juan Chagas. In his honor, the disease is called **Chagas' disease. Triatomid bugs** of the genera *Triatoma* and *Rhodnius* are essential to transmission of the trypanosomes. (The insects are also known as reduviid bugs.) The insects are found in the cracked walls of mud and adobe houses. They feed at night and bite where the skin is thin, such as on the lips, face, or forearms. For this reason, they are called "kissing bugs." The insects deliver nitric oxide to the wound via their saliva to keep the blood vessel open while they complete their blood meal.

In humans, South American sleeping sickness is characterized by fever and widespread tissue damage, especially in the **heart**. The trypanosomes destroy the cardiac nerves so thoroughly that the victim experiences sudden heart failure. Organisms may also reach the brain, where they induce coma and death. A recent

MicroFocus 15.3

CLOSE, BUT NO CIGAR

In the late 1800s, new trade routes opened in Africa, and travel increased substantially into the hitherto unknown equatorial belt. Among the most adventurous explorers were the British, but they regularly fell ill with the "sleeping sickness." Therefore, in 1894, the British government sent a medical team headed by David Bruce to investigate the disease and find its cause. In several types of animals, the researchers located a new parasite (later named *Trypanosoma brucei* for the team leader), but they could not find it in human victims. Interestingly, they also found the parasite in tsetse flies.

As it turned out, the British were not the only ones interested in sleeping sick-

ness. The Italians also had a medical team in Africa, and a group headed by Aldo Castellani found Bruce's parasite in the nervous system of infected humans. Bruce read Castellani's report and began a search for parasites in human blood, for if they could reach the nervous system, the blood would be the logical route. And sure enough, they were in the blood—in scores of thousands. But how did they get there? The tsetse flies, of course! All the pieces of the puzzle seemed to fit: The sickness is transmitted among animals by tsetse flies, which also bite humans and inject the parasites into the blood. Passage to the brain follows.

The solution was obvious: Stop the tsetse flies and thereby stop the sleeping

sickness. After all, that's what Gorgas and Reed were doing with mosquitoes and yellow fever in the Caribbean islands and Central America. But it was not to be. Yellow fever is primarily a human disease, but sleeping sickness affects numerous wild animals, and the animals could not be kept away from human populations. Moreover, tsetse flies breed everywhere, from water-logged river banks to arid deserts to savannas and grasslands (mosquitoes breed only where water collects). The effort to stop the disease was valiant, but it was doomed to failure. To this day, sleeping sickness remains a threat to human life in Africa.

---

estimate put the number of cases in South and Central America at 12 million. Although there is no completely effective treatment for the disease, some relief is experienced with nifurtimax (also known as Bayer 2502). **MicroFocus 15.4** explores an avenue to prevention.

ni-fur'ti-max

An interesting theory emerged in the 1980s to explain why victims of trypanosomiasis suffer waves of blood invasion of parasites and accompanying waves of fever. Researchers found that proteins on the membrane surface of the trypanosome were different as each new blood invasion occurred. Thus, the antibodies formed against the preceding parasites were ineffective against the new variants. The change in the

MicroFocus 15.4

GENE ENGINEERS TO THE RESCUE

Dealing with Chagas' disease in Latin and South America has always been difficult: Health-care workers have plastered the walls of native homes to try and eliminate the triatomid (reduviid) bugs that spread the disease. And they have used insecticides at various formulations to kill the intermediary insect. Still the epidemic continues to rage.

Now, gene engineers have entered the picture. Yale University researchers have isolated *Rhodococcus rhodnii*, a bacterium living harmlessly in the gut of

the insect. Within the triatomid bug (genus *Rhodnius*), the bacterial rod lives a peaceful, unassuming existence, deriving nutrients from the insect and contributing a natural defense against invading bacteria. The relationship is an example of mutualism in nature.

Researchers have cultivated *R. rhodnii* and altered its genome so it produces a powerful drug called cecropin A. This peptide compound is extremely active against *Trypanosoma cruzi*, the agent of Chagas' disease. When produced within the insect's gut, the drug kills the para-

site and prevents its transmission to the next individual. Researchers next hope to introduce to the environment a number of triatomid bugs with their built-in medical arsenal. In the best-case scenario, the new insects will replace the traditional ones and bring the drug to where it is needed most—the insect gut. The insect will survive, the human will survive, and the most dangerous member of the triumvirate, the protozoal parasite, will be eliminated.

FIGURE 15.13

A Photomicrograph of *Leishmania tropica*

L. tropica is shown in the rosette patterns, in which long, thin flagellates are clustered, giving the appearance of petals on a flower. The rosette pattern is found in older culture media. Some researchers believe that the organisms are in a feeding frenzy at this point, but there is no evidence to support this theory.

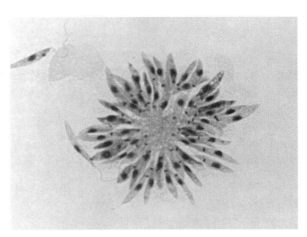

Insertion sequences: segments of chromosomal DNA that produce copies, which insert at other places on the chromosomes.

trypanosome's surface proteins is apparently due to chromosomal **insertion sequences**, which produce copies of themselves and move along the DNA, changing the genetic codes for membrane proteins (Chapter 6). Charles Darwin was one of the prominent sufferers of the disease (**MicroFocus 15.5**).

LEISHMANIASIS

lēsh'mah-ni'ah-sis

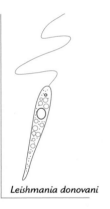

Leishmania donovani

Leishmaniasis is a rare disease in the United States, but it occurs worldwide in large-scale epidemics. (An estimated 12 million people in the tropics and subtropics suffer from the disease annually.) The responsible protozoa include several species of *Leishmania*, such as **Leishmania donovani** and **L. tropica** (**FIGURE 15.13**). Transmission is by the **sandfly** of the genus *Phlebotomus*.

One form of leishmaniasis is a visceral disease called **kala-azar**, meaning "black fever." This disease is characterized by infection of the body's white blood cells and is accompanied by irregular bouts of fever, swollen spleen and liver, progressive anemia, and emaciation. A second form of leishmaniasis is a disfiguring, cutaneous disease, less severe because the parasites remain in the skin, as shown in **FIGURE 15.14**. This disease is often referred to as **Oriental sore** ("Oriental" because epidemics have been documented in China). It is also known in the Middle East as the "rose of Jericho" disease from the flowery appearance of the skin lesion. (In some Israeli communities, it is called shoske, after the Hebrew *shoshana*, meaning "rose.") Estimated to be endemic in 88 countries worldwide, leishmaniasis is usually fatal if untreated.

Control of the sandfly remains the most important method for preventing outbreaks of leishmaniasis. Several drugs, including antimony compounds, are available

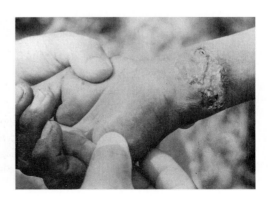

FIGURE 15.14

The Leishmaniasis Sore

A cutaneous sore on the wrist of a man with leishmaniasis. Note the shallow, circular nature of the ulcer.

MicroFocus 15.5

CHAGAS AND DARWIN

In 1909, Carlos Chagas was a young Brazilian doctor of 29 when he arrived in a small town north of Rio de Janeiro. Chagas was there to study malaria, but another problem caught his attention: Many of the local people were suffering from lethargy, shortness of breath, and irregular heartbeat. And no one knew what was the cause.

Chagas set aside his interest in malaria and began a search for the parasite of this strange new disease. He quickly tracked down the vector, a cricketlike triatomid bug that lived in the walls of thatched houses and sucked the blood of sleeping inhabitants. From the bug he extracted a whiplike protozoan similar to the trypanosome of African sleeping sickness. In rapid succession, Chagas proved that the trypanosome could infect monkeys; he found it in a cat in a bug-infested house, and he isolated it from the blood of a young girl displaying the symptoms of the disease (now recognized as Chagas' disease).

To be sure, the disease had not been described previously, but neither was it a new disease. Unbeknown to Chagas, it had probably claimed the life of Charles Darwin many years before. Historians record that Darwin's health declined perceptibly on his return to England from South America (during his famous voyage aboard HMS *Beagle*). Some writers maintain that the illness was psychosomatic—Darwin took a public battering on publication of his theory of natural selection—but Saul Adler, a tropical medicine researcher, believes otherwise. Adler believes that Darwin suffered from Chagas' disease. Indeed, while in Argentina, Darwin wrote: ". . . at night I experienced an attack (for it deserves no less a name) of *Reduvius*, the giant black bug of the Pampas. It is most disgusting to feel soft, wingless insects about an inch long, crawling over one's body. Before sucking they are quite thin, but afterwards they become round and bloated with blood."

The bug that Darwin describes is probably *Triatoma infestans*, the vector that Chagas would identify generations later. Furthermore, Darwin's symptoms matched those in Chagas' patients. The disease would linger in Darwin's tissues for 40 years and reduce the vigorous adventurer to a shell of his former self.

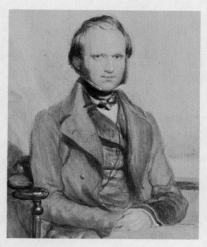

■ *Charles Darwin*

for treating established cases. At least 7 cases of visceral leishmaniasis and 16 cases of cutaneous leishmaniasis occurred in military personnel associated with Operation Desert Storm, in 1991 (FIGURE 15.15). In 1993, visceral leishmaniasis broke out in epidemic proportions in civil war-torn regions of Sudan. In 1997, investigators identified a transposon in the genome of *Leishmania* (appropriately called *mariner*) that moves about, changing the organism's genetic character, and thereby rendering it unaffected by the immune response.

lēsh-ma'ne-ah

To this point . . .

We have considered seven protozoal diseases caused by amoebas or flagellates. Amoebiasis is a disease of the intestinal tract that has become fairly widespread in the United States since it was introduced from tropical areas. The cyst form may be contracted from contaminated food or water or by contact with infected individuals. A similar situation holds for giardiasis. Sewage leaks are another community problem that may lead to giardiasis.

We also studied trichomoniasis, a sexually transmitted disease that is among the most common illnesses in Americans. Women are particularly susceptible to this disease, but men can be carriers. The discussion then moved to arthropodborne protozoal diseases, in which species of Trypanosoma and Leishmania rely on insects to complete their life cycles. The arthropod represents the "weak link" in the transmission of these diseases, and control can be effected by eliminating the arthropod. This is one reason leishmaniasis and sleeping sickness are not prevalent where sanitation methods are established. The diseases are uncommon in the United States also because the necessary arthropods are not usually found here.

We shall now focus our attention on a disease caused by a ciliate and several diseases due to apicomplexans (sporozoa). In this group we shall find rapidly emerging problems in medical microbiology, as well as one illness, malaria, that is the most widespread human disease recognized today.

FIGURE 15.15

An Outbreak of Leishmaniasis

This outbreak occurred among military personnel who fought in Operation Desert Storm during 1991.

TEXTBOOK CASES

1. During 1991, approximately 500,000 military personnel took part in Operation Desert Storm in Saudi Arabia, Kuwait, and other countries of the Persian Gulf region.

2. While stationed in the Middle East during and after the fighting, many individuals were subjected to the bites of sandflies, the arthropods that transfer the protozoan *Leishmania tropica.*

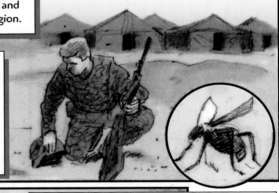

3. On returning to the United States after several months' duty, seven men displayed the symptoms of leishmaniasis, including high fever, chills, malaise, liver and spleen involvement, and gastrointestinal distress. Several had low-volume watery stools and abdominal pain.

4. When bone marrow samples from the seven patients were examined, the tissue yielded evidence of *L. tropica*, the agent of leishmaniasis. The men were treated over a period of weeks with an antimony compound called sodium stibogluconate. All recovered.

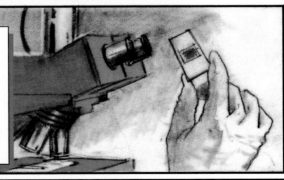

15.4

Protozoal Diseases Caused by Ciliates & Apicomplexans (Sporozoa)

Only one serious human disease is associated with a ciliated protozoan, but numerous diseases are related to the second group in this section. Moreover, the roster of diseases caused by apicomplexans (sporozoa) continues to grow, partly because of their association with a weakened immune system. Compromised immunity can be related to a disease such as AIDS, as well as to immunosuppressant cancer therapy or treatment following an organ transplant. In these cases, the protozoal disease may present a serious challenge to the patient.

BALANTIDIASIS

Balantidiasis is an intestinal disease caused by **Balantidium coli**. The protozoan is among the largest organisms to infect humans. It measures up to 100 μm in length by 70 μm in width, with cilia over its entire surface, and has a large kidney-shaped nucleus as well as a small micronucleus. Trophozoite and cyst stages exist.

bal'an-tĭ-di'ah-sis
bal'an-tid'e-um

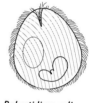

Balantidium coli

Balantidiasis is a rare disease in temperate climates. It is spread by contaminated water or food, especially pork. Cysts pass through the stomach, and the ciliated trophozoites emerge in the intestines, where they cause mild ulceration. Profuse diarrhea, nausea, and rapid weight loss are characteristic signs of disease. Often the disease is chronic, since cysts remain in the intestinal wall. Metronidazole or paromomycin are used for treatment. Though cases are uncommon in the United States, some concern has been voiced about symptomless carriers returning from tropical regions of the world.

TOXOPLASMOSIS

Toxoplasmosis was first recognized as a clinical disease in 1909 by **Charles Nicolle**, the French investigator who associated lice with epidemic typhus. Nicolle assumed that toxins were a factor in the disease and named it accordingly, but no evidence exists for this involvement. Instead, the symptoms arise from tissue damage caused by the growth of protozoa.

The cause of toxoplasmosis is **Toxoplasma gondii**. *T. gondii* exists in three forms: the trophozoite, the cyst, and the oocyst. **Trophozoites** are crescent-shaped or oval organisms without evidence of locomotor organelles (**FIGURE 15.16a**). Located in tissue during the acute stage of disease, they force their way into all mammalian cells (**FIGURE 15.16b**), with the notable exception of erythrocytes. To enter cells, the parasites form a ring-shaped structure of the host cell membrane, then pull the membrane over themselves, much like pulling a sock over the foot. **Cysts** develop from the trophozoites within host cells and may be the source of repeated infections. Muscle and nerve tissue are common sites of cysts. **Oocysts** are oval bodies that develop from the cysts by a complex series of asexual and sexual reproductive processes.

toks'o-plaz'mah gon'de-e
o'o-sist

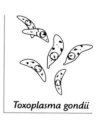

Toxoplasma gondii

Toxoplasma gondii exists in nature in the cyst and oocyst forms. Grazing animals acquire these forms from the soil and pass them to humans via **contaminated beef, pork, or lamb**. Rare hamburger meat is a possible source. **Domestic cats** acquire the

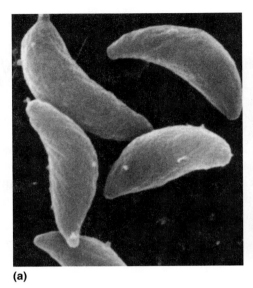

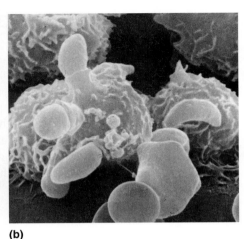

(a)   **(b)**

FIGURE 15.16

Toxoplasma gondii, the Cause of Toxoplasmosis

(a) A scanning electron micrograph of numerous parasites in the crescent-shaped trophozoite stage (×31,000). (b) A white blood cell simultaneously attacked by several trophozoites (×13,500). There are at least three sites where invasion of the white blood cells is taking place.

cysts from the soil or from infected birds or rodents. Oocysts then form in the cat. Humans are exposed to the oocysts when they forget to wash their hands after contacting cat feces while changing the cat litter or working in the garden. Touching the cat can also bring oocysts to the hands, and contaminated utensils, towels, or clothing can contact the mouth and transfer oocysts.

Toxoplasmosis develops after trophozoites are released from the cysts or oocysts in the host's gastrointestinal tract. *T. gondii* invades the intestinal lining and spreads throughout the body via the blood. Patients develop fever, malaise, sore throat, and swelling of the spleen, liver, and lymph nodes. In these respects the disease resembles **infectious mononucleosis**. Lesions may also occur on the retina, and virtually any organ may be involved. Complications, however, are rare. Diagnosis may be made by isolating trophozoites from the blood or other body fluids. Sulfonamide drugs are commonly used in therapy.

Pregnant women are at risk of developing toxoplasmosis because the protozoa may cross the placenta and infect the fetal tissues, as FIGURE 15.17 illustrates. Neurological damage, lesions of the fetal visceral organs, or spontaneous abortion may result. **Congenital infection** is least likely during the first trimester, but damage may be substantial when it occurs. By contrast, congenital infection is more common if the woman is infected in the third trimester, but fetal damage is less severe. Lesions of the **retina** are the most widely documented complication in congenital infections. The T in the **TORCH** group of diseases refers to toxoplasmosis (the others are rubella, cytomegalovirus, and herpes simplex; O is for other diseases, such as syphilis).

Toxoplasma gondii is also known to cause severe disease in **immunosuppressed individuals**. For example, in patients with **AIDS**, the normal immune defenses that prevent the spread of disease have been destroyed, and *T. gondii* attacks the **brain**

Retina:
the layer of light-sensitive nerve cells along the rear periphery of the eye.

AIDS:
a serious viral disease characterized by destruction of cells of the immune system.

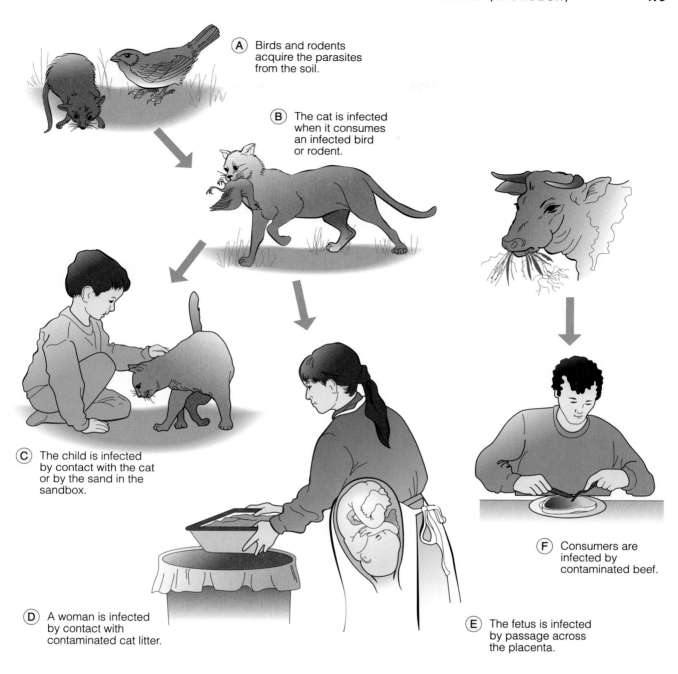

A Birds and rodents acquire the parasites from the soil.

B The cat is infected when it consumes an infected bird or rodent.

C The child is infected by contact with the cat or by the sand in the sandbox.

D A woman is infected by contact with contaminated cat litter.

E The fetus is infected by passage across the placenta.

F Consumers are infected by contaminated beef.

FIGURE 15.17

The Cycle of Toxoplasmosis in Nature

tissue. The infected tissue attracts immune system components, and the resulting inflammation and swelling often result in cerebral lesions, seizures, and death. Often the disease stems from opportunistic parasites already in the body. Patients receiving immunosuppressant therapy for cancer, or to prevent organ transplant rejection, are similarly at risk.

Toxoplasma gondii is regarded as a universal parasite. Some researchers suggest that it is the most common parasite of humans and other vertebrates. It is important to ranchers, dairy product producers, pet breeders, and anyone who comes in contact with a domestic cat. Indeed, evidence indicates that where there are no cats, toxoplasmosis is rare. Hundreds of millions of humans worldwide are estimated to be infected.

MALARIA

Though the disease malaria has been known to exist since at least 1000 B.C., the word *malaria* has been used only since the 1700s. Before that time, the disease was known as ague, from the French *aigu*, meaning "sharp" (a reference to the sharp fever that accompanies the disease). During the 1700s, however, Europeans began using the Italian word for "bad air" (*mal-aria*), reflecting the theory that the disease was somehow related to an unknown atmospheric influence called miasma. Wave after wave of malaria swept over the world during that century, and few regions were left untouched. American pioneers settling in the Mississippi and Ohio valleys suffered great losses from the disease.

More than 250 million of the world's population now suffer the chills, fever, and life-threatening effects of **malaria**. The disease exacts its greatest toll in Africa, where the WHO estimates that over 1 million children under the age of 5 die from malaria annually. No infectious disease of contemporary times can claim such a dubious distinction. Though progress has been made in the control of malaria, the figures remain appallingly high. (Even the United States is involved in the malaria pandemic—over 1000 cases are diagnosed annually.)

Malaria is caused by four species of ***Plasmodium:*** *P. vivax, P. ovale, P. malariae,* and *P. falciparum*. All are transmitted by the female ***Anopheles*** **mosquito**, which consumes human blood to provide chemical components for her eggs. The life cycle of the parasites has three important stages: the sporozoite, the merozoite, and the gametocyte. Each is a factor in malaria.

The mosquito sucks human blood and acquires **gametocytes**, the form of the protozoan found in red blood cells (FIGURE 15.18). Within the insect a transition to sporozoites takes place, and the **sporozoites** then migrate to the salivary gland. When the mosquito bites another human, several hundred sporozoites enter the person's bloodstream and quickly migrate to the liver. After several hours, the transformation of one sporozoite to 25,000 merozoites has been completed, and the **merozoites** emerge from the liver to invade the **red blood cells**. While in the red blood cells (RBCs), the merozoites synthesize about 150 proteins that attach to RBC membranes and anchor the RBCs to the blood vessels. By constantly switching among 150 genes (for 150 proteins), the malarial parasite avoids detection by the body's immune system.

Within the human red blood cells, the merozoites undergo another series of transformations that result in several gametocytes and thousands of new merozoites. In response to a biochemical signal, thousands of RBCs rupture simultaneously, thereby releasing the parasites and their toxins. Now the excruciating **malaria attack** begins. First, there is intense cold, with shivers and chattering teeth. The temperature then rises rapidly to 104°F, and the sufferer develops intense fever, headache, and delirium. After 2 or 3 hours, massive perspiration ends the hot stage, and the patient often falls asleep, exhausted.

During this quiet period, the merozoites enter a new set of red blood cells and repeat the cycle of transformations. *P. vivax* and *P. ovale* spend about 48 hours in the

---

Vertebrates: animals with backbones.

a'gu

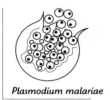

Plasmodium malariae

ah-nof'e-lēz

spor-o-zo'ī t
mer-o-zo'ī t
gam-e'to-cī t

Merozoite: an intermediate stage in the life cycle of malaria parasites.

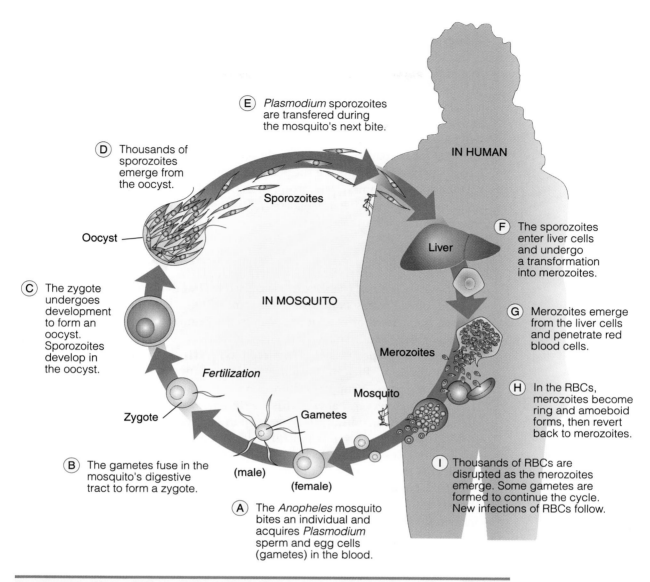

E) *Plasmodium* sporozoites are transfered during the mosquito's next bite.

D) Thousands of sporozoites emerge from the oocyst.

Sporozoites

IN HUMAN

Oocyst

Liver

F) The sporozoites enter liver cells and undergo a transformation into merozoites.

C) The zygote undergoes development to form an oocyst. Sporozoites develop in the oocyst.

IN MOSQUITO

G) Merozoites emerge from the liver cells and penetrate red blood cells.

Merozoites

Fertilization

Mosquito

H) In the RBCs, merozoites become ring and amoeboid forms, then revert back to merozoites.

Zygote

Gametes

B) The gametes fuse in the mosquito's digestive tract to form a zygote.

(male)

(female)

I) Thousands of RBCs are disrupted as the merozoites emerge. Some gametes are formed to continue the cycle. New infections of RBCs follow.

A) The *Anopheles* mosquito bites an individual and acquires *Plasmodium* sperm and egg cells (gametes) in the blood.

FIGURE 15.18

The Malaria Cycle

Malaria continues to be among the most widespread infectious diseases in the world.

red blood cells, so that 48 hours pass between malaria attacks. This is **tertian malaria** (*tertian* is from the Latin for "three-day," based on the Roman custom of calling the day the event happened the first day of the cycle). For *P. malariae*, the cycle takes 72 hours, and the disease is called **quartan malaria** ("four-day" malaria). The cycle of *P. falciparum* is not defined, and attacks may occur at widely scattered intervals. This type of malaria, the most lethal, is known as **estivo-autumnal malaria**, referring to the summer-fall periods when mosquitoes breed heavily.

Death from malaria may be due to a number of factors related to the loss of red blood cells. Substantial anemia develops, and the hemoglobin from ruptured blood cells enters the urine; malaria is, therefore, sometimes called **blackwater fever**. Cell fragments accumulate in the small vessels of the brain, kidneys, heart, liver, and

Quartan malaria:
a type of malaria in which attacks occur every 4 days.

Anemia:
a condition characterized by a notable lack of red blood cells.

other vital organs and cause clots to form. Heart attacks, cerebral hemorrhages, and kidney failure are common. The intense fever leads to convulsions.

Since its discovery about 1640, **quinine** has been the mainstay for treating malaria. When the trees used as a source of this drug fell into the hands of the Japanese in World War II, American researchers developed chloroquine for the active stage of malaria and primaquine for the dormant stage. Chloroquine remained an important mode of therapy until recent years, when drug resistance began emerging in *Plasmodium* species. Since 1989, an alternative drug called mefloquine has been recommended for individuals entering malaria regions of the world. Another drug called proguanil is recommended if the person cannot tolerate mefloquine. Since 1991, the CDC has also recommended using quinidine gluconate, a quinine derivative, for treating complicated *P. falciparum* infections. Prospects for a malaria vaccine emerged in the 1990s (**MicroFocus 15.6**).

klor′o-kwin
prim′ah-kwin

mef′lo-kwin

pro-guan′il

BABESIOSIS

Babesiosis is a malarialike disease caused by ***Babesia microti***. The protozoa live in **ticks** of the genus ***Ixodes***, and are transmitted when these arthropods feed in human skin. Areas of coastal Massachusetts, Connecticut, and Long Island, New York, have experienced outbreaks in recent years.

Babesia microti penetrates human **red blood cells**. As the cells disintegrate, a mild anemia develops. Piercing headaches accompany the disease and, occasionally, meningitis occurs. A suppressed immune system appears to favor establishment of the disease. However, babesiosis is rarely fatal, and drug therapy is not recommended. Carrier conditions may develop in recoverers, and spread by blood transfusion is possible. Travelers returning from areas of high incidence are therefore advised to wait several weeks before donating blood to blood banks. Tick control is considered the best method of prevention.

Babesia has a significant place in the history of American microbiology because in the late 1800s, **Theobald Smith** located *B. bigemina* in the blood of cattle suffering from Texas fever (Chapter 1). His report was one of the first linking protozoa to disease, and, in part, it necessitated that the then-prevalent "bacterial" theory of disease be modified to the "germ" theory of disease.

bah-be′ze-o′sis
bah-be′ze-ah
iks-o′dēz

Babesia microti

CRYPTOSPORIDIOSIS

Before 1976, **cryptosporidiosis** was recognized as a cause of diarrhea in animals but was unknown in humans. Since that year, however, microbiologists have observed the disease in humans, and the number of cases has risen markedly.

Cryptosporidiosis is caused by ***Cryptosporidium parvum*** and other species of *Cryptosporidium* such as **C. coccidi**. The organism is similar to *Toxoplasma gondii* in that it has a complex life cycle involving trophozoite, sexual, and oocyst stages (**FIGURE 15.19**). Patients with competent immune systems appear to suffer limited diarrhea that lasts 1 or 2 weeks and does not require hospitalization. However, individuals with suppressed immune systems, such as **AIDS** patients, experience choleralike, profuse **diarrhea** that is severe and often irreversible. These patients undergo dehydration and emaciation, and often die of the disease.

Cryptosporidiosis has an incubation period of about 1 week, which explains why few cases are diagnosed properly because most people relate their nausea and diarrhea to something they ate a day or two before. In healthy adults, the infection usually lasts

krip′to-spor-id′e-o′sis

krip′to-spor-id′e-um
kok-sid′e

MicroFocus 15.6

EUPHORIA TO DESPONDENCY AND BACK AGAIN

Early in the 1960s, international health authorities thought they had malaria licked. Drugs such as quinine and chloroquine, and insecticides such as DDT, had reduced the incidence dramatically, and some officials were bold enough to speak of eradication.

But then reality dawned: *Plasmodium falciparum*, the most lethal of the malaria species, showed signs of resistance to chloroquine; mosquitoes with DDT resistance began emerging; Third World countries became complacent about malaria and relaxed their vigilance; and the campaign to control the disease in remote parts of the globe failed. Between 1972 and 1976, the worldwide number of malaria cases doubled, and by various estimates, the incidence is now over 300 million cases per year, with an estimated 2 million deaths.

New hope exists, however, that a vaccine for malaria may be in the near future. The vaccine's story began in 1967 when Ruth Nussenzweig and her coworkers at New York University showed that irradiated sporozoites provoke an immune response in mice. A vaccine with whole sporozoites was not feasible, though, because sporozoites were impossible to obtain in quantity. The advent of genetic engineering in the

1970s solved this problem. Nussenzweig's group first isolated large amounts of the antibodies that react with sporozoites. Then they used the antibodies to track down the immune-stimulating antigen on the sporozoite surface. By 1984, they located the antigen. The next step was to pinpoint the gene that codes for the antigen; by 1985, this also was accomplished.

Now the scene shifts to Colombia and a research group led by Manuel Elkin Patarroyo. In the late 1980s, Patarroyo's group developed a vaccine containing four different and synthetic protein antigens derived from *P. falciparum*. One antigen is from the sporozoite stage (similar to Nussenzweig's antigen), and the other three are from the merozoite stage, the stage in which plasmodia actually infect red blood cells. In March 1993, the Colombian researchers announced in *Lancet* the results of a clinical trial in which 738 volunteers received the vaccine—the result was a 39 percent reduction of malaria cases. Later that year, a second trial in 468 Ecuadorian volunteers resulted in 68 percent fewer cases among vaccine recipients. The scientific community noted that reductions of 39 percent and 68 percent are not extraordinary for a vaccine; nevertheless, when

2 million people die of malaria annually, these reductions constitute significant numbers. The vaccine has been named SPf66.

Research into a malaria vaccine continues today (with 2-year field trials ongoing in Thailand and Tanzania), and Patarroyo's vaccine stands as the prototype for other vaccines. When he began his research, Patarroyo pledged that if his vaccine proved effective, he would donate his patent rights to the United Nations. In May 1995 he made good on the pledge, signing over all vaccine rights to the U.N. and its public health agency, the World Health Organization.

There are problems with the agreement, however. The agreement specifies that the WHO must select a nonprofit manufacturer suitable to Patarroyo; the field trials have yielded mixed results, and some pessimism regarding the vaccine's efficacy has surfaced; and still to be settled is who determines when the vaccine is ready for large-scale production. There is also the Nussenzweig factor—Ruth Nussenzweig and her collaborators have continued their research into vaccine development, and in 1995 they announced a peptide vaccine that is highly effective in mice. Stay tuned.

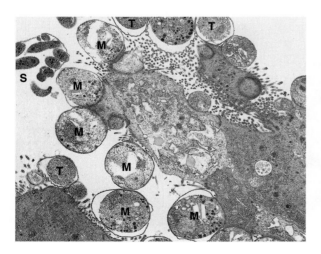

FIGURE 15.19

Cryptosporidium coccidi

A transmission electron micrograph of the intestinal lining of an animal infected with *Cryptosporidium* (×9000). Many aspects of the complex life cycle are visible, including the trophozoite stage (T), and the schizont stage (S) releasing eight merozoites. The macrogametes (M) are large cells that fuse in the sexual reproductive cycle of the organism. Dense dotlike areas within the macrogametes are polysaccharide granules.

about 10 days, but the diarrhea may remain for up to 2 months. A fecal-oral route is the major mode of transmission (as noted in the chapter opening), but physical contact can also transmit *Cryptosporidium* (children in day-care centers are at risk). Experiments indicate that the **dose** level to establish infection is very low (as low as 30 organisms), and no drug is widely accepted to treat the disease at this writing, although paromomycin and azithromycin have showed promise. High-level infections can be detected in patients by performing the **acid-fast test** (Chapter 3) on stool specimens and noting the presence of acid-fast oocysts.

pa-ro'mo-my'sin
a-zith'ro-my'sin

CYCLOSPORIASIS

Beginning in 1996 and continuing through 1997 and 1998, public health officials noted a series of clusters of intestinal disease related to raspberries imported from Guatemala. In all cases, the outbreaks were related to the protozoan *Cyclospora cayetanensis*, shown in FIGURE 15.20.

si-clo-spor'ah cay'e-tan-en'sis

In Americans, ***Cyclospora cayetanensis*** was first observed in 1986 in travelers returning from Mexico and Haiti. The organism is a coccidian parasite, previously found only in reptiles and limited species of mammals. The organisms produce oocysts, each containing two sporocysts; they appear microscopically as spheres 8 to 10 μm in diameter, with a cluster of membrane-enclosed globules. In this regard, they are similar to but larger than the oocysts of another coccidian parasite, *Cryptosporidium*. Differential diagnosis is important because *C. cayetanensis* responds to the drug combination of trimethoprim-sulfamethoxazole, whereas *Cryptosporidium* does not.

Cyclosporiasis has an unusually long incubation period of 1 week. This lengthy period can be a clue to identifying the disease (but it also impairs the ability of people to recall how they were exposed, and the responsible food may have been dis-

FIGURE 15.20

The Source and Cause of Cyclosporiasis

(a) During 1996, 1997, and 1998, raspberries imported from Guatemala were identified as a source of cyclosporiasis, an intestinal disease caused by an apicomplexan protozoan. (b) The agent of cyclosporiasis is *Cyclospora cayetanensis*, shown in the photomicrograph in the oocyst stage after acid-fast staining.

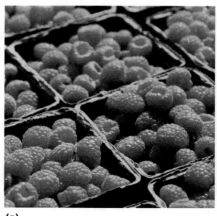

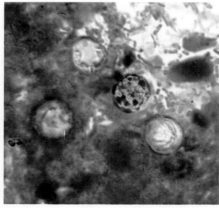

(a)   (b)

carded so it cannot be tested). Symptoms of the disease include watery diarrhea, nausea, abdominal cramping, bloating, and vomiting. Treatment is successful with the drugs noted above, but the symptoms often return. Moreover, the symptoms often remain for over 1 month during the first illness.

How raspberries become contaminated during outbreaks is not clear. Public health officials believe that tainted water used for washing the berries may be the source; or the berries may be handled by someone whose hands are contaminated; or they may be contaminated during shipping. Regardless of the source, the CDC and FDA have insisted that Guatemalan growers and exporters of raspberries introduce control measures focusing on improved water quality and better sanitation methods on local farms. Transmission from person to person is unlikely. An earlier link of cyclosporiasis to strawberries (MicroFocus 15.7) proved erroneous.

PNEUMOCYSTOSIS

Pneumocystosis is currently the most common cause of nonbacterial pneumonia in Americans with suppressed immune systems. The causative organism, ***Pneumocystis carinii***, was first observed in 1910 by John Carini in studies with rats. It remained in relative obscurity until the 1980s, when it was recognized as the cause of death in over 50 percent of patients dying from the effects of **AIDS**.

Pneumocystis carinii has a complex life cycle that takes place entirely in the alveoli of the lung. The trophozoite stage swells to become a precyst stage, in which up to eight sporozoites develop. When the cyst is mature, it opens and liberates the sporozoites, which enlarge and undergo further reproduction and maturation to trophozoites. It should be noted that although this life cycle is reminiscent of a protozoan,

nu'mo-sis-to'sis
nu'mo-sis'tis car-in'e-e

Alveoli:
the air sacs of the lungs.

MicroFocus 15.7

THE BEST NEWS SINCE SHORTCAKE

Strawberry growers and distributors were about to take a hit. A serious outbreak of diarrheal illness was being blamed on their livelihood, and they were shaking in their boots. The outbreak was developing in Houston, Texas, where 62 cases were confirmed. All indications pointed to the strawberries. Already the government memos were being prepared: People should avoid California strawberries. Clearly, 1996 was not shaping up as a banner year.

Then news of another outbreak reached them, this time in Charleston, South Carolina. Intestinal illness had developed after a luncheon attended by 64 people; 37 of the 64 were sick with abdominal cramping, vomiting, and

diarrhea. For dessert, the management had served strawberries.

But, they learned, the management had also served raspberries at the same dessert. And there was another luncheon at the same restaurant that same day. Ninety-five people had attended that second luncheon, and nobody got sick! And the only fruit the management served was strawberries. Hmmm. Maybe it wasn't the strawberries after all. Maybe it was the raspberries?

The ensuing weeks would be considerably brighter for the strawberry growers, but nightmarish for the raspberry producers. *Cyclospora*-related illness broke out in New York City, New Jersey, Toronto, and a host of other locales. In

each case, raspberries were implicated, but strawberries were nowhere to be seen. The strawberry industry had dodged the bullet. Whew! Bring on the shortcake.

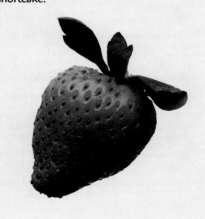

a recent body of evidence points to the possibility that *P. carinii* is a fungus. Analysis of its ribosomal RNA, for example, shows a closer relationship to fungal RNA than to protozoal RNA. However, *P. carinii* has historically been considered a protozoan, and we shall consider it here until the evidence for reclassification becomes conclusive.

Present evidence indicates that *P. carinii* is transmitted by droplets from the respiratory tract. A wide cross section of individuals harbor the organism without symptoms, mainly because of the control imposed by T-lymphocytes. However, when the immune system is suppressed, as in AIDS patients, *Pneumocystis* tropho-

TABLE 15.1

A Summary of Protozoal Diseases in Humans

ORGANISM	TYPE	ORGANS OF MOTION	DISEASE	TRANSMISSION
Entamoeba histolytica	Amoeba	Pseudopodia	Amoebiasis	Water Food
Naegleria fowleri	Amoeba	Pseudopodia	Primary amoebic meningoencephalitis	Water
Giardia lamblia	Flagellate	Flagella	Giardiasis	Water Contact
Trichomonas vaginalis	Flagellate	Flagella	Trichomoniasis	Sexual contact
Trypanosoma brucei	Flagellate	Flagella	African sleeping sickness	Tsetse fly (*Glossina*)
Trypanosoma cruzi	Flagellate	Flagella	South American sleeping sickness	Triatomid bug (*Triatoma*)
Leishmania donovani	Flagellate	Flagella	Leishmaniasis (Kala-azar)	Sandfly (*Phlebotomus*)
Balantidium coli	Ciliate	Cilia	Balantidiasis	Food Water
Toxoplasma gondii	Apicomplexan	None in adult	Toxoplasmosis	Domestic cats Food
Plasmodium species	Apicomplexan	None in adult	Malaria	Mosquito (*Anopheles*)
Babesia microti	Apicomplexan	None in adult	Babesiosis	Tick (*Ixodes*)
Cryptosporidium parvum	Apicomplexan	None in adult	Cryptosporidiosis	Water, food
Cyclospora cataynensis	Apicomplexan	None in adult	Cyclosporiasis	Food
Pneumocystis carinii	Apicomplexan	None in adult	Pneumocystosis	Droplets

zoites and cysts fill the alveoli and occupy all the air spaces. A nonproductive cough develops, with high fever and difficult breathing. Progressive deterioration leads to consolidation of the lungs and, eventually, death. The disease is commonly referred to as *Pneumocystis carinii* pneumonia (**PCP**).

The current treatment of choice for PCP is **pentamidine isethionate**. Another drug, trimetrexate, is also used. These drugs, however, have limited value in immunosuppressed individuals, as evidenced by the high death rate in AIDS patients.

pen-tam′ĭ-dēn i-se-thī′o-nāt
tri-meh-trex′ate

TABLE 15.1 summarizes the protozoal diseases of humans.

ORGAN AFFECTED	DIAGNOSIS	TREATMENT	COMMENT
Intestine Liver Lungs	Stool examination	Paromomycin Metronidazole	Deep intestinal ulcers
Brain	Spinal fluid examination	None effective	Uncommon in U.S.
Intestine	Stool examination Gelatin capsule	Quinacrine Furazolidine	Incidence increasing in U.S.
Urogenital organs	Urine or swab examination	Metronidazole Tinidazole	May result in sterility
Blood Brain	Blood smear	Various drugs	Two types, depending on region
Blood Brain Heart	Blood smear	Various drugs	Common in South America
White blood cells Skin Intestine	Tissue examination	Antimony	Ulcers yield skin disfiguration
Intestine	Stool examination	Paromomycin Metronidazole	Symptomless carriers common
Blood Eyes Tissue cells	Blood examination	Sulfonamide drugs	Congenital damage possible Associated with AIDS
Liver Red blood cells	Blood examination	Quinine Mefloquine Proguanil	World's most urgent public health problem
Red blood cells	Blood examination	None recommended	Carrier state possible
Intestine	Stool examination	None effective	Associated with AIDS
Intestine	Stool examination	Trimethoprim Sulfamethoxazole	Long incubation period
Lungs	Lung examination	Pentamidine isethionate	Associated with AIDS

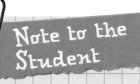

Note to the Student

On an October day in 1983, a local medical laboratory notified the Los Angeles Department of Health Services of a large number of stool samples containing *Entamoeba histolytica*, the protozoan of intestinal amoebiasis. The laboratory had also reported 38 cases of amoebiasis during the previous 2 months. Department officials were mystified because there had been no increase in the number of specimens the laboratory examined, no clustering of cases of amoebiasis, few patients in high-risk categories (tourists, immigrants, or institutionalized patients), and no instances of increased reporting from other laboratories. When Health Department investigators reexamined 71 slides of fecal material from the 38 cases, they found only 4 with *Entamoeba histolytica*. Officials concluded that the laboratory was in error, and that the bodies thought to be amoebas were in fact white blood cells.

Diagnostic methods for protozoal diseases have not changed fundamentally for many generations, and the sophisticated devices used for bacterial and viral detection have not yet reached the parasitology laboratory. Cultivation methods for pathogenic protozoa are difficult, and a correct diagnosis often depends on direct observation of tissue specimens, together with a sense of intuition and understanding of the patterns of disease. In the Los Angeles case described above, these were apparently lacking.

With the increasing prevalence of protozoal diseases in recent years, parasitologists have strengthened their role in the health-care delivery system. Giardiasis has become a well-known intestinal disease, and trichomoniasis remains among the most common sexually transmitted diseases. Diseases such as cryptosporidiosis, toxoplasmosis, and pneumocystosis were relatively new in the 1990s, and increasing coverage in media reports is testimony to their importance. Even malaria is still encountered in travelers and immigrant groups.

It takes years of training and experience to be a good parasitologist. A keen and discriminating eye is essential, and the right questions must be asked to distinguish between organisms and tissue debris. If your future goals are not yet established, you might wish to consider parasitology as a career.

Summary

Protozoa are of interest to microbiologists because they are unicellular, have a microscopic size, and cause infectious disease. They are usually very large organisms, and the functions of their cells bear a resemblance to the functions of multicellular organisms. The majority of protozoa are heterotrophic, and some exist in the trophozoite and cyst forms, the latter a very resistant form.

While a new classification system emerges, protozoa are divided into four broad categories according to the method of locomotion they display. Protozoa such as amoebas move by means of pseudopodia. Flagellated protozoa and ciliated protozoa are also recognized, and the nonmotile protozoa are termed apicomplexans, or sporozoa. Chlorophyll-containing protozoa, species that undergo sexual recombinations, and various other interesting forms are found within the groups.

The most serious amoeba-related disease is amoebiasis, due to *Entamoeba histolytica*. Intestinal ulcers and sharp, appendicitislike pain accompany the disease. Giardiasis is also an intestinal disease, but the protozoa do not penetrate the tissue. The agent, a flagellate named *Giardia lamblia*, is acquired from contaminated food and water. Trichomoniasis, a sexually transmitted disease caused by a flagellate, is among the most common diseases in the United States.

Arthropod vectors can play a role in protozoal disease. Sleeping sickness (trypanosomiasis) and leishmaniasis are transmitted by tsetse flies and sandflies, respectively. Blood invasion and tissue involvement characterize both diseases. Among the ciliates, *Balantidium coli* is known as an intestinal parasite acquired by a fecal-oral route. An apicomplexan, *Toxoplasma gondii*, causes serious disease in AIDS patients, as do other apicomplexans named *Cryptosporidium coccidi* and *Pneumocystis carinii*. *Toxoplasma* affects various organs, especially those of the nervous system. *Cryptosporidium* causes choleralike diarrhea, and *Pneumocystis* is an agent of pneumonia. Another nonmotile protozoan, *Plasmodium*, is the cause of malaria, one of the most serious global health problems. Transmitted by mosquitoes, *Plasmodium* species destroy the red blood cells and often bring on death. A similar disease called babesiosis is tickborne and more localized in occurrence.

Questions for Thought and Discussion

1. *Giardia lamblia* has been imaginatively described as a "cross-eyed tennis racket." From the margin diagram and electron micrograph of this organism, can you think of any other such descriptions? Considering the other protozoa in this chapter, what innovative descriptions can you give of them?

2. A newspaper article written in the 1980s asserted that parasitology is a "subject of low priority in medical schools, largely because the diseases are considered as exotic infections that occur in remote parts of the world." Do you agree with the contention that they are "exotic infections that occur in remote parts of the world"? Would you favor increased attention to protozoal diseases and more study of the general field of parasitology in the medical school curriculum? Why?

3. In the early part of this century, quinine syrup was taken to prevent malaria during visits to tropical regions of the world. To most people, the taste of quinine is very bitter, but the British found a way to make it less objectionable by mixing it with a type of alcoholic liquor. What do you suppose was that liquor, and how did the drink come to be known?

4. On returning from the Persian Gulf War, American servicemen were not accepted as blood donors because there was concern about their having been exposed to *Leishmania* species. What is the connection?

5. The incidence of malaria is said to be skyrocketing in Africa, in part because of the antidrought measures being used in certain regions and the agricultural

improvements being developed in other areas. Why is the malaria increase related to these measures?

6. The term *irritable bowel syndrome* is often used when a physician cannot explain why a patient is suffering long-lasting diarrhea, abdominal pain, and fatigue. (Such a diagnosis is euphemistically called a wastebasket diagnosis.) What candidates for this syndrome might be found in this chapter, and what is the description of each organism sought out in the cases you mention?

7. Recent outbreaks of waterborne protozoal disorders of the intestinal tract have raised the possibility that municipalities may have to begin filtering their water instead of just chlorinating

it. Cost estimates for the filtering technology could reach into the millions or billions of dollars. Do you think the average taxpayer will consider the money well spent?

8. An anonymous CDC epidemiologist once said in an interview: "Day-care centers are the open sewers of the twentieth century." Would you agree? Why or why not?

9. You and a friend who is 3 months pregnant stop at a hamburger stand for lunch. Based on your knowledge of toxoplasmosis, what helpful advice can you give your friend? On returning home, you notice that she has two cats. What additional information might you be inclined to share with her?

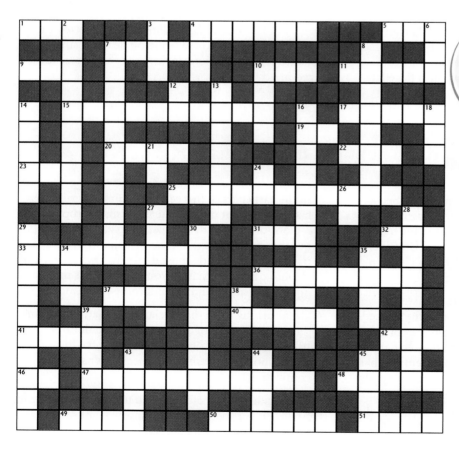

Review

A major theme of this chapter has been the protozoal diseases that affect humans. To review the chapter contents, solve the following crossword puzzle. The answers to the puzzle are in Appendix D.

■ ACROSS

1. Pet that is a reservoir for *Toxoplasma gondii*.
4. One of the species that causes malaria (abbr).
5. *Trichomonas* has _____ posterior flagellum.
7. Discovered the agent of African sleeping sickness.
9. Pregnant women should not clean an animal's litter _____.
10. Agency that summarizes protozoal disease statistics.
11. Specimen examined to detect *Trichomonas* infection.
15. Genus of apicomplexans involved in malaria.
17. Possible mode of transmission of *Giardia lamblia*.

10. Malaria is widely accepted as a contributing factor to the downfall of Rome. Over the decades, the incidence of malaria seemed to increase with expansion of the Roman Empire, which stretched from the Sahara desert to the borders of Scotland, and from the Persian Gulf to the western shores of Portugal. How do you suspect the disease and the expansion are connected?

11. The flagellated protozoan *Giardia lamblia* is named for Alfred Giard, French biologist of the late 1800s, and Vilem Dusan Lambl, Bohemian physician of the same period. Unfortunately, this information does not tell us much about the organism (except who did much of the descriptive work). Quite to the contrary, the names of other protozoa in this chapter tell us much. What are some examples of the more informative names?

12. It has been said that until recent times, many victims of a particular protozoal disease were buried alive because their life processes had slowed to the point where they could not be detected with the primitive technology available. Which disease was probably present?

13. In 1989, giardiasis was the most reported disease in the state of Vermont. Assuming that Vermont residents have reasonably good standards of hygiene, how is it that a disease like giardiasis can top the list of reported diseases in that state?

14. The outbreak of infections due to *Cryptosporidium* has prompted a reevaluation of drinking water purification systems in the United States. Of particular concern is the observation that *Cryptosporidium* species are unaffected by chlorine, the major

---

19. Amoeba (initials) that may cause nervous system illness.
20. Arthropod that transmits *Babesia microti*.
22. Climate where malaria is commonly found.
23. Emitted from intestine during cases of giardiasis.
25. Sexually transmitted flagellated protozoan.
31. Type of cell (abbr) infected by *Toxoplasma gondii*.
32. Number of malaria attacks possible before death.
33. Induces intestinal ulcers and sharp pains after water transmission.
36. Arthropod that transmits *Plasmodium* species.
37. System (abbr) affected during cases of trypanosomiasis.
40. Mode of locomotion of ciliates.
41. How a protozoan is able to _____ determines its group designation.
42. Once believed to transmit malaria.
46. There are _____ flagella in *Balantidium coli*.
47. Genus of protozoa involved in sleeping sickness.
48. Extraordinarily high during cases of malaria.

49. Resistant form present in *Entamoeba* and *Giardia*.
50. Insect fluid that contains malarial parasites.
51. Number of classes of protozoa.

■ DOWN

2. Causes a disease that resembles infectious mononucleosis.
3. *Triatoma* species live in the _____ walls of South American huts.
4. Can be infected by *Toxoplasma*.
6. Body organ infected by *Acanthamoeba* species.
7. Ciliated protozoan that causes intestinal illness.
8. Genus of arthropod that transmits *T. cruzi*.
10. Possible complication of trypanosomiasis.
12. Sporozoa display _____ evidence of locomotion in the adult form.
13. Mastigophora species with two nuclei and eight flagella.
14. Symptom present in people with *Pneumocystis* infection.
16. Causes a lung disease that is common in AIDS patients.

18. Cell (abbr) in which *Plasmodium* undergoes its life cycle.
21. Apicomplexan (initials) that induces choleralike diarrhea.
24. Trichomoniasis is associated with an elevated vaginal _____.
26. State (abbr) where babesiosis is known to occur.
27. Fly that transmits protozoan that causes trypanosomiasis.
28. Stage in the life cycle of *Plasmodium*.
29. Flagellated protozoan that causes kala-azar and Oriental sore.
30. Group to which amoebas belong.
34. Number of recognized forms of trypanosomiasis.
35. Serious human disease complicated by protozoal infection.
38. Protozoan (initials) that causes a life-threatening lung disease.
39. Rare hamburger _____ can be a mode of transmission for *Toxoplasma*.
43. Resistant form present in *Entamoeba* and *Giardia*.
44. Environment from which amoebic cysts can be obtained.
45. The motion of *Giardia* resembles that of a falling _____.

disinfectant used in drinking water. Indeed, in a 1995 interview, the head of a research team studying the chlorine resistance of *Cryptosporidium* said, "You can wash these things in Clorox and they will smile right back at you." And an earlier CDC study showed that *Cryptosporidium* could actually grow on Clorox powder. In view of these findings, what alternatives might be available for safeguarding the nation from *Cryptosporidium*-contaminated water?

15. African herdsmen know that to prevent trypanoso-miasis, cattle should be driven across the "fly belt" from one grazing ground to another only at night. What does this bit of folk knowledge tell you about tsetse flies?

16. In 1991, cardiologists at a Los Angeles hospital hypothesized that a few patients with a certain pro-tozoal disease could easily be lost among the far larger population of heart disease sufferers patroniz-ing county clinics. They proved their theory by find-ing 25 patients with this protozoal disease among patients previously diagnosed as having coronary heart disease. Which protozoal disease was involved?

17. In the 1950s, this African country was called the Bel-gian Congo. Then in the 1960s, it became Zaire. Cur-rently it is the Democratic Republic of the Congo. Through all these political changes and episodes of civil strife, the epidemic of African sleeping sickness has remained. Why?

http://microbiology.jbpub.com

The site features **eLearning,** an on-line review area that provides quizzes and other tools to help you study for your class. You can also follow useful links for in-depth information, read more MicroFocus stories, or just find out the latest microbiology news.

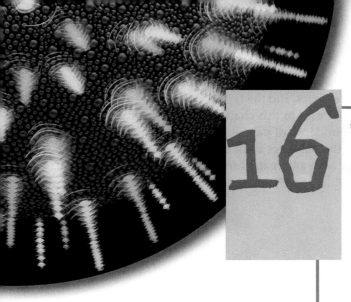

16 The Multicellular Parasites

Pass the Sushi, Carefully

—Headline to an article alerting consumers to the possible parasites in raw fish

O N FEBRUARY 13, 1984, A GROUP of 18 students from the United States arrived in Kenya for various purposes of study. The weather was hot and humid, so the students decided to improvise a small swimming pool. They carefully placed rocks and branches across a small stream and within a few hours, they had their pool. The water was cool and refreshing, and they congratulated themselves on their ingenuity.

But soon a problem developed. Several students broke out with an itchy rash, and subsequently, 14 of the group became acutely ill with fever, diarrhea, malaise, and weight loss. Two of the students developed paralysis of the lower extremities and had to return home for treatment. Stool examinations revealed the eggs of *Schistosoma mansoni*, a parasitic worm. Apparently the water had been contaminated. What had begun as a pleasant day turned into a nightmare.

shis-to-so'mah

Schistosomiasis is one of the diseases caused by the multicellular parasites we shall study in this chapter. Multicellular parasites, including the flatworms and roundworms, probably infect more people worldwide than any other group of organisms. They range in size from the tiny flukes, which must be studied with a microscope, to the tapeworms, which sometimes reach 20 feet in length. In the strict sense, flatworms and roundworms are animals, but they are also studied in microbiology because of their small size and ability to cause disease. Together with the protozoa discussed in Chapter 15, they are the subject of study of the biological discipline known as **parasitology**.

shis'to-so-mi'a-sis

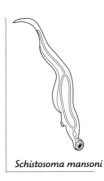

Schistosoma mansoni

Our review of the multicellular parasites will be a brief one. We shall include descriptions of the parasites, their life cycles, and the types of organisms and tissues they infect. You may note that the diseases in this chapter have few unique symptoms and are characterized by an abundance of parasites in a particular area of the body. Often the body will tolerate the parasites until the worm burden becomes immense. At that point, interference with an organ's function develops, and disease symptoms follow.

16.1
Flatworms

plat′e-hel-min′thēz

Flatworms belong to the animal phylum **Platyhelminthes**, a name derived from the Greek *platy-* for "flat" and *helminth* for "worm." All the parasites in this phylum have flattened bodies that are slender and broadly leaflike, or long and ribbonlike (FIGURE 16.1). The animals exhibit **bilateral symmetry**, meaning that when cut in the longitudinal plane, the body yields identical halves.

As multicellular animals, flatworms have tissues functioning as organs in organ systems. Many species have a gut consisting of a sac with a single opening. Complex reproductive systems are found in many animals of the group, and a large number of species have both male and female reproductive organs. These organisms are termed **hermaphroditic**.

her-maf′ro-dit′ik
tur′be-la′re-ah

Flatworms are divided into three classes. The first class, Turbellaria, includes free-living flatworms that do not cause disease and therefore will not be covered here. The common planarian studied in general biology programs is a typical member of the Turbellaria. The second class, Trematoda, includes the flukes. We shall begin our coverage with this group of parasites. The third class, Cestoda, consists of tapeworms. These parasites will be discussed after the flukes.

trem′ah-to′dah

A GENERAL DESCRIPTION OF FLUKES

Flukes are leaflike parasitic worms of the class **Trematoda**. Generally, flukes have complex life cycles that may include encysted egg stages and temporary larval forms. Sucker devices are commonly present to enable the parasite to hold fast to its host. In many cases, two hosts exist: an **intermediate host**, which harbors the larval form, and a **definitive host**, or final host, which harbors the sexually mature adult form. In this chapter, we shall be concerned with parasites whose definitive host is a human.

FIGURE 16.1

Two Examples of Flatworms

(a) A scanning electron micrograph of the fluke *Fasciola hepatica*. Note the flattened, broad, and leaflike shape of this parasite. *F. hepatica* thrives in the liver of humans. The ventral and oral suckers used for attachment to the tissue can be seen.
(b) An unmagnified view of the tapeworm *Taenia saginata*. This flatworm is long and ribbonlike, and consists of hundreds of visible segments. *T. saginata* infects the human intestinal tract.

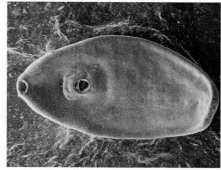
(a)

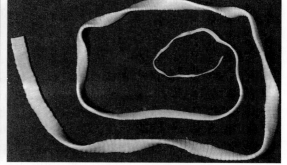
(b)

The life cycle of a fluke often contains several phases. In the human host, the parasite produces **fertilized eggs** generally released in the feces. When the eggs reach water, they hatch and develop into tiny ciliated larvae called **miracidia** (sing., miracidium). The miracidia penetrate **snails** (the intermediate host) and go through a series of asexual reproductive stages, often including **sporocyst** and **redia** stages. Rediae become tadpolelike **cercariae**, which are released to the water. Now the cercariae develop into encysted forms called **metacercariae**, which make their way back to humans. We shall see variations on this basic life cycle in the discussions of fluke diseases that follow.

Miracidia: tiny, ciliated larvae of flukes.

Cercariae: tadpolelike stages in the life cycles of flukes.

BLOOD FLUKE DISEASE

Three important species of flukes invade the bloodstream in humans: ***Schistosoma mansoni, S. japonicum***, and ***S. haematobium***. The first is distributed throughout Africa and South America, the second in the Far East, and the third mainly in Africa. The WHO estimates that 250 million people worldwide are infected with *Schistosoma*, including about 400,000 individuals in the United States. The disease is called **schistosomiasis**. In some regions, the term **bilharziasis** is still used; it comes from the older name for the genus, *Bilharzia*.

*shis-to-so'mah
jah-pon'ĭ-kum
hēm'ah-tōb'e-um*

*bil'har-zi'ah-sis
bil-har'zi-ah*

Species of *Schistosoma* measure about 10 mm in length. Male and female species mate in the human liver and produce eggs that are released in the feces (FIGURE 16.2). The eggs hatch to miracidia in water, and the miracidia make their way to snails, where conversions to sporocysts and cercariae take place. The cercariae escape

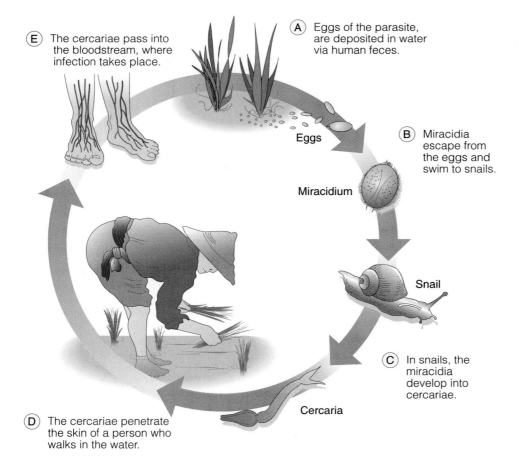

E The cercariae pass into the bloodstream, where infection takes place.

A Eggs of the parasite, are deposited in water via human feces.

Eggs

B Miracidia escape from the eggs and swim to snails.

Miracidium

Snail

C In snails, the miracidia develop into cercariae.

Cercaria

D The cercariae penetrate the skin of a person who walks in the water.

FIGURE 16.2

The Life Cycle of the Blood Fluke, *Schistosoma mansoni*

from the snails and attach themselves to the bare skin of humans. Cercariae become young schistosomes, which infect the blood and cause fever and chills. The major effects of disease are due to eggs formed in the liver. Liver damage is usually substantial. Eggs also gather in the intestinal wall causing ulceration, diarrhea, and abdominal pain. Bladder infection is signaled by bloody urine and pain on urination. Outbreaks may have substantial consequences, as MicroFocus 16.1 explains.

Certain species of *Schistosoma* penetrate no farther than the skin because the definitive hosts are birds instead of humans. The cercariae of these schistosomes cause dermatitis in the skin and a condition commonly known as **swimmer's itch**. After penetration, the cercariae are attacked and destroyed by the body's immune system, but they release allergenic substances that cause the itching and body rash (FIGURE 16.3). The condition, not a serious threat to health, is common in northern lakes in the United States.

Swimmer's itch:
a skin condition caused by allergenic substances released by *Schistosoma* species.

FIGURE 16.3

An Outbreak of Schistosomiasis in Delaware

TEXTBOOK CASES

1. On October 19, 1991, a group of 37 students from a local high school biology class visited a shellfishing area at Cape Henlopen State Park in Delaware. The tide was low, the water was calm, and the weather was sunny and unseasonably warm. Several ducks and geese were nearby.

2. The students and their teacher spent about 2 hours wading in the water collecting specimens. There were many clams, oysters, and snails in the water, as well as other marine specimens of interest.

3. Within 10 days of the trip, 29 of the 37 students developed pruritic dermatitis, an itching skin condition. Eleven of the affected students visited their doctors for treatment. Eventually, 36 of the 37 individuals developed pruritis; the only unaffected student was one who did not go into the water.

4. Public health investigators examined snails from the seawater. Schistosomes normally associated with ducks, geese, and other birds were found in a small percentage of snails examined. Also, it is known that thousands of schistosomes can be released from a single snail, and the release is favored by weather conditions seen that day.

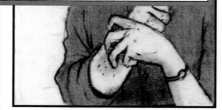

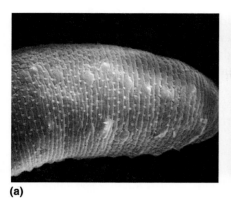

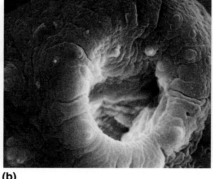

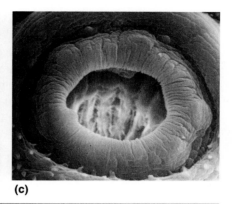

(a)

(b)

(c)

FIGURE 16.4

The Chinese Liver Fluke

Scanning electron microscope views of *Clonorchis sinensis*, the Chinese liver fluke. (a) A whole mount showing the anterior aspect of the parasite (×2400). (b) The oral sucker device (×7000). (c) The ventral sucker device (×4800).

CHINESE LIVER FLUKE DISEASE

The **Chinese liver fluke** is so named because it infects the liver and is common in many regions of the Orient, especially China, southern Asia, and Japan. The organism is named *Clonorchis sinensis*. It has oral and ventral sucker devices (**FIGURE 16.4**) and is hermaphroditic, with a complex reproductive system.

klo-nor′kis si-nen′sis

Eggs of *C. sinensis* contain complete miracidia, which emerge after the eggs enter water. The miracidia penetrate snails and change into sporocysts, which then produce a generation of elongated rediae. These rediae become cercariae, which escape from the snail and bore into the muscles of fish, the second intermediary host. Now the cercariae develop into encysted metacercariae, and humans acquire the metacercariae by consuming raw or poorly cooked fish. Public health officials recommend heating fish to a minimum of 50°C for 15 minutes to destroy the cysts. In

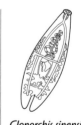

Clonorchis sinensis

MicroFocus 16.1

INVASION

In the late 1940s, clashes between the nationalist Chinese, headed by Chiang Kai-Shek, and the communist Chinese, led by Mao Tse Tung, heated up to the point of open warfare. After months of fighting, the communist forces drove Chiang's troops off the Chinese mainland and onto the island of Taiwan (then called Formosa). It soon became apparent to world leaders that a communist invasion of Taiwan was imminent.

But invading an island takes a certain type of training. Therefore, communist generals gathered their troops by the hundreds of thousands in a swampy area near the southern coast of mainland China to learn the methods of amphibious warfare. Unbeknown to them, however, the area was infested with parasites and snails, and within days, over 30,000 men were infected with *Schistosoma*. The troops suffered severe fever, liver damage, and intestinal distress, and Chinese leaders were forced to postpone their assault on Taiwan for several months.

The delay was critical because it gave the nationalist Chinese precious extra time to prepare for invasion. In addition, intelligence reports of the impending invasion reached U.S. President Harry Truman, and he sent ships from the Seventh Naval Fleet to the waters off Taiwan to preserve the neutrality of Chiang's forces. Eventually, these and other factors persuaded the communist Chinese to abandon their assault, and the republic of Taiwan was left intact.

We shall never know whether the invasion would have succeeded or what the political ramifications might have been. Indeed, some historians point out that the United States was preparing to back the nationalist Chinese, while the former Soviet Union was readying itself to support the communists. One thing does appear certain: A worm played a significant role in the turn of world events.

humans, the metacercariae become adults and migrate from the small intestine up the bile duct to the gall bladder and liver, where infection takes place.

The effect of *C. sinensis* on humans depends on the extent of infection. Substantial infection in the gall bladder may lead to duct blockage and poor digestion of fats. There may also be damage to the liver as eggs accumulate in the tissues of this organ (FIGURE 16.5). Often the patient is without symptoms because of the low number of parasites. Cats, dogs, and pigs may also carry the metacercaria cysts.

OTHER FLUKE DISEASES

The **intestinal fluke** of humans is known as ***Fasciolopsis buski***, a large fluke that can be as long as 8 cm. The parasite lives in the duodenum, where it causes diarrhea and intestinal blockage. From the feces, eggs enter water in such places as rice paddies and drainage ditches, and miracidia emerge. Snails are the next host for the

Gall bladder:
the pouch on the underside of the liver that stores bile.

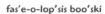

fas'e-o-lop'sis boo'ski

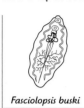

Fasciolopsis buski

FIGURE 16.5

The Life Cycle of the Chinese Liver Fluke, *Clonorchis sinensis*

The photograph shows eggs of *C. sinensis* in human tissue. The thick protective covering of the eggs is evident.

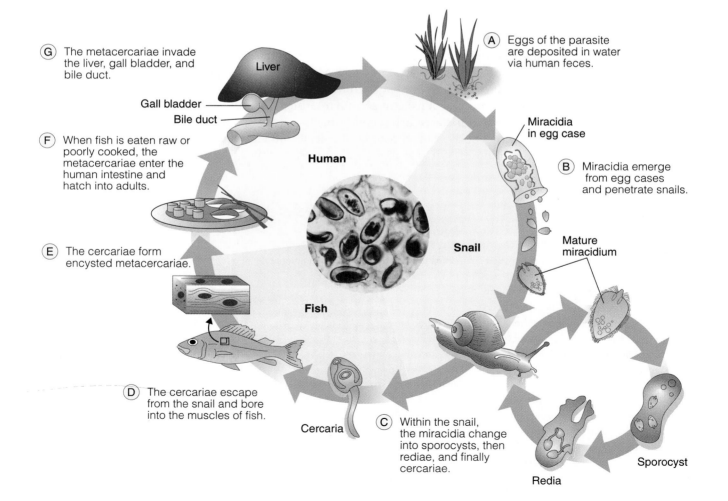

(G) The metacercariae invade the liver, gall bladder, and bile duct.

(F) When fish is eaten raw or poorly cooked, the metacercariae enter the human intestine and hatch into adults.

(E) The cercariae form encysted metacercariae.

(D) The cercariae escape from the snail and bore into the muscles of fish.

(A) Eggs of the parasite are deposited in water via human feces.

(B) Miracidia emerge from egg cases and penetrate snails.

(C) Within the snail, the miracidia change into sporocysts, then rediae, and finally cercariae.

Liver

Gall bladder
Bile duct

Human

Snail

Fish

Cercaria

Miracidia in egg case

Mature miracidium

Sporocyst

Redia

miracidia, and cercariae escape from the snail and swim to blades of grass and vegetation where metacercariae form. Such plants as water chestnuts and water bamboo are likely to be contaminated. Consumption of these vegetables raw or poorly cooked leads to human infection.

The human **lung fluke** is *Paragonimus westermani*. This parasite is common in the Orient and South Pacific. Its eggs are coughed up from the lung, swallowed, and then excreted in the feces. Cercariae develop in snails, and metacercariae later form in crabs. Infection follows when people eat the poorly cooked crabmeat, and the flukes pass from the intestine to the blood to the lungs. Difficult breathing and chronic cough develop as the parasites accumulate in the lungs. Fatalities are possible.

The human **liver fluke** is *Fasciola hepatica*, a leaflike flatworm common in sheep and cattle. Eggs from the animal reach the soil in feces, and if snails are present, the conversions to cercariae and encysted metacercariae follow. Parasite cysts gather on vegetation such as watercress, and ingestion by humans follows. The parasites penetrate the intestinal wall and migrate to the liver, where tissue damage may be substantial, especially if fluke numbers are high.

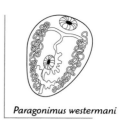

Paragonimus westermani

par'ah-gon'ĭ-mus wes'ter-man-i fah-si-o'lah

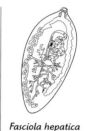

Fasciola hepatica

A GENERAL DESCRIPTION OF TAPEWORMS

Tapeworms belong to the third class of flatworms, **Cestoda**. These worms have long, flat bodies consisting of a head region and a ribbonlike series of segments called **proglottids**. The head region, called the **scolex**, contains hooks or suckerlike devices that enable the worm to hold fast to infected tissue. Behind the scolex is a neck region in which new proglottids are formed. These new proglottids constantly push the mature proglottids to the rear. The most distant ones, called **gravid proglottids**, are filled with fertilized eggs. As they break free, they spread the eggs of the tapeworm.

Tapeworms generally live in the intestines of a host organism. In this environment they are constantly bathed by nutrient-rich fluid, from which they absorb their food. Tapeworms have adapted to a parasitic existence and have lost their intestines, but they still retain well-developed muscular, excretory, and nervous systems.

Tapeworms are widespread parasites that infect practically all mammals, as well as many other vertebrates. Since they are more dependent on their hosts than flukes, tapeworms have precarious life cycles. Tapeworms have a limited range of hosts, and the chances for completing the cycle are often slim. With rare exceptions, tapeworms require at least two hosts, as we shall see in the following examples of tapeworm diseases.

Scolex:
the head region of a tapeworm.

Gravid proglottids:
segments filled with fertilized eggs at the back end of a tapeworm.

BEEF AND PORK TAPEWORM DISEASES

Humans are the definitive hosts for both the **beef tapeworm** *Taenia saginata* and the **pork tapeworm** *Taenia solium*. People infected with one of these tapeworms expel numerous gravid proglottids daily. The proglottids accumulate in the soil and are consumed by cattle or pigs. Embryos from the eggs travel to the animal's muscle, where they encyst. Humans then acquire the cysts in poorly cooked beef or pork.

The beef tapeworm may reach 25 feet in length, while the pork tapeworm length averages 20 feet. Each tapeworm may have up to 2000 proglottids. Attachment via the scolex occurs in the small intestine, and obstruction of this organ may result. In most cases, however, there are few symptoms other than mild diarrhea, and a mutual

tā'ne-ah saj-in-ah'tah

so'le-um

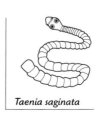

Taenia saginata

tolerance may develop between parasite and host. The notion that a tapeworm causes severe emaciation is largely unfounded.

FISH TAPEWORM DISEASE

di-fil'o-both're-um

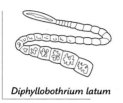

Diphyllobothrium latum

The **fish tapeworm** is the longest human parasite, some species measuring 60 feet in length. The parasite is named ***Diphyllobothrium latum***. Its life cycle is complex and includes two intermediate hosts: a small shrimplike crustacean called a **copepod** and a fish (FIGURE 16.6). The copepod acquires tapeworm embryos from proglottids excreted into water by humans. Next the copepod is eaten by fish such as minnows, and the embryo finds its way to the fish muscle. Minnows may be eaten by larger fish such as trout, perch, and pike, and the embryos are passed along. Consumption of raw or poorly cooked fish by humans completes the cycle.

Infections with fish tapeworms occur throughout the world. In the United States, infections are most common in the Great Lakes region. Obstruction of the

FIGURE 16.6

The Life Cycle of the Fish Tapeworm, *Diphyllobothrium latum*

The photograph shows *D. latum* isolated from a human patient.

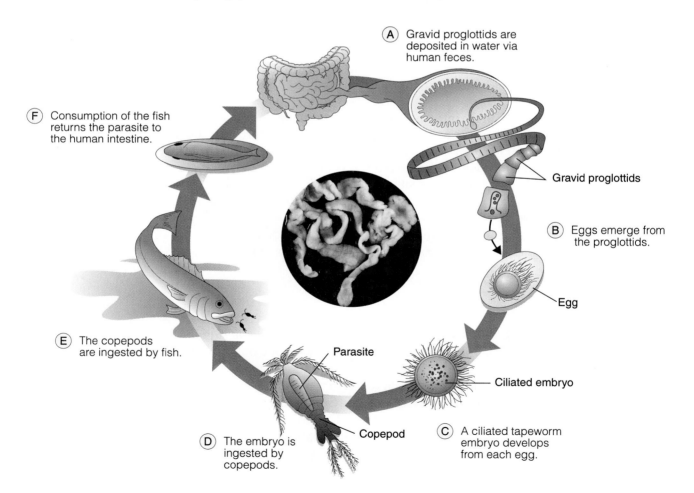

(A) Gravid proglottids are deposited in water via human feces.

Gravid proglottids

(B) Eggs emerge from the proglottids.

Egg

(C) A ciliated tapeworm embryo develops from each egg.

Ciliated embryo

Parasite

Copepod

(D) The embryo is ingested by copepods.

(E) The copepods are ingested by fish.

(F) Consumption of the fish returns the parasite to the human intestine.

small intestine may occur, and anemia may develop in the patient, possibly due to the parasite's consumption of vitamin B_{12} needed for red blood cell formation. Cooking at 50°C for 15 minutes is generally sufficient to destroy the cysts, but the recent popularity of raw fish dishes has contributed to a rise in the incidence rates of the disease.

OTHER TAPEWORM DISEASES

The **dwarf tapeworm** *Hymenolepis nana* is so named because it is only 25 mm long. The most common tapeworm in humans worldwide, *H. nana* lives in the small intestine, where it holds fast with four sucker devices and a row of small hooks. Eggs released in the feces spread among humans by contaminated food or contact with objects or an infected individual. People living in the southeastern United States often experience infections.

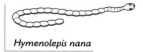

Hymenolepis nana

Dogs and other canines such as wolves, foxes, and coyotes are the definitive hosts for the **dog tapeworm** called ***Echinococcus granulosus*** (FIGURE 16.7). Eggs reach the soil in feces and spread to numerous intermediary hosts, one of which is humans. Contact with a dog may also account for transmission. In humans, the parasites travel by the blood to the liver, where they form thick-walled **hydatid cysts**. Surgery may be necessary for their removal. Completion of the life cycle takes place when a dog consumes infected animal liver, such as after a kill. Dog food is another possible source of cysts. The adult tapeworm then emerges to parasitize the dog.

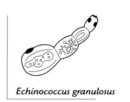

Echinococcus granulosus

The flatworm diseases of humans are summarized in TABLE 16.1.

FIGURE 16.7

The Dog Tapeworm

Two views of the dog tapeworm *Echinococcus granulosus*, as seen by phase-contrast microscopy. (a) The head region, or scolex, of *E. granulosus*. The hooks at the end of the scolex are used to attach to the infected tissue; the indentations at the base of the scolex emphasize its presence. (b) The hydatid cyst of *E. granulosus* isolated from a lung section of a 31-year-old woman immigrant from the Sudan. (Both magnifications ×580.)

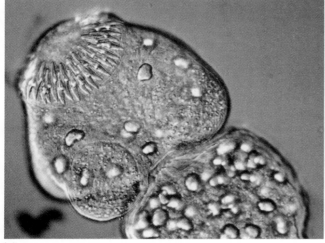

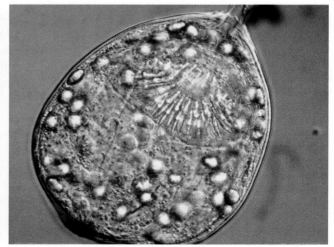

(a)

(b)

TABLE 16.1

A Summary of Flatworm Parasitic Diseases in Humans

ORGANISM	DISEASE	TRANSMISSION	ORGANS AFFECTED	CHARACTERISTIC SIGN	ANIMAL HOST
Schistosoma mansoni S. japonicum S. haematobium	Blood fluke disease	Water contact	Skin Liver Blood	Rash Liver damage Fever	Snail
Clonorchis sinensis	Chinese liver fluke disease	Fish consumption	Gall bladder Liver	Liver damage Poor fat digestion	Snail Fish
Fasciolopsis buski	Intestinal fluke disease	Consumption of water plants	Intestine	Diarrhea	Snail
Paragonimus westermani	Lung fluke disease	Consumption of crabs	Lungs	Cough Poor breathing	Snail Crab
Fasciola hepatica	Liver fluke disease	Consumption of water plants	Liver	Liver damage	Snail Cattle
Taenia saginata	Beef tapeworm disease	Beef consumption	Intestine	Diarrhea	Cattle
Taenia solium	Pork tapeworm disease	Pork consumption	Intestine	Diarrhea	Pig
Diphyllobothrium latum	Fish tapeworm disease	Fish consumption	Intestine	Diarrhea Anemia	Copepod Fish
Hymenolepis nana	Dwarf tapeworm disease	Food Contact	Intestine	Diarrhea	None significant
Echinococcus granulosus	Dog tapeworm disease	Contact	Liver	Liver damage	Dog, other canines

To this point . . .

We have surveyed many of the flatworm parasites that infect humans. The flatworms include flukes, which are slender and broadly leaflike, and tapeworms, which are long and ribbonlike. Flukes belong to the class Trematoda. They have complex life cycles, with snails serving as an intermediate host. Stages in the life cycle include the miracidium, cercaria, and metacercaria, among others. The blood fluke is acquired by contact with water, while the Chinese liver fluke is ingested in raw or poorly cooked fish. Intestinal flukes and lung flukes are also acquired in foods.

We then discussed the tapeworms of the class Cestoda. These parasites generally live in the human intestinal tract. Proglottids carry tapeworm eggs to the soil or water, from which they are consumed by animals or fish. Human infection is reestablished when contaminated meat or fish is eaten. Beef, pork, and fish tapeworm diseases are passed along in this way. Contaminated food or objects may be the source of dwarf tapeworm disease, and dogs may pass dog tapeworms to humans. In dog tapeworm disease, humans are an intermediary host.

We shall now focus on the roundworms. Roundworms are anatomically more complex than flatworms and are classified in a completely different phylum of animals. We shall see how the life cycles of roundworms are considerably more simple than the cycles of flatworms, and how infection is spread much more easily. Among the roundworms are those that cause pinworm disease and trichinosis, two diseases that are common in the United States.

Roundworms

Roundworms occupy every imaginable habitat on Earth. They live in the sea, in freshwater, and in soil from polar regions to the tropics. Good topsoil, for example, may contain billions of roundworms per acre. They parasitize every conceivable type of animal and plant, causing both economic damage and serious disease.

The roundworms are a subgroup of the phylum **Aschelminthes**, from the Greek *asc-* for "sac" and *helminth* for "worm." The sac refers to a digestive tract set apart from the internal muscles in a saclike or pouchlike arrangement, a feature not found in flatworms. In reality, the sac is a tubular intestine open at the mouth and anus. Food can thus move in one direction, a substantial improvement over the blind sac arrangement in Platyhelminthes. This is one reason the Aschelminthes are considered to be more evolutionarily advanced than the Platyhelminthes.

Roundworms have separate sexes. Following fertilization of the female by the male, the eggs hatch to larvae that resemble miniature adults. Growth then occurs by cellular enlargement and mitosis. Damage in hosts is generally caused by large worm burdens in the intestines, blood vessels, or lymphatic vessels (FIGURE 16.8). Also, the infestation may result in nutritional deficiency or damage to the muscles.

Roundworms have been traditionally known as **nematodes** because they are threadlike (*nema* is Latin for "thread"). Indeed, in some texts the phylum of roundworms is called **Nematoda**, and in other books it is referred to as **Nemathelminthes**.

ask'hel-min'thēz

plat'e-hel-min'thēz

Nematode: an alternate name for a roundworm.

ne-mah-to'dah
ne'mat-hel-min'thēz

PINWORM DISEASE

The widely encountered **pinworm** is a roundworm called *Enterobius vermicularis*. This worm is the most common helminthic parasite in the United States, with an estimated 30 percent of children and 16 percent of adults serving as hosts. The male and female worms live in the distant part of the small intestine and in the large intestine, where the symptoms of infection include diarrhea and itching in the anal region. The female worm is about 10 mm long, and the male is about half that size.

The life cycle of the pinworm is relatively simple. Females migrate to the anal region at night and lay a considerable number of eggs. The area itches intensely, and scratching contaminates the hands and bed linens with eggs. Reinfection may then take place if the hands are brought to the mouth or if eggs are deposited in foods by the hands. The eggs are swallowed, whereupon they hatch in the duodenum and mature in the regions beyond.

en'ter-o'be-us ver'mik-u-la'ris

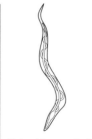

Enterobius vermicularis

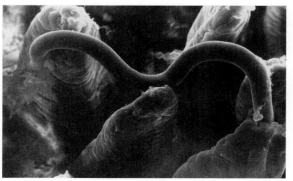

FIGURE 16.8

The Roundworm *Trichinella spiralis*

A scanning electron micrograph of the roundworm *Trichinella spiralis* in human intestinal tissue. This parasite is the cause of trichinosis. In the photograph, the worm is emerging from one intestinal villus and entering another villus.

Diagnosis of pinworm disease may be accurately made by applying the sticky side of cellophane tape to the area about the anus and examining the tape microscopically for pinworm eggs (FIGURE 16.9). Several drugs are effective for controlling the disease, and all members of an infected person's family should be treated because transfer of the parasite has probably taken place. Even without medication, however, the worms will die in a few weeks, and the infection will disappear as long as reinfection is prevented.

WHIPWORM DISEASE

trik-u'ris trik-e-u'rah

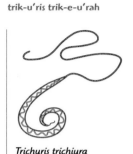

Trichuris trichiura

The **whipworm** ***Trichuris trichiura*** acquired its name from the observation that its anterior end is long and slender like a buggy whip. Infection takes place in the human intestine, especially near the junction of the small and large intestines, as shown in FIGURE 16.10. Damage to the intestinal lining may be severe, and appendicitislike pain is sometimes experienced, with some anemia resulting from ingestion of blood by the parasite.

The female whipworm is approximately 40 mm long; the male is shorter with a characteristically curled tail. Eggs eliminated in the human feces hatch to larvae after

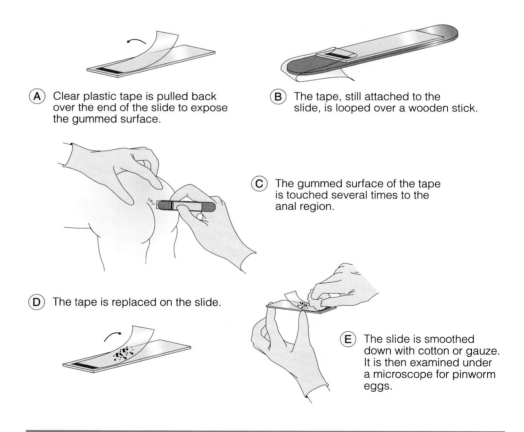

(A) Clear plastic tape is pulled back over the end of the slide to expose the gummed surface.

(B) The tape, still attached to the slide, is looped over a wooden stick.

(C) The gummed surface of the tape is touched several times to the anal region.

(D) The tape is replaced on the slide.

(E) The slide is smoothed down with cotton or gauze. It is then examined under a microscope for pinworm eggs.

FIGURE 16.9

Diagnosing Pinworm Disease

The transparent tape technique used in the diagnosis of pinworm disease.

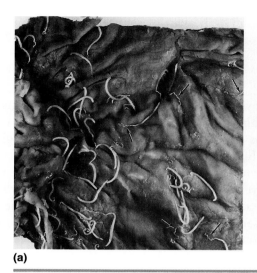

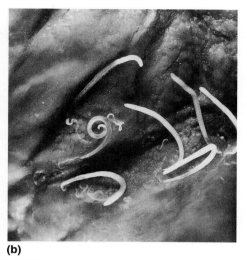

(a) **(b)**

FIGURE 16.10

The Whipworm *Trichuris trichiura*

(a) A view of the whipworm *Trichuris trichiura* in human intestinal tissue. The worms are relatively small compared to other roundworms discussed in this chapter. Whipworms have a long slender form resembling a buggy whip. (b) A closer view.

about two weeks in the soil. Transmission occurs by soil-contaminated food and water as well as by contact with soiled hands. Whipworm disease is encountered where the environment is hot and moist (such as in the tropics), and where poor sanitary facilities exist. Patients often have concurrent infections with other parasites. Diagnosis depends on the identification of eggs in the feces.

ROUNDWORM DISEASE

Infection with "roundworms" usually implies infection with ***Ascaris lumbricoides***. One of the largest intestinal nematodes, the female *A. lumbricoides*, may be up to 1 foot long, and the male, 8 inches long. The parasite resembles an earthworm and is the most wormlike of the helminthic parasites.

A female *Ascaris* is a prolific producer of eggs, sometimes generating over 200,000 per day. The eggs are fertilized and passed to the soil in the feces, where they hatch to larvae. The larvae then attach to plants and are ingested. In many parts of the world, human feces, or nightsoil, is used as fertilizer for crops. This adds to the spread of the parasite. Contact with contaminated fingers and consumption of water containing soil runoff are other possible modes of transmission.

After the larvae have been consumed, the tiny worms grow in the small intestine. Abdominal symptoms develop as the worms reach maturity in about 2 months. Intestinal blockage may be a consequence when tightly compacted masses of worms accumulate, and perforation of the small intestine is possible. In addition, roundworm larvae may pass to the blood and infect the lungs, causing pneumonia. If the larvae are coughed up and then swallowed, intestinal reinfection occurs.

Except for pinworms, *A. lumbricoides* is the most prevalent multicellular parasite in the United States. The WHO estimates that hundreds of millions of people are infected worldwide. Tropical and subtropical regions are the primary foci of disease,

as'kah-ris lum'brĭ-koid'ēz

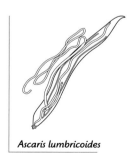

Ascaris lumbricoides

Pneumonia:
a disease of the lung tissues.

but areas of the southwestern United States are heavily infested because eggs remain viable in the moist clay soil of this region.

TRICHINOSIS

Trichinosis is a term familiar to anyone who enjoys pork and pork products, because packages of pork usually contain warnings to cook the meat thoroughly to avoid this disease. Ironically, trichinosis is common where living standards are high enough for pork to be eaten routinely, but the disease is rare where pork is a luxury.

Trichinosis is caused by the small roundworm *Trichinella spiralis*. The worm lives in the intestines of pigs and several other mammals. Larvae of the worm migrate through the blood and penetrate the pig's skeletal muscles, where they remain in cysts. When raw or **poorly cooked pork** is consumed, the cysts pass into the human intestines and the worms emerge. Intestinal pain, vomiting, nausea, and constipation are common symptoms.

Complications of trichinosis occur when *T. spiralis* larvae migrate to the muscles and form cysts. The patient commonly experiences pain in the breathing muscles of the ribs, loss of eye movement due to cyst formation in the eye muscles, swelling of the face, and hemorrhaging in various body tissues. Some sufferers also develop a cough and skin lesions, and the larvae may invade the brain, where they cause paralysis. Paralysis and death occurred in a man in New York in 1985 after he contracted trichinosis by consuming pork inadvertently ground with beef. The man had a habit of nibbling the meat while preparing hamburgers.

The cycle of trichinosis is completed as cysts are transmitted back to nature in the human feces (FIGURE 16.11). Consumption of human waste and garbage then brings the cysts to the pig. Modern methods of agriculture provide standardized feed for pigs, but many pigs are still exposed to the cysts. Consumers should be aware that poorly cooked pork is the principal source of the approximately 150 cases of trichinosis reported in the United States annually. Pickling, smoking, and heavy seasoning are not adequate substitutes for thorough heating, but freezing greatly reduces larval viability. Routine inspection of pigs for *T. spiralis* cysts is not common practice in slaughterhouses, and thus the burden for the prevention of trichinosis falls to the consumer. In 1986, the U.S. government approved the use of low-dose irradiation of fresh pork to combat trichinosis.

HOOKWORM DISEASE

Hookworms are roundworms that have a set of hooks or sucker devices for firm attachment to tissues of the host. Two hookworms, both about 10 mm in length, may be involved in human disease. The first is the **Old World hookworm,** *Ancylostoma duodenale*, which is found in Europe, Asia, and the United States; the second is the **New World hookworm,** *Necator americanus*, which is prevalent in the Caribbean islands (where it may have been brought by slaves from Africa).

Hundreds of millions of people around the globe are believed to be infected by hookworms. These parasites live in the human intestine, where they suck blood from the tissues. Hookworm disease is therefore accompanied by blood loss and is generally manifested by anemia. Cysts may also become lodged in the intestinal wall, and ulcerlike symptoms may develop.

The life cycle of a hookworm involves only a single host, the human (FIGURE 16.12). Hookworm eggs are excreted to the soil, where the larvae emerge as long,

trik′ĭ-nel′ah spir-al′is

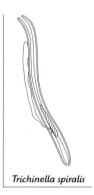

Trichinella spiralis

Cyst:
a dormant, highly resistant form of an organism such as a protozoan or multicellular parasite.

an′kĭ-los′to-mah du-od-in-al′e

ne-ka′tor a-mer-i-ca′nus

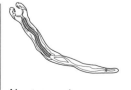

Necator americanus

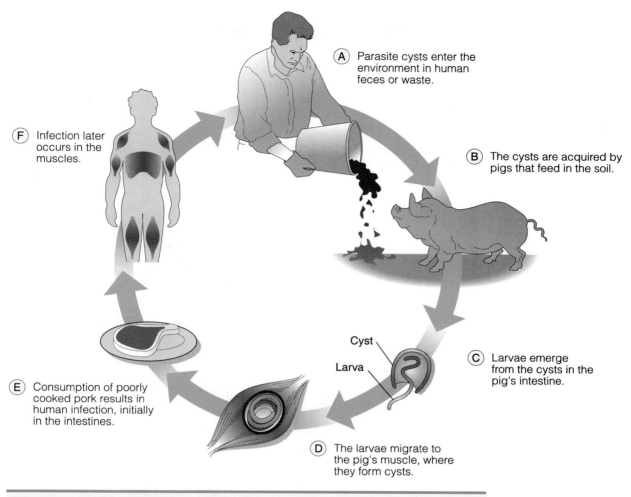

A Parasite cysts enter the environment in human feces or waste.

B The cysts are acquired by pigs that feed in the soil.

F Infection later occurs in the muscles.

C Larvae emerge from the cysts in the pig's intestine.

Cyst

Larva

E Consumption of poorly cooked pork results in human infection, initially in the intestines.

D The larvae migrate to the pig's muscle, where they form cysts.

FIGURE 16.11

The Life Cycle of *Trichinella spiralis*

rodlike **rhabditiform** larvae. These later become threadlike **filariform** larvae that attach themselves to vegetation in the soil. When contact with bare feet is made, the filariform larvae penetrate the skin layers and enter the bloodstream. Soon they localize in the lungs and are carried up to the pharynx in secretions, then swallowed into the intestines.

Hookworms are common where the soil is warm, wet, and contaminated with human feces. The disease is prevalent where people go barefoot. Drugs may be used to reduce the worm burden, and the diet may be supplemented with iron to replace that lost in the loss of blood. It should be noted that dogs and cats also harbor hookworm eggs and pass them in the feces.

rab-dit'ĭ-form

fil-ar'ĭ-form

STRONGYLOIDIASIS

Strongyloidiasis is caused by ***Strongyloides stercoralis***, a parasite that resembles hookworms in appearance, distribution, and life cycle. Adult worms inhabit the small intestine, especially the duodenum, where they cause abdominal pain, nausea,

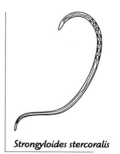

Strongyloides stercoralis

stron'jĭ-loi-di'ah-sis
stron'ji-loi'dez ster-ko-ral'is

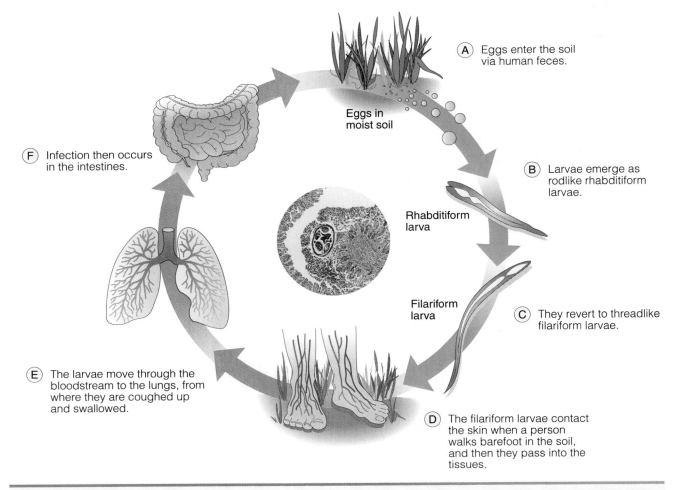

(A) Eggs enter the soil via human feces.

Eggs in moist soil

(F) Infection then occurs in the intestines.

Rhabditiform larva

(B) Larvae emerge as rodlike rhabditiform larvae.

Filariform larva

(C) They revert to threadlike filariform larvae.

(E) The larvae move through the bloodstream to the lungs, from where they are coughed up and swallowed.

(D) The filariform larvae contact the skin when a person walks barefoot in the soil, and then they pass into the tissues.

FIGURE 16.12

The Life Cycle of the Hookworms *Ancylostoma duodenale* and *Necator americanus*

The photograph shows an egg lodged in intestinal tissue.

vomiting, and diarrhea alternating with constipation. Pulmonary symptoms mimic the pneumonia induced by hookworms. A drug called thiabendazole provides effective therapy.

Strongyloidiasis is of importance to Americans because many Vietnam veterans were exposed to the parasites in Southeast Asia. In a 1981 study, for example, doctors tested 530 veterans of Pacific wars for the parasite and found that 43 harbored it in their stools. In some cases, this was almost 40 years after the initial infection. Many reported regular 5-day episodes of itchy skin rash, another sign of the disease.

FILARIASIS

Filariasis is a parasitic disease caused by a roundworm named ***Wuchereria bancrofti***. The worm breeds in the tissues of the human lymphatic system and causes extensive inflammation and damage to the lymphatic vessels and lymph glands. After years of infestation, the arms, legs, and scrotum swell enormously and become distorted with fluid. This condition is known as **elephantiasis** because of the gross

Wuchereria bancrofti

fil′ah-ri′ah-sis
voo′ker-e′re-ah ban-krof′ti

deformity of tissues and the resemblance of the skin to elephant hide (FIGURE 16.13).

The female form of *Wuchereria bancrofti* is about 100 mm long. Its fertilized eggs give rise to tiny eel-like microfilariae, which enter the human bloodstream. The microfilariae are then ingested by **mosquitoes** during a blood meal, where they develop into infective larvae passed along to another human during the next blood meal. The larvae subsequently grow to adults and infect the lymphatic system. Infection is limited to the number of larvae injected by the mosquito, since microfilariae cannot grow to adulthood without first passing through the mosquito.

Filariasis is prevalent where mosquitoes are plentiful, such as in the hot, humid climates of Central and South America and the Caribbean islands. Missionaries, emigrants, and visitors from these areas often carry the worms in their tissues.

GUINEA WORM DISEASE

The **Guinea worm** is a roundworm, thought to have been introduced to Africa, India, and the Middle East by navigators who plied the sealanes between these areas and South Pacific islands such as New Guinea. The worm's scientific name is ***Dracunculus medinensis.***

The male Guinea worm is small, but the female may be up to 80 cm in length. Often the worm lies just below the skin of humans and causes swellings that resemble varicose veins. It causes a skin ulcer through which larvae are discharged into water. A small shrimplike crustacean called a **copepod** picks up the larvae and transmits them to another human when the copepod is consumed in water. Alternately, the copepod is eaten by fish, which then transmit the larvae (MicroFocus 16.2). Once in humans, the larvae migrate to the human skin and grow to adults.

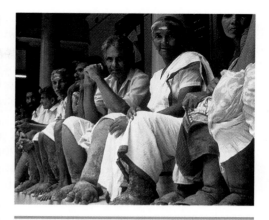

FIGURE 16.13

The Effect of Filariasis

Elephantiasis of the leg caused by the parasite *Wuchereria bancrofti*. The worm breeds in the tissues of the lymphatic vessels and damages them. As fluid accumulates, the legs swell and become distorted.

drah-kung'ku-lus med-i-nen'sis

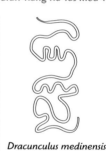

Dracunculus medinensis

MicroFocus 16.2

WELCOME TO NEW YORK CITY!

The Guinea worm had long been a parasite among Scandinavian fishermen and their families. Individuals acquired the worm by drinking water that contained infected crustaceans, or by eating fish that had previously eaten the crustaceans. For the Guinea worm, New York City appeared to be a long way off, but a somewhat circuitous route made the transition possible during the 1800s.

Scandinavians immigrated to the United States in substantial numbers during the nineteenth century. They settled along the shores of the Great Lakes, and, as their feces made their way into the lakes, the Guinea worm followed along. Eventually, fish from the Great Lakes became infected with larvae of the worm.

As the years passed, substantial commerce in fish developed between the Midwest and New York City. Jewish homemakers were particularly fond of pike, pickerel, and carp from the Great Lakes, and they used the fish to make a delicacy called gefilte fish. Carefully they pressed minced fish, eggs, and seasonings into balls and boiled the mixtures. During cooking, however, they often tasted the gefilte fish to see if it was done. While sampling the uncooked fish, they unwittingly acquired roundworm larvae and became new hosts for the Guinea worms. The transition was complete.

Guinea worm infection is now rare in New York City or elsewhere in the United States. Sanitary practices, fish inspection, and the commercial production of gefilte fish have limited the spread of the worm. Gefilte fish is still popular among Jewish people, but the unwanted hitchhikers have largely been eliminated.

The Guinea worm exposes itself through the skin ulcer and thus can be removed by careful winding on a stick. This primitive but time-honored method must be performed cautiously and slowly. The site of the ulcer burns intensely, and the fever and local burning are often described as "fiery." Partly because of this perception, it is believed that the "fiery serpents" mentioned in the Bible's Book of Numbers may have been Guinea worms. Also, the stick with worms wound around it may be the source of the serpent on a staff that is the symbol of healing used by the medical profession.

As of 1990, Guinea worm disease affected an estimated 5 million people in 17 African countries and parts of India and Pakistan. By that time, eradication programs had been established in Ghana and Nigeria to interrupt the spread of the disease by providing safe sources of drinking water, by teaching populations at risk to boil or filter contaminated water, and by treating drinking water with chemicals. By the end of the century, prospects were raised for complete eradication in the near future.

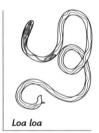

Loa loa

EYEWORM DISEASE

The **eyeworm** is a type of roundworm called *Loa loa*. This parasite, native to West and Central Africa, is about 60 mm long. It is often found in insects such as deerflies and horseflies and is injected into the subcutaneous tissues of humans during an insect bite. The parasite may remain in the connective tissues for many months.

Loa loa is called the eyeworm because it is often attracted to the surface of the eye by warm temperatures. Commonly, it appears on the cornea (FIGURE 16.14). Here it causes conjunctivitis and painful irritation of the eye muscles. Swellings of the extremities are also observed. The parasite returns to the subcutaneous tissues as the skin temperature cools.

TABLE 16.2 summarizes the human diseases caused by roundworms.

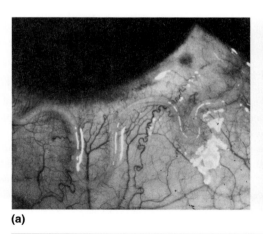
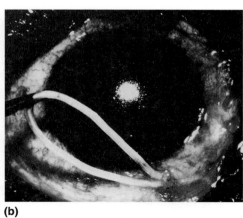

(a)　　　　　　　　　　　　　　　　(b)

FIGURE 16.14

The Eyeworm *Loa loa*

Two views of the human eye showing infection with *Loa loa*, the eyeworm. (a) The worm is seen below the conjunctiva along the white of the eye. (b) The worm is being removed from the eye.

TABLE 16.2

A Summary of Roundworm Parasitic Diseases in Humans

ORGANISM	DISEASE	TRANSMISSION	ORGANS AFFECTED	CHARACTERISTIC SIGN	ANIMAL HOST
Enterobius vermicularis	Pinworm disease	Contact Food, clothing	Intestine	Anal itching	None significant
Trichuris trichiura	Whipworm disease	Food Water	Intestine	Abdominal pain	None significant
Ascaris lumbricoides	Roundworm disease	Food, water Contact	Intestine Lungs	Emaciation Pneumonia	None significant
Trichinella spiralis	Trichinosis	Pork consumption	Intestine Muscles Eyes	Diarrhea Muscle pain Loss of eye movement	Pig
Ancylostoma duodenale Necator americanus	Hookworm disease	Contact with moist vegetation	Intestine Lungs Lymph	Anemia Abdominal pain	None significant
Strongyloides stercoralis	Strongyloidiasis	Contact with moist vegetation	Intestine Lungs	Anemia Abdominal pain	None significant
Wuchereria bancrofti	Filariasis	Mosquito	Lymph vessels	Edema Elephantiasis	Mosquito
Dracunculus medinensis	Guinea worm disease	Food Water	Skin	Skin ulcer	Copepod Fish
Loa loa	Eyeworm disease	Deerflies Horseflies	Eye Connective tissues	Conjunctivitis	Insects

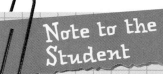

Note to the Student

When we think of commensalism, we often conjure thoughts of microorganisms living in our intestines, mouths, and other organs while causing no apparent harm. We sometimes discover that microorganisms such as certain bacteria actually benefit us.

Distasteful as it may be, we must now broaden our definition of commensalism to include certain multicellular parasites, for indeed, many of us harbor these worms in our organ menageries. As we have seen in this chapter, infection by multicellular parasites need not be fatal. Moreover, we should realize how widespread the parasites are. According to estimates by the World Health Organization, more people are infected with multicellular parasites than anyone previously imagined. With the emergence of Third World countries and travels by Americans to remote parts of the world, the parasites will continue to enter our society in ever-increasing numbers. They may represent an area of public health concern in the years ahead.

Summary

Multicellular parasites are worms of two general types: flatworms and roundworms. Flatworms are classified as flukes and tapeworms. Flukes are leaflike worms belonging to the class Trematoda in the animal phylum Platyhelminthes. Their life cycles include several phases, including miracidium, sporocyst, redia, cercaria, and metacercaria. Snails are intermediate hosts for flukes. The major fluke parasites of humans include the blood fluke (*Schistosoma*), the Chinese liver fluke (*Clonorchis*), the intestinal fluke (*Fasciolopsis*), and the lung fluke (*Paragonimus*).

Tapeworms are long, segmented worms belonging to the class Cestoda in the animal phylum Platyhelminthes. The worms consist of segments called proglottids and a head region called the scolex, often with hooks or sucker devices for attachment to the host tissue. Tapeworms can infect all mammals and are generally transmitted to humans in foods. Examples of foodborne tapeworms are the beef tapeworm (*Taenia*) and the fish tapeworm (*Diphyllobothrium*). Other tapeworms are acquired from the soil.

Roundworms belong to the animal phylum Aschelminthes. The life cycles of roundworms are relatively simple (compared to those of the flatworms), and include separate male and female sexes. Roundworm eggs from the soil are a common method of infection. The pinworm (*Enterobius*) is acquired this way, as are the whipworm (*Trichuris*) and the "roundworm" (*Ascaris*). An important human parasite is the pork roundworm (*Trichinella*) acquired in undercooked pork. Hookworms (*Necator* and *Ancylostoma*) are soilborne, and the filarial worm (*Wuchereria*) that causes elephantiasis is mosquitoborne. Arthropods also transmit the eyeworm (*Loa loa*). Most of the damage due to roundworms arises from the worm burden in the tissues.

Symptoms of disease generally emerge from the worm's interference with body functions, and the diseases caused by multicellular parasites are worldwide in scope.

Questions for Thought and Discussion

1. A diplomat visits a foreign country with which relations have recently been established. She observes that the people eat raw fish, wear no shoes, consume snails as a regular part of their diet, enjoy watercress and water chestnuts in their salads, and do not believe in pesticides. What report might she make on her return to the United States?

2. As of 1991, the World Health Organization reported that malaria was the most prevalent tropical disease (300 million cases per year). The next two were schistosomiasis and filariasis (200 million and 90 million annual cases, respectively). How do you believe the incidence of these diseases can be reduced on a global scale?

3. Because tapeworms have no intestines, they must obtain their nutrients by absorbing organic matter from the external environment in the intestines of humans or animals. How does this observation dispel the notion that evolution always yields animals more complex than their predecessors?

4. Federal law now stipulates that food scraps fed to pigs must be cooked to kill any parasites present. It is also known that feedlots for swine are generally more sanitary than they have been in the past. As a result of these and other measures, the incidence of trichinosis in the United States has declined, and the acceptance of "pink pork" has increased. Do you think this is a dangerous situation? Why?

5. In the 1960s, the Aswan High Dam was built in Egypt to retain the water of the Nile River for irrigation. The agricultural productivity of the region increased significantly but was accompanied by a dramatic increase in the snail population in the water. Before long, the number of cases of schistosomiasis in farmers had doubled. How are all these events related?

6. The Greek stems *di-* and *phyllo-* infer "double-thin" (filo dough is thin dough used in Greek pastry). *Bothros* is also a Greek word, meaning "dirty water." *Latum* is the Latin word for "broad" or "wide." How does this knowledge of classical languages help in remembering the description of the parasite *Diphyllobothrium latum*?

7. In Japan, eating raw fish is a traditional and honored custom. Are there any hazards involved in this practice?

8. Why are some veterinarians inclined to recommend that dog and cat owners avoid buying pet food that contains liver?

9. A person finds that he has difficulty digesting fats. Mayonnaise makes him ill, fried foods cause diarrhea, and he cannot eat salads made with oily salad dressings. However, he does enjoy raw fish dishes, such as sushi and sashimi. What might be his problem?

10. A group of campers was sitting around a fire on a chilly summer evening, when one noticed a threadlike body in the eye of another camper. What might the body have been, and what conditions might have led to its appearance at that time?

11. A newspaper report once indicated that for every case of cancer, the National Institutes of Health spends $209 annually on research. By contrast, for every case of blood fluke disease (schistosomiasis), the amout is $0.04. What factors might account for this sharp distinction in spending? Would you support increased expenditures for schistosomiasis research?

12. Trichinosis may occur in Italian, Polish, and German communities, but it is extremely rare in Jewish communities. Why is this so? How can the local butcher play a key role in preventing the spread of trichinosis among his customers?

13. It has been suggested that with fewer and fewer of the world's peoples walking barefoot, the possibility of infection by skin-penetrating parasites will continue to decline. How many other instances can you name where a change in living habits will bring about a decline in parasitic diseases? Now consider the reverse. How many instances can you name where changes in peoples' habits will bring an increasing incidence of parasitic disease?

14. Certain restaurants offer a menu item called steak tartare. Aficionados know that the beef in this dish is served raw. What hazard might this meal present to the restaurant patron?

15. A biologist, writing in a 1984 publication, stated: "Perhaps the most important reason for discussing parasitical diseases is that they highlight just how enmeshed we are in the web of life. . . ." How many examples can you find in this chapter to support this concept?

Review

Consider the characteristic on the left and the three possible choices on the right. Select the disease(s) or parasite name(s) that best apply to the characteristic, and place the letter(s) next to the characteristic. The answers are listed in Appendix D.

_____ 1. Transmitted by an arthropod.
   a. Filariasis
   b. Trichinosis
   c. Hookworm disease

_____ 2. Animal tapeworm.
   a. *Taenia piscium*
   b. *Taenia latum*
   c. *Taenia saginata*

_____ 3. Type of fluke.
   a. *Schistosoma*
   b. *Necator*
   c. *Fasciola*

_____ 4. Eggs are the mode of transmission.
   a. Dog tapeworm disease
   b. Lung fluke disease
   c. Whipworm disease

_____ 5. Infects the human intestines.
   a. *Trichinella spiralis*
   b. *Ascaris lumbricoides*
   c. *Fasciolopsis buski*

_____ 6. Type of tapeworm.
   a. *Paragonimus*
   b. *Hymenolepis*
   c. *Fasciola*

_____ 7. Snail is the intermediate host.
   a. Blood fluke
   b. Dog tapeworm
   c. Intestinal fluke

_____ 8. Attaches to host tissue by hooks.
   a. *Necator*
   b. *Diphyllobothrium*
   c. *Loa*

_____ 9. Affects pigs as well as humans.
   a. *Loa loa*
   b. *Trichinella spiralis*
   c. *Clonorchis sinensis*

_____ 10. Life cycle includes miracidium and cercaria.
   a. *Schistosoma*
   b. *Fasciola*
   c. *Paragonimus*

_____ 11. Acquired by consuming contaminated meat.
   a. *Taenia soleum*
   b. *Loa loa*
   c. *Necator americanus*

_____ 12. Classified in the phylum Aschelminthes.
   a. *Dracunculus*
   b. *Wuchereria*
   c. *Trichinella*

_____ 13. Infects tissues of the human eye.
   a. *Schistosoma*
   b. *Clonorchis*
   c. *Loa*

_____ 14. Male and female forms exist.
   a. *Hymenolepis*
   b. *Ascaris*
   c. *Trichuris*

_____ 15. Forms hydatid cysts.
   a. Fish tapeworm
   b. Guinea worm
   c. Dog tapeworm

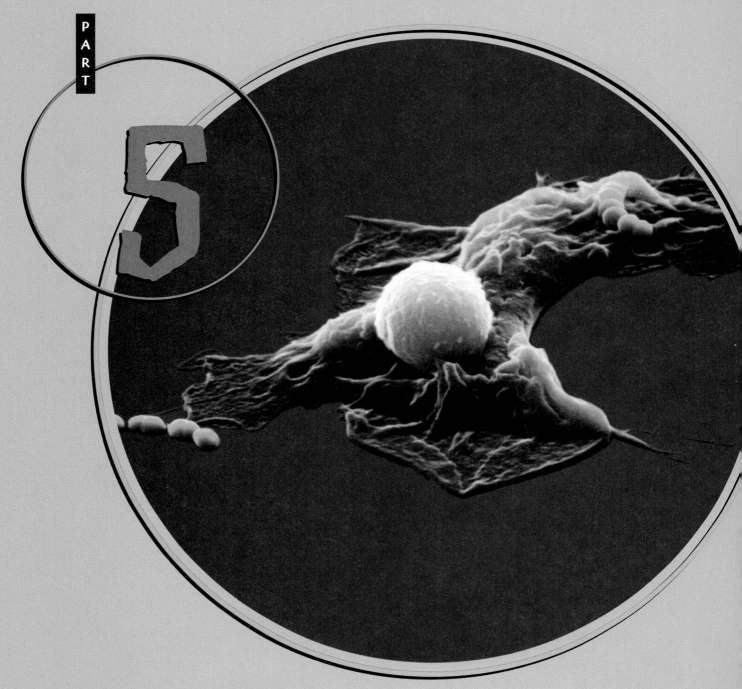

PART

S

Disease and Resistance

In past centuries, the spread of disease appeared to be willfully erratic. Illnesses would attack some members of a population while leaving others untouched. A disease that for many generations had taken small, steady tolls would suddenly flare up in epidemic proportions. And strange, horrifying plagues descended unexpectedly on whole nations.

Scientists now know that humans live in a precarious equilibrium with the microorganisms that surround them. Generally the relationship is harmonious, because humans can come in contact with most microorganisms and develop resistance to them. However, when the natural resistance is unable to overcome the aggressiveness of microorganisms, disease sets in. In other instances, the resistance is diminished by a pattern of human life that gives microorganisms the edge. For example, during the Industrial Revolution of the 1800s, many thousands of Europeans moved from rural areas to the cities. They sought new jobs, adventure, and prosperity. Instead, they found endless labor, unventilated factories, and wretched living conditions—and they found disease.

In Part 5 of this text, we shall explore the infectious disease process and the mechanisms by which the body responds to disease. Chapter 17 will open with an overview of the host–parasite relationship and the factors that contribute to the establishment of disease. In Chapter 18, the discussion turns to nonspecific and specific methods by which body resistance develops, with emphasis on the immune system. Various types of immunity are explored in Chapter 19, together with a survey of laboratory methods that utilize the immune reaction in the diagnosis of disease. In Chapter 20 the discussion centers on immune disorders that lead to serious problems in humans. In these chapters, we shall ferret out the roots of infectious disease and resistance and come to understand them at the fundamental level.

HEALTH AND MEDICINE

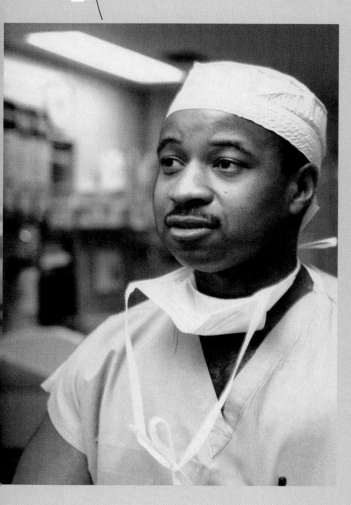

One of the givens of studying health and allied health is the importance of a course in microbiology. It should not be difficult to convince someone that the study of infectious diseases is central to the study of health and medicine. To have an appreciation of AIDS, tuberculosis, influenza, malaria, and other notable diseases is to have an appreciation of contemporary life itself.

But contemporary microbiology is more than infectious diseases. Over the past 25 years or so, the discipline of immunology has ingrained itself into modern health care. For instance, dealing with allergy is dealing with an immunological problem. Diseases such as lupus and rheumatoid arthritis are the domain of immunology, as is Rh disease of the newborn. Geriatric medicine is related to immunology because the immune systems of the elderly function less efficiently and therefore leave individuals more susceptible to infectious diseases.

Many microbiological tests performed in today's laboratories are based in immunology. Where older tests attempted to detect the presence of microorganisms, the newer tests detect antibodies produced in response to these organisms. Antibody tests are also being used to detect hormones in blood and urine (such as the hormone test for pregnancy). Before a transplant is performed, immunological tests are required to determine how compatible the recipient and donor tissues are. Antibody tests are even used in forensic medicine to identify blood types and other secretions.

As a subdiscipline of microbiology, immunology has emerged to become an important facet of the health-care system. Many health science curricula offer separate courses in immunology, but for many undergraduates, the exposure to immunology begins and ends with the microbiology course. For this reason, it is important to understand not only the philosophical significance of immunology, but also the practical benefit of studying the immune system.

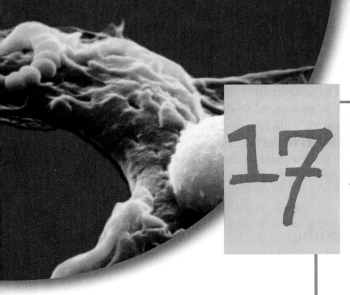

17 Infection and Disease

Tastes like swamp water.

—Australian physician Barry J. Marshall remarking to a colleague, as he secretly drank a culture of *Helicobacter pylori* to prove it causes peptic ulcers

CHOLERA BROKE OUT IN EUROPE in the 1840s and reached London in June 1849. One of the most severely affected areas was the district around Golden Square, where in a 10-day period in August, over 500 people died of the disease.

A physician named **John Snow** lived close to Golden Square. Snow had long been interested in cholera, and the outbreak provided an opportunity to continue and concentrate his study. The prevailing wisdom was that bad air and direct contact spread the disease, but Snow believed they played negligible roles. His beliefs would be strengthened by his observations.

Snow noted that most cholera patients in the Golden Square district drew their water from a well on Broad Street. The water was obtained by a hand-operated pump accessible to all. Snow discovered that the well was contaminated by the cesspool overflow from a tenement in which a cholera patient lived, and he concluded that water was the source of the disease. On September 7, 1849, he presented his findings to the local community council. Snow's study impressed the council members, and they inquired how he intended to stop the epidemic. Snow thought for a moment and replied with the now classic solution: "Take the handle off the Broad Street pump." By the following day, the handle was gone; shortly thereafter, the epidemic subsided.

Unfortunately, not all epidemics are quite as easy to interrupt. In this chapter, we shall discuss the complex mechanisms that underlie the spread and development of

533

infectious disease. Individual diseases are considered in many other chapters of this text, and our purpose here is to bring together many concepts of disease and synthesize an overview of the host–parasite relationship. We shall summarize much of the important terminology used in medical microbiology and focus on the methods used by microorganisms to establish themselves in the tissues. This study will prepare us for a detailed discussion of resistance mechanisms in the following chapters.

17.1

The Host–Parasite Relationship

The word **infection** is derived from Latin origins meaning "to mix with" or "to corrupt." The term refers to the relationship between two organisms, the host and the parasite, and the competition for supremacy that takes place between them. A host whose resistance is strong remains healthy, and the parasite is either driven from the host or assumes a benign relationship with the host. By contrast, if the host loses the competition, disease develops. The term **disease** appears to have originated from Latin stems that mean "living apart," a reference to the separation of ill individuals from the general population. Disease may be conceptualized as any change from the general state of good health. It is important to note that disease and infection are not synonymous; a person may be infected without becoming diseased.

THE NORMAL FLORA

The concept of infection in the host–parasite relationship is expressed in the body's normal flora. The **normal flora**, such as that shown in FIGURE 17.1, is a population of microorganisms that infect the body without causing disease. Some organisms in the population establish a permanent relationship with the body, while others are present for limited periods of time. In the large intestine of humans, for example, *Escherichia coli* and *Candida albicans* are almost always found, but streptococci are transient.

The relationship between the body and its normal flora is an example of a **symbiosis**. In some cases the symbiosis is beneficial to both the body and the microorganisms.

This relationship is called **mutualism**. For example, species of *Lactobacillus* live in the human vagina and derive nutrients from the environment while producing acid to prevent the overgrowth of other organisms. In other cases, the symbiosis is beneficial only to the microorganisms, in which case the symbiosis is called **commensalism**. *Escherichia coli* is generally presumed to be a commensal in the human intestine, although some evidence exists for mutualism because the bacteria produce certain amounts of vitamins B and K.

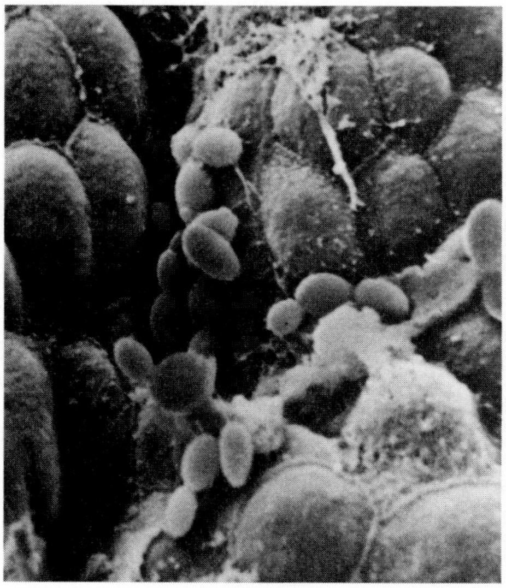

A normal flora may be found in several body tissues. On the **skin**, for instance, there are various forms of viruses, fungi, and bacteria, particularly staphylococci and

---

FIGURE 17.1

The Normal Flora

A scanning electron micrograph of an intestinal membrane showing *Candida albicans* attached to the surface. The yeast form of the cells is apparent.

Propionibacterium acnes. The **oral cavity** commonly contains members of the genera *Neisseria, Leptotrichia,* and *Bacteroides,* as well as many diphtherialike bacilli (diphtheroids), fungal spores, and streptococci. Many of the bacteria are related to bad breath, as MicroFocus 17.1 explores. The upper **respiratory tract** is the site of all these organisms, as well as pneumococci and species of *Haemophilus* and *Mycoplasma.* These organisms may cause respiratory disease if the body defenses are compromised.

The stomach in humans is generally without a normal flora, mainly because of the low pH of its contents. However, the latter part of the **small intestine** and the **large intestine** abound with microorganisms. *Bacteroides* species are numerous, together with *Clostridium* spores, various streptococci, and a number of Gram-negative rods, including species of *Enterobacter, Klebsiella, Proteus,* and *Pseudomonas.* In females, *Lactobacillus* is a notable component of the **vagina**; other organisms may be located near the urogenital orifices in both males and females. The blood and urine are usually sterile unless disease is in progress.

Organisms of the normal flora are introduced when the newborn passes through the birth canal. Additional organisms enter when breathing begins and upon first feeding, as FIGURE 17.2 illustrates. Within 2 to 3 days, most organisms of the flora

pro'pe-on'e-bak-te're-um
nī-se're-ah
lep'to-trik'e-ah
bak'te-roi'dēz

he-mof'ĭ-lus

klo-strid'e-um
kleb'se-el'lah
soo'do-mon'as

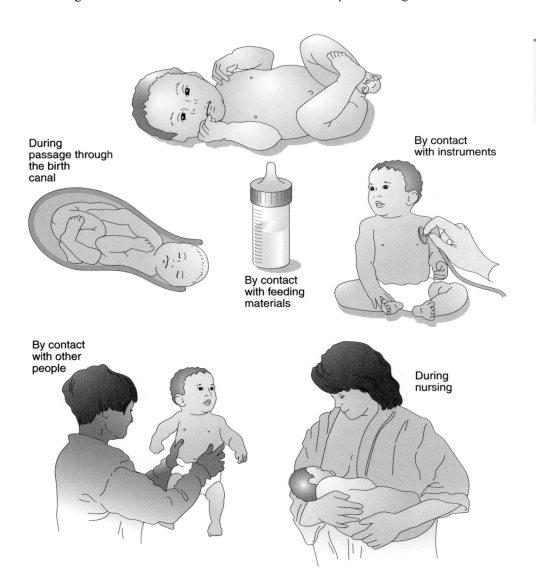

FIGURE 17.2

Five Possible Origins of the Normal Flora in a Newborn

During passage through the birth canal

By contact with feeding materials

By contact with instruments

By contact with other people

During nursing

MicroFocus 17.1

BIG BUSINESS

The newest wrinkle in the franchise business is the bad-breath clinic, the "halitosis heaven." Advertisements for these clinics promise cure rates of 98 percent, and, for those unable to visit in person, home treatment programs are available. People with a breath problem can even use the Internet to "talk" with halitosis experts and receive treatment—as long as a credit card is available. Even NBC's *Today Show* and ABC's *20/20* have featured segments on the perils of dragon mouth.

But is a breath makeover really necessary? Generally not, if you realize the cause. High on the list are the pungent foods we eat—for example, garlic seeps out of our digestive tract and comes back to haunt us through the lungs and skin. And there are numerous disease-associated bad breaths: the fruity odors of diabetes, the fishy odors from kidney problems, and the cheesy smells from tonsil inflammations.

Aside from these, 90 percent of halitosis cases are related to anaerobic bacteria breaking down the tiny particles of food between the teeth, under the gums, and beneath braces or dentures. As they multiply merrily in their myriad morsels of munchies, bacteria produce sulfur gases not unlike those in a swamp. (Indeed, a rotten egg and a rotten mouth find common ground in the same sulfur gases.) And the area at the back of the tongue is a notoriously good hang-out for bacteria, especially since everything we eat passes that way.

So what's a clean breath maven to do? First off, brush and floss vigorously and often to get rid of the bacteria and their meals. (It's a good idea to gently brush your tongue, especially the back part, as well.) Chew gum, preferably sugar-free, to increase saliva flow and keep saliva's natural antibacterial agents flowing. Snack on apples, carrots, and other fiber-rich foods that scrub the teeth between meals. And drink lots of water to reduce stagnation in the mouth and prevent bacteria from gaining a foothold.

The over-the-counter cures for bad breath (mints, sprays, and mouthwashes) have become a billion dollar industry. But we do not need to spend a penny if we use a bit of common sense. And a bit of microbiology.

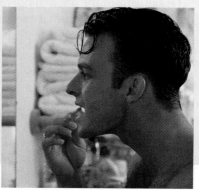

have appeared. During the next few weeks, contact with the mother and other individuals will expose the child to additional microorganisms. The normal flora remains throughout life, undergoing changes in response to the internal environment of the individual.

PATHOGENICITY

Pathogenicity:
the ability of a parasite to gain entry to host tissues and bring about disease.

Pathogenicity refers to the ability of a parasite to gain entry to the host's tissues and bring about a physiological or anatomical change, resulting in altered health and leading to disease. The word is derived from the Greek term *pathos*, meaning "suffering." The term **pathogen** has the same root and refers to an organism having pathogenicity. The symbiotic relationship between host and parasite is called **parasitism**. FIGURE 17.3 compares some of the most prolific pathogens.

Parasites vary greatly in their pathogenicity. Certain parasites, such as the cholera, plague, and typhoid bacilli, are well known for their ability to cause serious human disease. Other organisms, such as common cold viruses, are considered less pathogenic because they induce milder illnesses. Still other organisms are **opportunistic**.

Opportunistic organisms:
those that invade the tissues when body defenses are suppressed.

These organisms may be commensals in the body until the normal defenses are suppressed, at which time the commensals seize the "opportunity" to invade the tissues and express their pathogenicity. An example is observed in individuals with **acquired immune deficiency syndrome (AIDS)**. These patients are highly susceptible to opportunistic organisms such as *Pneumocystis carinii* and *Toxoplasma gondii*.

nu'-mo-sis'tis car-in'e-e

Another new pathogen is depicted in FIGURE 17.4.

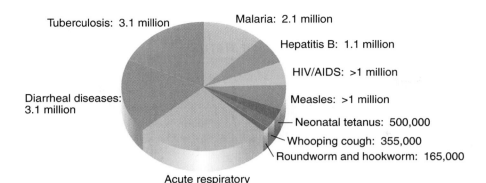

Tuberculosis: 3.1 million

Malaria: 2.1 million

Hepatitis B: 1.1 million

HIV/AIDS: >1 million

Measles: >1 million

Neonatal tetanus: 500,000

Whooping cough: 355,000

Roundworm and hookworm: 165,000

Diarrheal diseases: 3.1 million

Acute respiratory infections: 4.4 million

FIGURE 17.3

The Ten Most Prolific Killers

This pie chart depicts the ten most lethal infectious diseases and the number of worldwide deaths they caused in 1999, as reported by the World Health Organization.

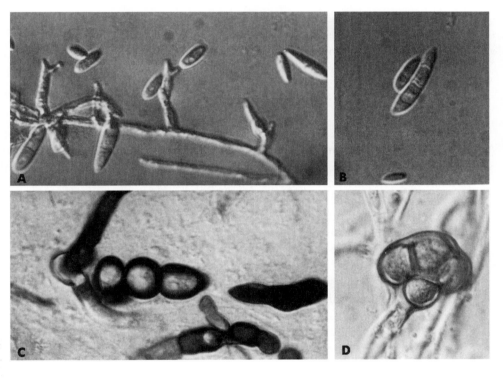

FIGURE 17.4

A New Pathogen

Microorganisms constantly undergo change in their genetic compositions, and sometimes, the change confers new pathogenic qualities on the organism. This is a series of photographs of the fungus *Fusarium chlamydosporum*. In 1998, investigators identified the organism in the tissues of a woman undergoing immunosuppressive therapy. It was the first report of disease related to this species of fungus. The photographs show various stages of the new pathogen, including (a) its hyphae, (b) its macroconidium containing four cells, and (c) and (d) its asexually produced chlamydospores.

Diseases caused by opportunistic organisms illustrate how a shift in the body's delicate balance of controls may convert "infection" to "disease." Another example happened in the 1950s when antibiotics came into widespread use. As bacteria in the intestine's normal flora disappeared, the biological controls exerted on **Candida albicans** vanished and candidiasis became common. Thus, a chance upset in resistance mechanisms or control shifts may enhance the ability of organisms to establish disease (MicroFocus 17.2).

Candida albicans:
a yeast fungus that can cause infection of the intestines, vagina, or oral cavity.

A sobering concept has emerged in recent years. Microbiologists once believed that organisms were either pathogenic or nonpathogenic. This distinction has been blurred by the realization that otherwise benign organisms may be pathogenic when body defenses weaken or fail. The AIDS epidemic points up this concept well. Transplant and cancer patients treated with radiation and immunosuppressant drugs are also affected. It is now recognized that pathogenicity is a function of the aggressive nature of the parasite, as well as the level of resistance in the host.

MicroFocus 17.2

UPSETTING THE BALANCE OF NATURE

An incident that took place on the South Pacific island of Borneo illustrates how an unthinking approach to the eradication of disease may have dire consequences.

In 1955, Borneo was in the throes of a malaria epidemic. With the specter of widespread death looming, the government issued an appeal for assistance to the World Health Organization. The WHO obliged by sending teams of technicians to spray the natives' huts with DDT and dieldrin, two powerful insecticides. The spraying successfully reduced the mosquito population and halted the spread of malaria.

But it also touched off a bizarre series of events. First, the insecticides killed massive numbers of houseflies. The houseflies were eagerly consumed by tiny lizards called geckos, which also died. Geckos, in turn, were eaten by the island's population of house cats, which likewise perished. Only then did ecologists realize that house cats had been keeping the rat population under control; within weeks, rats were everywhere. Now a new problem emerged because rats carry the fleas that transmit bubonic plague. Before long, everyone had plague.

But the World Health Organization was not about to admit defeat. It rounded up thousands of house cats, placed them in boxes, and parachuted the boxes into the island's remote villages. The project was labeled Operation Cat Drop. Eventually the cats established themselves on Borneo and brought the rat population (and the plague) under control. Looking back on the operation, one observer wryly noted: "That was the day it rained cats."

Virulence:
the degree of pathogenicity of a parasite.

Avirulent:
lacking the ability to cause disease.

The word **virulence** is used to express the degree of pathogenicity of a parasite. This term is derived from the Latin *virulentus*, meaning "full of poison." An organism that invariably causes disease, such as the typhoid bacillus, is said to be "highly virulent." By comparison, an organism that sometimes causes disease, such as *Candida albicans*, is labeled "moderately virulent." Certain organisms, described as **avirulent**, are not regarded as disease agents. The lactobacilli and streptococci found in yogurt are examples. However, it should be noted that any microorganism has the ability to change genetically and become virulent.

In recent years, a new term "pathogenicity islands" has been used to refer to the clusters of genes responsible for virulence. The genes encode many of the virulence factors (e.g., enzymes and toxins) discussed later in this chapter. These blocs of genetic information may move into a benign organism and convert it to a pathogen. In effect, they direct the host response in a way that suits the pathogen's survival better than the host's survival.

THE PROGRESS OF DISEASE

Disease is a dynamic series of events expressing the competition between parasite and host (although certain diseases, such as botulism, follow an ingestion of toxins). In most instances, there is a recognizable pattern in the progress of the disease following the entry of the parasite. (FIGURE 17.5 summarizes some entry methods for respiratory parasites.) Certain periods may be distinguished as follows.

The episode of disease begins with a **period of incubation**, reflecting the time that elapses between the entry of the parasite to the host and the appearance of symptoms. Incubation periods may be a short 1 to 3 days, as in cholera; a moderate 2 weeks, as in chickenpox; or a long 3 to 6 years, as in leprosy. Such factors as the number of parasites, their generation time and virulence, and the level of host resistance determine the incubation period's length. The location of entry may also be a determining factor. For instance, the incubation period for rabies may be as short as several days or as long as a year, depending on how close to the central nervous system the viruses enter the body.

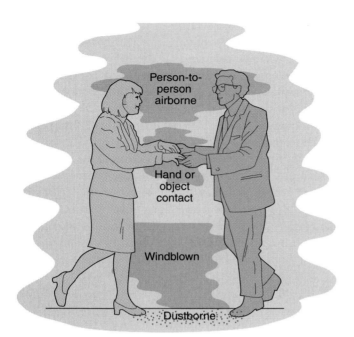

Person-to-person airborne

Hand or object contact

Windblown

Dustborne

FIGURE 17.5

Several Methods for Transmitting Microorganisms from the Respiratory Tract

The next phase in disease is the **period of prodromal symptoms**, also known as the **prodrome**. This period is characterized by general symptoms such as nausea, fever, headache, and malaise, which indicate that the competition for supremacy has begun. Although the patient feels miserable, there is some evidence that the symptoms are beneficial (**MicroFocus 17.3**).

The **period of acme** follows. This is the acute stage of the disease, when specific symptoms appear. Examples are the skin rash in scarlet fever, jaundice in hepatitis, teardrop-shaped vesicles in chickenpox, and swollen lymph nodes in infectious mononucleosis. Often, patients suffer high fever and chills, the latter reflecting differences in temperature between the superficial and deep areas of the body. Dry skin

MicroFocus 17.3

ILLNESS MAY BE GOOD FOR YOU

For most of the twentieth century, medicine's approach to infectious disease was relatively straightforward: Note the symptoms, and fix them. But that may change in the future, as Darwinian medicine gains a stronger foothold. Proponents of Darwinian medicine ask *why* the body has evolved its symptoms and question whether relieving the symptoms may leave the body at greater risk.

Consider coughing, for example. In the rush to stop a cough, we may be neu-

tralizing the body's mechanism for clearing pathogens from the respiratory tract. Nor may it be in our best interest to stifle a fever, since fever enhances the immune response to disease. Many physicians view iron insufficiency in the blood as a symptom of disease, yet many bacterial species (e.g., tubercle bacilli) require this mineral, and while iron is sequestered out of the blood in the liver, they cannot grow well. Even diarrhea can be useful—it helps propel pathogens from the intestine and assists the elimination of enterotoxins.

Darwinian biologists point out that disease symptoms have evolved over the vast expanse of time and probably have benefits that are waiting to be understood. They are not suggesting a major change in how doctors treat their patients, but they are pushing for more studies on whether symptoms are part of the body's natural defenses. It's not quite time to throw out the Nyquil, Tylenol, or Imodium. Not yet, at least.

and a pale complexion may result from constriction of the skin's blood vessels to conserve heat. FIGURE 17.6 depicts the phases of a disease's progress.

As the symptoms subside, the **period of decline**, or defervescence, sets in. This period may be preceded by a crisis period, after which recovery is often rapid. In other cases, the period of decline may last a long time. Sweating is common as the body releases excessive amounts of heat, and the normal skin color soon returns as the blood vessels dilate. The sequence comes to a conclusion during the **period of convalescence**. During this time, the body's systems return to normal.

Diseases may be described as clinical or subclinical. A **clinical** disease is one in which the symptoms are apparent, while a **subclinical** disease is accompanied by few obvious symptoms. Many people, for example, have experienced subclinical cases of mumps or infectious mononucleosis and have developed immunity to future attacks. By contrast, certain diseases are invariably accompanied by clearly recognized clinical symptoms. Measles and malaria are examples. MicroFocus 17.4 recounts how the remains of a disease can be used to resolve conflicts.

THE TRANSMISSION OF DISEASE

The agents of disease may be transmitted by a broad variety of methods conveniently divided into two general categories: direct methods and indirect methods, as illustrated in FIGURE 17.7.

Direct methods of transmission imply close or personal contact with one who has the disease. Hand-shaking, kissing, sexual intercourse, and contact with feces are

def'er-ves'ens

Subclinical disease:
a disease accompanied by few or no symptoms.

FIGURE 17.6

The Course of Disease, as Typified by Measles

(a) A child is exposed to measles viruses in respiratory droplets, and the period of incubation begins. (b) At the end of this period, the child experiences fever, respiratory distress, and general weakness as the period of prodromal symptoms ensues. (c) The period of acme begins with the appearance of specific measles symptoms, such as the body rash. (d) The period reaches a peak as the rash covers the body. (e) The rash fades first from the face and then the body trunk as the period of decline takes place. (e) With the period of convalescence, the body returns to normal. (f) The child later returns to school.

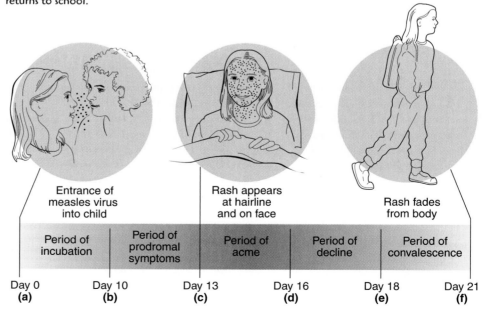

| Period of incubation | Period of prodromal symptoms | Period of acme | Period of decline | Period of convalescence |

Entrance of measles virus into child — Rash appears at hairline and on face — Rash fades from body

Day 0   Day 10   Day 13   Day 16   Day 18   Day 21
(a)   (b)   (c)   (d)   (e)   (f)

MicroFocus 17.4

THE TRUTH IN COAL DUST

The story is told of a rich man who died and left his considerable estate to his only son, whom he had not seen in many years. Some time later, two men showed up, each with credible documents and each claiming to be the man's son and heir.

The boy's pediatrician was called in to consult. He didn't recognize either man,

but after reviewing the son's medical records, he had an idea. He sent both men down to the cellar to shovel coal, telling them not to wipe away the coal dust. When they returned, one of the men had tiny bits of white showing through the coal dust on his face. This man, the pediatrician said, was the true son. The answer was in the medical

records: The son had had smallpox as a boy, and even though the scars disappeared, the doctor knew that dust would not stick to places on the skin where the smallpox scars had been. The impostor was exposed, and the son collected his fortune.

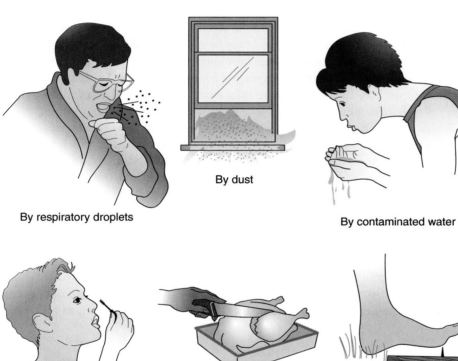

By dust

By respiratory droplets

By contaminated water

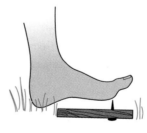

By contact with
contaminated objects

By contaminated food

By injection of
contaminated soil

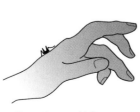
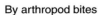

By arthropod bites

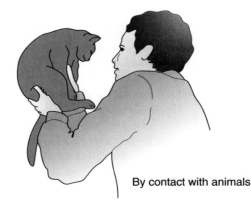

By contact with animals

FIGURE 17.7

Methods of Transmitting Disease

Droplets:
tiny particles of mucus expelled from the respiratory tract in a cough or sneeze.

fo′mī tz
Fomites:
inanimate objects that carry disease organisms.

Vectors:
living organisms that transmit disease organisms.

Reservoir:
organisms that harbor disease agents but show no sign of disease.

Carrier:
one who has recovered from a disease but continues to shed the disease agents.

Toxoplasmosis:
a protozoal disease of the blood characterized by mononucleosis-like symptoms.

examples. Such diseases as gonorrhea and genital herpes are spread by direct contact. Direct contact may also mean exposure to **droplets**, the tiny particles of mucus and saliva expelled from the respiratory tract during a cough or sneeze. Diseases spread by this method include influenza, measles, pertussis (whooping cough), and streptococcal sore throat. For some diseases, direct contact with an animal is necessary. Rabies, leptospirosis, and toxoplasmosis are typical.

Indirect methods of disease transmission include the consumption of contaminated food or water (**MicroFocus 17.5**), and contact with fomites. Foods are contaminated during processing or handling, or they may be dangerous when made from diseased animals. Poultry products, for example, are often a source of salmonellosis because *Salmonella* species frequently infect chickens; and pork may spread trichinosis because *Trichinella* parasites live in muscles of the pig. **Fomites** are inanimate objects that carry disease organisms. For instance, bed linens may be contaminated with pinworm eggs, and contaminated syringes and needles may transport the viruses of hepatitis B and AIDS.

Arthropods represent another indirect method of transmission. Living organisms that carry disease agents from one host to another, such as arthropods, are called **vectors**. In some cases, the arthropod may be a **mechanical vector** of disease because it transports microorganisms on its legs and other body parts. In other cases, the arthropod itself is diseased and serves as a **biological vector**. In malaria and yellow fever, for instance, disease organisms infect the arthropod and accumulate in its salivary gland, from which they are injected during the next bite.

For a disease to perpetuate itself, a continuing source of disease organisms in nature is necessary. These sources are called **reservoirs** (**FIGURE 17.8**). In smallpox, the sole reservoir of viruses is humans, and the World Health Organization was able to limit the spread of the virus and eradicate smallpox from the world by locating all human reservoirs (Chapter 12). A **carrier** is a special type of reservoir. Generally a carrier is one who has recovered from the disease but continues to shed the disease agents. For instance, people who have recovered from typhoid fever or amoebiasis become carriers for many weeks after the symptoms of disease have left. Their feces may spread the disease to others via contaminated food or water.

Animals may also be reservoirs of disease. Domestic house cats usually show no symptoms of toxoplasmosis but are able to transmit *Toxoplasma gondii* to humans, where the disease manifests itself. Cats can also transmit Q fever, as **FIGURE 17.9**

MicroFocus 17.5

DINNER AT LA CASA CUCARACHA

"We're having a wonderful time in this tropical wonderland. Last night, we went to a great restaurant. We walked down Cabeza de Vaca Boulevard, just as they told us, and there on the corner of Ponce de Leon square, we saw it—La Casa Cucaracha.

"The shrimp were so icy cold, we couldn't eat them fast enough. [Uh oh. Should never have cold seafood in that part of the world.] The salad was crisp and delicious, especially the lettuce. [Shouldn't have salad either; the fixins' were probably washed in the local water.] And the waiter was so helpful— he peeled the orange for me right there at the table. [Another no no; his hands probably touched the peeled fruit.]

"Dinner was superb. We had crab meat *au gratin* just warm enough to bring out the flavor. [It should have been steaming hot.] The local vegeta-bles were good enough to eat raw [Another mistake], but the potato was a run-of-the-mill baked potato. [Probably the only safe thing you ate.] For dessert we had local fruits on a lovely bed of crushed ice. [The water, again.]

"How am I feeling today? OK, I guess. On second thought, I do have this little pain in my stomach. . . ."

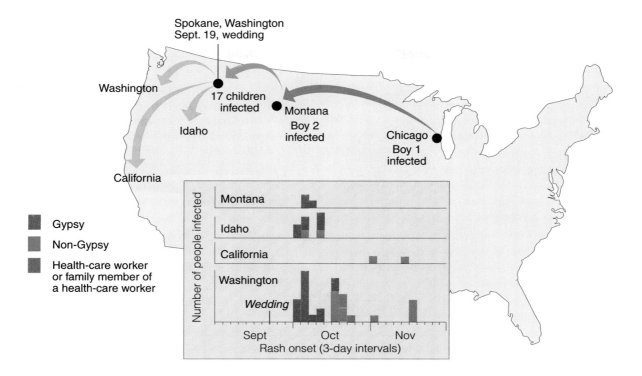

FIGURE 17.8

How a Reservoir May Introduce Disease to a Population

Measles broke out in a Chicago neighborhood late in August 1983. A 2-year-old Gypsy boy contracted the virus, and during the period of incubation, he returned home to Billings, Montana. On September 4, he broke out in a rash and infected boy number 2. The second boy developed a rash on September 19 while at a wedding in Spokane, Washington. The wedding was attended by about 375 people from Gypsy communities in Idaho, Montana, Oregon, and Washington. Seventeen children at the wedding were infected. They eventually spread measles to numerous individuals in non-Gypsy populations, as well as to health-care workers and families of health-care workers, as represented in the diagram. In all, 42 people contracted the disease from the initial reservoir.

indicates. Water and soil may likewise be considered reservoirs since they are often contaminated with disease agents.

Most diseases studied in this text are **communicable** diseases; that is, they are transmissible among hosts. Certain communicable diseases are further described as **contagious**, because they pass with particular ease among hosts. Chickenpox, measles, and genital herpes fall into this category. One reason for easy transmission is that the focus of disease is on or close to the body surface. **Noncommunicable** diseases are singular events in which the agent is acquired directly from the environment and is not easily transmitted to the next host. In tetanus, for example, penetration of soil containing *Clostridium tetani* spores to the anaerobic tissue of a wound must occur before this disease develops.

Diseases may also be described as endemic diseases, epidemic diseases, or pandemic diseases as they are tracked by the Centers for Disease Control and Prevention (FIGURE 17.10). An **endemic** disease is one that occurs at a low level in a certain geographic area. By comparison, **epidemic** diseases (or epidemics) break out in explosive proportions within a population, and **pandemic** diseases (pandemics) occur worldwide.

Contagious disease:
a disease that passes with particular ease among hosts.

Epidemic disease:
a disease that breaks out in explosive proportions in a population.

FIGURE **17.9**

An Outbreak of Q Fever Associated with a Cat

This incident happened in Halifax, Nova Scotia, during the winter months when windows in the home are usually closed and there is little circulation of outside air through the house.

TEXTBOOK CASES

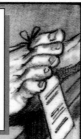
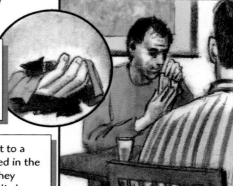
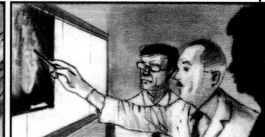

1. On February 14, 1987, a cat gave birth to a litter of kittens in a home in Halifax. The birth took place in the corner of the den. There were three kittens in the litter, and no complications were apparent.

2. Several days later, the family was distressed to see that one of the kittens had died. The mother appeared to be healthy, and there seemed to be no reason for the kitten's death.

3. The man living in the house was host to a regular poker game. The group gathered in the den at least once a week. That week they played poker the day after the kitten died.

4. Several weeks later, all six of the poker players began coughing, sneezing, and displaying respiratory distress. One man with a history of heart disease became seriously ill and died.

5. Physicians detected pneumonia in all the men, and health researchers began a search to discover the cause. They examined the cat and found evidence of *Coxiella burnetii* in its uterine tissue. Evidence of the same organism was found in blood samples from the five remaining men. The disease was identified as Q fever. All five men received doses of antibiotics and recovered.

TYPES OF DISEASES

The dictionary of medical microbiology contains numerous terms that describe types of disease. For example, the word "communicable" or "noncommunicable" is commonly applied to a disease to denote its ability to be transmitted, and "endemic" or "epidemic" indicates how widespread the disease is. We shall briefly summarize some other types of disease next.

The words "acute" and "chronic" are applied to diseases as relative measurements of their severity. An **acute** disease develops rapidly, is usually accompanied by severe symptoms, comes to a climax, and then fades rather quickly. Cholera, epidemic

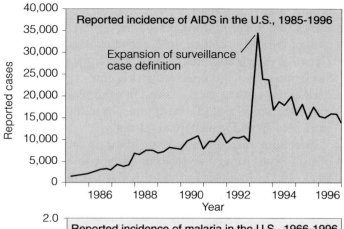

A This line graph shows actual number of cases over an extended period of time.

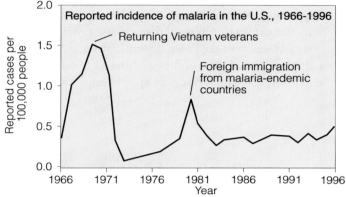

B This graph shows the number of cases per 100,000 people. It takes into account the growing population in the United States over the 30-year period. This factor affects the graph considerably.

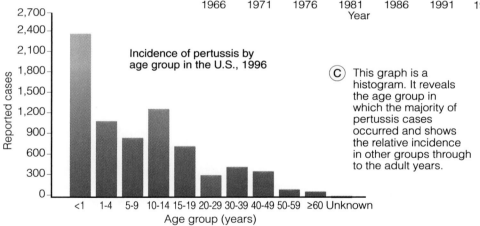

C This graph is a histogram. It reveals the age group in which the majority of pertussis cases occurred and shows the relative incidence in other groups through to the adult years.

Geographic distribution of cholera, 1996

D This map graphically shows the states in which cholera occurred. Different colors or shades can be used in maps such as these to indicate different frequencies of disease.

■ Reported cases

□ No reported cases

FIGURE 17.10

Four Methods for Analyzing Data Associated with a Disease

Chronic disease:
one that lingers for a long time, rarely reaches a climax, and disappears slowly.

typhus, and yellow fever are examples of acute diseases. **Chronic** diseases, by contrast, often linger for long periods of time. The symptoms are slower to develop, a climax is rarely reached, and convalescence may continue for several months. Hepatitis A, trichomoniasis, and infectious mononucleosis are chronic diseases. Sometimes an acute disease may become chronic when the body is unable to rid itself completely of the parasite. For example, one who has giardiasis or amoebiasis may experience sporadic symptoms for many years. FIGURE 17.11 shows how diseases may spread in a hospital setting.

Secondary disease:
one that develops in a weakened host.

Infections may develop as primary or secondary diseases. A **primary** disease occurs in an otherwise healthy body, while a **secondary** disease develops in a weakened individual. In the influenza pandemic of 1918 and 1919, hundreds of millions of individuals contracted influenza as a primary disease and many developed pneumonia as a secondary disease. Numerous deaths in the pandemic were due to pneumonia's complications.

Systemic disease:
a disease that disseminates to the deep organs and tissues.

As the names imply, **local** diseases are restricted to a single area of the body, while **systemic** diseases are those disseminating to the deeper organs and systems. Thus, a staphylococcal skin boil beginning as a localized skin lesion may become more serious when staphylococci spread and cause systemic disease of the bones,

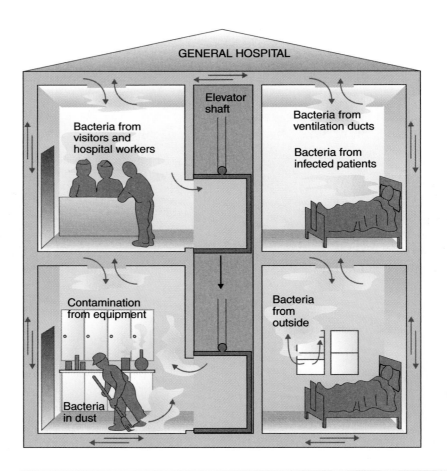

FIGURE 17.11

Numerous Methods for Transmitting Microorganisms in a Hospital meninges, or heart tissue. The word commonly used for dissemination of bacteria through the bloodstream is **bacteremia**. Another term, **septicemia**, means an infection spreading in the blood and is often used as a synonym. The "septicemia" or "blood poisoning" appearing in older textbooks is now regarded as streptococcal or staphylococcal blood disease. **Fungemia** refers to the spread of fungi, **viremia** to the spread of viruses, and **parasitemia** to the spread of protozoa and multicellular worms to the blood.

A word of caution might be appropriate at this juncture. We have used the word "disease" loosely to define a clinical condition initiated by an infectious microorganism. It should not be inferred, however, that this description is true of all diseases. For example, physiological diseases, such as diabetes mellitus, are due to a malfunction of a body organ or system; nutritional diseases, such as scurvy and beri-beri, are caused by a dietary insufficiency; and genetic diseases, such as sickle-cell anemia and cystic fibrosis, are traced to defects in human genes. In these cases, infectious agents or parasites are not involved. Therefore, as we use the word "disease," it is well to remember that we are referring to "infectious disease."

Viremia: dissemination of viruses into the bloodstream.

To this point . . .

We have begun our study of infection and disease by studying the host–parasite relationship. Infection refers to the relationship between the host and parasite, while disease results from the change in the state of the host's health brought about by damage caused by the parasite. We noted that the body is inhabited by a normal flora of organisms, some of which are commensals and opportunists. The term pathogenicity was explored in the general sense, and we noted how a shift in the delicate balance of body control can lead to disease. Virulence refers to the degree of pathogenicity of a parasite.

Next we surveyed the periods during the progress of disease and used many examples from various diseases to illustrate the basic concepts. Clinical and subclinical diseases vary on the basis of clinical symptoms, and the transmission of disease occurs by direct and indirect methods, including reservoirs and carriers. We defined communicable and noncommunicable diseases, acute and chronic diseases, primary and secondary diseases, and local and systemic diseases.

We shall now focus on the factors contributing to the establishment of disease. Portal of entry, dose, and tissue penetration are examples of these factors. We shall then survey some of the enzymes and toxins used by the parasite to overcome body defenses and interfere with vital metabolic processes. The section will end with a discussion of the blood, since the blood is often the site of infection and spread of parasites, and it is the organ where a major aspect of body resistance takes place.

17.2

The Establishment of Disease

A **parasite** must possess unusual abilities if it is to overcome host defenses and bring about the anatomical or physiological changes leading to disease. Before it can manifest these abilities, however, the parasite must first gain entry to the host in sufficient numbers to establish a population (FIGURE 17.12). Next, it must be able to penetrate the tissues and grow at that location. Disease is therefore a complex series of interactions between parasite and host. In this section,

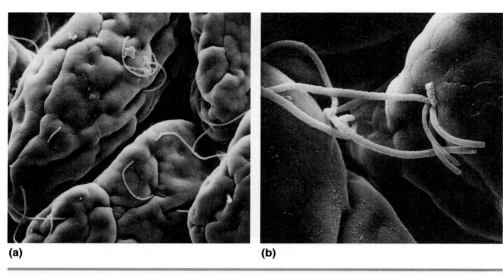

(a)   **(b)**

FIGURE 17.12

A Population of Intestinal Bacteria

Two scanning electron micrographs of the villi of the intestine showing filamentous bacteria. (a) In this view, the bacteria appear to emerge from clefts in the tissue and extend out onto the surface of the villus (×400). (b) When magnified 1800 times, the attachment in the cleft of tissue can be seen more clearly. Note the three-dimensional image afforded by the scanning electron microscope.

we shall examine some of the factors that determine whether disease can occur, with a focus on the parasite. The events are summarized in FIGURE 17.13.

PORTAL OF ENTRY

Portal of entry:
a site where microorganisms enter the body of a host in anticipation of disease.

Pili:
short hairlike appendages used by bacteria for attachment to the tissues.

Q fever:
a rickettsial disease due to *Coxiella burnetii* characterized by flulike symptoms.

Portal of entry refers to the site at which the parasite enters the host. It varies considerably for different organisms and is a key factor in the establishment of disease. For example, **tetanus** may occur if *Clostridium tetani* spores are introduced from the soil to the anaerobic tissue of a wound, but tetanus will not develop if spores are consumed with food because the spores do not germinate in the human intestinal tract. This is why one can eat a freshly picked radish without fear of tetanus. One reason offered for specific portals of entry is the presence of adhesive factors on the surface of parasites. For example, gonococci attach by means of pili to specific receptor sites on tissues of the urogenital system.

Certain parasites have multiple portals of entry. The **tubercle bacillus**, for instance, may enter the body in respiratory droplets, contaminated food and milk, and skin wounds. The **Q fever** organism enters by all these methods, as well as by an arthropod bite. The **tularemia bacillus** may enter the eye by contact, the skin by an abrasion, the respiratory tract by droplets, the intestines by contaminated meat, or the blood by an arthropod bite. Indeed, arthropodborne diseases will break out or disappear according to the extent of the arthropod population (MicroFocus 17.6).

It should be noted that upon entry to a host, a pathogen is confronted with a profoundly different environment than it is used to. Adaptation to this environment requires the genetic machinery that enables the pathogen to grow and multiply. Indeed, the expression of pathogenicity may be delayed until such time that the microorganism finds its favorite niche in the body.

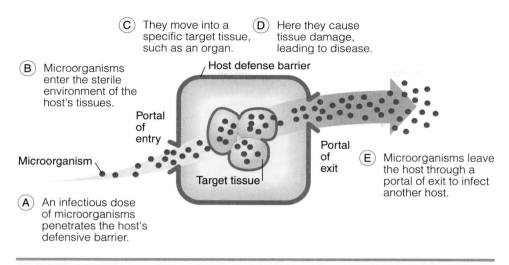

(B) Microorganisms enter the sterile environment of the host's tissues.

(C) They move into a specific target tissue, such as an organ.

(D) Here they cause tissue damage, leading to disease.

Host defense barrier

Portal of entry

Microorganism

Target tissue

Portal of exit

(E) Microorganisms leave the host through a portal of exit to infect another host.

(A) An infectious dose of microorganisms penetrates the host's defensive barrier.

FIGURE 17.13

The Generalized Events in the Establishment of Disease

At the conclusion of its pathogenicity cycle, a pathogen must be able to leave the body through some suitable **portal of exit**, as shown in FIGURE 17.14. This is of more than passing importance because easy transmission permits the pathogen to continue its pathogenic existence in the world. Modern microbiologists, such as Amherst College's Paul Ewald, have suggested that if a microorganism cannot find a suitable portal of exit or mode of transmission, it may be replaced by less pathogenic species. Ewald's theory is described in MicroFocus 17.7.

MicroFocus 17.6

AT HOME IN A TIRE

Each year, Americans discard about 200 million tires, most of which are buried in landfills or left to rot in vacant lots. In these settings, discarded tires make perfect homes for mosquitoes. The tires fill with water and garbage, and the mosquitoes grow larger, live longer, and complete their life cycles sooner than their relatives from swamps and drainage ditches.

Since 1963, the state of Ohio has recorded over 600 cases of La Crosse encephalitis. First observed in La Crosse, Wisconsin, in 1960, La Crosse encephalitis is endemic in a crescent-shaped area of the Great Lakes region extending from southeastern Minnesota to New York. A serious viral disease of the brain,

La Crosse encephalitis is transmitted by mosquitoes of the genus *Aedes.*

When the Ohio Department of Health investigated 69 cases of La Crosse encephalitis in the 1980s, it found that discarded tires were connected in some way with almost three-quarters of the cases. It also located *Aedes* mosquitoes in tires associated with half the cases. A notable episode of La Crosse encephalitis occurred in 1983 in the daughter of a rural Ohio businessman. His business was recycling tires.

Some years later, a case of La Crosse encephalitis was observed in a Milwaukee suburb, well outside the normal area for the disease. While pursuing leads, health officials noted that a neighbor of

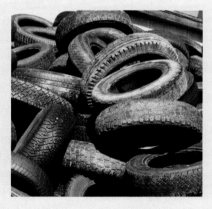

the patient had previously lived near La Crosse. They questioned the neighbor and learned that when he moved, he brought along one very significant item: his collection of old tires.

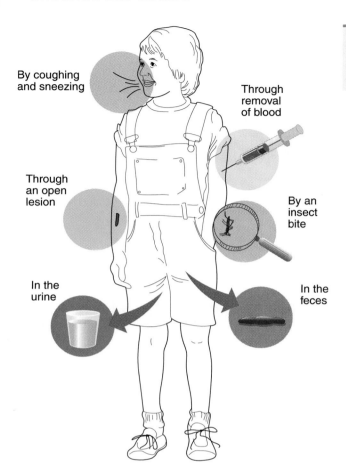

By coughing
and sneezing

Through
removal
of blood

Through
an open
lesion

By an
insect
bite

In the
urine

In the
feces

FIGURE 17.14

**Six Different Portals
of Exit from the Body**

DOSE

Dose refers to the number of parasites that must be taken into the body for disease to be established. Experiments indicate, for example, that the consumption of a few hundred thousand **typhoid bacilli** will probably lead to disease. By contrast, many million **cholera bacilli** must be ingested if cholera is to be established. One explanation is the high resistance of typhoid bacilli to the acidic conditions in the stomach, in contrast to the low resistance of cholera bacilli. Also, it may be safe to eat fish when the water contains hepatitis A viruses, but eating raw clams from that same water can be dangerous because clams are filter-feeders, and the concentration (or dose) of hepatitis A viruses is much higher in these animals.

Often the host is exposed to low doses of a parasite and, as a result, develops immunity. For instance, many people can tolerate low numbers of mumps viruses without exhibiting disease. They may be surprised to find that they are immune to **mumps** when it breaks out in their family at some later date. Other individuals have developed immunity to fungal pathogens after several low-grade exposures. Cases of **histoplasmosis**, for example, are regarded as a mild "summer flu" in the Ohio and Mississippi valleys, but histoplasmosis can be serious in an individual not previously exposed to the disease. **Blastomycosis** can be equally dangerous, as FIGURE 17.15 illustrates. It should be noted that immune people remain healthy because they enjoy strong resistance, again pointing to the notion that resistance and disease are fundamentally inseparable.

Mumps:
a viral disease characterized by swollen salivary glands.
his'to-plaz-mo'sis

MicroFocus 17.7

CONTROLLING THE PATHOGEN

What if we could control the destiny of a pathogen? What if we could make a virulent pathogen less virulent, or even induce it to become harmless? Suppose, for example, we could "tame" the human immunodeficiency virus (HIV), and thereby put an end to the AIDS epidemic?

It may be possible, says Paul Ewald, of Amherst College in Massachusetts. Ewald maintains that cutting off HIV from access to new hosts would induce milder strains, possibly even harmless strains, to evolve. Following this reasoning, it would make sense to take funds from anti-HIV drug programs and put them into transmission-prevention programs, as he suggests.

Ewald's novel approach to medicine is presented in his seminal book, *Evolution of Infectious Disease.* His theory is based on the observation that when a killer pathogen cannot spread from person to person, it cannot infect enough people to survive, and it will soon die out. But it will not leave a total void. Rather, its niche will be filled by a milder strain that will not make people sick enough to die. This milder strain can be passed among people because they leave their homes and make contact

with one another. Thus, it is in the interest of the pathogen to be mild, especially when it depends on the host to transmit it.

But sometimes the pathogen does not need its host for transmission, so it doesn't have to evolve to a mild form. (Consider, for instance, diseases such as malaria, sleeping sickness, yellow fever, and plague.) The common thread among these diseases is transmission by an arthropod. The pathogen can remain a killer because transmission is relatively easy, as long as the correct arthropod is available. In these cases, Ewald's transmission-prevention program (arthropod control) would be

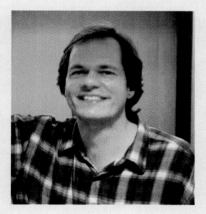

extremely beneficial in encouraging the pathogens to evolve to mild forms.

Much of Ewald's work has been with cholera. His research has shown that water heavily polluted with feces contains virulent *Vibrio cholerae*, but that milder strains inhabit clean water. The implication is that cholera bacilli evolve to milder forms when they cannot use water as a transfer vehicle. Once again, transmission prevention would appear not only to interrupt the epidemic but, more importantly, to force the pathogen into a more benign mode of existence.

Ewald's boldness and originality are hailed by some scientists, but viewed with skepticism by others who see a need for independent corroboration and much deeper study. Trying to understand a microorganism's evolution in response to its environment is difficult, the skeptics say, but trying to understand the evolution when another species (humans) is involved can complicate this issue much further. Still, Ewald's views have placed transmission-prevention programs in a new light, while encouraging epidemiologists to continue fighting the good fight.

TISSUE PENETRATION

Most knowledge of tissue penetration (FIGURE 17.16) has been developed from studies on histological preparations, tissue cultures, and animals, and an understanding of the penetration process is generally incomplete. Experiments reported by Stanley Falkow and his coworkers at Stanford University indicate that genes for cell penetration exist on the chromosome of certain bacteria. These genes appear to code for surface proteins that assist penetration. In the late 1980s, Falkow's group successfully isolated the penetration genes from *Yersinia pseudotuberculosis* and inserted them into *E. coli*, which then displayed penetration. Falkow has written that pathogens use their invasive tendencies to gain access to privileged niches denied to nonpathogens. For example, pathogenic ***E. coli* O157:H7** penetrates to sites in the small intestine tissue and urinary system that are not available to commensal *E. coli* strains remaining in the lumen of the small intestine. Other researchers have reported genes for penetration on the plasmids of *Shigella flexneri*.

Yersinia:
a genus of Gram-negative rods that display bipolar staining.

FIGURE **17.15**

An Outbreak of Blastomycosis

This outbreak occurred in Boulder, Colorado, during the summer of 1998. Growth of the responsible fungus may have been encouraged by the animal feces present, and unusually heavy rainfall may have contributed to the high humidity needed for fungal growth. Epidemiologists postulated that spores in the dust were inhaled by the men infected.

TEXTBOOK CASES

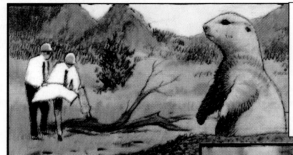

1. During June 1998, officials from the City of Boulder (Colorado) Open Space program decided to move ahead on a planned project to relocate a colony of prairie dogs from an area at the outskirts of the city to make way for a park.

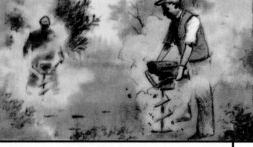

2. By early August, the animals had been relocated, and 15 workers were busy excavating the site, especially the abandoned prairie dog tunnels and burrows. Their gasoline-powered augers created a lot of dust. No protective clothing or facemasks were provided to the men at the site. As a result, they had an opportunity to breath much dust.

3. Within two weeks, one of the workers experienced fever, weight loss, fatigue, and a cough with much mucus. His doctor prescribed two antibiotics, but the symptoms worsened. He was hospitalized by September.

4. Laboratory technologists isolated *Blastomyces dermatitidis*, a yeastlike fungus, from nodules taken from the man's lung. The man received an antifungal antibiotic called amphotericin B and began a period of recovery.

5. Days later, another man from the project reported to the same hospital with identical symptoms. An alert doctor saw the similarities and tested the man for *B. dermatitidis*. When the test was positive, the doctor called epidemiologists.

Pertussis:
a bacterial disease accompanied by mucus accumulation in the respiratory tract.

The ability of a parasite to penetrate tissues and cause structural damage is a virulence factor called **invasiveness.** The bacilli of typhoid fever and the protozoa that cause amoebiasis are well known for their invasiveness. (A species of bacteria related to the typhoid bacillus is shown invading tissue in FIGURE 17.17.) By penetrating the tissue of the gastrointestinal tract, these organisms cause ulcers and sharp, appendicitislike pain characteristic of the respective diseases. In some cases, penetration may not be critical to disease. The **pertussis bacillus,** for example, remains on the surface layers of the respiratory tract while producing the toxins that lead to disease. The **cholera bacillus** does likewise in the intestine.

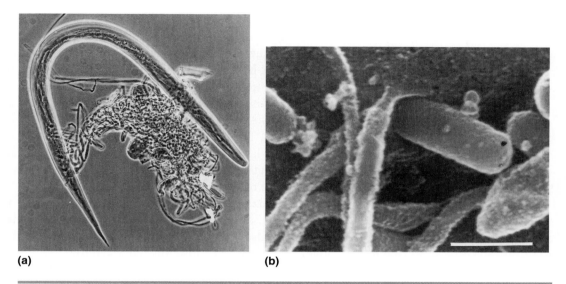

(a)   **(b)**

FIGURE 17.16

Two Examples of Tissue Penetration by Parasites

(a) The fungus *Dactylaria* attacking the roundworm *Panagreilus* in two places. The fungus penetrates the outer membranes of the worm and parasitizes its tissues. (b) An *Escherichia coli* cell experimentally reengineered to produce a surface protein that permits invasion of tissue calls. In this photograph, *E. coli* is invading a human lung cell. The fingerlike protrusions are part of the normal outer membrane of the lung cell.

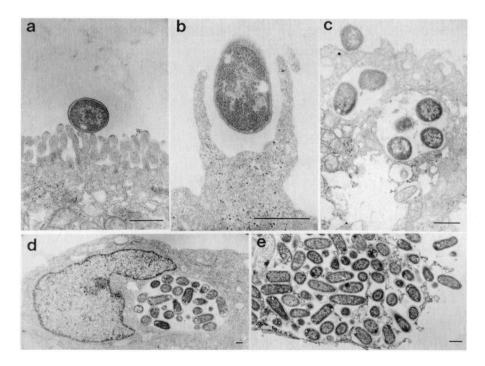

FIGURE 17.17

Tissue Invasion

A series of transmission electron micrographs displaying the interaction between invasive *Salmonella typhimurium* and epithelial cells of the human intestine. (a) At 30 minutes postinfection, bacteria are seen adhering to the tips of intestinal microvilli. (b) A bacterium is being engulfed by an epithelial cell. (c) At 1 hour postinfection, salmonellae can be observed within vacuoles in the cells. (d) At 12 hours postinfection, a number of vacuoles containing bacteria unite with one another, and bacteria multiply within this large vacuole. (e) At 24 hours postinfection, the epithelial cell is filled with salmonellae and is breaking down to release the bacteria. (Bar = 1 μm.)

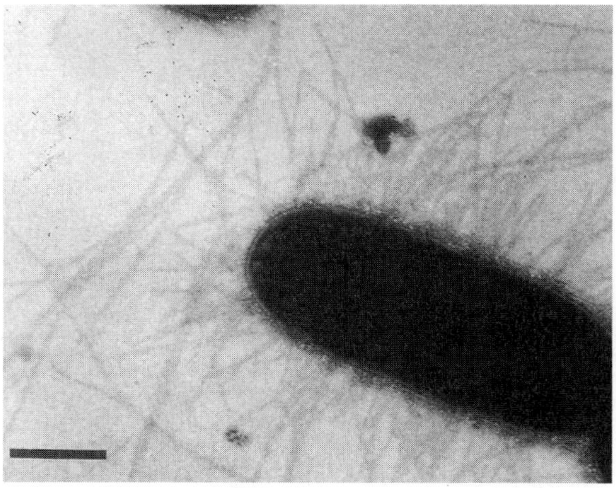

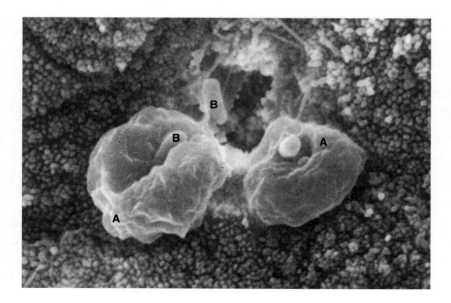

FIGURE 17.18

Adhesion Pili in *E. coli*

A scanning electron micrograph of *Escherichia coli* displaying the pili used for adhesion to the tissue. Adhesins in pili such as these increase the pathogenicity of the organism by encouraging it to localize at its appropriate tissue site. (Bar = 0.5 μm.)

Although penetration may not be essential to pathogenicity, **adhesion** is often a key factor. Adhesion localizes pathogens at appropriate tissue sites and may result in internalization by phagocytosis or bacterial-induced endocytosis. A variety of molecules and structures collectively known as **adhesins** are involved. Adhesins are often associated with pili (fimbriae), as shown in FIGURE 17.18, or they may act independently of these structures. The M protein of *Streptococcus* species is an example of the latter (Chapter 7). The host cell is often an active partner in the adhesion because the pathogen triggers it to express target receptor sites for adhesin binding.

Cell internalization by phagocytic cells (endocytosis) is well researched, but it has become apparent that bacterial pathogens can also induce nonphagocytic cells to take up the pathogens. This process allows the pathogen to enter a protective niche or to pass through otherwise impenetrable barriers, such as the blood-brain barrier. The pathogens seem to have the capacity to form a zipperlike mechanism binding host cell to the pathogen and a trigger mechanism in which the host cell membrane "ruffles" (like a flamenco dancer's skirt). As a result of this molecular cross-talk, wide channels form, thereby allowing the pathogen to enter the host cell. FIGURE 17.19 shows these changes.

Cell-to-cell transport is an equally interesting concept. Researchers have found that certain genera of bacteria (e.g., *Listeria* and *Shigella*) can use the host cell's actin to synthesize a type of tail that propels the organism through the cell's cytoplasm (MicroFocus 17.8). When the bacterium thuds against the cell membrane, it distorts and indents the adjacent cell. Using a molecule called **cadherin**, the pathogen bridges the junction between the two cells and enters the next cell (somewhat like moving from train car to train car through connecting doors). A remarkable photograph of *Listeria* moving from cell to cell is presented in Chapter 8, and another series is shown in FIGURE 17.20. The system allows bacterial invasion to occur without bacteria leaving the cellular environment.

FIGURE 17.19

Salmonella Penetration of Intestinal Cells

Researchers have discovered that microvilli of the intestinal epithelium undergo dramatic changes when *Salmonella* cells come into close contact. The microvilli themselves disappear, and tiny membrane blebs (or "ruffles") spring up in their place, engulfing the salmonellae. Some 2 hours later the microvilli reappear, but the bacteria are now within the cells. In this scanning electron micrograph, the membrane blebs (A) can be seen as puffy structures. A bacterium (B) is within the cavity of one bleb and another is adjacent to it.

MicroFocus 17.8

TRAVELING LIGHT

Rather than bringing along a personal source of intercellular motility, a *Shigella* bacterium uses what is available and designs it to its own specifications. The organism possesses a gene that allows it to take active protein from the scaffolding of a host cell and jerry-rig the protein to form a cometlike tail. Then the bacterium moves from cell to cell, avoiding body defenses and causing intestinal illness.

The gene for this opponent retooling has been identified by researchers from the Whitehead Institute in Massachu-

setts. A team led by Julie A. Therist isolated the gene and transferred it to nonmotile *E. coli* cells. When placed in a culture of tissue cells, the *E. coli* quickly grew *Shigella*-like tails and began thrusting about. What was first believed to be a very complicated system turned out to be quite simple.

Students of anatomy and physiology know actin as the major protein of thin filaments in the sliding-filament model of muscle contraction. (Can you name the protein of the thick filaments?) Students of general biology will recognize

actin as a component of the cytoskeleton. And now "actin" has come to microbiology. Welcome, actin.

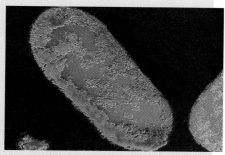

■ A Shigella *bacterium*

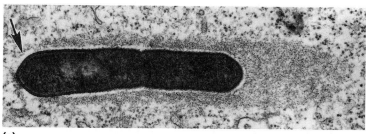

(a)

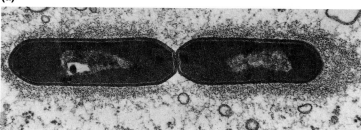

(b)

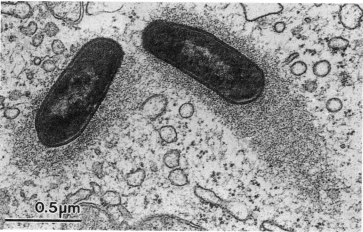

0.5μm

(c)

FIGURE 17.20

Movement in *Listeria monocytogenes*

Listeria monocytogenes is a Gram-positive rod responsible for outbreaks of a foodborne disease known as listeriosis (Chapter 8). After entering a host cell, the bacterium moves about by forming a polar tail composed of filaments of a protein called actin. (a) *Listeria* is seen in the cytoplasm of a host macrophage. A short tail is observed at the right pole but not the left pole (arrow). (b) A *Listeria* cell is dividing in the host cell cytoplasm, and actin filaments are seen at all surfaces except where division is occurring. (c) The two new rods are each producing their polar tails.

The genes that control such activities as these appear to cluster in bacterial cells. A so-called invasion complex has been identified in many *Shigella* species, and molecular geneticists refer to a "pathogenicity island" to denote the location of the virulence genes. While fascinating in itself, the study of microbial pathology is doubly important because it provides a glimpse of the biology of humans as well.

ENZYMES

The virulence of a parasite depends to some degree on its ability to produce a series of enzymes that help the parasite resist body defenses. The enzymes act on host cells and interfere with certain functions meant to retard invasion. TABLE 17.1 summarizes the activities of these enzymes.

An example of a bacterial enzyme is the **coagulase** produced by virulent staphylococci. Coagulase catalyzes the formation of a blood clot from fibrinogen proteins in human blood. The clot sticks to **staphylococci**, protecting them from phagocytosis. Part of the walling-off process observed in a staphylococcal skin boil is due to the clot formation. Coagulase-positive staphylococci may be identified in the laboratory by combining staphylococci with human or rabbit plasma. The formation of a clot in the plasma indicates coagulase activity.

Many streptococci have the ability to produce the enzyme **streptokinase**. This substance dissolves fibrin clots used by the body to restrict and isolate an infected area. Streptokinase thus overcomes an important host defense and allows further tissue invasion by the parasites.

Hyaluronidase is sometimes called the spreading factor because it enhances penetration of a parasite through the tissues. The enzyme digests hyaluronic acid, a polysaccharide that binds cells together in a tissue. The term *tissue cement* is occasionally applied to this polysaccharide. Hyaluronidase is an important virulence factor in pneumonococci and certain species of streptococci and staphylococci. In addition, gas gangrene bacilli use it to facilitate spread through the muscle tissues.

Leukocidins and hemolysins are enzymes that destroy blood cells. **Leukocidins** are products of staphylococci, streptococci, and certain bacterial rods. The enzymes disintegrate circulating neutrophils and tissue macrophages, both of which are active

Coagulase:
a bacterial enzyme that catalyzes the formation of a blood clot.

Streptokinase:
a bacterial enzyme that dissolves fibrin clots.

hi′ah-lu-ron′ĭ-dās

loo′ko-si′din
he-mol′ĭ-sin

TABLE 17.1			
A Summary of Enzymes That Add Virulence			
ENZYME	SOURCE	ACTION	EFFECT
Coagulase	Staphylococci	Forms a fibrin clot	Allows resistance to phagocytosis
Streptokinase	Streptococci	Dissolves a fibrin clot	Prevents isolation of infection
Hyaluronidase	Pneumococci Streptococci Staphylococci	Digests hyaluronic acid	Allows tissue penetration
Leukocidin	Staphylococci Streptococci Certain rods	Disintegrates phagocytes	Limits phagocytosis
Hemolysins	Clostridia Staphylococci	Dissolves red blood cells	Induces anemia and limits oxygen delivery

phagocytes. Usually disintegration occurs before phagocytosis has taken place, but occasionally it occurs after the phagocyte has engulfed the parasite. The enzymes attach to the phagocyte's membrane and trigger changes leading to the release of lysosomal enzymes in the cytoplasm. The phagocyte quickly disintegrates.

Hemolysins are a group of enzymes that dissolve red blood cells. Studies show that hemolysins combine with the membranes of erythrocytes and cause the formation of pores, after which lysis takes place as cytoplasmic contents spill out. During cases of gas gangrene, hemolysins lead to substantial anemia. Staphylococci and streptococci are also known to produce these virulence factors. In the laboratory, hemolysin producers can be detected by hemolysis, a destruction of blood cells in a blood agar medium.

Furthermore, if a pathogen exists in a biofilm, its virulence can be enhanced because here it can resist body defenses and drugs. A **biofilm** is a sticky layer of extracellular polysaccharides and proteins enclosing a colony of bacteria at the tissue surface (Chapter 4). Phagocytes and antibodies have difficulty reaching the microorganisms in this slimy conglomeration of armorlike material (FIGURE 17.21). Moreover, microorganisms often survive without dividing in a biofilm. This makes them impervious to the antibiotics that attack dividing cells. (Indeed, the antibiotics do not penetrate the biofilm easily.) And the target of the antibiotic may be hidden by a chemical reaction between target molecule and biofilm material. CDC officials have estimated that fully 65 percent of human infections involve biofilms.

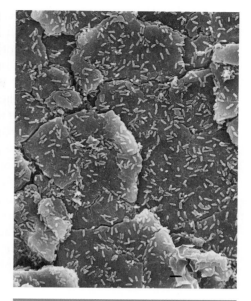

FIGURE 17.21

Bacteria in a Biofilm

A scanning electron micrograph of *Pseudomonas aeruginosa* found in a biofilm in a latex catheter in a hospital setting. Within biofilms like these, the bacteria can resist disinfectant treatment of the equipment. In the human body, biofilms add to the virulence of a pathogen by helping it resist drugs and natural body defenses. (Bar = 5 μm.)

TOXINS

Toxins are microbial poisons that profoundly affect the establishment and course of disease because a single toxin can make an organism virulent. Two types of toxins are recognized: exotoxins and endotoxins (TABLE 17.2).

Exotoxins are produced chiefly by Gram-positive bacteria. They are protein molecules, manufactured during the metabolism of bacteria. Exotoxins are released

TABLE 17.2

A Comparison of Exotoxins and Endotoxins

CHARACTERISTIC	EXOTOXINS	ENDOTOXINS
Usual source	Mainly Gram-positive bacteria	Mainly Gram-negative bacteria
Location in parasite	Cytoplasm	Cell wall
Chemical composition	Protein	Lipid-polysaccharide-peptide
Antibodies elicited	Yes	No
Conversion to toxoid	Possible	Not possible
Liberation of toxin	On production by the parasite	On disintegration of the parasite
Representative effects	Interfere with synaptic activity Interrupt protein synthesis Increase capillary permeability Increase water elimination	Increase body temperature Increase hemorrhaging Increase swelling in tissues Induce vomiting, diarrhea

into the surrounding environment of the tissue as they are produced (*exo-* is Greek for "outside"). They dissolve in the blood fluid and circulate to their site of activity. The symptoms of disease soon develop.

The exotoxin produced by the botulism bacillus ***Clostridium botulinum*** is among the most lethal toxins known. One pint of the pure toxin is believed sufficient to destroy the world's population. In humans, the toxin inhibits the release of acetylcholine at the synaptic junction, a process that leads to the paralysis seen in botulism (Chapter 8). Another exotoxin is produced by **tetanus** bacilli. In this case, the exotoxin blocks the relaxation pathway that follows muscle contraction, thereby permitting volleys of spontaneous nerve impulses and uncontrolled muscular contractions.

A third toxin is produced by ***Corynebacterium diphtheriae***, the diphtheria bacillus. The exotoxin interferes with the assembly of proteins in the cytoplasm of epithelial cells of the upper respiratory tract. Disintegrated cells then accumulate with mucus, bacteria, fibrous material, and white blood cells, resulting in life-threatening respiratory blockages. Other exotoxins are formed by the bacteria that cause scarlet fever, staphylococcal food poisoning, pertussis, and cholera.

When toxins function in a particular organ system, they are given more clearly defined names. For example, the botulism toxin is called a **neurotoxin** because of its activity in the nervous system, while the staphylococcal toxin is called an **enterotoxin** since it functions in the gastrointestinal tract.

The body responds to exotoxins by producing special antibodies called **antitoxins**. When toxin and antitoxin molecules combine with each other, the toxin is neutralized. This process represents an important defensive measure in the body. Therapy for people who have botulism, tetanus, or diphtheria often includes injections of antitoxins (immune globulin) to neutralize the toxins.

Because exotoxins are proteins, they are susceptible to the heat and chemicals that normally react with proteins. A chemical such as formaldehyde may be used to alter the toxin and destroy its toxicity without hindering its ability to elicit an immune response in the body. The result is a **toxoid**. When the toxoid is injected into the body, the immune system responds with antitoxins that circulate and provide a measure of defense against disease. Toxoids are used for diphtheria and tetanus immunizations in the diphtheria-tetanus-acellular pertussis (DTaP) vaccine.

Endotoxins are part of the cell wall of bacteria, and as such, they are released only upon disintegration of the parasite. They are present in the outer membrane (Chapter 4) in many Gram-negative bacilli and are composed of lipid-polysaccharide-protein complexes. The lipid portion of the lipopolysaccharide (LPS) of the outer membrane is the toxic portion. Endotoxins do not appear to stimulate an immune response in the body, nor can they be altered to prepare toxoids. They appear to function by activating a blood-clotting factor to initiate blood coagulation and by influencing the complement system (Chapter 18). The toxins of plague bacilli are especially powerful (MicroFocus 17.9).

Endotoxins manifest their presence by certain signs and symptoms. Usually an individual experiences an increase in body temperature, substantial body weakness and aches, and general malaise. Damage to the circulatory system and shock may also occur. In this case, the permeability of the blood vessels changes and blood leaks into the intercellular spaces, where it is useless. The tissues swell, the blood pressure drops, and the patient may lapse into a coma. This condition, commonly called **endotoxin shock**, may accompany antibiotic treatment of diseases due to Gram-negative bacilli because endotoxins are released as the bacilli disintegrate.

Endotoxins usually play a contributing rather than a primary role in the disease process. Certain endotoxins reduce platelet counts in the host and thereby hinder

---

as'e-til-ko'lēn
Acetylcholine:
a neurotransmitter released in the synapse, the junction of two nerves or a nerve and muscle.

ko-ri'ne-bac-te're-um
dif-the're-ā

Antitoxins:
antibodies that neutralize toxin molecules.

Toxoid:
an altered toxin used for immunization purposes.

Endotoxins:
microbial poisons released upon disintegration of the parasite cell.

Endotoxin shock:
a condition arising from the release of endotoxins and characterized by low blood pressure, swollen tissues, and shock.

MicroFocus 17.9

ENDEMIC TO EPIDEMIC

For centuries, nomadic Mongol tribesmen of Siberia observed well-established customs when dealing with marmots. These large, burrowing rodents could be shot but never trapped. A sluggishly moving animal was taboo. The lump of tissue under the animal's arm was not to be eaten because legend said it contained the soul of a dead hunter. And if a marmot colony was deemed sick, custom required that the tribesmen strike their tents and move away. Contemporary microbiologists know that prescriptions like these reduced the possibility of acquiring plague, a disease often carried by mar-

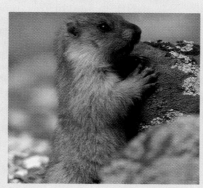

mots. As long as the laws were obeyed, the disease remained endemic.

But in 1910, furriers suddenly increased their demand for marmot skins. The skins were an ideal, low-cost substitute for sable used in women's coats. Thousands of greedy trappers invaded Siberia, led by inexperienced Chinese guides. Unaware of the local Mongol traditions, the hunters captured numerous sick marmots among the healthy ones. The results were predictable: Plague soon broke out among the hunters, and they brought the disease back to China. In a 7-month period during 1910 to 1911, an estimated 60,000 Chinese people died as the disease assumed epidemic proportions. Historians note that this was the last epidemic of plague ever recorded.

---

clot formation. Other endotoxins are known to increase hemorrhaging. Like exotoxins, endotoxins add to the virulence of a parasite and enhance its ability to establish disease.

17.3

The Human Circulatory System

The circulatory system of the human host serves as the principal vehicle for the dissemination of parasites and their toxins. Many important factors in the host defense systems also operate within the circulation. These two concepts add to the importance of a basic understanding of the circulatory system and its capabilities. Our outline of the system will also serve as a bridge between the disease process discussed in this chapter and the resistance process surveyed in the next chapter. The emphasis will be on the blood and its components.

BLOOD COMPONENTS

Blood consists of three major components: the fluid, the clotting agents, and the cells. The fluid portion, called **serum**, is an aqueous solution of minerals, salts, proteins, and other organic substances. When clotting agents, such as fibrinogen and prothrombin, are present, the fluid is referred to as **plasma**. The pH of arterial blood is about 7.35 to 7.45.

Three types of cells circulate in the blood: the red blood cells, or erythrocytes; the white blood cells, or leukocytes; and the platelets, or thrombocytes. **Erythrocytes** arise in the bone marrow and carry oxygen to the tissues loosely bound to the red pigment hemoglobin. A normal adult has about 5 million erythrocytes per cubic millimeter

Serum:
the fluid portion of the blood minus the clotting agents.
Plasma:
serum plus the clotting agents in blood.

Bilirubin:
a pigment derived from hemoglobin that gives bile a deep yellow color.

(mm³) of blood. After circulating for about 120 days, erythrocytes disintegrate in the spleen, liver, and bone marrow. The hemoglobin is then converted to bilirubin, a pigment that gives bile a deep yellow color. Normally, bilirubin is carried to the liver for degradation in a protein-bound form. However, if the liver is damaged by a disease, or if too many erythrocytes disintegrate, excess bilirubin and bile pigments may enter the bloodstream. This condition, called **jaundice**, is responsible for the yellow color of the complexion during cases of hepatitis and yellow fever.

The white blood cells, or **leukocytes**, have no pigment in their cytoplasm and therefore appear gray when unstained. These cells are also produced in the bone marrow. They number about 5000 to 9000 per mm³ of blood and have different lifespans, depending on the type of cell. TABLE 17.3 shows the different types of white blood cells, along with the other components of blood.

One type of leukocyte has a multilobed nucleus and is therefore referred to as a **polymorphonuclear cell**, or **PMN cell**. In its cytoplasm it has many lysosomes that contain digestive enzymes. One type of PMN cell is called a neutrophil, because its granules stain with neutral dyes. **Neutrophils** (FIGURE 17.22) function chiefly as phagocytes. They pass out of the circulation through pores in the vessels and squeeze into narrow passageways among the cells to engulf particles. Approximately 55 to 60 percent of the leukocytes are neutrophils. Their lifespan is about 12 hours.

pol'e-mor'fo-nu'kle-ar

Basophils are types of PMN leukocytes whose granules stain with basic dyes such as hematoxylin. The basophils number about 50 to 90 per mm³ of blood and represent about 1 percent of the total number of leukocytes. They function in allergic reactions, as their granules release physiologically active substances such as histamine. This process is discussed in detail in Chapter 20.

ba'so-fil

Eosinophils are the third type of PMN leukocyte, representing about 2 percent of the total number. These cells exhibit red cytoplasmic granules when an acidic dye such as eosin is applied. Substances in the granules are thought to neutralize the active chemicals in basophil granules. (Eosinophils, basophils, and neutrophils are often called granulocytes.) Eosinophils are postulated to have phagocytic activity.

e'o-sin'o-fil

Another major phagocyte of the circulatory system is the **monocyte**. This cell has a single, bean-shaped nucleus that takes up most of the area of the cytoplasm (a **mononuclear** cell). Monocytes lack granules and account for approximately 5 to 8 percent of the leukocytes. In the tissues, monocytes mature into a type of phagocyte called the **macrophage**. In contrast to the 2-week lifespan of monocytes, macrophages may live for several months.

Another type of leukocyte is the mononuclear **lymphocyte**. This cell arises in the bone marrow and migrates to the lymph nodes after modification. It has a single, large nucleus and no granules. (Monocytes and lymphocytes are often called agranulocytes.) Lymphocytes make up about 30 to 35 percent of the white blood cells in the human

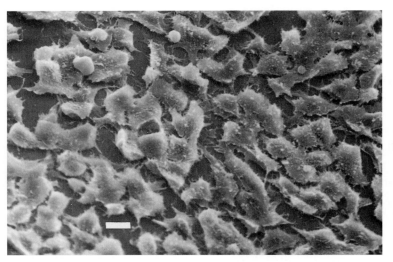

FIGURE 17.22

A View of Neutrophils

A scanning electron micrograph of neutrophils. Note the irregular shapes of the cells, demonstrating the amoebalike projections used in phagocytosis and motility. (Bar = 10 μm.)

TABLE 17.3

The Cellular Composition of Human Blood

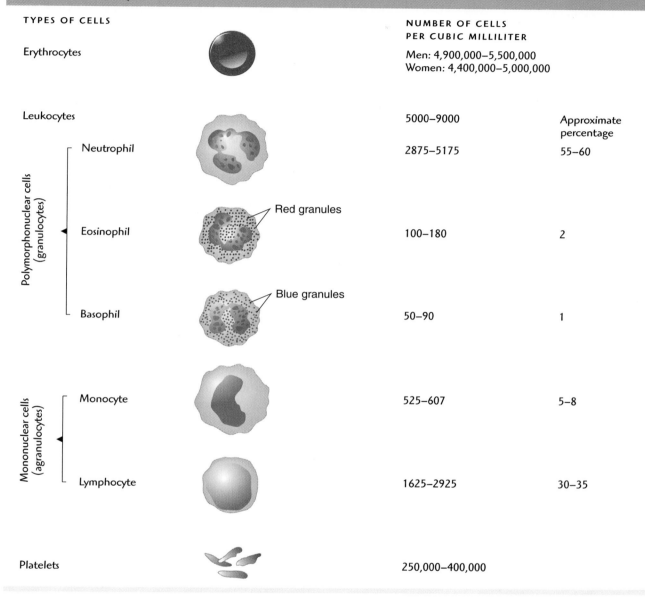

TYPES OF CELLS			NUMBER OF CELLS PER CUBIC MILLILITER	Approximate percentage
Erythrocytes			Men: 4,900,000–5,500,000 Women: 4,400,000–5,000,000	
Leukocytes			5000–9000	
Polymorphonuclear cells (granulocytes)	Neutrophil		2875–5175	55–60
	Eosinophil	Red granules	100–180	2
	Basophil	Blue granules	50–90	1
Mononuclear cells (agranulocytes)	Monocyte		525–607	5–8
	Lymphocyte		1625–2925	30–35
Platelets			250,000–400,000	

body. They function in the immune system as B-lymphocytes and T-lymphocytes (Chapter 18). Their numbers increase dramatically during the course of certain diseases, such as infectious mononucleosis.

Blood platelets, or **thrombocytes**, represent the third type of cell in the circulatory system. They are small, disk-shaped ("plate-let") cells that originate from cells in the bone marrow. Platelets have no nucleus and function chiefly in the blood-clotting mechanism.

THE LYMPHATIC SYSTEM

Lymph:
the cell-free fluid that surrounds tissue cells and fills the intercellular spaces.

The fluid that surrounds the tissue cells and fills the intercellular spaces is called tissue fluid, or **lymph**. Lymph is similar to serum except that lymph has fewer proteins. Lymph bathes the body cells, supplying oxygen and nutrients while collecting wastes. It is pumped along in tiny vessels by the contractions of skeletal muscle cells. Eventually the tiny lymph vessels unite to form large vessels that compose a lymphatic system. On the right side, the system empties into a large vein just before the heart. FIGURE 17.23 illustrates the interrelationship of the lymphatic system and the circulatory system in humans.

Lymph nodes:
pockets of lymphocytes, phagocytes, and lymphatic tissue along the lymph vessels.

Pockets of lymphatic tissue located along the lymph vessels are known as **lymph nodes**. Lymph nodes are prevalent in the neck, armpits, and groin. They are bean-shaped organs containing phagocytes, which engulf particles in the lymph, and lymphocytes, which respond specifically to substances in the circulation. Since resistance mechanisms are closely associated with the lymph nodes, it is not surprising that they become enlarged during periods of disease (sometimes they are called "swollen glands"). The tonsils, adenoids, spleen, Peyer's patches of the small intestine, and appendix are specialized types of lymph nodes. Their locations are noted in FIGURE 17.24.

Optimal functioning of the circulatory system is an essential prerequisite to good health. Parasites possess a wealth of virulence factors that add to pathogenicity, but hosts have an equally formidable array of defensive capabilities. For example, in the 1300s an estimated one-third of the population of Europe fell to bubonic plague. However, two-thirds survived, and without the benefit of antibiotics, antibody injections, or other treatments now used for disease. The nature and function of the defensive mechanisms that led to this survival and the resistance modes that operate in all humans are the major topics of Chapter 18.

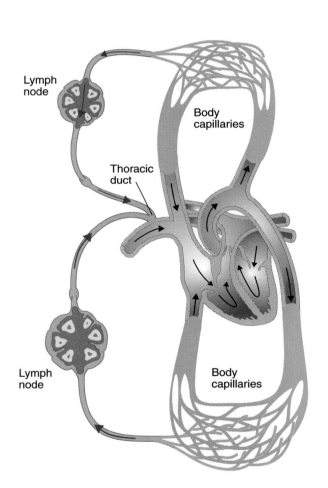

Lymph node

Body capillaries

Thoracic duct

Lymph node

Body capillaries

FIGURE 17.23

The Interrelationship of the Lymphatic System and the Circulatory System

Blood fluid passes out of the arteries in the upper and lower parts of the body. It enters a system of lymphatic ducts that arise in the tissues. The fluid, called lymph, passes through lymph nodes and on the right side makes its way back to the general circulation via the thoracic duct. The thoracic duct enters a main vein just before the vein enters the heart. A similar system exists on the left side.

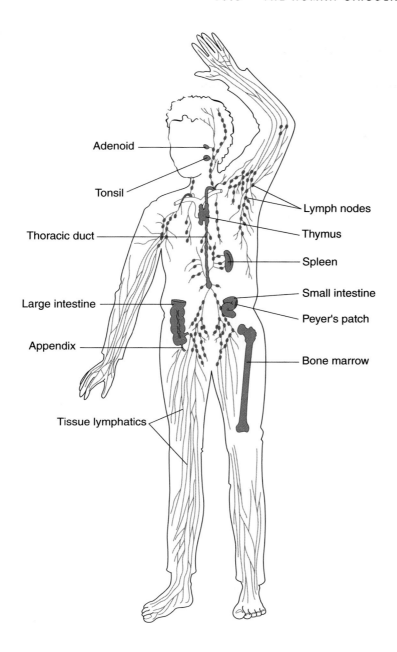

Adenoid

Tonsil

Lymph nodes

Thymus

Thoracic duct

Spleen

Small intestine

Large intestine

Peyer's patch

Appendix

Bone marrow

Tissue lymphatics

FIGURE 17.24

The Human Lymphatic System

The human lymphatic system consists of lymphocytes, lymphatic organs, lymph vessels, and lymph nodes located along the vessels. The lymphatic organs are illustrated, and the preponderance of lymph nodes in the neck, axilla, and groin is apparent.

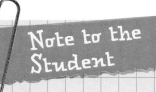

Note to the Student

You may have noted that infection, disease, and host death are widely separated phenomena with many intermediary steps. Consider, for example, what happens when cholera strikes. The bacillus, *Vibrio cholerae*, multiplies along the walls of the intestine and produces toxins. The toxins cause such massive diarrhea that up to 6 quarts of fluid may be lost over the next several hours. The blood thickens, urine production ceases, the skin becomes dry, wrinkled, and cold, and the sluggish flow of blood to the brain leads to shock, coma, and death.

Now consider where this leaves the cholera bacilli. After the host dies, the bacilli are pushed to the side by the enormous number and variety of other microorganisms normally found in the intestine. For the cholera bacilli, their source of nourishment is gone, and the environment is now filled with hostile predators. The situation has gotten thoroughly out of hand, and soon the cholera bacilli will perish just as the host perished.

It is clear that, in the long run, host death is rarely beneficial to the parasite. Is it possible that the death of the host is, in fact, a biological accident?

Summary

A review of certain concepts about infection and disease, and the factors leading to the establishment of disease, are the two principal focal points of this chapter. Infection refers to the relationship between two organisms, the host and the parasite, and the competition taking place between them. Disease may be considered a change from a general condition of good health arising from the parasite's victory in the competition. Pathogenicity, the ability of the parasite to cause disease, is fundamentally inseparable from the host's ability to resist disease. Thus, disease and resistance go hand-in-hand. Virulence refers to the degree of pathogenicity that a parasite displays.

The progress of disease follows a regular pattern that includes periods of incubation, prodrome, acme, decline, and convalescence. Diseases may be transmitted by direct or indirect methods; and a disease may be communicable, such as measles, or noncommunicable, such as tetanus. A disease may also be classified as acute or chronic, primary or secondary, local or systemic.

A parasite must have unusual abilities in order to bring about disease, and certain conditions must exist if disease is to be established. For example, the correct portal of entry and dose must be fulfilled. The possibility of disease is enhanced if a parasite can penetrate tissue or produce enzymes to overcome body defenses or synthesize toxins to interfere with body processes. Toxins can be classified as exotoxins or endotoxins, depending on their physiological effects and activity. A consideration of factors like these helps us appreciate why a parasite is pathogenic. An understanding of the blood and circulation is important because the disease process often occurs here, and because resistance arises from factors in the circulatory system.

Questions for Thought and Discussion

1. In 1840, Great Britain introduced penny postage and issued the first adhesive stamps. However, politicians did not like the idea because it deprived them of the free postage they were used to. Soon, a rumor campaign was started, saying that these gummed labels could spread disease among the population. Can you see any wisdom in their contention? Would their concern "apply" today?

2. A woman takes an antibiotic to relieve a urinary tract infection caused by *Escherichia coli*. The infection resolves, but in 2 weeks, she develops a *Candida albicans* infection of the vaginal tract. What conditions may have caused this to happen? What nonantibiotic course of treatment might a doctor prescribe to solve this problem?

3. In his classic book *The Mirage of Health* (1959), the French scientist René Dubos develops the idea that health is a balance of physiological processes, a balance that takes into account such things as better nutrition and better living conditions. (Such a view opposes the more short-sighted approach of locating an infectious agent and developing a cure.) From your experience, describe several other things that Dubos might add to his list of "balancing agents."

4. The transparent windows placed over salad bars are commonly called "sneeze bars" because they help prevent nasal droplets from reaching the salad items. What other suggestions might you make to prevent disease transmission via the salad bar?

5. In 1892, a critic of the germ theory of disease named Max von Pettenkofer sought to discredit Robert Koch's work by drinking a culture of cholera bacilli diluted in water. Von Pettenkofer suffered nothing more than mild diarrhea. What factors may have contributed to the failure of the bacilli to cause cholera in his body?

6. Between 1982 and 1992, the number of Americans dying of infectious diseases rose 58 percent. That rise continues to this day. Population shifts, modern travel patterns, and microbial evolution are three of the many reasons given for the emergence and reemergence of infectious diseases. How many other reasons can you name?

7. While slicing a piece of garden hose, a certain textbook author cut himself with a sharp knife. The wound was deep, but it closed quickly. Shortly thereafter, he reported to the emergency room of the community hospital, where he received a tetanus shot. What did the tetanus shot contain, and why was it necessary?

8. In the early 1970s, the Egyptian demographer Abdul Waheed Omran observed that in many modern industrial nations, the major killers no longer were infectious diseases. As people lived longer, he maintained, they succumbed to "diseases of civilization," such as cancer, heart disease, diabetes, obesity, and osteoporosis. Omran was among the first to recognize what he called an "epidemiological transition." Scientists now recognize that a new epidemiological transition is taking place in our era. What is this new transition, and what evidence do you think the scientists cite for the transition?

9. It has been estimated that in a sneeze, 4600 droplets are shot forth with a muzzle velocity of 152 feet per second. Scientists believe that the droplets from a single sneeze hang suspended in the air for up to 30 minutes, and collectively may contain over 35 million viruses. How many diseases can you name that are transmitted by droplets such as these?

10. An environmental microbiologist has created a stir by maintaining that a plume of water is aerosolized when a toilet is flushed, and that the plume carries bacteria to other items in the bathroom, such as toothbrushes. Assuming this is true, what might be two good practices to follow in the bathroom?

11. You are a microorganism hunter assigned to make a list of the ten worst "hot zones" in your home. The title of your top-ten list will be "Germs, Germs Everywhere." What places will make your list, and why?

12. A man takes a roll of dollar bills out of his pocket and "peels" off a few to pay the restaurant tab. Each time he peels, he wets his thumb with saliva. What is the hazard involved?

13. In your opinion, would an epidemic disease or an endemic disease pose a greater threat to public health in the community? Why? Given the choice, would you rather experience a chronic disease or an acute disease?

14. While touring a day-care center, a visitor notices that a nail brush is next to each sink. When asked why, the center director replies that all personnel are requested to use the brush after they wash their hands, especially after changing a child's diaper. Why is this a good idea?

15. When Ebola fever broke out in Africa in 1995, public health epidemiologists noted how quickly the responsible virus killed its victims and guessed that the epidemic would end shortly. Sure enough, within 3 weeks it was over. What was the basis for their prediction? What other conditions had to apply for them to be accurate in their guesswork?

Review

Test your knowledge of this chapter's contents by determining whether the following statements are true or false. If the statement is true, write "True" in the space. If false, substitute a word for the underlined word to make the statement true. The answers are listed in Appendix D.

_____ 1. An epidemic disease is one that occurs at a low level in a certain geographic area.

_____ 2. A parasite that is invasive has the ability to penetrate tissues and cause structural damage.

_____ 3. Among the microbial enzymes that are able to destroy blood cells are hemolysins and leukocidins.

_____ 4. The term disease refers to the living together of two organisms and the competition that takes place between them for supremacy.

_____ 5. Organs of the human body that do not have a normal flora include the blood and the small intestine.

_____ 6. A commensalism is a form of symbiosis in which only one organism benefits but no damage occurs to the other.

_____ 7. An organism with high virulence is generally unable to cause disease in the body.

_____ 8. The period of decline follows the period of prodromal symptoms in the progress of a disease.

_____ 9. A biological vector is an arthropod that carries pathogenic microorganisms on its feet and body parts.

_____ 10. Those organisms that cause disease when the immune system is depressed are known as opportunistic organisms.

_____ 11. A reservoir is one who has recovered from a disease but continues to shed the disease agents.

_____ 12. The human body responds to the presence of toxins by producing endotoxins.

_____ 13. The term bacteremia refers to the spread of bacteria through the bloodstream.

_____ 14. A pathogenic staphylococcus is able to form a fibrin clot through its production of hyaluronidase.

_____ 15. A toxoid is an immunizing agent prepared from an exotoxin.

_____ 16. Few symptoms are exhibited by a person who has a subclinical disease.

_____ 17. Among the indirect methods of disease transmission are kissing, hand-shaking, and contact with feces.

_____ 18. Certain parasites, such as the bacterium that causes tuberculosis, have multiple portals of entry.

_____ 19. A chronic disease is one that develops rapidly, is usually accompanied by severe symptoms, and comes to a climax.

_____ 20. The period of acme is the time between the entry of the parasite to the host and the appearance of symptoms.

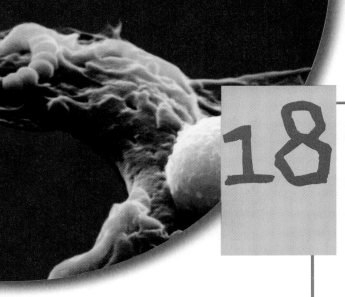

18 Resistance and the Immune System

> Interlopers are vigorously attacked and their molecular signatures are memorized so that next time they can be carded and stopped at the door.
>
> —*New York Times* reporter George Johnson describing the immune system's activity

THINK OF THE HUMAN BODY as a doughnut. Just as the hole passes through the center of the doughnut, so too the gastrointestinal tract passes through the center of the human body. The body secretes enzymes out into the hole, digests the food we eat, absorbs what it needs, and lets the remainder pass out of the hole. There is no natural opening to the internal tissues in the gastrointestinal tract, and the fact that something is in the GI tract does not mean that it is in the body.

The same is true for the respiratory and urinary tracts. The respiratory tract leads to dead-end pouches of the alveoli, while the urinary tract leads first to the urinary bladder and then to the kidneys, where it terminates at cup-shaped structures called Bowman's capsules. In both instances, a layer of cells shields the blood and the body's internal organs from the outside environment. Close examination of other parts of the body reveals similar dead-ends, and it becomes clear that the body, like the doughnut, is a closed container. Only after the walls of this container are penetrated can most diseases be established.

The skin and its extensions into the gastrointestinal, respiratory, and urinary tracts represent a major form of resistance to infection and disease. This form is **nonspecific**, because it exists in all humans and is present from birth. Also, it protects against all parasites. (The immunity is also said to be "innate.") Other forms of resistance are **specific**, because they come about in response to a particular parasite and are directed solely at that parasite

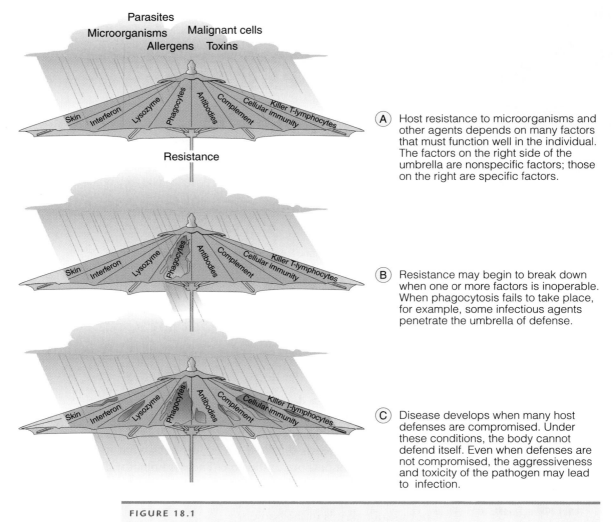

(A) Host resistance to microorganisms and other agents depends on many factors that must function well in the individual. The factors on the right side of the umbrella are nonspecific factors; those on the right are specific factors.

(B) Resistance may begin to break down when one or more factors is inoperable. When phagocytosis fails to take place, for example, some infectious agents penetrate the umbrella of defense.

(C) Disease develops when many host defenses are compromised. Under these conditions, the body cannot defend itself. Even when defenses are not compromised, the aggressiveness and toxicity of the pathogen may lead to infection.

FIGURE 18.1

The Relationship Between Host Resistance and Disease

(FIGURE 18.1). The focus of this chapter will be to examine both forms of resistance and to show how good health depends upon their proper functioning. The discussion is related to the previous chapter's study of disease, except that the emphasis switches from the parasite to the host.

18.1

Nonspecific Resistance

Nonspecific resistance to disease involves a broad group of factors, many of which are still not defined. It depends upon the general well-being of the individual and proper functioning of the body's systems. Accordingly, it takes into account such determinants as nutrition, fatigue, age, sex, and climate. Specific examples of these factors are highlighted in discussions of individual diseases, and therefore we shall not pause to delineate them here.

One form of nonspecific resistance is called **species immunity**. This genetically determined resistance implies that diseases affecting one species will not affect another. For example, humans do not contract hog cholera, while hogs do not contract AIDS (their cells lack the necessary receptor sites for HIV). Similarly, cattle plague is unknown in humans, while gonorrhea does not occur in cattle. Immunities such as these are probably based on physiological, anatomical, and biochemical differences. MicroFocus 18.1 presents an interesting offshoot of species immunity.

Behavioral immunities exist among various races and peoples of the world. Many of these immunities are due to nonspecific factors related to a people's way of life. For example, in the 1700s, Tamil laborers were brought from southern India to work on plantations in Malaya. The laborers continued the custom of bringing water into their houses only once a day and not storing it between times. This deprived mosquitoes of indoor breeding places and reduced the incidence of malaria among the laborers.

Racial immunities reflect the evolution of resistant humans. For instance, black Africans affected by the genetic disease sickle-cell anemia do not contract malaria, presumably because the parasite cannot penetrate distorted red blood cells. Some investigators hold to the theory that **population immunities** exist because parasites have adapted to the body's environment. Americans, for example, generally view measles as a mild disorder, but when the disease was introduced to Greenland in the early 1960s, it exacted a heavy toll of lives in a population that had no previous exposure to the virus. A similar event took place when the Spanish conquistadors arrived in the New World in the 1500s (MicroFocus 18.2).

In addition to species and other immunities, the body possesses a number of identifiable processes for nonspecific resistance. Like the immunities explored previously, they are present in the body from birth, but they differ because they

Species immunity:
immunity existing in one species of organism but not others.

Racial immunity:
immunity existing in one racial group but not others.
Sickle-cell anemia:
an inherited disease in which a defect in the genetic code leads to distorted red blood cells.

MicroFocus 18.1

"THANKS, BUT I'LL PASS!"

There are probably many reasons for avoiding cannibalism, but research reported in 1998 offers another disincentive: Animals that practice cannibalism will probably ingest lethal microorganisms.

The research was performed at the University of North Carolina by David Pfennig and his colleagues. Pfennig's group raised four groups of naturally cannibalistic salamanders, giving each group one of the following menus: healthy salamanders of another species, ill salamanders of another species (ill because they were exposed to bacteria-contaminated water), healthy salamanders of their own species, or ill salamanders of their own species. Of the four groups, three did very well; the one that did poorly were the sala-

manders that ate ill members of their own species. Nearly half died of bacterial infection.

The results point to the concept that bacteria specialize in particular species. If cannibalism takes place among members of the same species, the bacteria are easily transferred, and the salamanders die. But bacteria infecting a different species are not necessarily able to infect the cannibalistic species. Thus, the salamanders eating the sick animals of another species do not themselves become ill.

In the cold calculus of biology, it can make sense for an animal to reabsorb crucial energy when it consumes its young during periods of starvation ("crisis cannibalism"). But evolutionary history seems to show that animals rejecting cannibalism do better in the

long run. Perhaps they avoid self-injury by refusing to attack one another. Then again, perhaps they are really avoiding species-specific microorganisms. After all, if microbes target the dinner, why shouldn't they target the diner as well?

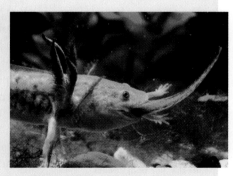

■ *A tiger salamander larva eating a member of its species.*

MicroFocus 18.2

CONQUEST BY DISEASE

History books teach that Spain's conquest of the Aztec nation of Central America was due to horses, gunpowder, and the superior force of Spanish arms. But conquest meant overcoming millions of people and overturning long-standing traditions of religion and culture, and there were only 800 men with Hernando Cortez the day he landed in Mexico in 1518. Cortez and the Spanish eventually toppled the Aztec nation, but their strongest ally was not gunpowder and arms; it was disease.

Mexico was totally unprepared for smallpox. The disease was new to the country, and the Aztec population was without any trace of immunity. The Spanish, on the other hand, had contended with European outbreaks of smallpox for generations, and they were relatively immune. Little thought was given to the consequences when slaves sick with smallpox arrived with the Spaniards. Soon the Aztec community was infected.

By April 1521, Cortez had established a colony on Mexican soil and marched inland to attack Mexico City, the stronghold of the Aztec nation. The siege continued for four months, until the city finally fell on August 13, 1521. Expecting to plunder the city, the Spanish rushed in, but were shocked to find the houses filled with the dead. A smallpox epidemic was raging. Half the population had succumbed.

Nor did it end here. Eleven years later, Spanish invaders introduced another epidemic of disease, believed to be measles. Thousands of Aztecs died. In 1545, disease broke out again. Contemporary writings describing the symptoms indicate that it was either epidemic typhus or typhoid fever. In one province 150,000 people are estimated to have died. Influenza raged in 1558 and 1559, and mumps broke out with fatal consequences in 1576.

By the end of the century, the Aztec nation was battered into submission. Native authority figures succumbed, and the surviving Aztecs dutifully obeyed the commands of Spanish landowners, tax collectors, and missionaries. To both the conqueror and the conquered, the divine and natural orders had spoken out loudly against the native beliefs; the Aztecs would offer no further resistance. By one historian's account, almost 19 million of the original population of 25 million died of disease by 1595.

---

operate against all foreign substances and organisms. We shall review a number of these processes next.

MECHANICAL AND CHEMICAL BARRIERS

As noted in the chapter's introduction, the intact **skin** and the **mucous membranes** that extend into the body cavities are among the most important resistance factors. The skin's epidermis is constantly being sloughed off, and with it go microorganisms. The keratin in skin is a poor source of carbon for microorganisms; the fatty acids in sebum and sweat are antimicrobic; and, from the viewpoint of a microorganism, the low water content of the skin presents a veritable desert. Toxins notwithstanding, unless penetration of these barriers occurs, disease is rare.

But penetration of the skin barrier is a fact of everyday life. A cut or abrasion, for example, allows staphylococci to enter the blood, and an arthropod bite acts as a hypodermic needle permitting many different organisms to enter. Yellow fever viruses, malaria parasites, most species of rickettsiae, and plague bacilli are but a few examples. Other means of penetrating the barrier include splinters, tooth extractions, burns, shaving nicks, war wounds, and injections.

Certain features of the mucous membranes provide resistance to parasites. For instance, cells of the mucous membranes along the lining of the respiratory passageways secrete **mucus**, which traps heavy particles and microorganisms. The **cilia** of other cells then move the particles along the membranes up to the throat, where they are swallowed. Stomach acid now destroys any microorganisms.

Resistance in the vaginal tract is enhanced by the low pH. This develops when *Lactobacillus* **species** in the normal flora break down glycogen to various acids. Many

Mucus:
a thick fluid secreted by membranes that line body cavities opening to the exterior.

researchers believe that the disappearance of lactobacilli during antibiotic treatment encourages diseases such as candidiasis and trichomoniasis to develop. In the urinary tract, the slightly acidic pH of the urine promotes resistance to parasites, and the flow of urine flushes microorganisms away.

A natural barrier to the gastrointestinal tract is provided by **stomach acid**, which has a pH of approximately 2.0. (A cotton handkerchief placed in stomach acid would dissolve in a few short moments.) Most organisms are destroyed in this environment. Notable exceptions include typhoid and tubercle bacilli, protozoal cysts, and polio and hepatitis A viruses and *Helicobacter pylori*, a major cause of peptic ulcers. **Bile** from the gallbladder enters the system at the duodenum and serves as an inhibitory substance. In addition, duodenal enzymes digest the proteins, carbohydrates, fats, and other large molecules of microorganisms.

A chemical inhibitor of a nonspecific nature is the enzyme **lysozyme**. This protein was described in the early 1920s by Alexander Fleming, who later gained recognition for the discovery of penicillin. Lysozyme is found in human tears and saliva. It disrupts the cell walls of Gram-positive bacteria by digesting peptidoglycan. Another inhibitor is **interferon**. Interferon is actually a group of substances (interferons) produced by body cells in response to invasion by viruses. Interferons trigger the production of inhibitory substances that "interfere" with viral reproduction. A thorough account of the interferons is presented in Chapter 11.

TABLE 18.1 summarizes many of the nonspecific mechanical and chemical resistance mechanisms.

PHAGOCYTOSIS

Shortly after the germ theory of disease was verified by Koch, a native of Ukraine named **Elie Metchnikoff** made a chance discovery that clarified how living cells could protect themselves against microorganisms. Metchnikoff noted that motile cells in the larva of a starfish gathered around a wooden splinter placed within the cell mass. He suggested that the cells actively sought out and engulfed foreign particles in the environment to provide resistance. Metchnikoff's theory of **phagocytosis**, published in

kan′dĭ-di′ah-sis
trik′o-mo-ni′ah-sis

Bile:
the yellow-brown mixture of acids, salts, pigments, and other substances produced by the liver and stored in the gallbladder for fat digestion.

li′so-zīm

in′ter-fēr′on

Metch′ni-koff

fag′o-sī-to′sis

TABLE 18.1

Nonspecific Mechanical and Chemical Barriers to Disease

RESISTANCE MECHANISM	ACTIVITY
Skin layers	Provide a protective covering to all body tissues
Mucous membranes of body cavities	Trap airborne particles in mucus Sweep particles along by cilia
Acidity in the vagina and stomach	Acidic pH toxic to microorganisms
Bile	Inhibitory to most microorganisms
Duodenal enzymes	Digest structural and metabolic chemical components of microorganisms
Lysozyme in tears, saliva, secretions	Digests cell walls of Gram-positive bacteria
Interferons	Inhibit replication of viruses
Peristalsis	Moves materials along in GI tract to limit attachment

Antitoxins:
antibodies produced specifically
against toxins.

Monocytes:
large, phagocytic white blood
cells having a single, bean-shaped
nucleus.

Lysosome:
a saclike organelle in eukaryotic
cells that contains digestive
enzymes and other factors to aid
digestion.

Complement:
a series of proteins that function
in resistance mechanisms.

1884, was received with skepticism, because it appeared to conflict with the antitoxin theory then in vogue. Many investigators believed that antitoxins produced by the body were the sole basis for resistance, but in succeeding years they came to appreciate phagocytosis as equally important. Metchnikoff later became an associate of Pasteur and was a corecipient of the 1908 Nobel Prize in Physiology or Medicine.

In contemporary microbiology, phagocytosis ("cell-eating") is viewed as a major form of nonspecific defense in the body. The cells involved are called **phagocytes** (FIGURE 18.2). They are polymorphonuclear (PMN) cells and monocytes of the circulatory system (Chapter 17), as well as cells of the **reticuloendothelial system (RES)**. This system, also called the **mononuclear phagocyte system**, is a collection of monocyte-derived cells that leave the circulation and undergo modification in the tissues. They include Kupffer cells of the liver and **macrophages** of the spleen, bone marrow, lymph nodes, brain, and connective tissues. RES cells are larger than monocytes and have more lysosomes and a longer lifespan. Some phagocytes are termed **resting cells** because they are stationary, while other phagocytes are **wandering cells** because they are actively motile.

Phagocytosis begins with an invagination, or folding in, of the cell membrane to form a phagocytic vesicle, or **phagosome** (FIGURE 18.3). The phagosome then pinches off and fuses with a **lysosome**, an organelle that contributes digestive enzymes, lysozyme, and an acidic pH to the digestion process. Lysosomal substances also increase the permeability of capillaries, which brings more phagocytes to the area. The process is completed as waste materials are egested from the phagocyte.

A chemical attraction called a **chemotaxis** exists between parasite and phagocyte. This attraction is mediated by several substances released by the parasite. One substance is the end of a methionine-containing protein clipped off by a prokaryote during the protein's maturation. The interaction between parasite and phagocyte is also enhanced by the presence of **antibodies**. These protein molecules attach to parasites and increase adherence to the phagocytic cell at specific receptor sites. In other situations, components of the complement system (discussed shortly) bind the parasite to the phagocyte. Enhanced phagocytosis is called **opsonization**, and the antibodies or complement components that encourage it are termed **opsonins**, from Latin stems meaning "to prepare for." Opsonins were first described in 1903 by Almroth Wright, who imagined them as serum proteins increasing the susceptibility of

FIGURE 18.2

Phagocytosis

A transmission electron micrograph of a dividing bacillus being engulfed by a polymorphonuclear cell. The extensions of the PMN cell surround the bacilli, and membranes of the phagocytic vesicle follow the contours of the organism engulfed.

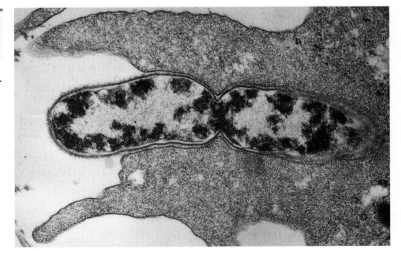

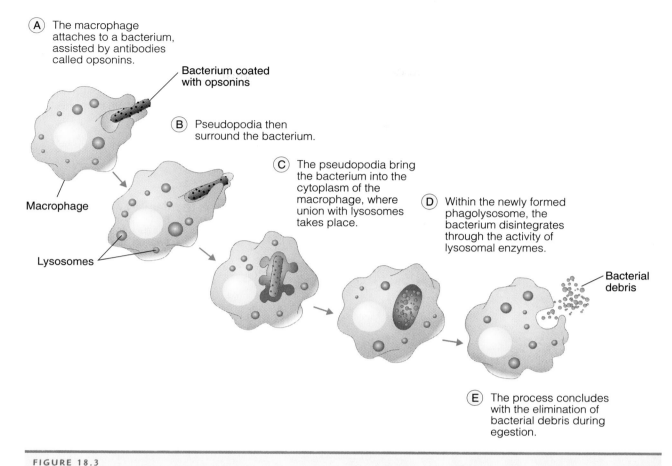

(A) The macrophage attaches to a bacterium, assisted by antibodies called opsonins.

Bacterium coated with opsonins

Macrophage

(B) Pseudopodia then surround the bacterium.

(C) The pseudopodia bring the bacterium into the cytoplasm of the macrophage, where union with lysosomes takes place.

(D) Within the newly formed phagolysosome, the bacterium disintegrates through the activity of lysosomal enzymes.

Lysosomes

Bacterial debris

(E) The process concludes with the elimination of bacterial debris during egestion.

FIGURE 18.3

The Mechanism of Phagocytosis

parasites to phagocytosis. At the time, it was a way of unifying Metchnikoff's phago-cytosis theory with the antitoxin theory.

INFLAMMATION

Inflammation is a nonspecific defensive response by the body to an injury in the tissue. It develops after a mechanical injury, such as an injury or blow to the skin, or from exposure to a chemical agent, such as acid or bee venom. It may also be due to a physical agent, such as heat or ultraviolet radiation, or to a living organism, such as a parasite.

The irritant sets into motion a process that limits the extent of the injury (FIGURE 18.4). Dilation of the blood vessels leads to increased capillary permeability, fol-lowed by a flow of plasma into the tissue and fluid accumulation at the site of irri-tation. Neutrophils adhere to the vessels close to the injury and migrate through the wall (diapedesis) to begin phagocytosis of the irritant. Soon, macrophages replace the neutrophils. The area will exhibit four characteristic signs of inflammation: **rubor**, a red color from blood accumulation; **calor**, warmth from the heat of the blood; **tumor**, swelling from the accumulation of fluid; and **dolor**, pain from injury to the local nerves.

Neutrophils:
phagocytic white blood cells
having a multilobed nucleus.

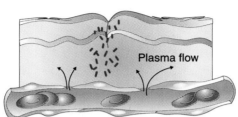

(A) A thorn pierces the skin, causing a mechanical injury and bringing bacteria into the tissue.

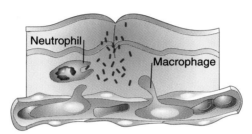

(B) Capillary walls open (dilate), and plasma flows to the site of injury, making it red, swollen, and warm.

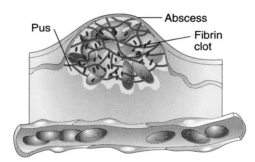

(C) Neutrophils arrive and begin phagocytosis, and macrophages follow to continue the process.

(D) A fibrin wall accumulates around the mixture of plasma, leukocytes, bacteria, and tissue cells, collectively called pus. An abscess becomes apparent.

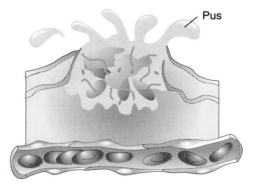

(E) Lancing of the abscess releases the pus.

FIGURE 18.4

The Process of Inflammation

A product of phagocytosis during inflammation is the mixture of plasma, dead tissue cells, leukocytes, and dead bacteria known as **pus**. When pus becomes enclosed in a wall of fibrin through activation of the clotting mechanism, a sac may form. This sac is an **abscess**, or **boil**, often due to staphylococci. When several abscesses accumulate, an enlarged structure called a **carbuncle** results.

Inflammation and phagocytosis are thus interrelated. Their purpose is to confine the irritant to the site of entry and to repair or replace the tissue that has been injured.

Abscess:
a fibrin-enclosed sac of pus.

FEVER

Fever is an abnormally high body temperature that may provide a nonspecific mechanism of defense against disease. Scientists believe that bacteria, viruses, and other microorganisms affect a region at the base of the brain called the **hypothalamus** and stimulate it to raise the body temperature several degrees. The rise is mediated by a substance called interleukin-1, which is generated by phagocytes engulfing the parasites. As this takes place, cell metabolism increases and blood vessels constrict, thus denying blood to the skin and keeping its heat within the body. Patients thus experience cold skin and chills along with the fever.

Fever may be beneficial because it appears to inhibit the growth of certain organisms. The increased metabolism in cells also encourages rapid tissue repair and raises the level of phagocytosis, while reducing the amount of bloodborne iron needed by parasites. However, if the temperature rises above 40.6°C (105°F), convulsions and death may result.

NATURAL KILLER CELLS

Natural killer (NK) cells are a unique group of defensive cells that roam the body in blood and lymph and kill cancer cells and virus-infected cells before the immune system is enlisted. NK cells were originally believed to be lymphocytes involved in the immune response, but this theory has proven untrue, because NK cells act spontaneously and without any involvement of the immune system. The name "natural" killer cells reflects the nonspecific nature of the killing activity.

NK cells contain on their surfaces a set of special receptor sites that must form a complex with the target cells before a cell-cell interaction takes place. The receptor sites match with a group of class I MHC proteins (to be discussed presently), which are found on all body cells. When the normal class I MHC proteins are present, the NK cell recognizes the target cell as one of the body's own, and spares it. However, when the MHC proteins are absent or in reduced amounts (as on a cancer cell or virus-infected cell), then the NK cell binds to the target cell, damages its cell membrane, and induces lysis.

COMPLEMENT

Complement (also called the complement system) is a series of over 20 proteins that circulate in the bloodstream. Though complement is better known for its relationship to the immune system (it "complements" antigen–antibody activity), the protein series is also a nonspecific deterrent to disease. One of the complement proteins is the so-called **C3 molecule**. This protein binds to microbial proteins protruding from the cell walls of bacteria and other microorganisms. Once bound, the C3 molecule activates other complement components to bind as well, and soon the organism is enclosed in a layer of proteins and destroyed.

Complement also works nonspecifically through its interaction with phagocytes. After engulfing bacteria, phagocytes release a substance called **interleukin-6**. Transported through the bloodstream, interleukin-6 causes the liver to secrete a protein that binds to the carbohydrate mannose in the capsule of the bacterium. The binding triggers other complement components to react on the surface of the bacterium, and the latter is soon destroyed. By acting without intervention of the immune system, complement represents a form of nonspecific defense. We shall encounter the complement system once again in the next section.

To this point . . .

We have begun the study of resistance to disease by outlining some nonspecific mechanisms that defend against all parasites from the time of birth. Species and racial immunities are examples. Other examples are mechanical and chemical barriers, including the barriers presented by the skin and mucous membranes, the acidity in the stomach and vagina, and the antimicrobial substances lysozyme and interferon.

We examined phagocytosis in depth since this process is a major form of nonspecific defense. The process may involve particles as well as dissolved materials. Chemotaxis and antibodies increase the efficiency of phagocytosis. We also noted the value of inflammation, fever, and natural killer cells in nonspecific resistance. The complement system was formerly believed to be solely a part of the specific mechanism of resistance, but scientists now realize its nonspecific role.

We shall now focus on specific resistance as reflected by the immune system. After a brief discussion of the beginnings of immunology, we shall survey antigens, the substances that stimulate the immune response. From there, we shall explore the origin of the immune system and see how it is established in the body. The system is actually dual in nature, although the processes are interlocking. The discussion will therefore diverge, first to study the system of cell-mediated immunity and later to examine antibody-mediated immunity. In a sense, this is the most important section in the entire textbook because it outlines the processes by which specific resistance to specific parasites takes place. How well the resistance operates largely dictates whether a person will remain free of infectious disease or will recover from disease.

18.2

Specific Resistance and the Immune System

In the late 1800s, the mechanisms of specific resistance to infectious disease were largely obscure because no one was really sure how the body responded when infected. However, medical bacteriologists were aware that certain proteins of the blood unite specifically with chemical compounds of microorganisms. The blood proteins were named **Bence Jones proteins** after Henry Bence Jones, a British physician who identified them in the urine of a patient. In 1922, researchers from Johns Hopkins University showed that Bence Jones proteins (later found to be parts of antibodies) were unlike normal serum proteins, but the nature of the proteins remained a matter of conjecture.

Until the 1950s, specific resistance to disease was virtually synonymous with immunity. By that time, vaccines were available for numerous diseases, and immunologists saw themselves as specialists in disease prevention. But the explosion of interest in the biological sciences after World War II spilled over to immunology, and soon it became apparent that **specific resistance** is a phenomenon with broader implications, including organ transplantation, allergic reactions, and resistance to cancer. In addition, the groundwork was laid for deciphering the nature and function of the Bence Jones proteins. This work would lead to the elucidation of antibody structure in the 1960s, and the maturing of immunology to one of the key scientific disciplines of our times.

In this section, we shall study the immune system as it relates to specific resistance to disease. But it should be noted that the immune system also relates to the cancer patient, transplant recipient, laboratory diagnostician, and hay fever sufferer. Some of these topics are explored in detail in Chapters 19 and 20. Research in immunology provides an important window to the disease process, as well as many other processes of life. Our study will begin with a survey of the substances that stimulate the immune response.

ANTIGENS

Antigens are chemical substances capable of mobilizing the immune system and provoking an immune response. Most antigens are large, complex molecules (macromolecules), which are not normally found in the body and are consequently referred to as "nonself." Antigens exhibit two important properties: **immunogenicity**, the ability to stimulate cells of the immune system; and **reactivity**, the ability to react with products of immune system cells, or with the cells themselves. Antigens are often called **immunogens**.

The list of antigens is enormously diverse. It includes milk proteins, substances in bee venom, hemoglobin molecules, bacterial toxins, and chemical substances found in bacterial flagella, pili, and capsules (FIGURE 18.5). The most common antigens are proteins, polysaccharides, and the chemical complexes formed between these substances and lipids or nucleic acids. Proteins are the most potent antigens because their amino acids have the greatest array of building blocks, an array leading to a

Antigens:
any foreign substances that elicit a response by the body's immune system.

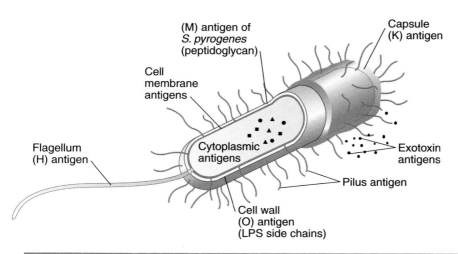

FIGURE 18.5

The Various Antigens Possible on a Bacterial Cell

Each different antigen in this idealized bacterium is capable of stimulating the immune system.

Dalton:
a unit of weight equal to the
weight of one hydrogen atom.

huge variety of combinations and hence, diversity in three-dimensional structures. Polysaccharides are less potent antigens than proteins because they lack chemical diversity and rapidly break down in the body. Lipids can also be antigenic, as exemplified by the cell wall lipids (mycolic acid) of tubercle bacilli.

Antigens usually have a molecular weight of over 10,000 daltons. Because of this large size, the antigen molecule is easily phagocytized by macrophages, the necessary first step in the immune process. Antigens do not stimulate the immune system directly. Rather, the stimulation is accomplished by a small part of the antigen molecule called the **antigenic determinant**, or **epitope**. An antigenic determinant (epitope) contains about six to eight amino acid molecules or monosaccharide units. Each antigenic determinant has a characteristic three-dimensional shape and a molecular weight of about 350 daltons. An antigen may have numerous antigenic determinants, and a structure such as a bacterial flagellum may have hundreds of these molecules. Antigenic determinants are unique microbial fingerprints to which the immune system responds (FIGURE 18.6).

Small nucleotides, hormones, peptides, and other molecules usually are not capable of stimulating the immune system by themselves. However, when they link to proteins in the body, the immune system may recognize the combination as foreign and respond to it. Allergy reactions (Chapter 20) are examples of immune responses to these combinations. The small molecule in the combination provides the key

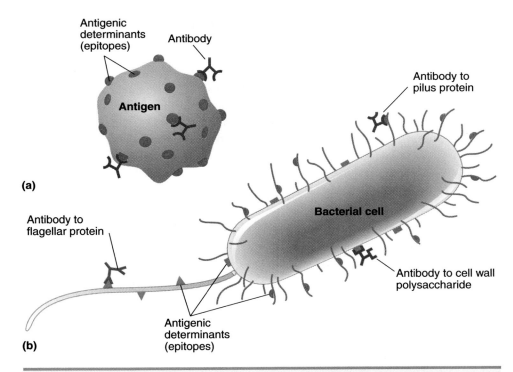

(a)

(b)

FIGURE 18.6

Antigens and Antigenic Determinants

(a) A large antigen molecule showing a number of antigenic determinants, also called epitopes. These are the sites where products of the immune system, such as antibodies, will interact. The reaction between antigenic determinants and antibodies neutralizes the antigen. (b) A bacterium with various sources of antigens and the antibodies that react with the antigenic determinants on these antigens. Note the variations in structure of the antigenic determinants and the corresponding antibodies that unite specifically with them.

functional unit and is known as a **hapten** (*haptein* is Greek for "grasp," a reference to the interactions between the hapten molecule and the immune system's antibody). Examples of haptens are penicillin molecules, molecules in poison ivy plants, and molecules in certain cosmetics and dyes.

Under normal circumstances, one's own chemical substances do not stimulate an immune response. This failure to stimulate the immune system occurs because the substances are interpreted as "self." Immunologists believe that prior to birth, the body's proteins and polysaccharides inactivate the immune system cells that otherwise might respond to them. In the fetal stage, these responsive cells are easily paralyzed. The individual thereby develops a tolerance of "self" and remains able to respond only to "nonself." This theory, known as **specific immunologic tolerance**, was advanced in the late 1950s by Frank MacFarlane Burnet (a 1960 Nobel laureate) and David Talmage. Cells responding to self are also destroyed in the thymus, as we shall see shortly.

Antigens enter the body through a variety of portals such as the mucous membranes of the respiratory tract, a wound, an arthropod bite through the skin, or an injury to the gastrointestinal tract. **Autoantigens** are a person's own chemical substances that stimulate an immune response when self-tolerance breaks down (as in lupus erythematosus, Chapter 20). **Alloantigens** are antigens existing in certain but not all members of a species. The A, B, and Rh antigens of humans are typical alloantigens. **Heterophile** antigens are antigens found in unrelated species. Other types of antigens that we shall encounter later in this chapter are T-dependent antigens, T-independent antigens, and superantigens. Any of these antigens are responsible for eliciting the immune response, as we shall see next.

THE ORIGIN OF THE IMMUNE SYSTEM

The **immune system** is a general term for the complex series of cells, factors, and processes providing an adaptive and specific response to antigens associated with microorganisms, or with potentially harmful molecules such as microbial toxins. As such, the system lends specific resistance against infection and disease.

The cornerstones of the immune system are a set of body cells known as **lymphocytes**. These cells are distributed throughout the body, where they comprise the lymphoid system (Chapter 17). Lymphocytes are small cells, about 10 to 20 μm in diameter, each with a large nucleus taking up almost the entire space of the cytoplasm. Under the microscope, all lymphocytes look similar. However, two types of lymphocytes can be distinguished on the basis of developmental history, cellular function, and unique biochemical differences. The two types are B-lymphocytes and T-lymphocytes. **B-lymphocytes** are largely responsible for antibody-mediated immunity (AMI), while **T-lymphocytes** are primarily responsible for cell-mediated immunity (CMI). In AMI, antibodies provide resistance to disease, while in CMI, cytotoxic T-lymphocytes provide resistance through direct cell-to-cell contact.

The immune system arises in the fetus about 2 months after conception (FIGURE 18.7). At this time, lymphocytes originate from primitive cells in the yolk sac and bone marrow known as **stem cells**. Stem cells differentiate into two types of cells: **erythropoietic cells** (myeloid cells), which become red blood cells; and **lymphopoietic cells**, which become lymphocytes of the immune system. (The Greek word *poien* means "to make"; thus, lymphopoietic cells are "lymphocyte-making cells.") We shall now follow the fate of the lymphopoietic cells.

Lymphopoietic cells take either of two courses. Some of the cells proceed to an organ of the thoracic cavity called the **thymus**. This flat, bilobed organ lies below the

Hapten:
a small molecule that complexes with a protein or polysaccharide to form an antigen.

Autoantigens:
a person's own chemical substances that elicit an immune response.

het′er-o-fil′
Heterophile antigens:
identical antigens found in apparently unrelated species.

ĕ-rith′ro-poi-et′ik
lim-fo′poi-et′ik

FIGURE 18.7

The Origin of the Immune System

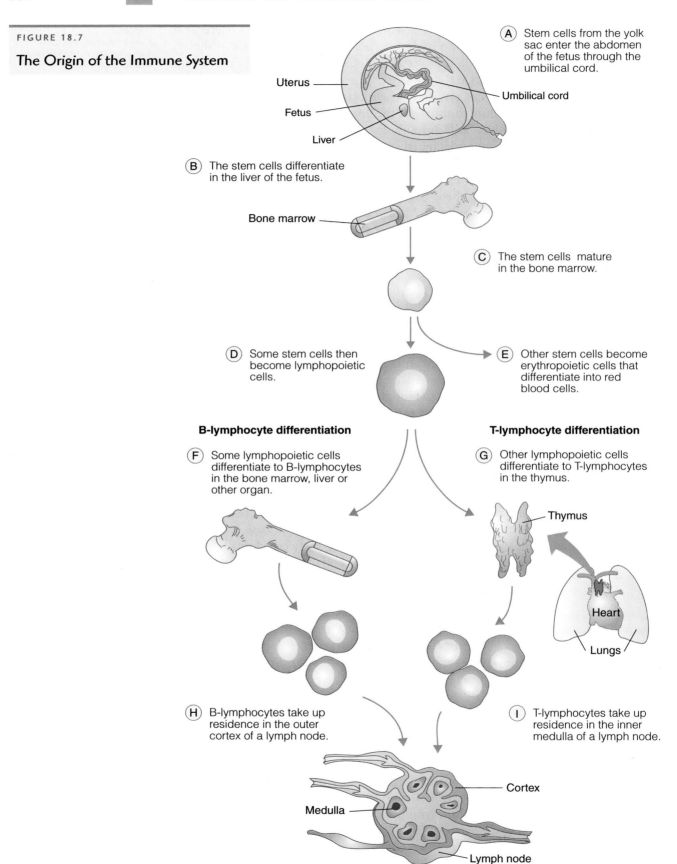

A Stem cells from the yolk sac enter the abdomen of the fetus through the umbilical cord.

Uterus

Umbilical cord

Fetus

Liver

B The stem cells differentiate in the liver of the fetus.

Bone marrow

C The stem cells mature in the bone marrow.

D Some stem cells then become lymphopoietic cells.

E Other stem cells become erythropoietic cells that differentiate into red blood cells.

B-lymphocyte differentiation

T-lymphocyte differentiation

F Some lymphopoietic cells differentiate to B-lymphocytes in the bone marrow, liver or other organ.

G Other lymphopoietic cells differentiate to T-lymphocytes in the thymus.

Thymus

Heart

Lungs

H B-lymphocytes take up residence in the outer cortex of a lymph node.

I T-lymphocytes take up residence in the inner medulla of a lymph node.

Cortex

Medulla

Lymph node

thyroid gland near the top of the heart. The thymus is large in size at birth and increases in size until the age of puberty, when it begins to shrink. Within the thymus, the lymphopoietic cells mature over a 2- or 3-day period and are modified by the addition of surface receptor proteins. They emerge from the organ as T-lymphocytes (T for thymus). Mature T-lymphocytes, or **T-cells**, are ready to engage in cell-mediated immunity and are said to be **immunocompetent**. The T-lymphocytes colonize the lymph nodes, spleen, tonsils, and other lymphoid organs, and they become a major portion of the lymphoid system.

Thymus:
a flat bilobed organ in the upper thorax of humans where T-lymphocytes are modified.

It should be noted that a large percentage of lymphopoietic cells are destroyed in the thymus (a type of "programmed cell death"). These cells would normally react with self antigens. Therefore, the mature T-lymphocytes emerging are the cells able to interact with nonself antigens.

The B-lymphocytes mature and become immunocompetent in a site that has not been determined with certainty in humans. Much evidence suggests that the bone marrow is the maturation site, but some immunologists favor the liver, spleen, or gut-associated tissue as the site. In the embryonic chick, the maturation site has been identified as the bursa of Fabricius (MicroFocus 18.3). For this reason, the lymphocyte is known historically as the bursa-derived or B-lymphocyte (although the letter B can be related to bone marrow). Like the T-lymphocytes, B-lymphocytes mature with surface receptor proteins on their membranes and become immunocompetent. Once they are **immunocompetent**, the B-lymphocytes, or **B-cells**, move through the circulation to colonize organs of the lymphoid system, where they join the T-lymphocytes.

Bursa of Fabricius:
a gland in the gastrointestinal tract of chicks where B-lymphocytes are formed.

As noted, the maturation of both T-lymphocytes and B-lymphocytes is accompanied by the insertion of **surface receptor proteins** spanning the width of the cell membrane. The receptor protein enables the lymphocyte to recognize a specific

MicroFocus 18.3

"YOU GAVE ME BAD CHICKENS!"

For a young graduate student studying poultry science at Ohio State University, it was a rather embarrassing end to a routine laboratory experiment.

Timothy S. Chang had been assigned to show some younger students how chickens develop immunity when injected with *Salmonella* bacilli. For the demonstration, he borrowed a dozen healthy chickens from Bruce Glick, a fellow graduate student. Glick had been using the chickens to study the functions of a mysterious gland in their intestines. Chang and his students carefully inoculated the chickens with *Salmonella*, waited a week, and then drew blood samples to test for evidence of *Salmonella* antibodies. To Chang's surprise and chagrin, 10 of the 12 chickens failed to show any sign of antibodies.

Chang went down the hall to Glick's lab and asked if he were playing some kind of joke. Puzzled at his friend's results, Glick checked his lab records and found he had removed the mysterious gland from the 10 "bad" chickens. The two animals that developed antibodies still had the gland intact.

The year was 1954. The gland was the bursa of Fabricius, named for Hieronymus Fabricius, a seventeenth-century anatomist who discovered it. Glick had developed an interest in the obscure gland after observing it in the intestine of a goose and learning that its function was unknown. He had removed the gland in newborn chicks and found there was no effect on growth. His research was at a dead-end until Chang's experiment gave him a clue to the true function of the gland. Glick and Chang

repeated the experiment and published their results in 1956 in *Poultry Science*, a specialty journal.

The accidental discovery might have gone unnoticed except that zoologists at the University of Wisconsin spotted it and confirmed the findings. As word spread to immunologists, Robert A. Good at the University of Minnesota assigned a team of colleagues to develop the theory of "bursa-derived immunity." In 1965, Good's team delivered its report before the American Academy of Pediatrics. Several immunologists cautioned against drawing conclusions about humans from work with chickens, but many saw the discovery as an important first step to understanding the origin of antibodies.

antigenic determinant (epitope) and bind to it. After this recognition and binding has occurred, the lymphocyte is said to be **committed**. In T-lymphocytes, the receptor protein at the cell surface is composed of two chains of glycoproteins linked to one another by sulfur-sulfur chemical bonds. In B-lymphocytes, the receptor protein is an antibody molecule believed to be IgD. About 100,000 surface receptors are found on each T- or B-lymphocyte.

The location of highly specific receptor proteins on the lymphocyte surface is one of the more remarkable discoveries of contemporary immunology. The implication is that even before an antigen enters the body, an immunocompetent cell is already waiting for it. Moreover, the genetic code for synthesizing the surface receptor is present in an individual even though that individual has not ever been exposed to an antigen. We may never experience malaria, for example, yet we already have surface receptor proteins for recognizing and binding to the antigens of malaria parasites. This concept is engaging and thought-provoking.

The recognition between antigenic determinants and lymphocytes depends on surface receptor proteins plus another set of glycoprotein molecules called the **major histocompatibility complex proteins**, or **MHC proteins**. (These proteins are sometimes called MHC antigens because they stimulate an antibody response in other individuals.) MHC proteins are embedded in the membranes of all cells of the body. At least 20 different genes encode MHC proteins, and at least 50 different forms of the genes exist. Thus, the variety of MHC proteins existing in the human population is enormous, and the chance of two individuals having the same MHC proteins is incredibly small. (The notable exception is identical twins.) The MHC proteins define the uniqueness of the individual and play a role in the immune response.

There are two important classes of MHC proteins, and both help define the individual as self. **Class I MHC proteins** are found on virtually all cells of the body, but **class II MHC proteins** can be found only on B-lymphocytes and macrophages and a few other types. These class II proteins function in the immune response. There is also evidence that certain human diseases are associated with the MHC proteins (Chapter 20).

The actual immune response originates with the entry of antigens into the body and the penetration into the lymphatic or cardiovascular system. Here the antigens are phagocytized by **macrophages** and other phagocytic cells, and the antigens are broken down to release the antigenic determinants, or epitopes (FIGURE 18.8). The macrophages display the antigenic determinants on their surface and transport

Glycoprotein:
a protein molecule having a number of attached carbohydrate molecules.

MHC proteins:
proteins on the surface of body cells that define the uniqueness of an individual.

FIGURE 18.8

Phagocytosis

This colored scanning electron micrograph shows a macrophage (gray) engulfing a species of *Leishmania* (purple), the protozoan that causes leishmaniasis (Chapter 15). Note the highly irregular fluid nature of the surface of the macrophage.

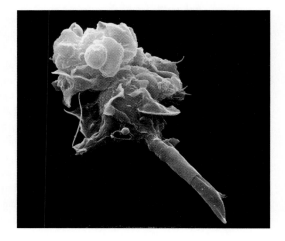

them to the lymphoid organs, where T-lymphocytes and B-lymphocytes are waiting. Another important antigen transporter is the **dendritic cell**, a cell with long, fingerlike extensions that form lacy networks in virtually all tissues and phagocytize infected cells nearby. The phagocytosis and transport are extremely important because research evidence indicates that unprocessed antigens stimulate the immune system poorly.

Within the tissues of the lymphoid organs (spleen, lymph nodes, tonsils, and so on), the T-lymphocytes and B-lymphocytes are waiting to implement either of the two arms of the immune system. **Antibody-mediated immunity** (previously known as **humoral immunity**) will result in antibodies that react with microorganisms (e.g., free bacteria and viruses), soluble antigens, and nonself cells within the body's environment. **Cell-mediated immunity** will result in activated T-lymphocytes for direct interaction with eukaryotic pathogens, as well as antigen-marked cells (such as virus-infected and transplanted cells). In the next section, we shall discuss both types of immunity, beginning with cell-mediated immunity.

But before discussing these processes, we must make note of a newly emerging theory of how the immune system works. This is the so-called **danger model of immunity**. To this point, we have been developing the notion that the immune system fights anything that is not part of our body, the self/nonself model of immunity. The danger model suggests that the immune system ignores harmless materials, while fighting dangerous ones. Thus, the system would not react to the foods we eat (allergies notwithstanding) but would react to invading parasites. While the self/nonself model requires the immune system to educate itself as to what's good and what's not, the danger model maintains that the immune system can tolerate antigens at any time and does not need to distinguish self from nonself. Instead, it will spring into action only when an antigen is associated with harm.

The origin of the danger model traces to three papers published in 1996 in the highly respected journal *Science*. Research teams from various laboratories found that the immature immune systems of mice can produce an immune response when confronted with viruses. (The conventional wisdom is that immature systems cannot respond because they are busy learning how to tolerate themselves by "weeding out" the appropriate cells.) They also discovered that adult, mature mice can be taught to tolerate cells they never before encountered (theoretically, that tolerance should have existed before birth). Some of the researchers see the results as modifications to the self/nonself model, but others envision an immune system that does not discriminate between self and nonself. And if that is the case, then perhaps the system is discriminating between dangerous and nondangerous.

At this writing, the danger model remains controversial, especially since it questions a theory that has been entrenched for a half-century. However, some immunologists are willing to admit that the immune system may be capable of doing both: developing a basic sense of self early in life (through the careful winnowing of cells), and responding to danger later on. How the controversy will play out is anyone's guess. Meanwhile, we shall continue on.

CELL-MEDIATED IMMUNITY

The body's defense against microorganisms infecting its cells is centered in **cell-mediated immunity (CMI)**, sometimes called cellular immunity. Cell-mediated immunity responds to cells that have been infected with pathogens such as viruses, rickettsiae, and certain bacteria, including *Mycobacterium tuberculosis*. The pathogens announce their presence by altering the infected cells and changing the

Tuberculosis: an airborne bacterial disease of the lungs, characterized by severe cough and lesion formation.

molecular architecture of the cell's surface. The infected cells therefore act as sign-posts and become objects of an attack by cells of CMI. Protozoa and fungi also stimulate CMI, as do cancer cells and the cells of transplanted tissue.

The T-lymphocytes participating in CMI are of four major types in two categories. The first category contains the **effector T-lymphocytes**, so named because they bring about or "effect" CMI. The effector T-lymphocytes include cytotoxic T-lymphocytes

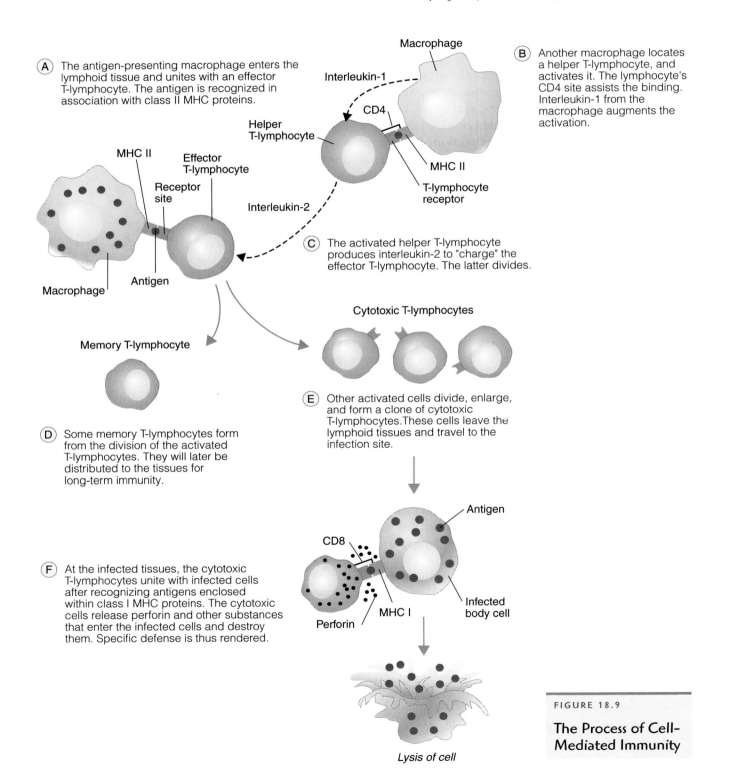

(A) The antigen-presenting macrophage enters the lymphoid tissue and unites with an effector T-lymphocyte. The antigen is recognized in association with class II MHC proteins.

(B) Another macrophage locates a helper T-lymphocyte, and activates it. The lymphocyte's CD4 site assists the binding. Interleukin-1 from the macrophage augments the activation.

(C) The activated helper T-lymphocyte produces interleukin-2 to "charge" the effector T-lymphocyte. The latter divides.

(D) Some memory T-lymphocytes form from the division of the activated T-lymphocytes. They will later be distributed to the tissues for long-term immunity.

(E) Other activated cells divide, enlarge, and form a clone of cytotoxic T-lymphocytes. These cells leave the lymphoid tissues and travel to the infection site.

(F) At the infected tissues, the cytotoxic T-lymphocytes unite with infected cells after recognizing antigens enclosed within class I MHC proteins. The cytotoxic cells release perforin and other substances that enter the infected cells and destroy them. Specific defense is thus rendered.

FIGURE 18.9

The Process of Cell-Mediated Immunity

and delayed hypersensitivity T-lymphocytes (Chapter 20). The second category of T-lymphocytes are **regulator T-lymphocytes**. These cells oversee the immune process. They include helper T-lymphocytes and suppressor T-lymphocytes.

The process of cell-mediated immunity is shown in FIGURE 18.9. It begins this way: In the body where infected tissue exists, a series of macrophages (as well as dendritic cells, and other phagocytic cells) have engulfed viruses, virus-infected cells, or other microorganisms and released their antigens. In the macrophage's cytoplasm, the antigens have been broken down to antigenic determinants (epitopes), and the latter have been captured and returned to the macrophage's surface, nestled within class II MHC proteins (FIGURE 18.10). The macrophage now has a series of "red

Regulator T-lymphocytes: the helper and suppressor T-lymphocytes that oversee the immune process.

FIGURE 18.10

Two Mechanisms for Uniting an Immunocompetent T-Lymphocyte with an Infected Cell

(a) In both the dual recognition and altered self mechanisms, the normal body cell is altered by infection with viruses. In the dual recognition mechanism, the virus-associated antigen is displayed on the cell surface alongside the MHC protein. In the altered self mechanism, the MHC protein has been altered by the viral antigen, and a single receptor site now exists. (b) When the T-lymphocyte unites with the infected cell, the union may involve two separate components for recognition (dual recognition), or a single recognition site with the MHC protein modified by the foreign viral antigen (altered self).

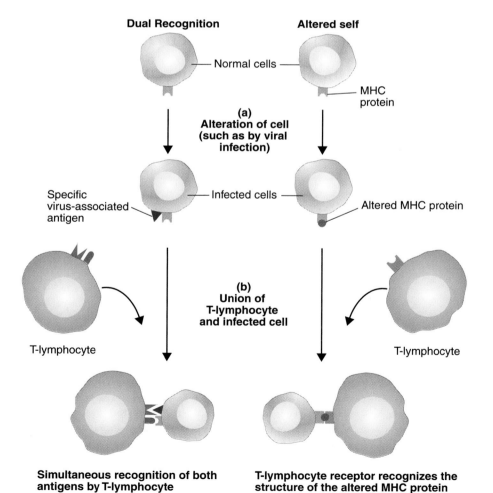

flags" on its surface; it is an **antigen-presenting cell**. (At this point, the infected cell or microorganism also is displaying the "red flags.") The antigen-presenting cell travels to an organ of the lymphoid system, and CMI is ready to continue.

When the antigen-presenting cell enters the lymphoid organ, a hunt begins. With its exposed antigenic determinants, the macrophage mingles among the myriad groups of inactive effector T-lymphocytes, searching for the cluster having the surface receptor proteins corresponding to its antigenic determinants. This process requires considerable time and energy because only one cluster of T-lymphocytes will have receptors that match the antigenic determinants. Soon the correct cluster is found.

But the match is not yet complete. For the T-lymphocyte and macrophage to bind, another recognition must take place. This recognition is between the class II MHC proteins on the macrophage surface and class II MHC receptors on the T-lymphocyte surface. (Remember that the antigenic determinants are nestled within the MHC proteins.) Indeed, the T-lymphocyte will recognize the antigenic determinants only within the spatial context of the MHC proteins, as described by 1996 Nobel laureates Peter Doherty and Rolf Zinkernagel (MicroFocus 18.4). It is as if the T-lymphocyte must first ascertain that it and the macrophage are from the same body before it will respond. Once the recognition has been made, the inactive T-lymphocyte becomes an activated **cytotoxic T-lymphocyte**.

While all this is going on, the macrophages must also locate "regulator" T-lymphocytes to assist the response. These regulators are **helper T-lymphocytes**. The correct helper cells will be selected out because the chemical complex on the macrophage matches receptors on the helper cells as well. Another surface receptor protein on the helper T-lymphocyte is the **CD4 receptor**. This receptor enhances binding of the helper cell to the macrophage because the CD4 protein is attracted to the class II MHC protein. (Incidentally, the CD4 receptor is where HIV binds to T-lymphocytes.) Eventually the search is completed, and the matching

MicroFocus 18.4

COMPELLING

They were assigned to the same cramped lab because there was no room elsewhere: Peter Doherty, the native Australian, and Rolf Zinkernagel, the visiting researcher from Switzerland. It was the early 1970s, and research space at the John Curtin School of Medical Research in Canberra was limited. But they would make do.

Both researchers were interested in how the brain is affected by the virus of lymphocytic choriomeningitis (LCM). The duo infected a mouse with LCM virus and collected its activated cytotoxic T-lymphocytes. As they anticipated, the latter killed the virus-infected brain cells when the cells were combined in a test tube. What

happened next, however, perplexed them: The same activated T-lymphocytes failed to kill virus-infected cells from another strain of mice.

Doherty and Zinkernagel scratched their heads. Then they remembered a report by Harvard immunologist Hugh McDevitt linking immune activities to the major histocompatibility complex (MHC) proteins at body cell surfaces. The MHC proteins are a sort of "molecular identification card" unique to the cells of a particular individual. At that time, they were known to be involved in the rejection of organs transplanted between unrelated people. The researchers wondered whether they might also be involved in T-lymphocyte activity.

Then followed many years of work with T-lymphocytes and infected cells bearing various combinations of MHC proteins. Time after time, the T-lymphocyte attacked only the cell with matching MHC proteins. The theory was gradually emerging: An attacking T-lymphocyte must recognize two signals, a signal from the virus and a signal from the infected cell (i.e., the antigenic determinant and the MHC protein).

Doherty and Zinkernagel proposed the model that turned out to be correct. Their theory was compelling, and so was their prize: the 1996 Nobel Prize in Physiology or Medicine.

sites are found (i.e., all the square pegs have fit into the square holes and the round pegs into the round holes).

Now the antigen-presenting cell (the macrophage) interacts with the helper T-lymphocyte (the regulator), and things become more lively: The helper cell is activated and forms a clone of helper T-lymphocytes. The latter secrete a series of highly charged glycoproteins known as **lymphokines** (also called **cytokines**). One lymphokine (cytokine) is **interleukin-2**. It stimulates the helper cell to become more active, and it charges the cytotoxic T-lymphocytes to become killer cells. Another lymphokine called **interleukin-1** is produced by the macrophage to further mature the helper cell.

The cytotoxic T-lymphocytes are key participants in cell-mediated immunity. Under the influence of lymphokines (cytokines), they enlarge and divide dramatically to form a clone of cytotoxic T-lymphocytes capable of killing infected cells (some books call the cytotoxic cells killer T-lymphocytes). The T-lymphocytes leave the lymphoid tissue and enter the lymph and blood vessels. They circulate until they come upon their **target cells**, the infected cells displaying telltale antigenic determinants (the "red flags") on their surface. What has happened in the interim is this: A cell infected by an indwelling microorganism has been producing microbial proteins. Class I MHC proteins have picked up some of these proteins and transported them to the cell surface, displaying them within the class I MHC proteins. These are the "red flags" detected by the cytotoxic T-lymphocyte as it arrives on the scene; they are the antigenic determinants with which the cell will react.

Now the cell-cell interaction begins. The cytotoxic T-lymphocyte joins its receptor proteins with the antigenic determinants and uses one of its surface receptors called **CD8** to bind to class I MHC protein on the infected cell surface. Then the cytotoxic T-lymphocyte releases a number of active substances, including a toxic protein called **perforin**. Perforin inserts into the membrane of the infected cell and dissolves the membrane. Ions, fluids, and cell structures escape, thereby bringing about lysis and the so-called "lethal hit." Cell death not only deprives the parasite of a place to live, but it also exposes the parasite to antibodies in the extracellular fluid. (A similar type of action is brought about by natural killer (NK) cells, but there is no response to antigenic determinants involved in this nonspecific defense.)

Cytotoxic T-lymphocytes are also active against tumor cells because these cells display distinctive molecules on their surfaces (FIGURE 18.11). The molecules are not present in other body cells, so they are viewed as antigenic determinants. Harbored within class I MHC proteins at the cell surface, the antigenic determinants react with receptors on cytotoxic T-lymphocytes, and the tumor cells are subsequently killed. Those cancer agents that reduce the level of class I MHC proteins at the cell surface reduce the reactivity of the cell and encourage immunologic escape and survival.

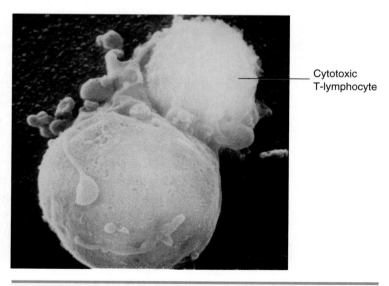

Cytotoxic T-lymphocyte

FIGURE 18.11

A "Lethal Hit"

A scanning electron micrograph of a cytotoxic T-lymphocyte attacking a tumor cell. The activity of T-lymphocytes represents a key defensive mechanism by the immune system.

lim'fo-kīn'
Lymphokine:
a protein produced by
lymphoblasts that increases
the efficiency of phagocytosis.

Cytotoxic T-lymphocytes are also the source of **lymphokines (cytokines)**, the low-molecular-weight glycoproteins used to enhance the defensive capabilities of the body. One lymphokine (cytokine) is the **macrophage activating factor (MAF)**. MAF attracts macrophages to the infection site and activates their enzymes to encourage cellular digestion. Another lymphokine, known as **migration inhibitor factor (MIF)**, prevents macrophages from leaving the infection site. A third, called **transfer factor (TF)**, mobilizes other T-lymphocytes in the area and encourages their conversion to cytotoxic cells. The latter continue the destruction of infected cells and augment the process of immunity.

Clone:
a colony of identical cells.

When the infected cells have been eliminated, a special clone of T-lymphocytes forms, one that will provide resistance in the event the antigen reenters the body any time in the future. These lymphocytes are called **memory T-lymphocytes**. They distribute themselves to virtually all parts of the body and remain in the tissues to provide a type of long-term immunity. Should the antigens be detected once again in the tissues, the memory T-lymphocytes will multiply rapidly, interact with the infected cells quickly, secrete lymphokines without delay, and set into motion the process of providing instantaneous CMI. This is one reason we enjoy long-term immunity to a given disease after having contracted and recovered from that disease.

To this point . . .

We have delved into specific resistance by describing the antigens that stimulate the immune system. The list of possible antigens is enormously diverse, but most are polysaccharides and proteins with a series of antigenic determinants. Haptens may function as antigenic determinants, but first they must complex with protein or polysaccharide. We saw why the immune system will not usually respond to the body's own substances (self) in the theory of specific immunologic tolerance. Among the identifiable antigens are autoantigens, alloantigens, and heterophile antigens.

The discussion then moved on to the immune system. We explored the origin of the system in terms of B-lymphocytes and T-lymphocytes, and noted how each colonizes the lymphoid tissues to form the immune system. The process of immunity generally begins with the phagocytosis of antigens and delivery of antigenic determinants to the lymphoid tissues. The immune process then diverges to either of two systems. The focus next turned to cell-mediated immunity, the complex process in which cytotoxic T-lymphocytes migrate to the antigen site and interact with cells, while stimulating phagocytosis through a series of lymphokines. The roles of other forms of T-lymphocytes were also mentioned briefly.

We shall now explore the second form of immunity, called antibody-mediated immunity. Here the B-lymphocytes play a central role, and antibodies function in the immune response. We shall examine the structures and types of antibodies, how they are related to the genes of B-lymphocytes, and the processes by which they interact with antigens and provide specific resistance. Together with cell-mediated immunity, antibody-mediated immunity represents the key to continued good health.

ANTIBODY-MEDIATED (HUMORAL) IMMUNITY

Cell-mediated immunity (CMI) is provided by attacking cells, but **antibody-mediated immunity (AMI)** is centered in antibodies, a series of protein molecules circulating in the body's fluids. (A body fluid is also known as a "humor," and antibody-mediated immunity has traditionally been called **humoral immunity**, but we shall use the more contemporary name.) In AMI, antibodies react with such things as toxin molecules in the bloodstream, as well as with antigens on microbial surfaces or microbial structures (e.g., flagella, pili, capsules), and with viruses in the extracellular fluid. The interaction of antibody and antigen leads to elimination of the antigen by various means, as we shall discuss in this section.

Antibody-mediated immunity, the second arm of the immune system, is well known because its origins trace back to the 1890s. In that period, Emil von Behring and Shibasaburo Kitasato determined that animals surviving a serious bacterial infection have "protective factors" in their blood to increase resistance to future attacks of the same infection. Today, these protective factors are known to be **antibodies**. Antibody formation and activity are the major topics of this section.

Like cell-mediated immunity, antibody-mediated immunity begins with an encounter between phagocytes bearing antigenic determinants and cells of the immune system. In this case, however, the major participating cell is the **B-lymphocyte**. The antigenic determinants stimulating the process are usually derived from antigens free in the bloodstream, such as those associated with bacteria, viruses, and certain organic substances as we have noted. The antigenic determinants interact with B-lymphocytes, as shown in FIGURE 18.12.

Activation of the B-lymphocytes begins when macrophages and other phagocytes find their way to the lymphoid organ and bring the antigenic determinants close to the appropriate B-lymphocytes that can respond. As with CMI, a considerable search process is involved as the antigenic determinants attempt to match with surface receptor proteins on the B-lymphocytes, as Figure 18.12 illustrates. The surface proteins on B-lymphocytes are antibodies of the type IgD. Activation of the B-lymphocytes requires that multiple antigenic determinants bind simultaneously with multiple antibody molecules and pull the antibodies into a continuous cluster, a process called **capping**. Small haptens may be poor stimulators of B-lymphocytes because of their inability to perform capping.

The selection of a single cluster of B-lymphocytes by a particular antigenic determinant is the underlying basis for the **theory of clonal selection**, shown in Figure 18.12. First proposed in the 1950s by Nobel laureates Frank MacFarlane Burnet and Peter Medowar, the updated theory of clonal selection explains how antigenic determinants "select out" the B-lymphocytes that will function in the immune process from the enormous variety of possible types available in the lymphoid tissue. A detailed discussion of the contemporary theory follows.

Once the antigenic determinant has bound with its corresponding surface receptor protein, and after capping has occurred, the combination of receptor protein and antigenic determinant is taken into the cytoplasm of the B-lymphocyte. Then the B-lymphocyte displays the antigenic determinants on its surface. While these processes have been going on, macrophages and other phagocytes bearing the antigenic determinants have contacted **helper T-lymphocytes**, and the macrophages have been recognized as belonging to the human body (self). This recognition occurs because the antigenic determinants are cradled within the correct class II MHC proteins on the macrophage surface. Now the helper T-lymphocyte is activated, and it forms a clone of helper T-lymphocytes keyed to the particular antigenic determinant. Lymphokines (cytokines) such as interleukin-2 are produced by the helper cells to stimulate the helper cell to become more active. These **activated helper T-lymphocytes** then recognize the same antigenic determinant–MHC molecule complex on the B-lymphocyte surface, and they bind to the B-lymphocytes

Antigenic determinant: a small part of an antigen that stimulates the immune system.

FIGURE 18.12

Clonal Selection

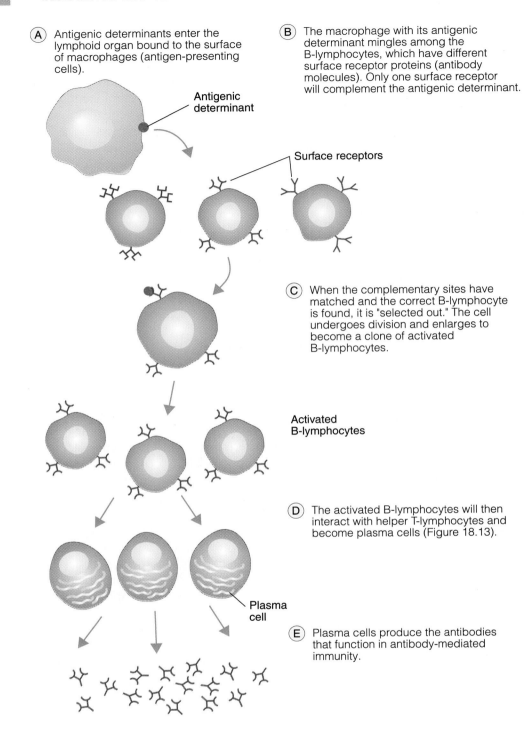

(A) Antigenic determinants enter the lymphoid organ bound to the surface of macrophages (antigen-presenting cells).

(B) The macrophage with its antigenic determinant mingles among the B-lymphocytes, which have different surface receptor proteins (antibody molecules). Only one surface receptor will complement the antigenic determinant.

Antigenic determinant

Surface receptors

(C) When the complementary sites have matched and the correct B-lymphocyte is found, it is "selected out." The cell undergoes division and enlarges to become a clone of activated B-lymphocytes.

Activated B-lymphocytes

(D) The activated B-lymphocytes will then interact with helper T-lymphocytes and become plasma cells (Figure 18.13).

Plasma cell

(E) Plasma cells produce the antibodies that function in antibody-mediated immunity.

(FIGURE 18.13). This immunologic cooperation between the macrophage, the B-lymphocyte, and the helper T-lymphocyte continues the immune response. Interleukin-2 assists the B-lymphocyte activation.

At this point, antibody-mediated immunity has been initiated, and B-lymphocytes bearing certain receptors have been selected by their reaction with specific antigenic determinants. Antigens that evoke this sort of response are called **T-dependent antigens** because they require the services of helper T-lymphocytes. We should note that

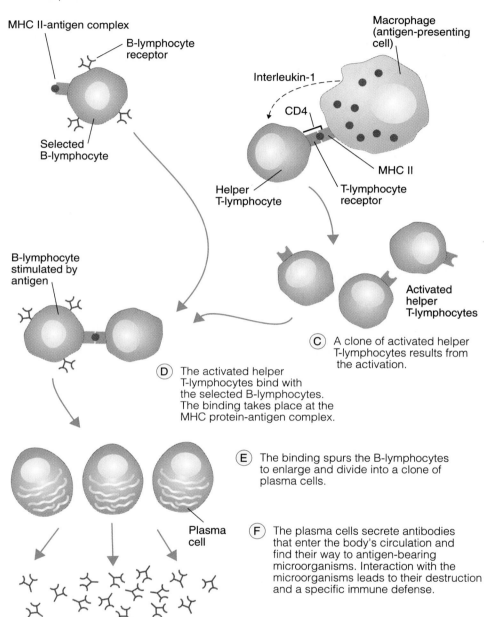

(A) The antigen-receptor complex has been taken into the selected B-lymphocyte, and the antigenic determinant is now displayed on the B-lymphocyte's surface within the MHC protein.

(B) Meanwhile, an antigen-presenting macrophage has activated a helper T-lymphocyte. Interleukin-1 from the macrophage assists the activation.

FIGURE 18.13

The Process of Antibody–Mediated Immunity

MHC II-antigen complex

B-lymphocyte receptor

Selected B-lymphocyte

Macrophage (antigen-presenting cell)

Interleukin-1

CD4

Helper T-lymphocyte

MHC II

T-lymphocyte receptor

B-lymphocyte stimulated by antigen

Activated helper T-lymphocytes

(C) A clone of activated helper T-lymphocytes results from the activation.

(D) The activated helper T-lymphocytes bind with the selected B-lymphocytes. The binding takes place at the MHC protein-antigen complex.

(E) The binding spurs the B-lymphocytes to enlarge and divide into a clone of plasma cells.

Plasma cell

(F) The plasma cells secrete antibodies that enter the body's circulation and find their way to antigen-bearing microorganisms. Interaction with the microorganisms leads to their destruction and a specific immune defense.

some antigens are **T-independent antigens**. These substances (such as in bacterial capsules and flagella) do not require the intervention of helper T-lymphocytes. Instead, they bind directly with the receptor proteins on the B-lymphocyte surface and stimulate the cells. However, the immune response is generally weaker, and no memory cells are produced. Indeed, when T-independent antigens are used in vaccines, scientists must find ways to bind the antigens to substances that will stimulate T-lymphocyte intervention. Chapter 19 explores this problem in more detail.

Superantigens:
Antigens that do not require processing before initiating an immune response, and that stimulate an extremely vigorous response.

Plasma cells:
antibody-producing cells derived from B-lymphocytes.

Immunoglobulin:
an alternate term for an antibody.

Memory B-lymphocytes:
stimulated B-lymphocytes that remain in the lymphoid tissues anticipating the reappearance of a certain antigen.

Another group of antigens worth mentioning are the **superantigens.** "Regular" antigens must be broken down and processed to antigenic determinants before they are ushered by the macrophage's MHC proteins to the T-lymphocyte surface, but superantigens bind directly to the MHC proteins without any internal processing. The binding to MHC proteins is unique, and when the superantigen is displayed on the macrophage's surface, it stimulates massive numbers of activated helper T-lymphocytes to form, through an unusually high secretion of lymphokines (cytokines). The result is an extremely vigorous immune response. Superantigens are associated with the staphylococcal toxins of toxic shock syndrome and scalded skin syndrome (Chapter 10), and possibly with immune system diseases such as arthritis, multiple sclerosis, and psoriasis. Having digressed for these exceptions, we now return to our survey of antibody-mediated immunity.

Once activated by helper T-lymphocytes and lymphokines, the B-lymphocytes multiply and give rise to a clone of **plasma cells.** Plasma cells are large, complex cells having no surface protein receptors. Their sole purpose is to produce **antibodies.** A plasma cell lives about 4 to 5 days, during which time it produces an incredible 2000 antibody molecules per second. Each antibody molecule has the same antigen-binding property as the receptor on the B-lymphocyte, and all the antibody molecules eventually reach the circulation. In a matter of several hours, the body becomes saturated with antibodies. Antibody molecules fill the blood, lymph, saliva, sweat, and all other body secretions. By sheer force of numbers they come upon the original site of antigens, bind to the antigens, and mark them for destruction. (In many cases, however, they are too late to prevent the initial surge of infection, and symptoms may already be present when they arrive to provide their specific defense.)

At any one time, antibody molecules represent about 17 percent of the total protein in a person's blood fluid. Antibodies are extremely diverse, and the cells of a single species of bacterium may elicit the formation of hundreds of different kinds of antibodies corresponding to hundreds of different kinds of bacterial antigens. Each unique antibody molecule is then capable of uniting with the unique antigen molecule. The term **immunoglobulin (Ig)** is used interchangeably with *antibody* because antibodies exhibit the properties of *globulin* proteins and are used in the *immune* response. In this text, we shall use the terms antibody and immunoglobulin as synonyms.

We shall study the interaction of antibodies and antigens shortly, but at this point it is important to note that certain B-lymphocytes do not become plasma cells. Instead, they become a clone of **memory B-lymphocytes.** Memory B-lymphocytes remain in the lymphoid tissues for many years, in some cases for a person's lifetime. Should the parasite and its antigens reenter the body, the memory cells will immediately revert to plasma cells and produce antibodies without delay. The antibodies rapidly flood the bloodstream and bring about an immediate neutralization of the antigens. The symptoms of infection rarely occur this time.

STRUCTURE AND TYPES OF ANTIBODIES

Details about the nature of antibodies began to emerge in the late 1950s and early 1960s, with the union of immunology and molecular biology. Research focused on the Bence Jones proteins, identified a century earlier by Henry Bence Jones. A substantial body of information and numerous theories existed about the functions and origins of these proteins, but little was known about their detailed chemical composition. Investigators expected that an understanding of the structure of the proteins (now known to be antibodies) would provide an understanding of their unique specificity for antigens. The answers were provided by **Gerald M. Edelman** and **Rodney M. Porter**, who described the chemical composition and structure of the proteins and received the 1972 Nobel Prize in Physiology or Medicine for their work.

The basic antibody molecule consists of four polypeptide chains: two identical **heavy (H) chains** and two identical **light (L) chains**. These chains are joined together by sulfur-to-sulfur (disulfide) linkages to form a Y-shaped structure, illustrated in FIGURE 18.14. Each heavy chain consists of about 400 amino acids, while each light chain has about 200 amino acids. The antibody molecule formed is called a **monomer**. It has two identical halves, each half consisting of a heavy chain and a light chain.

Constant and variable regions exist within each polypeptide chain. The amino acids in the **constant regions** of both light and heavy chains are virtually identical among different types of antibodies. However, the amino acids of the **variable region** differ across the hundreds of thousands of antibody types. Thus, the variable

Polypeptide: a chain of amino acids.

Variable region: the region of an antibody molecule where the amino acid composition varies among antibodies.

FIGURE 18.14

Details of an Antibody Molecule

(A) The antibody molecule consists of four chains of protein: two light chains and two heavy chains connected by disulfide (S-S) linkages. The heavy chains bend at a hinge point.

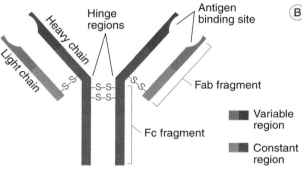

(B) The variable region is where the amino acid compositions of various antibodies differ. In the constant region, the amino acid compositions are similar in different antibodies.

(C) On treatment with papain enzyme, cleavage occurs at the hinge point, and three fragments result: two Fab fragments and one Fc fragment.

(D) This detailed view shows the disulfide linkages and the loops that form domains. All light chains have a single variable domain (V_L) and a single constant domain (C_L). Heavy chains contain a variable domain (V_H) and three or four constant domains.

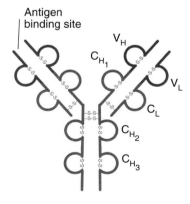

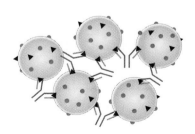

Immobilized clump of antigens

(E) The reaction between antibody molecules and the antigenic determinants of an antigen shows the specificity that occurs. Note that the antibody molecules unite with the triangular antigenic determinants but not with the circular ones.

regions of a light and heavy chain combine to form a highly specific, three-dimensional structure somewhat analogous to the active site of an enzyme. This portion of the antibody molecule is uniquely shaped to "fit" a specific antigen or antigenic determinant. Moreover, the "arms" of the antibody are identical so that a single antibody molecule may combine with two antigen molecules. These combinations may lead to a complex of antibody and antigen molecules.

When an antibody molecule is sectioned with papain, an enzyme from the papaya fruit, the molecule separates at the hinge joint, and two functionally different segments are isolated (Figure 18.14). One segment, called the **Fab fragment**, for *f*ragment-*a*ntigen-*b*inding, is the portion that will combine with the antigenic determinant. The second segment, called the **Fc fragment**, for *f*ragment able to be *c*rystallized, performs various functions: it is the part of the antibody molecule that combines with phagocytes in opsonization; it appears to neutralize viral receptor sites; it attaches to certain cells in allergic reactions; and it activates the complement system in resistance mechanisms.

At present, five types of antibodies have been identified, based on differences in the heavy chains in the constant region. Using the abbreviation Ig (immunoglobulin), the five classes are designated IgM, IgG, IgA, IgE, and IgD. The structures of these antibodies are illustrated in FIGURE 18.15. IgM consists of a **pentamer** (five monomers), whose tail segments are connected by a glycoprotein called a joining (J) chain. IgA is a **dimer** (two monomers), with the segments also connected by a J chain. In addition, a secretory component of IgA enables the molecule to leave secretory epithelial cells (MicroFocus 18.5). The remaining three antibodies are monomers.

IgM is the first antibody to appear in the circulation after the stimulation of B-lymphocytes. It is the principal component of the **primary antibody response** (FIGURE 18.16) and the largest antibody molecule (M stands for macroglobulin). Because of its size, most IgM remains in the circulation. Research indicates that IgM is formed

Fab fragment:
the portion of an antibody molecule that combines with the antigenic determinant.

J chain:
a glycoprotein in IgM and IgA molecules that connects the subunits of an antibody.

Primary antibody response:
the first antibody reaction of the immune system to the presence of antigens.

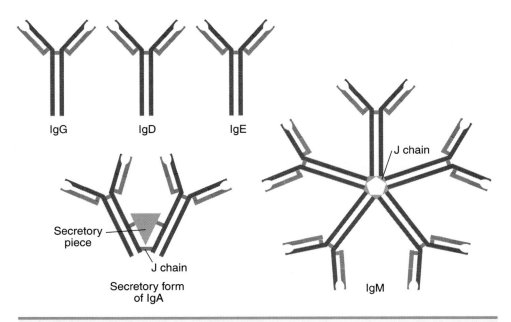

FIGURE 18.15

The Structures of Five Types of Antibodies

Note the complex structures of IgM (a pentamer) and IgA (a dimer). IgG, IgE, and IgD consist of monomers, each composed of two heavy chains and two light chains of amino acids.

during fetal infections with rubella or toxoplasmosis, indicating that a certain immunological competence exists in the fetus. About 5 to 10 percent of the antibody components of normal serum consists of this antibody. IgM is one of the antibodies bound to the B-lymphocyte surface as a receptor protein.

IgG is the classical **gamma globulin**. This antibody is the major circulating antibody, comprising about 80 percent of the total antibody content in normal serum. IgG appears about 24 to 48 hours after antigenic stimulation and continues the

Serum: the straw-colored fluid portion of the blood minus the clotting agents.

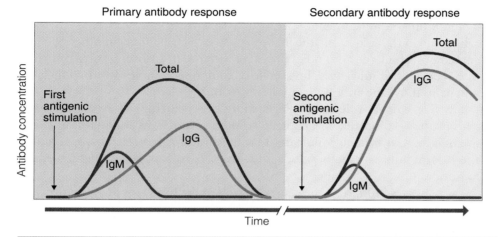

FIGURE 18.16

The Primary and Secondary Antibody Responses

After the initial antigenic stimulation, IgM is the first antibody to appear in the circulation. It is the principal component of the primary antibody response. Later, IgM is supplemented by IgG. On second exposure to the same antigen, the production of IgG is more rapid, and the concentration in the serum reaches a higher level than previously. Thus, the IgG antibody is more concentrated in the secondary antibody response.

MicroFocus 18.5

THE OTHER ARMY

Most people are familiar with the body's army, headquartered downtown—the antibodies and T-lymphocytes that constitute the blood-centered system of immunity. Few, however, know much about the army of the suburbs—the specialized cells and antibodies that protect the body at its vulnerable entryways in locations, such as its respiratory, gastrointestinal, and urinary tracts. The cells and antibodies in the fragile mucous membranes lining these systems constitute a network now known as the mucosal immune system.

The extent of communication between the blood and mucosal systems is uncertain at this writing. Injected vaccines, for example, rarely evoke IgA production for mucosal immunity. However, stimulating one region of mucosal tissue to elicit IgA appears to produce an immune response at a distant mucosal surface. Thus, a vaccine in a nasal spray can elicit an antibody response along the gastrointestinal tract. This interrelatedness has led immunologists to think in terms of a single mucosal system.

Studies in mucosal immunity have lagged behind those of bloodborne immunity in part because tissue samples from the mucosa are difficult to work with. But studies are being encouraged because stopping infection at its point of entry is highly desirable. Also, vaccine research would benefit considerably because oral vaccines are preferred to injectable types, and developing an oral vaccine requires a basic understanding of mucosal immunity. Indeed, the output of the mucosal system appears to outdistance that of the bloodborne system. It has been estimated, for instance, that over 3 grams of IgA are secreted, as compared to only 1 gram of IgA released into the bloodstream. On this basis alone, the "suburban army" merits a greater share of attention.

Maternal antibodies:
antibodies from a pregnant woman that cross the placenta and provide protection to the fetus.

antigen–antibody interaction begun by IgM. It is thus the principal antibody of the **secondary antibody response**. In addition, it provides long-term resistance to disease as a product of the memory B-lymphocytes. Booster injections of a vaccine raise the level of this antibody considerably in the serum. IgG is also the **maternal antibody** that crosses the placenta and renders immunity to the fetus until the child is able to make antibodies at about 6 months of age after it is born.

Approximately 10 percent of the total antibody in normal serum is **IgA**. One form of this antibody, called **serum IgA**, exists in the serum and is similar to IgG. A second form accumulates in body secretions and is referred to as **secretory IgA**. This antibody provides resistance in the respiratory and gastrointestinal tracts, possibly by inhibiting the attachment of parasites to the tissues. It is also located in tears and saliva, and in the colostrum, the first milk secreted by a nursing mother. When consumed by a child, the antibodies provide resistance to gastrointestinal disorders, as MicroFocus 18.6 indicates. The secretory component comes from epithelial cells and helps move the antibody into the secretions.

IgE plays a major role in allergic reactions by sensitizing cells to certain antigens. This process is discussed in Chapter 20. Both the functions and significance of **IgD** are unclear, but evidence indicates that the antibody is a cell surface receptor on the B-lymphocytes together with IgM. For this reason, it is called a membrane antibody.

TABLE 18.2 summarizes the characteristics of the five types of antibodies.

ANTIBODY DIVERSITY

For decades, immunologists were puzzled as to how an enormous variety of antibodies (perhaps a million or more different types) could be encoded by the limited

---

MicroFocus 18.6

THE BENEFITS OF BREAST-FEEDING

Ironically, the literature from a major baby formula company says it best: "Breast-feeding is the most natural and satisfying conclusion to the normal cycle of pregnancy and birth." Years of research have bolstered the truth of this statement.

The immune system of a child is primitive at birth, and its intestinal wall is poorly developed. These factors make the infant easy prey for the bacteria that cause diarrhea. Breast-feeding may help solve this problem because the milk contains IgA, which accumulates in the intestines and provides surveillance against intestinal pathogens. Indeed, studies show that epidemics of diarrhea can be limited by feeding infants with colostrum, the antibody-rich "pre-milk"

of nursing mothers. Moreover, up to 80 percent of the cells in colostrum are macrophages, the leukocytes that perform phagocytosis.

Nursing may also limit allergies later in the child's life. Immunologists postulate that the IgA in mother's milk blocks the entry into the circulation of allergenic materials that would otherwise pass through the immature intestinal wall. Freedom from allergenic substances in the newborn may portend freedom from allergy in the years ahead.

It has also been suggested that a nursing mother's immune system may be programmed to provide specific antibodies for the child. During contact with her child, the mother is exposed to antigens such as those from disease organ-

isms. She may then produce antibodies that would return to the child via the milk. Obviously these antibodies could not be provided by cow's milk. Some immunologists even foresee the day when women may be immunized against diseases that commonly infect newborns. After giving birth, they could serve as personalized immunological factories for their offspring.

Certain manufacturers have researched the possibility of adding antibodies to artificial formulas to simulate mother's milk. However, data gathered for decades indicate that bottle-feeding is a pale substitute for a process that has withstood the test of centuries. As the sage puts it, "Human milk is for humans; cow's milk is for calves."

TABLE 18.2

Properties of Five Types of Antibodies

DESIGNATION	PERCENTAGE OF ANTIBODY IN SERUM	LOCATION IN BODY	MOLECULAR WEIGHT (DALTONS)	NUMBER OF FOUR-CHAIN UNITS	CROSSES PLACENTA	CHARACTERISTICS
IgM	5–10	Blood Lymph	900,000	5	No	Principal component of primary response
IgG	80	Blood Lymph	150,000	1	Yes	Principal component of secondary response
IgA	10	Secretions Body cavities	400,000	2	No	Protection in body cavities
IgE	<1	Blood Lymph	200,000	1	No	Role in allergic reactions
IgD	0.05	Blood Lymph	180,000	1	No	Possible receptor sites on B-lymphocytes

number of genes associated with the immune system. Because antibodies, like all proteins, are specified by genes, it would be reasonable to assume that an individual must have a million or more genes for antibodies. But geneticists point out that human cells have only about 100,000 genes for all their functions.

The antibody diversity problem apparently has been resolved in recent years by showing that embryonic cells contain about 300 genetic segments that can be shuffled (like transposons) and combined in each B-lymphocyte as it matures. The process, known as **somatic recombination**, is a random mixing and matching of gene segments to form unique antibody genes. Information encoded by these genes is then expressed in the surface receptor proteins of B-lymphocytes and in the antibodies later expressed by the stimulated clone of plasma cells.

Transposons: segments of DNA that carry functional genes from one chromosomal location to another.

The process of somatic recombination was first postulated in the late 1970s by **Susumu Tonegawa**, winner of the 1987 Nobel Prize in Medicine or Physiology. According to the process, the gene segments coding for the light and heavy chains of an antibody are located on different chromosomes. The light and heavy chains are synthesized separately, then joined to form the antibody. One of five constant genes, one of four joiner genes, one of three diversity genes, and one of up to 80 variable genes can be used to form a heavy chain. One variable gene is selected and combined with one joiner gene, one diversity gene, and a constant gene to form the active light-chain gene. After deletion of intervening genes, the new gene can function in protein synthesis, as shown in FIGURE 18.17. For the heavy chain of the antibody, the process is similar but even more complex because there is a greater variety of variable genes and more possible combinations.

Tonegawa's discovery was revolutionary because it questioned two dogmas of biology: that the DNA for a protein needs to be one continuous piece (for antibody synthesis, the gene segments are separated); and that every body cell has exactly the same DNA (the antibody genes for different B-lymphocytes differ). Current evidence suggests that no more than 600 different antibody gene segments exist per cell. From this relatively small collection, however, the cell can generate over 200 million different antibody molecules through somatic recombination.

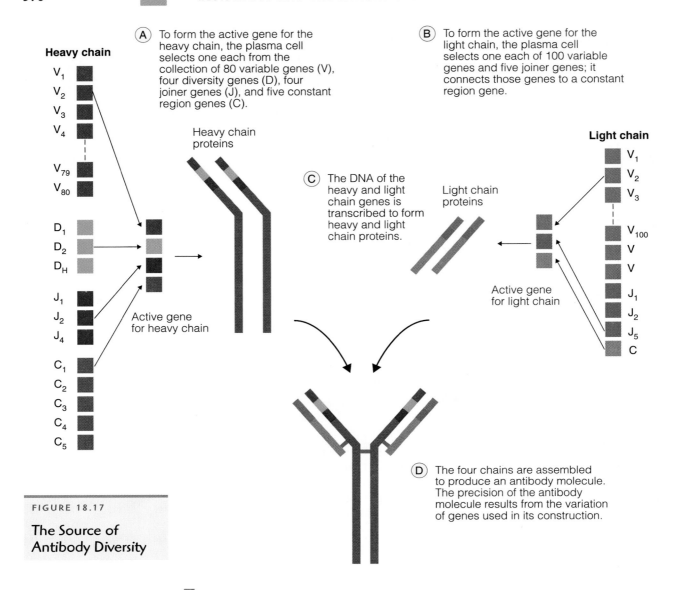

Heavy chain

(A) To form the active gene for the heavy chain, the plasma cell selects one each from the collection of 80 variable genes (V), four diversity genes (D), four joiner genes (J), and five constant region genes (C).

(B) To form the active gene for the light chain, the plasma cell selects one each of 100 variable genes and five joiner genes; it connects those genes to a constant region gene.

Heavy chain proteins

(C) The DNA of the heavy and light chain genes is transcribed to form heavy and light chain proteins.

Light chain proteins

Light chain

Active gene for heavy chain

Active gene for light chain

(D) The four chains are assembled to produce an antibody molecule. The precision of the antibody molecule results from the variation of genes used in its construction.

FIGURE 18.17

The Source of Antibody Diversity

ANTIGEN–ANTIBODY INTERACTIONS

In order for specific resistance to develop, antibodies must interact with antigens in such a way that the antigen is altered. The alteration may result in death to the microorganism that possesses the antigen, inactivation of the antigen, or increased susceptibility of the antigen to other body defenses.

Certain antibodies, called **neutralizing antibodies**, react with viral capsids and prevent viruses from entering their host cells. Influenza viruses are inhibited by neuraminidase antibodies in this way (FIGURE 18.18). Neutralizing antibodies also bind viruses together in clumps, thereby encouraging phagocytosis. Moreover, neutralizing antibodies represent a vital mechanism of defense against toxins. The antibodies, known as **antitoxins**, alter the toxin molecules near their active sites and mask their toxicity. Neutralization of toxin molecules also increases their size, thus encouraging phagocytosis while lessening their ability to diffuse through the tissues.

Antibodies called **agglutinins** react with antigens on the surface of organisms such as bacteria. This action causes clumping, or agglutination, of the organisms and

Antitoxins: antibodies that combine with and neutralize toxin molecules.

ah-gloo'tĭ-nin

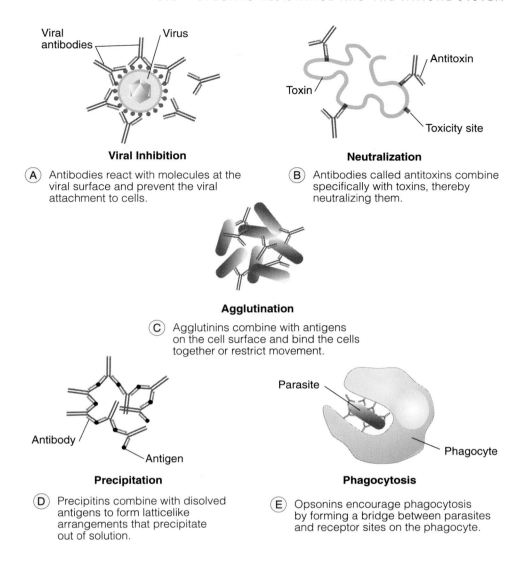

Viral antibodies
Virus

Viral Inhibition

(A) Antibodies react with molecules at the viral surface and prevent the viral attachment to cells.

Antitoxin
Toxin
Toxicity site

Neutralization

(B) Antibodies called antitoxins combine specifically with toxins, thereby neutralizing them.

Agglutination

(C) Agglutinins combine with antigens on the cell surface and bind the cells together or restrict movement.

Antibody
Antigen

Parasite
Phagocyte

Precipitation

(D) Precipitins combine with disolved antigens to form latticelike arrangements that precipitate out of solution.

Phagocytosis

(E) Opsonins encourage phagocytosis by forming a bridge between parasites and receptor sites on the phagocyte.

FIGURE 18.18

Five Mechanisms by Which Antibodies Interact with Antigens

enhances phagocytosis. Movement is inhibited if antibodies react with antigens on the flagella of microorganisms, and the organisms may even be clumped together by their flagella. The reaction of antibodies with pilus antigens prohibits attachment of an organism to the tissues while agglutinating them and increasing their susceptibility to phagocytosis.

Another form of antibodies is the **precipitins**. These antibodies react with dissolved antigens and convert them to solid precipitates. In this form, antigens are usually inactive and more easily phagocytized.

Opsonins are antibodies that stimulate phagocytosis by direct intervention. The antigen attaches to the Fab fragment of the antibody while the Fc portion inserts into a receptor site on the phagocyte. An example occurs in the inactivation of *Streptococcus pneumoniae*, the pneumococcus. Normally the organism resists phago-

Precipitins: antibodies that react with dissolved antigens to yield precipitates.

cytosis, but when antibodies react with the M protein in the bacterial capsule, phagocytosis takes place quickly.

A final example of antigen–antibody interaction involves the **complement system** (complement), introduced earlier in the chapter. Originally described in 1895 by Jules Bordet at the Pasteur Institute, the complement system is a series of over 20 proteins that function in a cascading set of reactions. It includes components designated C1 to C9, as well as many other proteins. The complement system exists in all normal sera and is activated by IgM or IgG. Complement works with antibodies to cause opsonization, chemotaxis, and lysis of bacterial cells.

The **classical pathway** for complement activation is set into motion by the interaction of antigen and antibody molecules, as shown in FIGURE 18.19. Usually the

bor-dā'

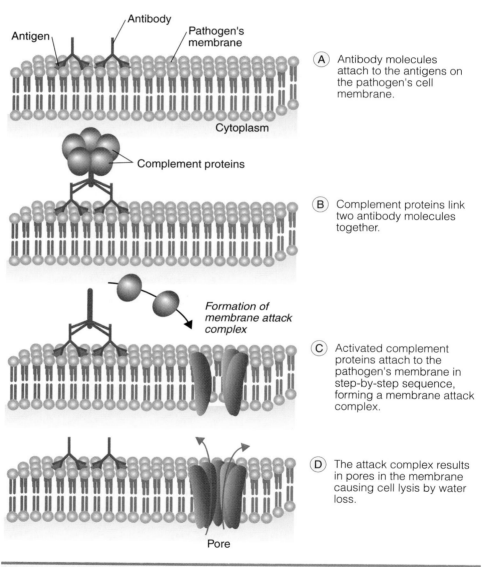

A Antibody molecules attach to the antigens on the pathogen's cell membrane.

B Complement proteins link two antibody molecules together.

C Activated complement proteins attach to the pathogen's membrane in step-by-step sequence, forming a membrane attack complex.

D The attack complex results in pores in the membrane causing cell lysis by water loss.

FIGURE 18.19

The Classical Pathway of Complement Activity

interaction takes place on the surface of a cell, such as a bacterium. The cascade results in several substances, one of which is a **membrane attack complex** (C5b, C6, C7, C8, C9). This complex increases cell membrane permeability and induces the cell to undergo lysis through the leakage of water from its cytoplasm (in a process reminiscent of cytotoxic T-lymphocyte activity with perforin). Another substance in the cascade (C5a) attracts phagocytes through chemotaxis, while another substance (C2a, C3b, C4b) facilitates phagocytosis by binding the cell to the phagocyte. Still other fragments (C3 and C5a) are **anaphylatoxins**. These substances react with tissue cells called mast cells (Chapter 20) and induce the release of histamine, which contracts smooth muscles and thereby increases the movement of phagocytes out of the blood vessels at the infection site.

an'ah-fī'lah-tok'sin
Anaphylatoxins: substances that react with mast cells and cause the release of histamine, which contracts smooth muscles.

Complement activity may also take place through an **alternative pathway**. In this system, several complement components are bypassed, and an antigen–antibody reaction is not required for stimulation. A serum protein named **properdin** functions in the process, together with several newly discovered factors. The alternative pathway is stimulated by endotoxins as well as by capsular polysaccharides in streptococci and by certain fungi. It functions to prevent intravascular invasion occurring before the development of antibodies. A membrane attack complex forms at its conclusion, and cell lysis occurs.

Immunologists have recently discovered a third pathway called the **lectin pathway**. Lectin is a liver protein that binds to mannose, a carbohydrate found in the cell walls of bacteria and, in a few cases, in the envelopes of viruses. Production of lectin is stimulated by cytokines produced by macrophages after phagocytosis of pathogens. The lectin binds to the bacterial wall and viral envelope and stimulates phagocytosis. It also activates the alternative pathway and, in some instances, the classical pathway. Note, however, that an antigen–antibody reaction is not necessary to cause the lectin pathway to spring into action.

The complement system is particularly useful against Gram-negative bacteria because it alters their cell walls and makes them susceptible to lysozyme. Moreover, studies show that a complement component encourages the release of lysozyme from local macrophages. In Gram-positive bacteria, the peptidoglycan of the cell wall resists the attack complex, but lysozyme from macrophages degrades the cell wall, thereby leading to cell disintegration. Moreover, enhanced phagocytosis of all bacteria occurs, regardless of their type.

Lysozyme: an enzyme that degrades the cell walls of certain bacteria.

THINKING WELL

The idea that mental states can influence the body's susceptibility to and recovery from disease has a long history. The Greek physician Galen asserted that cancer struck more frequently in melancholy women than in cheerful women. During the twentieth century, the concept of mental state and disease was researched more thoroughly, and a firm foundation was established linking the nervous system and the immune system (MicroFocus 18.7).

One such link exists between the hypothalamus and the T-lymphocytes. The **hypothalamus** is a portion of the brain located beneath the cerebrum. It produces a chemical-releasing factor that induces the pituitary gland, positioned just below the hypothalamus, to secrete the hormone ACTH, which targets the adrenal glands. The adrenal glands, in turn, secrete steroid hormones (glucocorticoids) that influence the activity of T-lymphocytes in the thymus gland.

glu'co-cort'i-coids

MicroFocus 18.7

SICK OVER EXAMS

At the end of every semester, medical students at Ohio State University suffer through the Day of the Big Bleed. First, they "bleed" over their final exams; then they bleed, quite literally, for psychologist Janice Kiecolt-Glaser and immunologist Ronald Glaser, her husband. The Glasers are attempting to learn whether the stress of final exams diminishes the activity of the immune system.

The "thinking well" phenomenon has been known for years—a positive attitude can help the immune system's

activities, while stress can place a burden on the system. Providing proof of this phenomenon has been difficult, but the Glasers are among those determined to show that a correlation exists between stress and reduced immune activity. Already, they have demonstrated reduced activity in natural killer cells in blood taken from students during exam week. Also, they have shown that in herpes-infected students, the virus is more active when exams are going on (a reflection of reduced body defense).

In their latest study, the Glasers gave the Ohio State students hepatitis B vaccinations and then tested them for antibody responses. Not surprisingly, the more stressed-out and anxious students consistently responded with lower antibody levels. Perhaps these students might have contracted hepatitis B more readily if the virus were present, but that would be difficult to test. The lessons appear straightforward: Prepare thoroughly for exams, think of clear mountain streams, and stay healthy.

thy′mo-sins

Pituitary gland:
a pea-sized gland at the base of the brain that stores and secretes hormones.

Another link is established by branches of the **autonomic nervous system** that extend into the lymph node and spleen tissues. The autonomic nervous system automatically regulates the functioning of such organs as the heart, stomach, and lungs through myriad nerve fibers. The direct anatomical link between the immune and nervous systems allows a direct two-way communication.

A third link between the nervous and immune systems starts with **thymosins**, a family of substances originating in the thymus gland. When experimentally injected into brain tissue, thymosins stimulate the pituitary gland via the hypothalamus to release hormones, including the one that stimulates the adrenal gland. Although the precise functions of thymosins are yet to be determined, it appears that they serve as specific molecular signals between the thymus and the pituitary gland. A circuit is apparently present that stimulates the brain to adjust immune responses and the immune system to alter nerve cell activity.

The outcome of these discoveries is the emergence of a strong correlation between a patient's mental attitude and the progress of disease. Rigorously controlled studies conducted in recent years have shown that the aggressive determination to conquer a disease can increase one's lifespan. Therapies can consist of relaxation techniques, as well as mental imagery that disease organisms are being crushed by the body's stalwart defenses. Behavioral therapies of this nature can amplify the body's response to disease and accelerate the mobilization of its defenses.

Few reputable practitioners of behavioral therapies believe that such therapies should replace drug therapy. However, the psychological devastation associated with many diseases such as AIDS cannot be denied, and it is this intense stress that the "thinking well" movement attempts to address. Very often, for instance, a person learning of a positive HIV test goes into severe depression, and because depression can adversely affect the immune system, a double dose of immune suppression ensues. Perhaps by relieving the psychological trauma, the remaining body defenses can adequately handle the virus.

As with any emerging treatment method, there are numerous opponents of behavioral therapies. Some opponents argue that naive patients might abandon conventional therapy; another argument is that therapists might cause enormous guilt to develop in patients whose will to live cannot overcome failing health. Proponents counter with the growing body of evidence showing that patients with strong commitments and a willingness to face challenges—signs of psychological hardiness—have relatively greater numbers of T-lymphocytes than passive, nonexpressive patients. To date, no study has proven that mood or personality has a life-prolonging effect on immunity. Still, doctors and patients are generally inspired by the possibility that one can use his or her mind to help stave off the effects of infectious disease. Though unsure of what it is, they generally agree that *something* is going on.

Note to the Student

It may have occurred to you that an episode of disease is much like a war. First, the invading microorganisms must penetrate the natural barriers of the body; then they must escape the phagocytes and other chemicals that constantly patrol the body's waterways and tissues. Finally, they must elude the antibodies or T-lymphocytes that the body sends out to combat them. How well we do in this battle will determine whether we survive the disease.

Obviously, we have done very well, because most of us are in good health today. As it turns out, most infectious organisms are stopped at their point of entry to the body. Cold viruses, for example, get no farther than the upper respiratory tract. Many parasites come into the body by food or water, but they rarely penetrate beyond the intestinal tract. The staphylococci in a wound may cause inflammation at the infection site, but this is usually the extent of the problem.

To be sure, drugs and medicines help in those cases where diseases pose life-threatening situations. In addition, sanitation practices, vector control, care in the preparation of food, and other public health measures prevent microorganisms from reaching the body in the first place. However, in the final analysis, body defense represents the bottom line in protection against disease, and, as history has shown, body defenses work very well. Indeed, as Lewis Thomas has suggested in *The Lives of a Cell*, a microorganism that catches a human is in considerably more danger than a human who has caught a microorganism.

http://microbiology.jbpub.com

The site features **eLearning,** an on-line review area that provides quizzes and other tools to help you study for your class. You can also follow useful links for in-depth information, read more MicroFocus stories, or just find out the latest microbiology news.

Summary

The body's resistance to disease takes two forms: nonspecific resistance and specific resistance. Nonspecific resistance exists in all humans and protects against all parasites. It involves species and population immunities and such mechanical and chemical barriers as the skin surface, mucus secretions, stomach acid, lysozyme, and interferon. Phagocytosis is a nonspecific mechanism in which macrophages and other phagocytes engulf and destroy microorganisms. Fever and inflammation are other forms of this resistance.

Specific resistance develops from the response by the body's immune system to substances called anti-gens. Antigens are large, complex molecules interpreted as nonself. Proteins, polysaccharides, and an enormous list of substances containing these molecules are antigenic. A small part of the antigen called the antigenic determinant performs the actual stimulation of the immune system. A person's own chemical substances are nonantigenic because they are interpreted as self.

The immune system originates with bone marrow cells that undergo differentiation to form B-lymphocytes and T-lymphocytes. These cells comprise the tissue of the spleen, lymph nodes, and other lymphoid organs, and they are the major underpinnings

Review

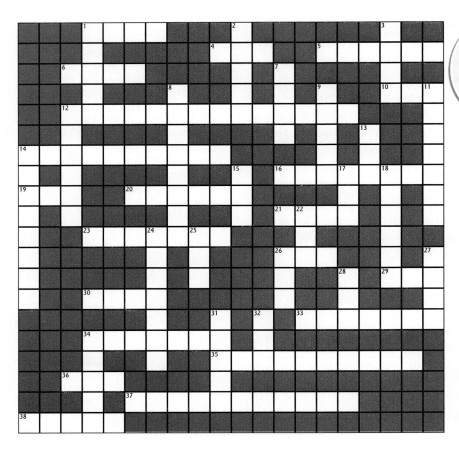

A major theme of this chapter is antigens and antibodies, two key aspects of the immune system. To test your knowledge of antigens and antibodies, solve the following puzzle. The answers are given in Appendix D.

■ ACROSS

1. Does not induce an immune response.
4. Type of immunity (abbr) where T-lymphocytes function.
5. Antigenic on rare occasions.
6. Immunity related to antibodies is also said to be hum-_____.
10. Small molecules may act as antigens called _____-tens.
12. Alternate name for antibody.
14. Protein group; functions in antigen–antibody reaction.
16. End of antibody molecule where antigen reacts.

of the immune system. When T-lymphocytes are stimulated by antigenic determinants, they leave the immune system as cytotoxic cells and travel to the infection site. Here they kill the infecting organisms in a process called cell-mediated immunity. Memory T-lymphocytes remain in the tissue to provide long-lasting protection.

A second process is antibody-mediated (humoral) immunity. In this case, B-lymphocytes are stimulated to form antibody-producing cells called plasma cells.

Antibodies are formed in the lymph nodes and are protein molecules composed of light and heavy chains of amino acids. The antibodies enter the circulation and reach the infection site, where they react with and neutralize microorganisms by various mechanisms. Five types of antibodies are recognized, each with its own function and structure. Together with cytotoxic T-lymphocytes, the antibodies impart specific resistance during times of disease, and they remain in the body for long-lasting resistance.

19. Antigenic materials are classified as _____-self.
20. Cells that produce antibody molecules.
21. Number of monomeric units in IgM.
23. Antibody response in which IgM is the principal component.
26. Largest antibody.
29. Number of heavy chains in a monomeric antibody molecule.
30. A person's own chemical substance is an _____-antigen.
33. Alternate name for an antigenic determinant.
34. Reaction in which IgE functions.
35. Cell that phagocytizes microorganisms and begins immune response.
36. Number of amino acid molecules possible in an antigenic determinant.
37. White blood cells involved in immune response.
38. In the embryonic chick, B-lymphocytes mature in the _____ of Fabricius.

■ DOWN
1. Medium for transport of antibodies.
2. Type of acid in antibody molecule.
3. Antigens generally have a _____ molecular weight.
7. Numbers of chains in a monomeric antibody molecule.
8. Nobel Prize for study of antibody diversity.
9. Structure of IgA.
11. Sole organic material in antibody molecule.
12. Body system depending on antibody activity.
13. Secretory antibody.
14. Region of identity among antibody molecules.
15. Fragment of antibody that combines with antigenic determinant.
17. Sensitizes cells to certain antigens.
18. Proposed theory of clonal selection.
22. Major antibody of the secondary antibody response.
24. Antibody molecule with two identical halves.

25. Type of blood cell (abbr) containing alloantigens.
26. Antibody at the surface of B-lymphocytes.
27. An antibody molecule reacts with an epi-_____.
28. Type of immunity (abbr) based on activity of B-lymphocytes.
31. Nodes where immune system cells gather.
32. Molecules functioning in recognition reactions between cells.
34. Nucleic _____ usually are poor antigens.

Questions for Thought and Discussion

1. The opening of this chapter suggests that for many diseases, a penetration of the walls surrounding the human body must take place. Can you think of any diseases where penetration is not a prerequisite to illness?

2. It has been said that no other system in the human body depends and relies on signals as greatly as the immune system. What evidence can you offer to support or reject this concept?

3. Lysozyme is a valuable natural enzyme for the control and destruction of Gram-positive bacteria. Can you postulate why this substance is not a commercially available pharmaceutical product?

4. The ancestors of modern humans lived in a sparsely settled world where communicable diseases were probably very rare. Suppose that by using some magical scientific invention, one of those individuals was thrust into the contemporary world. How do you suppose he or she would fare in relation to infectious disease? What is the immunological basis for your answer?

5. In the book and movie *Fantastic Voyage*, a group of scientists is miniaturized in a submarine (the *Proteus*) and sent into the human body to dissolve a blood clot. The odyssey begins when the miniature submarine carrying the scientists is injected into the bloodstream. Can you think of any natural opening to the body interior they could have used instead of the injection?

6. One of the most intriguing aspects of dental research is that a vaccine may eventually be produced to protect against tooth decay. A study in the 1980s, for example, showed that reduced incidence of decay correlated with high levels of salivary IgA specific for *Streptococcus mutans*. What problems do you foresee in the development of such a vaccine, and what advantages and disadvantages might there be in its use?

7. A University of Cincinnati immunologist has demonstrated that cockroaches injected with small doses of honeybee venom can develop resistance to future injections of venom that would ordinarily be lethal. Does this finding imply that cockroaches have an immune system? Which might be the next steps for the research to take? What does this research tell you about the cockroach's ability to survive for 3 or 4 years, far longer than most other insects?

8. Cattle are known to have the alcoholic carbohydrate erythritol in their placentas. When brucellosis occurs in pregnant cattle, the causative agent *Brucella abortus* metabolizes the erythritol and grows in the placenta, causing abortion of the fetal calf. Humans, by contrast, have no erythritol in the placenta and therefore do not suffer similar effects when they contract brucellosis. What type of immunity does this exemplify?

9. The botulism toxin is the most powerful toxin known to science; the tetanus toxin is the second most powerful. Despite this, the botulism toxin may be less dangerous than the tetanus toxin. Why is this so?

10. Why is it a good idea to cry when something gets into your eye?

11. Phagocytes have been described as "bloodhounds searching for a scent" as they browse along the walls of blood vessels. The scent they usually seek is a chemotactic factor, a peptide released by a bacterium. Does it strike you as unusual that a bacterium should release a substance to attract the "bloodhound" that will eventually lead to the bacterium's demise?

12. One of the earliest symptoms of disease in the body is swollen lymph nodes (erroneously referred to as "swollen glands"). Why?

13. A microbiology professor has suggested that an antigenic determinant arriving in the lymphoid tissue is like a parent searching for the face of a lost child in a crowd of a million children. Would you agree with this analogy? Why or why not?

14. A 1989 high school biology text contains the following statement: "T cells do not produce circulating antibodies. They carry cellular antibodies on their surface." What is fundamentally incorrect about this statement, and what would you say in your letter to the publisher after reading the statement?

15. Some years ago, a novel entitled *Through the Alimentary Canal with Gun and Camera* appeared in bookstores. The book described a fictitious account of travels through the human body. What perils, microbiologically speaking, would you encounter if you were to take such an adventure?

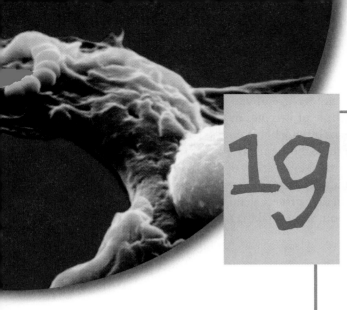

19 Immunity and Serology

"Ouch!"

—The plaintive cry of a child receiving yet another vaccination

TRADITION TELLS US THAT as early as the eleventh century, Chinese doctors ground up smallpox scabs and blew the powder into the noses of healthy people to protect them against the ravages of smallpox. Modern vaccines work less haphazardly. They are composed of chemically altered toxins, treated microorganisms, or chemical parts of microorganisms. Such vaccines work by exploiting the immune system's ability to recognize antigens and respond with antibodies and other factors that remain in the body and later attack the toxins or microorganisms should they appear.

And the technology continues to improve. Using the techniques of genetic engineering, researchers are now striving to eliminate all but the absolutely necessary material required to stimulate the immune system. Scientists identify the antigen that triggers the immune response, clone the genes that encode the antigen's production, and insert the genes into organisms such as yeasts and *Escherichia coli*. These biological factories promptly churn out millions of copies of the antigen. The antigens are then extracted from the culture media, purified, and concentrated to form the new vaccine. A synthetic vaccine for hepatitis B is now available, and laboratories are working on synthetic vaccines for such diseases as genital herpes, rabies, AIDS, typhoid fever, diphtheria, malaria, and cholera. They are also exploring new

esh-er-ik′e-ah

607

methods for administration, as MicroFocus 19.1 explores. In the view of many scientists, the current era represents a golden age of vaccine technology.

In this chapter, we shall study the role of vaccines in the immune response while examining the four major mechanisms by which immunity comes about. Antibodies occupy a central position in each of these mechanisms. We shall also study how antibodies may be detected in a disease patient by a variety of laboratory tests. These diagnostic procedures help the physician understand the disease and prescribe a course of treatment. Immune mechanisms generally protect against disease, but when they fail, the laboratory tests provide a clue about what is taking place in the patient.

19.1 Immunity to Disease

The word *immune* is derived from the Latin *immuno*, meaning "safe" or "free from." In its most general sense, the term implies a condition under which an individual is protected from disease. This does not mean, however, that one is immune to all diseases, but rather to a specific disease or group of diseases.

MicroFocus 19.1

PINCUSHION PARANOIA

The crying starts as you round the corner and little Michael realizes that he's on the way to the doctor's office. At 2 months of age, he got his hepatitis B shot, then his DTaP, then Hib, then polio, then another and another. At 4 months, they started all over—DTaP, polio, Hib, hepatitis B—and they even threw in a rotavirus shot. Back to the doctor's at 6 months for another series. And now he was a year old, and he was hearing new words: varicella and MMR. It was just no fun being a kid!

It may be too late for Michael, but the future looks brighter for Michael Junior. Researchers are experimenting with diphtheria and tetanus immunizations using a skin patch carrying toxoids. The patch contains 400 microscopic needles that introduce vaccines just beneath the skin layers but above the nerve endings, so there is no pain.

Moreover, a California company is experimenting with a nasal spray (Flu-Mist) that delivers active influenza viruses to the mucosal surfaces of the nose. The device looks like a syringe (Michael, beware), but instead of a needle it has a sprayer that squirts an aerosol mist into each nostril. By encouraging antibody production in the nasal passageways, the vaccine encourages defense at the portal of entry for flu viruses. The principal antibody stimulated is IgA.

And if things go well, Michael Junior may even be offered a banana for his hepatitis B immunization. Researchers at New York's Boyce Thompson Institute have already spliced *E. coli* genes into potato plants and produced potatoes containing *E. coli* antigens. Although the "veggie vaccine" is not especially tasty (it must be eaten raw to avoid destroying the antigens), the process has been deemed a success, and experiments are continuing to introduce the same genes to banana plants. Bananas are attractive because children like them (and children are the main recipients of vaccines); the fruit grows in tropical countries (where vac-

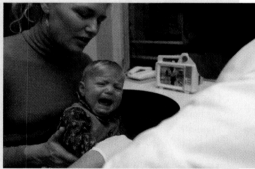

cines are widely used); and the fruit does not have to be cooked. On the down side, there is the matter of transporting the antigens through the stomach's hydrochloric acid and past the duodenum's enzymes. Unfortunately, many years of tinkering lie ahead before the banana replaces the needle.

So for the time being, Michael must bear it as best he can. But someday he'll be off to college, and they will send his tuition bill home. Ah, revenge is sweet.

Two general types of immunity are recognized: innate immunity and acquired immunity. **Innate immunity** is an inborn capacity for resisting disease. It begins at birth and depends on genetic factors expressed as physiological, anatomical, and biochemical differences among living things. Examples of innate immunity are the lysozyme found in tears, saliva, and other body secretions; the acidic pH of the gastrointestinal and vaginal tracts; and the interferon produced by body cells to protect against viruses. Innate immunity is synonymous with nonspecific resistance, discussed in Chapter 18.

Acquired immunity, by contrast, begins after birth. It depends on the presence of T-lymphocytes, antibodies, and other factors originating in the immune system. Four types of acquired immunity are generally recognized, as the following discussions will explore (FIGURE 19.1). Although the emphasis will be on antibodies and antibody-mediated immunity, it should be remembered that cell-mediated immunity is also an important consideration in the total spectrum of resistance to infectious disease.

Innate immunity:
an inborn capacity to resist disease.

Acquired immunity:
immunity that develops after the interaction of antigens with the immune system.

FIGURE 19.1

The Four Types of Acquired Immunity

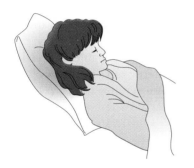

(A) Naturally acquired active immunity arises from an exposure to antigens and often follows a disease.

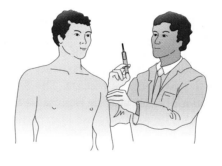

(B) Artificially acquired active immunity results from an inoculation of toxoid or vaccine.

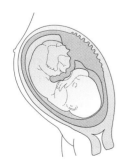

(C) Naturally acquired passive immunity stems from the passage of IgG across the placenta from the maternal to the fetal circulation.

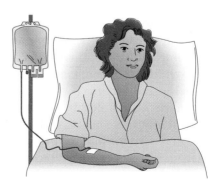

(D) Artificially acquired passive immunity is induced by an injection of antibodies taken from the circulation of an animal or another person.

NATURALLY ACQUIRED ACTIVE IMMUNITY

Active immunity:
immunity derived from an exposure to antigens and subsequent production of antibodies.

Active immunity develops after antigens enter the body and the individual's immune system responds with antibodies. The exposure to antigens may be unintentional or intentional. When it is unintentional, the immunity that develops is called naturally acquired active immunity.

Naturally acquired active immunity usually follows a bout of illness and occurs in the "natural" scheme of events. However, this is not always the case, because subclinical diseases may also bring on the immunity. For example, many people have acquired immunity from subclinical cases of mumps or from subclinical fungal diseases such as cryptococcosis. This is the **primary antibody response** (Chapter 18).

krip'to-kok-o'sis

Memory cells residing in the lymphoid tissues are responsible for the production of antibodies that yield naturally acquired active immunity. The cells remain active for many years and produce IgG immediately upon later entry of the parasite to the host. Such an antibody response is sometimes called the **secondary anamnestic response**, from the Greek *anamnesis*, for "recollection." It is also known as the **secondary antibody response**.

an'am-nes'tik

ARTIFICIALLY ACQUIRED ACTIVE IMMUNITY

Artificially acquired active immunity:
immunity that develops after an intentional exposure to antigens followed by an immune response.

Artificially acquired active immunity develops after the immune system produces antibodies following an intentional exposure to antigens. The antigens are usually contained in an immunizing agent such as a **vaccine** or **toxoid**, and the exposure to antigens is "artificial."

Viral vaccines consist of either **inactivated viruses**, incapable of multiplying in the body, or **attenuated viruses**, which multiply at low rates in the body but fail to cause symptoms of disease. The Salk polio vaccine typifies the former, while the Sabin oral polio vaccine represents the latter. Bacterial vaccines fall into similar categories. The formerly used pertussis (whooping cough) vaccine consisted of dead cells, while the tuberculosis vaccine is composed of attenuated bacteria (**MicroFocus 19.2**). Whole-microorganism viral and bacterial vaccines are commonly called **first-generation vaccines**.

First-generation vaccine:
one that contains whole microorganisms.

One advantage of vaccines made with attenuated organisms is that organisms multiply for a period of time within the body, thus increasing the dose of antigen administered. This higher dose results in a higher level of immune response than that obtained with the single dose of inactivated organisms. Also, attenuated organisms can spread to other people and reimmunize them, or immunize them for the first time. However, attenuated organisms may be a health hazard because of this same ability to continue multiplying. In 1984, for example, a recently immunized soldier spread vaccinia (cowpox) viruses to his daughter. She, in turn, infected seven young friends at a slumber party.

Attenuated:
weakened.

Currently, there are no widely used bacterial vaccines made with whole-organisms and used for long-term protection. The older **pertussis** vaccine was replaced by the acellular pertussis vaccine composed of *Bordetella pertussis* extracts. Some whole organism vaccines are used for temporary protection. For instance, bubonic plague and cholera vaccines are available to limit an epidemic. In these cases, the immunity lasts only for several months because the material in the vaccine is weakly antigenic. Weakly antigenic vaccines are also available for laboratory workers who deal with rickettsial diseases such as Rocky Mountain spotted fever, Q fever,

MicroFocus 19.2

TRAGEDY AT LUBECK

Albert Calmette and Camille Guérin were excited. Since 1908, they had been transferring a strain of tubercle bacillus to fresh media every 2 weeks, and now, after 13 long years, they found that the strain had lost most of its virulence. When test animals were inoculated, the bacillus failed to cause tuberculosis. Moreover, it apparently immunized animals to the disease and could be used as a vaccine. Their report, published in 1921, described the vaccine and gave it the name BCG, for bacille Calmette Guérin.

By 1929, physicians had immunized thousands of children throughout the world and established the value of BCG. Statistical data added to the confidence doctors had in the vaccine, even as reports began to filter in from the Public Health Laboratories at Lubeck.

Lubeck was a major city on the Baltic Sea in what is now western Germany. It had a rich history dating back to the medieval period and was once the capital of the Hanseatic League. Doctors in the bacteriology laboratory at the city hospital had prepared the vaccine as directed by Calmette, and administered it to 252 children. However, to their shock and dismay, 71 of the recipients soon died of tuberculosis. Subsequent studies showed that a contaminating tubercle bacillus had caused the deaths, but the damage was already done. World opinion soon turned against BCG.

In the following years, doctors continued to use BCG, but with caution and skepticism. Some confidence was restored by a 1937 Chicago study showing that in 20,000 vaccinated infants and schoolchildren, doctors found an 80 percent reduction of expected cases of tuberculosis. By 1964, about 200 million people worldwide had been immunized, and the safety of BCG once again was established. However, the United States had then, and still has today, a blind spot. Many American doctors argue that BCG would destroy the effectiveness of the tuberculin test and that most cases of tuberculosis can be controlled with drugs. Nevertheless, tuberculosis affects over 25,000 Americans, and it is plausible that physicians may rethink the use of BCG. No doubt the tragedy at Lubeck will continue to color their decision.

and typhus. The danger in these vaccines is that the residual egg protein in the cultivation medium for rickettsiae may cause allergic reactions in recipients. TABLE 19.1 presents a summary of currently available bacterial and viral vaccines.

Immunizing agents that stimulate immunity to toxins are known as **toxoids**. These agents are currently available for protection against diphtheria and tetanus, two diseases whose major effects are due to exotoxins. Toxoids are prepared by incubating toxins with a chemical, such as formaldehyde, until the toxicity is lost.

> Toxoid:
> an immunizing agent, consisting of chemically altered toxins, that provides protection against toxins.

To avoid multiple injections of immunizing agents, it is advantageous to combine vaccines into a **single-dose vaccine**. Experience has shown this possible for the diphtheria-pertussis-tetanus vaccine (DPT), the newer diphtheria-tetanus-acellular pertussis vaccine (DTaP), the measles-mumps-rubella vaccine (MMR), and the trivalent oral polio vaccine (TOP). There is even a vaccine that will immunize against four diseases simultaneously: In 1993, the FDA approved a combined vaccine which includes diphtheria and tetanus toxoids, pertussis vaccine, and *Haemophilus influenzae* b (Hib) vaccine. Marketed as Tetramune, the quadruple vaccine is used in children aged 2 months to 5 years to protect against the DPT diseases, as well as *Haemophilus* meningitis. FIGURE 19.2 outlines the recommendations for these vaccines in healthy infants and children. For other vaccines, however, a combination may not be useful because the antibody response is lower for the combination than for each vaccine taken separately. Immunologists believe that poor phagocytosis by macrophages is one reason. Activation of suppressor T-lymphocytes may be another reason.

> he-mof'i-lus

> Macrophages:
> large white blood cells that phagocytize antigens and begin the immune process.

Immunologists foresee the day when preparations called **subunit vaccines**, or **second-generation vaccines**, will be used exclusively. For example, pili from bacteria may be extracted and purified for use in a vaccine to stimulate antipili antibodies

> Second-generation vaccine:
> one that contains parts or subunits of microorganisms.

TABLE 19.1

The Principal Bacterial and Viral Vaccines Currently in Use

DISEASE	ROUTE OF ADMINISTRATION	RECOMMENDED USAGE/COMMENTS
Contain Killed Whole Bacteria		
Cholera	Subcutaneous (SQ) injection	For travelers; short-term protection
Typhoid	SQ and IM	For travelers only; variable protection
Plague	SQ	For exposed individuals and animal workers; variable protection
Contain Live, Attenuated Bacteria		
Tuberculosis (BCG)	Intradermal (ID) injection	For high-risk occupations only; protection variable
Subunit Bacterial Vaccines (Capsular Polysaccharides)		
Meningitis (meningococcal)	SQ	For protection in high-risk individuals, such as military recruits; short-term protection
Meningitis (H. influenzae)	Intramuscular (IM) injection	For infants and children; may be administered with DTaP
Pneumococcal pneumonia	IM or SQ	Important for people at high risk: the young, elderly, and immuno-compromised; moderate protection
Pertussis	IM	For newborns and children
Subunit Bacterial Vaccine (Outer Surface Lipoprotein)		
Lyme disease	IM	For protection in high-risk individuals living in tick-infested areas; three injections
Toxoids (Formaldehyde-Inactivated Bacterial Exotoxins)		
Diphtheria	IM	A routine childhood vaccination; highly effective in systemic protection
Tetanus	IM	A routine childhood vaccination; highly effective
Botulism	IM	For high-risk individuals, such as laboratory workers
Contain Inactivated Whole Viruses		
Polio (Salk)	IM	Routine childhood vaccine; highly effective; safer than Sabin vaccine
Rabies	IM	For individuals sustaining animal bites or otherwise exposed; highly effective
Influenza	IM	For high-risk individuals; requires constant updating for new strains
Hepatitis A	IM	Protection for travelers and anyone at risk; effectiveness not established
Contain Attenuated Viruses		
Adenovirus infection	Oral	For immunizing military recruits
Measles (rubeola)	SQ	Routine childhood vaccine; highly effective
Mumps (parotitis)	SQ	Routine childhood vaccine; highly effective
Polio (Sabin)	Oral	Routine childhood vaccine; highly effective; possible vaccine-induced polio
Rubella	SQ	Routine childhood vaccine; highly effective
Chickenpox (varicella)	SQ	Routine childhood vaccine; immunity can diminish over time; effectiveness not yet established
Yellow fever	SQ	For travelers, military personnel in endemic areas
Recombinant Viral Vaccine		
Hepatitis B	IM	Medical, dental, laboratory personnel; newborns, others at risk; highly effective
Rotavirus*	Oral	For young children, especially in developing countries

*temporarily withdrawn

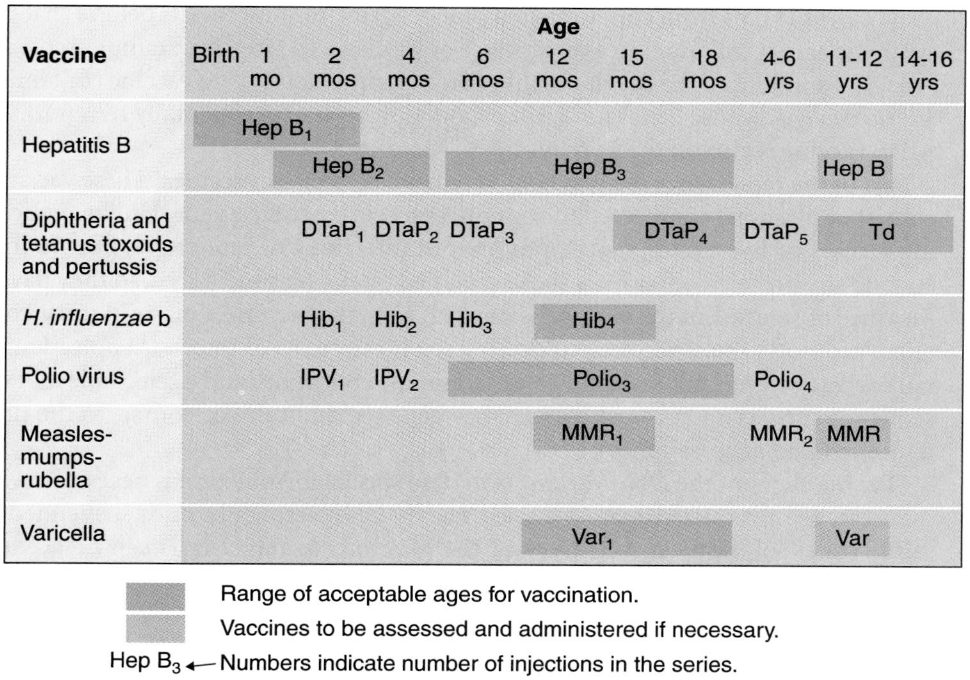
Vaccine
Age
Birth 1 mo 2 mos 4 mos 6 mos 12 mos 15 mos 18 mos 4-6 yrs 11-12 yrs 14-16 yrs
Hepatitis B
Hep B1
Hep B2
Hep B3
Hep B
Diphtheria and tetanus toxoids and pertussis
DTaP1 DTaP2 DTaP3
DTaP4 DTaP5
Td
H. influenzae b
Hib1 Hib2 Hib3
Hib4
Polio virus
IPV1 IPV2
Polio3
Polio4
Measles-mumps-rubella
MMR1
MMR2 MMR
Varicella
Var1
Var
Range of acceptable ages for vaccination.
Vaccines to be assessed and administered if necessary.
Hep B3 ← Numbers indicate number of injections in the series.

FIGURE 19.2

Childhood Immunization Schedule

Established in 1999 by the Advisory Committee on Immunization Practices of the CDC, this schedule indicates the recommended ages for routine administration of licensed childhood vaccines. "Catch-up" vaccination may be administered if a visit to the doctor is missed. Additional recommendations concerning the schedule are available from the CDC at www.cdc.gov.

(FIGURE 19.3). These would inhibit the attachment of bacteria to tissues and facilitate phagocytosis. Another example is the vaccine for **pneumococcal pneumonia**, licensed for use in 1983. The vaccine contains 23 different polysaccharides from the capsules of 23 strains of *Streptococcus pneumoniae.* Still another example is the **Hib vaccine** against *Haemophilus influenzae* b, the agent of *Haemophilus* meningitis (Chapter 7). Also composed of capsular polysaccharides, the vaccine has been available since 1988 and has been a critical factor in reducing the incidence of *Haemophilus* meningitis, from 18,000 cases annually (1986) to a few dozen cases in recent years (1999).

Another form of vaccine is the **synthetic vaccine**, or **third-generation vaccine.** This preparation represents a sophisticated and practical application of recombinant DNA technology. To produce the vaccine, three major technical problems must be solved: The immune-stimulating antigen must be identified, living cells must be reengineered to produce the antigens, and the size of the antigens must be increased to promote phagocytosis and the immune response.

The genetic engineering process has worked for a synthetic vaccine for **hepatitis B**. The vaccine is marketed by different companies as Recombivax or Engerix-B. Because the vaccine is not made from blood fragments (as the previous hepatitis B vaccine was), it relieves the fear of contracting human immunodefi-

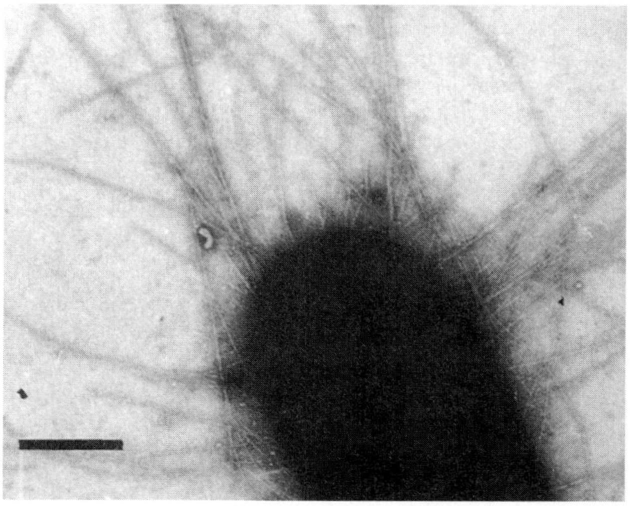

FIGURE 19.3

A Possible Approach to Antibody Use

A scanning electron micrograph of a cell of *Escherichia coli* showing the numerous pili at the pole of the cell. Pili are used to help the bacterium adhere to the infected tissue. A vaccine containing pilus antigens could be used to stimulate antipili antibodies, which bind to the pili and prevent the bacterium from adhering. (Bar = 0.5 μm.)

Third-generation vaccine:
one that contains microbial
fragments produced by genetic
engineering.

DNA vaccine:
a vaccine containing genetically
engineered plasmids.

ciency virus (HIV) from contaminated blood. Many immunologists believe that the synthetic agents will usher in a renaissance of vaccines. In 1993, for example, biotechnologists announced the development of an experimental cholera vaccine containing *Vibrio cholerae* whose genes for toxin production were experimentally removed. An AIDS vaccine is also on the horizon (MicroFocus 19.3).

Part of the renaissance is a group of vaccines called **DNA vaccines**. These vaccines consist of plasmids engineered to contain a protein-encoding gene. Unlike replicating viruses or live bacteria, plasmids are not infectious or replicative, nor do they encode any proteins other than those specified by the plasmid genes, so they have a measure of safety. But the vaccine is difficult to make because a plasmid must contain a promoter site, a convenient cloning site for the gene of interest, a polyadenine tail used as a termination sequence, an origin of replication, and a selectable marker sequence such as an ampicillin-resistance gene (in addition, of course, to the protein-encoding gene or genes).

One highlight of the DNA vaccine is that no special formulation is necessary. Animals can be immunized against disease merely by injecting plasmids suspended in saline (salt) solution. And delivery of the plasmids to target cells can be accomplished by nasal spray; injection into the muscle or vein, and under the skin; and by

MicroFocus 19.3

AN AIDS VACCINE—WHY THE WAIT?

Producing an AIDS vaccine might appear rather straightforward: Cultivate a huge batch of human immunodeficiency virus (HIV), inactivate it with chemicals, purify it, and prepare it for marketing. Unfortunately, things are not quite so simple when HIV is involved. For example, the effects of a bad batch of vaccine would be catastrophic; and people are generally reluctant to be immunized with whole HIV particles, no matter how reassuring scientists are.

Nevertheless, developing an AIDS vaccine is a major priority of modern scientists because about 20 million people are candidates to receive it. The cohort of candidates include anyone practicing high-risk behaviors (e.g., unprotected sexual intercourse) or using drugs intravenously or having contact with blood. The latter group includes doctors, surgeons, dentists, nurses, medical technologists, morticians, emergency medical technicians, police officers, and firefighters. All would welcome the vaccine when it becomes available.

The operative word is *when*, because an AIDS vaccine *will* be available one day. Already, biotechnologists have

cloned the genes for the gp120 and gp41 molecules in the HIV envelope, and they are producing these subunit molecules in vast quantities. Others are researching gp160, the precursor molecule to gp120 and gp41, for use as a vaccine subunit; still others are utilizing p17, an HIV core protein, in their candidate vaccine. There is a potential vaccine containing HIV minus its envelope, and another composed of simian immunodeficiency virus (SIV). Proponents of the latter vaccine hope to use it as cowpox viruses were once used against smallpox.

Before a vaccine reaches the human population, however, a number of problems must be resolved. For instance, HIV tends to mutate much as influenza viruses do, and a vaccine would have to take HIV variants into account. Then too, HIV remains within T-lymphocytes as a provirus, and antibodies elicited by a vaccine could not reach it here. There is also the problem of locating an animal model for testing purposes. (Chimpanzees are the only animals that display AIDS symptoms.)

When it comes to field trials, still other problems must be confronted. For exam-

ple, volunteers can be used only once, and there are many candidate vaccines to test. Also, volunteers will test positive for HIV antibodies after participating in a trial, and, should they contract HIV, the diagnostic test for antibodies would not work. Moreover, they might suffer discrimination (e.g., in obtaining medical insurance) when they test positive during and after the vaccine trial.

There is also the problem of counseling. When a person volunteers for a vaccine trial, the physician is ethically obliged to counsel the person on methods of avoiding HIV. It would then be difficult to assess whether the person remained free of HIV because of the counseling or because of the vaccine. And finally, once a person has developed antibodies from the vaccine, it is ethically unsound to inject that person with HIV to see if the antibodies are protective.

To be sure, the problems are daunting. However, the project is equally massive in scope and effort. No vaccine has appeared in the marketplace less than 10 years after the inception of development. For AIDS, no vaccine predates 1990, so if we add 10 years . . .

a so-called gene gun. A gene gun is a propulsion device that shoots DNA-coated gold beads into the skin. Furthermore, deploying plasmids as DNA vaccines has the added advantage of stimulating both antibody-mediated immunity (AMI) and cell-mediated immunity (CMI), because DNA vaccines encode proteins that are released from the cell (for AMI) and proteins that fix themselves to the target cell surface (for CMI). DNA vaccines also appear to elicit a strong immune response possibly due to an immune response to other genes in the plasmid, and the vaccines are more stable than conventional vaccines at low and high temperatures (which makes shipping easier). At this writing, DNA vaccines have been used experimentally to protect against influenza, *Salmonella typhi*, HIV infection, herpes simplex, and hepatitis B. MicroFocus 19.4 explores their discovery.

Vaccines for immunizations may be administered by injection, oral consumption, or nasal spray, as currently used for some respiratory viral diseases. **Booster immunizations** commonly follow as a way of raising the antibody level by stimulating the memory cells to induce the secondary anamnestic response. This is why a tetanus booster is given to anyone who sustains a deep puncture wound by a soil-contaminated object. TABLE 19.2 summarizes the vaccines universally recommended by the CDC as of 1999.

Substances called **adjuvants** increase the efficiency of a vaccine or toxoid by increasing the availability of the antigen in the lymphatic system. Common adjuvants include aluminum sulfate ("alum") and aluminum hydroxide in toxoid preparations, as well as mineral oil or peanut oil in viral vaccines. The particles of adjuvant linked to antigen are taken up by macrophages and presented to lymphocytes more efficiently than dissolved antigens. Experiments also suggest that adjuvants may stimulate the macrophage to produce interleukin-1, a lymphocyte-activating factor, and thereby reduce the necessity for helper T-lymphocyte activity. Moreover, adjuvants provide slow release of the antigen from the site of entry and provoke a more sustained immune response. MicroFocus 19.5 describes a new category of antibodies.

ad'ju-vant
Adjuvant:
a substance that increases the immunizing potential of a vaccine or toxoid by boosting the availability of the antigen.

MicroFocus 19.4

A HAPPENING

It was another of those remarkable moments in science, an unexpected observation that opened the door to a whole new type of vaccine. It happened in 1989 at Vical Inc., a California biotechnology company. Biochemist Philip Felgner and his research group were experimenting with plasmids, the ultramicroscopic ringlets of cytoplasmic DNA that carry many nonessential genes in bacteria. Felgner wished to learn whether the plasmids could carry genes into a mouse when wrapped in lipid-containing bodies called liposomes. He could hardly imagine what he was about to discover.

Felgner's protocol was simple. Some plasmids were packaged in the tiny, spi-ral liposomes, then injected into the muscle of a mouse. As a control, some unpackaged plasmids were injected into another mouse. The latter plasmids, by all expectations, should remain inert or be destroyed.

But they were not destroyed; nor did they remain inert. Instead, the cells receiving them began synthesizing the proteins encoded by the naked plasmids. Somehow, the plasmids had remained intact, found the necessary biochemical machinery, and induced the cell to begin sputtering protein. And, adding to the wild results, the proteins were stimulating the mouse's immune system to produce antibodies. The realization slowly dawned on Felg-ner and his group: They had discovered a new way to immunize an animal; they had produced a DNA vaccine.

Scientists are constantly taught never to anticipate their results when performing an experiment. The trick is to formulate a hypothesis, devise a reasonable set of experimental conditions, turn on the juice, and sit back while Mother Nature reveals her truths. Usually the process is slow and plodding. But every now and then, nature astounds us with a bit of knowledge that makes all the dreary days worthwhile. It has happened innumerable times in science, and it happened once again in 1989 in San Diego.

Oh, by the way, the plasmids packaged in liposomes also encoded protein.

TABLE 19.2

Universally Recommended Vaccinations for Children, Adolescents, and Adults

POPULATION	VACCINATION	DOSAGE
All young children	Measles, mumps, and rubella	2 doses
	Diphtheria-tetanus toxoid and pertussis vaccine	5 doses
	Polio	4 doses
	Haemophilus influenzae b	3–4 doses
	Hepatitis B	3 doses
	Rotavirus*	3 doses before first birthday
	Varicella	1 dose
Previously unvaccinated or partially vaccinated adolescents	Hepatitis B	3 doses, total
	Varicella	If no previous history of varicella, 1 dose for children <12 years, 2 doses for children ≥12 years
	Measles, mumps, and rubella	2 doses, total
	Tetanus-diphtheria toxoid	If not vaccinated during previous 5 years, 1 combined booster during ages 11–16
All adults	Tetanus-diphtheria toxoid	1 dose administered every 10 years
All adults ≥65 years	Influenza	1 dose administered annually
	Pneumococcal	1 dose

*temporarily withdrawn

NATURALLY ACQUIRED PASSIVE IMMUNITY

Passive immunity: immunity derived from an infusion of antibodies from an outside source.

Passive immunity develops when antibodies enter the body from an outside source (in contrast to active immunity, in which individuals synthesize their own antibodies). The infusion of antibodies may be unintentional or intentional, and thus, natural or artificial. When unintentional, the immunity that develops is called naturally acquired passive immunity.

Naturally acquired passive immunity is also called **congenital immunity**. It develops when antibodies pass into the fetal circulation from the mother's bloodstream via the placenta and umbilical cord. These antibodies, called **maternal antibodies**, remain with the child for approximately 3 to 6 months after birth and fade as the child's immune system becomes fully functional. Certain antibodies, such as measles antibodies, remain for 12 to 15 months. The process occurs in the "natural" scheme of events.

Maternal antibodies play an important role during the first few months of life by providing resistance to diseases such as pertussis, staphylococcal infections, and viral respiratory diseases. Because the antibodies are of human origin and are contained in human serum, they will be accepted without problem. The only antibody in the serum is IgG.

kŏ-los′trum

Maternal antibodies also pass to the newborn through the first milk, or **colostrum**, of a nursing mother, as well as during future breast-feedings. In this instance, IgA is the predominant antibody, although IgG and IgM have also been

MicroFocus 19.5

STAY TUNED

Just when you thought you had seen it all, something new pops onto the radar screen. This time it's plantibodies. That's right, plantibodies—corn plants that produce human antibodies.

The proud parents are scientists from Agracetus Inc., a biotechnology company in Wisconsin. Using a secret gene-delivery system, the researchers force genes that encode human antibodies into the genome of corn seeds. Then they plant the latter in an unpretentious cornfield. When harvested by conven-tional agricultural methods, the corn kernels yield human antibodies that can be used to ferry radioisotopes to human tumor cells and destroy them. As of 1999, the researchers were planning clinical trials of their new isotope delivery system.

But there's more. Already planted in the fields are soybeans that produce herpes simplex antibodies (for treating genital herpes), and tobacco plants that manufacture streptococcal antibodies. The latter might be added to a mouth-wash to fight tooth decay associated with *Streptococcus mutans*.

Many people see these innovative and imaginative products as the culmination of decades of biotechnology research. Others see them as the first offspring of a new family of biotechnology products. Indeed, researchers point to Winston Churchill's immortal words: "This is not the end; this is not even the beginning of the end; it is, perhaps, the end of the beginning." Don't turn off the radar screen just yet.

found in the milk. The antibodies accumulate in the respiratory and gastrointestinal tracts of the child and apparently lend increased disease resistance (Chapter 18).

ARTIFICIALLY ACQUIRED PASSIVE IMMUNITY

Artificially acquired passive immunity arises from the intentional injection of antibody-rich serum into the patient's circulation. The exposure to antibodies is thus "artificial." In the decades before the development of antibiotics, such an injection was an important therapeutic tool for the treatment of disease. The practice is still used for viral diseases such as Lassa fever and arthropodborne encephalitis, and for bacterial diseases in which a toxin is involved. For example, established cases of bot-ulism, diphtheria, and tetanus are treated with serum containing the respective antitoxins.

Various terms are used for the serum that renders artificially acquired passive immunity. **Antiserum** is one such term. Another is **hyperimmune serum**, which indicates that the serum has a higher-than-normal level of a particular antibody. If the serum is used to protect against a disease such as hepatitis A, it is called **pro-phylactic serum**. When the serum is used in the therapy of an established disease, is it called **therapeutic serum**. When serum is taken from the blood of a convalescing patient, physicians refer to it as **convalescent serum**. Another common term, **gamma globulin**, takes its name from the fraction of blood protein in which most antibodies are found. Gamma globulin usually consists of a pool of sera from dif-ferent human donors, and thus it contains a mixture of antibodies, including those for the disease to be treated.

Passive immunity must be used with caution because in many individuals, the immune system recognizes foreign serum proteins as antigens and synthesizes anti-bodies against them in an allergic reaction. When antibodies interact with the pro-teins, a series of chemical molecules called immune complexes may form (Chapter 20), and with the activation of complement, the person develops a disease called **serum sickness**. This is often characterized by a hivelike rash at the injection site, accompanied by labored breathing and swollen joints. To avoid the disease, it is

Artificially acquired passive immunity:
immunity that develops after an intentional exposure to antibodies.

Antiserum:
serum that is rich in a particular antibody.

Gamma globulin:
an alternate name for antiserum based on the fraction of blood protein in which antibodies are located.

Serum sickness:
a type of allergic reaction in which the immune system forms antibodies against proteins in antiserum.

imperative that the patient be tested for allergies before serum therapy is instituted. If an allergy exists, minuscule doses should be given to eliminate the allergic state, and then a large therapeutic dose can be administered.

Artificially acquired passive immunity provides substantial and immediate protection against disease, but it is only a temporary measure. The immunity that develops from antibody-rich serum usually wears off within days or weeks. Among the serum preparations currently in use are those for hepatitis A and chickenpox. Both are made from the serum of blood donors routinely screened for hepatitis A and chickenpox. The four types of immunity are summarized in TABLE 19.3.

To this point . . .

We have discussed four different types of acquired immunity with examples of each. Naturally acquired active immunity develops after a bout of illness or following a subclinical disease. The exposure to antigens is unintentional, and the immune system produces antibodies. By contrast, artificially acquired active immunity requires an intentional exposure to antigens, such as when one receives a vaccine or toxoid. Subunit vaccines, synthetic vaccines, and DNA vaccines contain no organisms and thus are an improvement over whole-organism vaccines. As before, immunity comes about when the immune system produces antibodies.

The third type of immunity is naturally acquired passive immunity. This develops from the passage of antibodies from mother to child across the placenta. The antibodies remain active for several months after birth, a time during which the immune system is not fully functional. An injection of antibodies brings about the fourth type of immunity, artificially acquired passive immunity. Allergic reactions in the recipient limit the use of this form of immunity.

In the next section, we shall shift our attention to the activity of antibodies in the laboratory. We will focus on serological reactions, in which antigen–antibody interactions are used for diagnostic purposes. We shall survey multiple forms of these tests and note the advances in technology that have made the serology laboratory a highly sophisticated environment for conducting practical immunology.

TABLE 19.3

Characteristics of the Four Types of Immunity

TYPE OF IMMUNITY	IMMUNIZING AGENT	EXPOSURE TO IMMUNIZING AGENT	EFFECTIVE DOSE REQUIRED	RELATIVE TIME UNTIL IMMUNITY	RELATIVE DURATION OF IMMUNITY
Naturally acquired active	Antigens	Unintentional	Small	Long	Long (lifetime)
Artificially acquired active	Antigens	Intentional	Small	Long	Long (months to years)
Naturally acquired passive	Antibodies	Unintentional	Large	Short	Short (4–6 months)
Artificially acquired passive	Antibodies	Intentional	Large	Short	Short (up to 6 weeks)

19.2 Serological Reactions

Antigen–antibody interactions studied under laboratory conditions are known as **serological reactions** because they commonly involve serum from a patient. In the late 1800s, serological reactions were first adapted to laboratory tests used in the diagnosis of disease. The principle was simple and straightforward: If the patient had an abnormal level of a specific antibody in the serum, a suspected disease agent was probably present. Today, serological reactions have diagnostic significance, as well as more broad-ranging applications. For example, they are used to confirm identifications made by other procedures and detect organisms in body tissues. In addition, they help the physician follow the course of disease and determine the immune status, and they aid in determining groupings below the species level.

Serological reaction: a laboratory reaction in which serum is involved.

CHARACTERISTICS OF SEROLOGICAL REACTIONS

The reactants in a serological reaction generally consist of an antigen and a serum sample. The nature of either must be known; the object is to determine the nature of the other. In some cases, the unknown can be determined merely by placing the reactants on a slide and observing the presence or absence of a reaction. However, serological tests are not always quite so direct. For example, an antigen may have only one antigenic determinant, and the combination with an antibody molecule on a one-to-one basis may be invisible. To solve this dilemma, a second-stage reaction using an indicator system may be required, or a contact signal may be necessary. We shall see how this works in several tests.

Another possible drawback to a successful serological reaction is that antigen or antibody solutions may require considerable dilution to reach a concentration at

Serum: the clear, cell-free fluid portion of the blood that contains no clotting agents.

USUAL ROUTE OF INTRODUCTION	SOURCE OF ANTIBODIES	FUNCTION	EFFECTIVENESS IN NEWBORN	EFFECTIVENESS IN ADULT	ORIGIN
Various tissues	Self	Therapeutic Prophylactic	Low	High	Clinical or subclinical disease
Intramuscular or intradermal	Self	Prophylactic	Low	High	Toxoid or vaccine
Intravenous	Other than self	Prophylactic	High	Low	Transplacental passage of antibodies
Intravenous	Other than self	Prophylactic Therapeutic	High	Moderate	Serum that contains antibodies

ti′ter
Titer:
the most dilute concentration of serum antibody that yields a detectable reaction with a specific antigen.

Hapten:
a partial antigen that complexes to carrier proteins or polysaccharides to form a complete antigen.

which a reaction will be most favorable. This may be used to the physician's advantage, however, because the dilution series is a valuable way of determining the titer of antibodies, as shown in FIGURE 19.4. The **titer** is the most dilute concentration of serum antibody that yields a detectable reaction with its specific antigen. This number is expressed as a ratio of antibody to total fluid (e.g., 1:50) and is used to indicate the amount of antibodies in a patient's serum. For instance, the titer of **influenza** antibodies may rise from 1:20 to 1:320 as an episode of influenza progresses, and then continue upward, stabilizing at 1:1280 as the disease reaches its peak. A rise in the titer of a certain antibody also indicates that an individual has a case of that disease, an important factor in diagnosis.

Haptens may pose a problem in a serological reaction because, as partial antigens, they usually have only a single antigenic determinant. Technologists have circumvented this problem by conjugating the haptens to carrier particles, such as polystyrene beads. When the hapten unites with an antibody, the entire bead is involved in the complex, and a visible reaction occurs.

Serology has become a highly sophisticated and often automated branch of immunology. As the following tests illustrate, the serological reactions have direct application to the clinical laboratory—not only in microbiology, but in other fields as well.

NEUTRALIZATION

Neutralization is a serological reaction in which antigens and antibodies neutralize each other. The reaction is used to identify toxins and antitoxins, as well as viruses and viral antibodies. Normally, little or no visible evidence of a neutralization reaction is present, and the test mixture must therefore be injected into a laboratory animal to determine whether neutralization has taken place.

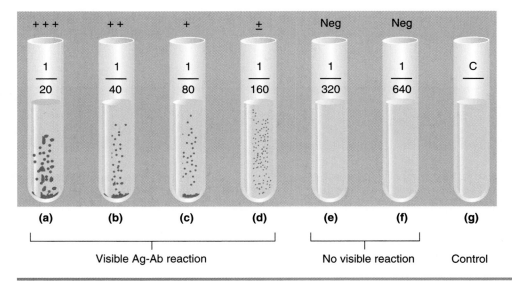

FIGURE 19.4

The Determination of Titer

A sample of antibody-containing serum was diluted in saline solution to yield the dilutions shown. An equal amount of antigen was then added to each tube, and the tubes were incubated. An antigen–antibody interaction may be seen in tubes (a) through (d), but not in tubes (e) or (f) or the control tube, (g). The titer of antibody is the highest dilution of serum antibody in which a reaction is visible—in this case, tube (d). The titer is therefore expressed as 1:160.

An example of a neutralization test is the one used to detect **botulism toxin** in food. Normally the botulism toxin is lethal to a laboratory animal, and if a sample of the food contains the toxin, the animal will succumb after an injection. However, if the food is first mixed with botulism antitoxins, the antitoxin molecules neutralize the toxin molecules, and the mixture has no effect on the animal. Conversely, if the toxin was produced by some other organism, no neutralization will occur, and the mixture will still be lethal to the animal. A similar test for diphtheria is the **Schick test**.

Botulism:
a foodborne bacterial disease in which toxins lead to muscular paralysis.

PRECIPITATION

Precipitation reactions are serological reactions involving thousands of antigen and antibody molecules cross-linked at multiple determinant sites to form a structure called a **lattice**. The lattices are so huge that particles of precipitate form, and the reaction product is visually observed.

Precipitation tests are performed in either fluid media or gels. In **fluid precipitation**, the antibody and antigen solutions are layered over each other in a thin tube. The molecules then diffuse through the fluid until they reach a zone of equivalence, the ideal concentration for precipitation. A visible mass of particles now forms at the interface or at the bottom of the tube. Fluid precipitation is frequently used in forensic medicine to learn the origin of albumin proteins in bloodstains.

Zone of equivalence:
the ideal concentration of reactants at which precipitation occurs.

In **gel precipitation**, the diffusion of antigens and antibodies takes place through a semisolid gel, such as agarose. (The tests are also called **immunodiffusion tests**.) The Oudin tube technique, described in 1946 by Jacques Oudin, is typical. A plug of gel is placed between solutions of antigen and antibody in a thin tube. As the molecules diffuse through the gel, they eventually reach the zone of equivalence, where they interact and form a visible ring of precipitate. This type of technique is called a **double diffusion process** because both reactants diffuse. Another application is in the Ouchterlony plate technique, named for Orjan Ouchterlony, who devised it in 1953. In this technique, antigen and antibody solutions are placed in wells cut into agarose in Petri dishes. The plates are incubated, and precipitation lines form at the zone of equivalence (**FIGURE 19.5**).

oo-deh'

ouk'ter-lōn'e

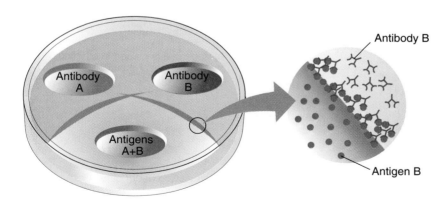

FIGURE 19.5

A Precipitation Test

Wells are cut into a plate of purified agar. Different known antibodies are then placed into the two upper wells, and a mixture of unknown antigens is placed into the lower well. During incubation, the reactants diffuse outward from the wells, and cloudy lines of precipitate form where the reactants happen to meet. The lines cross each other because each antigen has reacted only with its complementary antibody.

im'mu-no-e-lek'tro-fo-re'sis

In the procedure known as **immunoelectrophoresis**, the techniques of gel electrophoresis and diffusion are combined for the detection of antigens. A mixture of antigens is placed in a reservoir on an agarose slide, and an electrical field is applied to the ends of the slide. The different antigens then move through the agarose at different rates of speed, depending on their electrical charges. This process is **gel electrophoresis** (FIGURE 19.6). A trough is then cut into the agarose along the

FIGURE 19.6

The Technique of Gel Electrophoresis Applied to DNA

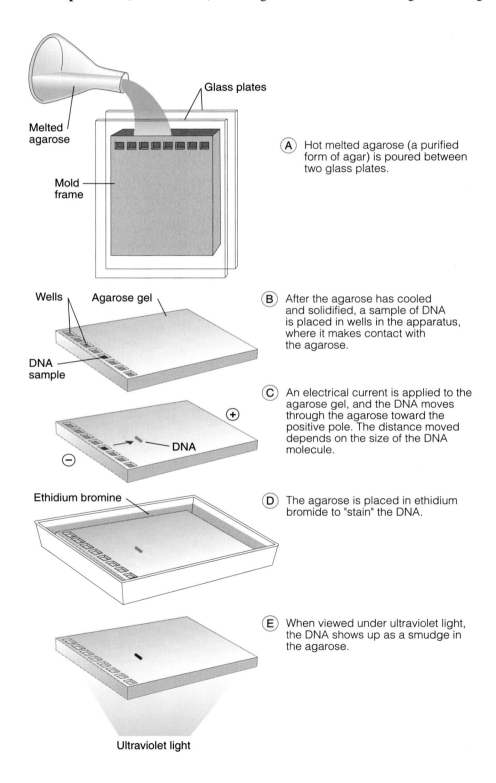

Glass plates

A Hot melted agarose (a purified form of agar) is poured between two glass plates.

Melted agarose

Mold frame

Wells   Agarose gel

B After the agarose has cooled and solidified, a sample of DNA is placed in wells in the apparatus, where it makes contact with the agarose.

DNA sample

C An electrical current is applied to the agarose gel, and the DNA moves through the agarose toward the positive pole. The distance moved depends on the size of the DNA molecule.

(+)

(−)

DNA

Ethidium bromine

D The agarose is placed in ethidium bromide to "stain" the DNA.

E When viewed under ultraviolet light, the DNA shows up as a smudge in the agarose.

Ultraviolet light

same axis, and a known antibody solution is added. During incubation, antigens and antibodies diffuse toward each other and precipitation lines form, as in the Ouchterlony technique.

AGGLUTINATION

Agglutination is a serological reaction in which antibodies interact with antigens on the surface of particular objects and cause the objects to clump together, or agglutinate. Agglutination techniques were among the earliest serological reactions adapted to the diagnostic laboratory. For example, until the 1960s, the diagnosis of typhoid fever was based on the agglutination of *Salmonella* cells by antibodies in the patient's serum. This test, called the **Widal test** after its developer Georges Fernand I. Widal, is now supplemented by more sophisticated procedures performed in plastic microtiter plates.

> Agglutination: an antigen–antibody interaction accompanied by clumping.

> ve-dahl'

Agglutination procedures are performed on slides or in tubes. For example, emulsions of unknown bacteria are added to drops of known antibodies on a slide, and the mixture is observed for clumping. If none occurs, different antibodies are tried until the correct one is found (**FIGURE 19.7**). This process is essentially a trial-and-error method, although the chances for success may be enhanced by using a **polyvalent serum**, that is, one containing a mixture of antibodies. Tube agglutinations may be performed with serum to determine the titer of antibodies present.

> Polyvalent serum: serum that contains a mixture of antibodies.

Passive agglutination is a modern approach to traditional agglutination methods. Antigens are adsorbed onto the surface of latex spheres, polystyrene particles, red blood cells, bacteria, or other carriers. Serum antibodies are then detected by observing agglutination of the carrier particle. **Hemagglutination** refers to the agglutination of red blood cells. This process is particularly important in the determination of blood types prior to blood transfusion (Chapter 20). In addition, certain viruses,

> hem'ah-gloo'tĭ-na'shun

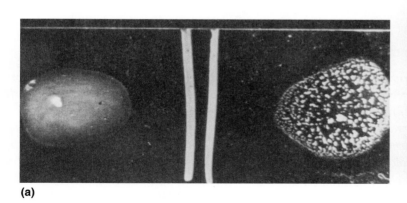

(a)

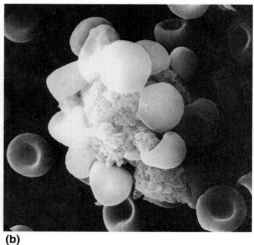

(b)

FIGURE 19.7

Two Views of Agglutination

(a) A slide agglutination procedure. *Salmonella* cells were mixed with *Salmonella* antibodies on the right side of the slide and with antibody-free saline solution on the left side. Clumps of cells are visible on the right side. (b) A scanning electron micrograph of human red blood cells agglutinated by a microcolony of *Mycoplasma pneumoniae*, the cause of primary atypical pneumonia.

such as measles and mumps viruses, agglutinate red blood cells. Antibodies for these viruses may be detected by a procedure in which the serum is first combined with laboratory-cultivated viruses and then added to the red blood cells. If serum antibodies neutralize the viruses, agglutination fails to occur. This test, called the **hemagglutination inhibition (HAI) test**, is discussed in Chapter 11.

A hemagglutination test called the **Coombs test** is used to detect **rh antibodies** involved in hemolytic disease of the newborn (discussed in Chapter 20). These rh antibodies will react with red blood cells (RBCs) bearing the corresponding Rh antigens. In the Coombs test, RBCs having the Rh antigen are combined with the patient's serum, which may or may not have rh antibodies. After a short incubation period, a sample of **antiglobulin antibodies** are added. These antibodies react with rh antibodies. If the rh antibodies were present in the serum, they have now gathered on the RBC surface, and when the antiglobulin antibodies are added, the RBCs will form a clump, yielding a positive test. However, if there were no rh antibodies in the serum, no gathering on the RBC surface took place, and when the antiglobulin antibodies are added, no clumping of the RBCs will take place. The absence of clumping indicates a negative test—the patient does not have rh antibodies in the serum.

FLOCCULATION

flok'u-la'shun

The **flocculation** test combines the principles of precipitation and agglutination. The antigen exists in a noncellular particulate form that reacts with antibodies to yield large, visible aggregates.

Cardiolipin:
an alcoholic extract of beef heart used in the flocculation test for syphilis.

VDRL test:
a flocculation test used for the rapid identification of syphilis antibodies.

An example of the flocculation test is the Venereal Disease Research Laboratory (VDRL) test used for the rapid screening of patients to detect **syphilis**. The antigen consists of an alcoholic extract of beef heart called cardiolipin. When diluted with buffer solution, the cardiolipin forms a milky-white precipitate. Serum from a patient is then added. If the serum contains syphilis antibodies, the particles of precipitate react with antibodies and cling together, yielding aggregates. Observation under the low-power objective of the microscope reveals the extent of aggregate formation and gives a clue to the amount of antibodies present. The **VDRL test** has been in use for many decades and is part of the "blood test" that couples may be required to take before obtaining a marriage license.

To this point . . .

We have surveyed a number of serological reactions used in the diagnostic laboratory to detect interactions between antigens and antibodies. In each case, the reaction is fairly simple and straightforward, and the laboratory technician can usually determine whether an interaction has occurred. For example, particles clump in agglutination, and precipitates form in precipitation. Many of the basic reactions have been adapted by modern technologists to improve on the fundamental theme of the process.

In the final section of this chapter, we shall explore another series of serological reactions and tests. Most of the tests involve a multistep procedure, and the visible manifestation of the reaction usually requires the participation of accessory factors, indicator systems, and specialized equipment. These diagnostic tests are more complicated to perform and require skilled technicians, but their development has ensured the position of laboratory immunology as a key link in the health-care delivery system.

Other Serological Reactions

Among the other serological reactions are a set of sophisticated procedures that detect antibodies in novel ways, including the use of radioactivity and gene probes. We begin the section, however, with a standard procedure used since the beginning of the 1900s.

COMPLEMENT FIXATION

The **complement fixation test** was devised by Jules Bordet and Octave Gengou in 1901. It was later adapted for syphilis by August von Wassermann in 1906, and for many decades it remained a mainstay for syphilis diagnosis. Technologists now use it for detecting antibodies for a variety of viruses, fungi, and bacteria.

The test is performed in two parts. The first part, the **test system**, utilizes the patient's serum, a preparation of antigen from the suspected pathogen, and complement derived from guinea pigs. The second part, the indicator system, requires sheep red blood cells and a preparation called hemolysin (antibodies against sheep red cells). Hemolysins cause lysis of red blood cells only in the presence of complement.

The first step in the test is to heat the patient's serum to destroy any complement present in the serum. Next, carefully measured amounts of antigen and guinea pig complement are added to the serum (FIGURE 19.8). This test system is then incubated at 37°C for 90 minutes. If antibodies specific for the antigen are present in the serum, an antibody–antigen interaction takes place, and the complement is used up, or "fixed." However, there is no visible sign of whether a reaction has occurred.

Now the **indicator system** (sheep red blood cells and hemolysin) is added to the tube, and the tube is reincubated. If the complement was previously fixed, none will be available to the hemolysin, and lysis of the sheep red blood cells cannot take place. The blood cells would therefore remain intact, and when the tube is centrifuged, the technician observes clear fluid with a "button" of blood cells at the bottom. Conclusion: The serum contained antibodies that reacted with the antigen and fixed the complement.

If the complement was not fixed in the test system, it will still be available to the hemolysin, and the hemolysin-complement mixture will lyse the sheep red blood cells. When the tube is centrifuged, the technician sees red fluid, colored by the hemoglobin of the broken blood cells, and no evidence of blood cells at the bottom of the tube. Conclusion: The serum lacked antibodies for the antigen tested.

The complement fixation test is valuable because it may be adapted by varying the antigen. In this way, tests may be conducted for such diverse diseases as encephalitis, Rocky Mountain spotted fever, meningococcal meningitis, and histoplasmosis. The versatility of the test, together with its sensitivity and relative accuracy, have secured its continuing role in diagnostic medicine.

FLUORESCENT ANTIBODY TECHNIQUES

The **fluorescent antibody technique** is a slide test performed by combining particles containing antigens with antibodies and a fluorescent dye (Chapter 3). When the three components react, the dye causes the complex to glow on illumination with

bor-dā′
shan-jou′

he-mol′ĭ-sin
Hemolysin:
antibodies that will lyse sheep red blood cells in the presence of complement.

Hemoglobin:
the red oxygen-carrying pigment in erythrocytes.

FIGURE 19.8

The Complement Fixation Test

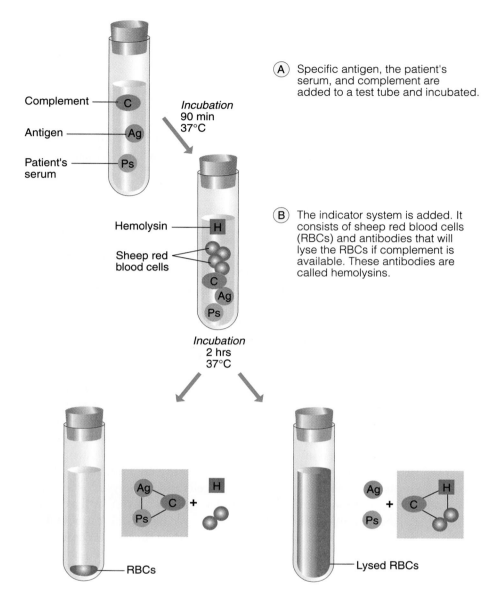

A Specific antigen, the patient's serum, and complement are added to a test tube and incubated.

Complement — C
Antigen — Ag
Patient's serum — Ps

Incubation 90 min 37°C

B The indicator system is added. It consists of sheep red blood cells (RBCs) and antibodies that will lyse the RBCs if complement is available. These antibodies are called hemolysins.

Hemolysin — H
Sheep red blood cells

Incubation 2 hrs 37°C

RBCs

C If specific antibodies are present in the serum, a reaction will take place between the antibodies, antigen, and complement. Because the complement has been used up, no lysis of the sheep RBCs will occur when the indicator system is added.

Lysed RBCs

D If specific antibodies are not present in the serum, no reaction occurs during the first incubation, and the complement is left free to unite with the sheep RBCs and hemolysins. Lysis of the red blood cells results.

Fluorescence microscope: a microscope that uses ultraviolet light to illuminate dye-coated particles.

ultraviolet light under a fluorescence microscope, as shown in FIGURE 19.9. Two commonly used dyes are fluorescein, which emits an apple-green glow, and rhodamine, which gives off orange-red light.

Fluorescent antibody techniques may be direct or indirect. In the **direct method,** the fluorescent dye is linked to known antibody molecules. The antibodies are then combined with particles that may contain complementary antigens, such as bacteria. If the presumption is correct, the tagged antibodies accumulate on the particle surface, and the particle glows under the microscope. In this way, an unknown antigen or unknown organism can be identified.

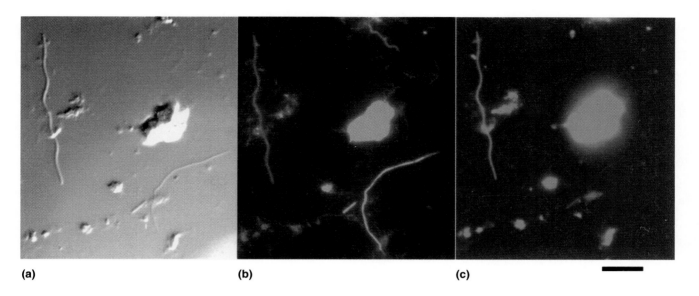

(a)   (b)   (c)

FIGURE 19.9

Fluorescent Antibody Staining

Three views of spirochetes in the hindgut of a termite. (a) An unstained area displayed by differential interference contrast microscopy. (b) The same viewing area seen by fluorescence microscopy using rhodamine B as a stain. (c) The same area viewed after staining with fluorescein. (Bar = 10 μm.)

The **indirect method** is illustrated by the FTA-ABS diagnostic procedure used for detecting **syphilis** antibodies in the blood of a patient (FIGURE 19.10). A sample of commercially available syphilis spirochetes is placed on a slide, and the slide is then flooded with the patient's serum. Next, a sample of fluorescein-labeled **antiglobulin antibodies** is added. These are antibodies that unite with human antibodies. They are produced by an animal injected with human antibodies. The slide is then observed under the fluorescence microscope.

The test is interpreted as follows. If the patient's serum contains syphilis antibodies, the antibodies bind to the surfaces of spirochetes, and the labeled antiglobulin antibodies are attracted to them. The spirochetes then glow from the dye. However, if no antibodies are present in the serum, nothing accumulates on the spirochete's surface, and labeled antiglobulin antibodies also fail to gather on the surface. The labeled antibodies remain in the fluid, and the spirochetes do not glow.

Fluorescent antibody techniques are adaptable to a broad variety of antigens and antibodies and are widely used in serology. Antigens may be detected in bacterial smears, cell smears, and viruses fixed to carrier particles. The value of the techniques is enhanced because the materials are sold in kits and are readily available to small laboratories.

RADIOIMMUNOASSAY (RIA)

Radioimmunoassay (RIA) is an extremely sensitive serological procedure used to measure the concentration of low-molecular-weight antigens, such as haptens. Since its development in the 1960s, the technique has been adapted for quantitating hepatitis antigens, as well as reproductive hormones, insulin, and certain drugs.

FTA-ABS:
fluorescent treponemal antibody absorption test; a diagnostic procedure for syphilis.

Antiglobulin antibodies:
antibodies that react with human antibodies in diagnostic tests; produced in animals after injection with human antibodies.

Radioimmunoassay:
a sensitive serological procedure in which radioactive antigens compete with nonlabeled antigens for reactive sites on antibody molecules.

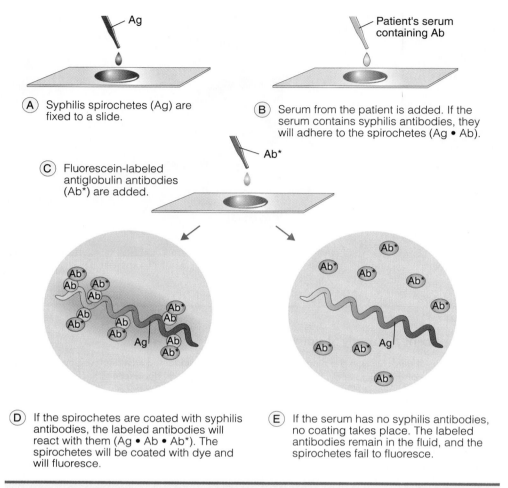

A Syphilis spirochetes (Ag) are fixed to a slide.

B Serum from the patient is added. If the serum contains syphilis antibodies, they will adhere to the spirochetes (Ag • Ab).

C Fluorescein-labeled antiglobulin antibodies (Ab*) are added.

D If the spirochetes are coated with syphilis antibodies, the labeled antibodies will react with them (Ag • Ab • Ab*). The spirochetes will be coated with dye and will fluoresce.

E If the serum has no syphilis antibodies, no coating takes place. The labeled antibodies remain in the fluid, and the spirochetes fail to fluoresce.

FIGURE 19.10

The Indirect Fluorescent Antibody Technique for Diagnosing Syphilis

One of its major advantages is that it can detect trillionths of a gram of a substance (**MicroFocus 19.6**).

The RIA procedure is based on the competition between radioactive-labeled antigens and unlabeled antigens for the reactive sites on antibody molecules. A known amount of the radioactive (labeled) antigens is mixed with a known amount of specific antibodies, and an unknown amount of unlabeled antigens. The antigen–antibody complexes that form during incubation are then separated out, and their radioactivity is determined. By measuring the radioactivity of free antigens remaining in the leftover fluid, one can calculate the percentage of labeled antigen bound to the antibody. This percentage is equivalent to the percentage of unlabeled antigen bound to the antibody because the same proportion of both antigens will find spots on antibody molecules. The concentration of unknown unlabeled antigen can then be determined by reference to a standard curve.

Radioimmunoassay procedures require substantial investment in sophisticated equipment and carry a certain amount of risk because radioactive isotopes are used. For these reasons, the procedure is not widely used in routine serological laboratories. However, immunologists with access to radioimmunoassay have discovered a wealth of information.

MicroFocus 19.6

SOMETHING SPECIAL FROM A SPECIAL SOMEONE

When the Nobel Prize in Physiology or Medicine was announced on October 14, 1977, the scientific community applauded a special person and a special technique. One of the recipients was Rosalyn Sussman Yalow, a developer of the radioimmunoassay (RIA) technique. This technique is one of the most highly regarded immunological procedures.

RIA has made possible the detection of incredibly small amounts of chemical substances in body fluids. One offshoot was the discovery of certain hormones not previously known to exist in the body. Another was the revelation that individuals receiving insulin injections produce antibodies against insulin. This finding put in serious doubt the contention that the insulin molecules were too small to be antigenic.

Radioimmunoassay also allows the detection of tumor viruses in the body before the appearance of a tumor. Moreover, it may be utilized to screen for hepatitis B viruses in blood used for transfusions. RIA is said to be sensitive enough to detect trillionths of a gram of a substance. This is equivalent to detecting a lump of sugar in Lake Erie.

Like the process she developed, Rosalyn Yalow is also special. She was educated during a time when opportunities for women were limited, and her work was done in restricted surroundings at the Veterans Hospital in the Bronx, New York. She was the sixth woman honored by the Nobel Committee and only the second in Physiology or Medicine. (She is also a product of the same New York City neighborhood as a certain textbook author.) Rosalyn Yalow remains one of the eminent immunologists of our time.

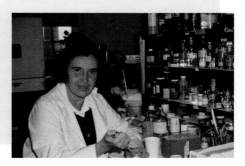

THE RADIOALLERGOSORBENT TEST (RAST)

The **radioallergosorbent test (RAST)** is an extension of the radioimmunoassay. Another sophisticated procedure, it may be used to detect IgE, other antibodies, or a variety of small antigens.

To detect **IgE** against penicillin, penicillin antigens are attached to a suitable particle. Serum that may contain penicillin IgE is then added. If the antibody is present, it will combine with the penicillin antigens on the surface of the particle. Now another antibody, one that will react with human antibodies, is added. This antiglobulin antibody carries a radioactive label. The entire complex will therefore become radioactive if the antiglobulin antibody combines with the IgE, as FIGURE 19.11 illustrates. By contrast, if no IgE was present in the serum, no reaction with the antigen on the particle surface will take place, and the radioactive antibody will not be attracted to the particle. When tested, the particles will not show radioactivity.

The RAST is commonly known as a **"sandwich" technique**. There is no competition for an active site as in RIA, and the type of unknown antibody, as well as its amount, may be learned by determining the amount of radioactivity deposited.

THE ENZYME-LINKED IMMUNOSORBENT ASSAY (ELISA)

The **enzyme-linked immunosorbent assay (ELISA)** has virtually the same sensitivity as radioimmunoassay and the RAST, but does not require expensive equipment or radioactivity. The procedure involves attaching antibodies or antigens to a solid surface and combining (immunosorbing) the coated surfaces with the test material. An enzyme system is then linked to the complex, the remaining enzyme is washed away, and the extent of enzyme activity is measured. This gives an indication that antigens or antibodies are present in the test material.

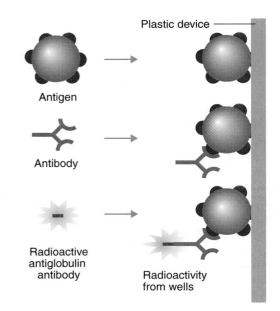

(A) The antigen to the suspected antibody is bound to a plastic device, such as a plastic plate with wells.

(B) The test solution, such as urine, is added to the device. The antibody may or may not be present in the solution.

(C) An antibody that reacts with a human antibody (an antiglobulin antibody) is added. The antiglobulin antibody carries a radioactive label. If radioactivity is detected in the wells, the technician concludes that the solution contained the suspected antibody.

Antigen

Antibody

Radioactive antiglobulin antibody

Plastic device

Radioactivity from wells

FIGURE 19.11

The Radioallergosorbent Test (RAST)

This technique provides an effective way of detecting very tiny amounts of antibody in a preparation. A known antigen is used. The objective is to determine whether the complementary antibody is present.

An application of the ELISA is found in the highly efficient laboratory test used to detect antibodies against the **human immunodeficiency virus (HIV)** (FIGURE 19.12). A serum sample is obtained from the patient and mixed with a solution of plastic or polystyrene beads coated with antigens from HIV. Antibodies present in the serum will adhere to the antigens on the surface of the beads. The beads are then washed and incubated with antiglobulin antibodies chemically tagged with molecules of the enzyme horseradish peroxidase. The preparation is washed, and a solution of substrate molecules for the peroxidase enzyme is added. Initially the solution is clear, but if enzyme molecules react with the substrate, the solution will become yellow-orange in color. The enzyme molecules will be present only if HIV antibodies are present in the serum. If no HIV antibodies are in the serum, no enzyme molecules could concentrate on the bead surface, no change in the substrate molecules could occur, and no color change would be observed.

ELISA procedures may be varied depending on whether one wishes to detect antigens or antibodies. The solid phase may consist of beads, paper disks, or other suitable supporting mechanisms, and alternate enzyme systems such as the alkaline phosphatase system may be used. In addition, the results of the test may be quantified by noting the degree of enzyme-substrate reactions as a measure of the amount of antigen or antibody in the test sample. The availability of inexpensive ELISA kits has brought the procedure into the doctor's office and routine serological laboratory, and broad applications of the test are expected in the future.

MONOCLONAL ANTIBODIES

Myeloma:
a mass of cells reproducing at an uncontrolled rate.

An antibody-secreting cell, like any other cell, can become cancerous. Unchecked, the cell proliferates to become a mass of cells called a **myeloma**. Because a myeloma

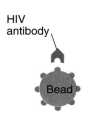
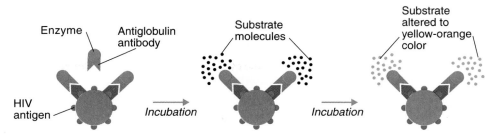

(A) Plastic beads coated with HIV antigens are combined with a serum sample from the patient. If the serum contains HIV antibodies, they combine with antigens on the bead surface.

(B) The beads are incubated with antiglobulin antibodies linked to the enzyme horseradish peroxidase. The antibodies combine with antibodies on the bead surface, and the enzyme accumulates.

(C) A substrate for the enzyme is added, and again the mixture is incubated.

(D) In a positive test, a yellow-orange color develops in the mixture as the enzyme changes the substrate to a colored compound. In a negative test, no color develops, implying that no antibodies were present on the bead surface at the beginning.

FIGURE 19.12

The ELISA, a Test for HIV Antibodies

The enzyme linked immunosorbent assay (ELISA) as it is used in the HIV antibody test to detect HIV antibodies.

begins as a single cell, all of its progeny constitute a clone with identical genetic characteristics. The remarkable feature of this clone is that the cells produce only a single type of antibody. Thus, the serum of an animal with a myeloma contains substantial amounts of one antibody, and a tissue culture of a myeloma produces only one antibody.

In 1975, **Georges J. F. Köhler** of West Germany and **Cesar Milstein** of Argentina developed a method for the laboratory production of antibodies from a single clone of myeloma cells. Antibodies from this clone were named **monoclonal antibodies**. Their method, now in widespread use, begins with the injection of antigens into mice, followed by the extraction of plasma cells from the spleen of the mice (FIGURE 19.13). The plasma cells are then fused with unstimulated myeloma cells from another mouse to form a clone of hybrid cells. This fusion results in a **hybridoma** (a hybrid myeloma). The hybridoma is immortal, and it is programmed to produce a single antibody for the original antigen. The plasma cells supply the program for the antibody, the myeloma cells provide the immortality. In 1984, Köhler and Milstein shared the Nobel Prize in Physiology or Medicine for the development of the monoclonal antibody technique.

Monoclonal antibodies and the hybridoma technique have been hailed as one of our era's most important methodological advances in biomedicine. The antibodies differ from ordinary antibodies because they are far more pure and uniform, and exquisitely sensitized to probe for their antigenic targets. Monoclonal antibodies, for example, have been used to pinpoint the antigens on the surfaces of parasites, thereby enabling researchers to zero in on these antigens for vaccine production. In this regard, they are excellent research tools.

Monoclonal antibodies may also hold the key to the treatment of tumors. Scientists have developed a technique in which tumor cells are removed from a patient and injected into a mouse, whereupon the mouse's spleen begins producing tumor

ko'ler

hi'brĭ-do'mah
Hybridoma:
a clone of cells produced by the union of antibody-producing cells with myeloma cells.

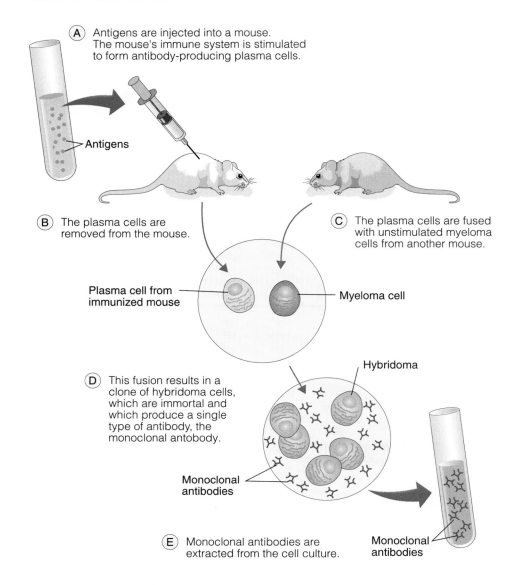

A) Antigens are injected into a mouse. The mouse's immune system is stimulated to form antibody-producing plasma cells.

Antigens

B) The plasma cells are removed from the mouse.

C) The plasma cells are fused with unstimulated myeloma cells from another mouse.

Plasma cell from immunized mouse

Myeloma cell

Hybridoma

D) This fusion results in a clone of hybridoma cells, which are immortal and which produce a single type of antibody, the monoclonal antobody.

Monoclonal antibodies

E) Monoclonal antibodies are extracted from the cell culture.

Monoclonal antibodies

FIGURE 19.13

The Production of Monoclonal Antibodies

antibodies. Spleen cells are then fused with myeloma cells to produce a hybridoma that produces antibodies for that specific tumor. When the antibodies are injected back into the patient, they react specifically with the tumor cells without destroying other tissue cells. The day is at hand when monoclonal antibodies are used to carry drugs to the tumor and destroy its cells.

Monoclonal antibodies are reproducible because of how they are manufactured; therefore, laboratories throughout the world can use identical antibodies. This allows comparisons of tests and research results that were previously impossible to obtain. Monoclonal antibodies are also used for cleansing bone marrow prior to transplantation, in treating disorders of the immune system, and for an assortment of basic studies and practical approaches to medicine. They represent one of the most elegant expressions of modern biotechnology.

GENE PROBES

Althouogh antibody tests are a valuable resource in the clinical laboratory, a new series of diagnostic tests permit the identification of an organism (MicroFocus 19.7) and its antigens. These tests are based on the use of a DNA fragment called the gene probe and a procedure known as the polymerase chain reaction (PCR). A **gene probe** is a relatively small, single-stranded DNA segment that can hunt for a complementary fragment of DNA within a morass of cellular material, much like a right hand searching for a left hand. When the probe locates its complementary fragment, it emits a signal such as a pulse of radioactivity. If the complementary fragment cannot be found, then no signal is sent. The procedure is remarkable for its accuracy. For example, if we were to line up the 46 human chromosomes as a two-lane highway, the highway would stretch around planet Earth 300 times. A gene probe can locate and unite with a few-mile stretch of this highway.

Gene probe:
a small DNA fragment having a single strand and uniting with its complementary DNA fragment.

MicroFocus 19.7

CAUGHT IN THE SPOTLIGHT

Current diagnostic tests for tuberculosis can take several weeks to complete because the tubercle bacillus *Mycobacterium tuberculosis* multiplies very slowly, a binary fission taking place every 24 hours or so. While waiting for a definitive diagnosis, physicians must make treatment decisions based on very limited information. It is therefore possible that ineffective drugs may be prescribed during this interval, and that the patient's illness will worsen; also, the patient may transmit the disease to others as the wait goes on.

With help from the firefly, researchers have developed an innovative and imaginative diagnostic test for tuberculosis that could shorten the time interval for detection considerably. Only a few days may be required, and the test could help determine whether that particular strain of *M. tuberculosis* is drug-resistant. The new approach relies on the firefly enzyme luciferase to produce a flash of light in living *M. tuberculosis*. The process works this way: A bacteriophage (a bacterial virus) specific for *M. tuber-*

culosis is genetically engineered to carry the gene for luciferase. A sample of phage is then mixed with a culture of bacteria. If the culture contains *M. tuberculosis*, the phage penetrates the bacterium and inserts itself into the bacterial chromosome, carrying the luciferase gene along. The bacterium promptly begins producing luciferase. Now luciferin, a compound attacked by luciferase, is added to the culture together with the high-energy molecule ATP (Chapter 5). If luciferase is present,

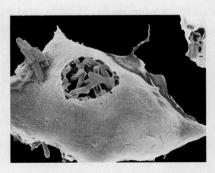

■ *A macrophage (yellow) phagocytizing Mycobacterium tuberculosis (green).*

the enzyme breaks down luciferin, and the reaction results in a flash of light. A sensitive instrument detects the light flash, and the culture is confirmed to contain *M. tuberculosis*. The report is made to the physician, and the diagnosis is complete.

To determine drug susceptibility or resistance, the same procedure is used, except a drug is added to the culture. If the bacteria are sensitive to the drug, they die and, quite literally, their "lights go out." If they are resistant, they continue to live, and they produce luciferase—and they give off light.

In the spring of 1993, scientists from New York's Albert Einstein College of Medicine and the University of Pittsburgh reported the test's development in *Science* magazine. As expected, headline writers from numerous publications had a field day as word of the successful test filtered through various journals and newspapers. The well-worn cliché is particularly appropriate in this instance—the future of tuberculosis diagnosis "appears bright."

Polymerase chain reaction: a biochemical procedure in which a small number of DNA molecules is amplified to a huge number.

To use a gene probe effectively, it is valuable to increase the amount of DNA to be searched. The **polymerase chain reaction (PCR)** accomplishes this task. The procedure takes a segment of DNA and reproduces it to a billion copies in a few short hours. Target DNA is mixed with polymerase (the enzyme that synthesizes DNA), short strands of primer DNA, and a mixture of nucleotides. The mixture is then alternately heated and cooled during which time the double-stranded DNA unravels, is duplicated, then reforms the double helix. The process is repeated over and over again in a highly automated PCR machine, which is the biochemist's equivalent of an office copier. Each cycle takes about 2 minutes, and each new DNA segment serves as a model for producing many additional copies, which in turn serve as models for producing more copies. Instead of looking for a needle in a haystack, the gene probe now has a huge number of needles.

One place where gene probes and PCR have been useful is in the detection of **human immunodeficiency virus (HIV)**. T-lymphocytes are obtained from the patient and disrupted to secure the cellular DNA. The DNA is then amplified by PCR and the gene probe is added. The probe is a segment of DNA that complements the DNA in the provirus synthesized from the genome of HIV (Chapter 13). If the person is infected with HIV, the probe will locate the proviral DNA, bind to it, and emit radioactivity. An accumulation of radioactivity thus constitutes a positive test. Because the test identifies viral DNA rather than viral antibodies, the physician can be more confident of the patient's health status.

A gene probe test is also available for detecting **human papilloma virus**, the virus that causes genital warts. The test utilizes a gene probe to detect viral DNA in a sample of tissue obtained from a woman's cervix. Because certain forms of human papilloma virus have been linked to cervical tumors, the test has won acceptance as an important preventive technique, and it has been licensed by the FDA. It is commercially available as the ViraPap test.

A similar technique can be used to conduct **water-quality tests** based on the detection of coliform bacteria such as *Escherichia coli* (Chapter 25). Traditionally, *E. coli* had to be cultivated in the laboratory and identified biochemically. With gene probe technology, a sample of water can be filtered, and the bacteria trapped on the filter can be broken open to release their DNA for PCR and gene probe analysis. Not only is the process time-saving (many days by the older method, but a few short hours by the newer method), it is also extremely sensitive: A single *E. coli* cell can be detected in a 100-ml sample of water. Moreover, the pathogens transmitted by water, rather than the "indicator" *E. coli*, can be detected by DNA analysis. Thus, the identification of *Salmonella*, *Shigella*, and *Vibrio* species will become more feasible in the future as gene probe analysis becomes more widely accepted.

Gene probe assays are widely available in kit forms for a variety of bacteria (e.g., streptococci, *Haemophilus*, *Listeria*, *Mycobacterium*, and *Neisseria*), as well as for fungi (e.g., *Blastomyces*, *Coccidioides*, and *Histoplasma*). In many cases, the tests are described as "exquisitely accurate," with a high degree of discrimination and reliability as strong as older identification methods. Since first introduced in the 1970s, gene probe tests have been met with periods of unbridled enthusiasm counterbalanced by periods of disappointment. The future value of gene probes will depend in part on the development of ways to minimize false-positive reactions due to contamination, on methods of increasing the sensitivity of tests, and on mechanisms for enhancing the signals from probes bound to their target molecules.

Ever consider that we are born too soon? Is 9 months in the womb enough? Or would 18 months be preferable?

Absurd you say? Why, then, is a baby born immunologically "unfinished"—that is, why is its immune system not fully functional until it is roughly 6 months old? And why is it so dependent on its parents that it probably could not lead an independent existence until it is 9 months old? Still not convinced? Then consider a newborn colt or a newly hatched chick. Each is able to walk about and gather food within hours of its birth. Certainly the colt and chick will survive better than a newborn human.

If we are willing to buy into the concept that we are born too soon, the next question is: Why does this happen? The answer, according to Stephen Jay Gould and other evolutionary biologists, is the size of our brain. In proportion to the remainder of our body, our brain is larger than any other animal's brain. To have this large brain, we must have a large head. After 9 months, our head can fit through the birth canal, but it could not fit if we stayed inside much longer. So it becomes a matter of give-and-take. Evolution has given us a large brain (and head), but it has also decreed that we must complete our development outside the comfortable confines of our mother. That development includes immunological development as well as physical development. It also increases our dependence on our parents, and perhaps that's not all so bad—it certainly helps us appreciate the ones who care for us. Thanks, guys.

Summary

Antibodies are the key element in the long-term resistance to infectious disease exhibited by the body. They are also important elements of diagnostic tests used to detect diseases. These two concepts are the major topics of this chapter.

Antibodies confer immunity to the body. If the body's immune system produces the antibodies, the immunity is said to be active. By contrast, if antibodies come from some source outside the body, then the immunity is passive. Both active and passive immunities may be natural or artificial. Natural immunity happens in the "natural" course of events, such as when a person becomes ill with disease (natural active immunity) or a fetus acquires antibodies from its mother (natural passive immunity). Artificial immunity occurs in an unnatural way, such as when a person receives an injection of vaccine (artificial active immunity) or an injection of antibodies (artificial passive immunity).

Laboratory reactions in which antibodies are the focus of attention are called serological reactions because serum is generally involved. A serological reaction may involve direct observation of an antigen–antibody interaction, such as in precipitation or agglutination reactions; or the reaction may involve indirect observation of an antigen–antibody interaction, such as in complement fixation or fluorescent antibody techniques. Several of the indirect reactions have become quite sophisticated and often use radioactive markers or complex enzyme reactions to denote whether a reaction has occurred. However, all share the property of detecting antibodies in the patient sample as a way of knowing whether a particular disease is present.

Questions for Thought and Discussion

1. It is estimated that when at least half the individuals in a given population have been immunized against a disease, the chances of an epidemic occurring are very slight. The population is said to exhibit "herd immunity," because members of the population (or herd) unknowingly transfer the immunizing agent to other members and eventually immunize the entire population. What are some ways by which the immunizing agent can be transferred?

2. The tendency of women in the present generation is to have children at an older age than in past generations. How might this present an immunological problem for the newborn?

3. A man is found murdered on the front seat of his automobile, and the police observe bloodstains on the floor. It is important to know whether this is the victim's blood, the murderer's blood, or the blood of the victim's dog, which was always with him. However, it could also be fish blood, since the man was an avid fisherman, or blood from the poorly wrapped chicken the man was bringing home from the supermarket. How might the medical examiner proceed?

4. In 1991, scientists first reported success in vaccinating women late in pregnancy to protect their newborns from *Haemophilus* meningitis. The researchers found that levels of meningitis antibodies in the newborns were far above those normally present. Would you favor this approach to protecting newborns? Why or why not?

5. When a child is born in Great Britain, he or she is assigned a doctor. Two weeks later, a social services worker visits the home, enrolls the child on a national computer registry for immunization, and explains immunization to the parents. When a child is due for an immunization, a notice is automatically sent to the home, and if the child is not brought to the doctor, the nurse goes to the home to learn why. Do you believe a method similar to this can work in the United States to achieve uniform national immunization?

6. For passive immunity, serum containing type G immunoglobulins is routinely used. Why do you suppose type M immunoglobulins are not used, especially since they are the important components of the primary antibody response? Do you believe that research in this direction would be fruitful?

7. Given a choice, which of the four general types of immunity would it be safest to obtain? Why? Ultimately, which would be the most helpful?

8. One of the hot research items of 1993 was that naked DNA molecules could conceivably be used to immunize an individual. The theory was that DNA from a virus could be made to penetrate to cells such as muscle cells, which would then display that virus' proteins on their surface. What do you suppose would happen next?

9. A complement fixation test is performed with serum from a patient with an active case of syphilis. In the process, however, the technician neglects to add the syphilis antigen to the tube. Would lysis of the sheep red blood cells occur at the test's conclusion? Why?

10. From 1980 to 1989, the incidence of pertussis increased in the United States, and the greatest incidence was found to be in adolescents and adults. Can you think of any reason why adolescents and adults should have been the targets of the bacillus, especially since these individuals were usually considered immune to the disease? Would you be in favor of using the new acellular pertussis vaccine to reimmunize these populations?

11. Suppose the titer of mumps antibodies from your blood was higher than that for your fellow student. What are some of the possible reasons that could have contributed to this? Try to be imaginative on this one.

12. Children between the ages of 5 and 15 are said to pass through the "golden age of resistance" because their resistance to disease is much higher than that of infants and adults. What factors may contribute to this resistance?

13. In 1985, a vaccine for meningococcal meningitis was licensed for use. The vaccine consists of capsular polysaccharides from four different strains of *Neisseria meningitidis*. What form of vaccine does this vaccine represent, and why is it safer to use than older vaccines made from whole meningococci?

14. The ability to keep the human body alive artificially, though brain dead, has stimulated the idea of keeping the organs functioning to produce vaccines for disease treatment. What arguments can be presented for and against this proposition?

15. In 1985, New York State dropped its requirement for a VDRL test prior to obtaining a marriage license. Why might you support this action? Can you think of any reasons to oppose it?

Review

On completing the section on immunity to disease, test your comprehension of the section's contents by filling in the following blanks with two terms that answer the description best. Appendix D contains the answers.

1. Two general forms of immunity:

   _____ and _____ .

2. Two types of natural immunity:

   _____ and _____ .

3. Two diseases that MMR is used against:

   _____ and _____ .

4. Two diseases that DPT is used against:

   _____ and _____ .

5. Two types of passive immunity:

   _____ and _____ .

6. Two adjuvants used in vaccines:

   _____ and _____ .

7. Two names for antibody-containing serum:

   _____ and _____ .

8. Two antibody types formed on antigen stimulation:

   _____ and _____ .

9. Two ways newborns have acquired maternal antibodies:

   _____ and _____ .

10. Two characteristics of serum sickness:

    _____ and _____ .

11. Two materials used in second-generation vaccines:

    _____ and _____ .

12. Two diseases for which synthetic vaccines are available:

    _____ and _____ .

13. Two factors that can determine innate immunity:

    _____ and _____ .

14. Two types of viruses in viral vaccines:

    _____ and _____ .

15. Two bacterial diseases for which toxoids are used:

    _____ and _____ .

16. Two methods for administering vaccines:

    _____ and _____ .

17. Two tracts in which IgA accumulates:

    _____ and _____ .

18. Two viral diseases where passive immunity is used:

    _____ and _____ .

19. Two functions of antibodies in antiserum:

    _____ and _____ .

20. Two bacterial diseases where passive immunity is used:

    _____ and _____ .

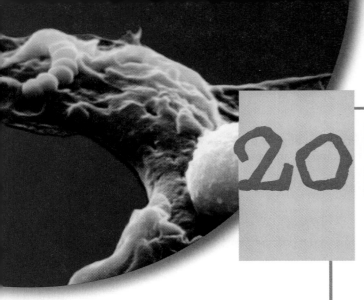

20 Immune Disorders

It is so overwhelming that it can leave virtually every body system in a state of collapse, and so ferocious that a patient can be dead in minutes despite the best medical treatment.

—Reporter Elizabeth Rosenthal describing anaphylactic shock in *Discover* magazine

DURING THE GOLDEN AGE of Microbiology, investigations were carried out on certain diseases that were not as dangerous as microbial diseases but were a source of great discomfort and inconvenience nevertheless. One such disease was **hay fever**. In the 1870s, British scientist Charles Harrison Blackley noted that crude pollen placed into the eyes of hay fever sufferers caused swelling of the membranes. Blackley also observed that pollen grains rubbed into a skin scratch produced a local reaction. Some of his critics suggested that the reaction was due to the mechanical injury inflicted by pollen grains, but in 1903, another British investigator, William Philipps Dunbar, supported Blackley's work by showing that saline extracts of pollen grains would cause the same reaction.

Research on hay fever has come a long way since the experiments of Blackley and Dunbar, and, as we shall see in this chapter, the disease is now regarded as a disorder of the immune system. About 35 million Americans currently suffer from hay fever, and thousands more are allergic to foods, cosmetics, leather, or metals. Many people cannot keep pets because of severe sensitivities, and between 2000 and 4000 Americans die of asthma annually. All told, an estimated 40 to 50 million people in the United States have some type of allergy.

The common denominator among these problems is a state of increased reactivity known as **hypersensitivity**. First reported in the early 1900s, hypersensitivity stems from activity of the immune system and involves both antibody-mediated and cell-mediated aspects of immunity. It represents a major topic of this chapter and is currently a subject of intense research in immunology.

Also included in the broad category of immune disorders are the autoimmune diseases and various immune deficiency diseases, as well as the principles of transplantation research and tumor immunology, as FIGURE 20.1 illustrates. We shall survey each of these in the sections that follow.

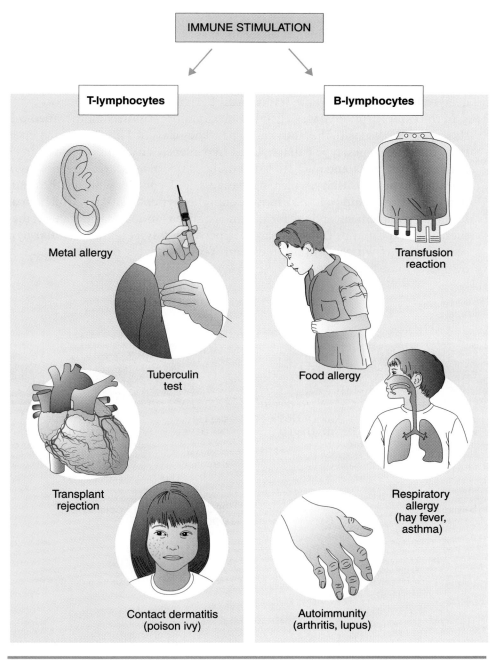

FIGURE 20.1

The Various Forms of Immune Disorders

Immune system disorders may be related to T–lymphocytes or B–lymphocytes. Stimulation of the immune system is the starting point for all these disorders.

Hypersensitivity

Hypersensitivity:
a state of increased sensitivity to
an antigen, arising from a previous exposure to that antigen.

ypersensitivity is a multistep phenomenon triggered by exposure to an antigen and consisting of a dormant (latent) stage, during which an individual becomes sensitized, and a reaction following a subsequent exposure to the antigen. The process may involve elements of antibody-mediated immunity or cell-mediated immunity, or sometimes both. The antibody response to the second dose of antigens often occurs within minutes, whereas the cell-mediated response develops over 2 to 3 days. For this reason, the terms **immediate hypersensitivity** and **delayed hypersensitivity** have traditionally been used to differentiate two types.

In the early 1970s, P. G. H. Gell and R. A. Coombs proposed another method for classifying hypersensitivities into four types. They classified immediate hypersensitivity into three types: **type I anaphylactic hypersensitivity**, a process involving IgE, mast cells, basophils, and mediators that induce smooth muscle contraction; **type II cytotoxic hypersensitivity**, which involves IgG, IgM, complement, and the destruction of host cells; and **type III immune complex hypersensitivity**, which involves IgG, IgM, complement, and the formation of antigen–antibody aggregates in the tissues. Gell and Coombs defined delayed hypersensitivity as **type IV cellular hypersensitivity**, in which lymphokines and T-lymphocytes function. TABLE 20.1 compares these four types.

TABLE 20.1

The Gell and Coombs Classification of Hypersensitivity Reactions

HYPERSENSITIVITY TYPE	ORIGIN OF HYPERSENSITIVITY	ANTIBODY INVOLVED	CELLS INVOLVED	MEDIATORS INVOLVED
Type I Anaphylactic	B-lymphocytes	IgE	Mast cells Basophils	Histamine Serotonin Leukotrienes Prostaglandins
Type II Cytotoxic	B-lymphocytes	IgG IgM	RBC WBC Platelets	Complement
Type III Immune complex	B-lymphocytes	IgG IgM	Host tissue cells	Complement
Type IV Cellular	T-lymphocytes	None	Host tissue cells	Lymphokines

TYPE I ANAPHYLACTIC HYPERSENSITIVITY

Anaphylactic hypersensitivity can be life-threatening. It is accompanied by **anaphylaxis**, a series of events in which chemical substances induce vigorous contractions of the body's smooth muscles. The term is derived from Latin stems that mean "against-protection," a reference to the dangerous nature of the condition.

Type I anaphylactic hypersensitivity begins with the entry of an antigenic substance into the body. This antigen, referred to as an **allergen**, may be any of a wide variety of materials such as bee venom, serum proteins, or a drug, such as penicillin. In the case of penicillin, the drug molecule itself is the allergen, but the molecule does not stimulate the immune system until after it has combined with tissue proteins to form an allergenic complex. Doses of antigen as low as 0.001 mg have been known to sensitize a person. Allergists refer to this first dose of antigen as the **sensitizing dose**.

The immune system responds to the allergen, and B-lymphocytes revert to plasma cells, which produce IgE (**MicroFocus 20.1**). This antibody, formerly known as reagin, enters the circulation and fixes itself to the surface of mast cells and basophils. **Mast cells** are connective tissue cells numerous in the respiratory and gastrointestinal tracts and near the blood vessels. They measure about 10 μm to 15 μm in diameter and are filled with 500 to 1500 granules containing histamine and other physiologically active substances. **Basophils** are circulating leukocytes, also rich in granules. They represent about 1 percent of the total leukocyte count in the circulation and measure about 15 μm in diameter. Mast cells and basophils each have over 100,000 receptor sites where IgE antibodies can attach.

an'ah-fĭ-lak'sis

Allergen:
an antigenic substance that induces an allergic reaction.

IgE:
a monomeric antibody produced by stimulated plasma cells.

ba'so-fĭl
Basophils:
granulated, circulating white blood cells that participate in anaphylactic reactions.

TRANSFER OF SENSITIVITY	EVIDENCE OF HYPERSENSITIVITY	SKIN REACTION	EXAMPLES
By serum	30 minutes or less	Urticaria	Anaphylaxis Atopic disease
By serum	Hours to days	Usually none	Transfusion reactions Hemolytic disease of newborns Thrombocytopenia Agranulocytosis Goodpasture syndrome
By serum	Hours to days	Usually none	Serum sickness Arthus phenomenon SLE Rheumatic fever LCM Organ rejection
By lymphoid cells	Days	Induration Tissue death	Contact dermatitis Infection allergy Skin graft rejection

MicroFocus 20.1

ITCHES AND ANTIBODIES

In the early 1960s, scientists knew that pollen and other allergens cause mast cells and basophils to release histamine. What they did not know was how allergens induced the cells to spill their contents. The immune system appeared to be involved, but researchers were ignorant of the nature or function of the immune mechanism.

At a hospital in Denver, Colorado, two Japanese doctors, Teruko Ishizaka and her husband, Kimishige, set out to find an antibody that would stimulate the allergic reaction. Neither scientist had any observable allergies, so they decided to use themselves as guinea pigs. When they injected an extract of ragweed pollen under their skin, no reaction took place. But if they first injected serum from an allergy patient and followed it with an injection of pollen extract, a raised itchy welt appeared. It was apparent that something in the patient's serum was responsible for the allergy.

The Ishizakas went to the next step. They separated the serum into as many different components as possible and repeated the skin test with each component. When a particular component caused welts, they purified it further and reinjected themselves. After four years of experiments (and lots of itching), they finally isolated their elusive substance. The substance was an antibody. The Ishizakas named it immunoglobulin E (or IgE) because the antibody was directed against antigen E of ragweed pollen. Then they breathed a sigh of relief that the investigation was over.

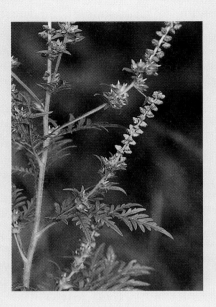

As IgE accumulates on mast cells and basophils, the individual becomes sensitized, as FIGURE 20.2 illustrates.

Sensitization usually requires a minimum of one week, during which time millions of molecules of IgE attach to thousands of mast cells and basophils. The attachment occurs at the Fc end of the antibody, leaving the Fab ends pointing outward from the cell. Multiple stimuli by allergen molecules may be required to sensitize a person fully. This is why penicillin often must be taken several times before a penicillin allergy manifests itself.

The symptoms of anaphylaxis occur rapidly on subsequent exposure to the allergen. Allergen molecules unite with IgE on the surfaces of sensitized mast cells and basophils and appear to form a bridge between adjoining combining sites, as shown in FIGURE 20.3. This union causes inhibition of the enzyme **adenyl cyclase**, which leads to a reduction of cyclic adenosine monophosphate (cAMP). As this takes place, the cells swell and the 500 to 1500 granules move to the cell surface, where they are released. An understanding of this biochemistry is important because anaphylaxis inhibitors (e.g., epinephrine) increase the activity of adenyl cyclase. This leads to an increase in cAMP, and the cAMP inhibits the further release of granules.

As granules flow into the extracellular fluid, they emit a number of mediator substances having substantial pharmacologic activity. The most important preformed mediator of allergic reactions is **histamine**, a derivative of the amino acid histidine. It is released within minutes of the cross-linking between IgE and its corresponding antigen. Once in the bloodstream, histamine circulates to the body cells and attaches to histamine receptors called **H-1 receptors**, present on most body cells. The principal effect will be on smooth muscle cells, as we shall see presently. **Heparin, serotonin, bradykinin**, and **tryptase** are other preformed mediators.

Adenyl cyclase:
an enzyme that digests adenosine triphosphate to adenosine monophosphate and phosphate ions.

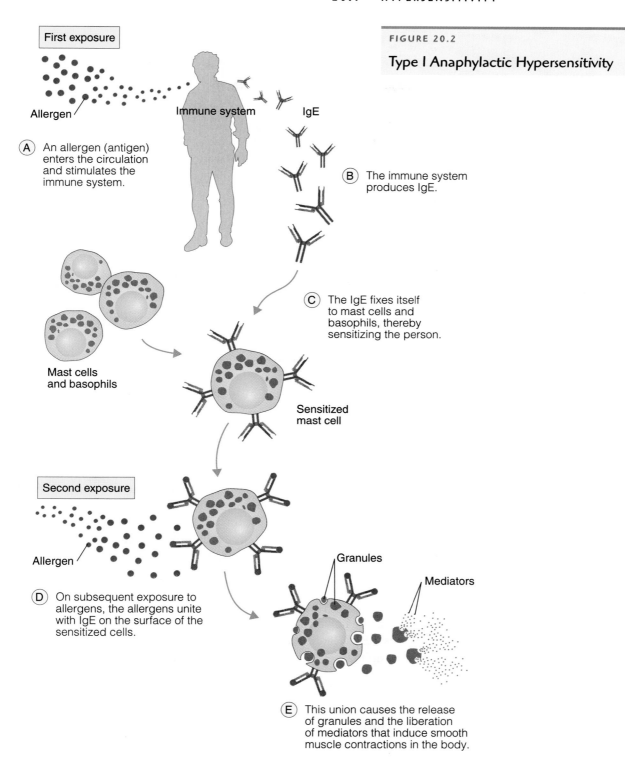

FIGURE 20.2

Type I Anaphylactic Hypersensitivity

First exposure

Allergen

Immune system

IgE

(A) An allergen (antigen) enters the circulation and stimulates the immune system.

(B) The immune system produces IgE.

(C) The IgE fixes itself to mast cells and basophils, thereby sensitizing the person.

Mast cells and basophils

Sensitized mast cell

Second exposure

Allergen

(D) On subsequent exposure to allergens, the allergens unite with IgE on the surface of the sensitized cells.

Granules

Mediators

(E) This union causes the release of granules and the liberation of mediators that induce smooth muscle contractions in the body.

Still other mediators must be synthesized after the antigen-IgE reaction. One example is a series of substances called **leukotrienes** (so named because they are derived from *leuko*cytes and have a *triene* chemical structure). Leukotrienes (once called "slow-reacting substance of anaphylaxis," or SRS-A) result from a complex set of interactions as follows. Histamine from the cellular granules of white blood cells

leu'ko-tri-ene'

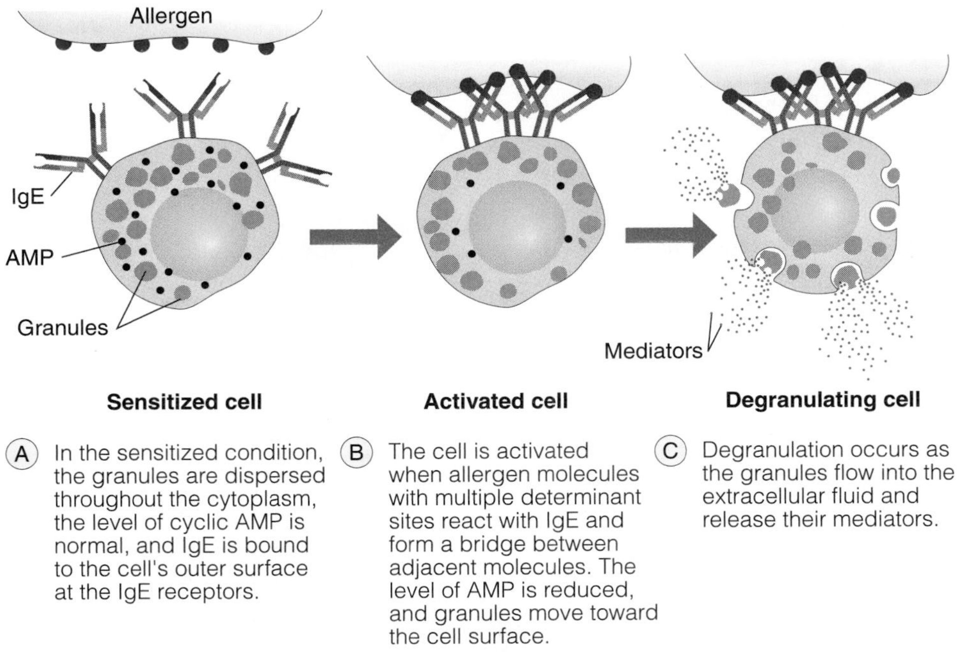

Sensitized cell

(A) In the sensitized condition, the granules are dispersed throughout the cytoplasm, the level of cyclic AMP is normal, and IgE is bound to the cell's outer surface at the IgE receptors.

Activated cell

(B) The cell is activated when allergen molecules with multiple determinant sites react with IgE and form a bridge between adjacent molecules. The level of AMP is reduced, and granules move toward the cell surface.

Degranulating cell

(C) Degranulation occurs as the granules flow into the extracellular fluid and release their mediators.

FIGURE 20.3

The Involvement of Mast Cells and Basophils in Anaphylaxis

a-rak'a-don'ik

activates an enzyme (phospholipase A), which in turn releases from the cell membrane a 20-carbon fatty acid called **arachidonic acid**. The arachidonic acid is acted on by another enzyme (5-lipoxygenase) and converted to leukotriene A, which is immediately converted to other leukotrienes. The latter, especially leukotriene D4, is extremely potent as a smooth muscle contractor. It also causes leakage in blood vessels and attracts eosinophils to continue the inflammatory reaction.

The second family of synthesized mediators are **prostaglandins**. These substances are well known as human hormones. They also result from reactions on arachidonic acid. In this case, however, the fatty acid is converted by a different enzyme (cyclooxygenase), and various prostaglandins result. One prostaglandin, prostaglandin D2, is a powerful constrictor of the bronchial tubes.

Lymphokines (also called **cytokines**) are also thought to be involved in the allergic response. Lymphokines are produced by numerous types of body cells (Chapter 18) and have actions that both stimulate and inhibit inflammation. One lymphokine, called **interleukin-4**, promotes IgE production; another, called **interleukin-5**, encourages the maturation and activity of eosinophils; and a third, called **tumor necrosis factor alpha**, is released from mast cells after the antigen-IgE reaction has occurred.

The principal activity of the mediators is to contract smooth muscles in the body. One effect is constriction of the small veins and the expansion of capillary pores, forcing fluid out and into the tissues. The skin becomes swollen around the eyes, wrists, and ankles, a condition called **edema**. The edema is accompanied by a hive-like rash, along with burning and itching in the skin, as the sensory nerves are excited. Contractions also occur in the gastrointestinal tract and bronchial muscles, leading to sharp cramps and shortness of breath, respectively. The individual inhales

Edema:
swelling of the body tissues.

rapidly without exhaling and traps carbon dioxide in the lungs, an ironic situation in which the lungs are fully inflated but lack oxygen. Death may occur in 10 to 15 minutes as a result of asphyxiation if prompt action is not forthcoming (hence the name "immediate" hypersensitivity). MicroFocus 20.2 describes the emergency treatment that may be given in such a case.

Some people experience a **late-phase anaphylaxis**. In this case, it takes several hours for the tissue to become hot, tender, red, and swollen. The mast cells induce this reaction by releasing chemical attractors (called chemotactic factors) that attract other cells to the site to bring about the changes. For example, **eosinophils** exist in unusually high numbers in allergic individuals, and they arrive at the site and release leukotrienes, as well as toxic substances that contribute to tissue damage. **Neutrophils** are normally the phagocytes of the bloodstream, but in allergic reactions, they liberate a number of enzymes that bring about local tissue damage. And **helper T-lymphocytes** are involved because they produce interleukin-4, which augments the allergic response. Many of these reactions are still under investigation.

A person sensitized to an allergen may undergo **desensitization** therapy to reduce the possibility of anaphylaxis. This procedure involves injections of tiny but increasing amounts of allergen over a period of hours or weeks, to effect a gradual reduction of granules in sensitized mast cells and basophils. Such treatment prevents a massive degranulation later. One who is sensitive to the immune serum used in disease therapy may need to undergo desensitization before the serum is used in large therapeutic doses.

Desensitization:
a process in which antigens are injected to relieve sensitivity to that antigen.

Another approach to desensitization is to give a series of injections of allergens over a period of weeks. Allergists believe that these exposures cause the immune system to produce IgG antibodies, which circulate and neutralize allergens before they contact sensitized cells. The **blocking antibodies**, as they are called, appear to be an effective device for individuals sensitized to bee stings. They may also be used for people who have food allergies (MicroFocus 20.3). A promising alternative is to inject Fc fragments of IgE to fill the receptor sites on mast cells and basophils, thereby making the sites unavailable to the person's IgE. TABLE 20.2 summarizes six cases of anaphylaxis in which desensitization procedures were not performed and death resulted.

Blocking antibodies:
IgG antibodies that neutralize allergens before they can induce hypersensitivity.

MicroFocus 20.2

WHEN ANAPHYLAXIS STRIKES

Anaphylaxis is a terrifying experience. The skin itches intensely and breaks into hives, the eyes and joints become red and puffy, and the person doubles over with abdominal pains. Breathing becomes difficult, then belabored, and finally is reduced to life-sucking gasps. The symptoms develop within minutes, and the individual usually faints and quickly lapses into a coma.

The key to survival is swift action. Epinephrine (adrenalin) is the highest priority drug. Within minutes of injection, it stabilizes basophils and mast cells to prevent further mediator release. It also dilates the bronchioles to reopen the air passageways, and constricts the capillaries to keep fluid in the circulation.

A smooth muscle relaxant such as aminophylline may also be used. This drug helps dilate the bronchial tubes and pulmonary blood vessels. An antihistamine such as diphenhydramine (Benadryl) may be valuable. This drug competes with histamine for the active sites on smooth muscle receptors, thereby inhibiting the action of histamine. Hydrocortisone may be used to reduce swelling in the tissue, and an expectorant may help clear laryngeal edema.

If the patient does not respond rapidly to the drugs, it may be necessary to insert a tube into the respiratory passageway or perform a tracheostomy. Either must be done quickly, because life is now reduced to a scant few minutes.

TABLE 20.2

Data from Six Cases of Human Anaphylaxis

CASE NO.	SEX	AGE (YR)	AGENT	DOSE (ML)	ROUTE OF ADMINISTRATION
1	F	39	Penicillin	1.5	Intramuscular
2	F	21	Guinea pig hemoglobin	0.2	Subcutaneous
3	M	52	Bee venom	—	Subcutaneous
4	M	45	Penicillin	—	Intramuscular
5	M	56	Hay fever desensitization vaccine	0.0625	Subcutaneous
6	F	38	Penicillin and streptomycin	—	Intramuscular

MicroFocus 20.3

THE PEANUT DILEMMA

Americans love peanuts—salted, unsalted, oil-roasted, dry-roasted, Spanish, honey-crusted, in shells, out of shells, and on and on.

But as declared peanut fanatics know, there is also the risk of a rather nasty allergic reaction: One can break out in hives, develop a serious headache, experience a racing heartbeat, or double over with intestinal cramps.

And, if that's not bad enough, research reported in 1996 indicates that feeding peanut butter to very young children increases their sensitivity to the legumes when they reach adulthood. Moreover, a 1997 report in the *New England Journal of Medicine* indicates that peanut-specific antibodies can be transferred from an organ donor to an organ recipient. (In the recipient, the skin reaction is not threatening, but it does complicate matters.)

The answer to all those miseries can best be summed up as "V plus V." The

first V is for vigilance. Vigilance means avoiding peanuts or peanut butter; but it also means being cautious about egg roll wrappers, chili fillers, and protein extenders in cake mixes, all of which may contain peanuts in one form or another. And it means vigilance that manufacturers clearly label their products and insistence that peanut-detection tests be performed routinely.

The second V is for vaccine. In 1999, investigators from Johns Hopkins University tested a peanut vaccine and showed that it protects sensitized mice against peanut proteins. The vaccine consists of DNA segments that encode the peanut proteins. Encased in protective molecules and delivered orally, the vaccine decreased the mice's capacity for producing peanut-related IgE. The developers postulated that the vaccine

elicits the so-called "blocking antibodies" that bind the peanut antigens before they reach the animal's immune system.

So does that mean we can expect health officials to distribute vaccine injections where we buy peanut butter, peanut brittle, or beer nuts? Not likely, say the researchers, at least not in the immediate future. But check back soon. You never know.

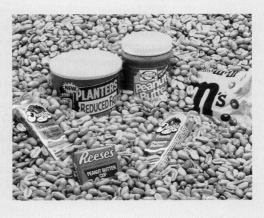

ESTIMATED TIME FROM CHALLENGE TO DEATH (MIN)	SYMPTOMS AND SIGNS	KNOWN PRIOR EXPOSURE	"ALLERGIC HISTORY"
60	Generalized warmth, tightness of throat, respiratory distress, cyanosis, convulsion, respiratory failure	Yes	"Hives" 2 weeks before death; allergen unknown
16	Headache, wheezing; cyanosis	No	"Asthma"; skin sensitivity to dog hair, kapok, shellfish, ragweed, timothy, orris root, and house dust
20	Unknown	Yes	Severe local reaction to bee sting 20 years previously
60	Dyspnea	Unknown	Unknown
45	Difficulty breathing	Yes	"Hay fever"—injection was 11th in series of weekly desensitization injections
120	Chest pain, cough, collapse, hypotension, cardiac arrest	Unknown	Unknown

A novel approach to desensitization is to develop monoclonal antibodies (Chapter 19) that recognize and react with IgE. These **anti-IgE antibodies** can be used to dislodge IgE from the surfaces of mast cells and basophils, thereby disarming the cells and preventing the allergic reaction from occurring. To date, research on these monoclonal antibodies has shown that they can be administered safely and effectively reduce the circulating levels of IgE. The treatment can be used to reduce both the immediate and the late-phase anaphylaxis, especially in asthma patients, as we shall see in the next section.

ATOPIC DISEASES

Type I hypersensitivity reactions need not result in the whole-body involvement that accompanies anaphylaxis. Indeed, the vast majority of hypersensitivity reactions are accompanied by limited production of IgE and the sensitization of mast cells in localized areas of the body. The result is an **atopic disease**, or **common allergy**. *a-top'ik*

An example of an atopic disease is **hay fever**, technically referred to as **allergic rhinitis**. This condition develops from springtime inhalations of tree and grass pollens, and summer and fall exposures to grass and weed pollens (FIGURE 20.4). Fall exposures coincide with the haying season, from which the disease first acquired its name (although there is no fever associated with the condition). Immune stimulation by pollen antigens leads to IgE production, and a sensitization of mast cells follows in the eyes, nose, and upper respiratory tract. Subsequent exposures bring on sneezing, tearing, swollen mucous membranes, and other well-known symptoms. In addition, hay fever symptoms may be caused by house dust, mold spores, dust mites, detergent enzymes, and the particles of animal skin and hair called dander. (Dander itself is not the allergen; the actual allergens are proteins deposited in the dander from the animal's saliva when it grooms itself.)

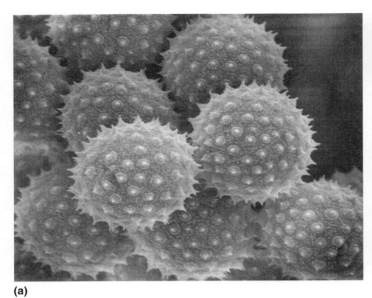

(a)

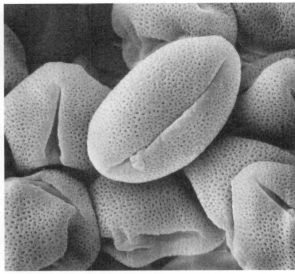

(b)

FIGURE 20.4

Scanning Electron Micrographs of Two Types of Pollen Grains

(a) Pollen grains of *Sphaeralcea munroana*, a desert plant (×1000). (b) Pollen grains from *Penstemon pruinosus*, a flowering plant that grows wild in the mountains of southern California (×2000). Antigens in pollen grains such as these stimulate allergic reactions.

az'mah

Leukotrienes:
white blood cell products that act as mediators in type I hypersensitivity reactions.

ur'tĭ-ka're-ah

Allergic reactions also are responsible for triggering the great majority of asthmatic attacks. **Asthma** is characterized by wheezing and stressed breathing, and appears to be caused by the same allergens that are associated with hay fever. The condition resembles late-phase anaphylaxis. Preceded by inflammation and constriction of the bronchial tubes, the hypersensitivity is set off by triggers such as dust mites, pollen, and molds. Leukotrienes seem to play a significant role. About 15 million Americans suffer from asthma, including about 3.7 million children and adolescents (**FIGURE 20.5**). Bronchodilators have been traditionally used to widen the bronchioles by relaxing the surrounding muscles, but newer evidence indicates that asthma is due to inflammation of the air passageways, so many physicians now prescribe anti-inflammatory agents such as inhaled steroids or nonsteroidal cromolyn sodium. Antileukotriene medications are also prescribed in some instances.

Food allergies are accompanied by symptoms in the GI tract, including swollen lips, abdominal cramps, nausea, and diarrhea. The skin may break out in a rash containing **hives**, each hive consisting of a central puffiness, called a wheal, surrounded by a zone of redness known as a flare. Such a rash is called **urticaria**, from the Latin *urtica* for "stinging needle." Allergenic foods include chocolate, strawberries, oranges, cow's milk, and fish (**MicroFocus 20.4**). A dry food such as flour may also cause respiratory allergy.

According to public health estimates, almost 20 percent of Americans have some type of atopic disease. An interesting avenue of research was opened when it was discovered that the lymphocytes responsible for IgE and IgA production lie close to one another in the lymphoid tissue, and that the IgA level and its corresponding lymphocytes are greatly reduced in atopic individuals. Immunologists have suggested

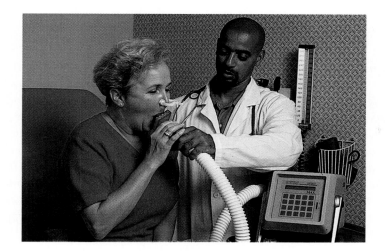

FIGURE 20.5

Testing for Asthma

A pulmonary function test measures the amount of air expelled from the bronchial tubes, as an indication of obstruction. Such a test enables the physician to determine whether the patient is allergic to an airborne antigen.

that in nonallergic individuals, IgA lymphocytes shield IgE lymphocytes from antigenic stimulation, but that atopic people may lack sufficient IgA lymphocytes to block the antigens.

Another theory of atopic disease maintains that allergy results from a breakdown of **feedback mechanisms** in the immune system. Research findings indicate that B-lymphocytes, which synthesize IgE, are controlled by suppressor T-lymphocytes, regulated in turn by IgE. Under normal conditions, IgE may limit its own production by stimulating suppressor T-lymphocyte activity. However, in atopic individuals the mechanism malfunctions, possibly because the T-lymphocytes are defective, and IgE is produced in massive quantities. Allergic people are known to possess almost 100 times the IgE level of people who do not have allergies. Radioimmunoassay (RAI) techniques and radioallergosorbent tests (RAST) are used to detect the nature and quantity of IgE in an individual (Chapter 19).

Some researchers postulate a **positive role** for the allergic response. They suggest, for example, that sneezing expels respiratory pathogens, and that contractions of the gastrointestinal tract force parasites out of the body. Others have theorized that allergy was once a survival mechanism, and that atopic individuals are the modern generation of people who developed this ability to resist pathogens and passed the trait along.

Suppressor T-lymphocytes:
T-lymphocytes that suppress the immune reaction to antigens.

MicroFocus 20.4

NOT THE REAL THING

"But I'm *not* allergic to crabs!" exclaimed the woman. "I've eaten shellfish all my life—clams, oysters, crabs—and I've never had a reaction. Why this time?"

"Let's go over it again," said the allergist. "You had the crabmeat egg rolls and within minutes you were wheezing."

"Yes."

"You're sure it was real crabmeat?"

"Well, the menu said 'egg rolls made with crabmeat.'"

"Could it have been surimi—you know, that processed fish used to make imitation crabmeat? They sell it in the supermarkets. It's artificially colored to look like crabmeat, but it's really processed pollack or some other inexpensive fish."

"I guess it could have been . . . ," her voice trailed off.

"Are you allergic to fish?"

"Yes, as a matter of fact, I am."

"I think we have the answer."

To this point . . .

We have spent considerable time discussing the process of type I anaphylactic hypersensitivity because it has substantial importance to the millions of people who have allergies. We noted how IgE plays a central role in the process, how mast cells, basophils, and numerous mediators are involved, and how smooth muscle contractions account for the symptoms in anaphylaxis and common allergy. Two forms of desensitization were outlined, and the discussion described two theories on why allergies develop. One theory has to do with the blockage of allergens by IgA lymphocytes; the second involves a defect in suppressor T-lymphocytes. We also explored some positive roles for the allergic reaction.

We shall continue the discussion of hypersensitivity by studying the salient features of the remaining three types of hypersensitivity. Type II involves a destruction of cells, type III leads to the formation of granular masses called immune complexes, and type IV depends upon the exaggeration of T-lymphocyte function. As the chapter progresses, you may note how phenomena of the immune system are helping to enlighten scientists on several disease conditions that were poorly understood in past decades.

20.2

Other Types of Hypersensitivity

TYPE II CYTOTOXIC HYPERSENSITIVITY

A **cytotoxic hypersensitivity** is a cell-damaging reaction that occurs when IgG reacts with antigens on the surfaces of cells, as FIGURE 20.6 depicts. Complement is often activated and IgM may be involved, but IgE does not participate, nor is there any degranulation of mast cells. The cells affected in cytotoxic hypersensitivity are known as **target cells.**

A well-known example of cytotoxic hypersensitivity is the **transfusion reaction** arising from the mixing of incompatible blood types. Four major human blood types are known: A, B, AB, and O. Each type is distinguished by unique antigens on the surface of erythrocytes and certain antibodies in the plasma that are directed against antigens not present in the individual's cells (TABLE 20.3). Before a transfusion is attempted, the laboratory technician must determine the **blood type** of all participants so that incompatible types are not mixed. For example, if a person with type A blood donates to a recipient with type O blood, the A antigens on the donor's erythrocytes will react with a antibodies in the recipient's plasma, and the cytotoxic effect will be expressed as agglutination of donor erythrocytes and activation of complement in the recipient's circulatory system. If the conditions are reversed, the donor's a antibodies will react with the recipient's A antigens, although to a lesser degree, because dilution in the recipient's plasma takes place. Most blood banks cross-match the donor's erythrocytes with the recipient's serum, as well as the reverse, to ensure compatibility (MicroFocus 20.5).

Another expression of cytotoxic hypersensitivity is **hemolytic disease of the newborn,** or **Rh disease.** This problem arises from the fact that erythrocytes of approximately 85 percent of Caucasian Americans contain a surface antigen, first described in rhesus monkeys and therefore known as the **Rh antigen.** Such individuals are said to be Rh-positive. The 15 percent who lack the antigen are considered Rh-negative. For African Americans, the figures are 90 percent and 10 percent, respectively. Evidence indicates that the antigen is really a group of antigens that vary among Rh-

Target cells:
cells against which cytotoxic hypersensitivity is directed.

Agglutination:
a clumping reaction.

Rh antigen:
a group of antigenic substances on the red blood cells of Rh-positive individuals.

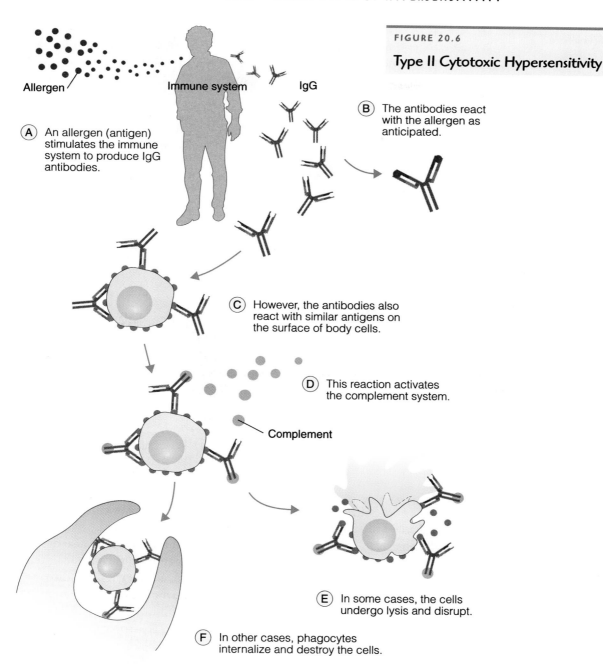

FIGURE 20.6

Type II Cytotoxic Hypersensitivity

Allergen   Immune system   IgG

(A) An allergen (antigen) stimulates the immune system to produce IgG antibodies.

(B) The antibodies react with the allergen as anticipated.

(C) However, the antibodies also react with similar antigens on the surface of body cells.

(D) This reaction activates the complement system.

Complement

(E) In some cases, the cells undergo lysis and disrupt.

(F) In other cases, phagocytes internalize and destroy the cells.

positive individuals, but we shall consider the group as a single factor for the purposes of discussion.

The ability to produce the Rh antigen is a genetically inherited trait. When an **Rh-negative woman** marries an **Rh-positive man**, there is a 3 to 1 chance (or 75 percent probability) that the trait will be passed to the child, resulting in an Rh-positive child. During the birth process, a woman's circulatory system is exposed to her child's blood, and if the child is Rh-positive, the Rh antigens enter the woman's blood and stimulate her immune system to produce rh antibodies (FIGURE 20.7). If a succeeding pregnancy results in another Rh-positive child, these antibodies will cross the placenta (along with other antibodies) and enter the fetal circulation.

TABLE 20.3

Some Characteristics of the Major Blood Groups

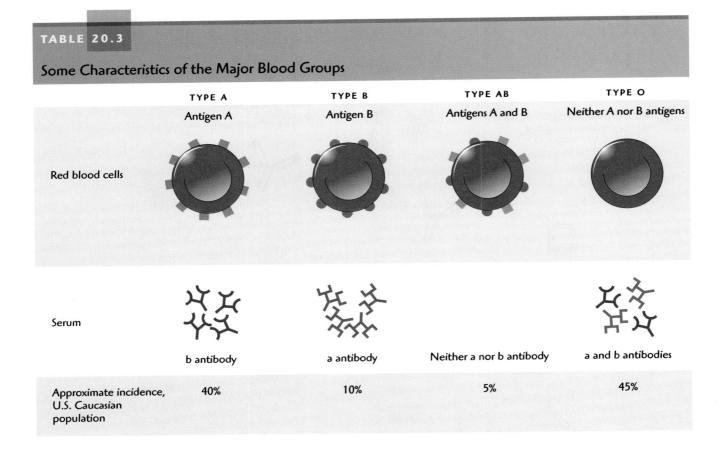

	TYPE A	TYPE B	TYPE AB	TYPE O
	Antigen A	Antigen B	Antigens A and B	Neither A nor B antigens
Red blood cells				
Serum	b antibody	a antibody	Neither a nor b antibody	a and b antibodies
Approximate incidence, U.S. Caucasian population	40%	10%	5%	45%

ĕ-rǐ'th'ro-blas-to'sis

throm'bo-si'to-pe'ne-ah
Thrombocytopenia:
a cytotoxic hypersensitivity in
which antidrug antibodies attack
thrombocytes.

There they will react with Rh antigens on the fetal erythrocytes and cause complement-mediated lysis of the cells. (The fetal circulatory system rapidly releases immature erythroblasts to replace the lysed blood cells, but these cells are also destroyed. From this observation, the disease acquired its older name, **erythroblastosis fetalis**.) The result may be stillbirth or, in a less extreme form, a baby with jaundice.

Modern treatment for hemolytic disease of the newborn consists of an injection of rh antibodies (**RhoGAM**). The injection is given within 72 hours of delivery of an Rh-positive child (no injection is necessary if the child is Rh-negative). Antibodies in the preparation interact with Rh antigens and remove them from the circulation, thereby preventing them from stimulating the woman's immune system. The success of this procedure has virtually eliminated expectant parents' concerns about disease in their newborns. It should be noted, however, that an Rh-negative woman may produce rh antibodies as a result of miscarriage or abortion of an Rh-positive fetus, or after a transfusion with Rh-positive blood.

Other examples of cytotoxic hypersensitivity are less familiar. One example, called **thrombocytopenia**, results from antibodies produced against such drugs as aspirin, certain antibiotics, or antihistamines. The antibodies combine with antigens and drug molecules adhering to the surface of thrombocytes (blood platelets), and as complement is activated, the thrombocytes undergo lysis. The effect is impaired blood clotting, and hemorrhages may occur on the skin and in the mouth. The symptoms subside as the drug is withdrawn. Another condition, referred to as

(A) Hemolytic disease of the newborn can develop when an Rh-positive man and an Rh-negative woman have a baby.

(B) When an Rh-negative woman gives birth to an Rh-positive baby, Rh antigens from the child's blood enter the woman's blood.

(C) The antigens stimulate her immune system to produce rh antibodies that circulate in her blood, but since the baby has already been born, there is no effect on the child.

(D) In a future pregnancy, if the baby is Rh-positive, the rh antibodies will cross the placenta and enter the baby's blood.

(E) The rh antibodies attack the baby's red blood cells by uniting with Rh antigens on their surface; they damage the cells, leading to severe anemia and hemolytic disease.

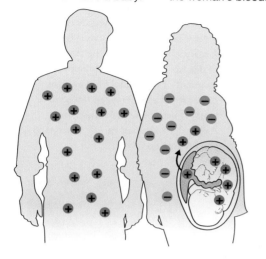
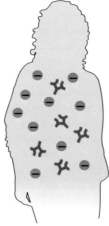
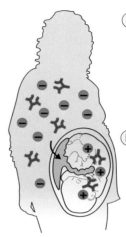

FIGURE 20.7

Hemolytic Disease of the Newborn

agranulocytosis, results from the destruction of neutrophils by antibodies. This problem, also stimulated by drugs, is manifested as a reduced capacity for phagocytosis. In both conditions, antibodies are directed toward the individual's own cells. The term **autoimmune disease** is therefore applied to the phenomenon.

A third autoimmune disease is **Goodpasture syndrome**. In this rare disease, antibodies combine with antigens on the membranes of glomeruli in kidneys. Antibody binding activates the complement system and, as the integrity of the membranes is destroyed, blood and proteins leak into the urine. Kidney failure may follow.

Antibodies reacting with antigens on cell surfaces do not always lead to cell destruction, but the reaction may alter the cellular physiology. In **myasthenia gravis**, for example, antibodies react with acetylcholine receptors on membranes covering the muscle fibers. This interaction reduces nerve impulse transfer to the fibers and results in a loss of muscle activity, manifested as weakness and fatigue. In **Graves' disease**, antibodies unite with receptors on the surfaces of thyroid gland cells, causing an overabundant secretion of thyroxine. The patient experiences goiter and a rise in the metabolic rate. A third example of altered cell physiology is **Hashimoto's disease**. This is a condition in which antibodies also attack thyroid gland cells, but the reaction changes their chemistry leading to a thyroxine deficiency. All three diseases are considered autoimmune diseases.

Although cytotoxic hypersensitivity is generally cast in a negative role with deleterious effects on the body, the cytotoxic activity may contribute to the body's resistance to disease. For example, the antigen–antibody interaction occurring on the surface of a parasite leads to destruction of the parasite. The interaction also may

a-gran'u-lo-si-to'sis

Autoimmune disease:
one in which the body produces antibodies against its own cells.
Glomeruli:
coils of capillaries in the kidneys through which blood fluid passes into the Bowman's capsules.

Acetylcholine:
a neurotransmitter acting in the synapse.

Thyroxine:
a thyroid hormone that regulates body metabolism.

MicroFocus 20.5

THE KEY TO TRANSFUSIONS

Since earliest times, people believed that blood contained mysterious powers of rejuvenation. The Romans, for example, would rush into the gladiatorial arena to drink the blood of dying gladiators because they thought that blood would restore youth.

Transfusions of blood came into popular use after 1667, when Jean Baptiste Denis, physician to King Louis XIV of France, temporarily restored a dying boy by transfusing lamb's blood into his veins. Transfusions, however, were a mixed blessing: Sometimes they worked, but often they proved fatal. Why this happened perplexed doctors, until Karl Landsteiner provided an answer in 1900.

Landsteiner was an 1891 graduate of the medical school at the University of Vienna. After graduation, he spent five years in Wurtzburg, Germany, working as a chemist with Emil Fischer, the 1902 Nobel laureate for the synthesis of sugars. Landsteiner was more interested in proteins, and he concluded that protein differences could be fruitfully revealed by studying interactions between serum proteins and the components of living

cells. In 1897 he became assistant at the Hygienic Institute in Vienna, and in 1900 he applied his method of protein analysis to blood cells.

Landsteiner observed that when erythrocytes from one person were mixed with the serum from another person, the cells sometimes clumped together. In other cases there was no clumping (as if a person's blood was being mixed with its own serum). By meticulous cross-comparisons, Landsteiner concluded that two markers, now called antigens, exist on the surface of the red blood cells. He labeled them with the first two letters of the alphabet, A and B. Landsteiner also surmised that a person's plasma contained antibodies against another person's antigens. These findings formed the basis of the familiar ABO blood groups and explained why some transfusions were successful and others fatal. It now became possible to work out the details for matching up blood groups for safe transfusions.

In World War I, physicians finally recognized the immense value of Landsteiner's work. Over 21 million men

were wounded during the war, and for many, a blood transfusion was life saving. More than 3 million Americans now receive safe transfusions annually during surgery, childbirth, or in the treatment of disease. In 1930, Landsteiner was the recipient of the Nobel Prize in Physiology or Medicine. Ten years later, while working with New York physician Alexander S. Weiner, he also discovered the Rh antigen.

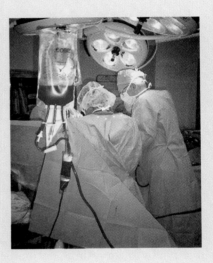

Chemotaxis:
a chemical attraction.

encourage chemotaxis or histamine release through the activity of C3a and C5a components of the complement system. Increased phagocytosis and membrane damage from the complement attack complex are other by-products of complement activation. These activities probably account for resistance to many disorders.

TYPE III IMMUNE COMPLEX HYPERSENSITIVITY

Neutrophils:
multilobed circulating white blood cells that function as phagocytes.

Immune complex hypersensitivity develops when antibodies combine with antigens and form aggregates that accumulate in blood vessels or on tissue surfaces (FIGURE 20.8). As complement is activated, the C3a and C5a components increase vascular permeability and exert a chemotactic effect on phagocytic neutrophils, drawing them to the target site. Here the neutrophils release lysosomal enzymes, which cause tissue damage. Local inflammation is common, and fibrin clots may complicate the problem. The antibodies are predominantly IgG, with IgM also found in certain cases.

Serum sickness:
a hypersensitivity reaction that follows injection of serum used for therapy.

Serum sickness is a common manifestation of immune complex hypersensitivity. It develops when the immune system produces IgG against residual proteins in serum preparations. The IgG then reacts with the proteins, and immune complexes

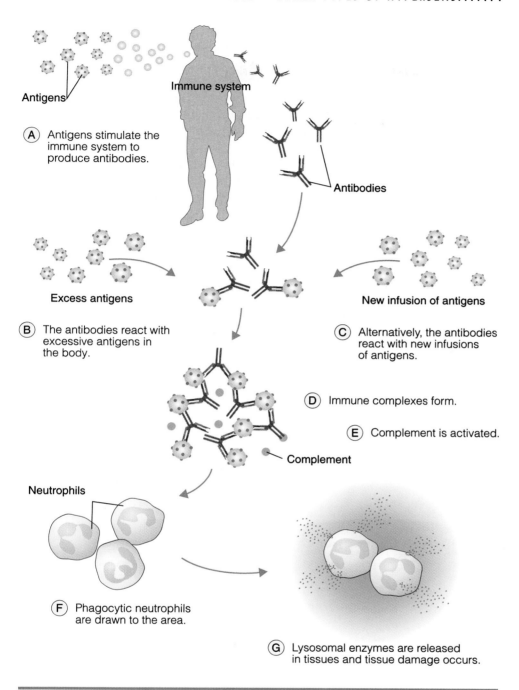

Antigens

(A) Antigens stimulate the immune system to produce antibodies.

Immune system

Antibodies

Excess antigens

(B) The antibodies react with excessive antigens in the body.

New infusion of antigens

(C) Alternatively, the antibodies react with new infusions of antigens.

(D) Immune complexes form.

(E) Complement is activated.

Complement

Neutrophils

(F) Phagocytic neutrophils are drawn to the area.

(G) Lysosomal enzymes are released in tissues and tissue damage occurs.

FIGURE 20.8

Type III Immune Complex Hypersensitivity

gather in the kidney over a period of days. The problem is compounded when IgE, also from the immune system, attaches to mast cells and basophils, thereby inducing a type I anaphylactic hypersensitivity. The sum total of these events is kidney damage, along with hives and swelling in the face, neck, and joints (TABLE 20.4 summarizes this and other immune disorders.)

Arthus phenomenon:
a type of hypersensitivity in which immune complexes form in blood vessels near the site of antigen entry.

Another form of immune complex hypersensitivity is the **Arthus phenomenon**, named for Nicolas Maurice Arthus, the French physiologist who described it in 1903. In this process, excessively large amounts of IgG form complexes with antigens, either in the blood vessels or near the site of antigen entry into the body. Antigens in dust from moldy hay and in dried pigeon feces are known to cause this phenomenon. The names **farmer's lung** and **pigeon fancier's disease** are applied to the conditions, respectively. Thromboses in the blood vessels may lead to oxygen starvation and cell death.

loo'pus er'i-them'ah-to'sis

Systemic lupus erythematosus (SLE) is another example of a type III hypersensitivity. SLE, also known as lupus, is an autoimmune disease in which B-lymphocytes produce IgG upon stimulation by nuclear components of disintegrating white blood cells. The terms "autoantigens" and "autoantibodies" apply because the antibodies are formed against the body's own molecules. When the autoantigens and autoantibodies react, immune complexes accumulate in the skin and body organs, and complement is activated. The patient experiences a **butterfly rash**, a facial skin condition across the nose and cheeks (FIGURE 20.9). Lesions also form in the heart, kidneys, and blood vessels. In **rheumatoid arthritis**, another autoimmune disease, immune complexes form in the joints.

glo-mer'u-lo-ně-fri'tis

Several microbial diseases are also complicated by immune complex formation. For example, the glomerulonephritis and rheumatic fever that follow **streptococcal diseases** (Chapter 7) appear to be consequences of immune complex formation in the kidneys and heart, respectively. In these cases, the deposit of complexes relates to common antigens in streptococci and the tissues. Other immune complex diseases

TABLE 20.4

A Summary of Some Immune Disorders

DISORDER	TYPE OF HYPERSENSITIVITY	TARGET TISSUE	STIMULATING ANTIGEN	EFFECT
Thrombocytopenia	Cytotoxic	Thrombocytes (blood platelets)	Aspirin Antibiotics Antihistamine	Impaired blood clotting Hemorrhages
Agranulocytosis	Cytotoxic	Neutrophils	Drugs	Reduced phagocytosis
Goodpasture syndrome	Cytotoxic	Kidneys	Own antigens (?)	Kidney failure
Myasthenia gravis	Cytotoxic	Membranes of muscle fibers	Not established	Loss of muscle activity
Graves' disease	Cytotoxic	Thyroid gland	Not established	Abundant thyroxine High metabolic rate
Hashimoto's disease	Cytotoxic	Thyroid gland	Not established	Thyroxine deficiency Low metabolic rate
Serum sickness	Immune complex	Kidney	Serum proteins	Kidney failure
Arthus phenomenon	Immune complex	Blood vessels Site of antigen entry	Environmental antigens	Thromboses in blood vessels
Systemic lupus erythematosus	Immune complex	Skin, heart, kidney, blood vessels	Own nucleo-proteins	Butterfly rash Heart, kidney failure
Rheumatoid arthritis	Immune complex	Joints	Own nucleo-proteins (?)	Swollen joints

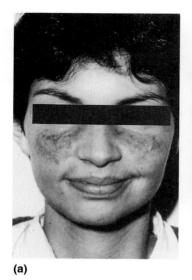
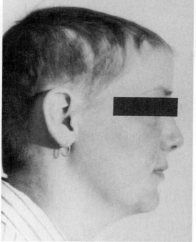
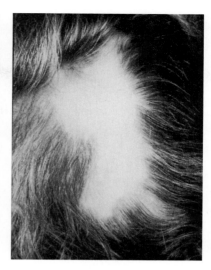

(a) (b)

FIGURE 20.9

Systemic Lupus Erythematosus

Two patients showing some of the symptoms of systemic lupus erythematosus (SLE). (a) The butterfly rash on the face. Note how the rash extends out to the cheeks like the wings of a butterfly. (b) A young girl displaying the loss of hair that accompanies some cases of SLE.

include hemorrhagic shock, which may accompany dengue fever; subacute sclerosing panencephalitis (SSPE), which follows cases of measles; and the slow-forming kidney deposits associated with lymphocytic choriomeningitis (LCM). Research evidence also suggests that Reye syndrome and Guillain-Barré syndrome may be related to immune complex formation.

ko're-o-men'in-ji'tis

ge-yan' bar-ra'

TYPE IV CELLULAR HYPERSENSITIVITY

Cellular hypersensitivity is an exaggeration of the process of cell-mediated immunity, discussed in Chapter 18. The adjective *cellular* was originally applied because contact between T-lymphocytes and antigens was thought to be necessary for the reaction. However, the later identification of lymphokines (cytokines) as mediators of the process challenged this assumption. The hypersensitivity cannot be transferred to a normal individual by serum lymphokines because their concentration is too low in transfused serum. Transfer is accomplished only with T-lymphocytes. TABLE 20.5 compares this **delayed hypersensitivity** with type I immediate hypersensitivity.

Type IV hypersensitivity is a delayed reaction whose maximal effect is not seen until 24 to 72 hours have elapsed (hence the name, delayed hypersensitivity). It is characterized by a thickening and drying of the skin tissue, a process called **induration**, and a surrounding zone of erythema (redness). Two major forms of type IV hypersensitivity are recognized: infection allergy and contact dermatitis.

Infection allergy develops when the immune system responds to certain microbial agents. Effector cells known as **delayed hypersensitivity T-lymphocytes** migrate to the antigen site and release lymphokines. The lymphokines attract phagocytes and encourage phagocytosis (Chapter 18). Sensitized lymphocytes then remain in the tissue and provide immunity to successive episodes of infection. Among the microbial agents that stimulate this type of immunity are the bacterial agents of

Lymphokines:
a series of lymphocyte-derived proteins that increases the efficiency of phagocytosis of antigens; also called cytokines.

Induration:
a thickening and drying of skin tissues in cellular hypersensitivity.

TABLE 20.5

Immediate and Delayed Hypersensitivities Compared

	TYPE I IMMEDIATE HYPERSENSITIVITY	TYPE IV DELAYED HYPERSENSITIVITY

Clinical state:	Hay fever
	Asthma
	Urticaria
	Allergic skin conditions
	Serum sickness
	Anaphylactic shock
		Drug allergies
		Infectious allergies
		   Tuberculosis
		   Rheumatic fever
		   Histoplasmosis
		   Trichinosis
		   Contact dermatitis

Onset:	Immediate	Delayed
Duration:	Short: hours	Prolonged: days or longer
Allergens:	Pollen Molds House dust Danders Drugs Antibiotics Soluble proteins and carbohydrates Foods	Drugs Antibiotics Microorganisms: bacteria, viruses, fungi, animal parasites Poison ivy and plant oils Plastics and other chemicals Fabrics, furs Cosmetics
Passive transfer of sensitivity:	With serum	With cells or cell fractions of lymphoid series

his′to-plaz-mo′sis

kan-dĭ-di′ah-sis

Tuberculosis:
a bacterial disease of the lungs and other tissues accompanied by tubercle formation.

tuberculosis, leprosy, and brucellosis; the fungi involved in blastomycosis, histoplasmosis, and candidiasis; the viruses of smallpox and mumps; and the chlamydiae of lymphogranuloma.

Infection allergy is demonstrated by injecting into the skin an extract of the microbial agent. As the immune response takes place, the area develops induration and erythema, and fibrin is deposited by activation of the clotting system. An important application of infection allergy is the **tuberculin skin test** for tuberculosis (FIGURE 20.10). A purified protein derivative (PPD) of *Mycobacterium tuberculosis* is applied to the skin by intradermal injection (the Mantoux test) or multiple punctures (tines). Individuals sensitized by a previous exposure to *Mycobacterium* species develop a vesicle, erythema, and induration.

FIGURE 20.10

A Positive Tuberculin Test

The raised induration and zone of inflammation indicate that antigens have reacted with T-lymphocytes, probably sensitized by a previous exposure to tubercle bacilli.

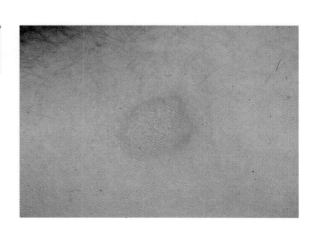

Skin tests based on infection allergy are available for many diseases. Immunologists caution, however, that a positive result does not constitute a final diagnosis. They note that sensitivity may have developed from a subclinical exposure to the organisms, from clinical disease years before, or from a former screening test in which the test antigens elicited a T-lymphocyte response.

Contact dermatitis develops after exposure to a broad variety of antigens, such as the allergens in clothing, insecticides, coins, cosmetics, and furs. The offending substances may also include formaldehyde, copper, dyes, bacterial enzymes, and protein fibers. In **poison ivy**, the allergen has been identified as **urushiol**, a low-molecular-weight chemical on the surface of the leaf. In the body, urushiol complexes with tissue proteins to form allergenic compounds. A poison ivy rash consists of very itchy pinhead-sized blisters usually occurring in a straight row (FIGURE 20.11).

The course of contact dermatitis is typical of the type IV reaction. Repeated exposures cause a drying of the skin, with erythema and scaling. Examples are on the scalp when allergenic shampoo is used, on the hands when contact is made with detergent enzymes, and on the wrists when an allergy to watchband chemicals exists. Contact dermatitis may also occur on the face where contact is made with cosmetics, on areas of the skin where chemicals in permanent press fabrics have accumulated, and on the feet when there is sensitivity to dyes in leather shoes. Factory workers exposed to photographic materials, hair dyes, or sewing materials may experience allergies. The list of possibilities is endless and includes the use of costume jewelry (MicroFocus 20.6). Applying a sample of the suspected substance to the skin (a patch test) and leaving it in place for 24 to 48 hours will help pinpoint the source of the allergy. Another method is illustrated in FIGURE 20.12. Relief generally consists of avoiding the inciting agents.

Contact dermatitis:
a cellular hypersensitivity of the skin that follows repeated exposure to certain antigens.

u-roo'she-ol

FIGURE 20.11

The Poison Ivy Rash

(A) When a sensitized person touches poison ivy, a substance called urushiol stimulates T-lymphocytes in the skin; within 24 hours, a type IV reaction takes place.

(B) The reaction is characterized by pinhead-sized blisters that usually occur in a straight row.

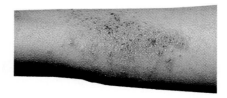

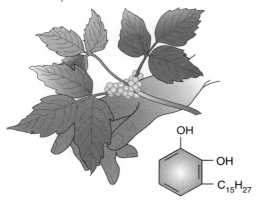

(C) The chemical structure of urushiol

MicroFocus 20.6

PIERCED PROBLEMS

He arrived at the office wearing studs and rings in his ears, eyebrows, nose, navel, and various other body parts. And he was scratching . . . and scratching . . . and scratching.

The doctor looked past the jewelry. She saw nickel. Not the coin, but the metal. Nickel is commonly used to make inexpensive costume jewelry.

Unfortunately, it also provokes contact dermatitis. (Other allergens in costume jewelry include chrome and palladium.)

What to do? The most obvious solution is to remove the jewelry and wait for the rash to fade. (Cortisone cream can be used to reduce the inflammation.) Furthermore, it's a good idea to substitute stainless steel or gold jewelry to pre-

vent a future recurrence. Most sterling silver is safe, but occasionally it may contain nickel or chrome, so a rash may still occur. If doubts persist, a skin test can pinpoint the allergy, and an allergist can offer helpful advice. Then, one's individual expression can continue.

FIGURE 20.12

The Test for Skin Allergies

The forearm is marked and injected with various test allergens. In a few minutes, the allergist notes where a skin wheal has occurred. This individual displays several positive reactions. The reaction can be assessed as slight, mild, moderate, or severe. In other instances, the skin of the back is used.

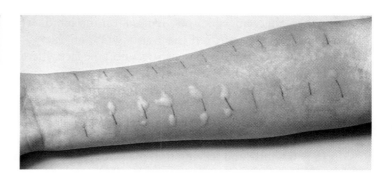

To this point . . .

We have completed a survey of the four types of hypersensitivity, and we have noted the salient differences among them. In type II cytotoxic hypersensitivity, there is an antigen–antibody interaction on the surface of cells that leads to cell destruction. Transfusion reactions and hemolytic disease of the newborn are symbolic of this cytotoxicity. Several autoimmune diseases, such as thrombocytopenia, myasthenia gravis, and Graves' disease, also result from the cytotoxic reaction. In type III hypersensitivity, immune complex formation takes place as antigens react with antibodies to form masses of granular material. With the activation of complement, a local destruction of body tissue ensues. The effects of serum sickness, the Arthus phenomenon, and systemic lupus erythematosus illustrate how tissue may be affected.

Type IV cellular hypersensitivity is substantially different from the other three types because it involves sensitized T-lymphocytes. An exaggeration of cell-mediated immunity is basic to type IV hypersensitivity. Infection allergy and contact dermatitis are two examples of this hypersensitivity. Poison ivy is an example.

In the final section of this chapter, we shall examine immune deficiency diseases, transplantation immunology, and tumor immunology. The immune deficiency diseases rob the body of its natural defenses against infection and demonstrate the vital role the immune system plays. In transplantation and tumor immunology, we shall encounter some of the most recent findings in immunology, and see how scientists are beginning to understand certain functions of the immune system unrelated to infectious disease. Studies in these areas represent major areas of concentration in modern immunological research.

20.3

Immune Deficiency Diseases

The spectrum of immune deficiency diseases ranges from major abnormalities that are life-threatening to relatively minor deficiency states. The latter may be serious in populations where malnutrition and frequent contact with pathogenic organisms are common. Diagnostic techniques for determining immune deficiency diseases include measurements of antibody types, detection tests for B-lymphocyte function, and enumeration of T-lymphocytes. Assays of complement activity and phagocytosis are also useful in diagnosis.

An example of an immune deficiency disease is **Bruton's agammaglobulinemia**, first described by Ogden C. Bruton in 1952 (MicroFocus 20.7). In this disease, B-lymphocytes fail to develop from pre-B-lymphocyte cells in the bone marrow. The patient's lymphoid tissues lack plasma cells, all five classes of antibodies are either low in level or absent, and antibody responses to infectious disease are undetectable.

a-gam'ah-glob'u-lĭ-ne'me-ah
Bruton's agammaglobulinemia: an immune deficiency disease characterized by the absence of B-lymphocytes.

MicroFocus 20.7

SOMETHING FROM NOTHING

In the 1940s and early 1950s, scientists frequently debated whether antibodies were essential to immunity. Amid this controversy, a pediatrician at Washington D.C.'s Walter Reed Hospital made a momentous discovery.

The story began when a U.S. Air Force officer's son was admitted to the hospital with acute streptococcal disease. The child's pediatrician, Ogden C. Bruton, used penicillin to control the infection, but 2 weeks later, the child was back, sick again. Wishing to determine the level of antibodies in the boy's system, Bruton sent a sample of blood for testing on a new machine recently acquired by the hospital.

The next day, the laboratory called Bruton to report that something must be wrong with the machine because it could not detect any antibodies in the blood. Bruton responded by sending over a second sample, but the results were the same: no antibodies. It occurred to Bruton that maybe the trouble was not in the machine but in the blood. Perhaps the blood had no

antibodies. Conceivably, this could account for the recurring infections. Bruton began giving the boy monthly injections of antibodies, with outstanding success.

In 1952, Bruton reported his remarkable findings. His report was a medical bombshell because it established the concept of immune deficiency disease, while helping to solidify the role played by antibodies in resistance to infection.

But the story was not finished, because certain patients with immune deficiency disease still produced the lymphocytes that immunize against skin grafts. This observation led to the notion that the immune system was actually a dual system—one branch centered in antibodies, a second branch centered in lymphocytes. The sources of antibodies and lymphocytes would be found almost simultaneously, 13 years later.

In 1965, at the meeting of the American Academy of Pediatrics, Robert A. Good's research group was presenting evidence on the importance of the bursa of Fabricius to antibody production. The audience was skeptical, but the evidence

appeared substantial. When the speaker finished, a Philadelphia pediatrician named Angelo DiGeorge stepped to the microphone to add a footnote. DiGeorge described how four children at his hospital were struck repeatedly with severe infections. The children had antibodies in their blood, but curiously, each lacked a thymus. DiGeorge's observation was lost in the shuffle, but a question arose in his mind: Were the children susceptible to skin grafts, or could they possibly be immune?

DiGeorge hurried back to the hospital and devised a set of experiments to determine whether the children could successfully receive skin grafts. After weeks of study, he found they could. The thymus was apparently the key to the production of lymphocytes and hence to graft immunity. Bruton's patient lacked the bursa type of immunity, but DiGeorge's patients lacked the thymus type of immunity. The duality of the immune system was thus strengthened, and a second immune deficiency disease, DiGeorge syndrome, entered the dictionary of microbiology.

Infections from staphylococci, pneumococci, and streptococci are common between the ages of 6 months and 2 years. Bruton's agammaglobulinemia is apparently a sex-linked inherited trait, much more frequently observed in males than in females. Artificially acquired passive immunity is used to treat infectious disease in patients with this form of immune deficiency.

DiGeorge syndrome is an immune deficiency disease in which T-lymphocytes fail to develop. The deficiency is linked to failure of the thymus gland to mature in the embryo. Cell-mediated immunity is defective in such individuals, and susceptibility is high to many fungal and protozoal diseases and certain viral diseases. Correction of the defect by grafts of thymus tissue has been reported. Partial thymus insufficiencies exist in some cases.

Perhaps the most dangerous immune deficiency disease is **severe combined immunodeficiency (SCID)**, which is characterized by defects in both antibody-mediated and cell-mediated immunity. The B-lymphocyte and T-lymphocyte areas of the lymph nodes are depleted of lymphocytes, and all immune function is suppressed. For many years immunologists believed that the syndrome resulted from a defect in stem cells of the bone marrow, but recent evidence indicates a failure in the normal development of both the thymus and the organ that results in B-lymphocytes.

The longest surviving victim of SCID was a boy known only as David (to protect his privacy). David lived for 12 years inside a sterile, plastic bubble at the Baylor College of Medicine in Houston (**FIGURE 20.13**). On October 21, 1983, he received a bone marrow transplant from his sister as doctors attempted to establish an immune system within his body. Three months later, David left the bubble, but on February 22, 1984, he died as a result of blood cancer traced to a virus apparently brought into his body by the transplant.

Other immune deficiency diseases are linked to the **neutrophils**, or polymorphonuclear (PMN) cells (Chapter 17). In these diseases, phagocytes fail to engulf and kill microorganisms because of defects in chemotaxis, ingestion, and/or intracellular digestion. For example, in the rare disease known as **Chédiak-Higashi syndrome**, a delayed killing of phagocytized microorganisms is traceable to the inability of lysosomes to release their contents. Another disease, called **Job syndrome**, is accompanied by defective chemotaxis. Scientists sometimes call this disease the "lazy leukocyte syndrome."

DiGeorge syndrome:
an immune deficiency disease characterized by the absence of T-lymphocytes.

Neutrophils:
phagocytic white blood cells with cytoplasmic granules and multi-lobed nuclei.

Job syndrome:
an immune deficiency disease in which defective chemotaxis leads to poor phagocytosis.

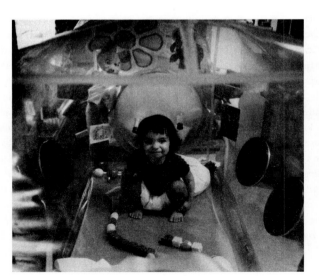

FIGURE 20.13

David, the Boy in the Plastic Bubble

David suffered from severe combined immunodeficiency (SCID) and lived for 12 years within the sterile confines of a plastic bubble. In 1983, he received a bone marrow transplant from his sister and left the bubble. Unfortunately, he developed a blood cancer and died some months thereafter.

Deficiencies in the **complement system** may be life-threatening. As noted in Chapter 18, complement is a series of proteins any of which the body may fail to produce. For reasons not currently understood, many patients with complement component deficiencies suffer systemic lupus erythematosus (SLE) or an SLE-like syndrome. Meningococcal and pneumococcal diseases are often observed in patients who lack C3, probably as a result of poor opsonization.

Although **acquired immune deficiency disease (AIDS)** is considered a viral disease (Chapter 13), we shall also mention it here. In patients with AIDS, cell-mediated immunity is severely weakened, while antibody-mediated immunity may also be altered. The number of T-lymphocytes is sparse, and a striking imbalance is observed between two subgroups of T-lymphocytes, the helper T-lymphocytes and the suppressor T-lymphocytes. Usually, the number of helper cells is twice that of suppressor cells, but in AIDS patients, the number of helper cells dramatically decreases. In scientific writing, the helper/suppressor ratio is expressed as the CD4/CD8 ratio because monoclonal antibody OkT4 identifies helper cells, and monoclonal antibody OkT8 identifies suppressor cells. The CD4/CD8 ratio in normal individuals is about 2:1, but in AIDS patients, it is permanently reversed.

20.4

Transplantation Immunology

Modern techniques for the transplantation of tissues and organs trace their origins to Jacques Reverdin, who in 1870 successfully grafted bits of skin to wounded tissues. Enthusiasm for the technique rose after his reports were published, but it waned when doctors found that most transplants were rapidly rejected by the body. Then in 1954, a kidney was transplanted between identical twins, and again, interest grew. The graft survived for several years, until ultimately it was destroyed by a recurrence of the recipient's original kidney disease. During that time, attempts to transplant kidneys between unrelated individuals were less successful.

Transplantation technology improved considerably during the next few decades, and today, four types of transplantations, or grafts, are recognized, depending upon the genetic relationship between donor and recipient. A graft taken from one part of the body and transplanted to another part of the same body is called an **autograft**. This graft is never rejected because it is the person's own tissue. A tissue taken from an identical twin and grafted to the other twin is an **isograft**. This, too, is not rejected because the genetic constitutions of identical twins are the same.

Rejection mechanisms become more vigorous as the genetic constitutions of donor and recipient cells become more varied (MicroFocus 20.8). For instance, grafts between brothers and sisters, or between fraternal twins, may lead to only mild rejection because many of their genes are similar. Grafts between cousins may be rejected more rapidly, and as the relationship becomes more distant, the vigor of rejection increases proportionally. **Allografts**, or grafts between random members of the same species, such as two humans, have variable degrees of success, while **xenografts**, or grafts between members of different species, such as a monkey and a human, are rarely successful. TABLE 20.6 summarizes this terminology.

Transplanted tissue is rejected by the body if the immune system interprets the tissue as nonself. The rejection mechanisms may take either of two forms. In the first

Autograft:
tissue grafted from one part of the body to another.

Allograft:
tissue grafted between members of the same species.
zen′o-graft

TABLE 20.6

A Summary of Transplantation Terminology

PREFIX	MEANING	COMBINING SUFFIXES	TRANSPLANTATION PARLANCE
Auto-	Self	-graft -geneic -antigen -antibody	An autograft is a self-graft, e.g., skin from one site of the patient's body moved to another site on the patient's body
Iso-	Equal; identical with another	"	An isograft is a graft between isogeneic individuals, i.e., between genetically identical individuals such as identical twins
Allo- (homo-)	Similar or like another	"	An allograft is a graft between allogeneic individuals, i.e., between nonidentical members of the same species
Xeno- (hetero-)	Dissimilar or unlike another; foreign	"	A xenograft is a graft between xenogeneics, i.e., between members of different species, as a graft from monkey to human

MicroFocus 20.8

ACCEPTANCE

Ordinarily a woman will reject a foreign organ, such as a kidney or heart, but she will accept the fetus growing within her womb. This acceptance exists, even though half the fetus' genetic information has come from a "foreigner"—namely, the father. Has her immune system failed?

Apparently not. It seems that the sperm carries an antigenic signal, which induces the woman's immune system to produce a series of so-called blocking antibodies. The blocking antibodies form a type of protective screen that sheaths the fetus and prevents its antigens from stimulating the production of rejection antibodies by the mother. So protected, the fetus grows to term and "escapes" before any immunological damage can be done to its tissues.

But sometimes a rejection in the form of a miscarriage occurs. A number of physicians now believe that at least cer-

tain miscarriages have an immunological basis. Their research indicates that the level of blocking antibodies in some pregnant women is too low to protect the fetus, and that the miscarriage is due to the woman's antibodies. Ironically, they have discovered the blocking antibody level may be low because the father's tissue is very similar to the mother's. In such a case, the sperm's antigens elicit a weak antibody response, too low to protect the fetus.

With this knowledge in hand, physicians are now attempting to boost the level of blocking antibodies as a way of preventing miscarriage. They inject white blood cells from the father into the mother, thereby stimulating her immune system to produce antibodies to the cells. These antibodies exhibit the blocking effect. In other experiments, injections of blocking antibodies are administered to augment the woman's

normal supply. Both approaches have been successful in trial experiments, and continuing research has given cause for optimism that fetal rejection will give way to acceptance.

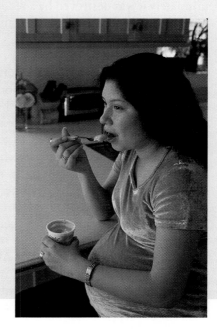

mechanism, cytotoxic T-lymphocytes aided by helper T-lymphocytes attack and destroy transplanted cells. The process is stimulated by the recognition of foreign MHC proteins (to be discussed next) on the surface of the graft cells. Class II MHC proteins stimulate helper T-lymphocytes, while class I MHC proteins are the sites that the cytotoxic cells recognize during their attack.

A second rejection mechanism involves helper T-lymphocytes alone. These lymphocytes are stimulated by class II MHC proteins, after which the lymphocytes release lymphokines (cytokines). The lymphokines stimulate phagocytes to enter the graft tissue. The phagocytes secrete lysosomal enzymes, which digest the tissues, leading to a dryness and thickening, as in type IV hypersensitivity. Cell death, or necrosis, follows.

Necrosis: cell death.

A rejection mechanism of a completely different sort is sometimes observed in bone marrow transplants. In this case, the transplanted marrow may contain immune system cells that form immune products against the host after the host's immune system has been suppressed during transplant therapy. Essentially, the graft is rejecting the host. This phenomenon is called a **graft-versus-host reaction (GVHR)**. It can sometimes lead to fatal consequences in the host body.

THE MAJOR HISTOCOMPATIBILITY COMPLEX

During the 1970s, immunologists determined that the acceptance or rejection of a graft depends largely on a relatively small number of genes called the major histocompatibility complex (MHC) genes. These genes encode a series of cell-surface glycoproteins called **major histocompatibility complex (MHC) proteins**, also known as **human leukocyte antigens (HLAs)**. The 1980 Nobel Prize in Physiology or Medicine was awarded to George Snell, Jean Dausset, and Baraj Benacerraf for their discoveries regarding MHC genes and proteins.

his'to-kom-pat'ĭ-bil'ĭ-te

The MHC genes are believed to exist on chromosome 6 in humans. The actual gene complex consists of four clusters of genes, each gene having multiple versions, or alleles. Two individuals chosen at random (a husband and wife, for example) are not expected to have many MHC genes in common. Identical twins, by contrast, have identical MHC genes. MHC proteins are of two types: class I and class II. Class II MHC proteins are important in the recognition of nonself antigens when T-lymphocytes combine with macrophages in cell-mediated immunity (Chapter 18). Class I MHC proteins are present on every cell in the human body and help define the uniqueness of a person's tissue. For this reason, they are important subjects of transplantation immunology.

Alleles: different versions of the same gene.

The nature of MHC proteins is a key element in transplant acceptance or rejection: The closer the match between donor and recipient MHC proteins, the greater the chance of a successful transplant. The matching of donor and recipient is performed by **tissue typing** (FIGURE 20.14). In this procedure, the laboratory uses standardized MHC antibodies for particular MHC proteins. Lymphocytes from the donor are incubated with a selected type of MHC antibodies. Complement and a dye, such as trypan blue, are then added. If the selected MHC antibodies react with the MHC proteins of the lymphocytes, the cell becomes permeable and dye enters the cells (living cells are not normally invaded by dye). Similar tests are then performed with recipient lymphocytes to determine which MHC proteins are present and how closely the tissues match one another. The blood types of donor and recipient must also be identical.

Tissue typing: a process used to determine how closely two tissues match genetically.

Studies of the MHC proteins also provide clues about the development of certain immune diseases. In **Graves' disease**, for example, antibodies appear to unite with

FIGURE 20.14

Tissue Typing for MHC Proteins

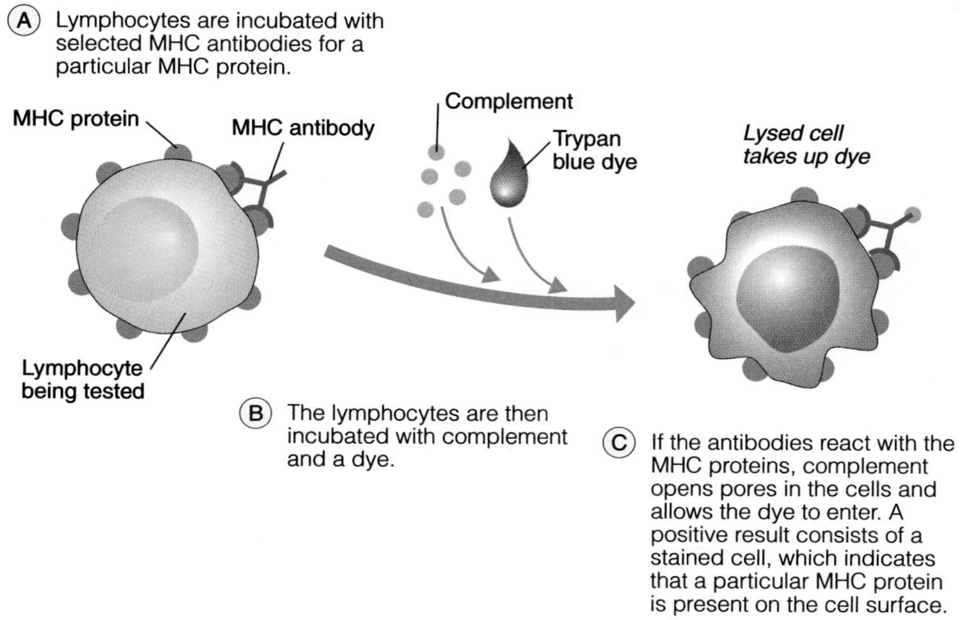

(A) Lymphocytes are incubated with selected MHC antibodies for a particular MHC protein.

MHC protein   MHC antibody   Complement   Trypan blue dye   Lysed cell takes up dye

Lymphocyte being tested

(B) The lymphocytes are then incubated with complement and a dye.

(C) If the antibodies react with the MHC proteins, complement opens pores in the cells and allows the dye to enter. A positive result consists of a stained cell, which indicates that a particular MHC protein is present on the cell surface.

ang'ki-lo'sing spon'di-li'tis

MHC proteins on the surface of thyroid gland cells and overstimulate the gland. Another example is seen in **ankylosing spondylitis**, a spinal disease in which adjacent vertebrae fuse and cause fixation and stiffness of the spine. The relative risk for this disease is far greater when individuals possess particular MHC proteins. A final possibility is that certain viruses, because of their similarity to MHC proteins, induce antibodies that attack body cells. This may be the source of Guillain-Barré syndrome and Reye syndrome that follow cases of influenza.

ANTIREJECTION MECHANISMS

a'zah-thi'o-prēn

Cyclosporin A: an antirejection drug that appears to suppress cell-mediated immunity.

Tissue typing and histocompatibility screening help reduce the rejection mechanism in allograft transfers, but they do not eliminate the mechanism completely. To inhibit rejection, it is necessary to suppress activity of the immune system. One method utilizes **antimitotic drugs**, which prevent multiplication of lymphocytes in the lymph nodes. The drug **azathioprine** is a nucleic acid antagonist used for this purpose. Another drug is **cyclosporin A**. Originally isolated from strains of fungi as an antimicrobial substance, this drug is now produced synthetically. It appears to suppress cell-mediated immunity without killing T-lymphocytes or interfering with antibody formation. Immunologists believe that cyclosporin A prevents the division of helper T-lymphocytes by blocking formation of the growth and division factor interleukin-2. Suppressor T-lymphocytes are apparently resistant to the drug.

Another means of diminishing the rejection mechanism is to introduce **antilymphocyte antibodies**. To obtain these antibodies, lymphocytes from the transplant recipient are injected into animals, and later, the animals are bled to obtain the antibody-rich serum. When introduced to the transplant recipient (serum sickness notwithstanding), the antibodies interact with the local lymphocytes, thereby slowing the rejection process and increasing the survival time of the transplant.

pred'nĭ-sōn

Additional methods of reducing rejection include the use of **prednisone**, a steroid hormone that suppresses the inflammatory response, and the bombardment of lymphocyte centers with **radiations** such as X rays. In another experimental treatment, the donor's bone marrow cells are injected into the recipient's bone marrow to induce lymphocytes that will recognize the transplant as self. It should be noted that virtually all treatments leave the recipient in an immunosuppressed condition, thereby increasing the susceptibility to a variety of infectious diseases. Immunosuppression is, at best, a poor expedient and is viewed as only a stopgap measure until the rejection mechanism can be understood and exploited.

20.5

Tumor Immunology

The alteration from a normal cell to a cell with tumor potential is accompanied by many physiological changes, including the change to an immature form, the loss of contact inhibition, and an increased rate of mitosis (Chapter 11). In addition, tumor cells contain antigens not found in surrounding cells, because they differentiate and revert to embryological cells. Since many of these antigens localize on the cell surface, they might be expected to induce an immune response and make the cancer cells vulnerable to destruction. However, the cells escape the resistance mechanisms of the body and proliferate to form the tumor. As the tumor breaks apart and spreads, a metastasizing cancer develops (FIGURE 20.15).

Host resistance to tumors depends on immune responses directed against the tumor antigens. This process is termed **immune surveillance**. It is considered an ongoing function of cytotoxic T-lymphocytes, which recognize the antigens as foreign and destroy the cells containing them in a manner analogous to graft rejection. Another cell thought to function in immune surveillance is the **natural killer (NK) cell**, which is a type of T-lymphocyte. NK cells exert a nonspecific, cytotoxic effect on other cells, including tumor cells. They kill cells in the absence of a prior sensitization and without the involvement of antibody. Interferon appears to regulate their activity and can increase it.

Cytotoxic T-lymphocyte: a T-lymphocyte that destroys cells displaying certain antigens.

Despite immune surveillance, tumors continue to occur in otherwise healthy people as tumor cells escape destruction. Various theories are offered to account for this **immunologic escape**. One possibility is such individuals learn to tolerate tumor cells before immunocompetence has developed, and then they express the tumors later in life. Another theory is that the majority of cancer cells are destroyed by NK cells, but that rapidly growing variants emerge and outpace the immune system. It is also possible that tumor antigens elicit antibodies that protect against natural killer cells by combining with antigens to form a complex to block NK cell activity. A final theory points to the release by tumor cells of substances that suppress the immune system, such as happens in **Hodgkin's disease** of the lymph nodes. Although experimental evidence exists for each theory, no one is universally accepted.

Immunotherapy for the management of cancer is developing along several lines. It has been suggested, for example, that killer lymphocytes specific for the tumor be injected into the patient or that monoclonal antibodies for tumor antigens be utilized (FIGURE 20.16). **Interferon** has also been investigated as a way of enhancing the activity of natural killer cells. In 1986, the FDA approved its use against **hairy cell leukemia**, a cancer of the white blood cells named for the hairlike appendages on malignant cells.

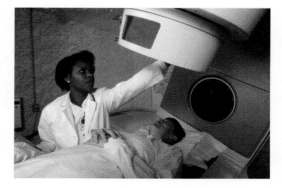

FIGURE 20.15

A Patient Being Treated with Radiation to Reduce a Tumor

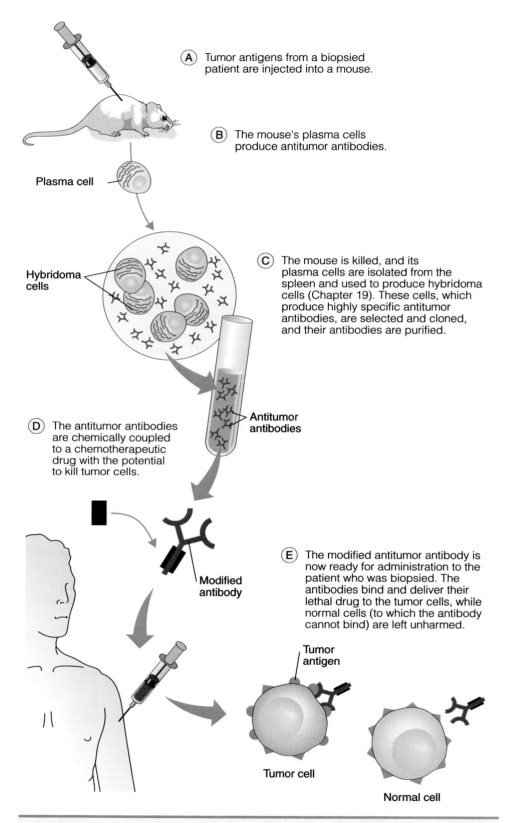

A Tumor antigens from a biopsied patient are injected into a mouse.

B The mouse's plasma cells produce antitumor antibodies.

Plasma cell

Hybridoma cells

C The mouse is killed, and its plasma cells are isolated from the spleen and used to produce hybridoma cells (Chapter 19). These cells, which produce highly specific antitumor antibodies, are selected and cloned, and their antibodies are purified.

Antitumor antibodies

D The antitumor antibodies are chemically coupled to a chemotherapeutic drug with the potential to kill tumor cells.

Modified antibody

E The modified antitumor antibody is now ready for administration to the patient who was biopsied. The antibodies bind and deliver their lethal drug to the tumor cells, while normal cells (to which the antibody cannot bind) are left unharmed.

Tumor antigen

Tumor cell

Normal cell

FIGURE 20.16

Monoclonal Antibodies in Tumor Therapy

Specific monoclonal antibodies are receiving clinical testing in new approaches to tumor therapy.

In the 1980s, interest grew in therapy with **interleukin-2**, a T-lymphocyte protein (a lymphokine) that stimulates the rapid multiplication of helper T-lymphocytes. In clinical trials, about 10 billion lymphocytes are removed from the cancer patient's blood and cultured for 3 days with interleukin-2. This process converts the resting lymphocytes to functional helper T-lymphocytes known as **lymphokine-activated killer (LAK) cells**. The LAK cells, along with additional amounts of interleukin-2, are then reinfused into the patient's bloodstream where they attack tumor cells. The gene for interleukin-2 has already been cloned, and biotechnology firms are now producing the lymphokine in volume by recombinant DNA techniques.

Another anticancer agent that has drawn attention is the **tumor necrosis factor (TNF)**. TNF, a protein product of macrophages, was discovered in 1975 by researchers at Memorial Sloan-Kettering Cancer Center in New York. The protein is currently produced by genetic engineering techniques and has been shown effective against more than 20 kinds of cancer cells grown in cultures. Combination with interferon appears to improve its anti-tumor abilities. At present, tumor immunology and treatment contain more questions than answers, but the prognosis remains positive.

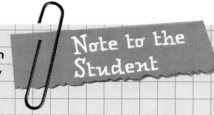

Note to the Student

The body's immunologic responses to transplants and tumors represent an ironic dilemma. Against transplants, the immune system responds vigorously (immunologists attempt to suppress the response); against tumors, the immune system responds weakly (immunologists attempt to enhance the response). Would that the situations could be reversed.

Summary

Among the immune disorders that affect humans are a series of hypersensitivity reactions categorized in four types. Type I hypersensitivity is accompanied by anaphylaxis, a whole-body reaction in which a series of mediators induce vigorous and life-threatening contractions by the smooth muscles of the body. The predominant antibody in anaphylaxis is IgE, produced in response to certain antigens and able to attach to the surfaces of mast cells and basophils. These cells release the mediators on subsequent exposure to the antigens. A localized anaphylaxis is a common allergy, such as hay fever or a food allergy.

The second type of hypersensitivity, type II, is called cytotoxic hypersensitivity. In this process, the immune system produces IgG and IgM, both of which react with the body's cells and often destroy the latter. The destruction of platelets in thrombocytopenia and neutrophils in agranulocytosis is typical of the immune disorder. No cells are involved in type III hypersensitivity. Rather, the body's IgG and IgM interact with dissolved antigen molecules to form visible masses of matter called immune complexes. The accumulation of immune complexes in various organs leads to local tissue destruction in such illnesses as serum sickness, Arthus phenomenon, and systemic lupus erythematosus. A final type of hypersensitivity involves no antibodies but is an exaggeration of the process of cell-mediated immunity based in T-lymphocytes. Contact dermatitis may be a manifestation of this hypersensitivity.

Immune disorders also include immune deficiency diseases in which important cells of the immune system, such as B- or T-lymphocytes, are not formed. Deficiencies in phagocytic cells or complement components may also be observed. The activity of the immune system is a key factor in the acceptance or rejection of transplanted tissue, and an understanding of immune system functions enhances our understanding of the development of tumors and how to deal with them.

Questions for Thought and Discussion

1. In December 1967, people throughout the world were startled to learn that Christiaan A. Barnard, a South African physician, had made the first successful heart transplant. The patient, Louis Washkansky, survived the rejection mechanism for 2 weeks before dying of pneumonia. Many scientists consider Barnard's surgery to signal the beginning of modern immunology. What evidence do you think might be offered to support this contention?

2. During war and under emergency conditions a soldier whose blood type is O donates blood to save the life of a fellow soldier with type B blood. The soldier lives, and after the war becomes a police officer. One day he is called to donate blood to a brother officer who has been wounded and finds that it is his old friend from the war. He gladly rolls up his sleeve and prepares for the transfusion. Should it be allowed to proceed? Why?

3. Coming from the anatomy lab, you notice that your hands are red and raw and have begun peeling in several spots. This was your third period of dissection. What is happening to your hands, and what could be causing the condition? How will you solve the problem?

4. Researchers have found that the powder in latex-powdered gloves has the ability to aerate and spread allergy-inducing latex proteins. Ordinarily, the powder helps hurried medical personnel don the gloves in emergency situations. Can you think of any substitute material that can be used to resolve the problem of "sticky gloves"?

5. A scientist observed ten men and noticed the following: All used an excessive amount of antihistamine, all were tall and had blond hair and a mustache, all were avid fishermen, and all enjoyed movies. Then she observed ten more men: All used less antihistamine than the first group, all were short and had black hair and no mustache, all were avid golfers, and all enjoyed fine dining. Which trait in the second group correlates with their tendency to use less antihistamine? What advice would the scientist give to men in the first group?

6. As part of an experiment, one animal is fed a raw egg, while a second animal is injected intravenously with a raw egg. Which animal is in greater danger? Why?

7. "He had a history of nasal congestion, swelling of his eyes and difficulty breathing through his nose. He gave a history of blowing his nose frequently, and the congestion was so severe during the spring he had difficulty running." The person in this description is a certain former President of the United States, and the writer is an allergist from Little Rock, Arkansas. What condition (technically known as allergic rhinitis) is probably being described?

8. When the skin of the feet becomes itchy, red, and scaly, many people assume they have athlete's foot, a fungal disease. However, allergists now know that the irritation could be a contact dermatitis resulting from chemicals in the insoles of sneakers. How might the distinction be made by physical examination of the feet and by laboratory testing?

9. A woman is having the fifth injection in a weekly series of hay fever shots. Shortly after leaving the allergist's office, she develops a flush on her face, itching sensations of the skin, and shortness of breath. She becomes dizzy, then faints. What is taking place in her body, and why has it not happened after the first four injections?

10. You may have noted that brothers and sisters are allowed to be organ donors for one another, but that a person cannot always donate to his or her spouse. Many people feel bad about being unable to help a loved one in time of need. How might you explain to someone in such a situation the basis for becoming an organ donor and why it may be impossible to serve as one?

11. Some years ago there was a commercial for a life insurance company that included this jingle: "There's nobody else exactly like you; nobody else like you." Why is this concept immunologically correct?

12. The story is told that in 1552, the distinguished physician Jerome Cardan of Pavia was called to England to advise treatment for Archbishop John Hamilton. Hamilton had suffered from asthma for 10 years. Cardan prescribed a carefully controlled diet, plenty of exercise and sleep, and the removal of feathers from the archbishop's mattress. Soon the asthma diminished. Which of Cardan's recommendations was the key to success? Why?

13. Paternity suits are often settled by determining the blood types of parents and child, and then concluding whether the man could be the father of the child. How could determining the major histocompatibility complex be used to replace the blood-typing procedure in paternity suits of the future?

14. In order to prevent hemolytic disease of the newborn, rh antibodies must be injected into an Rh-negative woman shortly after the birth of an rh-positive child. Where do you suppose these antibodies were obtained in the past, and what might be their source in the future?

15. The immune system is commonly regarded as one that provides protection against disease. This chapter, however, seems to indicate that the immune system is responsible for numerous afflictions. Even the title is "Immune Disorders". Does this mean that the immune system should be given a new name? On the other hand, is it possible that all these afflictions are actually the result of the body's attempts to protect itself? And finally, why can the phrase "immune disorder" be considered an oxymoron?

Review

This chapter has summarized some of the disorders associated with the immune system. To gauge your understanding, rearrange the scrambled letters to form the correct word for each of the spaces in the statements. The correct answers are in Appendix D.

1. The simple compound _____ is one of the major mediators released during allergy reactions.

   I T M E H I A S N

2. An immune deficiency called _____ syndrome is characterized by the failure of T-lymphocytes to develop.

   I D O G G E R E

3. In type IV hypersensitivity, a drying and thickening of the skin known as _____ is an observable symptom.

   A N U I R O N I D T

4. Cases of rheumatoid arthritis are accompanied by immune complex formation in the body's _____.

   N I S T J O

5. In cases of _____ disease, antibody molecules unite with receptors on the surface of thyroid gland cells.

   V S R E A G

6. In a _____ hypersensitivity, antibodies unite with cells and trigger a reaction that results in cell destruction.

   X Y O T C C I T O

7. Hay fever is an example of an _____ disease, one in which a local allergy takes place.

   O C T I A P

8. Immune complex hypersensitivities develop when antibody molecules interact with _____ molecules and form aggregates in the tissues.

   E N I G N A T

9. In people suffering from Bruton's agammaglobulinemia, the lymph nodes are noticeably deficient in _____ cells.

   S L M A A P

10. The skin test for _____ relies on a response by T-lymphocytes to PPD placed in the skin tissues.

    U U I C T R L S B E O S

11. Mast cells and _____ are the two principal cells that function in anaphylactic responses.

    S S B I O H P A L

12. During cases of thrombocytopenia, antibodies react with platelets and cause them to undergo _____.

    Y S S L I

13. Rh disease can develop in a fetus if the father's blood type was Rh-_____ and the mother's type was Rh-negative.

    O S I P I E T V

14. The glomerulonephritis that accompanies streptococcal disease may be due to immune complex formation in the _____.

    N I Y E K D

15. A key element in transplant acceptance or rejection is a set of molecules abbreviated as _____ proteins.

    H C M

16. Urticaria is a form of skin _____ that occurs in a person having an allergic reaction.

    A H S R

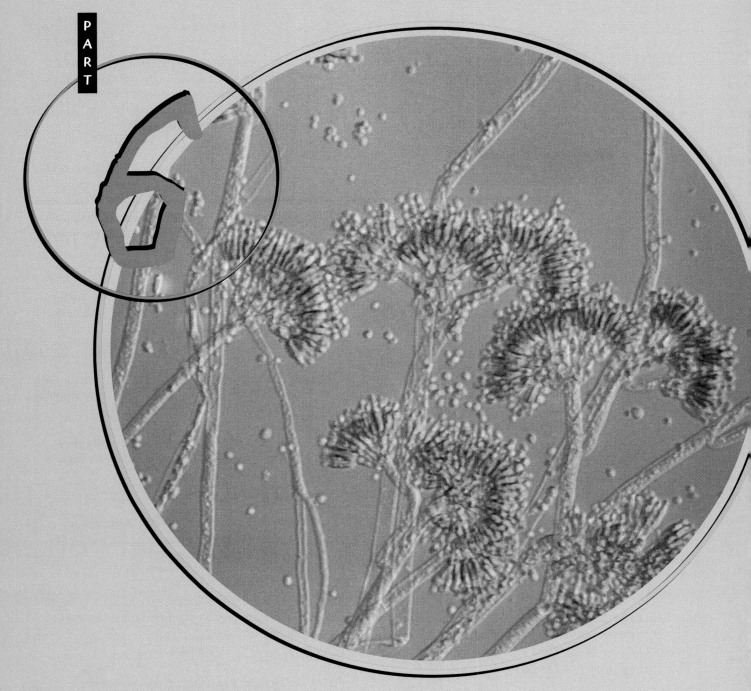

Control of Microorganisms

In the late 1800s and early 1900s, growing support for the germ theory of disease led to a dramatic reduction in the frequency of epidemics. Scientists reasoned that if microorganisms cause disease, then it was possible to control disease by controlling the microorganisms. The idea had been proposed by Pasteur decades before, but not until the turn of the century did it gather momentum and achieve a firm footing in the scientific community.

Two types of control gradually evolved: physical control and chemical control. To achieve physical control, scientists used heat, radiations, filters, and other physical agents to remove microorganisms from instruments, equipment, and fluids. Pasteurization of dairy products was in wide use by 1895, and food preservation methods were gradually updated. To achieve chemical control, doctors utilized antiseptics and disinfectants in medicine, surgery, and wound treatment. Moreover, municipalities began adding chlorine to their water supplies to protect citizens from waterborne diseases. As control methods became a way of life in public health, the chains of microbial transmission broke down, and disease outbreaks declined.

But little could be done for the patient who already was ill. Here, another type of control was necessary, one that supplemented the body's own natural defenses. That control device would emerge in the 1940s with the discovery and development of chemotherapeutic agents and antibiotics. Now, physicians could do something about diseases they could not hope to treat before. The new drugs and medicines ushered in a second dramatic reduction in the incidence of infectious disease.

The control of microorganisms is an essential factor in maintaining good health. In Part 6, we shall consider a variety of control methods and examine their uses and modes of action. Our survey will begin in Chapter 21 with an exploration of physical methods of control used for objects outside the body. It will continue in Chapter 22, where we examine chemical methods for objects that come in contact with the body (e.g., instruments) and on the body surface itself. Finally, in Chapter 23 we shall move inside the body environment to discuss chemotherapeutic agents and antibiotics. Applied on a broad scale, these control methods remain a major deterrent to infection and disease.

SALES AND RESEARCH

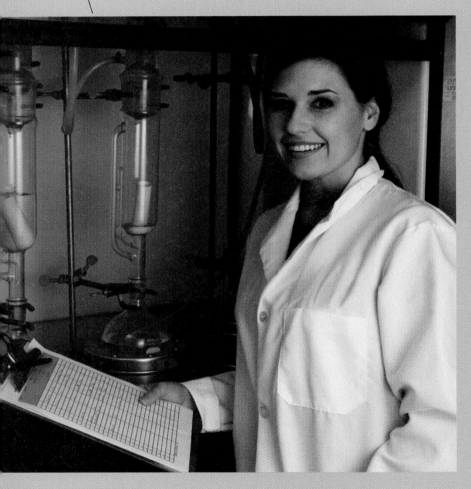

Not all salespeople sell vacuum cleaners or brushes. And not all microbiologists wear white coats and work in ultraclean laboratories. It is quite commonplace for a person trained in microbiology to find a comfortable and enjoyable future with a company that sells and distributes instruments, scientific chemicals, and pharmaceuticals. For example, it is valuable for a sterilizer salesperson to understand the microbiological basis for sterilizing such things as instruments, microbial media, and patient materials. Also, it makes sense for a disinfectant salesperson to realize why microorganisms must be eliminated from a particular surface. Finally, without question, an individual selling new antibiotics should have a strong familiarity with the microorganisms that the antibiotic is intended to eliminate. The bottom line is: Know your product, and know what to use it for.

Before a product is available for sale, however, it must be developed, and once again, the microbiologist is a member of the team. The microbiologist can appreciate why new methods must be developed for preserving dairy products and for storing foods. The microbiologist will be able to set the direction for developing new sterilizing instruments and can have significant input into the development of pharmaceuticals for treating infectious disease. The diagnostic lab will depend heavily on instruments produced under the guidance of microbiologists because the lab's objective is to detect microorganisms.

The contemporary health-care industry depends heavily on the talents of microbiologists for the development and sale of innovative and novel approaches to diagnosis and treatment. As you might suspect, a healthy dose of chemistry, physics, and mathematics is valuable, depending upon which road one chooses to follow. The ability to tinker with instruments is important to research and development, while strong interpersonal relationships are important for the sales phase. What may seem like services and sales is really microbiology at its core.

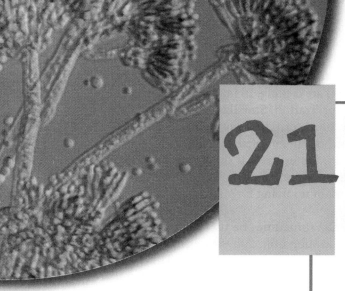

21 Physical Control of Microorganisms

I had difficulty believing anything like this could exist.

—A university microbiologist recalling his introduction to *Deinococcus radiodurans*, a bacterium that survives one-thousand times the radiation lethal to a human

BY THE BEST ESTIMATES of health officials, the problem began during the first week of July during 1988. Early that week, a person unintentionally contaminated the water while swimming in an indoor pool at a school in Los Angeles, California. The same week, the pool was used by a water polo team for its match against a local opponent. Shortly thereafter, a class of scuba divers used the pool to perfect their skills. A group of elementary schoolchildren also enjoyed the pool during a day-camp field trip.

Beginning in early August, doctors began receiving reports of watery diarrhea, abdominal cramps, and fever. Two members of the scuba class were hospitalized. Eleven patients were tested for stool microorganisms and in seven cases, the protozoan *Cryptosporidium* was located. Indeed, the attack rate was highest for those who were exposed to the water the longest. By the second week of August, 44 individuals were affected out of a total of 60 swimmers.

When CDC investigators arrived at the pool, they inquired about the water-purification methods. They were told that three filters were used to sterilize the water, and chlorine was added to maintain a low bacterial count. Their inspection revealed that the chlorination was adequate, but the filtration left much to be desired. One of the three filters was inoperative, and the flow rate of water through the remaining two filters was only 70 percent of the expected rate. It was clear that the water filtration had not worked.

krip'to-spor-id'e-um

675

Sterilization:
the destruction or removal of all forms of life.

Toxin:
a bacterial poison that can inflict damage on body tissues.

di'-pik-o-lin'ik

di'no-kok'us ra'di-o-dur'ans

The episode in Los Angeles illustrates how microorganisms can spread when proper methods of water purification are lacking. In many cases, these purification methods are designed to achieve sterilization. **Sterilization** is the destruction or removal of all life forms. It is an absolute term that cannot be qualified. Thus, one cannot assume "partial sterilization" or "incomplete sterilization," but must consider a material contaminated until it is sterilized. It should be pointed out, however, that material may remain harmful even though it is sterile. For example, a solution of bacterial toxin may contain no living forms but still cause physiological damage in the body.

Although filters and chemicals may sometimes be used to sterilize objects, the principal methods for achieving sterilization utilize physical agents, such as heat and radiation. These methods are not products of the modern era. They were used by Pasteur, Koch, and microbiologists of a century ago to prevent contamination of their materials and to ensure the accuracy of their work.

Microbiologists recognize that bacterial **spores** are among the most resistant forms of life (FIGURE 21.1). Anthrax spores, for example, have been found to remain viable after 60 years on dry silk threads. The spores are not metabolically inert. Rather, they carry on life processes at minimum rates and possess the necessary enzymes to transform from a dormant state to actively metabolizing vegetative cells. The extraordinary survival of spores is often attributed to their low water content, which yields a heat-resistant gel-like spore core. Another possible reason is the presence of **dipicolinic acid**, an organic compound that encourages heat resistance by linking to the spore proteins. Destruction of the bacterial spore is the principal aim of sterilization methods, especially those involving heat.

However, the bacterial spore is not necessarily the most resistant of all microorganisms. Recent research has focused on the bacterium ***Deinococcus radiodurans***, the organism mentioned in the opening quote to this chapter and pictured in FIGURE 21.2. *D. radiodurans* is notable for its resistance to radiation (the *Guinness Book of World Records* labels it the world's "toughest bacterium"). This resistance is

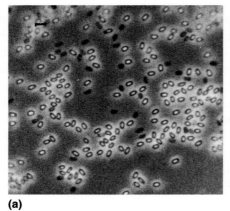
(a)

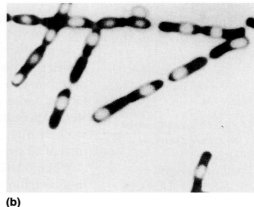
(b)

FIGURE 21.1

The Objectives of Physical Control

Two views of bacterial spores, the destruction of which is the objective of most physical control methods. (a) A phase contrast view of free spores of *Bacillus subtilis*. (Bar = 1 μm.) (b) Clear spores within the stained vegetative cells of *Bacillus anthracis* (×1000). Bacterial spores are among the most resistant forms of life known to science.

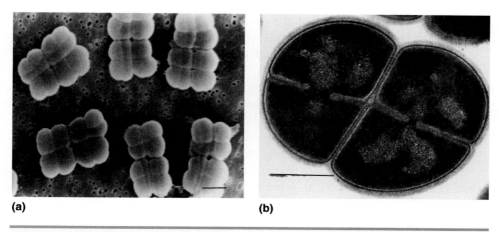

(a)   **(b)**

FIGURE 21.2

Extreme Radiation Resistance

Electron micrographs of *Deinococcus radiodurans*, a bacterium that can withstand a thousand times the radiation lethal to humans. (a) This organism is a tetracoccus, as shown in the scanning electron micrograph. (Bar = 2 μm.) (b) The transmission electron micrograph shows the complex cell wall of the four cells in the tetracoccus. (Bar = 1 μm.)

more substantial than for bacterial spores and may derive from the bacterium's unusually high ability to repair its DNA once radiation damage has occurred. In 1998, the complete genome of the organism was deciphered, and researchers began studying the genes for clues about the nature of the extreme radiation resistance. Indeed, the organism is being considered as a tool for detoxifying waste sites that contain radioactive materials, a process called bioremediation (Chapter 26).

21.1

Physical Control with Heat

he Citadel is a novel by A. J. Cronin that follows the life of a young British physician, beginning in the 1920s. Early in the story, the physician, Andrew Manson, begins his practice in a small coal-mining town in Wales. Almost immediately, he encounters an epidemic of typhoid fever. When his first patient dies of the disease, Manson becomes terribly distraught. However, he realizes that the epidemic can be halted, and in the next scene, he is tossing all of the patient's bedsheets, clothing, and personal effects into a huge bonfire.

Typhoid fever:
a serious waterborne and food-borne bacterial disease accompanied by intestinal ulcers and high fever.

The killing effect of **heat** on microorganisms has long been known. Heat is fast, reliable, and relatively inexpensive, and it does not introduce chemicals to a substance, as disinfectants sometimes do. Above maximum growth temperatures, biochemical changes in the cell's organic molecules result in its death. These changes arise from alterations in enzyme molecules or chemical breakdowns of structural molecules, especially in cell membranes. Heat also drives off water, and since all organisms depend on water, this loss may be fatal.

The killing rate of heat may be expressed as a function of time and temperature. For example, tubercle bacilli are destroyed in 30 minutes at 58°C, but in only 2 minutes at 65°C, and in a few seconds at 72°C. Each microbial species has a **thermal death time**,

Thermal death time:
the time required to kill a population of microorganisms at a given temperature.

the time necessary for killing it at a given temperature. Each species also has a **thermal death point**, the temperature at which it dies in a given time. These measurements are particularly important in the food industry, where heat is used for preservation (Chapter 24).

When determining the time and temperature for microbial destruction with heat, certain factors bear consideration. One factor is the type of organism to be killed. For example, if materials are to be sterilized, the physical method must be directed at bacterial spores. Milk, however, need not be sterile for consumption, and heat is therefore aimed at the most resistant vegetative cells.

Another factor is the type of material to be treated. Powder is subjected to dry heat rather than moist heat, because moist heat will leave it soggy. Saline solutions, by contrast, can be sterilized with moist heat but are not easily treated with dry heat. Other important factors are the presence of organic matter and the acidic or basic nature of the material. Organic matter may prevent heat from reaching microorganisms, while acidity or alkalinity may encourage the lethal action of heat.

THE DIRECT FLAME

Perhaps the most rapid sterilization method is the use of a **direct flame** in the process of incineration. The flame of the Bunsen burner is employed for a **few seconds** to sterilize the bacteriological loop before removing a sample from a culture tube and after preparing a smear (**FIGURE 21.3**). Flaming the tip of the tube also destroys organisms that happen to contact the tip, while burning away lint and dust.

In general, objects must be disposable if a flame is used for sterilization. Disposable hospital gowns and certain plastic apparatus are examples of materials that may be incinerated. In past centuries, the bodies of disease victims were burned to prevent spread of the pestilence (**FIGURE 21.4**). It is still common practice to incinerate the carcasses of cattle that have died of **anthrax** and to put the contaminated field to the torch because anthrax spores cannot adequately be destroyed by other means. Indeed, British law stipulates that anthrax-contaminated animals may not be autopsied before burning.

Saline:
salt or salty.

Anthrax:
a highly lethal bacterial disease of the blood and other organs caused by a sporeforming bacillus.

FIGURE 21.3

Use of the Direct Flame As a Sterilizing Agent

Laboratory use of the Bunsen burner. A few seconds in the flame is usually sufficient to effect sterilization.

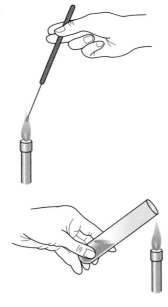

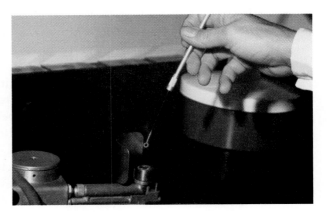

THE HOT-AIR OVEN

The **hot-air oven** utilizes radiating dry heat for sterilization. This type of energy does not penetrate materials easily, and therefore, long periods of exposure to high temperatures are necessary. For example, at a temperature of **160°C (320°F)**, a period of **2 hours** is required for the destruction of bacterial spores. Higher temperatures are not recommended because the wrapping paper used for equipment tends to char at 180°C. The hot-air method is useful for sterilizing dry powders and water-free oily substances, as well as for many types of glassware, such as pipettes, flasks, and syringes. Dry heat does not corrode sharp instruments as steam often does, nor does it erode the ground glass surfaces of nondisposable syringes.

The effect of **dry heat** on microorganisms is equivalent to that of baking. The heat changes microbial proteins by **oxidation** reactions and creates an arid internal environment, thereby burning microorganisms slowly. It is essential that organic matter such as oil or grease films be removed from the materials, because organic matter insulates against dry heat. Moreover, the time required for heat to reach sterilizing temperatures varies according to the material. This factor must be considered in determining the total exposure time.

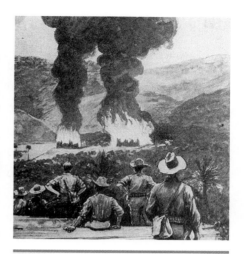

FIGURE 21.4

Incineration

A newspaper photograph from the Spanish-American War showing troops burning an evacuated yellow fever hospital in Cuba. Such methods were a drastic but accepted way of preventing the spread of yellow fever during that period.

BOILING WATER

Immersion in **boiling water** is the first of several moist-heat methods that we shall consider. **Moist heat** penetrates materials much more rapidly than dry heat because water molecules conduct heat better than air. Lower temperatures and a shorter exposure time are therefore required than for dry heat (FIGURE 21.5).

Moist heat kills microorganisms by denaturing their proteins. **Denaturation** is a change in the chemical or physical property of a protein. It includes structural alterations due to destruction of the chemical bonds holding proteins in a three-dimensional form. As proteins revert to a two-dimensional structure, they coagulate (denature) and become nonfunctional. Egg protein undergoes a similar transformation when it is boiled. (You might find reviewing the chemical structure of proteins in Chapter 2 helpful to understanding of this process.) The coagulation of proteins requires less energy than oxidation, and, therefore, less heat need be applied.

Boiling water is not considered a sterilizing agent because the destruction of bacterial spores and the inactivation of viruses cannot always be assured. Under ordinary circumstances, with microorganisms at concentrations of less than 1 million per milliliter, most species of microorganisms can be killed within 10 minutes. Indeed, the process may require only a few seconds. However, fungal spores, protozoal cysts, and large concentrations of hepatitis A viruses require up to 30 minutes' exposure. Bacterial spores often require 2 hours or more. Because inadequate information exists on the heat tolerance of many species of microorganisms, boiling water is not reliable for sterilization purposes.

If it is imperative that boiling water be used to destroy microorganisms, materials must be thoroughly cleaned to remove traces of organic matter, such as blood or feces. The minimum exposure period should be 30 minutes, except at high altitudes, where it should be increased to compensate for the lower boiling point of water. All materials should be well covered. Washing soda may be added at a 2 percent concentration to increase the efficiency of the process.

Denaturation:
a change in the usual nature of a substance, such as a structural alteration.

Hepatitis A:
a viral disease of the liver transmitted by contaminated food and water.

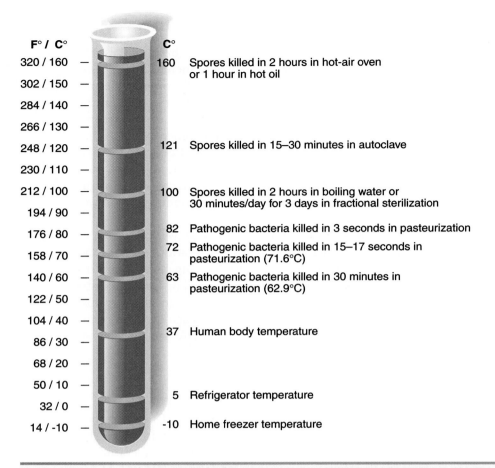

F° / C°   **C°**

320 / 160 —   160   Spores killed in 2 hours in hot-air oven
                      or 1 hour in hot oil

302 / 150 —

284 / 140 —

266 / 130 —

248 / 120 —   121   Spores killed in 15–30 minutes in autoclave

230 / 110 —

212 / 100 —   100   Spores killed in 2 hours in boiling water or
                      30 minutes/day for 3 days in fractional sterilization
194 / 90 —

176 / 80 —   82   Pathogenic bacteria killed in 3 seconds in pasteurization

               72   Pathogenic bacteria killed in 15–17 seconds in
158 / 70 —   pasteurization (71.6°C)

140 / 60 —   63   Pathogenic bacteria killed in 30 minutes in
                      pasteurization (62.9°C)
122 / 50 —

104 / 40 —
               37   Human body temperature
86 / 30 —

68 / 20 —

50 / 10 —
                5   Refrigerator temperature
32 / 0 —

14 / -10 —   -10   Home freezer temperature

FIGURE 21.5

Temperature and the Physical Control of Microorganisms

THE AUTOCLAVE

Moist heat in the form of pressurized steam is regarded as the most dependable method for the destruction of all forms of life, including bacterial spores. This method is incorporated into a device called the **autoclave**. Over 100 years ago, French and German microbiologists developed the autoclave as an essential component of their laboratories. MicroFocus 21.1 details some of the development.

A basic principle of chemistry is that when the pressure of a gas increases, the temperature of the gas increases proportionally. Because steam is a gas, increasing its pressure in a closed system increases its temperature. As the water molecules in steam become more energized, their penetration increases substantially. This principle is used to reduce cooking time in the home pressure cooker and to reduce sterilizing time in the autoclave. It is important to note that the sterilizing agent is the moist heat, not the pressure.

Most autoclaves contain a sterilizing chamber into which articles are placed and a steam jacket where steam is maintained, as shown in FIGURE 21.6. As steam flows from the steam jacket into the sterilizing chamber, cool air is forced out and a special valve increases the pressure to **15 pounds/square inch** (lb/in²) above normal atmospheric pressure. The temperature rises to **121.5°C**, and the superheated water

aw′to-klāv
Autoclave:
a pressurized steam device used
for sterilization purposes.

MicroFocus 21.1

A HEATED CONTROVERSY

Among the last defenders of spontaneous generation was the British physician Harry Carleton Bastian. Louis Pasteur had stated that boiled urine failed to support bacterial growth, but in 1876, Bastian claimed that if the urine were alkaline, microorganisms would occasionally appear. Pasteur repeated Bastian's work and found it correct. This led Pasteur to conclude that certain microorganisms could resist death by boiling. The spores of *Bacillus subtilis*, discovered coincidentally in 1876 by Ferdinand Cohn, were an example.

Pasteur soon realized that he would have to heat his broths at a temperature higher than 100°C to achieve sterilization. He therefore put his pupil and collaborator Charles Chamberland in charge of developing a new sterilizer. Chamberland responded by constructing a pressure steam apparatus patterned after a steam "digester" invented in 1680 by the French physician Denys Papin. The sterilizer resembled a modern pressure cooker. It attained temperatures of 120°C and higher, and established the basis for the modern autoclave. Chamberland would also

achieve fame in later years for his work with porcelain filters.

But Chamberland's invention was not universally accepted. A German group

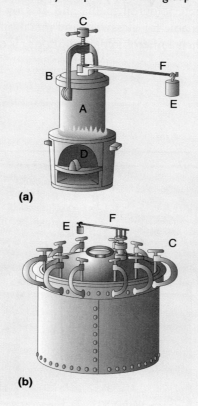

(a)

of investigators, led by Robert Koch, criticized the pressurized steam sterilizer because they believed its higher temperatures would destroy critical laboratory media. Instead they preferred an unpressurized steam sterilizer. In 1881, the German group developed a free-flowing steam sterilizer of the type used in tyndallization. In time, however, they came to appreciate the benefits of pressurized steam as a sterilizing agent, so much so that they modified Chamberland's device to an upright model. Ironically, the instrument became known as the Koch autoclave.

■ *(a) Origins of the autoclave. Denis Papin's steam digester, designed in 1680. The digester consisted of a vessel (A) into which food was placed. The lid (B) and screw (C) sealed the vessel. A furnace (D) raised the temperature, and a weight (E) and safety lever (F) controlled the pressure of steam in the vessel. (b) Chamberland's autoclave, built in 1880 according to the principles of Papin's digester. The lid is held in place by screws (C), and a weight (E) and safety lever (F) are used to control pressure. This autoclave is basically similar to a home pressure cooker.*

(b)

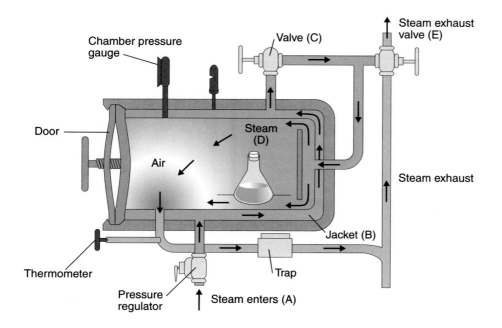

FIGURE 21.6

Operating an Autoclave

Steam enters through the port (A) and passes into the jacket (B). After the air has been exhausted through the vent, a valve (C) opens to admit pressurized steam (D) that circulates among and through the materials, thereby sterilizing them. At the conclusion of the cycle, steam is exhausted through the steam exhaust valve (E).

molecules rapidly conduct heat into microorganisms. The time for destruction of the most resistant bacterial spore is now reduced to about **15 minutes**. For denser objects, up to 30 minutes of exposure may be required. The conditions must be carefully controlled or serious problems could occur, as FIGURE 21.7 indicates.

The autoclave is used to control microorganisms in both hospitals and laboratories. It is employed for blankets, bedding, utensils, instruments, intravenous solutions, and a broad variety of other objects. The laboratory technician uses it to sterilize bacteriological media and destroy pathogenic cultures. The autoclave is equally valuable for glassware and metalware, and is among the first instruments ordered when a microbiology laboratory is established.

FIGURE 21.7

An Outbreak of *Pseudomonas* Infection Traced to a Contaminated Solution

This outbreak occurred in a Thailand hospital during 1992. It illustrates the need to carefully monitor the autoclave during use.

TEXTBOOK CASES

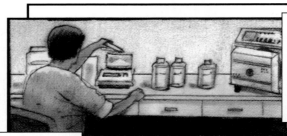

1. The problem began when hospital pharmacists prepared bottles of basal salts solution for use in the hospital operating rooms. To sterilize the solutions, the bottles were placed in the autoclave and left to run on its automatic cycle.

2. The bottles were then delivered to the surgery to be used to irrigate the eyes of patients undergoing cataract surgery. Some bottles were left unused.

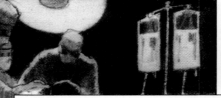

3. Within 30 hours, three cataract patients developed eye inflammations. The organism isolated from the patients was a pathogenic strain of *Pseudomonas*. The patients were treated with antibiotics.

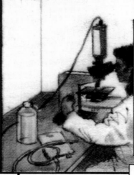

4. Health investigators tested the unused bottles of salt solution as well as the tubes that had been attached to the now empty bottles. The identical strain of *Pseudomonas* was found.

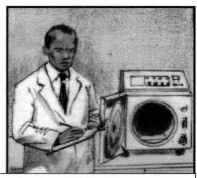

5. Examining the pharmacy records, investigators noted that the autoclave pressure had reached only 10 to 12 lb/in^2, rather than the required 15 lb/in^2. The salts solution apparently was not sterilized.

The autoclave also has certain limitations. For example, some plasticware melts in the high heat, and sharp instruments often become dull. Moreover, many chemicals break down during the sterilization process, and oily substances cannot be treated because they do not mix with water. To gauge the success of sterilization, a strip containing spores of a *Bacillus* species is included with the objects treated (FIGURE 21.8). At the conclusion of the cycle, the strip is placed in nutrient broth medium and incubated. If the sterilization process has been successful, no growth will occur, but growth indicates failure.

Bacillus:
a genus of sporeforming Gram-positive bacterial rods.

In recent years a new form of autoclave, called the **prevacuum autoclave,** has been developed for sterilization procedures. This machine draws air out of the sterilizing chamber at the beginning of the cycle. Saturated steam is then used at a temperature of **132°C to 134°C** at a pressure of **28 to 30 lb/in²**. The time for sterilization is now reduced to as little as **4 minutes.** A vacuum pump operates at the end of the cycle to remove the steam and dry the load. The major advantages of the prevacuum autoclave are the minimal exposure time for sterilization and the reduced time to complete the cycle.

FRACTIONAL STERILIZATION

In the years before the development of the autoclave, liquids and other objects were sterilized by exposure to free-flowing steam at 100°C for 30 minutes on each of 3 successive days, with incubation periods between the steaming. The method was called **fractional sterilization** because a fraction was accomplished on each day. It was also called **tyndallization** after its developer, John Tyndall (MicroFocus 21.2).

Fractional sterilization:
sterilization by exposure to free-flowing steam for 30 minutes on each of 3 successive days.

tyn′dal-ĭ-za′shun

Sterilization by the fractional method is achieved by an interesting series of events. During the first day's exposure, steam kills virtually all organisms except bacterial spores, and it stimulates spores to germinate to vegetative cells. During overnight incubation, the cells multiply and are killed on the second day. Again, the material is cooled and the few remaining spores germinate, only to be killed on the third day. Although the method usually results in sterilization, occasions arise when several spores fail to germinate. The method also requires that spores be in a suitable medium for germination, such as a broth.

Fractional sterilization has assumed renewed importance in modern microbiology with the development of high-technology instrumentation and new chemical substances. Often, these materials cannot be sterilized at autoclave temperatures, or by long periods of boiling or baking, or with chemicals. An instrument that generates free-flowing steam, such as the **Arnold sterilizer,** is used in these instances.

Arnold sterilizer:
an instrument that generates free-flowing steam.

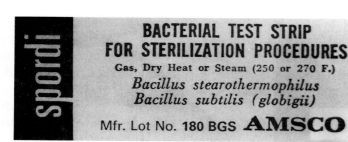

spordi

BACTERIAL TEST STRIP FOR STERILIZATION PROCEDURES
Gas, Dry Heat or Steam (250 or 270 F.)
Bacillus stearothermophilus
Bacillus subtilis (globigii)
Mfr. Lot No. **180 BGS AMSCO**

FIGURE 21.8

Testing Effective Sterilization

A bacterial test strip containing *Bacillus stearothermophilus* and *Bacillus subtilis (globigii)*. The strip inside the package is placed into broth medium at the conclusion of the sterilization cycle. If growth fails to appear on incubation, it may be assumed that the sterilization was successful. If growth occurs in the broth, then sterilization may not be assured.

TEDIOUS BUT WORTHWHILE

While Pasteur and Koch were setting down the foundations of microbiology in Europe, a British physicist named John Tyndall was developing a process for killing the most resistant forms of bacteria.

Tyndall believed that airborne microorganisms were associated with dust particles. In the early 1870s, he devised a wooden chamber with a glass front and glass side windows, and passed a beam of light through the chamber to visualize the dust. A beam of sunlight through a window displays dust particles the same way. Tyndall managed to prepare a sample of dust-free air and showed that it was free of microorganisms, thereby adding credence to Pasteur's theory that microorganisms were present in the air.

In 1876, Tyndall concluded that certain forms of bacteria were more resistant than other forms. His theory was based on observations that samples of old, dried hay were more difficult to sterilize than samples of fresh hay. Though unaware of the existence of spores, he resolved to develop a method to kill the "heat-resistant" bacteria.

Tyndall soon found that extended heating did not work well, but a stop-and-start method seemed useful. He heated hay samples to boiling on five consecutive occasions and allowed the samples to cool to room temperature

between heatings. Intervals of 10 to 12 hours between heatings were found most effective in the sterilization process. Tyndall's sterilization method preceded the development of the autoclave by several years. It showed that even the most heat-resistant forms of life could be eliminated, and it made possible the use of sterile broths for verifying the germ theory of disease. Today the method is known as tyndallization, for its developer.

■ *Tyndall's apparatus for observing dust particles and determining the presence of microorganisms. Dust-free air contained few microorganisms, and thus the sterile broths open to the air showed little evidence of growth on incubation. When dust was introduced through the tube, however, most broth tubes became cloudy on incubation, indicating that microorganisms were present in the dust.*

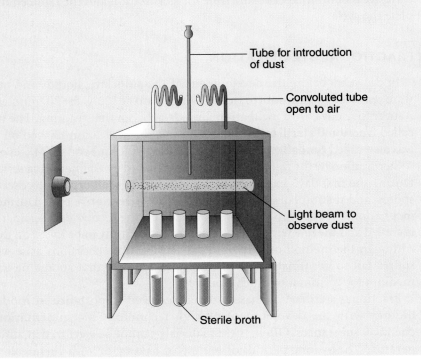

Tube for introduction of dust

Convoluted tube open to air

Light beam to observe dust

Sterile broth

PASTEURIZATION

Pasteurization:
a method of reducing microbial numbers in liquids by using heat.

therm-o-phil'ik

kok'se-el'lah bur-net'e-e

Pasteurization is not the same as sterilization. Its purpose is to reduce the bacterial population of a liquid such as milk and to destroy organisms that may cause spoilage and human disease (FIGURE 21.9). Spores are not affected by pasteurization.

One method for milk pasteurization, called the **holding method**, involves heating at 62.9°C for 30 minutes. Although thermophilic bacteria thrive at this temperature, they are of little consequence because they cannot grow at body temperature. For decades, pasteurization has been aimed at destroying *Mycobacterium tuberculosis*, long considered the most heat-resistant bacterium. More recently, however, attention has shifted to destruction of *Coxiella burnetii*, the agent of Q fever, because this organism has a higher resistance to heat. Since both organisms are eliminated by pasteurization, dairy microbiologists assume that other pathogenic bacteria are also destroyed.

Two other methods of pasteurization are the **flash pasteurization** method at 71.6°C for 15 seconds, and the **ultrapasteurization** method at 82°C for 3 seconds. These methods are discussed in detail in Chapter 24.

HOT OIL

Some dentists and physicians use **hot oil** at 160°C for the sterilization of instruments. A time period of 1 hour is usually recommended. Hot oil does not rust metals, and minimal corrosion takes place. However, once sterilization is complete, the instruments must be cleaned and dried for storage, and this step may reintroduce contamination. Silicone is sometimes used as an alternative to oil.

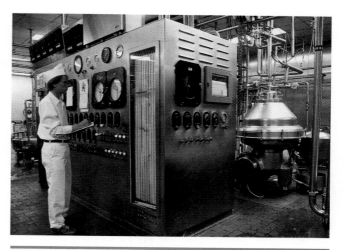

FIGURE 21.9

The Pasteurization of Milk

To this point . . .

We have surveyed a number of physical methods for controlling microorganisms that involve heat. These methods are generally aimed at sterilization, a term that denotes the destruction or removal of all life forms, including bacterial spores. Incineration with a direct flame is the most rapid heating method, but materials must be disposable. Dry heat is used in the hot-air oven where an exposure at 160°C for 2 hours achieves sterilization. A lower temperature of 100°C is used in boiling water, but sterilization cannot always be assured. The moist heat in boiling water is superior to the dry heat in the hot-air oven because moist heat penetrates better.

The autoclave is regarded as the most dependable instrument for sterilization. Moist heat in the form of steam under pressure is used in this instrument, and sterilization may be achieved in 15 to 30 minutes. The prevacuum autoclave utilizes a vacuum to draw out air at the beginning of the cycle and steam at the end, thereby reducing the cycle time. Higher pressures and temperatures are also used. We also noted how fractional sterilization is a useful tool under certain circumstances, and how pasteurization is not the same as sterilization. Hot oil was mentioned briefly.

We shall now direct our attention to physical methods that do not employ heat. These methods include filtration and the use of ultraviolet light, other radiations, and ultrasonic vibrations. Each method is of value under certain circumstances. For example, ultraviolet light is useful for sterilizing the air in a room. However, the destruction of all organisms may not be as thorough as with heating methods. The chapter will close with a review of certain preservation methods used in foods. Here, too, sterilization may not be achieved, but the number of microorganisms can be substantially reduced.

21.2

Physical Control by Other Methods

Although heat is a valuable physical agent for controlling microorganisms, sometimes it is impractical to use. For example, no one would suggest removing the microbial population from a tabletop by using a Bunsen burner, nor can heat-sensitive solutions be subjected to an autoclave. In instances such as these and numerous others, a heat-free method must be used. This section describes some examples.

FILTRATION

Filters came into prominent use in microbiology as interest in viruses grew during the 1890s. Previous to that time, filters had been utilized to trap airborne organisms and sterilize bacteriological media, but now they became essential for separating viruses from other microorganisms. Among the early pioneers of filter technology was **Charles Chamberland**, an associate of Pasteur. His porcelain filter was important to early virus research, as noted in Chapter 11. Another pioneer was **Julius Petri** (inventor of the Petri dish), who developed a sand filter to separate bacteria from the air.

The **filter** is a mechanical device for removing microorganisms from a solution. As fluid passes through the filter, organisms are trapped in the pores of the filtering material, as FIGURE 21.10 shows. The solution that drips into the receiving container is decontaminated or, in some cases, sterilized. Filters are used to purify such things as beverages, intravenous solutions, bacteriological media, toxoids, and many pharmaceuticals (FIGURE 21.11).

Several types of filters are available for use in the microbiology laboratory. **Inorganic filters** are typified by the Seitz filter, which consists of a pad of porcelain or ground glass mounted in a filter flask. **Organic filters** are advantageous because the organic molecules of the filter attract organic components in microorganisms. One example, the Berkefeld filter, utilizes a substance called **diatomaceous earth**. This material contains the remains of marine algae known as diatoms. Diatoms are unicellular algae that abound in the oceans and provide important foundations for the world's food chains. Their remains accumulate on the shoreline and are gathered for use in swimming pool and aquarium filters, as well as for microbiological filters used in laboratories.

The **membrane filter** is a third type of filter that has received broad acceptance. It consists of a pad of organic compounds such as cellulose acetate or polycarbonate, mounted in a holding device. This filter is particularly valuable because bacteria multiply and form colonies on the filter pad when the pad is placed on a plate of culture medium. Microbiologists can then count the colonies to determine the number of bacteria originally present. For example, if a 100-ml sample of liquid were filtered and 59 colonies appeared on the pad after incubation, it could be assumed that 59 bacteria were in the sample. FIGURE 21.12 demonstrates the process.

Air can also be filtered to remove microorganisms. The filter generally used is a **high-efficiency particulate air (HEPA) filter**. This apparatus can remove over 99 percent of all particles, including microorganisms with a diameter larger than 0.3 μm. The air entering surgical units and specialized treatment facilities, such as burn units, is filtered to exclude microorganisms. In some hospital wards, such as for respiratory

Cham'ber-land

Toxoid:
a chemically treated toxin used for immunization purposes.

sitz

di'ah-to-ma'shus

Membrane filter:
a filter composed of cellulose acetate on which bacterial colonies may form for enumeration.

FIGURE 21.10

The Principle of Filtration

Filtration is used to remove microorganisms from a liquid. The effectiveness of the filter is proportional to the size of its pores. (a) Bacteria-laden liquid is poured into a filter, and a vacuum pump helps pull the liquid through and into the flask below. But the bacteria are larger than the pores of the filter, and they become trapped. The liquid dripping into the flask is sterilized if all microbial forms, including viruses, are caught. Otherwise, the liquid will remain contaminated. (b) A view of *Escherichia coli* cells trapped in the pores of a 0.45 μm nylon membrane filter.

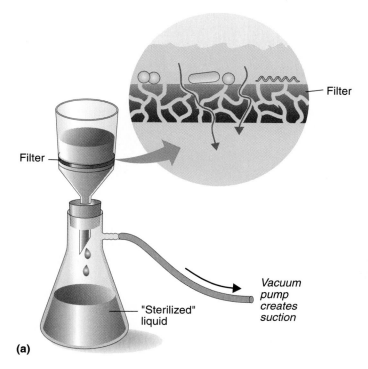

Filter

Filter

"Sterilized" liquid

Vacuum pump creates suction

(a)

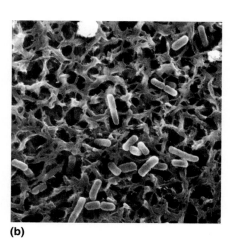

(b)

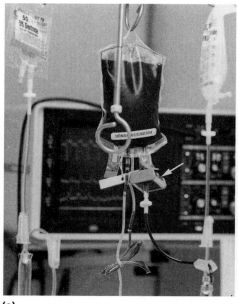

(a)

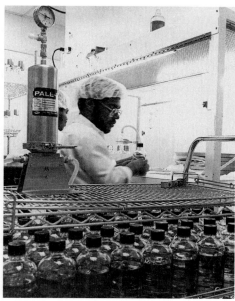

(b)

FIGURE 21.11

Industrial Fluid Filtration

Two examples of filters used in conjunction with fluids. (a) A filter of woven mesh dacron (arrow) is used to trap clumps of unwanted blood cells that might otherwise enter the recipient's circulation during a transfusion. (b) A cartridge filter removes contaminants from fluids to be used for intravenous injections or for other medical purposes.

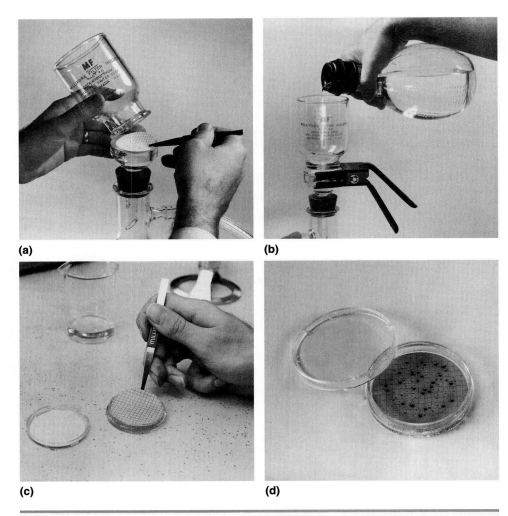

(a)

(b)

(c)

(d)

FIGURE 21.12

The Membrane Filter Technique

(a) The membrane filter consists of a pad of cellulose acetate, or similar material, mounted in a holding device. (b) The holding device is secured by a clamp, and a measured amount of fluid is filtered by pouring it into the cup. The solution runs through to a flask beneath, and bacteria are trapped in the filter material. (c) The filter pad is placed onto a plate of nutritious medium, and the plate is incubated. (d) After incubation, colonies appear on the surface of the filter pad. The colony count reflects the original number of bacteria in the fluid sample.

diseases, and in certain pharmaceutical filling rooms, the air is recirculated through HEPA filters to ensure its purity.

ULTRAVIOLET LIGHT

Nanometer:
a billionth of a meter.

Ultraviolet light:
a form of electromagnetic energy whose wavelength is between 100 and 400 nm.

Visible light is a type of radiant energy detected by the light-sensitive cells of the eye. The wavelength of this energy is between 400 and 800 nanometers (nm). Other types of radiation have wavelengths longer or shorter than that of visible light, and therefore they cannot be detected by the human eye.

One type of radiant energy, **ultraviolet (UV) light,** is useful for controlling microorganisms (MicroFocus 21.3). Ultraviolet light has a wavelength between 100 and 400 nm, with the energy at about 265 nm most destructive to bacteria. When microorganisms are subjected to UV light, cellular DNA absorbs the energy, and adjacent **thymine molecules** link together, as FIGURE 21.13 illustrates. Linked thymine molecules are unable to encode adenine on messenger RNA molecules during the process of protein synthesis. Moreover, replication of the chromosome in binary fission is impaired. The damaged organism can no longer produce critical proteins or reproduce, and it quickly dies.

Thymine:
one of the four nitrogenous bases of DNA.

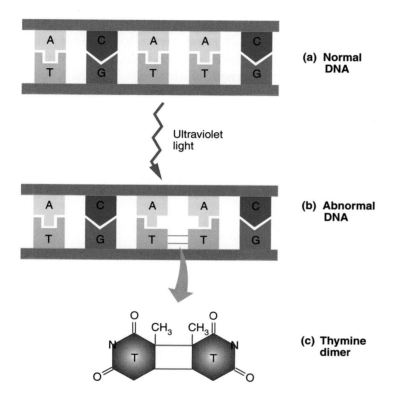

(a) Normal DNA

Ultraviolet light

(b) Abnormal DNA

(c) Thymine dimer

FIGURE 21.13

The Formation of Thymine Dimers

When bacteria are irradiated with ultraviolet light, the radiations affect the DNA of the cell. (a) A normal DNA molecule is converted to (b) an abnormal DNA molecule as the UV light binds adjacent thymine molecules within the DNA to form (c) a thymine dimer. With its thymine molecules bound in dimers, the DNA molecule cannot function properly and cannot replicate. The organism quickly dies.

MicroFocus 21.3

OUT OF HARM'S WAY

It has long been recognized that bacterial spores can resist the effects of ultraviolet light and survive where vegetative bacterial cells quickly die. The fact that spores remain alive for decades in soil exposed to the ultraviolet radiations of the sun is but one manifestation of the spore's resistance.

In the 1980s, scientists caught a glimpse of how this resistance works. Sporeformers, it seems, have the ability to produce a certain protein during the early stages of sporulation. The protein, referred to as a small, acid-soluble spore

protein (SASP), appears to protect the spore from UV light. In virtually all other bacteria, UV light affects adjacent thymine molecules in the cell's DNA and binds them together to form gnarled, double-looped structures. The disfigured DNA cannot replicate or be repaired. But in spores with SASP, there is no effect on the thymine molecules.

Then, in 1991, new light was shed on the process. Biochemists at the University of Connecticut and Boston University discovered that SASP can bind to DNA and untwist it ever so slightly. This

untwisting and change in DNA's geometry apparently makes the DNA resistant to the effects of UV light.

Earth-shattering news? Perhaps not. But that's how science works. We might expect scientific experiments to have profound effects on our lives, but the general rule is that scientific endeavors rarely have an immediate impact. More often, experimental findings (like those discussed here) elicit an "Aha!" from the scientist and from colleagues in the scientific community. Then the scientist goes back to work.

Ultraviolet light effectively reduces the microbial population where direct exposure takes place. It is used to limit airborne or surface contamination in a hospital room, morgue, pharmacy, toilet facility, or food service operation. It is noteworthy that ultraviolet light from the sun may be an important factor in controlling microorganisms in the air and upper layers of the soil, but it may not be effective against all bacterial spores. Ultraviolet light does not penetrate liquids or solids, and it may cause damage in human skin cells.

OTHER TYPES OF RADIATION

The spectrum of energies (FIGURE 21.14) includes two other forms of radiation useful for destroying microorganisms. These are **X rays** and **gamma rays**. Both have wavelengths shorter than the wavelength of ultraviolet light. As X rays and gamma rays pass through microbial molecules, they force electrons out of their shells, thereby creating ions. For this reason, the radiations are called **ionizing radiations**. The ions quickly combine with and destroy proteins and nucleic acids such as DNA, causing death. Gram-positive bacteria are more sensitive to ionizing radiations than Gram-negative bacteria. Ionizing radiations are currently used to sterilize such heat-sensitive pharmaceuticals as vitamins, hormones, and antibiotics, as well as certain plastics and suture materials.

Ionizing radiations: radiations that cause atoms to change to ions.

FIGURE 21.14

The Ionizing and Electromagnetic Spectrum of Energies

The complete spectrum is presented at the bottom of the chart, and the ultraviolet and visible sections are expanded at the top. Notice how the bactericidal energies overlap with the UV portion of sunlight. This may account for the destruction of microorganisms in the air and in upper layers of soil.

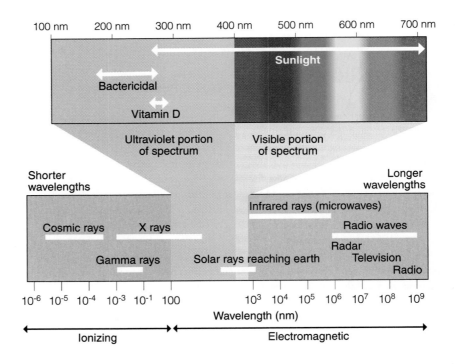

MicroFocus 21.4

"NO, THE FOOD DOES NOT GLOW!"

Manufacturers wrestling with the concept of food irradiation must constantly confront a leery public, some of whose members still have visions of Hiroshima and Nagasaki.

But food irradiation is entirely different. The irradiation comes from gamma rays produced during the natural decay of cobalt-60 or cesium-137. Alternately, it may come from the same type of X rays used in X-ray machines, or it may come from an electron beam not unlike that used in an electron microscope. Food technology plants using cobalt-60 store the pellets encapsulated twice in stainless steel pencil-like tubes arranged in racks under water. When food is to be irradiated, the racks are withdrawn from the water, and the food is passed through the radiation field.

During the radiation, the gamma rays penetrate the food, and, just as in cooking, cause molecular changes in the microorganisms, leading to their death. Nutritional losses are similar to those occurring in cooking and/or freezing. Otherwise, there are virtually no changes in the food, and there is no residue. And no, the food does not glow.

Ionizing radiations have also been approved for controlling microorganisms, and for preserving foods, as noted in MicroFocus 21.4. The approval has generated much controversy, fueled by activists concerned about the safety of factory workers and consumers. First used in 1921 to inactivate *Trichinella spiralis*, the agent of trichinosis, irradiation is now used as a preservative in more than 40 countries for over 100 food items, including potatoes, onions, cereals, flour, fresh fruit, and poultry (FIGURE 21.15). The U.S. Food and Drug Administration (FDA) approved cobalt-60 irradiation to preserve poultry in the early 1990s, and in 1997, it extended the approval to preserve red meats such as beef, lamb, and pork.

Trichinella spiralis:
a roundworm usually acquired in pork and the cause of intestinal and muscular infections.

Another form of energy, the **microwave**, has a wavelength longer than that of ultraviolet light. In a microwave oven, microwaves are absorbed by water molecules. The molecules are set into high-speed motion, and the heat of friction is transferred to foods, which become hot rapidly. Other than the heat generated, there is no specific activity against microorganisms (MicroFocus 21.5).

A final form of radiation we shall consider is light energy. When concentrated by sophisticated devices, light energy forms a **laser beam**. The word *laser* is an acronym for *light amplification by stimulated emission of radiation*. Recent experiments indicate that laser beams can be used to sterilize instruments and the air in operating rooms, as well as a wound surface. Microorganisms are destroyed in a fraction of a second, but the laser beam must reach all parts of the material to effect sterilization.

Laser beam:
a beam of light energy concentrated to considerably increase its energy.

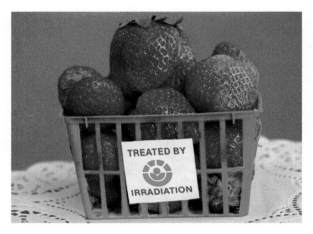

FIGURE 21.15

Food Irradiation

The FDA has approved irradiation as a preservation method for numerous foods, including many fruits and vegetables, as well as poultry and red meats.

MicroFocus 21.5

MICROWAVES: MYTHS AND FACTS

Myth: Microwaves cook food.

Fact: It's true that microwaves cook food, but in a somewhat indirect manner. Food is composed of a loosely woven nest of large proteins, fats, carbohydrates, and other organic materials. Water molecules float freely among the materials, and, like submicroscopic magnets, they have positive and negative ends. Alternating microwave fields (2.4 billion alternations per second) spin the water molecules about at implausibly high rates, thus creating friction. The heat of friction is transferred to the surrounding food molecules as heat, and the food cooks.

Myth: Microwaves cook from the inside out.

Fact: Not really. Microwaves excite all water molecules throughout the food simultaneously. However, some heat at the food surface is lost to the surrounding air, so the outside of the food cools more quickly than the inside, and the perception is that the inside has been heated more thoroughly.

Myth: There is no solution to soggy, limp pizza heated in a microwave oven.

Fact: Sure there is, but first you have to understand why the pizza gets soggy. In a regular oven, hot water molecules from the dough come to the surface where they meet the hot oven air and evaporate, leaving the pizza crust crisp and the inside moist. In the microwave oven, the

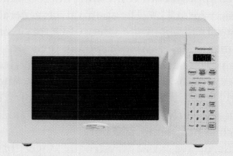

surrounding air is cool, so when the hot water molecules reach the surface, they condense to liquid and stay there or soak back into the pizza, creating a soggy mess. The answer to this problem is a metallic film mounted on a piece of cardboard. The metal heats up when exposed to microwaves, and the hot water molecules vaporize when they hit it, thereby forming a dry surface and a crisp pizza.

Myth: Microwaves are useless for sterilization.

Fact: Microwaves have potential as sterilizing agents. One company is experimenting with a process that shreds infectious waste, sprays it with water, and exposes it to microwaves until the temperature reaches near-boiling levels. Another company is testing a procedure that sterilizes instruments after sealing them within a vacuum in a glass container. Both methods show promise.

ULTRASONIC VIBRATIONS

Ultrasonic vibrations: high-frequency sound waves.

Ultrasonic vibrations are high-frequency sound waves beyond the range of human hearing. When directed against environmental surfaces, they have little value because air particles deflect and disperse the vibrations. However, when propagated in fluids, ultrasonic vibrations cause the formation of microscopic bubbles, or cavities, and the water appears to boil. Some observers call this "cold boiling." The cavities rapidly collapse and send out shock waves. Microorganisms in the fluid are quickly disintegrated by the external pressures. The formation and implosion of the

kav'ĭ-ta'shun

cavities are known as **cavitation.** FIGURE 21.16 illustrates this process.

Ultrasonic vibrations are valuable in research for breaking open tissue cells and obtaining their parts for study. A device called the **cavitron** is used by dentists to clean teeth, and ultrasonic machines are available for cleaning dental plates, jewelry, and coins. A major appliance company has also experimented with an ultrasonic washing machine.

As a sterilizing agent, ultrasonic vibrations have received minimal attention because liquid is required and other methods are more efficient. However, many research laboratories use ultrasonic probes for cell disruption and hospitals use ultrasonic devices to clean their instruments. When used with an effective germicide, an ultrasonic device may achieve sterilization, but the current trend is to use ultrasonic vibrations as a cleaning agent and follow the process by sterilization in an autoclave.

TABLE 21.1 summarizes the physical agents used for controlling microorganisms.

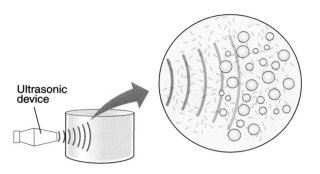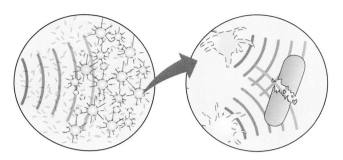

(A) High frequency sound waves cause microscopic bubbles to form in the fluid.

(B) As the bubbles collapse, shock waves are created in the fluid.

(C) Alternating high- and low-pressure areas impinge upon microorganisms and destroy them.

FIGURE 21.16

How Ultrasonic Vibrations Kill Microorganisms

TABLE 21.1

A Summary of Physical Agents Used to Control Microorganisms

PHYSICAL METHOD	CONDITIONS	INSTRUMENT	OBJECT OF TREATMENT	EXAMPLES OF USES	COMMENT
Direct flame	A few seconds	Flame	All microorganisms	Laboratory instruments	Object must be disposable or heat-resistant
Hot air	160°C for 2 hr	Oven	Bacterial spores	Glassware Powders Oily substances	Not useful for fluid materials
Boiling water	100°C for 10 min 100°C for 2 hr+	— —	Vegetative microorganisms Bacterial spores	Wide variety of objects	Total immersion and precleaning necessary
Pressurized steam	121°C for 15 min at 15 lb/in²	Autoclave	Bacterial spores	Instruments Surgical materials Solutions and media	Broad application in microbiology
Fractional sterilization	30 min/day for 3 successive days	Arnold sterilizer	Bacterial spores	Materials not sterilized by other methods	Long process Sterilization not assured
Pasteurization	62.9°C for 30 min 71.6°C for 15 sec	Pasteurizer	Pathogenic microorganisms	Dairy products	Sterilization not achieved
Hot oil	160°C for 1 hr	—	Bacterial spores	Instruments	Rinsing necessary
Filtration	Entrapment in pores	Berkefeld filter Membrane filter	All microorganisms	Fluids	Many adaptations
Ultraviolet light	265 nm energy	UV light	All microorganisms	Surface and air sterilization	Not useful in fluids
X rays Gamma rays	Short-wave length energy	Generator	All microorganisms	Heat-sensitive materials	Possible toxic chemicals
Ultrasonic vibrations	High-frequency sound waves	Sonicator	All microorganisms	Fluids	Few practical applications

PRESERVATION METHODS

Over the course of many centuries, various physical methods have evolved for controlling microorganisms in food. Though valuable for preventing the spread of infectious agents, these procedures are used mainly to retard spoilage and prolong the shelf life of foods, rather than for sterilization. Irradiation is an example of a preservation method.

Drying is useful in the preservation of various meats, fish, cereals, and other foods. Since water is necessary for life, it follows that where there is no water, there is virtually no life. Many of the foods in the kitchen pantry typify this principle. One example is discussed in MicroFocus 21.6.

Preservation by **salting** is based upon the principle of osmotic pressure. When food is salted, water diffuses out of microorganisms toward the higher salt concentration and lower water concentration in the surrounding environment. This flow of water, called **osmosis**, leaves the microorganisms to shrivel and die. The same phenomenon occurs in highly sugared foods such as syrups, jams, and jellies. However, fungal contamination may remain at the surface because aerobic molds tolerate high sugar concentrations.

Low temperatures found in the refrigerator and freezer retard spoilage by lowering the metabolic rate of microorganisms and thereby reducing their rate of growth. Spoilage is not totally eliminated in cold foods, however, and many microorganisms remain alive, even at freezer temperatures. These organisms multiply rapidly when food thaws, which is why prompt cooking is recommended.

Note in these examples that there are significant differences between killing microorganisms, holding them in check, and reducing their numbers. The preservation methods are described as bacteriostatic because they prevent the further multiplication of bacteria. A more complete discussion of food preservation as it relates to public health is presented in Chapter 24.

oz-mo′sis
Osmosis:
the diffusion of water molecules from a region of high water concentration to one of low water concentration.

MicroFocus 21.6

A DRY AND TWISTED TALE

The kitchen pantry usually contains many foods that resist microbial contamination simply because they are too dry to support life. In many pantries, one of these foods is the pretzel.

According to a major manufacturer, the origin of the pretzel dates back to the early 600s and a monk in southern France or northern Italy. Legend has it that the monk took leftover strips of bread and fashioned them into twisted loops, similar to the arms folded across the chest in prayer. He baked the loops and distributed them to children who performed good deeds, such as learning their prayers well. Each child received a "pretiola" or "little reward." The name was later shortened to pretzel.

It seems unfortunate that anyone would take issue with such an appealing tale, but Tom Burnam has done just that in *The Dictionary of Misinformation*. Burnam maintains that the word *pretzel* is derived from the German word for "branch," and is not Latin for "little reward." He points out that a pretzel looks like the intertwined branches of a tree, and he attempts to punch holes in the legend by noting that folding the arms across the chest is the conventional coffin arrangement, not the position for prayer. Some traditionalists might dispute this.

Whatever the true story, the pretzel was brought to America by European immigrants, especially the Pennsylvania Dutch (really "Deutsch," for German),

who settled in the northeastern states. Today, major pretzel factories are located in Lancaster and Lititz, Pennsylvania. Their products are as dry, twisted, and free of microbial contamination as the original pretzels of centuries ago.

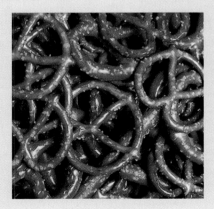

Note to the Student

As the science of microbiology evolved in the late 1800s, physicians were quick to grasp the notion that contaminated instruments, clothing, and similar articles were important to disease transmission. Also, researchers soon realized that contaminated growth media and materials could ruin their experiments and cast doubt on their findings. Physical methods for controlling microorganisms therefore attained acceptance rapidly, and steam and high-pressure sterilizers became commonplace in medical microbiology.

Over 100 years later, things have not changed substantially. The autoclave still occupies a prominent position in the clinical and research laboratory, and most physical methods for sterilization are essentially as they were a century ago. Even tyndallization, tedious as it is, has reemerged for use in decontaminating the products of modern biotechnology. To be sure, there are more blinking lights in today's sophisticated equipment, but it is reassuring to note that yesterday's principles are still valid. Perhaps this is one example of what is implied by the saying, "The more things change, the more they remain the same."

Summary

The physical methods for controlling microorganisms are generally intended to achieve sterilization. Sterilization is the destruction or removal of all life forms, with particular reference to the bacterial spore.

Microorganisms can be controlled by various methods. The direct flame, for example, achieves sterilization in a few seconds, while the hot-air oven requires exposure to hot air at 160°C for 2 hours. Exposure to boiling water at 100°C for 2 hours may also result in sterilization, but spore destruction cannot always be assured. By contrast, the autoclave uses pressurized steam at 121°C to sterilize objects in about 15 minutes. A prevacuum sterilizer shortens this time still further. Other heat methods for sterilization include fractional sterilization (30 minutes of exposure to steam on each of 3 successive days) and hot oil (160°C for 1 hour). Pasteurization reduces the microbial population in a liquid and is not intended to be a sterilization method.

Certain nonheat methods are also used to control microbial populations. Filters, for instance, use various materials to trap microorganisms within the pores of filtering material. Inorganic, organic, and membrane filters are used. Ultraviolet light is an effective way of killing microorganisms on a dry surface and in the air. X rays and gamma rays are two forms of ionizing radiations used to sterilize heat-sensitive objects. Laser beams and ultrasonic vibrations could also be useful for sterilization, but instruments that utilize these energies are not widely available in affordable forms.

For food preservation, drying, salting, and low temperatures can be used to control microorganisms, but sterilization is a virtual impossibility. However, for instruments, pharmaceuticals, medical apparatus, microbial media, and numerous other products, the physical methods noted are effective and widely used methods for achieving sterilization.

Questions for Thought and Discussion

1. Instead of saying that food has been irradiated, manufacturers indicate that it has been "cold pasteurized." Why do you believe they must use this deception? Do you think it is ethical? What will it take for food manufacturers to avoid the deception and use the correct term? Can you think of any place a euphemism like this one is used in foods?

2. When the local drinking water is believed to be contaminated, area residents are advised to boil their water before drinking. Often, however, they are not told how long to boil it. As a student of microbiology, what might be your recommendation?

3. The label on the container of a product in the dairy case proudly proclaims, "This dairy product is sterilized for your protection." However, a statement in small letters below reads: "Use within 30 days of purchase." Should this statement arouse your suspicion about the sterility of the product? Why?

4. Several days ago, you bought a steak and stored it in the refrigerator. Now you find that the surface of the steak has spots of bacterial contamination. You are certain that the bacteria have not penetrated deeply into the meat. Should you broil the steak, as you had planned, or discard it? Why?

5. In 1997, on approving irradiation as a preservation method for red meat, the Acting Commissioner of the U.S. Food and Drug Administration indicated that irradiated red meat might cost an extra 3 to 6 cents per pound. Opponents of irradiation point to this extra cost as a deterrent to irradiation. What other deterrents might they offer?

6. Early in the century, a prehistoric woolly mammoth was discovered in the tundra of Siberia. The meat of the animal was so well preserved that it was fed to hunters' dogs. What factors contributed to the meat's preservation?

7. Suppose a liquid needed to be sterilized. What methods could be developed using only the materials found in the average household?

8. Old metropolitan buildings often had hallway chutes in which garbage could be dumped. The garbage would drop into an incinerator and burn. How might this be of value to a budding microbiologist who happened to live in the building?

9. The Scope Shield is a patented device that covers a stethoscope and protects it from disease organisms sticking to these instruments during patient exams. The device is plastic, costs 10 cents, and is meant to be discarded after a single use. Do you think it will be widely used by physicians in the ensuing years? For which organisms will it interrupt transmission?

10. The Bunsen burner was invented in 1855 by the German chemist Robert W. Bunsen. In how many different ways can it be used to sterilize objects and materials under laboratory conditions?

11. The world's oldest known pottery was made in Japan almost 13,000 years ago. With this invention, people now had watertight containers to boil or steam foods. Archaeologists believe that a population explosion soon followed in Japan. One reason is that the Japanese could for the first time avail themselves of leafy vegetables. Can you think of any other reasons?

12. In view of all the sterilization methods we have reviewed in this chapter, why do you think none has been widely adapted to the sterilization of milk? Which, in your opinion, holds the most promise?

13. Why may sunlight be referred to as nature's great sterilizing agent?

14. The word *autoclave* is derived from stems that mean "self-closing." This is a reference to the fact that the chamber closes itself by the pressure of the steam. Would it be correct to equate the words *autoclave* and *sterilizer*? Why?

15. A liquid that has been sterilized may be considered pasteurized, but one that has been pasteurized may not be considered sterilized. Why not?

Review

Use the following syllables to form the term that answers the clue pertaining to sterilization. The number of letters in the term is indicated by the dashes, and the number of syllables in the term is shown by the number in parentheses. Each syllable is used only once. The answers are listed in Appendix D.

A A AU BA BER BRANE BUN CIL CLAVE CLEAN CRO CU DA DALL DE DER DI DRY GAM HOLD I IC IDS IN ING ING ING INS LET LO LUS MA MEM MENTS MI MO NA O OX OS PLAS POW PRES SEN SIS SIS SOL SON SPORE STRU SURE THIR TIC TION TION TO TOMS TOX TRA TRA TU TUR TY TYN UL UL VI WAVES

1. Instrument for sterilization   (3) __ __ __ __ __ __ __ __

2. Type of filter   (2) __ __ __ __ __ __

3. Sterilization in an oven   (2) __ __ __ __ __

4. Occurs in boiling water   (5) __ __ __ __ __ __ __ __ __ __ __

5. Developed fractional method   (2) __ __ __ __ __ __ __

6. Preserves meat, fish   (2) __ __ __ __ __ __

7. High-frequency vibrations   (4) __ __ __ __ __ __ __ __ __ __

8. Short-wavelength rays   (2) __ __ __ __

9. Most resistant life form   (1) __ __ __ __ __

10. Occurs in dry heat   (4) __ __ __ __ __ __ __ __

11. Raised in the autoclave   (2) __ __ __ __ __ __

12. Minutes for tyndallization   (2) __ __ __ __ __ __

13. Method of pasteurization   (2) __ __ __ __ __ __

14. Sterilized with hot oil   (3) __ __ __ __ __ __ __ __

15. Source of an organic filter   (3) __ __ __ __ __ __ __

16. Light for air sterilization   (5) __ __ __ __ __ __ __ __ __ __

17. Melts in the autoclave   (2) __ __ __ __ __ __

18. May remain after filtration   (2) __ __ __ __ __

19. Not penetrated by UV light   (2) __ __ __ __ __

20. Water flow from salting   (3) __ __ __ __ __ __ __

21. Used to heat water molecules   (3) __ __ __ __ __ __ __ __

22. Genus of sporeformers   (3) __ __ __ __ __ __ __

23. Direct flame burner   (2) __ __ __ __ __

24. Essential pretreatment   (2) __ __ __ __ __ __

25. Prevented by pasteurization   (5) __ __ __ __ __ __ __ __ __ __ __

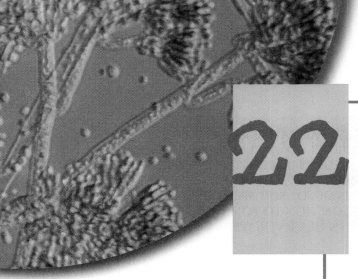

22 Chemical Control of Microorganisms

Please, wash your hands!

—A microbiologically astute mother to a young child
(on numerous occasions)

BEFORE THE 1900s, hospitals rarely had running water, and what water they had was usually contaminated. Garbage, human waste, and other hospital refuse were usually dumped into a pit in the courtyard; surgeons wiped their hands and instruments on their hospital jackets and trousers; bedclothes were rarely changed; and infection was rampant. Up to one-third of women giving birth died of puerperal (childbed) fever, a blood disease often caused by a species of *Streptococcus*.

As late as the mid-1800s, only a few visionaries recognized the relationship between filth and disease. One such person was the American physician, poet, and jurist, **Oliver Wendell Holmes**, author of an 1843 paper on the contagious nature of puerperal fever. Another was the Hungarian physician **Ignaz Semmelweis**.

In 1847, Semmelweis was working at a Vienna hospital's obstetrics clinic when he made a remarkable observation: An unusually high incidence of puerperal fever occurred in maternity wards tended by physicians fresh from dissecting cadavers. However, in the ward tended by midwives, the incidence was much lower. Semmelweis reasoned that disease was transmitted by infected hands, and he ordered all the attendants in his ward to wash their hands in chlorine water before ministering to patients. Soon the death rate among his patients fell significantly.

Semmelweis summarized his findings and presented his evidence for the transmission of disease to

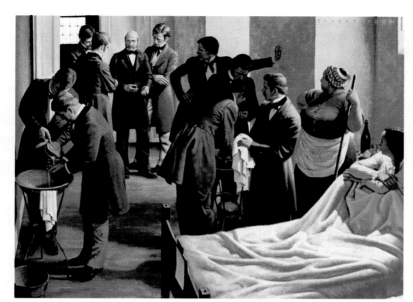

FIGURE 22.1

Ignaz Semmelweis

In this painting by Robert Thom, Ignaz Semmelweis is shown standing at the back of the delivery room encouraging other physicians to use disinfectants. Today, a monument to him stands in Budapest, Hungary, and refers to him as the "savior of mothers" because of his pioneering work in the maternity wards in Vienna hospitals.

hospital administrators. However, they rejected his conclusion that doctors were spreading disease because it cast doctors in a negative light. The debate became vehement, and Semmelweis insisted that rejecting his methods was tantamount to committing murder. Shortly thereafter, an anguished and frustrated Semmelweis left Austria for his native Hungary, where he died in 1865 (FIGURE 22.1).

Ironically, the death of Semmelweis paralleled Pasteur's landmark experiments in microbiology. As the germ theory of disease gained a foothold, the realization dawned that infectious microorganisms could move among individuals by clothing, utensils, instruments, and other objects. To interrupt the spread of organisms, doctors began using chemical antiseptics and disinfectants, and before long, they witnessed a substantial decline in the incidence of disease.

In this chapter, we shall examine a variety of chemical methods used for controlling the spread of microorganisms. Our study begins by outlining some general principles and terminology of disinfection practices, and then proceeds to a discussion of the spectrum of antiseptics and disinfectants. Whether for wounds, swimming pools, industrial machinery, or pharmaceutical products, antiseptics and disinfectants are fundamental to public health practices that ensure continued good health.

22.1 General Principles of Chemical Control

The notions of sanitation and disinfection are not unique to the modern era. **The Bible** refers often to cleanliness and prescribes certain dietary laws to prevent consumption of what was believed to be contaminated food. Egyptians used resins and aromatics for embalming even before they had a written language, and ancient peoples burned sulfur for deodorizing and sanitary purposes. Over the centuries, necessity demanded chemicals for food preservation, and spices were used as preservatives as well as masks for foul odors. Indeed, Marco Polo's trips to the Orient for new spices were made out of necessity as well as for adventure.

fahr'mah-ko-pe'ah

Mercury:
a toxic heavy metal that combines
with proteins to kill bacteria.

a-sep'tik

Medicinal chemicals came into widespread use in the 1800s. As early as 1830, for example, the **U.S. Pharmacopoeia** listed tincture of iodine as a valuable antiseptic, and soldiers in the Civil War used it in plentiful amounts. In the first decades of that century, people found copper sulfate useful for preventing fungal disease in plants, but unfortunately, this chemical was not well known during Ireland's great potato blight (Chapter 14). Mercury was sometimes used for treating syphilis, as first suggested by Arabian physicians centuries before. Moviegoers have probably noted that American cowboys practiced disinfection by pouring whiskey onto gunshot wounds between drinks.

In the 1860s, a physician at the University of Glasgow named **Joseph Lister** established the principles of aseptic surgery. Pasteur's references to airborne microorganisms convinced Lister that microorganisms were the cause of wound infections (MicroFocus 22.1). Lister experimented with several chemicals to kill microorganisms

MicroFocus 22.1

SURGERY WITHOUT INFECTION

While Louis Pasteur was speaking and writing about the germ theory of disease, the British physician Joseph Lister was doing his best to reform the practice of surgery.

Lister was an innovative and imaginative individual. He was, for example, among the earliest physicians to put the newly discovered anesthetics to use. By using carefully measured quantities of ether and air, Lister found he could perform operations without torture. But it distressed him that even though an operation could be painless and successful, the patient might still die of infection. Throughout Great Britain, roughly one out of every two amputations ended in death from "hospital gangrene," "blood poisoning," or other affliction.

Toward the end of 1864, Lister read Pasteur's reports on fermentation and successfully repeated many of Pasteur's experiments. The work convinced Lister that airborne microorganisms were responsible for postsurgical diseases. He decided to test Pasteur's suspicions that microorganisms cause disease.

While searching for an antimicrobial compound, Lister's attention was drawn to a newspaper account describing the use of carbolic acid (phenol) for the treatment of sewage in a town near Glasgow. After exploring the capabilities of this compound in laboratory cultures

and finding it effective, Lister was ready to proceed with human experiments.

The first recorded use of chemical disinfection in a surgical procedure occurred in March 1865 at the Glasgow Royal Infirmary. During surgery to repair a compound fracture, Lister sprayed the air with a fine mist of carbolic acid and soaked his instruments and ligatures in carbolic acid solution. Although the patient subsequently died of infection, Lister remained optimistic. He repeated the experiments, improved the procedures, and finally met with success. In 1867, he reported his results in an article in *The Lancet*, a British medical journal. Lister wrote that his antiseptic methods reduced the mortality

rate in postoperative surgery from 45 percent to 9 percent.

Lister's work was accomplished without a clear knowledge or understanding of pathogenic microorganisms, and in this regard, his achievements merit special note. Though hospital equipment and methods have changed, the principles he established are as valid today as they were over a century ago. Before his death in 1912, he was knighted by the British Crown and is remembered as Sir Joseph Lister.

■ *A painting by Robert Thom depicting Joseph Lister using antiseptic methods in the surgical treatment of a leg wound.*

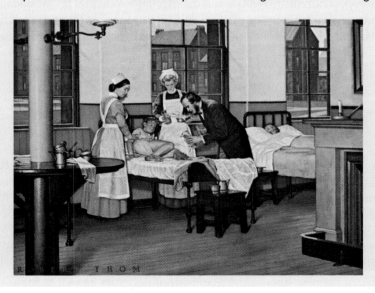

and finally settled on **carbolic acid** (**phenol**). He applied the chemical to wounds and instruments and sprayed it in the air near the operating table. Lister achieved brilliant success and was awarded many accolades as a pioneer microbiologist of his time, although he advocated the same principles recommended by Semmelweis years before.

TERMINOLOGY OF DISINFECTION

The chemical control of microorganisms extends into such diverse areas as hospital environments, food-processing plants, and everyday households. These broad fields have yielded an equally broad terminology that should be explored before we undertake a discussion of individual chemical agents.

The physical agents for controlling microorganisms (Chapter 21) are generally intended to achieve **sterilization**, the destruction of all forms of life, especially bacterial spores. Chemical agents, by contrast, rarely achieve sterilization. Instead, they are only expected to destroy the pathogenic organisms on or in an object. The process of destroying pathogens is called **disinfection**; the object is said to be disinfected. If the object is lifeless, such as a tabletop, the chemical agent is known as a **disinfectant**. However, if the object is living, such as a tissue of the human body, the chemical is an **antiseptic**. FIGURE 22.2 illustrates the fundamental difference between antiseptics and disinfectants. It is important to note that even though a particular chemical may be used as a disinfectant as well as an antiseptic (iodine, for example), the precise formulations are so different that the ability to kill microorganisms differs substantially in the two products.

Antiseptics and disinfectants are usually bactericidal, but occasionally they may be bacteriostatic. A **bactericidal agent** kills microorganisms, while a **bacteriostatic agent** temporarily prevents their further multiplication without necessarily killing them. For example, a bactericidal agent may inactivate the major enzymes of an

Sterilization:
the destruction or removal of all forms of life.

Disinfection:
the destruction or removal of pathogenic microorganisms.

bak-ter'-si'dal
bak-te're-o-stat'ik

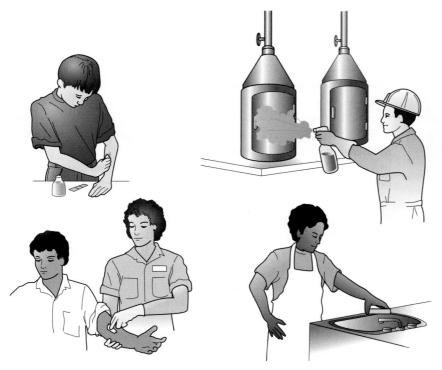

(a) Antiseptic   (b) Disinfectant

FIGURE 22.2

Sample Uses of Antiseptics and Disinfectants

(a) Antiseptics are used on body tissues, such as on a wound or before piercing the skin to take blood. (b) A disinfectant is used on inanimate objects, such as a tabletop or equipment used in an industrial process.

organism and interfere with its metabolism so that it dies. A bacteriostatic agent, by contrast, disrupts a minor chemical reaction and slows the metabolism, resulting in a longer time between cell divisions. Although a delicate difference sometimes exists between the bactericidal and bacteriostatic nature of a chemical agent, the terms indicate effectiveness in a particular situation.

The word **sepsis** is derived from the Greek *seps*, meaning "putrid." It refers to the contamination of an object by microorganisms and is the stem for *septicemia*, meaning "microbial infection of the blood," and *antiseptic*, which translates to "against infection." It is also the origin of the term **aseptic**, meaning "free of contaminating microorganisms."

Other expressions are associated with chemical control. To **sanitize** an object is to reduce the microbial population to a safe level as determined by local public health standards. For example, in dairy and food-processing plants, the equipment is usually sanitized (and the process is called sanitization). To **degerm** something is merely to remove organisms from its surface. Washing with soap and water degerms the skin surface but has little effect on microorganisms deep in the skin pores.

A final group of terms that deserves mentioning is the *-cidal* agents. These include the **fungicidal** agents, which kill fungi; the **virucidal** agents, for viruses; the **sporicidal** agents, for bacterial spores; and the **germicidal** agents, for various types of microorganisms.

SELECTION OF ANTISEPTICS AND DISINFECTANTS

To be useful as an antiseptic or disinfectant, a chemical agent must have certain properties, some of which are more desirable than others. The first prerequisite is that it must be able to kill microorganisms. It should also be nontoxic to animals or humans, especially if it is used as an antiseptic. It should be soluble in water and have a substantial shelf life during which its activity is retained. The agent should be useful in very diluted form and perform its job in a relatively short time. Both factors tend to minimize toxic side effects.

Other characteristics will also contribute to the value of a chemical agent: It should not separate on standing, it should penetrate well, and it should not corrode instruments. The chemical will have a distinct advantage if it does not combine with organic matter such as blood or feces, because the organic matter will bind and "use up" the chemical. Of course, the chemical should be easy to obtain and relatively inexpensive.

Since disinfection is essentially a chemical process, the **parameters of chemistry** should be considered when selecting an antiseptic or disinfectant. For example, the temperature at which the disinfection is to take place may be important because a chemical reaction occurring at 37°C (body temperature) may not occur at 25°C (room temperature). Also, a particular chemical may be effective at a certain pH but not another. Moreover, the chemical reaction may be very rapid with one agent and slower with another. Thus, if long-term disinfection is desired, the second agent may be preferable.

Two other considerations are the type of microorganism to be eliminated and the surface treated. For instance, the removal of bacterial spores requires more vigorous treatment than the removal of vegetative cells. Also, a chemical applied to a laboratory bench is considerably different from one used on a wound or for sterilizing an object (**FIGURE 22.3**). It is therefore imperative to distinguish the

Aseptic:
free of contaminating microorganisms.
Sanitize:
to reduce the microbial population to a safe level as determined by local public health standards.
Degerm:
to remove microorganisms from a surface.

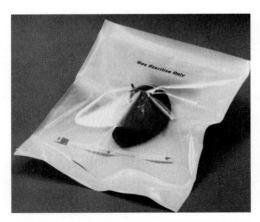

FIGURE 22.3

Packing for Chemical Sterilization

Various chemicals are available for disinfection, antisepsis, and in some cases, sterilization. The chemicals vary with the situation. In this case, a gas mask is to be sterilized, and it must be wrapped securely before being exposed to the sterilizing chemical. An antiseptic or disinfectant could not be used to sterilize this object.

antiseptic or disinfectant nature of a chemical before proceeding with its use. Indeed, chemical agents formulated as disinfectants are regulated and registered by the U.S. Environmental Protection Agency (EPA), while chemicals formulated as antiseptics are regulated by the U.S Food and Drug Administration (FDA).

EVALUATION OF ANTISEPTICS AND DISINFECTANTS

At the current time, the EPA lists over 8000 disinfectants for hospital use and thousands more for general use. Evaluating these chemical agents is a tedious process because of the broad diversity of conditions under which they are used.

A standard of effectiveness used for the chemical agents is the **phenol coefficient (PC)**. This is a number that indicates the disinfecting ability of an antiseptic or disinfectant in comparison to phenol under identical conditions (TABLE 22.1). A PC higher than 1 indicates that the chemical is more effective than phenol; a number less than 1 indicates poorer disinfecting ability than phenol. For example, antiseptic A may have a PC of 78.5, while antiseptic B has a PC of 0.28. These numbers are used relative to each other rather than to phenol, because phenol is allergenic and irritating to tissues and thus is rarely used.

The phenol coefficient is determined by a laboratory procedure in which dilutions of phenol and the test chemical are mixed with standardized bacteria, such as *Staphylococcus aureus* and *Salmonella typhi* or other species (FIGURE 22.4). The laboratory technician then determines which dilutions have killed the organisms after a 10-minute exposure but not after a 5-minute exposure. The test has many drawbacks, especially since it is performed in the laboratory rather than in a real-life situation. Nor does it take into account such factors as tissue toxicity, activity in the presence of organic matter, or temperature variations.

A more practical way of determining the value of a chemical agent is by an **in-use test**. For example, swab samples from a floor are taken before and after the application of a disinfectant to determine the level of kill. Another method is to dry standardized

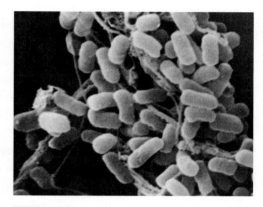

FIGURE 22.4

A Test Organism for the Phenol Coefficient Test

A scanning electron micrograph of a *Salmonella* species such as used in the phenol coefficient test ($\times$40,000). This Gram-negative rod is used to determine the efficiency of an antiseptic or disinfectant in comparison to phenol.

TABLE 22.1

Phenol Coefficients of Some Common Antiseptics and Disinfectants

CHEMICAL AGENT	STAPHYLOCOCCUS AUREUS	SALMONELLA TYPHI
Phenol	1.0	1.0
Chloramine	133.0	100.0
Tincture of iodine	6.3	5.8
Lysol	5.0	3.2
Mercury chloride	100.0	143.0
Ethyl alcohol	6.3	6.3
Formalin	0.3	0.7
Hydrogen peroxide	—	0.01

cultures of bacteria within small stainless steel cylinders and then expose the cylinders to the test chemical. After an established period of time, the bacteria are tested for survival rates. These methods of standardization have value under certain circumstances. However, it is conceivable that a universal test may never be developed, in view of the huge variety of chemical agents available and the numerous conditions under which they are used.

To this point . . .

We have examined some of the history and origins of disinfection practices, with emphasis on the works of Ignaz Semmelweis and Joseph Lister. We saw how chemicals have been used since ancient times and how increased use occurred in the 1800s as the germ theory of disease was widely propagated. We then outlined some of the important terms applied to chemical agents and distinguished disinfectants used on lifeless objects from antiseptics applied to the skin surface. Sterilization and disinfection were also compared. We explored certain specifications for selecting antiseptics and disinfectants, including characteristics of the chemical agent, the conditions under which it is used, and the type of microorganism it is intended to kill.

The discussion then turned to methods for evaluating the effectiveness of antiseptics and disinfectants, with emphasis on the phenol coefficient method. This method is limited because it is a laboratory test and does not necessarily reflect the conditions under which the chemical is to be used. Some in-use tests were briefly mentioned.

We shall now survey the broad spectrum of chemical agents used for disinfection. You will note an equally broad set of applications for these agents. We shall focus on the materials for which they are used and the mechanisms by which they kill microorganisms. Only a few agents in the first group are sterilizing agents.

22.2

Important Chemical Agents

The chemical agents currently in use for controlling microorganisms range from very simple substances, such as halogen ions, to very complex compounds, typified by detergents. Many of these agents in nature have been used for generations (MicroFocus 22.2), while others represent the latest products of chemical companies. In this section, we shall survey several groups of chemical agents and indicate how they are best applied in the chemical control of microorganisms.

HALOGENS

Halogen:
a highly reactive element whose atoms have seven electrons in the outer shell.

The **halogens** are a group of highly reactive elements whose atoms have seven electrons in the outer shell. Two halogens, chlorine and iodine, are commonly used for disinfection.

Chlorine is available in a gaseous form and as both organic and inorganic compounds. It is widely used in municipal water supplies, where it keeps bacterial populations at low levels. Chlorine combines readily with numerous ions in water; therefore, enough chlorine must be added to ensure that a residue remains for antibacterial activity. In municipal water, the residue of chlorine is usually about 0.2 to

MicroFocus 22.2

A CLOVE FOR ALL REASONS

Some people love it; some people loathe it. But nearly everyone has an opinion about the merits of garlic. Moreover, their opinions are often as strong as garlic itself.

The garlic controversy has been going on almost as long as garlic has been known to exist. The Egyptians had a love-hate relationship with the bulb. It was fed to slaves to build up their energy during construction of the pyramids, but people with garlic on their breath were forbidden to enter Egyptian temples because garlic was considered unclean. The Greeks perpetuated this attitude by feeding garlic to athletes, but they forbade anyone who ate it to enter holy places.

Garlic was also part of the pharmacopoeia of the Romans. Physicians applied it to wounds as an antiseptic and prescribed it for people who had respiratory problems, high blood pressure, or parasites. Moreover, Roman soldiers consumed it before going into battle to instill courage.

In recent years, a new group of garlic users has emerged. One scientist, for example, has suggested that joggers eat garlic to offset the pollutants in automobile exhaust fumes. His studies show that garlic binds up lead, mercury, and cadmium, allowing these minerals to pass in the feces. A West German doctor has written that in blood vessels, garlic helps break up the cholesterol that might lead to atherosclerosis. In China, researchers reported that 16 cases of meningitis due to *Cryptococcus neoformans* responded to treatment with

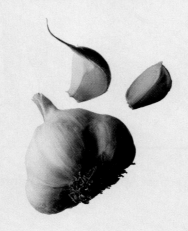

garlic alone. While the percentage of recoveries was lower than with drugs, nevertheless, the results of garlic treatment were said to be promising.

A central European superstition with blurred origins decrees that vampires cannot rise from their coffins if their mouths are crammed with garlic. For centuries, Asian peoples have eaten garlic to purify their complexions and strengthen their intellects, and in many cultures throughout the world, garlic is believed to have aphrodisiac powers. In addition, people in Balkan countries such as Bulgaria consume bulbs of garlic as a regular part of their diet, and their reputation for longevity is well known.

Garlic lovers should note that only fresh garlic achieves the desired medicinal effect. Garlic powder and garlic salt are pale substitutes. In Russia, a garlic extract named allicin is used as a type of antibiotic. The *Merck Index* lists allicin as an "antibacterial principle of garlic." Its odor quickly reveals its origin.

1.0 parts per million (ppm) of free chlorine. One ppm is equivalent to 0.0001 percent, an extremely small amount.

Chlorine is also available as **sodium hypochlorite (NaOCl)** or **calcium hypochlorite [Ca(OCl)$_2$]**. The latter, also known as chlorinated lime, was used by Semmelweis in his studies in Vienna. Hypochlorite compounds release free chlorine in solution. They are typified by the 0.5 percent sodium hypochlorite solution of H. D. Dakin, used extensively for wounds sustained in World Wars I and II. **Dakin's solution** remains popular in Europe, where it is used to treat athlete's foot.

Sodium hypochlorite is used as a bleaching agent in the textile industry; commercially available **bleach** contains about 5 percent of this compound. To disinfect clear water, the Centers for Disease Control and Prevention recommends a half-teaspoon of household chlorine bleach in 2 gallons of water, with 30 minutes of contact time before consumption. Hypochlorites are also useful in very dilute solutions for disinfecting swimming pools and sanitizing factory equipment (**FIGURE 22.5**).

The **chloramines**, such as chloramine-T, are organic compounds that contain chlorine. These compounds release free chlorine more slowly than hypochlorite solutions and are more stable. They are valuable for general wound antisepsis and root canal therapy.

hi-po-klor'ite

Athlete's foot:
a fungal disease accompanied by thin-walled blisters on the skin surface, usually of the feet.

klo'rah-měn
Chloramine:
a disinfectant compound containing chlorine and amino groups.

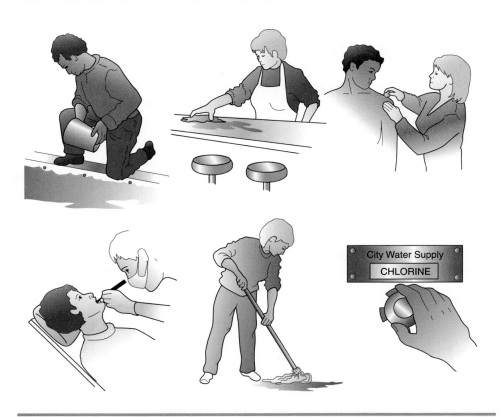

City Water Supply
CHLORINE

FIGURE 22.5

Some Practical Applications of Disinfection with Chlorine Compounds

Chlorine is effective against a broad variety of organisms, including most Gram-positive and Gram-negative bacteria, and many viruses, fungi, and protozoa. However, it is not sporicidal. In microorganisms, the halogen is believed to cause the release of atomic oxygen, which then combines with and inactivates certain cytoplasmic proteins, such as enzymes. Another theory is that chlorine changes the structure of cell membranes, thus leading to leakage.

The **iodine** atom is slightly larger than the chlorine atom and is more reactive and more germicidal. It is widely found in nature in such plants as marine seaweeds, where it is bound to chemical compounds. Iodine acts by halogenating tyrosine portions of protein molecules.

Tincture of iodine, a commonly used antiseptic for wounds, consists of 2 percent iodine and sodium iodide dissolved in ethyl alcohol. For the disinfection of clear water, the CDC recommends 5 drops of tincture of iodine in 1 quart of water, with 30 minutes of contact time before consumption. Iodine compounds in different forms are also valuable sanitizers for restaurant equipment and eating utensils.

Iodophors are iodine-detergent complexes that release iodine over a long period of time and have the added advantage of not staining tissues or fabrics. The detergent portion of the complex loosens the organisms from the surface, and the halogen kills them. Some examples of iodophors are Wescodyne, used in preoperative skin preparations; Ioprep, for presurgical scrubbing; Iosan, for dairy sanitation; and Betadine, for local wounds. Iodophors may also be combined with nondetergent carrier molecules. The best known carrier is **povidone**, which stabilizes the iodine

Tincture of iodine:
a 2 percent iodine solution in ethyl alcohol.

i-o'do-for

po'vĭ-dōn

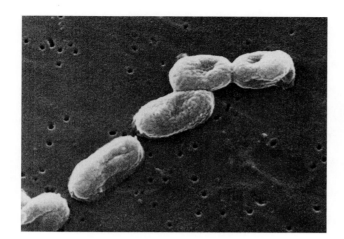

FIGURE 22.6

When Disinfectants Fail to Work

A scanning electron micrograph of *Burkholderia cepacia*. This species was found embedded in the interior surface of a pipe located in a manufacturing plant where iodine disinfectants were produced. Investigators located the bacteria in the pipe after a series of nosocomial diseases were traced to a contaminated iodine product made at the plant.

and releases it slowly. However, compounds like these are not self-sterilizing (FIGURE 22.6). In 1989, for example, four cases of peritoneal *Burkholderia* (*Pseudomonas*) *cepacia* infection were related to a contaminated povidone-iodine product.

burk'hold-er'i-a
se-pa'she-ah

PHENOL AND PHENOLIC COMPOUNDS

Phenol and phenolic compounds (phenolics) have played a key role in disinfection practices since Joseph Lister used them in the 1860s. Phenol remains the standard against which other antiseptics and disinfectants are evaluated in the phenol coefficient test. It is active against Gram-positive bacteria, but its activity is reduced in the presence of organic matter. Biochemists believe that phenol and its derivatives act by coagulating proteins, especially in the cell membrane.

Phenol is expensive, has a pungent odor, and is caustic to the skin; therefore, the role of phenol as an antiseptic has diminished. However, phenol derivatives called **cresols** have greater germicidal activity and lower toxicity than the parent compound. Mixtures of ortho-, meta-, and para-cresol (creosote) are used commercially as wood preservatives for railroad ties, fenceposts, and telephone poles. Another phenol derivative, **hexylresorcinol**, is used in a mouthwash and topical antiseptic (ST37) and in throat lozenges (Sucrets). It has the added advantage of reducing surface tension, thereby loosening bacteria from the tissue and allowing greater penetration of the germicidal agent.

Cresols:
phenol derivatives containing methyl groups.

hek'sil-rĕ-sor'sĭ-nol

Combinations of two phenol molecules called **bisphenols** are prominent in modern disinfection and antisepsis. **Orthophenylphenol**, for example, is used in Lysol, Osyl, Staphene, and Amphyl. Another bisphenol, **hexachlorophene**, was used extensively during the 1950s and 1960s in toothpaste (Ipana), underarm deodorant (Mum), and bath soap (Dial). One product, **pHisoHex**, combined hexachlorophene with a pH-balanced detergent cream. Pediatricians recommended it to retard staphylococcal infections of the scalp and umbilical stump, and for general cleansing of the newborn. However, a late 1960s study indicated that excessive amounts could be absorbed through the skin and cause neurological damage, and hexachlorophene was subsequently removed from over-the-counter products. The product pHisoHex is still available, but only by prescription.

hek'sah-klo'ro-fēn

An important bisphenol relative is **chlorhexidine** (FIGURE 22.7). This compound was approved in 1976 by the FDA for use as a surgical scrub, hand wash, and superficial skin wound cleanser. A 4 percent chlorhexidine solution in isopropyl alcohol

klor-heks'i-dēn

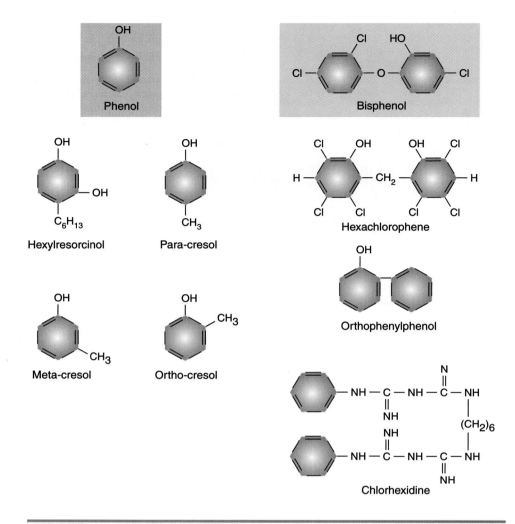

FIGURE 22.7

Phenol Derivatives

The chemical structures of some important derivatives of phenol used in disinfection and antisepsis.

is commercially available as Hibiclens. The chemical is believed to act on the cell membrane of Gram-positive and Gram-negative bacteria. Chlorhexidine in a concentration of 0.2 percent is also the most extensively tested and most effective antiplaque and antigingivitis agent. However, evidence indicates that bacteria may grow within it (FIGURE 22.8).

tri-klo'san

A bisphenol in widespread use is **trichlosan**, a broad-spectrum antimicrobial agent that destroys bacteria by disrupting cell membranes (and possibly, cell walls) by blocking the synthesis of lipids. Trichlosan, known commercially as Irgasan and Ster-Zac, is fairly mild and nontoxic, and it is effective against pathogenic bacteria (but only partially against viruses and fungi). The chemical is included in antibacterial soaps, lotions, mouthwashes, toothpastes, toys, food trays, underwear, kitchen sponges, utensils, and cutting boards. Products developed by Microban, Inc. incorporate trichlosan into the plastic and synthetic fibers of many of these items. The negative side to trichlosan use is that bacteria may develop resistance to the chemical, just

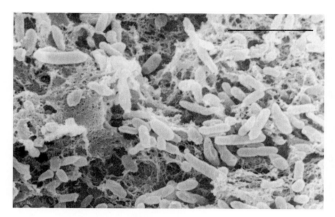

FIGURE 22.8

Contamination

A scanning electron micrograph of the inner surface of a plastic chlorhexidine bottle contaminated with *Serratia marcescens*. Epidemiologists located these bacilli following an outbreak of *S. marcescens* infections in a hospital. The study indicates that *S. marcescens* survives in chlorhexidine and may be transferred in the disinfectant. (Bar = 5 μm.)

as they have developed resistance to antibiotics. Indeed, a ninth-grade student presenting her experiment at a recent Massachusetts science fair was among the first to draw attention to this possibility.

HEAVY METALS

The term *oligodynamic action*, meaning "small power," expresses the activity of heavy metals, such as mercury, silver, and copper, on microorganisms. The elements are called **heavy metals** because of their large atomic weights and complex electron configurations.

Heavy metals are very reactive with proteins, particularly at the protein's sulfhydryl groups (—SH), and they are believed to bind protein molecules together by forming bridges between the groups. Because many of the proteins involved are enzymes, the cellular metabolism is disrupted, and the microorganism dies. However, heavy metals are not sporicidal.

Mercury is one of the traditional heavy metal antiseptics, having been used as **mercuric chloride (HgCl$_2$)** by the Greeks and Romans for treating skin diseases. However, mercury is very toxic to the host, and the antimicrobial activity of mercury is reduced when other organic matter is present. In such products as Mercurochrome, Merthiolate, and Metaphen, mercury is combined with carrier compounds and is less toxic when applied to the skin, especially after surgical incisions. Another mercury derivative is **thimerosal**, previously used as a preservative in vaccines. As of 1999, the U.S. Public Health Service recommended its removal and replacement as a safety measure.

Copper is active against chlorophyll-containing organisms and is a potent inhibitor of algae. As **copper sulfate (CuSO$_4$)**, it is incorporated into algicides and is used in swimming pools and municipal water supplies. Copper sulfate is also mixed with lime to form the bluish-white Bordeaux mixture used since 1882 to control the growth of fungi (**MicroFocus 22.3**).

Silver in the form of **silver nitrate (AgNo$_3$)** is useful as an antiseptic and disinfectant. For example, one drop of a 1 percent silver nitrate solution may be placed in the eyes of newborns to protect against infection by *Neisseria gonorrhoeae*. This Gram-negative diplococcus can cause blindness if contracted by a newborn during passage through the birth canal. In 1884, Karl S. F. Credé first used silver nitrate to prevent gonococcal eye disease; many states now require that Credé's

Heavy metal:
an electron-donating element whose atoms are large, with complex electron arrangements.

sul-fi′dril

thi-mer′o-sal

Algae:
simple green organisms that include cyanobacteria.

kra-dā′

MicroFocus 22.3

FROM OUT OF THE BLUE

One October day in 1882, Professor Alexis Millardet of the University of Bordeaux was strolling through a vineyard in Medoc, France. Downy mildew of grapes, a fungal disease, had been widespread that year, and Millardet was surprised to note that the grapevines beside his path were rather healthy. By contrast, those most everywhere else were diseased. He paused to examine the leaves and found them covered with a bluish-white deposit.

Millardet inquired of the owner what the deposit might be. The owner responded that it was customary to spray the vines with a mixture of copper sulfate (blue) and lime (white) to make them look poisonous. This would quickly deter any would-be thieves from helping themselves to the grapes.

Millardet's curiosity was aroused. It was clear that the pathway vines were greener and healthier than their counterparts farther off in the field. He therefore devised a set of experiments to test the antifungal properties of the copper sulfate and lime mixture. Within 3 years, he concluded that the combination of chemicals was an effective deterrent to mildew, and the now famous "Bordeaux mixture" came into being. Today the mixture is one of the most widely used fungicides in all the world.

The story has an ironic twist. While mildew was ravaging French vines, other Mediterranean countries hurriedly planted their own vines, anticipating the collapse of the French wine industry. But the collapse never came. The Bordeaux mixture saved French

vines and left the neophyte grape growers with lots of grapes but nowhere to sell them.

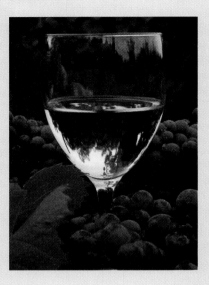

method be followed (although an erythromycin or tetracycline ointment is often substituted because silver nitrate can cause irritation). Silver compounds are also used to treat suturing threads.

ALCOHOLS

Ethyl alcohol:
a 2-carbon consumable alcohol used as an antiseptic and disinfectant.

Alcohols are effective skin antiseptics and valuable disinfectants for medical instruments. For practical use, the preferred alcohol is ethyl alcohol. **Ethyl alcohol** is active against vegetative bacterial cells, including the tubercle bacillus, but it has no effect on spores. It denatures proteins and dissolves lipids, an action that may lead to cell membrane disintegration. Ethyl alcohol also is a strong dehydrating agent.

Because ethyl alcohol reacts readily with any organic matter, medical instruments and thermometers must be thoroughly cleaned before exposure. Usually, a 50 to 80 percent alcohol solution is recommended because water prevents rapid evaporation and assists penetration into the tissues. A 10-minute immersion in 70 percent ethyl alcohol is generally sufficient to disinfect a thermometer or delicate instrument. Ethyl alcohol is used in many popular hand sanitizers.

i'so-pro'pil

Alcohol is used to preserve cosmetics, and to treat skin before a venipuncture or injection. It mechanically removes bacteria from the skin and dissolves lipids. **Isopropyl alcohol**, or rubbing alcohol, has high bactericidal activity in concentrations as high as 99 percent. Methyl alcohol is toxic to the tissues and is used infrequently.

To this point . . .

We have discussed four major groups of chemical agents used for disinfectant and antiseptic purposes. Halogen compounds, which include chlorine and iodine, are effective against most microorganisms. The halogens can be used either in elemental forms or as derivatives, such as chloramines and iodophors. Phenol is rarely used in modern disinfection practices, but the phenolic compounds, such as bisphenols, are valuable skin cleansers. The heavy metals include mercury, copper, and silver. Silver nitrate is often used to prevent the transmission of gonorrhea to newborns. Alcohols are valuable for the disinfection of instruments, especially as 70 percent ethyl alcohol.

Through the discussions of these chemical agents you may have noted certain general considerations that apply to all. For example, the chemical agent will usually combine with any organic matter present, so that cleanliness is an important prerequisite to disinfection. Also, the chemical agents react with a wide spectrum of organisms, not just one type. Moreover, they are generally useless against bacterial spores. Virtually no chemical agent is useful within the human body, but most are employed to interrupt the spread of organisms outside the body.

In the final section of this chapter, we shall discuss three chemical agents used for sterilization purposes. These agents are sporicidal if sufficient time is given for them to act and proper conditions are established. We shall also mention a group of other agents that are used on the skin surface and in wounds.

22.3

Other Chemical Agents

The chemical agents we discussed in previous sections are best recognized as disinfectants and antiseptics. In addition, there are some chemicals that can be used for sterilization purposes, especially for modern high-technology equipment (as well as the mundane but essential Petri dish). Three such agents are considered next.

FORMALDEHYDE

Formaldehyde is a gas at high temperatures and a solid at room temperatures. When 37 grams of the solid are suspended in 100 ml of water, a solution called **formalin** results. For over a century, formalin was used in embalming fluid for anatomical specimens (though rarely used any more) and by morticians, as well as for disinfecting purposes (MicroFocus 22.4). In microbiology, formalin is utilized for inactivating viruses in certain vaccines and producing toxoids from toxins.

In the gaseous form, formaldehyde is expelled into a closed chamber where it is a sterilizing agent for surgical equipment, hospital gowns, and medical instruments. However, penetration is poor, and the surface must be exposed to the gas for up to 12 hours for effective sterilization. Instruments can be sterilized by placing them in a 20 percent solution of formaldehyde in 70 percent alcohol for 18 hours. Formaldehyde, however, leaves a residue, and instruments must be rinsed

Formalin:
a 37 percent solution of
formaldehyde in water.

MicroFocus 22.4

FOR PEOPLE WHO WEAR SHOES

Here's some good news for people who can't bear to part with those extraordinarily comfortable but oh-so-smelly shoes: You can get rid of the smell and enjoy many more years with them. But before you do anything, you should understand what's going on.

The first thing you should know is that shoes become smelly when odors accumulate in the material of the shoe. The odors come from gases that bacteria produce while growing in the material. It seems that airborne cocci, recently identified as members of the genus *Micrococcus*, thrive in the sweat made by feet (about a gallon per week, in some people). This sweat is absorbed by the shoe's material. The bacteria break down the sweat's organic components and produce sulfur compounds not unlike the hydrogen sulfide in a swamp or landfill. These sulfur compounds gather in the material and produce the odor we turn up our nose at.

So what to do? First, try to rotate your shoes as often as possible, and let them air out as long as feasible between wearings. (Some of the gas will dissipate.) Try to wear cotton, silk, or other natural fiber socks rather than synthetic materials, because bacteria thrive better in synthetic materials. This is because synthetics retain more heat, increase sweating, and limit evaporation. And use a foot powder to absorb sweat to make life difficult for the micrococci.

Now, for those old shoes. Buy some formaldehyde at a local pharmacy, and try wiping the insides of the shoes with it. Be sure to follow all the precautions that come with the formaldehyde because it can be poisonous. You can also roll up rags, stuff them inside the shoes, and soak them with the formaldehyde. Place the shoes in a closed place, such as a box, and leave them for a few days in an airy environment where the fumes can disperse. Be sure to dry out the shoes before wearing them again. And if it works, score another one for the disinfectants.

---

before use. Many allergic individuals develop a contact dermatitis to this compound (Chapter 20).

Formaldehyde is an **alkylating agent**. It reacts with amino and hydroxyl groups of nucleic acids and proteins, and with carboxyl and sulfhydryl groups in proteins by inserting between them a small carbon fragment (an alkyl group) and forming bridges (FIGURE 22.9). This insertion changes the structures of the molecules and interferes with an organism's biochemistry, thereby leading to death. We shall discuss two other alkylating agents, ethylene oxide and glutaraldehyde, next.

Sulfhydryl group:
a chemical group consisting of a sulfur and a hydrogen atom.

ETHYLENE OXIDE

The development of plastics for use in microbiology required a suitable method for sterilizing these heat-sensitive materials. In the 1950s, research scientists discovered the antimicrobial abilities of **ethylene oxide (EtO)** and essentially made the plastic Petri dish and plastic syringe possible.

Ethylene oxide is a small molecule with excellent penetration capacity and sporicidal ability. However, it is both toxic and highly explosive. Its explosiveness is reduced by mixture with Freon gas in Cryoxide or carbon dioxide gas in Carboxide, but its toxicity remains a problem for those who work with it. The gas is released into a tightly sealed chamber where it circulates for up to 4 hours with carefully controlled humidity (FIGURE 22.10). The chamber must then be flushed with inert gas for 8 to 12 hours to ensure that all traces of EtO are removed, otherwise the chemical will cause "cold burns" on contact with the skin.

Ethylene oxide is utilized to sterilize paper, leather, wood, metal, and rubber products, as well as plastics. In hospitals, it is used to sterilize catheters, artificial heart valves, heart-lung machine components, and optical equipment. The National Aeronautics and Space Administration (NASA) uses the gas for sterilization of

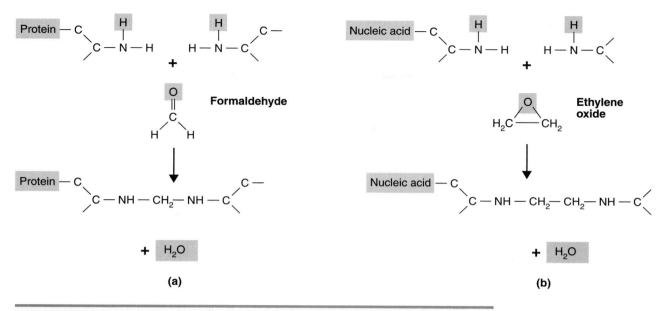

(a)   (b)

FIGURE 22.9

Alkylating Agents

The chemical reactions that take place between alkylating agents and other molecules. (a) Formaldehyde reacts with amino groups on protein molecules and forms bridges between adjacent groups. (b) Ethylene oxide reacts with nucleic acid molecules and forms bridges between adjacent groups. The effect in both cases is to alter the structure of the molecules and change the biochemistry of the microorganisms.

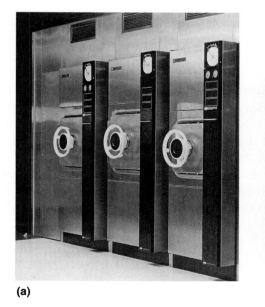

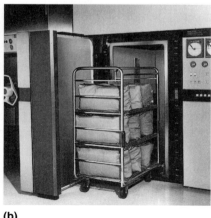

(a)   (b)

FIGURE 22.10

Sterilization with Ethylene Oxide

(a) A bank of ethylene oxide sterilizers used to achieve "gas sterilization" or "cold sterilization" of laboratory materials. (b) Materials are wheeled into the sterilizer and subjected to a multihour process, during which the most resistant microorganisms are destroyed. Plastic Petri dishes and other plastic items are sterilized by this method.

interplanetary space capsules. Ethylene oxide chambers have become chemical counterparts of autoclaves for sterilization procedures. Often they are called gas autoclaves.

A closely related gas, **beta-propiolactone (BPL)**, is less explosive than ethylene oxide, but its penetrating capacity is more limited. In liquid form, BPL is used to sterilize vaccines, sera, and surgical ligatures. However, scientists have shown it to be carcinogenic, and BPL is therefore used only under restricted circumstances.

GLUTARALDEHYDE

Glutaraldehyde has become one of the most effective chemical liquids for sterilization purposes. This small molecule destroys vegetative cells within 10 to 30 minutes and spores in 10 hours. Glutaraldehyde is an alkylating agent, usually employed as a 2 percent solution. To use it for sterilization purposes, materials have to be precleaned, immersed for 10 hours, rinsed thoroughly with sterile water, dried in a special cabinet with sterile air, and stored in a sterile container to ensure that the material remains sterile. If any of these parameters is altered, the materials may be disinfected but may not be considered sterile.

Because the activity of glutaraldehyde is not greatly reduced by organic matter, the chemical is recommended for use on surgical instruments where residual blood may be present. In addition, glutaraldehyde does not damage delicate objects, and therefore it can be used to sterilize optical equipment, such as the fiber optic endoscopes used for arthroscopic surgery. It gives off irritating fumes, however, and instruments must be rinsed thoroughly in sterile water. At pH 7.5, glutaraldehyde kills *S. aureus* in 5 minutes and *M. tuberculosis* in 10 minutes.

HYDROGEN PEROXIDE

Hydrogen peroxide (H_2O_2) is used as a rinse in wounds, scrapes, and abrasions. The area foams and effervesces, as **catalase** in the tissue breaks down hydrogen peroxide to oxygen and water. The furious bubbling removes microorganisms mechanically. Hydrogen peroxide decomposition also results in a reactive form of oxygen—the superoxide radical—highly toxic to microorganisms. Anaerobic bacteria are sensitive to hydrogen peroxide because the sudden release of oxygen gas inhibits their growth.

New forms of H_2O_2, such as Super D Hydrogen Peroxide, are more stable than traditional forms and therefore do not decompose spontaneously. Such inanimate materials as soft contact lenses, utensils, heat-sensitive plastics, and food-processing equipment can be disinfected within 30 minutes. Sterilization can also be achieved after 6 hours of exposure to a 6 percent solution. Microbiologists are currently researching the use of hydrogen peroxide for destroying bacteria in milk and milk products.

SOAPS AND DETERGENTS

A **soap** is a chemical compound of fatty acids combined with potassium or sodium hydroxide. The pH of the compound is usually about 8.0, and some microbial destruction is therefore due to the alkaline conditions established on the skin. However, the major activity of soap is as a degerming agent for the mechanical removal of microorganisms from the skin surface.

Soaps are **wetting agents**—that is, they emulsify and solubilize particles clinging to a surface. The surface tension is also reduced by the soap. In addition, soaps remove skin oils, further reducing the surface tension and increasing the cleaning action.

---

pro'pe-o-lak'tōn

Carcinogenic:
able to cause cancer.

gloo'tah-ral'dĕ-hīd

Hydrogen peroxide:
a simple chemical compound digested by catalase to water and oxygen.

Soap:
a compound of fatty acids and potassium or sodium hydroxide.

Surface tension:
the attraction between a surface and a particle lying on it.

Detergents are synthetic chemicals acting as strong wetting agents and surface tension reducers. Since they are actively attracted to the phosphate groups of cellular membranes, they also alter the membranes and encourage leakage from the cytoplasm. When used to clean cutting boards (MicroFocus 22.5), they can reduce the possibility of transmitting contaminants.

The **anionic detergents** yield negatively charged ions in solution. These detergents are somewhat active against Gram-positive bacteria, but the negative charges of bacteria usually repel them and limit their use to common laundry products. Anionic detergents such as Triton W-30 and Duponol find value as iodophors.

Other detergents are **cationic**. These derivatives of ammonium chloride contain four organic radicals in place of the four hydrogens, and at least one radical is a long-chain alkyl group (FIGURE 22.11). The positively charged ammonium group is counterbalanced by a negatively charged chloride ion. Such compounds are often called **quaternary ammonium compounds** or, simply, quats.

Anionic:
yielding negatively charged ions in solution.

Cationic:
yielding positively charged ions in solution.

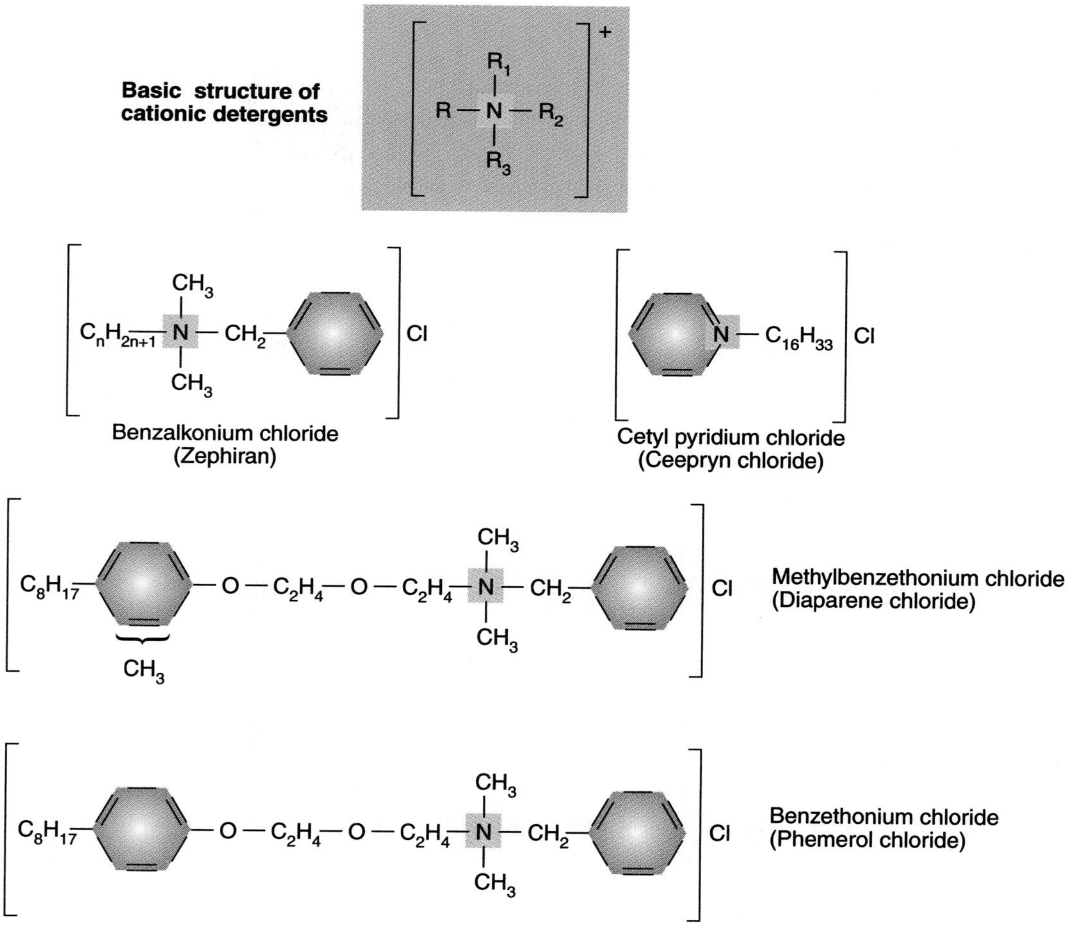

FIGURE 22.11

Cationic Detergents

The chemical structures of some important cationic detergents used in disinfection and antisepsis. Note that a long chain of carbon atoms, called an alkyl group, is included in each molecule, and that nitrogen is bonded to four radicals.

MicroFocus 22.5

CUTTING BOARD WARS

He: "I'll get out a cutting board to cut up the salad."

She: "You might want to use the plastic one instead of the wood one."

He: "Why's that?"

She: "Because bacteria get caught in the grooves of the wood."

He: "But I read somewhere that the wood draws moisture and bacteria so deep into the grooves they can't reach food. The article said that plastic lets

bacteria stay close to the surface so they get on the food."

She: "Well I heard that plastic cleans better than wood, so it's safer."

He: "Yeah, but wood has antibacterial powers that plastic doesn't have."

She: "Maybe so, but plastic doesn't have all those grooves and scars where bacteria can hide."

He: "How about this: I read about some guy in California who found

that Salmonella infections are more likely if a household uses a plastic board."

She: "Well, I don't know about anybody in California, but I do know that plastic is easier to dry thoroughly. Wood stays moist, and that lets bacteria stay alive."

He: "How about we forget the salad and go out to McDonald's?"

She: "How about Burger King?"

ben'zal-ko'ne-um
se'til pi'rid'i-um

The cationic detergents have rather long, complex names, such as **benzalkonium chloride** in Zephiran and **cetyl pyridium chloride** in Ceepryn. Other detergents are used in Phemerol and Diaparene. Cationic detergents are bacteriostatic on a broad range of bacteria, especially Gram-positive bacteria, and are relatively stable, with little odor. They are used as sanitizing agents for industrial equipment and food utensils, as skin antiseptics, in mouthwashes and in storage solutions for contact lenses, and for disinfecting hospital walls and floors. Their use as disinfectants for food-preparation surfaces can help reduce incidents (FIGURE 22.12). Mixing with soap, however, reduces their activity, and certain Gram-negative bacteria, such as *Burkholderia (Pseudomonas) cepacia*, can grow in them.

burk'hold-er'i-a se-pa'she-ah

DYES

tri-fen'il-meth'ān

Dyes are useful in microbiology as staining reagents and in laboratory media, where they help select out certain organisms from a mixture. A group of dyes called **triphenylmethane dyes** is also useful as antiseptics against species of *Bacillus* and *Staphylococcus*. The group includes malachite green and crystal violet. Crystal violet has also been used traditionally as **gentian violet** for trench mouth, and for *Candida albicans* infections such as thrush. Interference with cell wall construction appears to be the mode of activity. The dye is bactericidal at very weak dilutions of less than 1:10,000.

ak'ri-fla'vin

A second group of dyes, the **acridine dyes**, includes acriflavine and proflavine. Both dyes are used as antiseptics for staphylococcal infections in wounds. They apparently act by combining directly with DNA, thereby halting RNA synthesis.

ACIDS

un'dec-ĕ-len'ik

Certain acids are useful as antiseptics or disinfectants. The popular ones include **benzoic, salicylic**, and **undecylenic** acids for tinea infections of the skin. These infections are caused by various species of fungi, as noted in Chapter 14.

Organic acids are particularly valuable as food preservatives. Lactic and acetic acids, for example, are important preservatives in sour foods such as cheeses, sauerkraut, and pickled products. Propionic acid is added to bakery products to keep microbial populations low. Chapter 24 discusses these preservatives in more detail.

In general, acid enhances the effects of disinfectants and antiseptics and makes them more soluble. Also, heat is a more potent sterilizing agent if acid conditions are present, because hydrolysis is increased. Acid is therefore a valuable adjunct to disinfection, albeit in an indirect way.

TABLE 22.2 summarizes the chemical agents used in controlling microorganisms.

FIGURE **22.12**

A Case of *Plesiomonas* and *Salmonella* Infection

This incident occurred over a 5-day period in 1996. An unusually high number of people became ill as a result of food contamination traced to contaminated water.

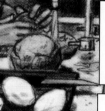

TEXTBOOK CASES

1. On June 19 and 20, it rained heavily in Livingston County, New York. The rain caused soil to run off from a local poultry farm into a stream adjoining the farm. The bacteria *Plesiomonas shigelloides* and *Salmonella* Hartford were probably in the soil, and they entered the water supply.

2. The stream ran into town and passed several feet over a well dug on the grounds of a local convenience store about 500 yards from the farm. The owner also sold pizza and catered neighborhood parties.

3. Two days later, on June 22, the caterer prepared food for a party. He made macaroni salad, potato salad, and a mixed green salad. He used the well water to wash and mix ingredients, and to clean his kitchen utensils. In doing so, he probably introduced contamination.

4. That evening, the caterer delivered the salads to the party along with a variety of other dishes and baked goods. Attending were 189 people who were celebrating the wedding anniversary of the host and hostess.

5. By June 24, 30 party guests were ill with diarrhea, nausea, abdominal cramps, and, in some cases, vomiting. Follow-up studies revealed that 43 of 56 people who ate macaroni salad became ill, and 36 of 49 guests who had potato salad were also sick. A total of 60 of the 189 attendees suffered illness.

6. Public health investigators examined the caterer's premises and were drawn to the well. The chlorinator was not operating, and there was no filtration mechanism. Lab tests revealed *Plesiomonas* and *Salmonella* in the water. They concluded that well water was the probable culprit in the outbreak.

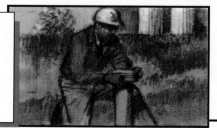

TABLE 22.2

Summary of Chemical Agents Used to Control Microorganisms

CHEMICAL AGENT	ANTISEPTIC OR DISINFECTANT	MECHANISM OF ACTIVITY	APPLICATIONS	LIMITATIONS	ANTIMICROBIAL SPECTRUM
Chlorine	Chlorine gas Sodium hypochlorite Chloramines	Protein oxidation Membrane leakage	Water treatment Skin antisepsis Equipment spraying Food processing	Inactivated by organic matter Objectionable taste, odor	Broad variety of bacteria, fungi, protozoa, viruses
Iodine	Tincture of iodine Iodophors	Halogenates tyrosine in proteins	Skin antisepsis Food processing Preoperative preparation	Inactivated by organic matter Objectionable taste, odor	Broad variety of bacteria, fungi, protozoa, viruses
Phenol and derivative	Cresols Trichlosan Hexachlorophene Hexylresorcinol Chlorhexidine	Coagulates proteins Disrupts cell membranes	General preservatives Skin antisepsis with detergent	Toxic to tissues Disagreeable odor	Gram-positive bacteria Some fungi
Mercury	Mercuric chloride Merthiolate Metaphen	Combines with —SH groups in proteins	Skin antiseptics Disinfectants	Inactivated by organic matter Toxic to tissues Slow acting	Broad variety of bacteria, fungi, protozoa, viruses
Copper	Copper sulfate	Combines with proteins	Algicide in swimming pools Municipal water supplies	Inactivated by organic matter	Algae Some fungi
Silver	Silver nitrate	Binds proteins	Skin antiseptic Eyes of newborns	Skin irritation	Organisms in burned tissue Gonococci
Alcohol	70% ethyl alcohol	Denatures proteins Dissolves lipids Dehydrating agent	Instrument disinfectant Skin antiseptic	Precleaning necessary Skin irritation	Vegetative bacterial cells, fungi, protozoa, viruses
Formaldehyde	Formaldehyde gas Formalin	Reacts with functional groups in proteins and nucleic acids	Embalming Vaccine production Gaseous sterilant	Poor penetration Allergenic Toxic to tissues Neutralized by organic matter	Broad variety of bacteria, fungi, protozoa, viruses
Ethylene oxide	Ethylene oxide gas	Reacts with functional groups in proteins and nucleic acids	Sterilization of instruments, equipment, heat-sensitive objects	Explosive Toxic to skin Requires constant humidity	All microorganisms, including spores
Glutaraldehyde	Glutaraldehyde	Reacts with functional groups in proteins and nucleic acids	Sterilization of surgical supplies	Unstable Toxic to skin	All microorganisms, including spores
Hydrogen peroxide	Hydrogen peroxide	Creates aerobic environment Oxidizes protein groups	Wound treatment	Limited use	Anaerobic bacteria
Cationic detergents	Commercial detergents	Dissolve lipids in cell membranes	Industrial sanitization Skin antiseptic Disinfectant	Neutralized by soap	Broad variety of microorganisms
Triphenyl-methane dyes	Malachite green Crystal violet	React with cytoplasmic components	Wounds Skin infection	Residual stain	Staphylococci Some fungi Gram-positive bacteria

Summary of Chemical Agents Used to Control Microorganisms (continued)

CHEMICAL AGENT	ANTISEPTIC OR DISINFECTANT	MECHANISM OF ACTIVITY	APPLICATIONS	LIMITATIONS	ANTIMICROBIAL SPECTRUM
Acridine dyes	Acriflavine Proflavine	React with cytoplasmic components	Skin infection	Residual stain	Staphylococci Gram-positive bacteria
Acids	Benzoic acid Salicylic acid Undecylinic acid Lactic and propionic acids	Alter pH	Skin infections Food preservatives	Skin irritation	Many bacteria and fungi

Note to the Student

In this chapter, we have focused on a broad variety of antiseptics and disinfectants but few, you will note, are of significant value on the body surface and virtually none are used to treat internal disease. Most chemical agents are used for equipment, instruments, materials, and other related purposes. The major reason so few are available as antiseptics is simple: Chemicals will often do more harm to the human body than to the microorganisms they are intended to kill.

Witness the spectacular rise and fall of hexachlorophene during the 1960s and 1970s. This compound's antimicrobial capabilities, residual activity, and lack of side effects appeared too good to be true. Eventually, though, it was found to be hazardous to the tissues. Similarly, many thousands of possible antiseptics have fallen by the wayside. If you have a background in chemistry, then you know of the dazzling array of available chemicals. Yet how many are useful as antiseptics?

Summary

Chemical agents are effectively used to control the growth of microorganisms, even though they do not achieve sterilization. Instead, they are generally able to destroy pathogenic microorganisms, a process called disinfection. A chemical agent used on a living object, such as the body surface, is an antiseptic; one used on a nonliving object, such as a tabletop, is a disinfectant. Both antiseptics and disinfectants are selected according to certain criteria and are evaluated by the phenol coefficient method.

Among the important chemical agents for disinfection are the halogens and phenols. Halogens, such as chlorine and iodine, are useful for water disinfection, wound antisepsis, and for various forms of sanitation. Phenol derivatives, such as hexachlorophene and chlorhexidine, are valuable skin antiseptics and presurgical scrubs. In both cases, the chemical agent reacts with most types of organic matter (including microorganisms), so precleaning is necessary prior to disinfection. Other useful chemical agents are heavy metals, such as silver in silver nitrate and copper in copper sulfate, and alcohol, which is commonly used in a 70 percent solution of ethyl alcohol. Precleaning and complete immersion are required for alcohol use.

Chemical agents can also be used as sterilizing agents, as long as a closed chamber is employed for exposure. Formaldehyde, ethylene oxide, and glutaraldehyde are examples of small molecules that unite with amino and hydroxyl groups in proteins and nucleic acids to alter the biochemistry of microorganisms. Hydrogen peroxide acts by releasing oxygen to cause an effervescing cleansing action, and

detergents have a profound effect on microbial membranes. Other useful chemical agents include dyes and acids, the latter used as preservatives in foods. The broad variety of chemical agents usually ensures that an agent is available for each situation.

Questions for Thought and Discussion

1. Suppose you were in charge of a clinical laboratory where instruments are routinely disinfected and equipment is sanitized. A salesperson from a disinfectant company stops in to spur your interest in a new chemical agent. What questions might you ask the salesperson about the product?

2. Statistics compiled by the CDC indicate that between 5 and 10 percent of hospitalized patients (between 1.75 and 3.5 million patients per year) acquire infections during their stay. A significant percentage of these situations could be prevented, officials maintain, if hospital workers took more care in washing their hands. What reasons, do you suppose, are offered by workers for their negligence?

3. While on a camping trip, you find that a luxury hotel has been built near the stream where you once swam and from which you drank freely. Fearing contamination of the stream, you decide that before drinking the water, some form of disinfection would be wise. The nearest town has only a grocery store, pharmacy, and post office. What might you purchase? Why?

4. European manufacturers have included chlorhexidine in their toothpastes and mouthwashes for many years, but there has been resistance to this practice in the United States. Would you favor or oppose such a move? Why?

5. A study reported in 1992 in the *New England Journal of Medicine* recounted the reluctance of patients to ask their physician a vitally important question just before their examination began. Can you guess what that question is? (It is not "How much do you charge?")

6. A portable room humidifier can incubate and disseminate infectious microorganisms. If a friend asked for your recommendations on disinfecting the humidifier, what might you suggest?

7. With over 11 million children currently attending day-care centers in the United States, the possibilities for disease transmission among children has mounted considerably. Under what circumstances may antiseptics and disinfectants be used to preclude the spread of microorganisms?

8. Researchers at Virginia Polytechnic Institute have shown that apples infected with Gram-negative rods can be made safe for consumption by dipping the apples in a mixture of vinegar and hydrogen peroxide, both available at grocery stores. How does each component in the mixture work?

9. In 1912, J. W. Churchman coined the word *bacteriostasis* to indicate that certain dyes were inhibitory rather than destructive to bacteria. What does the word mean today, and how is it applied to the germicides?

10. A recently published brochure called *Operation Clean Hands* lists several instances where individuals should wash their hands thoroughly. One list entitled "Before you" includes "prepare food" and "insert contact lenses." A second list entitled "After you" includes "change a diaper" and "play with an animal." How many items can you add to each list?

11. A student has finished his work in the laboratory and is preparing to leave. He remembers the instructor's precautions to wash and disinfect his hands before leaving. However, he cannot remember whether to wash first then disinfect, or to disinfect then wash. What advice might you give?

12. Before taking a blood sample from the finger, the blood bank technician commonly rubs the skin with a pad soaked in alcohol. Many people think that this procedure sterilizes the skin. Are they correct? Why?

13. A Clorox advertisement published in 1993 carries the following message: "Raw foods like chicken can carry germs and bacteria that cause salmonella sickness. It's important to kill the bacteria on any surface raw foods touch with a little Clorox. Soap and water won't do the trick." Immediately above the statement was a photograph of a raw chicken, a green pepper, three carrots, and a red Bermuda onion. At the bottom of the page a box describes "a little Clorox" as a solution made by mixing a sink full of water with ⅛ cup of Regular Clorox Liquid Bleach. How many things can you find wrong with this advertisement? Suppose you were the company microbiologist. What would you say in your version of the advertisement?

14. Suppose you had just removed the thermometer from the mouth of your sick child and confirmed your suspicion of fever. Before checking the temperature of the next child, how would you treat the thermometer to disinfect it?

15. The water in your home aquarium always seems to resemble pea soup, but your friend's is crystal clear.

Not wanting to appear stupid, you avoid asking him his secret. But one day, in a moment of desperation, you break down and ask, whereupon he knowledgeably points to a few pennies among the gravel. What is the secret of the pennies?

Review

The chemical agents are a broad and diverse group, as this chapter has demonstrated. To test your knowledge of the chapter contents, match the chemical agent on the right to the statement on the left by placing the correct letter in the available space. A letter may be used once, more than once, or not at all. The answers are listed in Appendix D.

_____ 1. The halogen in bleach
_____ 2. Sterilizes heat-sensitive materials
_____ 3. Used to prevent gonococcal eye disease
_____ 4. Part of chlorhexidine molecule
_____ 5. Oxygen retards anaerobic bacteria
_____ 6. Seventy percent concentration recommended
_____ 7. Active ingredient in Betadine
_____ 8. Quaternary compounds, or quats
_____ 9. Can induce a contact dermatitis
_____ 10. Valuable food preservative
_____ 11. Often used as a tincture
_____ 12. Rinse for wounds and scrapes
_____ 13. Example of a heavy metal
_____ 14. Enhances antimicrobial activity of heat
_____ 15. Two molecules in hexachlorophene
_____ 16. Aids mechanical removal of organisms
_____ 17. Exerts an oligodynamic action
_____ 18. Used by Joseph Lister
_____ 19. Used for plastic Petri dishes
_____ 20. Benzoic and salicylic for tinea
_____ 21. Found in Zephiran and Diaparene
_____ 22. Used to purify waters
_____ 23 Derivatives of ammonium compounds
_____ 24. Active ingredient in Dakin's solution
_____ 25. Broken down by catalase

A. iodine
B. ethylene oxide
C. hydrogen peroxide
D. ethyl alcohol
E. acid
F. chlorine
G. glutaraldehyde
H. soap
I. phenol
J. silver
K. cationic detergent
L. dye
M. anionic detergent
N. formaldehyde

http://microbiology.jbpub.com

The site features **eLearning,** an on-line review area that provides quizzes and other tools to help you study for your class. You can also follow useful links for in-depth information, read more MicroFocus stories, or just find out the latest microbiology news.

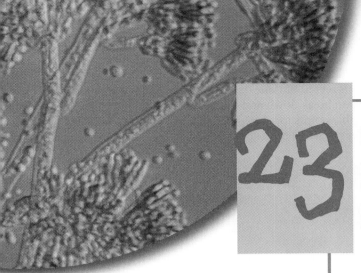

23 Chemotherapeutic Agents and Antibiotics

During the third and fourth years of [medical] school we also began to learn something that worried us all, although it was not much talked about. On the wards of the great Boston teaching hospitals . . . it gradually dawned on us that we could do nothing to change the course of the great majority of the diseases we were so busy analyzing, that medicine, for all its facade as a learned profession, was in real life a profoundly ignorant occupation.

—Lewis Thomas describing 1933 medicine in the preantibiotic era

FOR CENTURIES, PHYSICANS BELIEVED that heroic measures were necessary to save patients from the ravages of infectious disease. They prescribed frightening courses of purges and bloodlettings, enormous doses of strange chemical concoctions, blood-curdling ice water baths, deadly starvations, and other drastic remedies. These treatments probably complicated an already bad situation by reducing the natural body defenses to the point of exhaustion.

But a revolution in medicine took place about 1825 when a group of doctors in Boston and London experimented to see what would happen if such treatments were withheld from patients. Surprisingly, they found that the survival rate was essentially the same—and, in some cases, better. Over the next few decades, the lessons from their experiments spread, and as the worst features of heroic therapy disappeared, doctors adopted a more conservative, nonmeddling approach to disease. It became the doctor's job to diagnose the illness, explain it to the family, predict what would happen, and then stand by and care for the patient within the limits of what was known.

When the germ theory of disease emerged in the late 1800s, insights about microorganisms added considerably to the understanding of disease and increased the storehouse of knowledge available to the doctor. However, it did not change the fact that little, if anything, could be done for the infected patient (FIGURE 23.1). Tuberculosis continued to

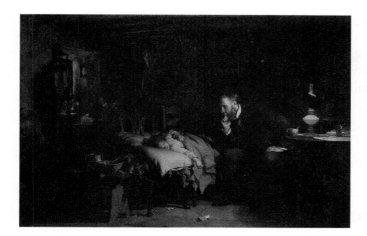

FIGURE 23.1

The Doctor

A painting depicting a physician in the 1800s caring for his patient. Physicians were expected to recognize an illness, distinguish it from other illnesses, and minister to their patients as best they could. Without antibiotics, their ability to treat infectious diseases was severely limited. This 1891 painting by Luke Fildes is entitled *The Doctor.*

kill one out of every seven people; and streptococcal disease was a fatal experience, as were pneumococcal pneumonia and meningococcal meningitis.

Then, in the 1940s, chemotherapeutic agents and antibiotics burst on the scene, and another revolution in medicine began. Doctors were astonished to learn that they could kill microorganisms in the body without doing substantial harm to the body itself. Medicine had a period of powerful, decisive growth, as doctors found they could successfully alter the course of infectious disease. The chemotherapeutic agents and antibiotics effected a radical change in medicine and charted a new course that has been followed to the present day.

In this chapter, we shall discuss the antimicrobial drugs that have become mainstays of our health-care delivery system. Some have been known for generations (MicroFocus 23.1), but most are of recent vintage. We shall explore their discovery

MicroFocus 23.1

THE FEVER TREE

Rarely had a tree caused such a stir in Europe. In the 1500s, Spaniards returning from the New World told of its magical powers for malaria patients, and before long, the tree was dubbed "the fever tree." The tall evergreen grew only on the eastern slopes of the Andes Mountains. According to legend, the Countess of Chinchón, wife of the Spanish ambassador to Peru, developed malaria in 1638 and agreed to be treated with its bark. When she recovered, she spread news of the tree throughout Europe, and a century later, Linnaeus named it *Cinchona* after her.

For the next two centuries, cinchona bark remained a staple for malaria treatment. Peruvian Indians called the bark *quina-quina* (bark of bark), and the

term *quinine* gradually evolved. In 1820, two French chemists, Pierre Pelletier and Joseph Caventou, extracted pure quinine from the bark and increased its availability still further. The ensuing rush

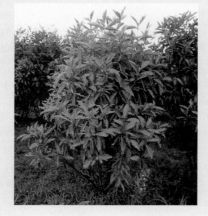

to stockpile the chemical led to a rapid decline in the supply of cinchona trees from Peru, but Dutch farmers made new plantings in Indonesia, where the climate was similar. The island of Java eventually became the primary source of quinine for the world.

During World War II, Southeast Asia came under Japanese domination, and the supply of quinine to the West was drastically reduced. Scientists synthesized quinine shortly thereafter, but production costs were prohibitive. Finally, two useful substitutes were synthesized in chloroquine and primaquine. Today, as resistance to these drugs is increasingly observed in malarial parasites, scientists are once again looking to the fever tree to help control malaria.

and examine their uses, while noting the important side effects attributed to many of them. When Louis Pasteur performed his experiments over 100 years ago, he implied that microorganisms could be destroyed and that some day, a way would be found to successfully treat many diseases. Only since the 1940s has Pasteur's prophecy become reality.

Chemotherapeutic Agents

Chemotherapeutic agent: a chemical agent used in the body for therapeutic purposes.

Chemotherapeutic agents are chemical substances used within the body for therapeutic purposes. The term generally implies a chemical that has been synthesized by chemists or produced by a modification of a preexisting chemical. By contrast, an **antibiotic** is a product of the metabolism of a microorganism. We shall maintain that distinction in this chapter, although many antibiotics are currently produced by synthetic or semisynthetic means and are more correctly "chemotherapeutic agents." Our discussion of chemotherapeutic agents will begin with a brief review of their development.

A BRIEF HISTORY OF CHEMOTHERAPY

Antibodies: highly specific protein products of the immune system that neutralize microorganisms. dif-thē're-ah

In the drive to control and cure infectious disease, the efforts of microbiologists in the early 1900s were primarily directed toward enhancing the body's natural defenses. Sera containing antibodies lessened the impact of diphtheria, typhoid fever, and tetanus; and effective antibody-inducing vaccines for smallpox and rabies (and later, diphtheria and tetanus) reduced the incidence of these diseases.

Among the leaders in the effort to control disease was an imaginative investigator named **Paul Ehrlich**. Ehrlich envisioned antibody molecules as "magic bullets" that seek out and destroy disease organisms in the tissues without harming the tissues. His experiments in stain technology indicated that certain dyes also had antimicrobial qualities, and by the early 1900s, his attention had turned to magic bullets of a purely chemical nature.

Syphilis: a sexually transmitted spirochete disease occurring in three stages and affecting organs of the skin, viscera, and nervous system.

ars-fen'ah-min

One of Ehrlich's collaborators was the Japanese investigator **Sahachiro Hata**. Hata wished to perform research on chemical control of the syphilis spirochete *Treponema pallidum*, and Ehrlich was happy to oblige. Previously, Ehrlich and his staff had synthesized hundreds of arsenic-phenol compounds, and Hata set to work testing them for antimicrobial qualities. After months of painstaking study, Hata's attention focused on **arsphenamine**, compound **#606** in the series. Hata and Ehrlich (FIGURE 23.2) successfully tested arsphenamine against *T. pallidum* in animals and human subjects, and in 1910, they made a derivative of the drug available to doctors for use against syphilis. Arsphenamine, the first modern chemotherapeutic agent, was given the common name **Salvarsan** because it offered *salv*ation from syphilis and contained *ars*enic.

Salvarsan met with mixed success during the ensuing years. Its value against syphilis was without question, but local reactions at the injection site, and indiscriminate use by some physicians, brought adverse publicity. Moreover, some church officials had used the threat of syphilis as a deterrent to immoral behavior, and they were less than enthusiastic about Salvarsan's therapeutic effect. Ehrlich's death in 1915, together with the general ignorance of organic chemistry and the impending

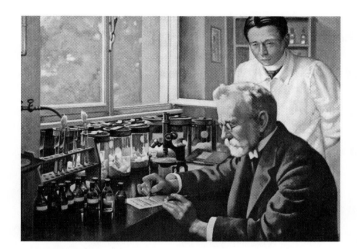

FIGURE 23.2

Ehrlich and Hata

A painting by Robert Thom depicting Paul Ehrlich and Sahachiro Hata, the two investigators who developed arsphenamine for the treatment of syphilis. Ehrlich is shown writing a work order with the stubby colored pencil he habitually used. He and Hata conducted their experiments at the Institute of Experimental Therapy in Frankfurt, Germany.

World War I, further eroded enthusiasm for chemotherapy. Instead, interest strengthened in serum and vaccine therapy for war-related diseases.

Significant advances in chemotherapy would not occur for another 20 years. During this interval, German chemists continued to synthesize and manufacture dyes for fabrics and other industries, and they routinely tested their new products for antimicrobial qualities. Among these products was a red dye, **prontosil**, synthesized in 1932.   pron'to-sil

Prontosil had no apparent effect on bacteria in culture. But things were different in animals. When **Gerhard Domagk** tested prontosil in animals, he found a pronounced inhibitory effect on staphylococci, streptococci, and other Gram-positive bacteria. In February 1935, Domagk injected the dye into his daughter Hildegarde, who was gravely ill with septicemia. (She had pricked her finger with a needle, and blood infection followed rapidly.) Hildegarde's condition gradually improved, and, to many historians, her recovery set into motion the age of modern chemotherapy. For his discovery, Gerhard Domagk was awarded the 1939 Nobel Prize in Physiology or Medicine (*in absentia*, however, because Chancellor Adolf Hitler prohibited him from accepting it).   do'mak

The next great leap occurred in 1935. A group at the Pasteur Institute, headed by **Jacques and Therese Tréfouël**, isolated the active principle in prontosil. They found it to be **sulfanilamide (SFA)**, a substance first synthesized by Paul Gelmo in 1908. Sulfanilamide was highly active against Gram-positive bacteria, and it quickly became a mainstay for treating wound-related diseases during World War II.   tref'oo-el   sul'fah-nil'ah-mīd

SULFANILAMIDE AND OTHER SULFONAMIDES

Sulfanilamide was the first of a group of chemotherapeutic agents known as **sulfonamides**. In 1940, the British investigators **D. D. Woods** and **E. M. Fildes** proposed a mechanism of action for sulfanilamide and other sulfonamides, and provided insights about how these substances interfere with the metabolism of bacteria without damaging body tissues. The mechanism came to be known as **competitive inhibition** (FIGURE 23.3).   sul-fon'ah-mīdz

Certain bacteria synthesize an important molecule called **folic acid** for use in nucleic acid production. Humans cannot synthesize folic acid and must consume it in foods or vitamin capsules. However, bacteria possess the necessary enzyme to manufacture folic acid. Indeed, they are incapable of absorbing folic acid from the surrounding environment.

Folic acid:
a chemical substance used by many types of living things in the synthesis of nucleic acids.

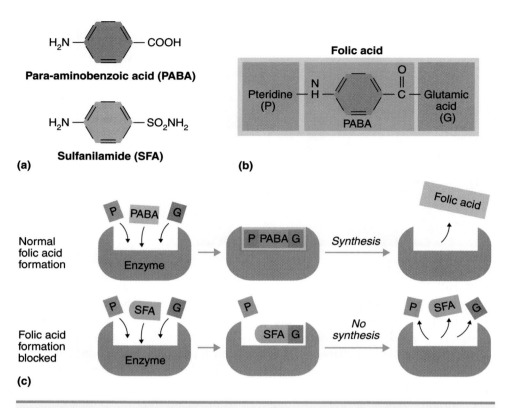

FIGURE 23.3

The Disruption of Folic Acid Synthesis by Competitive Inhibition

(a) The chemical structures of para-aminobenzoic acid (PABA) and sulfanilamide (SFA) are very similar. (b) Folic acid is made up of three components: pteridine, PABA, and glutamic acid. (c) In the normal synthesis of folic acid, a bacterial enzyme joins the three components to form folic acid. However, in competitive inhibition, the enzyme takes up SFA because it is abundant. The SFA assumes the position normally reserved for PABA, and folic acid cannot form. Without folic acid, nucleic acid metabolism is interrupted and the bacterium dies.

par'ah-am'ĭ-no-ben-zo'ik

In the production of folic acid, the bacterial enzyme joins together three important components, one of which is **para-aminobenzoic acid (PABA)**. This molecule is similar to sulfanilamide in chemical structure (Figure 23.3). Therefore, if the environment contains large amounts of sulfanilamide, the enzyme selects the sulfanilamide molecule instead of the PABA molecule for use in folic acid production. Once combined with the enzyme, the sulfanilamide binds tightly, and by the process of competitive inhibition interferes with the enzyme, thus making it unavailable for folic acid synthesis. As the production of folic acid is reduced, nucleic acid synthesis ceases, and the bacteria die.

sul'fah-meth-oks'ah-zōl

tri-meth'o-prim

Modern sulfonamides are typified by **sulfamethoxazole**. Doctors prescribe this drug against Gram-positive bacteria, as well as for urinary tract infections due to Gram-negative rods. Frequently the drug is combined with **trimethoprim**, an agent that inhibits another step in folic acid synthesis. Commercially the drug combination is known as Bactrim. It is frequently used to treat *Pneumocystis* pneumonia occurring in AIDS patients. Another common sulfonamide, **sulfisoxazole**, is marketed as Gantrisin cream for vaginal infections caused by Gram-negative bacteria. In some patients, a drug allergy to sulfonamides develops, with a skin rash, gastrointestinal distress, or type II cytotoxic hypersensitivity (Chapter 20).

sulf'is-oks'ah-zōl

OTHER CHEMOTHERAPEUTIC AGENTS

The discovery and development of sulfanilamide led to the development of numerous other chemotherapeutic agents, many of which are currently in wide use. One example is the antituberculosis drug **isoniazid** (isonicotinic acid hydrazide, or INH). Biochemists believe that isoniazid interferes with cell wall synthesis in *Mycobacterium* species by inhibiting the production of mycolic acid, a component of the wall (**MicroFocus 23.2**). Isoniazid is often combined in therapy with such drugs as rifampin and ethambutol. **Ethambutol** is a synthetic, well-absorbed drug that is tuberculocidal. Visual disturbances as a side effect limit its use to the treatment of tuberculosis.

i′so-ni′ah-zid

eth-am′bu-tol

Another chemotherapeutic agent, a quinolone called **nalidixic acid**, blocks DNA synthesis in certain Gram-negative bacteria that cause urinary tract infections. Synthetic derivatives of nalidixic acid called **fluoroquinolones** are also used in urinary tract infections, as well as for gonorrhea and chlamydia and for intestinal tract infections due to Gram-negative bacteria. Examples of the fluoroquinolone drugs are **ciprofloxacin** (Cipro), **enoxacin**, and **norfloxacin**.

nal-i-dĭks′ik

flu′ro-quin′o-lones

cip′ro-flox′a-cin
e-nox′a-cin
nor-flox′a-cin

Still another chemotherapeutic agent is **nitrofurantoin**, a drug actively excreted in the urine for treating urogenital infections. **Metronidazole** (Flagyl) has been used for decades against trichomoniasis, amoebiasis, and giardiasis. However, evidence that the drug causes tumors in mice has prompted physicians to use caution when prescribing it.

ni′tro-fu-ran′to-in
me′tro-ni′dah-zōl
trik′o-mo-ni′ah-sis
ji′ar-di′ah-sis

The treatment of malaria has long depended upon the use of **quinine**. When the tree bark used in its production became unavailable during World War II,

MicroFocus 23.2

THE TROJAN HORSE

In Greek mythology, the Trojan Horse was a colossal statue of a horse in which Greek soldiers hid to gain access to the city of Troy. Now, scientists have uncovered a similar plot used by the drug isoniazid to kill *Mycobacterium tuberculosis*, the bacterium that causes tuberculosis.

What happens is this: Isoniazid, a small, synthetic molecule, enters the bacterial cytoplasm as a benign, non-toxic chemical substance no different than any nutrient passing through the cell wall and membrane. But then the drug reveals its true identity. A common enzyme called catalase activates the isoniazid and converts it to a toxic form. The activated drug, now toxic, attacks a protein used by the bacterium to synthesize mycolic acid, a key component of its cell wall. Without a strong cell wall, the bacterium is left vulnerable to

destructive elements in the environment, and it quickly dies.

In the Greek tale, the city of Troy fell to invaders. But bacteria don't read books, and in some cases, the bacterium fights back and resists the drug. It stops producing catalase by switching off the gene that encodes the enzyme. Thus, the isoniazid remains inactivated. But the action also leaves the bacterium in a tenuous position because catalase breaks down hydrogen peroxide, a corrosive compound normally produced during its metabolism.

To resolve this dilemma, a second gene encodes a second enzyme (alkyl hydroperoxidase) that takes over the job of catalase and destroys the hydrogen peroxide.

In mythology, the Greeks carried the day and won the city of Troy. And in the early halcyon days of antibiotic use,

isoniazid was a prime weapon in the fight against tuberculosis. But in 1998, an estimated 8 million people developed tuberculosis worldwide, and about 3 million died. Tubercle bacilli are learning to resist the Trojan Horse. Let's hope the isoniazid has another trick up its sleeve.

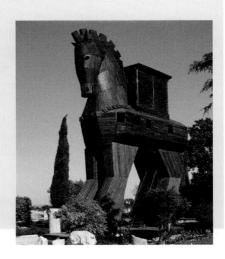

klor′o-kwin
prim′a-kwin

par′ah-am′ĭ-no-sal-ĭ-cil′ik
di-am′ĭ-no-di-fen′il-sul′fōn

researchers quickly set to work to develop two alternatives: chloroquine and primaquine. **Chloroquine** is effective for terminating malaria attacks; **primaquine** destroys the malaria parasites outside red blood cells.

Three other chemotherapeutic drugs, all inhibitory to *Mycobacterium* species, deserve a brief mention. The first two are **pyrazinamide (PZA)** and **para-amino-salicylic acid (PAS)**, both used for treating tuberculosis. The third agent is diamino-diphenylsulfone, or **dapsone**. This drug is used to treat leprosy.

To this point . . .

We have explored some of the events that led to the development of chemotherapeutic agents, first by Paul Ehrlich in the early 1900s and then by Gerhard Domagk in the 1930s. The landmark work of these investigators established the principle that chemical agents could be effective in the treatment of established diseases and encouraged other researchers to synthesize new compounds.

The focus next shifted to sulfanilamide. We described the mechanism of action of this compound and illustrated how a chemotherapeutic agent could interfere with an important metabolic process within a microorganism. Though sulfanilamide is rarely used any more, a number of modern derivatives, such as sulfamethoxazole, are often prescribed. We also mentioned several other chemotherapeutic agents and their uses in order to see the spectrum of these drugs. A variety of Gram-positive, Gram-negative, and acid-fast bacteria, as well as several protozoa and fungi, can be controlled with chemotherapeutic agents.

We shall now turn our attention to the antibiotics. These are naturally occurring products of the metabolism of microorganisms. As in the previous section, we shall examine the experiments leading to the discovery of antibiotics and then proceed to a discussion of the important groups of antibiotics. Because antibiotics are a key to successful recovery from a large number of diseases, many of the names in this section should be familiar. Antiviral agents are discussed in Chapter 11 and will be considered only briefly here.

23.2

Antibiotics

soo′do-mo′nas a′er-u-jin-o′sa

pi-o-si′ah-nin

Antibiotic:
an antimicrobial agent that is a naturally occurring product of the metabolism of microorganisms.

The word **antibiotic** is derived from Greek stems that mean "against life." In 1889, the French researcher **Paul Vuillemin** coined the term to describe a substance he isolated some years earlier from *Pseudomonas aeruginosa*. The substance, called pyocyanin, inhibits the growth of other bacteria in test tubes, but it was too toxic to be useful in disease therapy. Vuillemin's term has survived to the current era. Antibiotics are now considered to be chemical products or derivatives of microorganisms that are inhibitory to other microorganisms.

Scientists are uncertain as to how the ability to produce antibiotics arose in living things, but it is conceivable that random genetic mutations were responsible. Clearly, the ability to produce an antibiotic conferred an extraordinary evolutionary advantage on the possessor in the struggle for survival. In this section we shall discuss the sources of antibiotics, their modes of action, and side effects, and how they are used by physicians to control infectious disease. Our study will begin with Fleming's discovery of penicillin and the events that followed.

THE DISCOVERY OF ANTIBIOTICS

One of the first to postulate the existence and value of antibiotics was the British microbiologist **Alexander Fleming** (FIGURE 23.4). Fleming was a student of Almroth Wright, the discoverer of opsonins. During his early years, Fleming experienced the excitement of the Golden Age of Microbiology and spoke up for the therapeutic value of Salvarsan. In a series of experiments in 1921, he described **lysozyme**, the nonspecific enzyme that breaks down cell walls in Gram-positive bacteria. Micro-Focus 23.3 describes an ironic incident in Fleming's life.

The discovery of antibiotics is an elegant expression of Pasteur's dictum, "Chance favors the prepared mind." In 1928, Fleming was performing research on staphylococci at St. Mary's Hospital in London. Before going on vacation, he inoculated staphylococci onto plates of nutrient agar, and on his return, he noted that one plate was obviously contaminated by a green mold. His interest was piqued by the failure of staphylococci to grow near the mold. Fleming isolated the mold, identified it as a species of *Penicillium*, and found that it produces a substance that kills Gram-positive organisms. Though he failed to isolate the elusive substance, he named it **penicillin**. (A specimen of the *Penicillium* species in a Petri dish autographed by Fleming was sold at auction in 1998 for $13,121.)

Fleming was not the first to note the antibacterial qualities of *Penicillium* species. Joseph Lister had observed a similar phenomenon in 1871; John Tyndall did likewise in 1876; and a French medical student, Ernest Duchesne, wrote a research paper on the subject in 1896. Now, in 1928, Fleming proposed that penicillin could be used to eliminate Gram-positive bacteria from mixed cultures. Further, he unsuccessfully tried the filtered broth on infected wound tissue. At the time, vaccines and sera were

Opsonins:
antibodies from the immune system that enhance phagocytosis in microorganisms.

Penicillium:
a genus of molds belonging to the ascomycetes group of fungi.

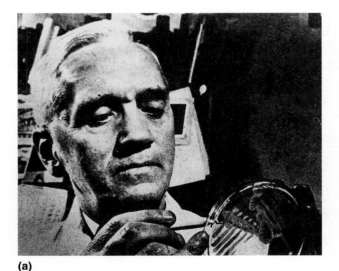

(a)

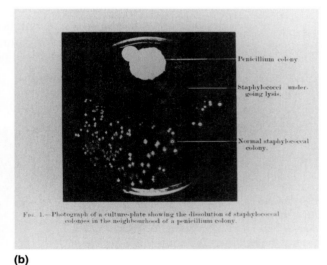

Penicillium colony

Staphylococci undergoing lysis.

Normal staphylococcal colony.

FIG. 1.—Photograph of a culture-plate showing the dissolution of staphylococcal colonies in the neighbourhood of a penicillium colony.

(b)

FIGURE 23.4

Penicillin and Its Discoverer

(a) Alexander Fleming, the British microbiologist who reported the existence of penicillin in 1928 but was unable to purify it for use as a therapeutic agent. (b) The actual photograph of Fleming's culture plate, originally published in the *British Journal of Experimental Pathology* in 1929. The photograph, taken by Fleming, shows how staphylococci in the region of the *Penicillium* colony have been killed (they are "undergoing lysis") by some unknown substance produced by the mold. Fleming called the substance penicillin. Ten years later, penicillin would be rediscovered and developed as the first modern antibiotic.

MicroFocus 23.3

COINCIDENCE OR FATE?

In August 1961, the *Bacteriological News*, a publication of the American Society for Microbiology, carried the following story.

In the 1870s, the son of a British nobleman became mired in a bog and was in danger of losing his life. Then a Scotsman happened along. The Scotsman waded into the bog and pulled the boy free.

When the nobleman learned of the deed, he offered money to the Scotsman, but the Scotsman politely refused. Instead, the Scotsman pointed out that he also had a son and perhaps the nobleman would be willing to educate the boy. The nobleman agreed, and the bargain was struck.

The Scotsman's son was Alexander Fleming. After some years, Fleming attended St. Mary's Hospital School of Medicine, and in the course of his research, he discovered penicillin. Meanwhile, the nobleman's son was also rising to a prominent position in British politics. During World War II, he was stricken with pneumonia but was treated with penicillin and survived. His name was Winston Churchill.

viewed as essential to disease therapy, and Fleming's request for financial support went unheeded. Moreover, biochemistry was not sufficiently advanced to make complex separations possible, and funds for research were limited since the Great Depression had begun. Fleming's discovery was soon forgotten.

In 1935, Gerhard Domagk's dramatic announcement of the antimicrobial effects of prontosil fueled speculation that chemicals could be used to fight disease in the body. Then, in 1939, **Rene Dubos** of New York's Rockefeller Institute reported that soil bacteria produce antibacterial substances. By that time, a group at England's Oxford University led by pathologist **Howard Florey** and biochemist **Ernst Boris Chain** (FIGURE 23.5) had reisolated Fleming's penicillin and were conducting trials with highly purified samples. An article in *The Lancet* in 1940 detailed their success. But England was deeply involved in World War II, so a group of American companies developed the techniques for the large-scale production of penicillin and made the drug available for commercial use (MicroFocus 23.4). Fleming, Florey, and Chain shared the 1945 Nobel Prize in Physiology or Medicine for the discovery and development of penicillin.

doo-bo'

FIGURE 23.5

The Developers of Penicillin

In 1940, Alexander Fleming (left, standing) learned that Howard Florey and Ernst Boris Chain (center and right, standing) had reisolated penicillin and were conducting tests on laboratory mice. He decided to visit them at the Sir William Dunn School of Pathology in Oxford, England. This painting by Robert Thom recalls the meeting of the three scientists who would share the Nobel Prize 5 years later. Norman Heatley, another member of the research group, is at the lower right.

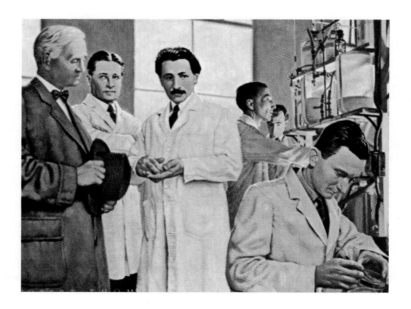

MicroFocus 23.4

TRANSPORTING A TREASURE

Their timing could not have been worse. Howard Florey, Ernest B. Chain, Norman Heatley, and others of the team had rediscovered penicillin, refined it, and proven it useful in infected patients. But it was 1939, and German bombs were falling on London. This was no time for research into new drugs and medicines.

There was hope, however. Researchers in the United States were willing to attempt the industrial produc-

tion of penicillin, so the British scientists would move their lab across the ocean. There were many problems, to be sure, but one was particularly interesting—how to transport the vital *Penicillium* cultures. If the molds were to fall into enemy hands or if the enemy were to learn the secret of penicillin, all their work would be wasted. Then Heatley made a suggestion: They would rub the mold on the inside linings of their coats, deposit the mold spores there, and

transport the *Penicillium* cultures across the ocean that way.

And so they did. On arrival in the United States, they set to work to reisolate the mold from their coat linings, and they began the laborious task of manufacturing penicillin. One of the great ironies of medicine is that virtually all the world's penicillin-producing mold has been derived from those few spores in the linings of the British coats. Few coats in history have yielded so noble a bounty.

PENICILLIN

Since the 1940s, penicillin has remained the most widely used antibiotic because of its low cost and thousands of derivatives. **Penicillin G**, or benzylpenicillin, is currently the most popular penicillin antibiotic and is usually the one intended when doctors prescribe "penicillin." Other types are penicillin F and penicillin V, all with the same basic structure of a **beta-lactam nucleus** and several attached groups (FIGURE 23.6).

The penicillins are active against a variety of Gram-positive bacteria, including staphylococci, streptococci, clostridia, and pneumococci (FIGURE 23.7). In higher concentrations, they are also inhibitory to the Gram-negative diplococci that cause gonorrhea and meningitis, and they are useful against syphilis spirochetes. Penicillin functions during the synthesis of the bacterial cell wall. It blocks the cross-linking of carbohydrates in the peptidoglycan layer during wall formation.

Beta-lactam nucleus: a distinctive chemical group central to the penicillin molecule.

pep'ti-do-gli'kan

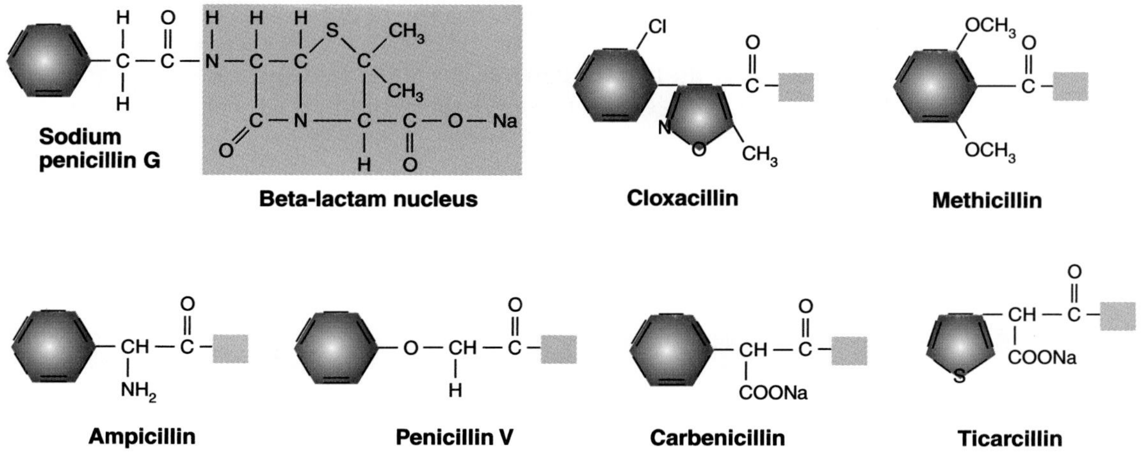

FIGURE 23.6

Some Members of the Penicillin Group of Antibiotics

The beta-lactam nucleus is common to all the penicillins. Different penicillins are formed by varying the side group on the molecule.

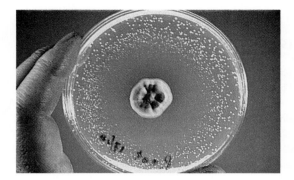

FIGURE 23.7

The Action of Penicillin on Bacteria

The *Penicillium* mold in the center of this petri dish is inhibiting the growth of the white *Staphylococcus* colonies around the perimeter.

Anaphylactic reaction: a whole-body allergic reaction accompanied by severe contractions of the smooth muscles.

pen'ĭ-sil-o'ik

nī-se're-ah

This results in such a weak wall that internal pressure causes the cell to swell and burst. Penicillin is therefore bactericidal in rapidly multiplying bacteria (as in an infection). Where bacteria are multiplying slowly or are dormant, the drug may have only a bacteriostatic effect, or no effect at all.

Over the years, two major drawbacks to the use of penicillin have surfaced. The first is the **anaphylactic reaction** occurring in allergic individuals (Chapter 20). This allergy applies to all compounds related to penicillin. Swelling around the eyes or wrists, flushed or itchy skin, shortness of breath, and a series of hives are signals that sensitivity exists and that penicillin therapy should cease immediately.

The second disadvantage is the evolution of penicillin-resistant bacteria. These organisms produce **penicillinase** (also called **beta-lactamase**), an enzyme that converts penicillin into harmless penicilloic acid (FIGURE 23.8). It is probable that the ability to produce penicillinase has always existed in certain bacterial mutants, but that the ability manifests itself when the organisms are confronted with the drug. Thus, a process of natural selectivity takes place, and the rapid multiplication of penicillinase-producing bacteria yields organisms over which penicillin has no effect. Recent years, for example, have witnessed an increase in penicillinase-producing *Neisseria gonorrhoeae* (PPNG), with the result that penicillin is now less useful for gonorrhea treatment. (Antibiotic resistance is discussed in depth later in this chapter.)

SEMISYNTHETIC PENICILLINS

In the late 1950s, the beta-lactam nucleus of the penicillin molecule was identified and synthesized, and scientists found they could attach various groups to this

Sodium penicillin G → Penicillinase, H_2O → **Sodium penicilloic acid**

FIGURE 23.8

The Action of Penicillinase on Sodium Penicillin G

The enzyme converts penicillin to harmless penicilloic acid by opening the beta-lactam nucleus and inserting a hydroxyl group to the carbon and a hydrogen to the nitrogen.

nucleus and create new penicillins. In the following years, thousands of penicillins emerged from this semisynthetic process.

Ampicillin exemplifies a semisynthetic penicillin. It is less active against Gram-positive cocci than penicillin G, but is valuable against several Gram-negative rods as well as gonococci and meningococci. The drug resists stomach acid and is absorbed from the intestine after oral consumption. **Amoxicillin**, a chemical relative of ampicillin, is also acid-stable and has the added advantage of not binding to food as many antibiotics do. Because ampicillin and amoxicillin are excreted into the urine, they are used to treat urinary tract infections.

ah-moks'ĭ-sil'in

Another semisynthetic penicillin, **carbenicillin**, is used primarily for infections of the urinary tract. Other semisynthetic penicillins include **methicillin, nafcillin, piperacillin**, and **oxacillin**. Still another is **ticarcillin**, a penicillin derivative often combined with **clavulanic acid** (the combination is called Timentin) for use against organisms resistant to other penicillins. The clavulanic acid inactivates penicillinase and thus overcomes the resistance. None of these drugs may be prescribed where allergy to the parent drug exists, and many have been implicated in gastrointestinal disturbances and kidney and liver damage.

car-ben'ĭsil'in

ti-car'cil-lin
clav'u-lan'ik

CEPHALOSPORINS

While evaluating seawater samples along the coast of Sardinia in 1945, an Italian microbiologist named Giuseppe Brotzu observed a striking difference in the amount of *E. coli* in two adjoining areas. Subsequently he discovered that a fungus, *Cephalosporium acremonium*, was producing an antibacterial substance in the water. The substance, named cephalosporin C, was later isolated and characterized by scientists, and eventually it formed the basis for a family of antibiotics known as **cephalosporins**.

sef'ah-lo-spōr'e-um
ak-re-mōn'e-um

sef'ah-lo-spōr'in

Cephalosporins are generally arranged in three groups, or "generations." **First-generation** cephalosporins are variably absorbed from the intestines and are useful against Gram-positive cocci and certain Gram-negative rods (**FIGURE 23.9**). They include cephalexin (Keflex) and cephalothin (Keflin). **Second-generation**

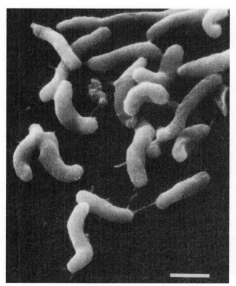
(a)

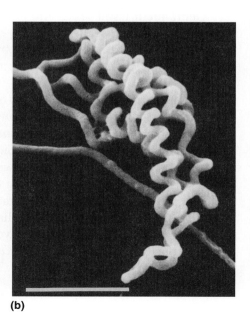
(b)

FIGURE 23.9

The Effects of Cephalexin on *Vibrio cholerae*

(a) A scanning electron micrograph of control cells grown in a medium free of antibiotic. The cells exhibit the typical vibrio shape with a short curve and an incomplete spiral. (Bar = 1 μm.) (b) Experimental cells treated with 3.13 μg of cephalexin per ml. The cells have elongated and formed right-handed spirals that are complete. (Bar = 5 μm.)

sef'ah-clor
sef-ox'i-tin
sef'u-rox'ime

sef'o-tax'ime
sef'tri-ax'on
sef-taz'i-dime

throm'bo-phle-bi'tis

am'i-no-gli'ko-sīd

strep-to-mī'cez

jen'tah-mi'sen

mi'kro-mo-no-spōr'ah

pol'e-mik'sin
bas'ī-tra'sin

par'o-mo-mi'sin

drugs are active against Gram-positive cocci as well as numerous Gram-negative rods (e.g., *Haemophilus influenzae*). They include cefaclor, cefoxitin, and cefuroxime (Zinacef). The **third-generation** cephalosporins are used primarily against Gram-negative rods (e.g., *Pseudomonas aeruginosa*) and for treating diseases of the central nervous system. Cefotaxime (Claforan), ceftriaxone (Rocephin), and ceftazidime (Fortaz) are in the group. A fourth generation of cephalosporins (e.g., cefepime) with improved activity against Gram-negative bacteria are in development.

Cephalosporins resemble penicillins in chemical structure, except that the beta-lactam nucleus has a slightly different composition. They are used as alternatives to penicillin where resistance is encountered, or in cases where penicillin allergy exists. Side effects appear to be minimal, but allergic reactions have been reported, and thrombophlebitis can occur. The drugs function by interfering with cell wall synthesis in bacteria.

AMINOGLYCOSIDES

The **aminoglycosides** are a group of antibiotic compounds in which amino groups are bonded to carbohydrate molecules (glycosides) that are bonded to other carbohydrate molecules. All aminoglycosides attach irreversibly to bacterial ribosomes, thereby blocking the reading of the genetic code on messenger RNA molecules. Since oral absorption is negligible, the antibiotics must be administered by injection. Their use has declined in recent years with the introduction of second- and third-generation cephalosporins, and with the introduction and development of quinolone drugs, such as the fluoroquinolones.

In 1943, the first aminoglycoside was discovered by researchers led by **Selman A. Waksman**, a soil microbiologist at Rutgers University. Waksman's group isolated an antibacterial substance from a moldlike bacterium named *Streptomyces griseus* and named the substance **streptomycin** (MicroFocus 23.5). At the time, the discovery was sensational because streptomycin was useful against tuberculosis and numerous diseases caused by Gram-negative bacteria. Since then it has been largely replaced by safer drugs, but streptomycin is still prescribed on occasion for such diseases as tuberculosis. The major side effect of therapy is damage to the auditory branch of the nerve extending from the inner ear. Deafness may result.

Gentamicin, a still-useful aminoglycoside, is administered for serious infections caused by Gram-negative bacteria, especially those causing urinary tract infections. The antibiotic is produced by species of *Micromonospora*, a bacterium related to *Streptomyces*. Damage to the kidney and the hearing mechanism has been reported.

Neomycin and kanamycin are two older antibiotics of the aminoglycoside group, having been isolated from *Streptomyces* species in 1949 and 1957, respectively. **Neomycin** is sometimes used to control intestinal infections because it is poorly absorbed, and it is prescribed as an ointment for bacterial conjunctivitis. Commercially, it is available in combination with polymyxin B and bacitracin as Neosporin. **Kanamycin** is used primarily against Gram-negative bacteria in wounded tissue. A derivative of kanamycin called **amikacin** is used for controlling numerous nosocomial diseases and for intestinal diseases. Physicians use **tobramycin** against *Pseudomonas* species, and **paromomycin** against *Entamoeba histolytica*. Both antibiotics are derived from *Streptomyces* species. In 1998, the FDA approved an aerosolized version of tobramycin (TOBI) for treating respiratory infections in patients with cystic fibrosis.

MicroFocus 23.5

SERENDIPITY

They met by chance on a ship sailing from France to the United States: Rene Dubos (doo-bo'), a 23-year-old French student interested in soil science, and Selman A. Waksman, a professor of soil microbiology at Rutgers University in New Jersey. The year was 1924. For the next two decades, their lives would intertwine as each carved out a niche in modern microbiology.

As they chatted aboard the ship, Waksman suggested that Dubos come to Rutgers to earn a doctorate in microbiology. Dubos took the advice, and by 1927, he had his Ph.D. and a job at Rockefeller Institute in New York City. There he discovered a bacterial enzyme that destroys the capsules of pneumococci and hastens their death.

But it was 1931, and Dubos' work stalled because biochemistry was still in a state of infancy. Soon, Domagk's work on prontosil burst on the scene, and Dubos began searching for ways to destroy whole organisms, not just capsules. He isolated a soil bacterium, *Bacillus brevis*, and in 1939 he extracted from it an antibiotic called tyrothricin. Further extractions yielded a second antibiotic, gramicidin. Both substances killed a variety of Gram-positive bacteria, but both were too toxic for use in the body.

Nevertheless, Dubos' discoveries encouraged Florey and Chain to continue their work with penicillin and showed that antimicrobial substances could be obtained from soil bacteria.

The lesson also had an impact on Selman Waksman. Over the years he had followed his former pupil's research, and in 1939 he began testing soil bacteria for antimicrobial compounds. The work was long, systematic, and plodding. In 1940, Waksman's group isolated the toxic antibiotic actinomycin, and in 1942, they found another antibiotic, streptothricin. But before this second drug could be thoroughly evaluated, streptomycin emerged.

The saga of streptomycin began in August 1943. Working with Albert Shatz and Elizabeth Bugie, Waksman isolated the moldlike bacillus *Streptomyces griseus* from the throat of a chicken. The bacillus produced streptomycin, an antibiotic with extraordinary capabilities. Preliminary studies showed its effectiveness against tubercle bacilli, and exhaustive tests at the Mayo Clinic in 1944 confirmed the results. Merck and Company soon began industrial production of the antibiotic, and within a decade, 26 companies throughout the world were manufacturing it. In 1952,

Waksman was awarded the Nobel Prize in Physiology or Medicine for his accomplishment.

Serendipity is a word derived from Horace Walpole's fairy tale *The Three Princes of Serendip*. In the tale, desirable things happen by accident or chance. Many antibiotics are the products of serendipity, but even more fundamental are the serendipitous meetings of two people such as once happened on a ship traveling from France to the United States.

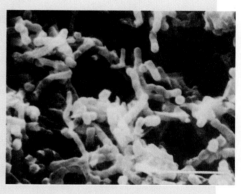

■ *A scanning electron micrograph of Streptomyces griseus, the organism isolated by Waksman, and one of the first species of bacteria to yield an antibiotic. (Bar = 5 μm.)*

CHLORAMPHENICOL

Chloramphenicol was the first **broad-spectrum antibiotic** discovered. Its isolation in 1947 by John Ehrlich, Paul Burkholder, and David Gotlieb was hailed as a milestone in microbiology because the drug was capable of inhibiting a wide variety of Gram-positive and Gram-negative bacteria, as well as several species of rickettsiae and fungi. During the next 30 years, however, physicians tempered their enthusiasm for chloramphenicol as side effects became apparent and new drugs appeared. Nevertheless, chloramphenicol still retains its importance in the treatment of many diseases.

Chloramphenicol is a small molecule that passes into the tissues, where it interferes with protein synthesis in microorganisms (FIGURE 23.10). It diffuses into the nervous system and is thus useful in treating meningitis. It also remains the drug of choice in the treatment of typhoid fever and is an alternative to tetracycline for

klo'ram-fen'ĭ-kol
Broad-spectrum antibiotic: one that is effective against a wide range of bacteria, rickettsiae, chlamydiae, and fungi.

Typhoid fever: a highly fatal foodborne and waterborne disease caused by *Salmonella typhi* and affecting numerous visceral organs.

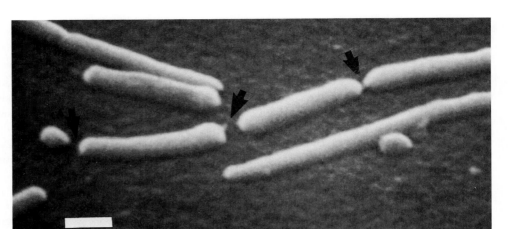

FIGURE 23.10

The Effect of Chloramphenicol on Bacteria

Escherichia coli was treated with chloramphenicol and photographed with the scanning electron microscope 20 minutes after the exposure. Note the formation of "minicells" and their threadlike attachments to the parent cells. Phenomena such as these are not usually found during normal cell division. They reflect the interference of the antibiotic with the organism's metabolism. (Bar = 0.5 μm.)

Aplastic anemia:
a condition in which red blood cells lack hemoglobin.

typhus fever and Rocky Mountain spotted fever. Originally isolated from the waste products of *Streptomyces venezuelae*, chloramphenicol became the first synthetic antibiotic when scientists at the Parke-Davis Company manufactured it from raw materials (its trade name is Chloromycetin). The drug has two major side effects: In the bone marrow, it prevents hemoglobin incorporation into the red blood cells and induces a condition called **aplastic anemia**; and it accumulates in the blood of newborns, causing a toxic reaction and sudden breakdown of the cardiovascular system known as the **gray syndrome**. For these reasons, chloramphenicol is not used to treat minor infections.

To this point . . .

We have surveyed four major groups of antibiotics and have noted their sources, modes of activity, and uses. We mentioned the side effects associated with each one, because they are a major consideration in determining which drug to prescribe. Penicillin and penicillin derivatives are primarily used for Gram-positive bacteria and have their activity at the cell wall of microorganisms. Penicillinase production and patient allergy limit their use. Cephalosporin antibiotics also function at the cell wall. The aminoglycoside group consists of numerous antibiotics that interfere with protein synthesis; physicians prescribe them for diseases caused by Gram-negative bacteria. Some are used on the skin, while others must be injected. Chloramphenicol is a broad-spectrum antibiotic with numerous uses but potentially lethal side effects.

As the discussion progressed, you may have noted how the antibiotics are products of microorganisms, especially Penicillium, Cephalosporium, *and* Streptomyces *species. Many of the original products are then modified to form semisynthetic antibiotics. In the case of chloramphenicol, the antibiotic is produced totally by synthetic means. This is why antibiotics are often placed under the umbrella of chemotherapeutic agents.*

We shall continue our discussion by examining the tetracycline antibiotics and a miscellaneous group of other drugs, including several that are used against fungi. Our survey will conclude with a description of the laboratory tests used to determine the effectiveness of antimicrobial agents under experimental conditions. Discussions of antibiotic resistance and abuse will also be presented.

23.3
Other Antibiotics

Some antibiotics, such as the penicillins, have withstood the test of time and have remained valuable adjuncts in the therapy for infectious diseases. Another "old-timer" is the tetracycline group of antibiotics that we discuss first in this section. Some of the newer antibiotics are then presented in the paragraphs that follow.

TETRACYCLINES

In 1948, scientists at Lederle Laboratories discovered chlortetracycline, the first of the tetracycline antibiotics. This finding completed the initial quartet of "wonder drugs": penicillin, streptomycin, chloramphenicol, and tetracycline.

Modern **tetracyclines** are a group of broad-spectrum antibiotics with a range of activity similar to chloramphenicols. They include naturally occurring **chlortetracycline** and **oxytetracycline** isolated from species of *Streptomyces* (FIGURE 23.11), and the semisynthetic **tetracycline, doxycycline, methacycline**, and **minocycline**. All have four benzene rings in their chemical structure. All interfere with protein synthesis in microorganisms by binding to ribosomes.

tet'ra-cy-cline
dox'e-cy-cline
min'o-cy-cline

Tetracycline antibiotics may be taken orally, a factor that led to their indiscriminate use in the 1950s and 1960s. The antibiotics were consumed in huge quantities by tens of millions, and in some people, the normal bacterial flora of the intestine

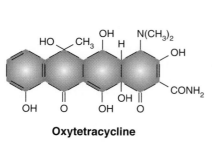

Oxytetracycline

(a)

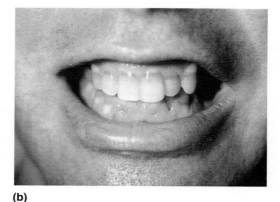

(b)

FIGURE 23.11

Oxytetracycline

(a) The chemical structure of oxytetracycline. Note the presence of four benzene rings, which characterizes all the tetracycline antibiotics. (b) The staining of teeth associated with tetracycline use.

nis'tah-tin

was destroyed. With these natural controls eliminated, fungi such as *Candida albicans* flourished. Patients then had to take an antifungal antibiotic such as nystatin, but because this drug was sometimes toxic, the preferred course was to replace the intestinal bacteria by consuming large quantities of bacteria-laden yogurt. Tetracyclines also cause a yellow-gray-brown discoloration of teeth and stunted bones in children. These problems are minimized by restricting use of the antibiotic in pregnant women and children through the teen years.

Despite these side effects, tetracyclines remain the drugs of choice for most rickettsial and chlamydial diseases, including the STD chlamydia (Chapter 10). They are used against a wide range of Gram-negative bacteria, and they are valuable for treating primary atypical pneumonia, syphilis, gonorrhea, pneumococcal pneumonia, and certain protozoal diseases. Although resistances have occurred, newer tetracyclines such as minocycline (Minocin) and doxycycline (Vibramycin) appear to circumvent these. Evidence indicates that tetracycline may have been present in the food of ancient people, as MicroFocus 23.6 points out.

MISCELLANEOUS ANTIBIOTICS

A miscellaneous group of antibiotics merits brief discussion because the drugs in this group are commonly used in modern therapy.

ĕ-rith'ro-mi'sin

mac'ro-līde

Erythromycin is a clinically important antibiotic in the group of substances called the macrolides. **Macrolides** consist of large carbon rings attached to unusual carbohydrate molecules. In the 1970s, researchers discovered that erythromycin was effective for treating primary atypical pneumonia and Legionnaires' disease. The antibiotic is a *Streptomyces* product and a protein synthesis inhibitor. It is recommended for use against Gram-positive bacteria in patients with penicillin allergy and against both *Neisseria* and *Chlamydia* species that can affect the eyes of newborns. Although it has few side effects, it sometimes interferes with gastrointestinal func-

---

MicroFocus 23.6

WONDER BREAD

In September 1980, a chance observation led to the discovery that antibiotics were protecting humans from disease long before anyone suspected.

The remarkable find was made by Debra L. Martin, a graduate student at Detroit's Henry Ford Hospital. After preparing thin bone sections for microscopic observation, Martin placed her slides under a fluorescent microscope because none other was available at the time. When illuminated with ultraviolet light, the sections glowed with a peculiar yellow-green color. Her colleagues identified the glow as that of the antibiotic tetracycline.

But these were no ordinary bone sections. Rather, they were from the mum-

mified remains of Nubian people excavated along the floodplain of the Nile River. Anthropologists from the University of Massachusetts, led by George Armelagos, had previously established that the Nubian population was remarkably free of infectious disease, and now Martin's discovery gave a possible reason why.

Streptomyces species are very common in desert soil, and the anthropologists postulated that bacteria may have contaminated the grain bins and deposited tetracycline. Bread made from the antibiotic-rich grain then conferred freedom from disease. The theory was strengthened when the amount of tetracycline in the ancient bone was shown to be equivalent to that in therapeutic doses used in medicine.

Another practice, reported in 1944, indicates that modern people were more deliberate in their use of contaminated bread. A doctor traveling in Europe noted that a loaf of moldy bread hung in the kitchens of many homes. He inquired about it and was told that when a wound or abrasion was sustained, a sliver of the bread was mixed with water to form a paste; the paste was then applied to the skin. A wound so treated was less likely to become infected. Presumably the modern bread, like the ancient bread, contained a chemical that would be recognized today as an antibiotic.

tions, presumably by combining with receptor sites used by body hormones to control nutrient transport in the GI tract.

Another macrolide antibiotic is **clarithromycin**, a semisynthetic drug. Clarithromycin (Biaxin) acts by binding to ribosomes to inhibit protein synthesis in Gram-negative bacteria, as well as the same Gram-positive bacteria inhibited by erythromycin. Still another macrolide called **azithromycin** (Zithromax) has a similar mode of action and spectrum of activity. Both antibiotics are dangerous to fetal tissue and should not be taken by pregnant women.

clar-ith′ro-mi′sin

a-zith′ro-mi′sin

Vancomycin, a cell wall inhibitor, is a product of a *Streptomyces* species. It is administered by intravenous injection against diseases caused by Gram-positive bacteria, especially severe staphylococcal diseases where penicillin allergy or bacterial resistance is found, as discussed later in the chapter. It is also used against *Clostridium* species, and against *Enterococcus* species (enterococci) that cause mild intestinal diseases. (In recent years, vancomycin resistant strains of enterococci termed VRE have emerged.) Its major side effects are damage to the ears and kidneys; the drug is not routinely prescribed for trivial conditions.

As drug resistance has developed and spread among staphylococci, the choice of antibiotics has gradually diminished, and vancomycin has emerged as a key treatment in therapy. Unfortunately, resistance to vancomycin has also been observed and substitute drugs have been sought. One possibility is Synercid, the trade name for the two-drug combination of **quinupristin** and **dalfopristin**. Approved by the FDA in 1999, Synercid is effective against resistant strains of *Staphylococcus aureus* and *Streptococcus pneumoniae*. It is the first of the streptogramin class of antibiotics to be approved. Both components interfere with bacterial reproduction, but the interference is enhanced when they are used together.

sin′er-cid

quin-u-pris′tin
dal-fo-pris′tin

strep′to-gram′in

Rifampin is a semisynthetic drug prescribed (in combinations with isoniazid and ethambutol) for tuberculosis and leprosy patients. It is also administered to carriers of *Neisseria* and *Haemophilus* species that cause meningitis and as a prophylactic when exposure has occurred. It acts by interfering with RNA synthesis in bacteria. Rifampin therapy may cause the urine, feces, tears, and other body secretions to assume an orange-red color and may cause liver damage. The drug is administered orally and is well absorbed. A related drug called **rifapentine** (Priftin) has been approved as a treatment for tuberculosis.

rif-am′pin

rif′a-pen′tin

Clindamycin and its parent drug, **lincomycin**, are alternatives in cases where penicillin resistance is encountered. Both are active against Gram-positive bacteria, including several anaerobic species (e.g., *Bacteroides* species). Use of the antibiotics is limited to serious infections, however, because the drugs eliminate competing organisms from the intestine and permit *Clostridium difficile* to overgrow the area. The clostridial toxins may then induce a condition called **pseudomembranous colitis**, in which membranous lesions cover the intestinal wall.

soo′do-mem′brah-nus

Both bacitracin and polymyxin B are polypeptide antibiotics produced by *Bacillus* species. These antibiotics are generally restricted to use on the skin because internally they may cause kidney damage and are poorly absorbed from the intestine. **Bacitracin** is available in pharmaceutical skin ointments and is effective against Gram-positive bacteria such as staphylococci. **Polymyxin B** is valuable against *Pseudomonas aeruginosa* and other Gram-negative bacilli, particularly those that cause superficial infections in wounds, abrasions, and burns. The two antibiotics are often combined with neomycin in Neosporin. Bacitracin inhibits cell wall synthesis, as FIGURE 23.12 indicates, while polymyxin B injures bacterial membranes.

bas′ĭ-tra′sin
pol′e-mik′sin

Spectinomycin is a *Streptomyces* product that shares chemical properties with the aminoglycosides. The antibiotic came into prominence in the 1970s for use against

spek-tin′o-mī′sin

gonorrhea caused by penicillin-resistant gonococci. It is given by intramuscular injection and appears to interfere with protein synthesis.

Monobactams are a group of antibiotics first synthesized by researchers at Squibb Laboratories in the early 1980s. The core of monobactam antibiotics is a beta-lactam nucleus isolated from *Chromobacter violaceum*, a purple-pigmented bacterium. One antibiotic, **moxalactam**, is active against a broad variety of Gram-negative bacteria, especially those involved in nosocomial diseases and bacterial meningitis. Resistance to penicillinase appears to be high, but interference with platelet function and severe bleeding have limited its use. Another set of beta-lactam drugs are the **carbapenems**. The representative of this group called **imipenem** (Primaxin) is effective against a variety of Gram-positive bacteria and Gram-negative rods, as well as anaerobes (e.g., *Bacteroides fragilis*). It is often prescribed in cases where resistances occur, and it appears to have minimal side effects.

ANTIFUNGAL ANTIBIOTICS

Fungal diseases pose a special problem for the medical mycologist because there are few drugs available for treatment. For infections of the intestine, vagina, or oral cavity due to *Candida albicans*, physicians often prescribe **nystatin** (MicroFocus 23.7). This product of *Streptomyces* is commercially available as Mycostatin or Achrostatin and is sold in ointment, cream, or suppository form. It acts by changing the permeability of the cell membrane by combining with fungal sterols. Often it is combined with antibacterial antibiotics to retard *Candida* overgrowth of the intestines during the treatment of bacterial diseases. Another antifungal product of *Streptomyces*, **candicidin**, has similar uses but is not as widely prescribed.

Griseofulvin is an antibiotic used for fungal infections of the skin, hair, and nails, such as ringworm and athlete's foot. Griseofulvin interferes with mitosis and causes the tips of molds to curl. It is a product of a *Penicillium* species and is taken orally.

For serious systemic fungal infections, the drug of choice is **amphotericin B**. This antibiotic degrades the cell membranes of fungal cells, and is effective for

mon'o-bak'tam

kro-mo-bak'ter vi'o-la'she-um moks-ah-lak'tam

car-ba-pen'ems im-i-pen'em

nis'tah-tin

gris'e-o-ful'vin

am'fo-tĕr'i-sin

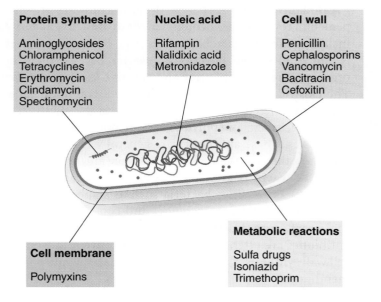

FIGURE 23.12

The Sites of Activity in a Bacterial Cell for Various Antibiotics

Protein synthesis
Aminoglycosides
Chloramphenicol
Tetracyclines
Erythromycin
Clindamycin
Spectinomycin

Nucleic acid
Rifampin
Nalidixic acid
Metronidazole

Cell wall
Penicillin
Cephalosporins
Vancomycin
Bacitracin
Cefoxitin

Cell membrane
Polymyxins

Metabolic reactions
Sulfa drugs
Isoniazid
Trimethoprim

MicroFocus 23.7

PERSISTENCE

The discovery of nystatin stems from the research of two scientists, Rachael F. Brown and Elizabeth Hazen. Their work was accomplished through persistent effort and the intelligent use of basic scientific principles. Sound research led them to a naturally occurring substance that would prove valuable in fighting fungal disease.

Rachael Brown was an organic chemist with a Ph.D. from the University of Chicago. Elizabeth Hazen was a mycologist. In the mid-1940s, the two scientists were employed at the New York State Department of Health where their interest was piqued by increasing reports concerning antibiotics. Penicillin was in widespread use by that time, and streptomycin had been discovered by Waksman in 1942. Both antibiotics were useful against bacteria, but none had yet been developed for fungal disease. Brown and Hazen would try to fill that gap.

In the 1940s, scientists knew that soil-borne bacteria of the genus *Streptomyces* were potential sources of antibiotics. Hazen therefore collected soil samples from various places and tested the waste products of soilborne microorganisms to determine whether they could inhibit fungal growth. A bacterium from soil on a farm owned by a certain Henry Nourse was especially promising. The organism was apparently unknown before Hazen isolated it, and she therefore named it *Streptomyces noursei* after the farmer. Now it was Brown's turn. Using her skills in chemistry, she isolated, purified, and characterized the active ingredient in the waste product. With Hazen, she demonstrated that minuscule amounts of the active principle were extraordinarily inhibitory to fungi. Hazen and Brown named the ingredient nystatin, for New York State.

Nystatin was introduced to the scientific community at the 1949 meeting of the National Academy of Sciences. Two years later, a patent was issued for production, and E. R. Squibb received exclusive license to manufacture the antibiotic. Before long, nystatin became a key treatment for various forms of candidiasis, and when the Arno River flooded Florence, Italy, in the 1970s, nystatin was used to combat fungi attacking the art treasures. Nystatin also has commercial value for preventing spoilage in foods, especially bananas, and it is used in surgery to preclude fungal infection.

For Brown and Hazen, the accolades were many, including several honorary degrees and awards. Students at Mount Holyoke College currently vie for the Rachael Brown Fellowship, and students at Mississippi University for Women are eligible for the Elizabeth Hazen Scholarship, both named for alumnae of the respective colleges.

treating serious diseases (Chapter 14). However, it causes a wide variety of side effects and therefore is used only in progressive and potentially fatal cases.

Other antifungal antibiotics are synthetic compounds. One example, **flucytosine**, is converted in fungal cells to an inhibitor that interrupts nucleic acid synthesis. The drug is used primarily with amphotericin B in systemic diseases. Another example, the **imidazoles**, include clotrimazole, miconazole, itraconazole, and ketoconazole. These compounds interfere with sterol synthesis in fungal cell membranes. **Clotrimazole** (Gyne-Lotrimin) is used topically for *Candida* skin infections, while the other drugs are used topically as well as internally for systemic diseases. Side effects are uncommon. **Miconazole** is commercially available as Micatin for athlete's foot and Monistat for yeast infections. **Itraconazole** is sold as Sporonox for athlete's foot.

flu-si'to-sēn

klo-tri'mah-zōl
mi-kon'ah-zōl
it'ra-kon'ah-zōl
ke'to-kon'ah-zōl

ANTIVIRAL ANTIBIOTICS

The inhibition and destruction of viruses present unique challenges for drug researchers because viruses are extraordinarily simple. They do not have the complex structures or the cell walls and membranes of other microorganisms, and they engage in few physiological activities other than replication. Thus, viruses have few places where researchers may focus their attention. Nevertheless, a number of antiviral antibiotics have emerged in recent years. They are discussed in depth in Chapter 11, but we shall review them here briefly.

ah-man'tah-dēn

a-zi'do-thi'mĭ-dēn
ri-ba-vi'rin

sa-quin'a-vir
ri-ton'i-vir

in'ter-fēr'on

Most antiviral antibiotics seek to interrupt an aspect of the viral replication cycle. For example, **amantadine** and **zanamivir** prevent the attachment of influenza viruses to host cell membranes. **Acyclovir** and **ganciclovir** are erroneously incorporated into viral DNA during the replication cycles of herpes simplex viruses and cytomegaloviruses, respectively. **Azidothymidine (AZT)** and **ribavirin** act in a similar way when DNA is synthesized using viral RNA as a template.

Two newer classes of antiviral antibiotics are inhibitors of enzymes used by viruses. The first class includes the anti-HIV drugs **nevirapine** and **delavirdine**. These drugs bind to and inhibit reverse transcriptase when HIV is replicating. In the second class are **saquinavir** and **ritonavir**. They bind to protease, the enzyme needed to form the viral capsid. The drugs are also used against HIV.

The **interferons** continue to attract attention because they are naturally produced by body cells. Now synthesized by genetic engineering methods, the interferons provoke host cells to produce antiviral proteins, and they stimulate natural killer cells into action. The FDA has approved interferons for treating hepatitis B, genital warts, and a type of leukemia.

NEW APPROACHES

As reports of antibiotic resistance and harmful side effects appear in the literature, scientists hasten their search for new approaches to antibiotic therapy. One approach centers on the **two-component signaling pathway** found in bacterial cells but not in animal cells. When infectious bacteria reach the human lung, for example, an enzyme called a **kinase** is activated. The kinase then signals a second protein called a **transcription factor,** which binds to the bacterial DNA and turns on the genes that will encourage infection. Scientists believe they can develop a chemical compound to prevent kinase activation and thereby interrupt the infection process. Evidence of their success was first reported in 1998.

Another approach is to focus on the lipid of the **outer membrane** in Gram-negative bacteria. This membrane, discussed in Chapter 4, includes a unique lipopolysaccharide (LPS) with several unusual carbohydrates that could be targets for new drugs. Indeed, researchers have already shown that bacteria with defective or disorganized LPS are susceptible to complement-mediated antibody activity. Furthermore, neutralizing the LPS would limit the release of endotoxins associated with LPS.

Interfering with regulatory systems might conceivably be another focus of research on antibiotic action. Almost all bacteria, for instance, use an enzyme protein called **DNA adenine methylase** to coat DNA with methyl groups and regulate DNA replication and repair. Researchers have significantly reduced the virulence of a *Salmonella* species by disabling the gene that encodes the enzyme. They now hope to develop a chemical compound to neutralize the enzyme (rather than the gene), thereby pinpointing a protein found only in the bacterium. At this point, however, they are not completely sure of the enzyme's activity.

Discovering a new class of antibiotic compounds might be another trail to follow. A number of researchers are investigating **peptide antibiotics,** a group of small proteins isolated from the immune system of various animals. The peptides are found in innumerable animal species; they guard against microbial entry at the body surface (e.g., the tongue of a cow, the stomach of a shark, the skin of a human). The antibiotics appear to disrupt cell membranes in bacteria, and their positive charge enhances binding to the negatively charged bacterial membrane. However, none have yet entered the pipeline as potential drugs, one reason being the estimated $300 million necessary to bring a new antibiotic to market.

23.4

Antibiotic Assays and Resistance

The substantial variety of antibiotics and chemotherapeutic agents developed since the 1930s (MicroFocus 23.8) necessitates that the physician determine which one is best for the patient under the circumstances of the infection. Accordingly, an antibiotic sensitivity assay is performed. The assay also helps determine whether a microorganism is resistant to a particular antibiotic, a problem that has developed into a major concern of modern medicine.

ANTIBIOTIC SUSCEPTIBILITY ASSAYS

Antibiotic susceptibility assays are used to study the inhibition of a test organism by one or more antibiotics or chemotherapeutic agents. Two general methods are in common use: the tube dilution method, and the agar disk diffusion method.

The **tube dilution method** determines the smallest amount of antibiotic necessary to destroy a population of a test organism. This amount is known as the **minimum inhibitory concentration (MIC)**. To determine the MIC, the microbiologist prepares a set of tubes with different concentrations of a particular antibiotic. The tubes are then inoculated with an identical population of the test organism, incubated, and examined for the growth of bacteria. The extent of growth diminishes as the concentration of antibiotic increases, and eventually an antibiotic concentration is observed at which growth fails to occur. This is the MIC.

The second method, the **agar disk diffusion method**, operates on the principle that antibiotics will diffuse from a paper disk or small cylinder into an agar medium containing test organisms. This method is shown in FIGURE 23.13a. Inhibition is observed as a failure of the organism to grow in the region of the antibiotic. A common application of the agar disk diffusion method is the **Kirby-Bauer test**, named after **W. M. Kirby** and **A. W. Bauer**, who developed it in the 1960s. This procedure determines the susceptibility of an organism to a series of antibiotics and is

MicroFocus 23.8

TRANSITION

The late Lewis Thomas was one of the remarkable individuals of the twentieth century. He was a well-known researcher, physician, professor, administrator, and writer. One of his notable books is a collection of essays entitled *The Youngest Science: Notes of a Medicine-Watcher* (1983). In an essay called "1933 Medicine," Thomas gives us an idea of what it was like to be a physician during the transition into the age of antibiotics:

"The two great hazards to life were tuberculosis and syphilis. These were feared by everyone in the same way that cancer is feared today. There was nothing to be done for tuberculosis except to wait it out, hoping that the body's own defense mechanisms would eventually hold the tubercle bacilli in check. . . . Then came the explosive news of sulfanilamide, and the start of the real revolution in medicine. I remember with astonishment when the first cases of

pneumococcal and streptococcal septicemia were treated in Boston in 1937. The phenomenon was almost beyond belief. Here were moribund patients, who would surely have died without treatment, improving in their appearance within a matter of hours of being given the medicine and feeling entirely well within the next day or so."

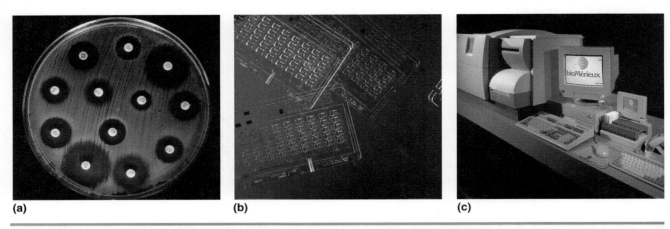

(a)   (b)   (c)

FIGURE 23.13

Antibiotic Susceptibility Testing

Two methods for determining an organism's antibiotic susceptibility are shown. (a) The more traditional method is the agar disk diffusion method. Bacteria are inoculated onto a plate of agar medium containing disks of various antibiotics. The plate is incubated, and the presence of a clear zone of inhibition shows susceptibility to a particular antibiotic. The absence of a zone or presence of a small zone indicates resistance. In a modern automated system, bacteria are automatically inoculated into wells on a card (b), each well containing a different antibiotic. The card is then incubated, and the presence or absence of growth is assayed by a computer (c). A printout relates the organism's susceptibility (no growth) to the antibiotic, or its resistance (growth).

performed according to standards established by the FDA. More sophisticated procedures are noted in Chapter 19.

ANTIBIOTIC RESISTANCE AND ABUSE

During the past 25 years, an alarming number of bacterial strains have evolved with resistance to chemotherapeutic agents and antibiotics. Public health microbiologists note that resistant organisms are increasingly responsible for human diseases of the intestinal tract, lungs, skin, and urinary tract. Those in intensive care units and burn wards are particularly vulnerable, as are infants, the elderly, and the infirm. Common diseases like bacterial pneumonia, tuberculosis, streptococcal sore throat, and gonorrhea that a few years ago succumbed to a single dose of antibiotics are now among the most difficult to treat.

One of the major concerns of public health officials is the bacterium *Staphylococcus aureus*. Capable of causing staphylococcal septicemia, pneumonia, endocarditis, and meningitis, *S. aureus* is involved in over 250,000 infections per year, primarily in hospitals and nursing homes. Over the years, strains of *S. aureus* have developed resistance to penicillin and numerous other drugs, and the term **MRSA**, for **multidrug-resistant *Staphylococcus aureus***, has often been used in hospital settings. Through those years, vancomycin remained a viable alternative for treating MRSA infections.

Then, in 1997, an MRSA strain evolved with intermediate (partial) vancomycin resistance; scientists named it **VISA**, for **vancomycin intermediately resistant *Staphylococcus aureus***. Although researchers have found useful alternatives in drug combinations, they are grappling with the possibility that nothing will be left in the antimicrobial arsenal to treat patients infected by this strain of staphylococci. At this writing, a strain of *S. aureus* with full vancomycin resistance (VRSA) has not emerged. However, the concern is acute because vancomycin-resistant enterococci (VRE) exist in the human intestine, and gene transfers to *S. aureus* strains are conceivable. Heightening the concern is the observation that genes for resistance are frequently found on easily transmitted plasmids.

Microorganisms may acquire resistance to antibiotics in a number of ways. In some cases, resistance arises from the microorganism's ability to destroy the antibiotic. The production of penicillinase by penicillin-resistant gonococci is an example. Other resistances are traced to changes in the permeability of the microbial cell wall and membrane, thus prohibiting passage of the antibiotic to the interior. In addition, resistance to the drug's activity may develop. An example of the latter takes place when sulfa drugs fail to unite with enzymes that synthesize folic acid because the enzyme's structure has changed. Moreover, drug resistance may be due to an altered metabolic pathway in the microorganism, a pathway that bypasses the reaction normally inhibited by the drug. An altered structural target for the drug may also evolve. For example, the structure of a pathogen's ribosome may change, thereby rendering a drug that unites with the ribosome useless.

Resistance may develop in bacteria during the normal course of events (FIGURE 23.14), but antibiotic abuse encourages the emergence of resistant forms. For example, drug companies promote antibiotics heavily, patients pressure doctors for quick cures, and physicians sometimes write prescriptions without ordering costly tests to pinpoint the patient's illness. In addition, people may diagnose their own illness and take leftover antibiotics from their medicine chests for ailments where antibiotics are useless. Moreover, many people fail to complete their prescription, and some organisms remain alive to evolve to resistant forms by gathering "genetic debris" from the local area. And the survivors proliferate well because they face reduced competition from susceptible organisms.

Hospitals are another forcing ground for the emergence of resistant bacteria. In many cases, physicians use unnecessarily large doses of antibiotics to prevent infection during and following surgery. This increases the possibility that resistant strains will overgrow susceptible strains and subsequently spread to other patients, thereby causing nosocomial disease. Antibiotic-resistant *Escherichia coli, Pseudomonas aeruginosa, Serratia marcescens,* and *Proteus* species are now widely encountered causes of illness in hospital settings.

Antibiotics are also abused in **developing countries** where they are often available without prescription, even though they have toxic side effects. Countries such as

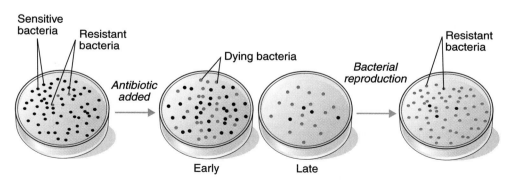

FIGURE 23.14

The Development of Drug Resistance

Drug resistance can occur widely in a population of bacteria as a result of natural selection during exposure to an antibiotic.

(A) Some members of the population have genes for drug resistance as a part of their genomes. In the absence of antibiotic, this resistance is not used.

(B) When the population of bacteria is treated with an antibiotic, the sensitive members gradually die off and the resistant ones thrive as the resistance genes become operative.

(C) The antibiotic-resistant bacteria now multiply and fill the environment with their enormous numbers. This antibiotic can no longer be used to control this population.

Mexico, Brazil, and Guatemala permit some of the most potent antibiotics to be sold over the counter, and large doses encourage resistance to develop. Between 1968 and 1971, some 12,000 people died in Guatemala from shigellosis attributed to antibiotic-resistant *Shigella dysenteriae*.

Moreover, the problem of antibiotic abuse is widespread in **livestock feeds**. An astonishing 40 percent of all the antibiotics produced in the United States finds its way into animal feeds to check disease and promote growth. By killing off less hardy bacteria, chronic low doses of antibiotics create ideal growth environments for resistant strains. Transferred to humans through meat, these resistant organisms may cause intractable illnesses. TABLE 23.1 summarizes the chemotherapeutic and antibiotic agents currently in use.

Allied to the problem of antibiotic resistance is the concern for transfer of the resistance. Researchers have amply demonstrated that plasmids and transposons account for the movement of antibiotic-resistant genes among bacteria (Chapter 6). Thus, the resistance in a relatively harmless bacterium may be passed to a pathogenic

TABLE 23.1

A Summary of Major Chemotherapeutic Agents and Antibiotics

CHEMOTHERAPEUTIC AGENT OR ANTIBIOTIC	SOURCE	ANTIMICROBIAL SPECTRUM	ACTIVITY IMPEDED	SIDE EFFECTS
Sulfonamides Sulfanilamide Sulfamethoxazole	Synthetic	Broad spectrum	Folic acid metabolism	Kidney and liver damage Allergic reactions
Isoniazid	Synthetic	Tubercle bacilli	Cell wall synthesis	Liver damage
Metronidazole	Synthetic	*Trichomonas vaginalis*	Cell metabolism	Tumors in mice
Chloroquine and primaquine	Synthetic	*Plasmodium* species	Cell metabolism	Eye damage
Fluoroquinolones Ciprofloxacin Enoxacin	Synthetic	Broad spectrum	DNA synthesis	Few reported
Penicillins Penicillin G Ampicillin Amoxicillin Nafcillin Oxacillin	*Penicillium notatum* and *Penicillium chrysogenum* Some semisynthetic Some synthetic	Broad spectrum, especially Gram-positive bacteria	Cell wall synthesis	Allergic reactions Selection of penicillinase-producing strains
Cephalosporins Cephalothin Cephalexin	*Cephalosporium* species Some semisynthetic	Gram-positive bacteria Broad spectrum	Cell wall synthesis	Occasional allergic reactions
Aminoglycosides Gentamicin Neomycin Amikacin Streptomycin	*Micromonospora* species *Streptomyces* species	Broad spectrum, especially Gram-negative bacteria	Protein synthesis	Hearing defects Kidney damage
Chloramphenicol	*Streptomyces venezuelae*	Broad spectrum, especially typhoid bacilli	Protein synthesis	Aplastic anemia Gray syndrome
Tetracyclines Chlortetracycline Oxytetracycline Doxycycline Minocycline	*Streptomyces* species Some semisynthetic	Broad spectrum, rickettsiae, chlamydiae, Gram-negative bacteria	Protein synthesis	Destruction of natural flora Discoloration of teeth Stunted bones

bacterium where the potential for disease is then increased by resistance to standardized treatment.

Dealing with the emerging antibiotic resistance is a major problem confronting contemporary researchers. One approach may lie in methods to boost the immune system, as noted in Chapter 18. Another approach may involve the use of bacteriophages (Chapter 11) to inhibit certain species of bacteria. Still another may involve innovative drugs and medicines that overcome the resistance. For example, biochemists have demonstrated that it is possible to prevent a bacterium from pumping an antibiotic out of its cytoplasm. Curbing the overuse of antibiotics through public and physician education and governmental regulation is a useful approach as well (although this approach will be particularly difficult, since the antibiotics market is currently worth about $23 billion). Increasing the research and development of effective vaccines and rapid diagnostic methods will also cut down on antibiotic needs. Indeed, all the principles that apply to the control of infection apply equally well to controlling the spread of antibiotic-resistant organisms.

CHEMOTHERAPEUTIC AGENT OR ANTIBIOTIC	SOURCE	ANTIMICROBIAL SPECTRUM	ACTIVITY IMPEDED	SIDE EFFECTS
Macrolides Erythromycin Clarithromycin Azithromycin	Streptomyces erythraeus Some semisynthetic	Gram-positive bacteria, Mycoplasma Broad spectrum	Protein synthesis	Gastrointestinal distress
Vancomycin	Streptomyces orientalis	Gram-positive bacteria, especially staphylococci	Cell wall synthesis	Ear and kidney damage
Rifampin Rifapentine	Streptomyces mediterranei Semisynthetic	Tubercle bacilli Gram-negative bacteria	RNA synthesis	Liver damage
Clindamycin Lincomycin	Streptomyces lincolnesis	Gram-positive bacteria	Protein synthesis	Pseudomembranous colitis
Bacitracin	Bacillus subtilis	Gram-positive bacteria, especially staphylococci	Cell wall synthesis	Kidney damage
Polymyxin	Bacillus polymyxa	Gram-negative bacteria, especially in wounds	Cell membrane function	Kidney damage
Spectinomycin	Streptomyces spectabilis	Gonococci	Protein synthesis	Few reported
Moxalactam Imipenem	Chromobacter violaceum	Gram-negative bacteria	Protein synthesis (?)	Few reported
Nystatin	Streptomyces noursei	Fungi, especially Candida albicans	Cell membrane function	Few reported
Griseofulvin	Penicillium janczewski	Fungi, especially in superficial infections	Nucleic acid synthesis	Occasional allergic reactions
Amphotericin B	Streptomyces nodosus	Fungi, especially in systemic infections	Cell membrane function	Fever Gastrointestinal distress
Imidazoles Clotrimazole Ketoconazole	Synthetic	Fungi, especially in superficial infections	Inhibit sterol synthesis	Few reported

Antibiotics have traditionally been known as miracle drugs, but there is a growing body of evidence that they are becoming overworked miracles. Some researchers suggest that antibiotics should be controlled as strictly as narcotics. The antibiotic roulette that is currently taking place should be a matter of discussion to all individuals concerned about infectious disease, be they scientist or student.

Note to the Student

In the last 100 years, there were two periods in which the incidence of disease declined sharply. The first period took place in the early 1900s. At this time an understanding of the disease process led to numerous social measures, such as water purification, careful food production, insect control, milk pasteurization, and patient isolation. Sanitary practices such as these made it possible to prevent virulent microorganisms from reaching their human targets.

The second period began in the 1940s with the development of antibiotics, and blossomed in the years thereafter when physicians found they could treat established cases of disease. Major health gains were made as serious illnesses came under control.

An outgrowth of these events has been the belief by many people that science can cure any infectious disease. A shot of this, a tablet of that, and then perfect health. Right? Unfortunately not.

Scientists may show us how to avoid infectious microorganisms and doctors may be able to control certain diseases with antibiotics, but the ultimate body defense depends upon the immune system and other natural measures of resistance. Used correctly, the antibiotics provide that extra something needed by natural defenses to overcome pathogenic microorganisms. The antibiotics supplement natural defenses; they do not replace them.

The great advances in chemotherapy should be viewed with caution. Antibiotics have undoubtedly relieved much misery and suffering, but they are not the cure-all some people perceive them to be. In the end, it is well to remember that good health comes from within, not from without.

Summary

Chemotherapeutic agents and antibiotics work with the body's natural defenses to stop the growth of bacteria and other microorganisms in the body. Chemotherapeutic agents are drugs produced by synthetic means in the laboratory. One group of such agents, the sulfonamides, interfere with the production of folic acid in bacteria. Other agents have various uses and various chemical compositions.

Although antibiotics are largely produced by synthetic means, they were originally derived from microorganisms. One example, penicillin, was first obtained from the green mold Penicillium. The antibiotic interferes with cell wall synthesis in Gram-positive bacteria and is available in numerous synthetic and semisynthetic derivatives such as ampicillin and amoxicillin. Where penicillin allergy or resistance is encountered, a cephalosporin antibiotic can be utilized. Certain cephalosporin drugs are first-choice antibiotics, and a wide variety of these drugs is currently in use.

For Gram-negative bacteria, the aminoglycoside antibiotics can be employed. Gentamicin, neomycin, and kanamycin are useful members of the aminoglycoside group. Chloramphenicol is a broad-spectrum antibiotic valuable against both Gram-positive and Gram-negative bacteria, but serious side effects limit its use. Less severe side effects accompany tetracycline use, and this antibiotic is recommended against Gram-negative bacteria as well as rickettsiae and chlamydiae. These and other antibiotics interfere with protein synthesis in bacteria. It is also possible that an antibiotic will interrupt nucleic acid or cell membrane metabolism. Certain antibiotics, such as amphotericin B and the imidazoles, are valuable against fungal infections.

A major problem attending antibiotic use is the development of antibiotic-resistant strains of microorganisms. Arising from any of several sources such as changes in microbial biochemistry, antibiotic resistance threatens to put an end to the cures of infectious disease that have come to be expected in contemporary medicine.

Questions for Thought and Discussion

1. In 1877, Pasteur and his assistant Joubert observed that anthrax bacilli grew vigorously in sterile urine but failed to grow when the urine was contaminated with other bacilli. What was happening?

2. Historians report that 2500 years ago, the Chinese learned to treat superficial infections such as boils by applying moldy soybean curds to the skin. Can you suggest what this implies?

3. During World War II, American soldiers were required to carry a full canteen of water. If they found it necessary to sprinkle a sulfa drug on a wound, they were instructed to drink the complete contents of the canteen. Why do you think this was necessary?

4. One of the novel approaches to treating gum disease is to impregnate tiny vinyl bands with antibiotic, stretch them across the teeth, and push them beneath the gumline. Presumably, the antibiotic would kill bacteria that form pockets of infection in the gums. What might be the advantages and disadvantages of this therapeutic device?

5. In May 1953, Edmund Hillary and Tenzing Norgay reached the summit of Mount Everest, the world's highest mountain. Since that time over 150 other mountaineers have reached the summit, and groups have gone to Nepal from all over the world on expeditions. The arrival of "civilization" has brought a drastic change to the lifestyle of Nepal's Sherpa mountain people. For example, half of all Sherpas used to die before the age of 20, but with antibiotics available for disease, the population has grown from 9 million to 15 million in three decades. Medical enthusiasts are proud of this increase in the life expectancy, but population ecologists see a bleaker side. What do you suspect they foresee, and what does this tell you about the impact that antibiotics have on a culture?

6. It was a crude remark, but during a discussion on the side effects of antibiotics, a student blurted out: "Better red than dead!" What antibiotic do you think was being discussed?

7. Most naturally occurring antibiotics appear to be products of the soil bacteria belonging to the genus *Streptomyces*. Can you draw any connection between the habitat of these organisms and their ability to produce antibiotics?

8. Bacitracin derives part of its name from Margaret Tracy, a patient from whom doctors isolated the *Bacillus subtilis* used in antibiotic production. Lincomycin is so named because it was first obtained from a bacterium isolated in Lincoln, Nebraska. From your knowledge of prefixes and suffixes, can you guess how other antibiotics in this chapter got their names?

9. Why would a synthetically produced antibiotic be more advantageous than a naturally occurring antibiotic? Why would it be less advantageous?

10. In 1994, researchers surveyed a number of emergency departments in urban hospitals to determine the top twenty drugs prescribed most often. Tylenol placed first. The top-rated antibiotic (fourth place) was amoxicillin. Why do you think this antibiotic was prescribed so often?

11. Of the thousands and thousands of types of organisms screened for antibiotics since 1940, only five genera appear capable of producing these chemicals. Does this strike you as unusual? What factors might eliminate potentially useful antibiotics?

12. History shows that over and over, creativity is a communal act, not an individual one. How does the 1945 Nobel Prize to Fleming, Florey, and Chain reflect this notion?

13. Ecologists tell us that by upsetting the balances in nature, a group of organisms may emerge with unusual characteristics. For instance, the continual use of rodenticides in the 1960s and 1970s permitted a variety of pesticide-resistant "super rat" to emerge in certain American cities. How does this principle relate to the appearance of PPNG?

14. Is an antibiotic that cannot be absorbed from the gastrointestinal tract necessarily useless? How about one that is rapidly expelled from the blood into the urine? Why?

15. The antibiotic issue can be argued from two perspectives. Some people contend that because of side effects and microbial resistance, antibiotics will eventually be abandoned in medicine. Others see the future development of a super antibiotic, a type of "miracle drug." What arguments can you offer for either view? Which direction in medicine would you support?

Review

On completing this chapter, you are invited to test your knowledge of its contents by completing the following crossword puzzle. The solution is in Appendix D.

■ ACROSS

1. Has a beta-lactam nucleus; most familiar antibiotic.
4. Four carbon _____ exist in certain antibiotic molecules.
6. Penicillinase is also known as _____-lactamase.
8. Erythromycin has relatively _____ activity against Gram-negatives.
9. Causes body secretions to assume a red-orange color.
13. An important antifungal drug is _____-conazole.
14. Drug of choice for rickettsial and chlamydial infections.
16. Country (intls) where penicillin developed after British discovery.
20. Number of major drawbacks to penicillin use.
22. An example of an aminoglycoside antibiotic is _____-tamicin.
23. Organ treated with neomycin to relieve infection.
24. Age group where tetracycline used for acne.

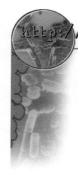

http://microbiology.jbpub.com

The site features **eLearning,** an on-line review area that provides quizzes and other tools to help you study for your class. You can also follow useful links for in-depth information, read more MicroFocus stories, or just find out the latest microbiology news.

25. Unit (abbr) to establish useful dose of antibiotic.
26. Macrolide antibiotic used as a penicillin substitute.
27. An antibiotic and its receptor are similar to a _____ and key.
30. Body organ possibly damaged by antibiotic use.
32. Bacterium (intls) from which bacitracin isolated.
34. The drug recommended for tuberculosis is _____L-niazid.
35. Disease (intls) treated with INH and rifampin.
36. Number of benzene rings in tetracycline molecule.
37. Antibiotic whose major side effect is damage to the auditory mechanism.
40. A desirable trait for antibiotics is _____ excretion to the urine.
41. Type of microorganism that produces certain antibiotics.
42. Organ affected by excessive streptomycin use.
45. A _____-day period of antibiotic use may be required.
46. Method for applying a topical antibiotic.
47. Number of beta-lactam nuclei in a penicillin molecule.

48. Body part where fungus infection may require antibiotic.
49. Bacterium (abbr) treated with penicillin or vancomycin.
50. Genus of fungus susceptible to nystatin therapy.

■ **DOWN**
1. Acidity level (abbr) that can influence antibiotic activity.
2. Penicillin has _____ effect on viruses.
3. Broad-spectrum antibiotic that interferes with protein synthesis.
4. Nucleic acid whose synthesis is inhibited by rifampin.
5. Many _____ cephalosporin antibiotics are available today.
7. Type of chemical group in gentamicin and neomycin.
9. Cell (abbr) having no hemoglobin following chloramphenicol use.
10. Fungus (intls) from which penicillin first isolated.
11. Antifungal drug to treat yeast infection.
12. Used in the eye for conjunctivitis.
15. After reaction with penicillinase, penicillin becomes _____-active.
17. Genus of antibiotic-producing bacteria.

18. Type of bacteria treated with aminoglycosides.
19. Method of introducing cephalosporins to body.
21. Used against penicillin-resistant bacteria.
22. Bacterial characteristic that often determines antibiotic use.
23. Where penicillin allergy exists, _____-thromycin is useful.
28. Function can be affected by antibiotic use.
29. Microorganism unaffected by many antibiotics.
31. Swollen during penicillin allergy.
33. Ampicillin and amoxicillin are _____-synthetic drugs.
38. Organic compound whose synthesis is inhibited by certain antibiotics.
39. Urinary _____ infections are treated with certain antibiotics.
43. Antibiotic synthesis is a multi-_____ process.
44. Part of body on which polymyxin is used.
48. Salt (abbr) of antibiotic that is often used.

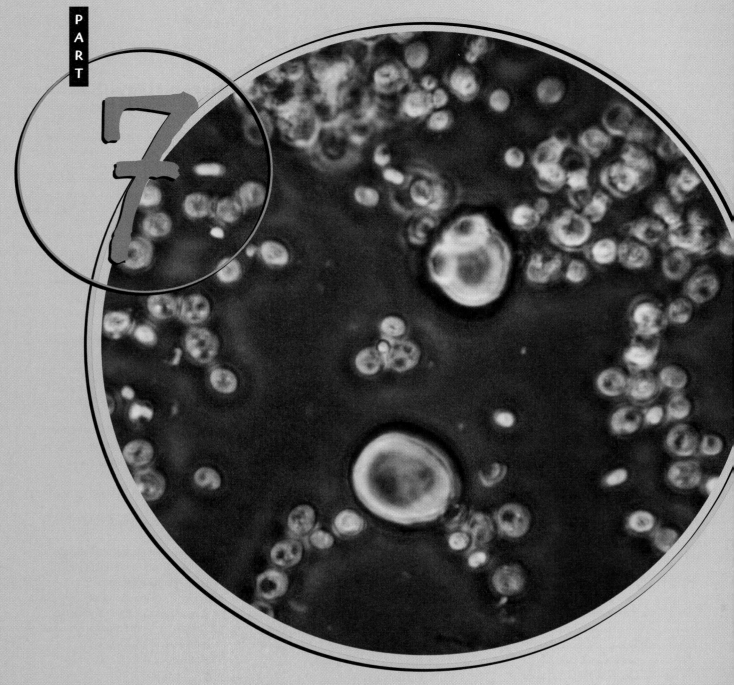

PART 7

Microbiology and Public Health

Public health has many facets. Several—such as mental health, nutritional health, and environmental health—lie outside the realm of this text. Other facets, however, are concerned with communicable disease and therefore fall within the scope of microbiology. Immunization, for example, is a public health measure because it creates a barrier within the individual that lessens susceptibility to infection. Case findings and antibiotic treatments are also under the umbrella of public health because they are used to limit the spread of communicable disease.

In Part 7, we shall be concerned with sanitation, a facet of public health designed to prevent microorganisms from reaching the body. The word *sanitation* is derived from the Latin *sanitas*, meaning "health." Sanitation came into full flower in the mid-1800s, and it is a relatively recent phenomenon. Before that time, living conditions in some Western European and American cities were almost indescribably grim: Garbage and dead animals littered the streets; human feces and sewage stagnated in open sewers; rivers were used for washing, drinking, and excreting; and filth was rampant.

The belief that filth was a catalyst to disease fueled the sanitary movement of the mid-1800s. As the Industrial Revolution sparked great population increases in the cities, health problems mounted, and sanitary reformers spoke up for effective sewage treatment, water purification, and food preservation. The germ theory of disease, developed in the 1870s, strengthened the movement and justified its actions because communicable disease could now be blamed on microorganisms in food and water. As sanitary reformers merged with bacteriologists, they issued loud calls for government support of public health and stimulated the development of sophisticated methods for dealing with food and water, which we shall study in Chapters 24 and 25.

But not all microorganisms are bad. Indeed, some contribute mightily to public health. For example, certain microorganisms are used to produce a broad assortment of foods and dairy products that make up a regular part of our diet. In addition, microorganisms play a dominant role in numerous cycles of elements in the environment and forge a link between what is useless and what is useful to other living things. Moreover, scientists employ microorganisms on industrial scales to synthesize a variety of products that we could not obtain otherwise. We shall see examples of these contributions in Chapters 24, 25, and 26.

PUBLIC HEALTH MICROBIOLOGY

I f you enjoy the adventure and excitement of travel, then a career in public health microbiology may be for you. Public health deals with the effects of the environment on community health. It involves strategic planning, the delivery of services, organization, marketing, and economics. Public health practitioners vary from individuals with 2-year college degrees to those with M.D. and Ph.D. degrees. Indeed, there is even a special degree for specialists in public health, the D.P.H. (Doctor of Public Health).

The public health microbiologist is often called an epidemiologist, that is, one who studies epidemics and the means to interrupt them. This individual is concerned with serious foodborne and waterborne diseases of the community, such as cholera and typhoid fever, and with worldwide diseases, such as AIDS. Even the less serious diseases, such as chickenpox and measles, are studied because large-scale outbreaks can exact heavy human tolls. Public health also takes into account the new and emerging epidemics occurring in various parts of the world. (Public health microbiologists were the doctors and researchers who arrived to study recent outbreaks of Ebola fever in Africa.)

Public health microbiologists are also involved with the sanitary treatment of water supplies, and they are constantly on the lookout to ensure conformity with public health standards. They oversee the proper disposal of sewage and industrial wastes and work to ensure the safety of milk, dairy products, and other foods we consume. The spread of disease by insects, rodents, and wildlife is also in the domain of the public health microbiologist working locally and in distant parts of the globe. Public health microbiologists attempt to prevent and control the spread of contagious diseases in the urban environment, as well as in the forest, open savanna, mountains, and deserts. There is virtually no place on Earth that the public health microbiologist will not put his or her talents to use.

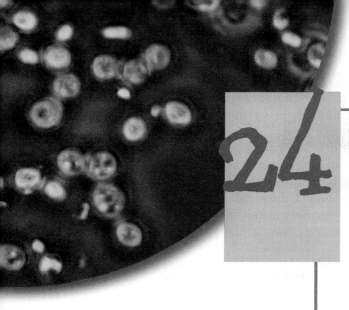

24 Microbiology of Foods

A dangerous quarter-pounder is as un-American as a murderous Mickey Mouse.

—A *Newsweek* writer commenting on the possibility of bacterial contamination in hamburger meat

THE IDEA WAS APPEALING and the price was right: a patty melt sandwich and a soft drink for lunch. The rye bread was toasted, the hamburgers were stacked and waiting to be cooked, the American cheese slices were lined up next to the grill, and the aroma from the sauteed onions was irresistible. It was October 1983, at the Skewer Inn, a restaurant at the Northwoods Mall in Peoria, Illinois. The stage was set for the third largest recorded outbreak of botulism in U.S. history.

Between October 14 and 16, numerous people stopped by the now-defunct restaurant and enjoyed patty melt sandwiches. Soon, however, 36 individuals began experiencing the paralyzing signs of botulism. They suffered blurred vision, difficulty swallowing and chewing, and labored breathing. One by one they called their doctors, and within a week, all were hospitalized. Twelve patients had to be placed on respirators. After many anxious hours, all but one recovered.

Investigators from the Centers for Disease Control and Prevention (CDC) arrived in Peoria shortly thereafter. They obtained detailed food histories from patients and from others who ate at the restaurant during the same 3-day period. First they identified patty melt sandwiches as the probable cause (24 of 28 patients interviewed specifically recalled eating the sandwiches); then they began a search to pinpoint the item that might be responsible. The data pointed to the onions. Investigators isolated *Clostridium botulinum* spores from the skins of fresh onions at the restaurant, and learned that once sauteed, the onions were left uncovered on the warm stove for hours. Furthermore, the onions were not reheated before serving. Spores had probably germinated within anaerobic mounds of warm onions and deposited their deadly toxins.

Incidents like this one highlight how most foods, even cooked foods, provide excellent conditions for the growth of microorganisms and the depositing of their toxins. The organic matter in food is plentiful, the water content is usually sufficient, and the pH is either neutral or only slightly acidic. To the food manufacturer or restaurant owner, the growth of microorganisms may spell economic loss or a reputation for bad business. To the consumer, it may mean illness or, in some cases, death.

The primary focus of this chapter will be to examine the types of microorganisms that contaminate various foods and to point out the consequences of contamination. We shall also examine food spoilage and the preservation methods used to prevent spoilage. Toward the end of the chapter, we shall see that some forms of microbial growth in food are actually desirable because they lead to numerous fermented foods we consume regularly.

24.1

Food Spoilage

Food spoilage has been a continuing problem ever since humans first discovered they could produce more food than they could eat in a single meal. Schoolchildren are taught that Marco Polo traveled to China in the thirteenth century to obtain spices and explore new trade routes. What many fail to realize is that spices were more than just a luxury at that time. They were essential for improving the smell and taste of spoiled food. Refrigeration was virtually unknown, and canning was yet to be invented.

Food is considered **spoiled** when it has been altered from the expected form. Usually, the food has an unpleasant appearance, aroma, and taste. Sometimes, however, these signs may be difficult to detect, such as when staphylococci deposit enterotoxins in food or when too few bacteria grow to cause a perceptible change. The consumption of toxins or microorganisms may cause a number of food poisonings or infections, including those noted in Chapter 8.

Contaminating microorganisms enter foods from a variety of sources. Airborne organisms, for example, fall onto fruits and vegetables, then penetrate the product through an abrasion of the skin or rind. Crops carry soilborne bacteria to the processing plant. Shellfish concentrate organisms by straining contaminated water and catching the organisms in their filtering apparatus. And rodents and arthropods transport microorganisms on their feet and body parts as they move about among foods.

Human handling of foods also provides a source of contamination. For example, bacteria from an animal's intestine contaminate meat handled carelessly by a butcher. Of even more concern are raw vegetables such as those obtained at salad bars. In March 1983, for instance, 107 Maryland residents contracted shigellosis after eating from the salad bar in the cafeteria at a military hospital. Earlier that year, 123 cases of hepatitis A were diagnosed in patients who dined at a salad bar restaurant in Lubbock, Texas. In both cases, investigators believed that food handlers were the source of pathogenic microorganisms.

Enterotoxins:
toxins that affect the gastrointestinal tract.

Shigellosis:
a bacterial disease of the intestine, caused by a Gram-negative rod and characterized by extensive diarrhea.

THE CONDITIONS OF SPOILAGE

Since food is basically a culture medium for microorganisms, the chemical and physical properties of food have a significant bearing on the type of microorganisms growing on or in it (FIGURE 24.1). **Water**, for instance, is a prerequisite for life, and therefore the food must be moist, with a minimum water content of 18 to 20 percent. Microorganisms do not grow in foods such as dried beans, rice, and flour because of their low water content.

Another important factor is **pH**. Most foods fall into the slightly acidic range on the pH scale, and numerous species of bacteria multiply under these conditions. In foods with a pH of 5.0 or below, acid-loving molds often replace the bacteria. Citrus fruits, for example, generally escape bacterial spoilage but yield to mold contamination.

A third property of a food is its **physical structure**. A steak, for example, is not likely to spoil quickly because microorganisms cannot penetrate the meat easily. However, an uncooked hamburger can deteriorate rapidly, since microorganisms exist within the loosely packed ground meat as well as on the surface.

The **chemical composition** of the food may be another determining factor in the type of spoilage possible. Fruits, for instance, support organisms that metabolize carbohydrates, whereas meats attract protein decomposers. Starch-utilizing bacteria

pH:
a measure of the acidity or alkalinity of a substance.

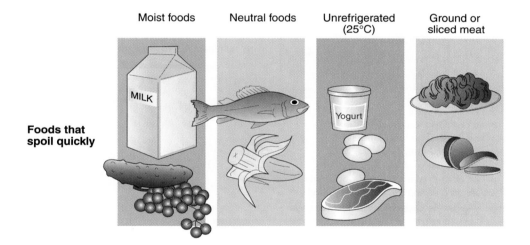

Moist foods   Neutral foods   Unrefrigerated (25°C)   Ground or sliced meat

Foods that spoil quickly

Dry foods   Acidic foods   Refrigerated (5°C)   Whole meat

Foods that resist spoilage

FIGURE 24.1

Food Spoilage

These drawings show the conditions under which foods are likely to spoil quickly or resist spoilage.

and molds are often found on potatoes, corn, and rice products. The presence of certain vitamins encourages particular microorganisms to proliferate, while the absence of other vitamins provides natural resistance to decay.

Oxygen and **temperature** are other considerations. Vacuum-sealed cans of food do not support the growth of aerobic bacteria, nor do vegetables or most bakery products support anaerobes. Similarly, the refrigerator is usually too cold for the growth of human pathogens, but the warm hold of a ship or a humid, hot warehouse storeroom is an environment conducive to the growth of these pathogens. It is common knowledge that contamination is more likely in cooked food at warm temperatures than in refrigerated cooked food (FIGURE 24.2).

Anaerobes:
microorganisms that live in the absence of oxygen.

FIGURE 24.2

A Case of *Vibrio parahaemolyticus* Food Poisoning

This outbreak occurred in Port Allen, Louisiana, in June 1978. *Vibrio parahaemolyticus* was subsequently found in the leftover shrimp, as well as in a major number of stool specimens from patients.

TEXTBOOK CASES

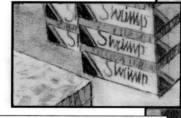

1. On the morning of June 21, a large amount of shrimp was cooked for a dinner by bringing the water to a "rolling boil." The gas was then turned off.

2. The shrimp were repackaged in the boxes in which they came, and covered with aluminum foil to keep them warm.

3. The shrimp were transported 40 miles in an unrefrigerated truck to the site of the dinner. The food was held unrefrigerated until 7:30 p.m., when served. A total of almost 8 hours had passed since preparation. Microorganisms proliferated during this extended period.

4. A group of 1700 people attended the dinner that evening. Shrimp were served to all as an appetizer in shrimp cocktail.

5. About 16 hours later, 1100 of the 1700 guests reported diarrhea, cramps, nausea, and vomiting. The diagnosis was food poisoning.

The food industry recognizes three groups of foods loosely defined on the basis of their chemical and physical properties. **Highly perishable** foods are those that spoil rapidly. They include poultry, eggs, meats, most vegetables and fruits, and dairy products. Foods such as nutmeats, potatoes, and some apples are considered **semi-perishable**, because they spoil less quickly. Orange juice is usually considered semi-perishable because of its high acidity, but in 1999, a major outbreak of *Salmonella* infection was linked to unpasteurized orange juice distributed to 15 states by an Arizona producer. **Nonperishable** foods are often stored in the kitchen pantry. Included in this group are cereals, rice, dried beans, macaroni and pasta products, flour, and sugar. FIGURE 24.3 summarizes the three groups.

THE CHEMISTRY OF SPOILAGE

Spoilage in foods is often due to the naturally occurring chemistry of contaminating microorganisms. Yeasts, for instance, live in apple juice and convert the carbohydrate into **ethyl alcohol**, a product that gives spoiled juice an alcoholic taste. Certain bacteria convert food proteins into amino acids, then break down the amino acids into foul-smelling end-products. Cysteine digestion, for example, yields hydrogen sulfide, which imparts a rotten egg smell to food. Tryptophan digestion yields **indole** and **skatole**, which give food a fecal odor.

sis-te'in

Indole:
a foul-smelling product of the breakdown of tryptophan.

Two other possible products of the microbial metabolism of carbohydrates are **acid**, which causes food to become sour, and **gas**, which causes sealed cans to swell. Moreover, when fats break down to fatty acids as in spoiled butter, a rancid odor or taste may evolve. **Capsule** production by bacteria causes food to become slimy, and **pigment** production imparts color. In numerous historical incidents, the red pigment from *Serratia marcescens* in bread has been interpreted as a sign of blood (MicroFocus 24.1).

sĕ-ra'-she-ah mar-ses'ens

Some foods resist spoilage naturally because they contain antimicrobial chemicals. The white of an egg has **lysozyme**, an enzyme that digests the cell wall of Gram-positive bacteria. Garlic contains certain compounds that inhibit many bacteria (MicroFocus 22.2). Oil of cloves appears to have healing tendencies, while radish and onion extracts both retard bacterial growth.

li'so-zime

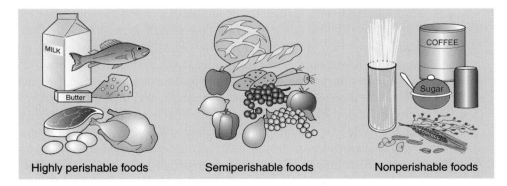

Highly perishable foods   Semiperishable foods   Nonperishable foods

FIGURE 24.3

The Perishability of Foods

Examples of highly perishable, semiperishable, and nonperishable foods. The physical and chemical properties of these foods are reliable indicators of their rate of perishability.

THE BLOOD OF HISTORY

Because of its characteristic blood-red pigment and propensity for contaminating bread, *Serratia marcescens* has had a notable place in history. For example, the dark, damp environments of medieval churches provided optimal conditions for growth on sacramental wafers used in Holy Communion. At times, the appearance of "blood" on the Host was construed to be a miracle. One such event happened in 1264 when "blood dripped" on a priest's robe. The event was later commemorated by Raphael in his fresco *The Mass of Bolsena*. Unfortunately, religious fanatics used such episodes to institute persecu-

tions because they believed that heretical acts caused the "blood" to flow.

It was not until 1819 that Bartholemeo Bizio, an Italian pharmacist, demonstrated that the bloody miracles were caused by a living organism. Bizio thought the organism was a fungus. He named it *Serratia* after Serafino Serrati, a countryman whom he considered the inventor of the steamboat. The name *marcescens* came from the Latin word for decaying, a reference to the decaying of bread.

In 332 B.C., Alexander the Great and his army of Macedonians laid siege to the city of Tyre in what is now Lebanon. The

siege was not going well. Then one morning, blood-red spots appeared on several pieces of bread. At first it was thought to be an evil omen, but a soothsayer named Aristander pointed out that the "blood" was coming from within the bread. This suggested that blood would be spilled within Tyre and that the city would fall. Alexander's troops were buoyed by this interpretation and with renewed confidence they charged headlong into battle and captured the city. The victory opened the Middle East to the Macedonians. Their march did not stop until they reached India.

MEATS AND FISH

Meats and fish are originally free of contamination because the muscle tissues of living animals are normally sterile. Spoilage organisms enter during handling, processing, packaging, and storage. For example, if a piece of meat is ground for **hamburger**, microorganisms from the surface accumulate in the teeth of the grinder along with other dustborne organisms. Bacteria from preparers' hands or from a sneeze compound the problem. The grinder may be cleaned well and refrigerated, but rarely is it sterilized. The importance of foodborne infection in ground meat is pointed up by the 1993 outbreak of hemolytic diarrhea traced to hamburger meat contaminated by *Escherichia coli* O157:H7. Over 500 patrons of Jack-in-the-Box restaurants were involved. A 1998 outbreak of the same disease necessitated a recall of 25 million pounds of hamburger meat (Chapter 8).

There is also the problem of the so-called "choke points," or places where animals come together and epidemics spread. In the United States, for instance, about 9000 farms produce calves for beef; the animals are then sent to about 46,000 feedlots for developing, and then, to about 80 plants for slaughter. Microorganisms can spread at any of these points. Moreover, animal feeds often contain the entrails of poultry as added protein sources, and another opportunity for bacteria to spread is presented.

Processed meats, such as luncheon meats, sausages, and frankfurters, represent special hazards because they are handled often. A 1999 listeriosis outbreak in Oklahoma was linked to hot dogs and deli meats (Chapter 8). Also, natural sausage and salami casings made from animal intestines may contain residual bacteria, especially botulism spores. When preparers pack such casings tightly with meat, *Clostridium botulinum* may multiply and produce its powerful toxins. As early as the 1820s, people recognized the symptoms of "sausage poisoning" and coined the name botulism, which translates loosely to sausage.

Organ meats, such as livers, kidneys, and sweetbreads (thymus and pancreas), are less compact tissue than muscle and thus spoil more quickly. Moreover, because

Clostridium botulinum:
a Gram-positive sporeforming rod that causes botulism.

the organs contain many natural filtering tissues, bacteria tend to be trapped here. Foods like these should therefore be cooked as soon as possible after purchase.

The extent of contamination in meats often consists of a harmless "greening" seen on the surface of a steak. This discoloration is commonly due to the Gram-positive rod **Lactobacillus**, or the Gram-positive coccus **Leuconostoc**. The green color results from pigment alteration in the meat and represents no hazard to the consumer. Slime formation on the outer casings and souring in frankfurters, bologna, or processed meats may also result from these organisms as well as from the *Streptococcus* species.

lac'to-ba-cil'lus
loo'ko-nos'tok

Microbiologists can often trace spoilage in **fish** to the water from which it is taken or held. Fish tissues deteriorate rapidly and the filleting of fish on a blood-stained block encourages contamination. It is also interesting to note that bacteria in fish are naturally adapted to the cold environment that fish live in and thus, cooling will not affect them so thoroughly; freezing is preferred. Shellfish are of particular concern because they commonly obtain their food by filtering particles from the water. Clams, oysters, and mussels therefore concentrate such pathogens as hepatitis A viruses, typhoid bacilli, cholera vibrios, or amoebic cysts. Many cases of cholera have been related to raw oysters.

POULTRY AND EGGS

Contamination in poultry and eggs may reflect human contamination (FIGURE 24.4), but it usually stems from microorganisms that have infected the bird. Members of the genus *Salmonella*, with over 2400 pathogenic serotypes, may cause diseases in **chickens** and **turkeys**, then pass to consumers via poultry and egg products. For example, an outbreak of **salmonellosis** in New York was traced to contaminated eggs used to make cheese lasagna and stuffed shells. Processed foods such as chicken pot pies, whole egg custard, mayonnaise, egg nog, and egg salad may also be sources of salmonellosis. **Psittacosis** is another problem because *Chlamydia psittaci* infects poultry. In one instance, 27 employees in a turkey-processing plant contracted psittacosis while preparing consumer products from diseased turkeys.

Salmonella:
a genus of Gram–negative nonsporeforming rods.

sit-ah-ko'sis
kla-mid'e-ah sit'ah-sī

Eggs are normally sterile when laid, but the outer waxy membrane, as well as the shell and inner shell membrane, may be penetrated by bacteria after several hours. *Proteus* species cause **black rot** in eggs as hydrogen sulfide gas accumulates from the breakdown of cysteine. This gives eggs a rotten odor. Other spoilages in eggs include **green rot** from *Pseudomonas* species and **red rot** from the growth of *Serratia marcescens*. Green rot results from a fluorescent pigment that causes the egg to glow when placed in front of an ultraviolet light. Red rot gives the yolk a blood-red appearance.

sis-te'in
soo'do-mo'nas

The primary focus of contamination in an egg is the yolk rather than the white. This is because of the nutritious quality of the yolk and because the white has a pH of approximately 9.0. Also, the lysozyme in egg white is inhibitory to Gram-positive bacteria. However, *Salmonella enteritidis* (FIGURE 24.5) is a common problem.

Lysozyme:
an enzyme that breaks down the cell walls of Gram-positive bacteria.

BREADS AND BAKERY PRODUCTS

In the production of bakery products, ingredients such as flour, eggs, and sugar are generally the sources of spoilage organisms. Although most contaminants are killed during baking, some bacterial and mold spores survive because **bread** is heated

FIGURE 24.4

A Case of *Staphylococcus aureus* Food Poisoning

This incident took place in Sussex County, Delaware, between March 8 and 10, 1979. Analysis showed that *S. aureus* phage type 95 was present in the nasal swab from the person who ground the chicken, as well as in the meat grinder and in the leftover chicken salad.

TEXTBOOK CASES

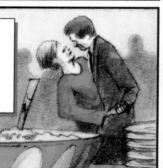

1. On March 8, 1979, chicken was cooked for chicken salad for a wedding reception to be held 2 days later.

2. The chicken was deboned and refrigerated overnight in a large washtub.

3. On March 9, the chicken was ground in a meat grinder by a person who had toxigenic *Staphylococcus aureus* in his nose.

4. The chicken was then mixed with celery, onions, and mayonnaise and refrigerated overnight in the same washtub.

5. On March 10, the chicken salad was delivered, unrefrigerated, to the wedding reception. A total of 7 hours passed before it was consumed.

6. Some hours later, 64 of the 107 guests at the wedding experienced nausea, diarrhea, intestinal cramps, and other symptoms of food poisoning.

FIGURE 24.5

Salmonella enteritidis

This Gram-negative rod is one of the most widely found contaminants in poultry and egg products.

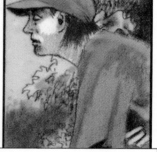
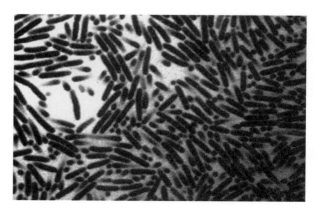

internally to 100°C for only about 9 minutes. Members of the sporeforming genus *Bacillus* commonly survive, and as they proliferate, their capsular material accumulates, giving the bread a soft cheesy texture with long, stringy threads. The bread is said to be **ropy**.

Cream fillings and toppings in **bakery products** provide excellent chemical and physical conditions for bacterial growth. For example, custards made with whole eggs may be contaminated with *Salmonella* species, and whipped cream may contain dairy organisms such as species of *Lactobacillus* and *Streptococcus*. The acid produced by these bacteria results in a sour taste. High sugar environments of chocolate toppings and sweet icings support the growth of fungi. Most bakery products should be refrigerated during warm summer months.

Ropy bread:
bread that is soft and stringy from the presence of capsular material.

Lactobacillus:
a genus of Gram–positive rods known for its production of acid in foods.

GRAINS

Two types of grain spoilage are important in public health microbiology. The first type of spoilage is caused by the ascomycete *Aspergillus flavus*. This mold produces **aflatoxins**, a series of toxins that accumulate in stored grains such as wheat as well as peanuts, soybeans, and corn. Scientists have implicated aflatoxins in liver and colon cancers in humans. The toxins are consumed in grain products, as well as meat from animals that feed on contaminated grain.

The second type of grain spoilage is caused by *Claviceps purpurea*, the cause of **ergot poisoning** (ergotism). Rye plants are particularly susceptible to this type of spoilage (MicroFocus 24.2), but wheat and barley grains may also be affected. The toxins deposited by *C. purpurea* may induce convulsions and hallucinations when consumed. The drug LSD is derived from the toxin.

klav′ĭ-seps pur-pu′re-ah

MicroFocus 24.2

OF PILGRIMS AND WITCHES

The first descriptions of ergot poisoning appeared in the Middle Ages, although it is probable that the disease was prevalent long before that time. Ergot poisoning was accompanied by burning pain in the extremities, and in the 1100s the disease was often called the Holy Fire (*Ignis Sacer*). For some strange reason, though, it would disappear if people made a pilgrimage to the hospital of St. Anthony, founded in 1039 near Vienne, France. Thus, the disease was also called St. Anthony's Fire.

Microbiologist now believe that ergot-contaminated rye was the cause of disease, and that people became ill from poisoned rye bread. The cure of St. Anthony probably resulted from a change of diet en route to the hospital

because the pilgrims ate uncontaminated bread. Also, the monks at the hospital served wheat bread, not rye bread.

An equally serious story related to ergot poisoning began in December 1691. That month, eight girls from the town of Salem, Massachusetts, developed disorderly speech, odd postures and gestures, and convulsive fits. Observers suggested that perhaps the girls were bewitched, since no other cause for their symptoms could be found. The girls were given a "witch cake" made from rye flour to determine if witchcraft was involved.

Now the symptoms worsened: The girls experienced burning pain in the extremities, buzzing in the ears, and sensations of flying through the air "out of the body." Diaries from that time record

that the winter of 1690–1691 was very cold, and that rye grains flourished where other crops failed. In retrospect, it is conceivable that ergot-contaminated grain was in the witch cakes and since children and teenagers ingest more food per unit of body weight, the poison may have affected them the most.

The infamous Salem witch trials began on June 2, 1692, and lasted through May of the following year. Nineteen young people were executed for witchcraft. The role of ergot poisoning is minimized by some historians, but it is possible that a mild form of poisoning may have initiated the incident, and that the social and psychological climate of the day made an already bad situation even worse.

MILK AND DAIRY PRODUCTS

Milk is an extremely nutritious food. It is an aqueous solution of proteins, fats, and carbohydrates that contains numerous vitamins and minerals. Milk has a pH of about 7.0 and is an excellent growth medium for humans and animals, as well as microorganisms.

About 87 percent of the substance of milk is water. Another 2.5 percent is a protein called **casein**, actually a mixture of three long chains of amino acids suspended in fluid. A second protein in milk is **lactalbumin**. This protein forms the surface skin when milk is heated to boiling. Lactalbumin is a whey protein, one that remains in the clear fluid (the whey) after the casein curdles during milk spoilage or fermentation. Carbohydrates make up about 5 percent of the milk. The major carbohydrate is **lactose**, sometimes referred to as milk sugar (*lactus* is Latin for "milk"). Rarely found elsewhere, lactose is a disaccharide that can be digested by relatively few bacteria, and these are usually harmless. The last major component of milk is **butterfat**, a mixture of fats that can be churned into butter. Butterfat comprises about 4 percent of the milk and is removed in the preparation of nonfat (skim) milk or low-fat milk. When bacterial enzymes digest fats into fatty acids, the milk develops a sour taste and becomes unfit to drink.

A common type of milk spoilage often takes place in the kitchen refrigerator or dairy case at the supermarket. Here, *Lactobacillus* or *Streptococcus* species multiply slowly and ferment the lactose in milk. Soon, large quantities of lactic and acetic acids accumulate. Enough acid may develop to change the structure of the protein and cause it to solidify as a curd. Dairy microbiologists refer to such an acidic curd as a **sour curd**. The lactobacilli and streptococci causing it have usually survived the pasteurization process.

Sweet curdling in milk may result when enzymes from species of *Bacillus, Proteus, Micrococcus*, or certain other bacteria attack the casein. As weak hydrogen bonds break, casein loses its three-dimensional structure and curdles. The reaction is said to be sweet because little acid production occurs. It is an essential step in the production of cheese. The clear liquid is **whey**, an aqueous solution of lactose, minerals, vitamins, lactalbumin, and other milk components. Whey is used to make processed cheeses and "cheese foods."

Milk may also be contaminated by Gram-negative rods of the coliform group of bacteria, including *Escherichia coli* and *Enterobacter aerogenes*. These bacteria produce acid and gas from lactose. The acid curdles the protein, and the gas forces the curds apart, sometimes so violently that they explode out of the container. The result is a **stormy fermentation**. *Clostridium* species also cause this reaction.

Ropiness in milk is similar to that in bread. It develops from capsule-producing organisms, such as *Alcaligenes, Klebsiella*, and *Enterobacter*. These Gram-negative rods multiply in milk, even at low temperatures, and deposit gummy material that appears as stringy threads and slime.

Another form of spoilage is caused by species of *Pseudomonas* and *Achromobacter* that produce the enzyme **lipase**. This enzyme attacks butterfats in milk and digests them into glycerol and fatty acids, giving milk a sour taste and a putrid smell. A similar problem may develop in butter.

Additional types of milk spoilage result from the red pigment deposited in dairy products by **Serratia marcescens**, the blue or green pigment of **Pseudomonas** species, and the gray rot caused by certain **Clostridium** species. In gray rot, hydrogen sulfide (H_2S) from cysteine imparts a rotten-egg smell to milk, and the H_2S

Whey:
the clear liquid portion of milk remaining after the protein curd has been removed.

Lactose:
a disaccharide composed of a glucose molecule and a galactose molecule covalently linked.

Streptococcus:
a genus of Gram-positive cocci in chain formation.

Hydrogen bonds:
weak bonds resulting from attractions between oppositely charged poles of adjacent molecules.

al′kah-lij′e-nēz
kleb′se-el′ah

soo′do-mo′nas
ah-kro′mo-bak′ter

sĕ-ra′she-ah mar-ses′ens

reacts with minerals to yield a gray or black sulfide compound. Spoilage due to wild yeasts is usually characterized by a pink, orange, or yellow coloration in the milk. Acid conditions stimulate mold decay in cheese products.

Milk is normally sterile in the udder of the cow, but contamination occurs as it enters the ducts leading from the udder, as well as from other unlikely sources (MicroFocus 24.3). The colostrum, or first milk, is laden with organisms. Species of soilborne *Lactobacillus* and *Streptococcus* are acquired during the passage, together with various coliform bacteria from dust, manure, and polluted water. The milk may derive other organisms from dairy plant equipment and unsanitary handling of dairy products by plant employees.

To this point . . .

We have discussed the problem of food spoilage and have indicated how various conditions may contribute to the type of spoilage observed. Among these conditions are the amount of water present, the pH of the food product, the physical structure of the food and its chemical composition, and the oxygen content and temperature of the environment in which the food is found. We also noted how the chemistry of spoilage leads to the deposit of certain end-products in foods. For example, hydrogen sulfide production from cysteine gives a rotten smell to eggs, and pigment production imparts color to foods.

The discussion then turned to various foods and the spoilage that takes place within them. We examined the sources and types of spoilage within meats and fish, poultry and eggs, breads and bakery products, grains, and milk and dairy products. In each case, some examples of the microbial flora were noted.

We shall now move on to the topic of food preservation. This section will outline various methods for preventing microorganisms from reaching food and causing spoilage. Food preservation is also an essential prerequisite to sanitation and public health because preservation methods halt the spread of infectious microorganisms. We will explore several traditional methods of preservation, and a number of contemporary methods used in food technology.

MicroFocus 24.3

GOOD AND NOT-SO-GOOD

In parts of Great Britain, milkmen still visit homes regularly and deliver bottles of fresh milk. That's good. Magpies, crows, and other birds arrive shortly thereafter and use their strong beaks to peck through the foil caps of the bottles and take a drink. That's not-so-good.

The birds use the milk to feed their young broods in the nest. That's good. But while taking a drink, they transmit *Campylobacter* species to the milk. That's not-so-good.

By having their milk delivered, British families save a trip to the market. That's good. Unfortunately, they also spend extra time in the bathroom suffering the misery of diarrhea. And that's not-so-good.

The moral of the story? "Bewildered Brits better beware bacteria-bearing birds."

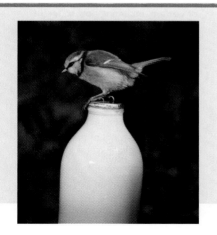

24.2

Food Preservation

Centuries ago, humans battled the elements to keep a steady supply of food at hand. Sometimes there was a short growing season; at other times, locusts descended on their crops; at still other times, they underestimated their needs and had to cope with scarcity. However, experience taught humans they could overcome these difficult times by preserving foods. Among the earliest methods was drying vegetables and strips of meat and fish in the sun. Foods could also be preserved by salting, smoking, and fermenting. Individuals could now trek far from their native habitat, and soon they took to the sea and moved overland to explore new lands.

ah-pehr'

The next great advance did not come until the mid-1700s. In 1767, **Lazaro Spallanzani** attempted to disprove spontaneous generation by showing that beef broth would remain unspoiled after being subjected to heat. **Nicholas Appert** applied this principle to a variety of foods (MicroFocus 24.4). Neither Appert nor any of his contemporaries was quite sure why food was being preserved, but it was clear that the spoilage could be retarded by prolonged heating. The significance of microorganisms as agents of spoilage awaited Pasteur's classic experiments with wine several generations later.

Through the centuries, preservation methods have had a common objective: to reduce the microbial population and maintain it at a low level until food can be consumed. Modern preservation methods are mere extensions of these principles. Though today's methods are sophisticated and technologically dynamic, advances in preservation processes are counterbalanced by the great volumes of food that must be preserved and the complexity of food products. Thus, the problems that early humans faced do not differ fundamentally from those confronting modern food technologists. In this section, we shall examine the methods of food preservation currently in use.

MicroFocus 24.4

TO FEED AN ARMY

Part of Napoleon's genius was understanding the finer points of warfare, including how to feed an army. Recognizing that thousands of men-at-arms were a glut on the countryside, he broke up his army into smaller units that foraged on their own as they moved. When the time for battle neared, he reassembled his forces and engaged the enemy.

The shortcomings of this system became painfully clear when Napoleon crossed into northern Italy in 1800 and engaged the Austrians at the Battle of Marengo. Aware that the French army was scattered about, the Austrians

charged before Napoleon could bring his forces together. Disaster was averted only when units arrived on the flanks to repel the Austrians. Napoleon had learned an important lesson: The next time he went to war, food would go with him.

Included in Napoleon's plan to resurrect France was a ministry that encouraged industry by offering prizes for imaginative inventions. A winemaker named Nicholas Appert attracted attention with his process of preserving food. Appert placed fruits, vegetables, soups, and stews in thick bottles, then boiled the bottles for several hours. He used

wax and cork to seal the bottles and wine cages to prevent inadvertent opening of the bottle. By 1805, Appert had set up a bottling industry outside Paris and had a thriving business.

The Ministry of Industry encouraged Appert to publish his methods and submit samples of bottled foods for government testing. The French navy took numerous bottles on long voyages and reported excellent food preservation. In 1810, Appert was awarded 12,000 francs for his invention. Two years later, Napoleon assembled hundreds of cannons, thousands of men, and countless bottles of food, and marched off to war with Russia.

HEAT

Heat kills microorganisms by changing the physical and chemical properties of their proteins. In a moist heat environment, proteins are denatured and lose their three-dimensional structure, reverting to a different three-dimensional form or a two-dimensional form. As structural proteins and enzymes undergo this change, the organisms die. Chapter 21 explores various forms of moist heat and their applications. You might find a brief review helpful in relating heat to food preservation.

The most useful application of heat is in the process of **canning**. Shortly after Appert established the use of heat in preservation, an English engineer named Bryan Donkin substituted iron cans coated with tin for Appert's bottles. Soon he was supplying canned meat to the British navy. In the United States, the tin can was virtually ignored until the Civil War period. In the years thereafter, mass production began and soon the tin can became the symbol of prepackaged convenience.

Modern canning processes are complex (FIGURE 24.6). Machines wash, sort, and grade the food product, then subject it to steam heat for 3 to 5 minutes. This last process, called **blanching**, destroys many enzymes in the food product and prevents any further cellular metabolism from taking place. The food is then peeled and cored, and its diseased sections are removed. Canning comes next, after which the air is evacuated and placed in a pressured steam sterilizer similar to an autoclave at a temperature of 121°C or lower, depending on the pH, density, and heat penetration rate.

The sterilizing process is designed to eliminate the most resistant bacterial spores, especially those of the genera *Bacillus* and *Clostridium*. However, the process is considered **commercial sterilization**, which is not as rigorous as true sterilization, and some spores may survive. Moreover, should a machine error lead to improper heating temperatures, a small hole allow airborne bacteria to enter, or a proper seal not form, contamination may result.

Denaturation:
a change in the usual nature of a substance, such as the structural alteration occurring in heated protein.

Blanching:
treatment with heat for a short period of time to destroy cellular enzymes.

Clostridium:
a genus of Gram-positive anaerobic sporeforming rods.

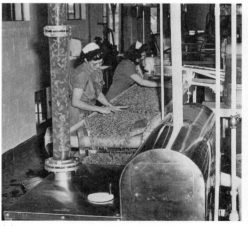
(a)

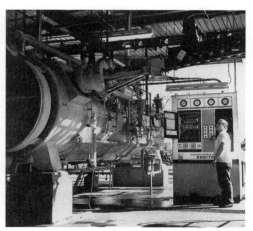
(b)

FIGURE 24.6

Two Steps in the Industrial Canning Process

(a) Initial inspection of green beans is made after cutting and sieve sizing. The beans are washed in the apparatus in the foreground and then conveyed through sanitary glass piping (at the left) to the blanching machine. (b) A continuous cycle orbital cooker used by modern vegetable processors to reduce cooking time of the product.

Contamination of canned food is commonly due to facultative or anaerobic bacteria that produce gas and cause the ends of the can to bulge. Food microbiologists call a can a **flipper** if the bulge can be flattened easily. It is a **springer** if pushing the bulge pushes out the opposite end of the can. A **soft swell** occurs when both ends bulge. If neither end can be pushed in because of the large amount of gas, a **hard swell** is present. The organisms often responsible for gas production are *Clostridium* species as well as coliform bacteria, a group of Gram-negative nonsporeforming rods that ferment lactose to acid and gas. Contamination is usually obvious since the spoiled product generally has a putrid odor.

Coliform bacteria:
a group of Gram-negative rods commonly found in the human and animal intestine.

Growth of acid-producing bacteria presents a different problem because spoilage cannot be discerned from the can's shape. Food has a **flat-sour** taste from the acid and has probably been contaminated by a *Bacillus* species, a coliform, or another acid-producing bacterium that survived the heating.

The process of **pasteurization** was developed by Louis Pasteur in the 1850s to eliminate bacteria in wines. His method was first applied to milk in Denmark about 1870, and by 1895 the process was widely employed. Although the primary object of pasteurization is to eliminate pathogenic bacteria from milk, the process also lowers the total number of bacteria and thereby reduces the chance of spoilage (Chapter 21). The more traditional method involves heating the milk in a large bulk tank at 62.9°C (145°F) for 30 minutes. This is the **holding method**, also known as the **LTLT method** for "low temperature, long time." Machines stir the milk constantly during the pasteurization to ensure uniform heating, and cool it quickly when the heating is completed. More concentrated products, such as cream, are often heated at the higher temperature of 69.5°C (155°F) to ensure successful pasteurization. An innovative method of egg pasteurization has recently been introduced, as MicroFocus 24.5 explains.

Holding method:
a method of pasteurization that uses heat at 62.9°C for 30 minutes.

MicroFocus 24.5

"BRING ON THE CAESAR SALAD!"

Some people have it Hawaiian-style with pineapple and ham; some have it Italian-style with pasta and tomatoes; and some enjoy it Southwestern style with roasted chili peppers. Some toss it with grilled chicken or flank steak or grilled calamari or Cajun scallops. Regardless of the addition, however, the salad remains the same—Caesar salad.

For history buffs, the first Caesar salad is reported to have evolved on July 4, 1924, in the mind of Caesar Cardini, the proprietor of a restaurant (Caesar's Place) in Tijuana, Mexico. Cardini was desperate for a fill-in during a particularly busy day, so he threw together some Romaine lettuce, Parmesan cheese, lemon, garlic, oil, and raw eggs. His customers were enchanted.

Over the years, the reputations of the salad and its inventor grew. There was only one problem, however—the eggs. For true Caesar salad, raw eggs are used to add creaminess to the dressing. But that became a problem when increasing cases of *Salmonella* infections were traced to raw eggs. Eggless Caesar dressings (with mayonnaise or heavy cream) were tried, but it just wasn't the same.

Caesar salad aficionados, take heart—the pasteurized egg is on the way. Purdue University microbiologists have found that *Salmonella* can be eliminated by heating eggs in hot water or a microwave oven, then maintaining them at 134°F in a hot-air oven for 1 hour. And a New Hampshire company (Pasteurized Eggs L.P.) is touting the benefits of its new machine for destroying egg-borne *Salmonella*. The machine heats eggs slowly, then directs them to successive baths in water ranging from 62°C to 72°C. Indeed, the process works so well that the U.S. Department of Agriculture (USDA) has issued a new stamp certifying that eggs treated by the company meet standards for egg pasteurization established by the Food and Drug Administration (FDA).

Agricultural officials estimate that almost 50 billion eggs are produced for American consumption each year, and that over 2 million are infected with *Salmonella*. In the years ahead, that second number should dwindle considerably as egg pasteurization becomes standard practice (as milk pasteurization already has). Then it will be safe to sample the cookie dough; or to have eggs over easy; or to enjoy Caesar salad the way it was meant to be enjoyed.

The more modern method of pasteurization is called the **flash method**. In this process, raw milk is first warmed using the heat of previously pasteurized milk. Machines then pass the milk through a hot cylinder at 71.6°C (161°F) for a period of 15 to 17 seconds. Next, the milk is cooled rapidly, in part by transferring its heat to the incoming milk. This is the **HTST method**, for "high temperature, short time." It is useful for high-quality raw milk, in which the bacterial count is consistently low. A new method called **ultrapasteurization** is used in some dairy plants. In this process, milk and milk products are subjected to heat at 82°C (180°F) for 3 seconds. Following pasteurization, a set of laboratory tests is performed to assay the quality of the milk and the success of pasteurization (TABLE 24.1).

The bacteria that survive pasteurization may be involved in spoilage. *Streptococcus lactis*, for instance, grows slowly in refrigerated milk, and when its numbers reach 20 million per milliliter, enough lactic acid has been produced to make the milk sour. Organisms that survive the heat of pasteurization are described as **thermoduric**. Pasteurization is virtually useless against **thermophilic bacteria**, since they grow naturally at 60°C to 70°C. These organisms generally do not grow at refrigerator temperatures or cause human disease because conditions are too cool. Pasteurization also has no effect on spores.

Although milk in the United States is normally pasteurized and refrigerated, exposure to steam at 140°C for 3 seconds can sterilize it. This **ultra-high temperature (UHT)** results in milk (e.g., Parmalat) with an indefinite shelf life as long as the container remains sealed. Small containers of coffee cream are often prepared this way.

Flash method: a method of pasteurization that uses heat at 71.6°C for 15 to 17 seconds.

Thermoduric: heat-enduring.
Thermophilic: heat-loving.

TABLE 24.1

Laboratory Tests Used to Assay the Quality of Milk

TEST	PURPOSE	IMPORTANCE
Phosphatase test	Determines whether phosphatase is present. Phosphatase is an enzyme normally destroyed during pasteurization.	To determine whether sufficient heat was used during pasteurization. If phosphatase is present, pathogens also might be present.
Reductase test	Estimates the number of bacteria in milk. The rate at which methylene blue is reduced to its colorless form is proportional to the number of bacteria present in a milk sample.	High-quality milk contains so few bacteria that a standard concentration of methylene blue will not be reduced in 6 hours. Low-quality milk has many bacteria, and methylene blue is reduced in 2 hours or less.
Standard plate count	Determines the total number of viable bacteria per ml of milk. Diluted milk is mixed with nutrient agar and incubated 48 hours; colonies are counted and the number of bacteria in the original sample is calculated.	The number per milliliter may not exceed 100,000 in raw milk before being pooled with other milk. It may not exceed 20,000 after pasteurization.
Test for coliforms	Determines the number of viable coliform bacteria per ml of milk. Similar to the standard plate count except that special media for coliform bacteria are used.	A positive coliform test indicates contamination with fecal material. The number per ml may not exceed established standards.
Test for pathogens	Detects the presence of pathogens. Methods depend on the pathogens suspected.	Helps locate the source of infectious agents that may be present in milk.

LOW TEMPERATURES

By lowering the environmental temperature, one can reduce the rate of enzyme activity in a microorganism and thus lower the rate of growth and reproduction. This principle underlies the process of refrigeration and freezing. Although the organisms are not killed, their numbers are kept low and spoilage is minimized. Ironically, the food is preserved by preserving the microorganisms.

Well before contemporary humans developed refrigerators, the Greeks and Romans had partially solved the problem of keeping things cold. They simply dug a snow cellar in the basements of their homes, lined the cellar with logs, insulated it with heavy layers of straw, and packed it densely with snow delivered from far-off mountaintops ("The iceman cometh!"). The compressed snow turned to a block of ice, and foods would remain unspoiled for long periods when left in this makeshift refrigerator. The modern **refrigerator** at 5°C (41°F) provides a suitable environment for preserving food without destroying its appearance, taste, or cellular integrity (FIGURE 24.7). However, psychrotrophic microorganisms survive and cause green meat surfaces, rotten eggs, moldy fruits, and sour milk. Pathogens such as *Listeria monocytogenes* and *Yersinia enterocolitica* also grow at low temperatures.

When food is placed in the **freezer** at –5°C (23°F), ice crystals form rapidly. These crystals tear and shred microorganisms and kill a significant number. However, many microorganisms survive, and the ice crystals are equally destructive to food cells. Therefore, when the food thaws, bacteria multiply quickly. Organisms such as staphylococci produce substantial amounts of enterotoxins, and *Salmonella* serotypes

si'kro-trof'ik
Psychrotrophic:
tolerating cold conditions but
preferring warmer ones.

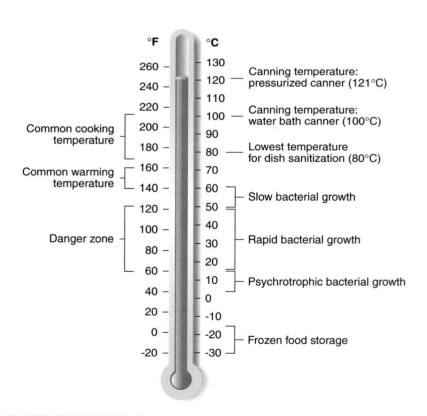

FIGURE 24.7

Important Temperature Considerations in Food Microbiology

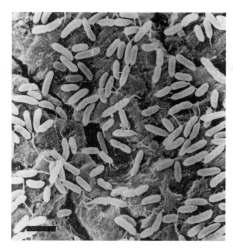

FIGURE 24.8

Food Contamination

A scanning electron micrograph of unidentified flagellated bacteria growing on the skin of a chicken carcass. Bacteria such as these contaminate frozen food and grow to large numbers when the food is thawed and held for long periods before cooking. (Bar = 2 μm.)

and streptococci and other bacteria grow to large numbers (FIGURE 24.8). Rapid thawing and cooking are thus recommended. Moreover, food should not be refrozen, because during thawing and refreezing, bacteria deposit sufficient enterotoxin to cause food poisoning the next time the food is thawed. Microwave cooking, which requires minimal thawing, may eliminate some of these problems.

Deep freezing at −60°C results in smaller ice crystals, and although the physical damage to microorganisms is less severe, their biochemical activity is reduced considerably. Small ice crystals do not damage food cells as severely as do the larger crystals formed at higher temperatures. Some food producers blanch their product before deep freezing, a process that further reduces the number of microorganisms.

A major problem in freezing is **freezer burn**, which may occur over long periods of time as food dries out from moisture evaporation. Another disadvantage is that the energy cost of freezing is considerable. Nevertheless, freezing has been a mainstay of preservation since Clarence Birdseye first offered frozen foods for retail purchase in the 1920s. Approximately 33 percent of all preserved food in the United States is frozen.

Freezer burn:
the drying of foods subjected to long periods of freezing.

MicroFocus 24.6

FOREVER IMMORTALIZED

They say it began in 1878 at Moon's Lake House Restaurant in fashionable Saratoga Springs, New York. Cornelius Vanderbilt, the wealthy entrepreneur, was visiting the resort, and one evening he took issue with the fried potatoes. They were too thick, it seemed, and the chef, a certain George Crum, should have known better. But Vanderbilt was magnanimous—Crum would have another chance to make a more acceptable potato dish.

Crum did not take the criticism well at all, and he plotted revenge. If Vanderbilt wanted thin potatoes, then thin potatoes he would get. Apparently trying for overkill, Crum sliced the potatoes superthin, dropped them into boiling oil, and fried them to a crisp. Then he sent the potatoes out to his picky patron, fully expecting to be working elsewhere the next day. You can imagine his surprise when he heard sounds of delight from the dining room—Vanderbilt loved the crunchy potatoes. Soon everyone was coming from miles around to sample the "Saratoga chips," as they were called. The chips later became famous as potato chips. Unfortunately, few people knew

about their inventor George Crum—until now, that is.

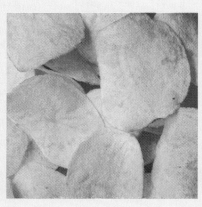

DRYING

The advantage of drying foods is best expressed by the phrase "Where there is no water, there is no natural life." Indeed, dry foods cannot support microbial growth (**MicroFocus 24.6**). In past centuries, people used the sun for drying, but modern technologists have developed sophisticated machinery for this purpose. For example, the **spray dryer** expels a fine mist of liquid such as coffee into a barrel cylinder containing hot air. The water evaporates quickly, and the coffee powder falls to the bottom of the cylinder.

Another machine for drying is the **heated drum**. Machines pour liquids such as soup on the drum, and the water evaporates rapidly, leaving dried soup to be scraped off the drum. A third machine utilizes a **belt heater** that exposes liquids such as milk to a stream of hot air. The air evaporates any water and leaves dried milk solids. Unfortunately, sporeforming and capsule-producing bacteria are problems because they resist drying.

During the past 20 years, freeze-drying, or **lyophilization**, has emerged as a valuable preservation method. In this process, food is deep frozen, and then a vacuum pump draws off the water in a machine like the one pictured in FIGURE 24.9. (Water passes from its solid phase [ice] to its gaseous phase [water vapor] without passing through its liquid phase [water].) The dry product is sealed in foil and easily reconstituted with water. Hikers and campers find considerable value in freeze-dried food because of its light weight and durability. However, there is a disquieting note: Lyophilization is also a useful method for storing, transporting, and preserving bacterial cultures.

OSMOTIC PRESSURE

When living cells are immersed in large quantities of a compound such as salt or sugar, water diffuses out of cells through cell membranes and into the surrounding environment, where it dilutes the high concentration of the compound. The flow of water is called **osmosis**, and the force that drives the water is termed **osmotic pressure**.

Osmotic pressure can be used to preserve foods because water flows out of microorganisms as well as food cells. For example, in highly salted or sugared foods, microorganisms dehydrate, shrink, and die. Jams, jellies, fruits, maple syrups, honey, and similar products typify foods preserved by **high sugar** concentrations. **Salted foods** include ham, cod, bacon, and beef, as well as certain vegetables such as sauerkraut, which has the added benefit of large quantities of acid. It should be noted, however, that staphylococci tolerate salt and may survive to cause staphylococcal food poisoning.

CHEMICAL PRESERVATIVES

In order for a chemical preservative to be useful in foods, it must be inhibitory to microorganisms while easily broken down and eliminated by the body without side effects. These requirements have limited the number of available chemicals to a select few.

A major group of chemical preservatives are organic acids, such as sorbic acid, benzoic acid, and propionic acid. Microbiologists believe that these compounds damage microbial membranes and interfere with the uptake of certain essential organic substances such as amino acids. Chemicals are used primarily against molds and yeasts, but their acidity is also a deterrent to bacterial growth.

Spray dryer:
a device that dries liquid foods by spraying a fine mist from which the water is evaporated.

li-of'ĭ-li-za'shun
Lyophilization:
the process of freeze-drying.

Osmotic pressure:
the force that drives water through a membrane in osmosis.

Staphylococci:
Gram-positive irregular clusters of aerobic cocci.

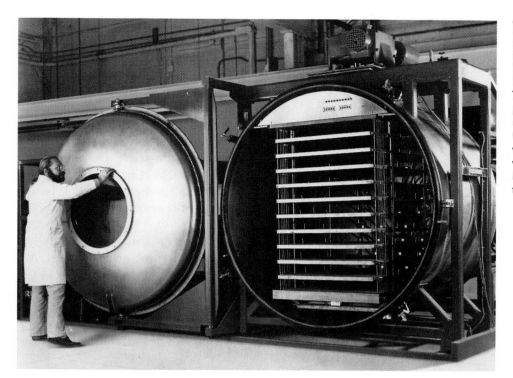

FIGURE 24.9

An Industrial Model Lyophilizer

This model removes 500 pounds of product moisture in 24 hours of freeze-drying. Using vacuum and heat, water is drawn off from ice without passing through the liquid phase to produce the freeze-dried product.

Sorbic acid, which came into use in 1955, is added to syrups, salad dressings, jellies, and certain cakes. **Benzoic acid**, the first chemical (1908) to be approved by the Food and Drug Administration (FDA), protects beverages, catsup, margarine, and apple cider. **Propionic acid** is incorporated in wrappings for butter and cheese, and is added to breads and bakery products, where it inhibits the ropiness commonly due to *Bacillus* species and prevents the growth of fungi. Other natural acids in food add flavor while serving as preservatives. Examples are **lactic acid** in sauerkraut and yogurt, and **acetic acid** in vinegar.

The process of **smoking** with hickory or other woods accomplishes the dual purposes of drying food and depositing chemical preservatives. By-products of smoke, such as aldehydes, acids, and certain phenol compounds, effectively inhibit microbial growth for long periods of time. Smoked fish and meats have been staples of the diet for many centuries.

Sulfur dioxide has gained popularity as a preservative for dried fruits, molasses, and juice concentrates. Used in either gas or liquid form, the chemical retards color changes on the fruit surface and adds to the aesthetic quality of the product. Another gas, **ethylene oxide**, is employed for the preservation of spices, nuts, and dried fruits, especially those packaged in cellophane bags. This same gas is used for the chemical sterilization of packaged Petri dishes and other plastic devices.

Some foods contain their own natural preservatives. Examples are the antimicrobial substances in garlic, the lysozyme in egg white, and the benzoic acid of cranberries.

Benzoic acid:
a phenyl-containing organic acid used as a food preservative.

Sulfur dioxide:
a chemical used as a preservative in foods.

RADIATION

Though much of the public is apprehensive about foods exposed to radiation, various forms of radiation are used to sterilize foods. Taste and appearance have been

Ultraviolet light:
a form of energy whose wavelength is shorter than that of visible light.

preserved by freezing food in liquid nitrogen and exhausting oxygen from the package before irradiation. Meat storage facilities use **ultraviolet light** to reduce surface contamination, and water can be treated with UV light when chlorine is not useful.

Gamma rays are utilized to extend the shelf life of fruits, vegetables, fish, and poultry from several days to several weeks. This form of radiation also increases the distances fresh food can be transported and significantly extends the storage time for food in the home. Gamma rays are high-frequency forms of electromagnetic energy emitted by a radioactive isotope called **cobalt-60**. The radiations are not radioactive, and they cannot cause food to become radioactive. They kill microorganisms by reacting with and destroying microbial DNA (Chapter 21). Opponents to their use point out, however, that the radiations also break chemical bonds in foods and cause new ones to form, thereby raising the possibility of new and toxic chemical compounds.

Interest in gamma radiation for food preservation grew during the 1950s under President Eisenhower's Atoms for Peace program. For the next quarter-century, the FDA conducted extensive tests to determine whether the process was safe. In March 1981, the FDA approved radiated foods such as spices, condiments, fruits, and vegetables for sale to American consumers. Gamma radiation of pork to prevent trichinosis won approval in 1985, and irradiated strawberries made it to market in 1992. Irradiation of red meat was approved in 1997, as further explored in Chapter 21.

Trichinosis:
a disease of the muscles, caused by a roundworm and transmitted by pork.

PREVENTING FOODBORNE DISEASE

Food may be a mechanical vector for infectious microorganisms or a culture medium for growth. People are then affected by the organism or the toxin it has produced in the food. In the former case, a food infection is established; in the latter, a food poisoning or intoxication occurs.

Food infections are typified by typhoid fever, salmonellosis, cholera, and shigellosis, all of which are of bacterial origin. The protozoal infections amoebiasis, balantidiasis, and giardiasis represent foodborne diseases. Viral infections are exemplified by hepatitis A. **Food intoxications** include botulism, staphylococcal food poisoning, and clostridial food poisoning. Since full discussions of these diseases are presented elsewhere in this text (Chapters 8, 13, and 17), we shall not examine them individually here.

am'e-bi'ah-sis
bal'an-ti'-di'ah-sis
ji'ar-di'ah-sis

In the United States, public health microbiologists estimate that between 2 and 10 million people are affected by foodborne disease annually. Many episodes require medical attention, but the vast majority of patients recover rapidly without serious complications. In many cases, the incident might have been avoided by taking some basic precautions. For example, unrefrigerated foods are a prime source of staphylococci and *Salmonella* serotypes (MicroFocus 24.7), and perishable groceries such as meats and dairy products should not be allowed to warm up while other errands are performed. Also, a thermometer should be used to ensure that the refrigerator temperature is below 40°F at all times.

Another way to avoid foodborne disease is to cover any skin boils while working with foods, since boils are a common source of staphylococci. The hands should always be washed thoroughly before and after handling raw vegetables or salad fixings to avoid cross-contamination of other foods. It is wise to cook meat from a frozen or partly frozen state; if this is impossible, the meat should be thawed in the refrigerator. Cutting boards should be cleaned with hot, soapy water after use, and old cutting boards with cracks and pits should be discarded (MicroFocus 22.5).

MicroFocus 24.7

FOWL PLAY

It was the annual company picnic and the softball game was finally over. Now the serious eating could begin. There were salads, stuffed eggs, barbecued chickens, lots of desserts, and a picnic table overflowing with goodies. Unfortunately, there was also an unwelcome guest at the picnic: a serotype of *Salmonella*. During the next 3 days, over half the attendees would suffer abdominal cramps, diarrhea, headaches, and fever. The common thread was the bar-

becued chicken—all the sick attendees had eaten it.

Public health inspectors questioned the woman in charge of the chickens. She led inspectors back to a local supermarket, where the barbecued chickens were sold "ready to eat." It seemed that store employees cooked the birds, then put them back in the original trays where the uncooked birds had been stored. Investigators found evidence of *Salmonella* in the trays. Further ques-

tioning revealed that the woman had bought the chickens in the morning and stored them for the next 7 hours in the trunk of her car, believing they would remain cool. They did not. In fact, they reached incubator temperatures quickly and by dinner time, at 7:00 P.M., they were teeming with *Salmonella*.

The lessons are clear: Keep meats cold; store them in clean, fresh trays after cooking; and play softball *after* dinner, not before.

Studies indicate that leftovers are implicated in most outbreaks of foodborne disease (FIGURE 24.10). It is therefore important to refrigerate leftovers promptly and keep them no more than a few days. Thorough reheating of leftovers, preferably to boiling, also reduces the possibility of illness.

Many instances of foodborne disease occur during the summer months, when foods are taken on picnics where they cannot be refrigerated. As a general principle, dairy foods, such as custards, cream pies, pastries, and deli salads should be excluded from the picnic menu. For outdoor barbecues, one dish should be used for carrying hamburgers to the grill and another dish for serving them. Many of these principles apply equally well to fall and winter tailgate parties.

Over 90 percent of **botulism** outbreaks reported to the CDC are traced to home-canned food. To prevent this sometimes fatal foodborne disease, health officials urge that homemakers use the pressure method to can foods. Reliable canning instructions should be obtained and followed stringently. Foods suspected of contamination should not be tasted to confirm the suspicion, but should be discarded immediately. When in doubt, boiling the food for a minimum of 10 minutes and thoroughly washing the utensil used to stir the food are recommended. Bulging or leaking cans must be discarded in a way that will not endanger other people or animals.

Botulism:
a foodborne disease of the nervous system characterized by paralysis.

Milk is an unusually good vehicle for the transmission of pathogenic microorganisms because its fat content protects organisms from stomach acid, and, being a fluid, it remains in the stomach a relatively short period of time. The diseases of cows transmitted by milk include bovine tuberculosis, brucellosis, and Q fever (Chapter 8). Since the 1980s, several outbreaks of milkborne disease have been linked to *Salmonella* serotypes. In 1984, for example, 16 cases of **salmonellosis** due to *Salmonella typhimurium* occurred in nuns at a convent in Kentucky. A failure in milk pasteurization accounted for the episode.

Brucellosis:
a bacterial disease caused by a Gram-negative rod and characterized by recurring fever.

Another milkborne organism of significance is ***Campylobacter jejuni,*** the cause of **campylobacteriosis**. In 1984, this Gram-negative curved rod was isolated from nine kindergarten children and adults who sampled raw milk at a bottling plant in southern California while on a school field trip. Scientists estimate that *Campylobacter jejuni* is present in the intestinal tracts of about 40 percent of dairy cattle.

kam'pĭ-lo-bak'ter jĕ-joo'ne
kam'pĭ-lo-bak'ter-e-o'sis

FIGURE 24.10

A Case of Botulism Due to Leftover Food

This incident happened in California in August 1984. Because the stew was discarded, it could not be tested for *Clostridium botulinum*. However, the 16-hour interval during which the stew remained at room temperature was sufficient for the germination of clostridial spores. The first man was unaffected because he ate the stew immediately after cooking.

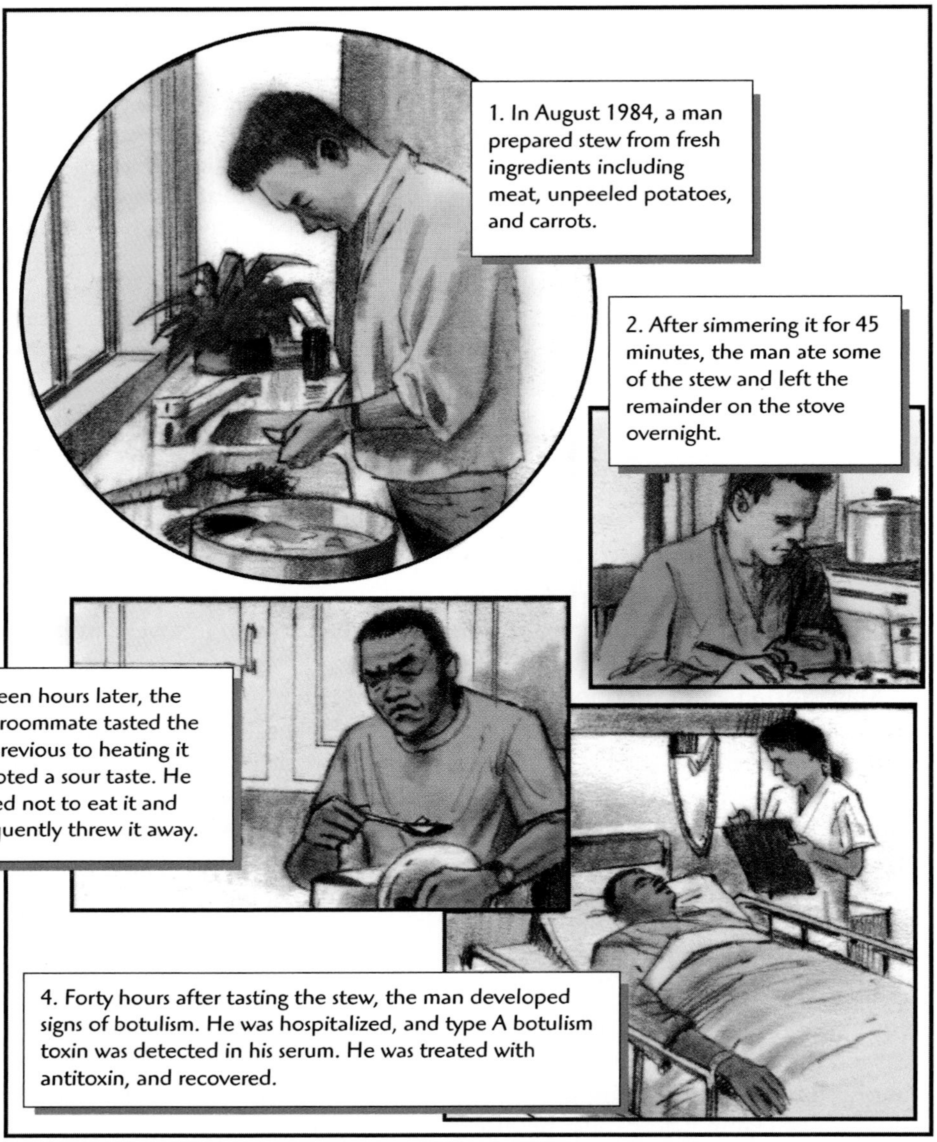

1. In August 1984, a man prepared stew from fresh ingredients including meat, unpeeled potatoes, and carrots.

2. After simmering it for 45 minutes, the man ate some of the stew and left the remainder on the stove overnight.

3. Sixteen hours later, the man's roommate tasted the stew previous to heating it and noted a sour taste. He decided not to eat it and subsequently threw it away.

4. Forty hours after tasting the stew, the man developed signs of botulism. He was hospitalized, and type A botulism toxin was detected in his serum. He was treated with antitoxin, and recovered.

TEXTBOOK CASES

Public health microbiologists seek to limit milkborne disease by inspecting food and dairy plants regularly, and making recommendations on improved sanitary practices. In the field, sick animals are treated with antibiotics and immunized. The success of mass brucellosis immunizations in the 1970s showed their effectiveness as a public health measure. New methods for immunizing poultry are explored in Chapter 8.

HACCP SYSTEMS

Fueled by consumer awareness, the entire food industry has been placed under a food-safety spotlight. Among the most important food safety systems is **Hazard Analysis Critical Control Points (HACCP)**, a set of scientifically based safety regulations now federally enforced in the seafood, meat, and poultry industries. In an HACCP system, manufacturers identify individual processing points that could affect the safety of a product. These points are called **critical control points**, or **CCPs** (in the jargon of food technology). The CCPs are supervised to ensure that any hazards associated with the operation are contained or, preferably, eliminated (the key concept is prevention). When all possible hazards are controlled at the CCPs, the safety of the product can be assumed without further testing or inspection.

HACCP systems are overseen by the U.S. Food and Drug Administration (FDA) and the U.S. Department of Agriculture (USDA). The systems are developed by each food establishment and tailored to its individual product, processing, or distribution conditions. The standard regulations require food processors to monitor and control eight key sanitation areas: (1) the safety of water that contacts food or used to make ice; (2) the condition and cleanliness of utensils, gloves, outer garments, and other food contact surfaces; (3) the prevention of cross-contamination from raw products and unsanitary objects to foods; (4) the maintenance of hand-washing and toilet facilities; (5) the protection of foods and food surfaces from adulteration with lubricants, fuel, pesticides, sanitizing agents, and other contaminants; (6) the proper labeling, storage, and use of toxic compounds; (7) the control of employee health conditions that could result in food contamination; and (8) the exclusion of pests from the food plant.

The HACCP system is a risk-reduction system originally developed in the 1960s for foods used in space travel ("space foods"), but not applied to the food industry until the 1990s. It places the responsibility for food safety on the shoulders of industry, but it also focuses consumer attention on food handling and safety issues. Several well-publicized foodborne disease outbreaks and product recalls have raised questions about the safety and quality of foods, and HACCP systems will attempt to restore consumer confidence. Improved epidemiological investigations and increased surveillance will add to that confidence in the ensuing years. Indeed, January 26, 1998, was an important date for consumers. On that day, HACCP systems began at 312 of the largest meat and poultry processing plants in the United States (**FIGURE 24.11**); by the time you read this, the remaining 6100 plants will have been phased in.

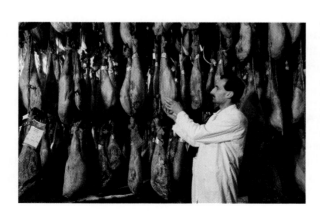

FIGURE 24.11

Meat Inspections

A meat inspector checks beef prior to sale. The long-standing "sniff-and-poke" method of inspection is being replaced by a newly instituted HACCP system of ensuring meat safety.

To this point...

We have focused on the topic of food preservation and have outlined the various ways in which preservation can be achieved. One of the most widespread methods of preservation is by using heat in the canning process. Another method is by employing low temperatures in the refrigerator and freezer. A third is by drying food through various industrial modes, and a fourth is by drawing fluid out of microorganisms by osmotic pressure.

Two additional methods of preservation are chemical preservatives and radiation. Chemicals currently utilized include sorbic, benzoic, and propionic acid, as well as sulfur dioxide and various chemicals in wood smoke. Gamma rays are a type of radiation shown to be an excellent food preservative under experimental conditions. We pointed out some advantages to the use of gamma rays, but extensive testing still needs to be completed, and consumer acceptance remains an obstacle to acceptance. Prevention of illness from food and dairy products can be effected by consumers, however, and we noted several methods.

The discussion up to this point has cast microorganisms in a negative role as spoilers of food and objects of preservation methods. But microorganisms may also play a positive role in the food and dairy product industries because their chemical activities result in numerous food products. We shall briefly discuss some of these products in the chapter's final section.

24.3 Foods from Microorganisms

Over the centuries, social customs and traditions have brought acceptance of a variety of foods produced by microorganisms. Some individuals regard these foods as "spoiled," but to many people, the food is "fermented" (FIGURE 24.12).

Fermented foods have three things in common: They are less vulnerable to extensive spoilage than unfermented foods; they are less likely to be vectors of foodborne illness than unfermented foods; and they have been accepted by the cultures in which they were developed (indeed, in some cases, they are considered delicacies). It is conceivable that ancient peoples were first attracted to the preservative qualities of fermented foods and coincidentally learned to appreciate their tastes.

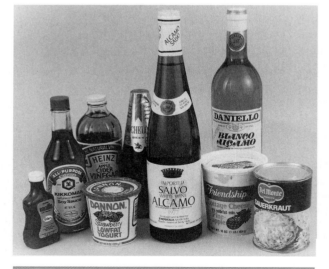

FIGURE 24.12

An Array of Foods and Beverages Produced by Microorganisms

SAUERKRAUT

Sauerkraut (German for "sour cabbage") is not only a well-preserved and tasty form of cabbage but also nutritionally sound. For instance, the vitamin C content of sauerkraut is equivalent to that of citrus fruits, and sauerkraut was often taken on British sea voyages to prevent scurvy because citrus fruits were too expensive.

Sauerkraut is prepared commercially by adding salt to shredded cabbage and packing the cabbage tightly to encourage anaerobic conditions. The first organisms to multiply are species of **Leuconostoc**, a Gram-positive coccus found naturally in the cabbage. These bacteria ferment carbohydrates in the plant cells and produce acetic and lactic acids. After some days, the acids lower the pH of the cabbage to about 3.5. Species of **Lactobacillus** then proliferate, and the additional lactic acid they produce by fermentation further reduces the pH to about 2.0. The salt helps retard mold contamination while drawing juices out of the plant cells. A compound called **diacetyl** (the flavoring agent in butter) is produced by *Leuconostoc*, adding aroma and flavor.

Sauerkraut:
fermented cabbage.

loo'ko-nos'tok

Diacetyl:
a compound that gives flavor to butter.

PICKLES

In the United States, "pickle" is practically synonymous with "pickled cucumber." Over 37 types of dill, sour, and sweet **pickles** have been categorized, but essentially the fermentations are similar. Cucumbers are placed in a salt solution of 8 percent or higher, at which point the cucumber changes color from bright green to olive green. Next comes curing.

Three groups of microorganisms are important to the fermentation and curing of cucumbers. **Enterobacter aerogenes**, a Gram-negative rod, produces large amounts of CO_2, which takes up all the air space and establishes anaerobic conditions. **Lactobacillus** and **Leuconostoc** species then dominate and form abundant amounts of acid that softens the tissues and sours the cucumbers (**FIGURE 24.13**). Finally, certain **yeasts** grow and establish many flavors associated with ripe pickles. Dill, garlic, and other herbs and spices are added to finish the product. Pickled pepper, tomatoes, and other vegetables undergo a somewhat similar process. Most pickles are heat-pasteurized or further acidified to increase their shelf life, but "kosher-style" pickles are given no further treatment.

a'er-oj'en-ēz

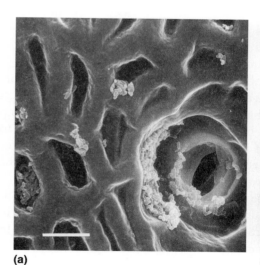
(a)

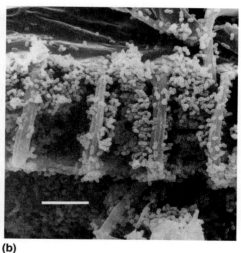
(b)

FIGURE 24.13

A Cucumber and Its Bacterial Flora

(a) A scanning electron micrograph of *Lactobacillus plantarum* on the surface of the cucumber. The openings are stomata, through which gases pass for the cucumber's metabolism. Note the accumulation of lactobacilli at these stomata. (Bar = 10 μm.) (b) A longitudinal section through the vascular tissue of a brined cucumber showing *Leuconostoc* species along the tubular walls. (Bar = 10 μm.)

VINEGAR

Vinegar is a fermented food that traditionally has been made by the spontaneous souring of wine. Indeed, the word is derived from the French *vinaigre*, which means "sour wine."

A widely used method for industrial vinegar production follows a procedure first devised in Germany in the early 1800s. **Yeasts** ferment the fruit juice to alcohol until the alcohol concentration is about 10 to 20 percent. Machines then spray the alcoholic juice into a tank containing the bacterium ***Acetobacter aceti*** growing on the surface of wood shavings, gravel, or other substrate. As alcohol percolates through, bacterial enzymes convert it to acetaldehyde and then acetic acid. The vinegar recirculates several times before collection at the bottom of the tank. Residual alcohol evaporates in the heat, and the product usually has an acetic acid content of about 3 to 5 percent. The flavor of vinegar is determined by oils, sugars, and other compounds produced by the bacteria, plus the residue of organic compounds in the wine from which it was made.

ah-se′to-bak′ter

as′et-al′dĕ-hīd

OTHER FERMENTED FOODS

Several other fermented foods are also worthy of note. One example, **soy sauce**, is made from roasted soybeans and wheat inoculated with the fungus *Aspergillus oryzae* and allowed to stand for 3 days (**FIGURE 24.14**). The fungus-covered product, called **koji**, is then added to a solution of salt and microorganisms, and aged for about a year. During this time, lactobacilli produce acid, and yeasts produce small amounts of alcohol. Together with the fungal products, the acid and alcohol determine the flavor. The liquid pressed from the mixture is soy sauce.

as′per-gil′lus o-ri′zā

ko′je

Another example is **fermented sausages**. These are generally produced as dry or semidry products and include pepperoni from Italy, thuringer from Germany, and polsa from Sweden. Curing and seasoning agents are first added to ground meats, followed by stuffing into casings and incubation at warm temperatures. Mixed acids produced from carbohydrates in the meat give the sausage its unique flavor and aroma.

Cocoa and coffee also owe their flavor in part to microorganisms. **Cocoa** derives some of its taste from the microbial fermentation that helps remove cocoa beans from the pulp covering them in the pod. Likewise, **coffee** is believed to obtain some of its flavor from the fermentation of coffee berries when the beans are soaked in water to loosen the berry skins before roasting.

The influence of microorganisms on animal nutrition is evident in the animal food called **silage**. Silage is made in huge, cylindrical silos that commonly stand adjacent to barns. The farmer packs the silo with corn, grain stalks, grass, potatoes, and virtually anything that can be fermented. During storage, various bacteria ferment the plant carbohydrates in a process similar to that for sauerkraut and pickles. Fermentation yields a broad mixture of acids, aldehydes, and ketones, as well as **diacetyl**, which is relished by cattle. After several weeks, the well-preserved plant material is sweet smelling, succulent, and nutritious to animals. It is also inexpensive to the farmer.

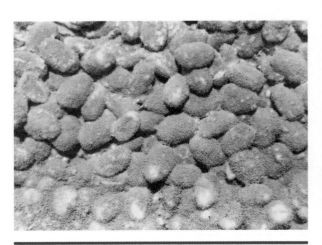

FIGURE 24.14

The Production of Soy Sauce

Roasted soybeans are inoculated with *Aspergillus oryzae* to produce the koji used for soy sauce. Fungi cover the beans and begin the fermentation later completed by bacteria during aging.

SOUR MILK PRODUCTS

Over the centuries, fermented milk products have assumed a key place in our diet. The sour milks are typical examples of fermented milk products. **Buttermilk** is made by adding starter cultures of *Streptococcus cremoris* and *Leuconostoc citrovorum* to vats of skim milk. The *Streptococcus* ferments lactose to lactic and acetic acids, and the *Leuconostoc* continues the fermentation to yield various aldehydes and ketones, and the compound **diacetyl**. These substances, especially diacetyl, give buttermilk its flavor, aroma, and acidity. For **sour cream**, the same process is used, except that pasteurized light cream is the starting point.

loo′ko-nos′tok sit′ro-vor′um

Acidophilus milk is produced in much the same way as buttermilk, except that the skim milk is inoculated with *Lactobacillus acidophilus*. This bacterium is a normal member of the human intestinal flora. Many health-care practitioners believe that the lactobacilli in acidophilus milk augment naturally occurring lactobacilli and help the digestion process, while keeping molds in check. A newer type of acidophilus milk, **sweet acidophilus milk**, lacks the sour taste. It is prepared by adding *Lactobacillus acidophilus* to pasteurized milk do.

as′ĭ-dof′ĭ-lus

Yogurt is a form of sour milk (**MicroFocus 24.8**), made by adding dry milk solids to boiled milk to achieve a custardlike consistency. The two starter cultures are *Streptococcus thermophilus* and *Lactobacillus bulgaricus*. Yogurt is sometimes called Bulgarian milk because it was popular among peasants in Bulgaria and other Balkan countries. After World War I, many Americans became health-conscious, and Elie Metchnikoff (the discoverer of phagocytosis) took note of the longevity of Bulgarian peasants and attributed it to the yogurt they drank. Metchnikoff believed that the streptococci and lactobacilli in yogurt assume residence in the intestine and replace organisms that contribute to aging. Although the aging theory has largely been discounted, many microbiologists hold that bacteria in yogurt support good health much as the bacteria in acidophilus milk do.

Yogurt:
a thick, sour milk product produced by bacterial action on lactose.

CHEESE

Cheese production begins when the casein curdles out of milk (**FIGURE 24.15**). Usually this accompanies a souring of the milk by streptococci, but the process may be accelerated by adding **rennin**, an enzyme obtained from the stomach lining of a

Rennin:
an animal enzyme that accelerates curdling in milk.

MicroFocus 24.8

MAKING YOUR OWN YOGURT

The popularity of yogurt as a nutritious low-calorie food has prompted many to try their hand at making it at home. Here is a recipe that works well.

Heat one quart of milk to about 170°F (77°C), stirring often and using a thermometer to check the temperature. This heating will evaporate some of the liquid and reduce the bacterial population. Let the milk cool to about 130°F (about 55°C), then add one cup of powdered milk and one-third cup of unflavored commercial yogurt. Mix thoroughly and pour into small containers with lids. Styrofoam coffee cups may be used.

For the incubation step, you will need a small cooler of the type used for picnics. Fill the cooler with several inches of water at 130°F (55°C). Now place the containers in the cooler, close the lid tightly, and let the containers stand for about 6 to 8 hours. (A large pan of hot water in the oven also works well, or the cups can be wrapped with hot towels.) During this time, the bacteria will multiply and the yogurt will thicken. Refrigerate, add fresh or frozen fruit, and enjoy.

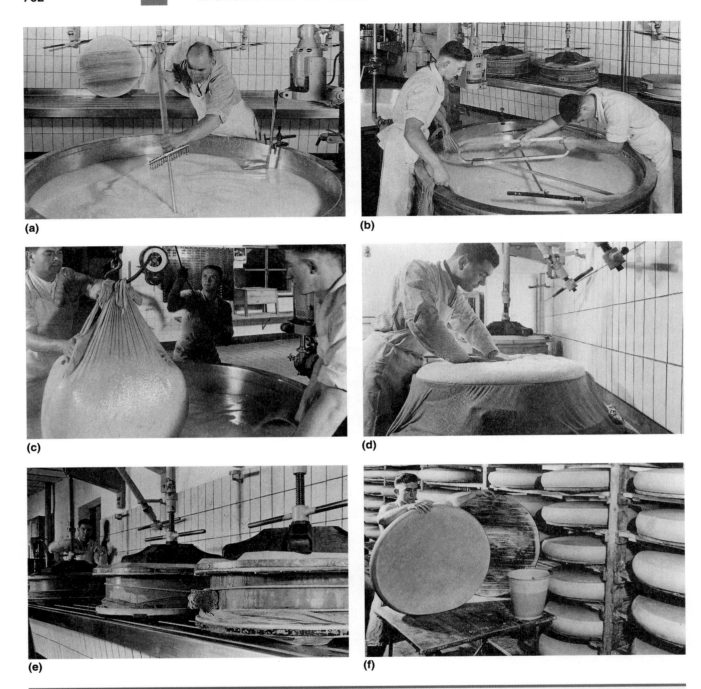

FIGURE 24.15

Steps in the Production of Swiss Cheese

(a) The milk is mixed with rennet and heated in a large kettle. After the curds form, the cheesemaker cuts the curds into small pieces using a series of copper wires called a cheese harp. This speeds the expulsion of the whey and ensures uniform heating of the curds by increasing the surface area. (b) About 2½ hours after adding the rennet, a square piece of cheesecloth composed of coarse-weave hemp is drawn down along the wall of the vat and passed under the curds. (c) The four corners of the cheesecloth are tied together, and the curds are removed by a block and tackle. (d) The curds are deposited on a wooden hoop, and the surface is kneaded lightly with the palms of the hands. (e) Press boards are placed on top of the cheese mass until no more whey emerges. This process, which usually requires a day, forms the familiar wheels of cheese. (f) The cheese is then transported to a warm cellar, where it is salted and set aside to ripen. Bacteria ferment the cheese for about 2 weeks at a temperature of 50°C to 57°C and a relative humidity of 90 percent. The cheese is then inspected, graded, and sold for consumption.

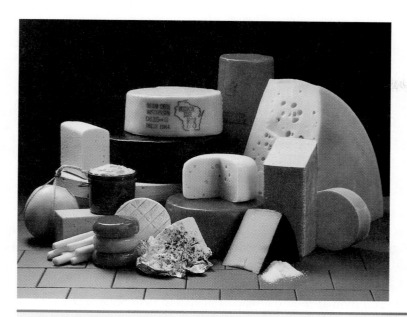

FIGURE 24.16

An Array of Cheeses Produced by Microorganisms

calf. The milk curd is essentially an unripened cheese. It may be marketed as **cottage cheese**, or pot cheese. **Cream cheese** is also unripened cheese with a butterfat content of up to 20 percent.

To prepare ripened cheese, the milk curds are washed, pressed, sometimes cooked, and cut to the desired shape. Often the curds are salted to add flavor, control moisture, and prevent contamination by molds. If **Swiss cheese** is to be made, two types of bacteria grow within the cheese: *Lactobacillus* species, which ferment the lactose to lactic acid; and *Propionibacterium* species, which produce organic compounds and carbon dioxide, which seeks out weak spots in the curd and accumulates as holes, or eyes (FIGURE 24.16). **Cheddar cheese** is scalded at a lower temperature than Swiss. Cheddar and Swiss are examples of cheese ripened internally by bacteria. Provolone, Edam, and Gouda are others. *(pro′pe-on′e-bak-te′re-um)*

Another group of cheeses are somewhat softer in texture, a characteristic deriving from the partial breakdown of the protein curds by microbial enzymes. Growth takes place primarily at the surface of these cheeses, and the products tend to be pungent. Within the group of **soft cheeses** are Muenster, Port du Salut, and Limberger. **Yeasts** and species of the Gram-positive rod *Brevibacterium* are among the surface flora. The rind of the cheese is derived from microbial pigments. *(brev′e-bak-te′re-um)*

The **mold-ripened** cheeses are represented by Camembert and Roquefort. **Camembert cheese** is made by dipping salted curds into *Penicillium camemberti* spores to stimulate a surface growth. The fungus grows on the outside of the curd and digests the proteins, thus softening the curd. **Roquefort** is a blue-veined cheese produced by *Penicillium roqueforti*. The mold penetrates cracks within the curd, creating the distinctive veins within the cheese. Most people, however, would rather remain blissfully ignorant of this fact.

Note to the Student

Since 1925, only five deaths from botulism have been attributed to commercially canned food in the United States. During this period, almost 100 billion cans of food were produced for sale to consumers.

I believe that these figures are a testament to the high standards achieved by the canning industry. They represent an achievement of which we consumers can be justifiably proud. I say "we consumers" because we are the ones who understand that foods can be a vehicle for disease, and we refuse to tolerate a manufacturer's ignorance. Working through our representatives in government agencies, we exact heavy penalties from companies whose products are tainted. Witness the 25 million pounds of hamburger meat recalled in 1988 (Chapter 8) and the 36,000 pounds of ham recalled in 1983 (this chapter). Both incidents were due to the possibility of microbial contamination.

The next time you shop at the supermarket, stop and take note of the broad variety of foods we consume, and consider that we buy and eat these foods with full confidence that none will make us ill. It is a confidence that is not shared by peoples in other parts of the world.

Summary

The microbiology of foods is concerned with the spoilage that occurs in foods, with methods for preserving foods, and with the activities of microorganisms in the formation of certain foods.

Food spoilage has been a continuing problem since ancient times. Certain conditions, such as water content, pH, physical structure, and chemical composition, determine the extent of food spoilage because they influence the growth of microorganisms. In meats and fish, spoilage organisms enter during processing; in fish, water is often the source. In poultry, the spoilage may reflect human contamination, but often it is due to members of the genus *Salmonella* that infect the bird. Bakery ingredients generally bring contaminants to bread, and grains may be spoiled by toxin-producing fungi. Dairy products are spoiled by microorganisms surviving pasteurization such as curd, capsule, and pigment producers.

To preserve food from spoilage, a number of methods are used including heat, low temperatures, drying, chemical preservatives, and radiation. The most useful application of heat is in the process of canning, while low temperatures are achieved in the refrigerator and freezer. Pasteurization is used for milk and dairy products. Drying is useful because water is an absolute necessity for life, and dried foods are therefore unable to support microbial life. Various chemicals, such as propionic, sorbic, and benzoic acids, are used to preserve foods, and ultraviolet light and gamma rays typify the radiations used in processing certain foods.

Certain foods "spoiled" by microorganisms have come to be accepted as the norm. Among these microbial products are sauerkraut, vinegar, and fermented sausages. The spoilage in these foods causes no harm to consumers, and the foods reflect the helpful activities that microorganisms perform to add to the quality of our lives. Numerous dairy products, such as cheeses, are also products of microorganisms.

Questions for Thought and Discussion

1. A writer in a food technology magazine once suggested that refrigerators be fitted with ultraviolet lights to reduce the level of microbial contamination in foods. Would you support this idea?

2. In 1997, the USDA approved the spraying of steam followed by vacuuming for the removal of microorganisms from the surface of meats. What are the advantages of this method over the previously used hand trimming? Can you think of any other useful methods for decontaminating meats?

3. Chicken and salad are two items on the dinner menu at home, and you are put in charge of preparing both. You have a cutting board and knife for slicing up the salad items and cutting the chicken into pieces. Which task should you perform first? Why? What other precautions might you take to ensure that the meal is not remembered for the wrong reason?

4. Tradition has it that Peruvian Incas of the Andes Mountains preserved their potatoes and other foodstuffs by placing them for several weeks on high mountain sides exposed to the air. Which method of food preservation were they practicing?

5. On January 12, 1996, the author opened a container of sour cream that had become lost in the back of the refrigerator some 9 months before (the expiration date listed on the bottom was April 27, 1995). The sour cream appeared satisfactory, and there was no unusual smell. The author proceeded to spoon it onto a baked potato and dig in. What factors might have contributed to the sour cream's preservation so long after the expiration date?

6. It is a hot Saturday morning in July. You get into your car at 9:00 A.M. with the following list of chores: Pick up the custard eclairs for tonight's dinner party, drop off clothes at the cleaners, buy the ground beef for tomorrow's barbecue, deliver the kids to the Little League baseball game, pick up a broiler at the poultry farm. Microbiologically speaking, what sequence should you follow?

7. Suppose you had the choice of purchasing "yogurt made with pasteurized milk" or "pasteurized yogurt." Which would you choose? Why? What are the "active cultures" in a cup of yogurt?

8. How would you answer a child who asks, "Who puts the holes in Swiss cheese?" Why might blue (Roquefort) cheese pose a possible threat to someone who has an acute allergy to penicillin?

9. It is 5:30 P.M. and you arrive on campus for your evening college class. You stop off at the cafeteria for a bite to eat. Which foods might you be inclined to avoid purchasing?

10. To avoid *Salmonella* infection when preparing eggs for breakfast, the operative phrase is "scramble or gamble." How many foods can you name that use uncooked or undercooked eggs and that can represent a health hazard?

11. The local fish market occasionally receives an unusually large order of fish, and it offers a special sale to customers. Whole fish are piled high on a bed of ice, and signs are put out advertising a one-time-only reduced price. However, smart consumers know that it might be better to pass up the sale, especially if they cannot pick out the individual fish they want to purchase. Why? If you could not resist the temptation to buy the sale fish, which ones would you purchase?

12. Which principles of preservation ensure that each of the following remains uncontaminated on the pantry shelf: vinegar, olive oil, brown sugar, tea bags, spaghetti, hot cocoa mix, pancake syrup, soy sauce, rice?

13. On Saturday, a man buys a steak and a pound of calves' liver and places them in the refrigerator. On Monday, he must decide which to cook for dinner. Microbiologically, which is the better choice? Why?

14. Certain fruits, such as oranges and cantaloupes, are peeled before they are eaten. For this reason, many people believe it unnecessary to wash them. Why might they be wrong?

15. One day in 1997, the students in a microbiology class presented the instructor with a basket of "microbial cheer" in recognition of his efforts on their behalf. From your knowledge of this and other chapters, can you guess some of the things that the basket contained?

16. Foods from tropical nations such as Mexico tend to be very spicy, with lots of hot peppers, spices, garlic, and lemon juice. By contrast, foods from cooler countries such as Norway and Sweden tend to be much less spicy. Why do you think this pattern has evolved over the ages?

17. You and a friend are going to an orchard to pick apples with the intention of pressing them in your new cider mill. However, you are aware of the recent outbreaks of infection with *E. coli* O157:H7 that were traced to fresh apple cider. What precautions can you take to ensure a "healthy" experience?

18. A standard set of recommendations and regulations exists for individuals who work in restaurants and cook food for customers (i.e., food handlers). However, very few regulations exist for individuals who pick fruits or vegetables in the fields. How many recent incidents can you identify where fresh-picked fruits or vegetables were linked to infectious disease? What regulations would you recommend for such workers?

Review

On completing this chapter on food microbiology, test your knowledge of its contents by using the following syllables to compose the term that answers the clue. Each term is a genus of microorganism important in food microbiology. The number of letters in the genus is indicated by the dashes, and the number of syllables in the genus is shown by the number in parentheses. Each syllable is used only once, and the answers are listed in Appendix D.

A A A AS AS BA BA BAC BAC CE CEPS CHLA CIL CIL CIL CLAV CLO CLO CO COC CUS DI DO EN GIL I I I LA LAC LEU LUS LUS LUS MO MON MY NEL NOS O PER PRO PSEU RA SAL SER STREP STRID STRID TE TER TER TER TI TO TO TO TOC UM UM US

1. Common poultry contaminant (4) ___ ___ ___ ___ ___ ___ ___ ___ ___

2. Discolors meat surface (5) ___ ___ ___ ___ ___ ___ ___ ___ ___ ___ ___ ___

3. Destroyed in canning (4) ___ ___ ___ ___ ___ ___ ___ ___

4. Red pigment in bread (4) ___ ___ ___ ___ ___ ___ ___ ___

5. Causes psittacosis (4) ___ ___ ___ ___ ___ ___ ___

6. Black rot in eggs (3) ___ ___ ___ ___ ___ ___

7. Sours dairy products (4) ___ ___ ___ ___ ___ ___ ___ ___ ___ ___

8. Sporeforming contaminant (3) ___ ___ ___ ___ ___

9. Used to make vinegar (5) ___ ___ ___ ___ ___ ___ ___ ___ ___

10. Sauerkraut producer (4) ___ ___ ___ ___ ___ ___ ___

11. Causes ergot poisoning (3) ___ ___ ___ ___ ___ ___

12. Produces potent exotoxins (4) ___ ___ ___ ___ ___ ___ ___ ___ ___

13. Green rot in foods (4) ___ ___ ___ ___ ___ ___ ___ ___

14. Used to cure cucumbers (5) ___ ___ ___ ___ ___ ___ ___ ___ ___ ___

15. Aflatoxins in grains (4) ___ ___ ___ ___ ___ ___ ___

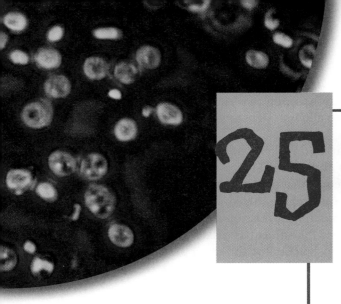

25 Environmental Microbiology

Milwaukee may happen again.

—Microbiologist Rita Colwell describing the urgency to develop safe drinking water standards to avoid repeating the epidemic that struck Milwaukee, Wisconsin, in 1993

I N THE EARLY 1800s, the steam engine and its product, the Industrial Revolution, brought crowds of rural inhabitants to European cities. To accommodate the rising tide, row houses and apartment blocks were hastily erected, and owners of existing houses took in tenants. Not surprisingly, the bills of mortality from typhoid fever, cholera, tuberculosis, dysentery, and other diseases mounted in alarming proportions.

As the death rates rose, a few activists spoke up for reform. Among them was an English lawyer and journalist named **Edwin Chadwick**. Chadwick subscribed to the then novel idea that humans could shape their environment and could eliminate diseases of filth by doing away with filth. In 1842, he published a landmark report indicating that poverty-stricken laborers suffered a far higher incidence of disease than people from middle or upper classes. Chadwick attributed the difference to the abominable living conditions of workers, and he declared that most of their diseases were preventable. His report established the basis for the Great Sanitary Movement, a wave of reform that began in Europe and spread to developed countries.

Chadwick was not a medical man, but his ideas captured the imagination of both scientists and social reformers. He proposed that sewers be constructed using smooth ceramic pipes, and that enough water be flushed through the system to carry waste to some distant depository. In order to work, the system required the installation of new water and sewer pipes, the devel-

787

opment of powerful pumps to bring water into homes, and the elimination of older sewage systems. He foresaw intrusions upon private property to permit water mains and extensive construction to allow straight sewer pipes. The cost would be formidable.

Chadwick's vision eventually came to reality, but it might have taken decades longer without the intervention of **cholera**. In 1849, a cholera epidemic broke out in London and terrified so many people that public opinion began to form in favor of Chadwick's proposal. Another epidemic occurred in 1853, during which John Snow proved that water was involved in transmission of the disease (Chapter 17). In both outbreaks, the disease reached the affluent as well as the poor, and the mortality rate exceeded 50 percent. Construction of the sewer system began shortly thereafter, with John Simon, London's first Medical Officer of Health, in command of the project.

The proverbial "icing on the cake" came in 1892 when a devastating epidemic of cholera erupted in Hamburg, Germany. For the most part, Hamburg drew its water directly from the polluted Elbe River. Adjacent to Hamburg lay Altona, a city where the German government had previously installed a water filtration plant. Altona remained free of cholera. The contrast was further sharpened by a street that divided Hamburg and Altona. On the Hamburg side of the street, multiple cases of cholera broke out; across the street, none occurred. Chadwick and his fellow sanitarians could not have imagined a more clear-cut demonstration of the importance of water purification and sewage treatment.

Dealing with water pollution and treating sewage are but two of the myriad activities that involve microbiology in public health. Concerns about water pollution and sewage treatment are environmental in scope. Other environmental issues involve the place of microbiology in biogeochemical cycles, whose microorganisms are critical to the recycling of nitrogen, sulfur, and carbon. Thus, the focus in environmental microbiology is to study microorganisms as they affect the natural environment.

Cholera:
a bacterial disease of the intestine characterized by unrelenting diarrhea.

25.1

Water Pollution

For purposes of simplification, scientists classify water into two major types: groundwater and surface water. **Groundwater** originates from deep wells and subterranean springs, and, because of the filtering action of soil, deep sand, and rock, it is virtually free of microorganisms. As the water flows up along channels, contaminants may enter it and alter its quality. **Surface water** is found in lakes, streams, and shallow wells. Its microbial population may reflect the air through which rain has passed, the meat-packing plant near which a stream flows, or the sewage-treatment facility located along a riverbank.

Certain terms are significant in water microbiology. For example, water is considered **contaminated** when it contains a chemical or biological poison, or an infectious agent. In water that is **polluted**, the same conditions apply, but the poison or agent is obvious. Polluted water carries an unpleasant taste, smell, or appearance. **Potability**, by contrast, refers to the drinkability of water. Potable water is fit for consumption, while unpotable water is unfit.

Surface water:
rainwater accumulating in lakes, streams, and shallow wells.

po'ta-bl

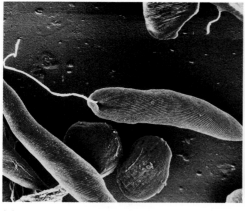
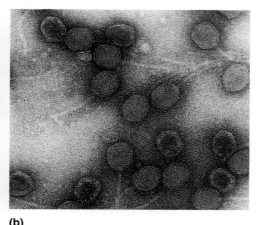

(a)   (b)

FIGURE 25.1

Microorganisms in Water Environments

(a) A scanning electron micrograph of the protozoan *Euglena*, a common inhabitant of unpolluted water. (b) A transmission electron micrograph of bacteriophages that replicate in *Vibrio parahaemolyticus* ($\times$150,000). Bacteriophages like these are commonly found in sewage-contaminated polluted water.

VARIOUS WATER ENVIRONMENTS

A body of **unpolluted** water, such as a mountain lake or stream, is usually low in organic nutrients, and thus, only a limited number of bacteria are present, perhaps a few thousand per milliliter. Most bacteria are soil organisms that have run off into the water during a rainfall. An example are the **actinomycetes**, a group of moldlike bacteria that give a musty odor to soil. Other inhabitants include yeasts, and bacterial and mold spores. **Cellulose digesters** such as members of the genus *Cellulomonas* are also found. These bacteria digest cellulose in plant cell walls. **Autotrophic bacteria** are also common, and free-living protozoa such as *Paramecium, Euglena, Tetrahymena,* and *Amoeba* abound (**FIGURE 25.1a**).

A **polluted** body of water, such as a polluted lake or river, presents a totally different picture (**FIGURE 25.1b**). The water contains large amounts of organic matter from sewage, feces, and industrial sources, and the population of microorganisms is usually **heterotrophic**. A major type of bacteria in polluted water is **coliform bacteria**, a group of Gram-negative nonsporeforming bacilli usually found in the human intestine. Coliform bacteria ferment lactose to acid and gas. Included in this group are *Escherichia coli* and species of *Enterobacter*. Noncoliform bacteria also common in polluted water include *Streptococcus, Proteus,* and *Pseudomonas* species.

In polluted water, microorganisms contribute to a chain of events that drastically alters the ecology of the environment, as **FIGURE 25.2** illustrates. When phosphates accumulate in the water, algae bloom. The algae supply nutrients to microorganisms, which multiply rapidly and use up the available oxygen. Soon, other protozoa, small fish, crustaceans, and plants die and accumulate on the bottom. Anaerobic species of

ak′tĭ-no-mi-se′tēz

Autotrophic:
able to synthesize its own food from simple inorganic compounds.

Heterotrophic:
obtains its food from preformed organic compounds.
Coliform bacteria:
Gram-negative intestinal rods that ferment lactose to acid and gas.

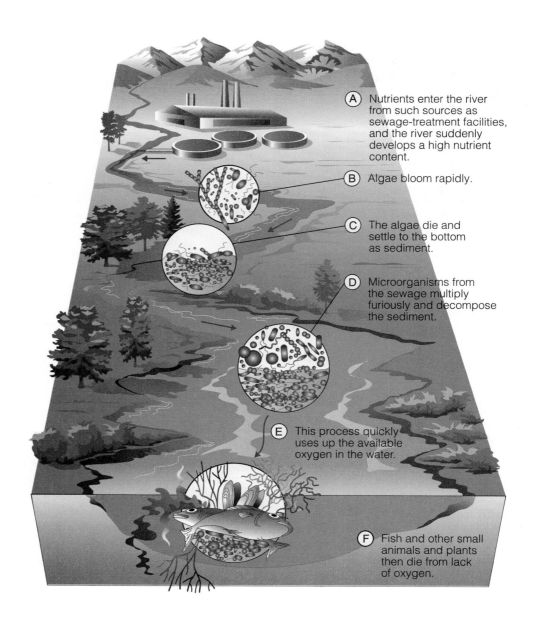

Ⓐ Nutrients enter the river from such sources as sewage-treatment facilities, and the river suddenly develops a high nutrient content.

Ⓑ Algae bloom rapidly.

Ⓒ The algae die and settle to the bottom as sediment.

Ⓓ Microorganisms from the sewage multiply furiously and decompose the sediment.

Ⓔ This process quickly uses up the available oxygen in the water.

Ⓕ Fish and other small animals and plants then die from lack of oxygen.

FIGURE 25.2

The Death of a River

de-sul'fo-vib're-o

bacteria such as *Desulfovibrio* and *Clostridium* then thrive in the mud and produce gases that give the water a stench reminiscent of rotten eggs. The organisms in mud may also pose a hazard to health, as MicroFocus 25.1 points out.

The **marine environment** of the oceans illustrates another view of microbial populations in water. In the high salt concentration of ocean water, **halophilic**, or salt-loving, microorganisms survive. In addition, the organisms must be **psychrophilic** since it is very cold below the surface. Those at the bottom must also withstand

Halophilic:
salt-loving.

MicroFocus 25.1

JELLO PREFERRED

Jello-wrestling may not be quite as chic as mud-wrestling, but it is presumably safer. At least, that is the opinion of physicians confronted with students suffering from skin rashes after a mud-wrestling contest.

The "contest" occurred in the spring of 1992 on Seattle's University of Washington campus. Within hours of participating, seven students experienced tiny red and pus-filled bumps on their skin.

The rash was heaviest on their arms and legs. Cultures of pus yielded species of *Enterobacter*, a common soil bacterium associated with fecal matter and manure. Other intestinal bacteria were also found. One student was treated with antibiotics, and no serious after-effects accompanied any of the cases.

For the record, microbiologists gave the new disease a name—*dermatitis* (skin inflammation) *palaestrae* (the

Greek arena for wrestling events) *limosae* ("pertaining to mud"). Translated literally, the name means "dermatitis-of-mud-wrestling." Doctors also recommended that if Jello were not available for future "events," the students might consider investing in sterilized potting soil.

great pressure and are therefore **barophilic**, or pressure-loving. The organisms in these environments pose no threat to humans because they cannot grow in the body tissues.

Marine microorganisms are vital to ecological cycles because they form the foundations of many food chains. For example, marine algae such as **diatoms** (**FIGURE 25.3**) and organisms such as the **dinoflagellates** capture the sun's energy and, using carbon dioxide, convert the energy to chemical energy in carbohydrates. The microorganisms are then consumed by other animals in the food chain. Dinoflagellates have made the news in recent years because certain species of *Gonyaulax* and *Gymnodinitum* are responsible for the red tide.

di'ah-tomz

gon'e-aw'laks
jim'no-din'e-um

Most marine microorganisms are found along the shoreline, or **littoral zone**, because this is where nutrients are plentiful. Certain unusual types of microorganisms have also been found on the ocean floor in the **benthic zone** and even at the bottom of 6-mile-deep trenches, the **abyssal zone**. Two types of protozoa, the foraminiferans and radiolarians, are of special interest to oil companies because these protozoa were dominant species during formation of the oil fields, and their fossils serve as markers for oil-bearing layers of rock.

a-bis'al

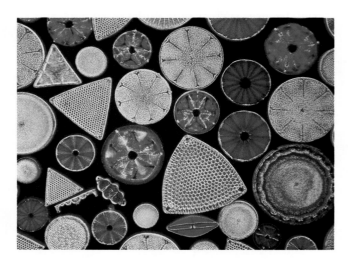

FIGURE 25.3

Marine Microorganisms

A scanning electron micrograph of a collection of diatoms. Note the broad variety of shapes and sizes of microorganisms in this group. Diatoms trap the sun's energy in photosynthesis and use it to form carbohydrates that are passed on to other marine organisms as food.

TYPES OF WATER POLLUTION

Water is vital to such industries as food processing, meat packing, and paper manufacturing. It is also used extensively in pharmaceutical plants and mines, and for cooling purposes in power-generating units. It irrigates agricultural lands and provides the focus for many recreational facilities. Uses such as these, however, commonly add to contamination and pollution of water.

Physical pollution of water occurs when particulate matter such as sand or soil makes the water cloudy, or when cyanobacteria bloom during midsummer and their remains give water the consistency of pea soup. **Chemical pollution** results from the introduction of inorganic and organic waste to the water. For example, water passing out of a mine contains large amounts of copper or iron. Other chemical pollutants in water include phosphates and nitrates from laundry detergents, as well as acids such as sulfuric acid.

The third type of pollution, **biological pollution**, is the main concern of our discussion. This type of pollution develops from microorganisms that enter water from human waste, food-processing and meat-packing plants, medical facilities, and similar sources (**FIGURE 25.4** shows a common pollutant). Normally, water can handle biological material because heterotrophic microorganisms digest organic matter to carbon dioxide, water, and useful ions (phosphates, nitrates, and sulfates). With the rapid movement of the water, aeration is constant, and waste is soon diluted and eliminated. However, when water stagnates or is overloaded with waste, it cannot deal with biological material and becomes polluted.

A critical measurement in polluted water is the **biochemical oxygen demand**, or **BOD**. This refers to the amount of oxygen that microorganisms require to decompose the organic matter in water. As the number of microorganisms increases, the demand for oxygen increases proportionally. In the laboratory, the BOD is determined by measuring the dissolved oxygen content of water immediately after collection and then after incubation at 20°C for 5 days. The difference in oxygen content represents the amount used up by microorganisms in the water sample. Results are generally expressed as parts per million (ppm), with a BOD of several hundred ppm usually considered high.

DISEASES TRANSMITTED BY WATER

Water consumption may be the vehicle for transfer of a broad variety of intestinal diseases, including **bacterial diseases** such as typhoid fever, cholera, shigel-

Cyanobacteria:
prokaryotes with photosynthetic capabilities.

BOD:
the amount of oxygen required by metabolizing microorganisms during a 5-day period of incubation.

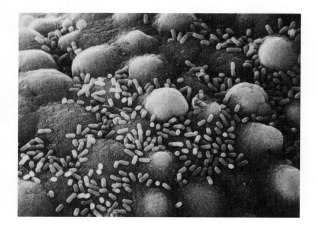

FIGURE 25.4

A Coliform Bacterium

A scanning electron micrograph of *E. coli* on the microvilli of an animal's small intestine (×3900). *E. coli* is commonly found in water that is biologically polluted. The bacillus represents the coliform group of bacteria and is often used as an indicator of bacterial pollution of water.

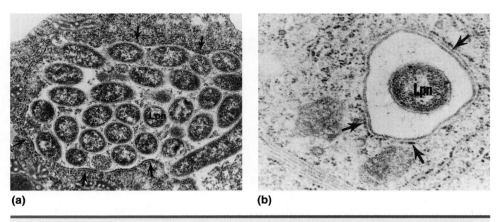

(a) **(b)**

FIGURE 25.5

Legionella in the Environment

Legionella pneumophila is the Gram-negative rod responsible for Legionnaires' disease. It infects the respiratory passages when it is inhaled in airborne droplets of water. In nature, the bacterium lives within the cytoplasm of the waterborne protozoan *Hartmanella*. (a) Numerous bacterial rods (labeled Lpn) are seen in a transmission electron micrograph of the cytoplasm of a *Hartmanella* cell (×15,000). (b) A closeup of a cross section of the bacterium (Lpn) is seen in the cytoplasm. The bacterium exists within a clear body known as a vacuole. The arrows point out the multilayered bordering membranes of the vacuole (×50,000).

losis, and others described in Chapter 8. Waterborne epidemics of these diseases, however, are rare because of continual surveillance. Many illnesses transmitted by drinking water are due to less familiar bacteria such as species of *Legionella* (**FIGURE 25.5**), *Yersinia*, and *Campylobacter*, and toxin-producing strains of *Escherichia coli*. Septicemia, necrotizing fasciitis, and gangrene may develop from the initial infection. An emerging pathogen associated with contaminated water is *Vibrio vulnificus*, a Gram-negative bacterium that can cause serious intestinal illness and septicemia in individuals with preexisting liver disease or compromised immune systems. In the 10-year period preceding 1993, 125 persons became infected with *V. vulnificus* and 44 died. Raw oyster consumption was implicated in the majority of deaths.

kam′pĭ-lo-bak′ter

vul-nif′i-cus

Several species of marine bacteria also contribute to **wound infections** when contaminated seawater has contacted the exposed tissue. Among the marine pathogens is *Erysipelothrix rhusiopathiae*, a Gram-negative pleomorphic rod that causes erysipeloid. Infections usually occur on the hands or feet and are accompanied by a bright red, well-demarcated lesion that burns or itches. Another pathogen is *Mycobacterium marinum*, an acid-fast rod that causes a small papular lesion at the wound site, particularly near the knuckles of the hand. The lesion often progresses to a nodule, and infection may spread via the lymphatic system. Fish handlers, seafood workers, and aquatic sports enthusiasts may suffer infection from these organisms, and antibiotics are used to limit the growth of both. The marine bacterium, *Vibrio vulnificus* (mentioned above) can cause wound infections with gangrene and necrotizing fasciitis; a fourth bacterium, *Aeromonas hydrophila*, is discussed in Chapter 8.

Viral diseases transmitted by water include hepatitis A, rotavirus disease, gastroenteritis due to Coxsackie or Norwalk virus, and in rare instances, polio. These diseases are generally related to fecal contamination of water. Many **protozoa** form cysts that survive for long periods in water. For this reason, water may be a vehicle

cook-sak′e

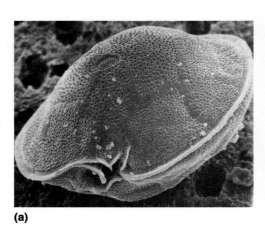 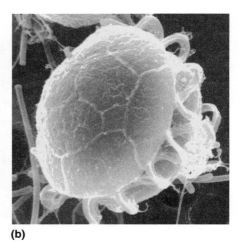

(a)   **(b)**

FIGURE 25.6

The Dinoflagellates of Human Poisonings

(a) *Gambierdiscus toxicus*, a cause of ciguatera fish poisoning. (b) *Pfiesteria shumwayae*, a species related to the *Pfiesteria* linked to human illness in 1997.

je-ar'de-ah

gon'e-aw'laks

gam'be-er-dis'cus

se'gwah-ta'rah

for the transfer of *Entamoeba histolytica* and *Giardia lamblia*. A notable outbreak of *Cryptosporidium* infection occurred in 1993 when the municipal water supply of Milwaukee, Wisconsin, became contaminated (Chapter 15).

Three **dinoflagellates** bear mention because of their involvement in human poisonings. The first, *Gonyaulax catanella*, produces a toxin that may cause muscular paralysis and death from asphyxiation. The toxin is ingested from shellfish that feed on the dinoflagellate. The second dinoflagellate is *Gambierdiscus toxicus* (**FIGURE 25.6**). This marine microorganism is consumed by small fish that concentrate the toxin and pass it to larger fish, such as sea bass and red snapper. Human consumption of the fish leads to neurological and muscular intoxication and a condition called **ciguatera fish poisoning** (from *cigua* for "poisonous snail," originally thought to be the cause).

The third dinoflagellate is *Pfiesteria piscicida*. This organism was observed in heavy concentrations in 1997 in waters near Maryland's Chesapeake Bay. It was linked to massive fish kills and human illnesses characterized by skin rash, memory loss, and difficult breathing. Researchers believe that agricultural runoff was the source of the extremely complex dinoflagellate (over 20 stages in its life cycle have been observed, including amoeboid and flagellated forms). Eutrophication in the waters may have encouraged the protozoal bloom. At least two *Pfiesteria* toxins are being studied, and the role of a secondary fungus invader is also being investigated, as MicroFocus 15.1 explains. The dinoflagellate was named for Lois Pfiester, a University of Oklahoma marine microbiologist.

To this point . . .

We have explored the microbial floras of various water environments to illustrate the differences that exist among them. In unpolluted and polluted waters, the amount and type of nutrients are important determining factors in the microbial population, while in marine environments, the salt, temperature, and pressure conditions regulate the population.

The focus was then on water pollution. We compared the physical, chemical, and biological sources of pollution, and we discussed the biochemical oxygen demand (BOD) as a way of determining the extent of biological pollution. We also outlined the types of diseases that could be transmitted by water, and referred to bacterial, viral, and protozoal diseases. Three dinoflagellates were noted because their poisons can cause human illness.

In the next section, we shall examine methods used for water purification and sewage treatment where the chain of transmission of waterborne diseases can be broken. We shall see how water is prepared for drinking purposes and how microorganisms can be used effectively to digest organic matter in sewage. The discussion will then pass to the laboratory, where the water-quality bacteriologist seeks to detect water pollution by a series of laboratory tests. The monitoring of water supplies by bacteriologists is an essential feature of environmental health for all of us.

25.2

The Treatment of Water and Sewage

Some years ago, health-care workers in Africa asked villagers to name their single greatest need. The answer was almost unanimous: "Water." A startling survey by the World Health Organization indicates that three of every four humans alive today do not have enough water to drink, or, if water is available, the supplies are contaminated.

Water is unfit to drink when it contains human sewage, animal waste, or other pollutants (FIGURE 25.7). However, the situation can be reversed through the proper management of water resources. Water-purification procedures prevent pathogenic microorganisms from reaching the body, while sewage-treatment processes remove pathogens from body waste products. In this section, we shall examine how these are accomplished.

WATER PURIFICATION

Three basic steps are included in the preparation of water for drinking: sedimentation, filtration, and chlorination. In the **sedimentation** step, leaves, particles of sand

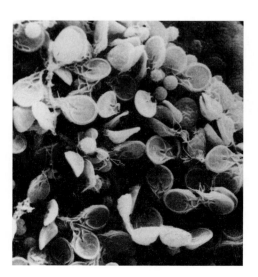

FIGURE 25.7

From Water to the Intestine

A mass of waterborne *Giardia lamblia* along the intestinal walls of an infected animal (×1958). This protozoan has a flat shape, with numerous flagella. A disklike sucker apparatus is seen on the ventral surface of several organisms. Since the 1970s, *Giardia lamblia* has been recognized as the most widespread protozoal cause of human intestinal disease in the United States. Most cases are related to consumption of contaminated water.

Flocs:
jellylike masses of coagulated material.
Flocculation:
the formation of jellylike masses of coagulated material.

shmoots'dek-ě
Schmutzdecke:
a layer of microorganisms that forms in a slow sand filter.

and gravel, and other materials from the soil are removed in large reservoirs or settling tanks. Chemicals such as aluminum sulfate (alum) or iron sulfate are dropped as a powder onto water and they form jellylike masses of coagulated material called **flocs**. The flocs fall through the water and cling to organic particles and microorganisms, dragging a major portion to the bottom sediment in the process of **flocculation**.

The **filtration** step is next. Although different types of filtering material are available, most filters utilize a layer of sand and gravel to trap microorganisms. A **slow sand filter**, containing fine particles of sand several feet deep, is efficient for smaller scale operations. Within the sand, a layer of microorganisms acts as a supplementary filter. This layer is called a **schmutzdecke**, or dirty layer. A slow sand filter may purify over 3 million gallons of water per acre per day. To clean the filter, the top layer is removed and replaced with fresh sand.

A **rapid sand filter** contains coarser particles of gravel. A schmutzdecke does not develop in this filter, but the rate of filtration is much higher, with over 200 million gallons purified per acre per day. This type of filter is commonly used in municipal water systems. It must be cleaned more often than the slow sand filter, a process accomplished by forcing water back through the filter by mechanical pressure. Both slow and rapid sand filters remove approximately 99 percent of the microorganisms from water.

The final step is **chlorination**, in which chlorine gas is added to the water. Chlorine is an active oxidizing agent that reacts with any organic matter in water. It is important, therefore, to continue adding chlorine until a residue is present. A residue of 0.2 to 1.0 parts of chlorine per million (ppm) of water is often the standard used. Under these conditions, most remaining microorganisms die within 30 minutes. FIGURE 25.8 illustrates the steps in the water-purification process.

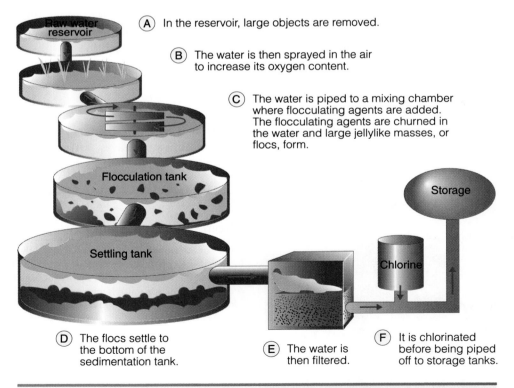

(A) In the reservoir, large objects are removed.

(B) The water is then sprayed in the air to increase its oxygen content.

(C) The water is piped to a mixing chamber where flocculating agents are added. The flocculating agents are churned in the water and large jellylike masses, or flocs, form.

Raw water reservoir

Flocculation tank

Settling tank

Storage

Chlorine

(D) The flocs settle to the bottom of the sedimentation tank.

(E) The water is then filtered.

(F) It is chlorinated before being piped off to storage tanks.

FIGURE 25.8

Steps in the Purification of Municipal Water Supplies

At this point, some communities **soften** water by removing magnesium, calcium, and other salts. Softened water mixes more easily with soap, and soap curds do not form. Water may also be fluoridated to help prevent tooth decay. Scientists believe that fluoride strengthens tooth enamel and makes it more resistant to the acid produced by anaerobic bacteria in the mouth.

SEWAGE TREATMENT

Systems for the treatment of human waste range from the primitive outhouse, which is nothing more than a hole in the ground, to the sophisticated sewage-treatment facilities used by many large cities. All operate under the same basic principle: Water is separated from the waste, and the solid matter is broken down by microorganisms to simple compounds for return to the soil and water.

In many homes, human waste is emptied into underground **cesspools**. These are concrete cylindrical rings with pores in the wall. Water passes into the soil through the bottom and pores of the cesspool, while solid waste accumulates on the bottom. Microorganisms, especially anaerobic bacteria, digest the solid matter into soluble products that enter the soil and enrich it. Some hardware stores sell enzymes and dried bacteria, usually *Bacillus subtilis* spores, to accelerate sludge digestion.

Cesspool:
a concrete cylindrical ring with pores, used for waste disposal.

Certain homes use a **septic tank**, an enclosed concrete box that collects waste from the house. Organic matter accumulates on the bottom of the tank, while water rises to the outlet pipe and flows to a distribution box. The water is then separated into pipes that empty into the surrounding soil. Since digested organic matter is not absorbed into the ground, the septic tank must be pumped out regularly.

Septic tank:
an enclosed concrete box with fluid outlet pipes, used for waste disposal.

Sewers are at least as old as the Cloaca Maxima of Roman times. Until the mid-1800s, however, sewers were simply elongated cesspools with overflow pipes at one end. They collected filth and had to be pumped out regularly. Finally, in 1842, Edwin Chadwick's report raised the possibility that sewage spreads disease, and soon thereafter a movement (fueled by a cholera outbreak) sprang up to sanitize European cities.

Small towns collect sewage into large ponds called **oxidation lagoons**. Here, the sewage is left undisturbed for up to 3 months. During that time, aerobic bacteria digest organic matter in the water, while anaerobic organisms break down sedimented material. Under controlled conditions, the waste may be totally converted to simple salts such as carbonates, nitrates, phosphates, and sulfates. At the cycle's conclusion, the bacteria die naturally, the water clarifies, and the pond may be emptied into a nearby river or stream.

Oxidation lagoon:
a large pond into which sewage is piped for natural digestion of organic matter.

Large municipalities rely on a mechanized sewage-treatment facility to handle the massive amounts of waste and garbage generated daily (FIGURE 25.9). The first step in the process, **pretreatment**, involves grit and insoluble waste removal. Next comes **primary treatment**, in which raw sewage is piped into huge open tanks for organic waste removal. This waste, called **sludge**, is passed into sludge tanks for further treatment. Flocculating materials, such as aluminum and iron sulfate, are then added to the raw sewage to drag microorganisms and debris to the bottom.

The **secondary treatment** of sewage has two phases, a liquid phase and a solid phase. The **liquid phase** involves aeration of the water portion to encourage aerobic growth of microorganisms. As they grow, microorganisms digest proteins into simple amino acids, carbohydrates into simple sugars, and fats into fatty acids and glycerol. Acids and alcohols are also produced, and carbon dioxide evolves. The water then is passed through a clarifier and filter to remove the microorganisms and remaining organic matter, after which it flows into a stream or river.

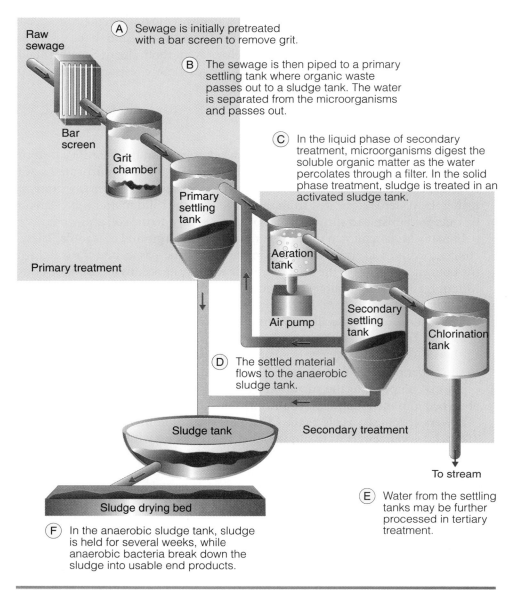

A Sewage is initially pretreated with a bar screen to remove grit.

B The sewage is then piped to a primary settling tank where organic waste passes out to a sludge tank. The water is separated from the microorganisms and passes out.

C In the liquid phase of secondary treatment, microorganisms digest the soluble organic matter as the water percolates through a filter. In the solid phase treatment, sludge is treated in an activated sludge tank.

D The settled material flows to the anaerobic sludge tank.

E Water from the settling tanks may be further processed in tertiary treatment.

F In the anaerobic sludge tank, sludge is held for several weeks, while anaerobic bacteria break down the sludge into usable end products.

Raw sewage

Bar screen

Grit chamber

Primary settling tank

Primary treatment

Aeration tank

Air pump

Secondary settling tank

Chlorination tank

Secondary treatment

To stream

Sludge tank

Sludge drying bed

FIGURE 25.9

A Sewage-Treatment Facility

Sludge tank:
a tank in which bacteria digest sedimented organic matter from primary sewage treatment.

zo'o-gle'ah ra-me'jer-ah

The **solid phase** of secondary treatment is carried on in a **sludge tank**. Within the tank, microbial growth is encouraged by either an aerobic or an anaerobic process. In the aerobic process, compressed air is forced into the sludge, and the suspended particles form tiny gelatinous masses swarming with microorganisms, which thrive on the organic matter. *Zoogloea ramigera*, a Gram-negative rod, produces the slime to which other microorganisms attach and congregate. The **activated sludge**, as it is termed, gathers to itself much of the microorganisms, organic material, color, and smell of the sewage. The activated sludge is drawn off and dried.

In the anaerobic method of sludge digestion, sewage is held in the tank for up to 30 days while the sludge ferments. Gases such as methane, carbon dioxide, and nitrogen are derived from this process. The methane may be captured and used to run the machinery of the sewage facility. Other gases, such as ammonia and hydrogen sulfide, are of value to chemical industries. The digested sludge, together with the dried activated sludge, may be used as agricultural fertilizer since it contains many valuable salts, or the sludge may be carted to landfill sites or offshore dumping grounds.

The separation of solid sludge leaves a certain amount of water that may be further processed in **tertiary treatment** by purifying the water. Sedimentation is followed by filtration and chlorination, after which the water is placed back into circulation and made available to consumers. In many municipalities, it is also important to remove salts such as phosphates from the water because they may spark blooms of algae.

Tertiary treatment: purification of the water remaining after the sludge has been removed.

Agricultural waste poses still another problem for sanitary microbiologists. Most animal waste is currently handled through systems in which manure is piped into clay-lined oxidation lagoons and allowed to remain while bacteria decompose the waste. The accumulation of ammonia nitrogen from urine is a problem, however, as is the buildup of phosphorus in the soil. Moreover, the stench tends to be overpowering, except during the late summer when photosynthetic bacteria thrive and turn the water a deep purple. Microbiologists have isolated a species of *Rhodobacter* from the purple water, and they have shown that the bacteria can break down many odoriferous (odor-causing) compounds, including volatile fatty acids and phenols. In the future, seeding such bacteria in the lagoons may help increase their efficiency and minimize their noxious odors.

BIOFILMS

For decades, microbiologists have focused on free-floating bacteria growing in laboratory cultures. In recent years, however, they have come to realize the importance of bacteria living in biofilms. A **biofilm** is an immobilized population of bacteria (or other microorganisms) caught in a sticky web of tangled polysaccharide fibers adhering to a surface. Biofilms develop on virtually all surfaces in contact with a watery environment (an example is depicted in FIGURE 25.10). Examples of such environments are the surfaces of catheter tubes, teeth, aquatic plants or animals, the urinary tract, water pipes, and stones. Contact with a fluid environment ensures a plentiful supply of nutrients, and as the bacteria grow, they secrete the polysaccharides characteristic of the slimy layer.

Bacteria behave much differently in a biofilm than in a culture tube. Within their microcosm, for example, aerobic bacteria coexist with anaerobic bacteria as they share passageways and interact metabolically. In this state, they form communities that store nutrients, benefit from each other's metabolic by-products, and resist predators such as protozoa and bacteriophages. By contrast, planktonic bacteria living as individuals do not enjoy these benefits and tend to be of smaller size, with a lower metabolic rate of respiration. Thus, the members of a biofilm often are morphologically and physiologically distinct from their free-floating neighbors.

And they apparently communicate. Researchers have studied *Pseudomonas aeruginosa* in their mushroomlike biofilms and noted that at least two extracellular signals exist: one for cell-to-cell communication and one for cell-density determination. The latter signal governs the pattern of the so-called quorum sensing discussed in a MicroFocus box in Chapter 4.

Biofilms carry both positive and negative connotations. Among the benefits of biofilms are their uses in **bioremediation**, where

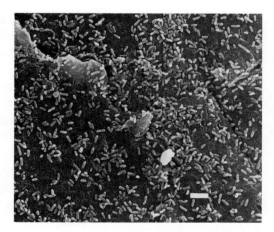

FIGURE 25.10

Biofilm Contamination

A scanning electron micrograph of a biofilm of *Pseudomonas aeruginosa* adhering to material used in urinary catheters in hospital settings. Experiments indicated that large numbers of these cells remained alive after exposure to high concentrations of tobramycin, an antibiotic to which the bacillus is normally susceptible. (Bar = 5 μm.)

biofilm populations are used to degrade toxic wastes and other synthetic products of industry. They are also employed in the **oil industry** to fill empty spaces after oil has been pumped out. And in natural settings, they degrade organic compounds, thus retarding pollutant buildup.

On the negative side, concern continues to mount about the tendency of biofilms to form on contact lens surfaces and cause eye infections. Moreover, biofilms form on catheters and medical implements (e.g., artificial hearts), and biofilms are important considerations in the development of dental caries and urinary tract infections (both Chapter 10). The concern is particularly acute because the bacteria in biofilms resist phagocytosis by white blood cells, display enhanced resistance to antibiotics, and withstand the destructive action of disinfectants and antiseptics.

In the industrial setting, biofilms pose problems when their sulfate-reducing members anaerobically convert sulfur compounds to hydrogen sulfide. The latter corrodes water pipes, especially those that carry seawater (where sulfate abounds). When they contaminate computer chips, biofilms act as conductors and thereby interfere with electronic signals. Indeed, one researcher has called biofilms the "venereal disease of industry." Some scientists estimate that in nature, 99 percent of all microbial activities occur in biofilms.

THE BACTERIOLOGICAL ANALYSIS OF WATER

Many methods are available for detecting the bacterial contamination of water, and various ones are selected according to the resources of the testing laboratory. Since it is impossible to test for all pathogenic microorganisms, water-quality bacteriologists have adopted the practice of testing for certain indicator bacteria normally found in the human intestinal tract. If these bacteria are present, fecal contamination has probably taken place.

Among the most frequently used indicator organisms are the coliform bacteria. **Coliform bacteria** are normally found in the intestinal tracts of humans and many warm-blooded animals. They are able to survive for extensive periods of time in the environment, and they are relatively easy to cultivate in the laboratory. *Escherichia coli* is the most important indicator organism within the group.

The **membrane filter technique** is a popular laboratory test in water microbiology because it is straightforward and can be used in the field. A technician holds a specially designed collecting bottle against the current and takes a 100-ml sample (FIGURE 25.11). The water is then passed through a membrane filter, and the filter pad is transferred to a plate of bacteriological medium, as outlined in Chapter 21. Bacteria trapped in the filter will form colonies, and by counting the colonies, the technician may determine the original number of bacteria in the sample.

Another method for testing water is the **standard plate count (SPC) technique**. Samples of water are diluted in sterile buffer solution, and carefully measured amounts are pipetted into Petri dishes. Agar medium is added, and the plates are set aside at incubation temperatures. A count of the colonies multiplied by the reciprocal of the dilution (the dilution factor) yields the total number of bacteria per ml of the original sample.

A third test is a statistical evaluation called the **most probable number (MPN) test**. In this procedure, a technician inoculates water in 10-ml, 1-ml, and 0.1-ml amounts into lactose broth tubes. The tubes are incubated and coliform organisms are identified by their production of gas from lactose. Referring to an MPN table, a statistical

Standard plate count:
a technique for determining the total number of bacteria per ml of fluid.

MPN test:
a statistical evaluation of the number of coliform bacteria in a water sample.

range of the number of coliform bacteria is determined by observing how many broth tubes showed gas.

DNA-based analysis can also be used to conduct water-quality tests based on the detection of indicator bacteria such as *Escherichia coli*. With DNA technology, a sample of water is filtered, and the bacteria trapped on the filter are broken open to release their DNA for amplification by the polymerase chain reaction (Chapter 19). Analysis for *E. coli* genes is then performed using **DNA probes** (Chapter 19). Not only does the process save time, it is extremely sensitive; for instance, a single *E. coli* cell can be detected in a 100-ml sample of water. Moreover, the pathogens transmitted by water (rather than the indicator organism) can be detected by DNA analysis. The identification of *Salmonella, Shigella*, and *Vibrio* species will become more feasible in the future as probe analyses become more widely accepted. The same principles hold for identifying viruses and virtually all other microorganisms.

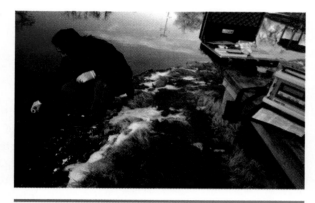

FIGURE 25.11

Collection of Water for Analysis

Ensuring the safety of potable waters is one of the high priorities of public health officials. The use of DNA probes and amplification methods represents a revolutionary and exciting era in water-quality testing. Where the previous procedures required many days of waiting, the DNA-based procedures often are complete within a few short hours. Quickly determining whether a health risk exists allows the introduction of health measures when they can benefit the most people.

To this point . . .

We have given close scrutiny to water pollution and the methods used in water purification and sewage treatment. We noted the three basic steps in the preparation of water for drinking: sedimentation, to remove bulky objects; filtration, to eliminate the vast majority of microorganisms; and chlorination, to destroy the last remnants of microbial life. We also saw how sewage treatment may involve something as simple as the outhouse, cesspool, or septic tank, or a highly sophisticated operation such as is used in metropolitan centers. Primary treatment involves screening the sewage, while secondary treatment is more concerned with the microbial decomposition of organic waste. Sludge tanks are used in the secondary treatment. Tertiary treatment is also practiced in some communities.

We then surveyed some of the tests used by bacteriologists to determine the fitness of water for consumption. We emphasized coliform bacteria as indicators of water pollution. The membrane filter technique, standard plate count, and most probable number procedure were outlined to illustrate the range of available tests. We also explored the DNA-based analyses that will become more commonplace in the future.

In the next section of this chapter, we shall shift gears and examine the important positions occupied by microorganisms in the cycles of elements. We shall use three examples—the carbon, sulfur, and nitrogen cycles—to show how microorganisms contribute to the quality of life. Working in their countless numbers in the environment, microorganisms effect a series of chemical changes fundamental to all life processes on Earth.

The Cycles of Elements in the Environment

The thought of microorganisms usually conjures a negative reaction because of their disease implication, and the contents of this chapter have undoubtedly supported that notion. It would be unwise, however, to neglect the positive role of microorganisms in the environment, because it is a substantial one. We have alluded to their role in the decay of organic matter, and we shall expand the idea by briefly examining the place of microorganisms in three vital cycles of nature: the carbon, sulfur, and nitrogen cycles. Indeed, the number of microorganisms in the environment is almost beyond belief. In 1998, microbiologists at the University of Georgia took a census of the various environments (i.e., ocean, air, soil, subsurface, and within other living things), and they calculated the number of microorganisms inhabiting the Earth to be an astounding 5 million trillion trillion, or enough to cover the top 3 feet of France!

THE CARBON CYCLE

Planet Earth is composed of numerous elements, among which is a defined amount of **carbon** that must constantly be recycled to allow the formation of organic compounds, of which all living things are made. **Photosynthetic organisms** take carbon in the form of carbon dioxide and convert it into carbohydrates using the sun's energy and chlorophyll pigments. The vast jungles of the world, the grassy plains of the temperate zones, and the plants of the oceans show the results of this process. Photosynthetic organisms, in turn, are consumed by grazing animals, fish, and humans, who use some of the carbohydrates for energy and convert the remainder to cell parts. To be sure, some carbon dioxide is released back to the atmosphere in respiration, but a major portion of the carbon is returned to the ground when the animal or plant dies (FIGURE 25.12).

It is here that the microorganisms exert their influence, for they are the **primary decomposers** of dead organic matter. Working in their countless billions in the water and soil, bacteria, fungi, and other microorganisms consume the organic substances and release carbon dioxide for reuse by the plants. This activity results from the concerted action of a huge variety of microorganisms, each with its own nutritional pattern of protein, carbohydrate, or lipid digestion (FIGURE 25.13). Without microorganisms, the Earth would be a veritable garbage dump of animal waste, dead plants, and organic debris accumulating in implausible amounts.

Microorganisms accomplish a similar goal in compost, where they decompose manure and other natural materials and convert them to compost for crop fertilization. Although both conventional and **organic agriculture** use manure as part of regular farm soil fertilization programs, only certified organic farmers are required to have a plan detailing the methods for building soil fertility using raw or aged manure. Furthermore, certified organic farmers are prohibited from using raw manure for at least 60 days prior to harvesting crops for human consumption.

But there is more. Microorganisms also break down the carbon-based chemicals produced by **industrial processes**, including herbicides, pesticides, and plastics. In addition, they produce methane, or natural gas, from organic matter and are

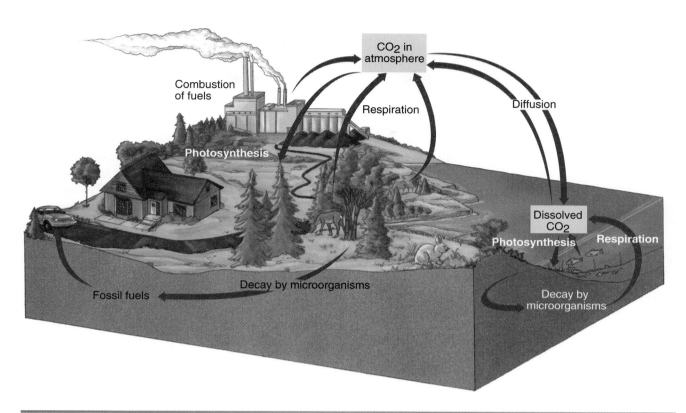

FIGURE 25.12

A Simplified Carbon Cycle

Photosynthesis represents the major method for incorporating carbon dioxide to organic matter, and respiration accounts for its return to the atmosphere. Microorganisms are crucial to all decay in soil and ocean sediments.

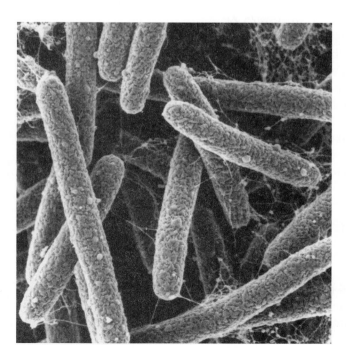

FIGURE 25.13

A Soil Bacterium

A scanning electron micrograph of the soil bacterium *Myxococcus xanthus*. This bacterium belongs to a group that displays gliding motility, complex social interactions, and under certain circumstances, a resistant spore called the myxospore. In this view, the fibrils connecting the cells at the surface can be seen.

probably responsible for the conversion of plants to petroleum and coal deep within the recesses of the Earth. Moreover, many microorganisms trap CO_2 from the atmosphere and form carbohydrates to supplement the results of photosynthesis. In these activities, the microorganisms represent a fundamental underpinning of organic creation.

THE SULFUR CYCLE

The sulfur cycle may be defined in more specific terms than the carbon cycle. **Sulfur** is a key constituent of such amino acids as cystine, cysteine, and methionine, all of which are important components of proteins. Proteins are deposited in water and soil as living things die, and bacteria decompose the proteins and break down the sulfur-containing amino acids to yield various compounds, including hydrogen sulfide. Sulfur may also be released in the form of sulfate molecules commonly found in organic matter. Anaerobic bacteria, such as those of the genus ***Desulfovibrio***, subsequently convert sulfate molecules to hydrogen sulfide.

The next set of conversions involves several genera of bacteria, including members of the genera ***Thiobacillus, Beggiatoa***, and ***Thiothrix***. These bacteria release sulfur from hydrogen sulfide during their metabolism and convert it into sulfate. The sulfate is now available to plants, where it is incorporated into the sulfur-containing amino acids. Consumption by animals and humans completes the cycle.

THE NITROGEN CYCLE

The cyclic transformation of nitrogen is of paramount importance to life on Earth. **Nitrogen** is an essential element in nucleic acids and amino acids. Although it is the most common gas in the atmosphere (about 80 percent of air), animals cannot use nitrogen in its gaseous form, nor can any but a few species of plants. The animals and plants thus require the assistance of microorganisms to trap the nitrogen. Among the first to recognize this relationship was **Martinus Beijerinck**, who did his work at the end of the 1800s (**MicroFocus 25.2**).

The nitrogen cycle begins with the deposit of dead plants and animals in the soil. In addition, nitrogen reaches the soil in urea contained in urine. A process of digestion and putrefaction by soil bacteria and other microorganisms follows, thus yielding a mixture of amino acids (**FIGURE 25.14**). Amino acids are further broken down by microbial metabolism, and the ammonia that accumulates may be used directly by plants.

Next, **mineralization** takes place. In this process, complex organic compounds are finally converted to inorganic compounds and additional ammonia. Much of the ammonia is converted to nitrite ions by ***Nitrosomonas*** species, a group of aerobic Gram-negative rods. In the process, the bacteria obtain energy for their metabolic needs. The nitrite ions are then converted to nitrate ions by species of ***Nitrobacter***, another group of aerobic Gram-negative rods, which obtain energy from the process. Nitrate is a crossroads compound: it can be used by plants for their nutritional needs, or it can be liberated as atmospheric nitrogen by certain microorganisms.

For the nitrogen released to the atmosphere, a reverse trip back to living things is an absolute necessity for life to continue as we know it. The process is called **nitrogen fixation**. Once again microorganisms in water and soil play a key role because they possess the enzyme systems that trap atmospheric nitrogen and convert it to

---

Cystine:
a sulfur-containing amino acid found in many proteins.

de-sul′fo-vib′re-o

thi′o-bah-sil′us
bei′je-ah-to′ah
thi′o-thricks

Urea:
the nitrogen–containing product of amino acid decomposition that comprises the main component of urine.

ni-tro-so-mo′nas

ni-tro-bak′ter

Nitrogen fixation:
the chemical process by which atmospheric nitrogen is incorporated to organic compounds.

MicroFocus 25.2

OF LUMPS AND BUMPS

The man from the Delft laboratory had an audacious proposal to the assembled farmers: "Don't plant your crops in the same field as last year," he said. "Leave the field alone for the next two years; let it lie fallow." The year was 1887. The man was Martinus Willem Beijerinck (bi′jer-ink). The country was The Netherlands. And, because agricultural land was at a premium, the proposal was revolutionary.

Beijerinck was a local bacteriologist. While his medical colleagues were investigating the germ theory of disease and its implications, Beijerinck was out in the fields. He was observing that fields are very productive when the land has just been cleared and freshly planted. He was noting that fields yield bountiful crops when the farmer is away for a couple of

years. And now he thought he had the answer: great populations of bacteria.

Beijerinck was an expert on plants, but he also had something that most other botanists lacked: a solid background in chemistry. He was of the opinion that nitrogen is essential for plant growth, but he had no idea how nitrogen bridges the gap between atmosphere and plant. Then it dawned on him that bacteria were the bridge. And the little lumps and bumps were the key. Time and again he observed great hordes of bacteria in the little lumps and bumps ("nodules") on plant roots. He didn't see the nodules as often on tended crops, but they always seemed to be on wild plants growing in untended fields.

Now Beijerinck performed the laboratory experiments that strengthened

his views: He took bacteria from the nodules and inoculated them to seedlings of various plants. In many cases, the plants developed nodules, and when he planted the seedlings, the nitrogen content of the soil rose dramatically. So, his advice that 1887 day was straightforward: Leave the field alone for a spell; plant elsewhere; let the wild plants thrive; and when the field is finally planted, the crop yield will be worth the wait.

And indeed he was right. Modern farmers know that every now and then, it is important to let a field lie fallow and "refresh" itself. To the macrobiologist, the lumps and bumps on the roots of wild plants are the important parts. To the microbiologist, it's what's inside that counts. Either way, we all benefit.

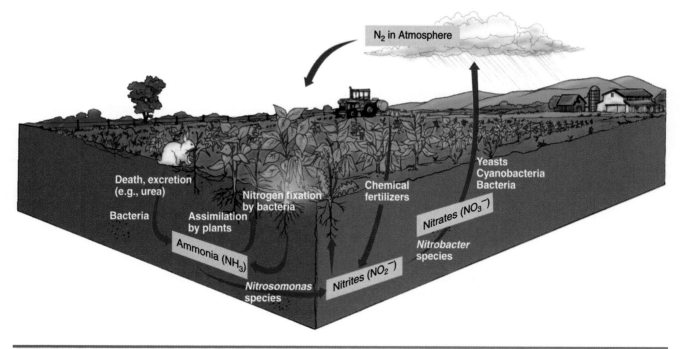

FIGURE 25.14

A Simplified Nitrogen Cycle

Plant and animal protein and metabolic wastes are decomposed by bacteria into ammonia. The ammonia may be utilized by plants, or it may be converted by *Nitrosomonas* and *Nitrobacter* species to nitrate, which is also used by plants. Some nitrate is broken down to atmospheric nitrogen. This nitrogen is returned to the leguminous plants by nitrogen-fixing microorganisms as nitrate, which is converted to ammonia. Animals consume the plants to obtain proteins that contain the nitrogen.

FIGURE 25.15

Metabolic Cycling in Cyanobacteria

Scanning electron micrographs of the cyanobacterium *Cyanothece*, showing the cycling of its metabolic functions. (a) During light periods (D0), nitrogen fixation is at a minimum. At this time, a series of carbohydrate granules (Carb) appears in the cytoplasm of the cell, indicating that photosynthesis is taking place. The granules are plentiful near the cell wall (CW). (b) When the cell enters a dark period (D6), nitrogen fixation occurs at a high rate, but photosynthesis slows. As the figure shows, most of the carbohydrate granules have disappeared, possibly because their contents are used as an energy source to fuel the reactions of nitrogen fixation. An empty granule (C) and some thylakoid membrane (T) can be seen. Also visible is a granule containing a cyanobacterial pigment called cyanophycin (CyG).

Legume:
a plant that bears its seeds in pods.

ri-zo'be-um

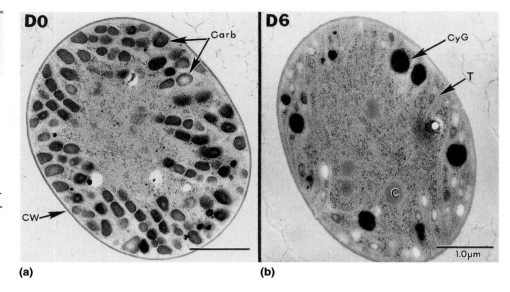

(a)   (b)

compounds useful to plants (FIGURE 25.15). In nitrogen fixation, gaseous nitrogen is incorporated to ammonia that fertilizes plants.

Two general types of microorganisms are involved in nitrogen fixation: free-living species and symbiotic species. **Free-living species** include bacteria of the genera *Bacillus, Clostridium, Pseudomonas, Spirillum,* and *Azotobacter,* as well as types of cyanobacteria and certain yeasts. Generally, the free-living species fix nitrogen during their growth cycles. The nitrogen-fixing ability of these species cannot be overemphasized.

Symbiotic species of nitrogen-fixing microorganisms live in association with plants that bear their seeds in pods. These plants, known as **legumes**, include peas, beans, soybeans, alfalfa, peanuts, and clover. Species of Gram-negative rods known as **Rhizobium** infect the roots of the plants and live within swellings, or nodules, in the roots. Although complex factors are involved, the central theme of the relationship is that *Rhizobium* fixes nitrogen and makes nitrogen compounds available to the plant while taking energy-rich carbon compounds in return. The bulk of the nitrogen compounds accumulates when *Rhizobium* cells die. Legumes then use the compounds to construct amino acids and, ultimately, protein. Animals consume the soybeans, alfalfa, and other legumes and convert plant protein to animal protein, thereby completing the cycle.

Humans have long recognized that soil fertility can be maintained by rotating crops and including a legume. The explanation lies in the ability of rhizobia to fix nitrogen within the nodules of legumes (FIGURE 25.16). So much nitrogen is captured, in fact, that the net amount of nitrogen in the soil actually increases after a crop of legumes has been grown. When cultivating legumes, there is no need to add nitrogen fertilizer to the soil. In addition, when crops such as clover or alfalfa are plowed under, they markedly enrich the soil's nitrogen content. Thus, humans are indebted to microorganisms for such edible plants as peas and beans, as well as for the indirect products of nitrogen fixation—namely, steaks, hamburgers, and milk.

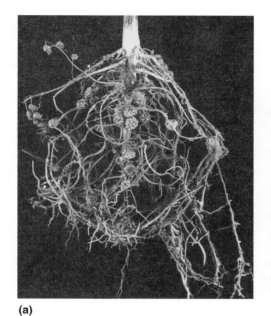

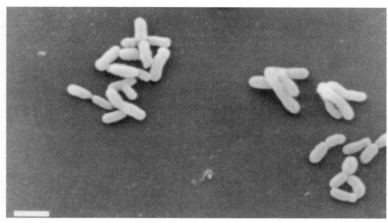

(a) (b)

FIGURE 25.16

Nitrogen Fixation

(a) Nodules on the roots of a cowpea, a legume plant. Species of *Rhizobium* live within the nodules and fix nitrogen to nitrogen-containing compounds. When the bacteria die, the compounds are utilized by the legume to synthesize amino acids. (b) A scanning electron micrograph of a *Rhizobium* species. (Bar = 2 μm.)

Note to the Student

In many chapters of this text, we have studied the negative role of microorganisms in disease, and I would not blame you for becoming paranoid about taking a breath of air, bite of food, or drink of water.

However, there is another side to the story of microorganisms, a side that reflects the positive roles they play in our lives. These roles are highlighted by the foods and dairy products manufactured by microorganisms (Chapter 24), and by the industrial products derived from their growth (Chapter 26).

The positive role of microorganisms is further exemplified by their activity in the treatment of sewage. Through a complex network of processes, microorganisms transform the devilish cocktail of sewage into simple compounds that can be handled by the environment. Working with quiet competence, they break down the vile mixture of human and animal feces, urine, hair, oily filth from roads, bloody effluent from slaughterhouses, and as ugly a profusion of grot as can be imagined. The mammoth and unceasing task is accomplished unfailingly and efficiently.

Nor does it end here. In the carbon, nitrogen, and sulfur cycles, the microorganisms convert the basic elements of life on Earth to usable forms and replenish the soil to nourish all living things. By far, the great majority of microorganisms are engaged in constructive, cooperative, healthy, and wholesome activities. It is well to remember that microorganisms represent the most efficient way of breaking down organic matter, and, in the general scheme of things, this happens after death, not before.

Summary

Environmental microbiology is concerned in large measure with the pollution brought on by microorganisms. An unpolluted water environment is inhabited by limited numbers of soil bacteria, but a polluted environment contains a huge variety of heterotrophic organisms from sewage, feces, and industrial sources. Coliform bacteria, the Gram-negative rods of human and animal intestinal tracts, abound in polluted water. By contrast, a marine environment has halophilic microorganisms, as well as psychrophilic and barophilic organisms.

Of the three types of pollution, biological pollution is of primary interest to the water microbiologist. The biochemical oxygen demand (BOD) is a measure of the amount of biological pollution, and concern exists for a variety of bacterial, viral, and protozoal diseases transmitted by water. To prepare the water for drinking purposes, municipalities employ various levels of water purification, including sedimentation, filtration, and chlorination. Sewage can also be treated by different steps according to the needs of the municipalities. Cesspools and septic tanks are used for local treatment, and variations of oxidation lagoons and secondary and tertiary treatments are used on larger scales. To test the effectiveness of purification procedures, several bacteriological tests are available, including the membrane filter technique, the standard plate count, the most probable number test, and a number of DNA-based analyses.

In the biosphere of the water and soil, microorganisms are positive factors in the cycles of carbon, sulfur, and nitrogen. In the carbon cycle, bacteria and fungi are essential to the breakdown of organic matter and the release of carbon back to the atmosphere for recycling. Anaerobic bacteria fill a similar niche in the sulfur cycle. In the nitrogen cycle, many microorganisms release nitrogen from urea, amino acids, and nitrogenous organic matter. Many types of nitrogen-based conversions are performed by microorganisms, and bacteria are essential in the steps of nitrogen fixation where nitrogen is brought back into the cycle. Indeed, the processes performed by nitrogen-fixing bacteria are so essential that life as we know it would probably not exist without bacterial intervention.

Questions for Thought and Discussion

1. When sewers were constructed in New York City in the early 1900s, engineers decided to join storm sewers carrying water from the streets together with sanitary sewers bringing waste from the homes. The result was one gigantic sewer system. In retrospect, was this a good idea? Why?

2. In the 1970s, a popular bumper sticker read: "Have you thanked a green plant today?" The reference was to photosynthesis taking place in plants. Suppose you saw this bumper sticker: "Have you thanked a microorganism today?" What might the owner of the car have in mind?

3. The English scientist John Harrington is credited with the invention of the first functional water closet (toilet) for the disposal of human waste. Why was this a significant advance in sanitation and water microbiology?

4. A student notes in her microbiology class that a particular species of bacteria actively dissolves fats, greases, and oils. Her mind stirs, and she wonders whether such an organism could be used to unclog the cesspool that collects waste from her house. What do you think she is considering? Will it work?

5. The water in a particular bay is relatively free of bacteria in the wintertime but generally polluted with bacteria in the summer. One reason is that summer boaters illegally empty their holding tanks into the bay before docking. Another is that fishermen clean their catch along the docks and dump the refuse into the bay. How many other reasons can you suggest for the summertime pollution?

6. The victims of disease, both animals and people, are buried underground, yet the soil is generally free of pathogenic organisms. Why?

7. In August 1989, two men were tragically killed while working in an industrial septic tank during cleaning. The cause of death was listed as methane poisoning. What was the source of the methane, and how was it related to the septic tank?

8. What information might you offer to dispute the following four adages common among campers and hikers? (1) Water in streams is safe to drink if there are no humans or large animals upstream. (2) Melted ice and snow is safer than running water. (3) Water gurgling directly out of the ground or running out from behind rocks is safe to drink. (4) Rapidly moving water is germ-free.

9. In 1978, Legionnaires' disease broke out in the garment district of New York City and was given front-page treatment in the press. During that same period, the coliform count rose dramatically in water in the Murray Hill section of the city, but this was given minor coverage in the papers. Many public health officials believed that the Murray Hill problem posed the more substantial threat. Do you agree? Why?

10. Your family is building a new home and has the choice of installing a cesspool or a septic tank. Which might you be inclined to choose? Why?

11. In his classic book *Rats, Lice, and History,* Hans Zinsser writes: "As soon as a state ceases to be mainly agricultural, sanitary knowledge becomes indispensable for its maintenance." What evidence can you provide to support this statement? Can you think of any evidence to refute it?

12. Some years ago, the syndicated columnist Erma Bombeck wrote a humorous book entitled *The Grass Is Always Greener Over the Septic Tank.* (The title was an adaptation of the expression "The grass is always greener on the other side of the fence.") Indeed, the grass is often greener over the septic tank. Why is this so? How can you locate your home's cesspool or septic tank in the days following a winter snowfall?

13. The author of a biology textbook writes: "Because the microorganisms are not observed as easily as the plants and animals, we tend to forget about them, or to think only of the harmful ones . . . and thus overlook the others, many of which are indispensable to our continued existence." How do the carbon, sulfur, and nitrogen cycles support this outlook?

14. A park in a local community has two swimming pools: an Olympic-sized pool for swimmers, and a small wading pool for toddlers. In which pool does the greater potential for disease transmission exist, and what precautions may be taken to limit the transmission of microorganisms?

15. Clamming and mussel gathering are often prohibited in contaminated waters even though fishing is permitted. What is the reason for this apparent discrepancy?

Review

Using your knowledge of environmental microbiology, consider each characteristic and the three possible choices below. In the space, place the letter or letters of the most appropriate choice(s). The answers are listed in Appendix D.

_____ 1. Genus (genera) of coliform bacteria
    a. *Escherichia*
    b. *Staphylococcus*
    c. *Enterobacter*

_____ 2. Where halophilic bacteria live
    a. lake
    b. ocean
    c. mountain stream

_____ 3. Used as markers for oil drilling
    a. bacteriophages
    b. radiolaria
    c. foraminifera

_____ 4. Waterborne microbial disease(s)
    a. hepatitis A
    b. amoebiasis
    c. hepatitis B

_____ 5. Step(s) in water purification
    a. filtration
    b. chlorination
    c. sedimentation

_____ 6. Found in polluted water
    a. *Proteus* species
    b. *E. coli*
    c. AIDS virus

_____ 7. Test(s) for oxygen consumption in water
    a. SPC
    b. BOD
    c. MPN

_____ 8. Type(s) of pollution when microorganisms are present
    a. biological
    b. physical
    c. chemical

_____ 9. Toxin-producing dinoflagellate(s)
    a. *Entamoeba*
    b. *Gambierdiscus*
    c. *Gonyaulax*

_____ 10. Produce(s) flocs in water
    a. iron sulfate
    b. copper sulfate
    c. aluminum sulfate

_____ 11. Needed to perform the standard plate count
    a. Petri dishes
    b. pipettes
    c. agar medium

_____ 12. Possible cause(s) of red tide
    a. *Gonyaulax*
    b. *Streptococcus*
    c. *Gymnodinium*

_____ 13. Found in anaerobic mud at lake bottom
    a. *Giardia*
    b. diatoms
    c. *Clostridium*

_____ 14. Release(s) carbon in carbon cycle
    a. viruses
    b. fungi
    c. bacteria

_____ 15. Function(s) in nitrogen cycle
    a. *Thiobacillus*
    b. *Nitrobacter*
    c. *Thiothrix*

http://microbiology.jbpub.com

The site features **eLearning,** an on-line review area that provides quizzes and other tools to help you study for your class. You can also follow useful links for in-depth information, read more MicroFocus stories, or just find out the latest microbiology news.

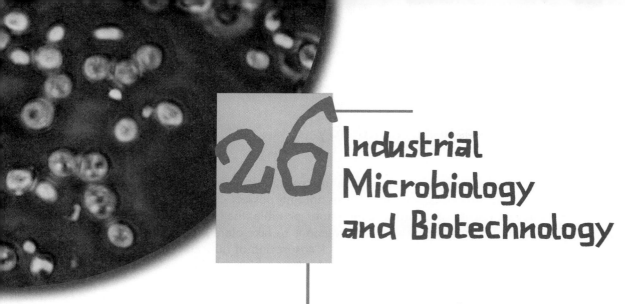

26 Industrial Microbiology and Biotechnology

Never underestimate the power of the microbe.

—Microbiologist Jackson W. Foster of the
University of Texas

HUMANS PROBABLY DISCOVERED alcoholic beverages by accident. It is conceivable that sunlight warmed some sort of fallen grape or other fruit and accelerated the fermentation of its juices by yeasts. Humans must have sampled this "spoiled" fruit with curiosity, and if the taste of the aromatic concoction was not especially pleasing, the euphoric feeling that followed probably brought them back for more. By trial and error, humans discovered the important factors in fermentation and soon learned to control the process. In doing so, they became the first industrial microbiologists.

But industrial microbiology is not restricted to alcoholic fermentations. It includes bread baking and cheese production, as well as the synthesis of organic compounds, antibiotics, insecticides, and the myriad products of genetic engineering. Basically, industrial microbiology refers to the uses of microorganisms in commercial enterprises.

Many products of industrial microbiology contribute to public health as aids to nutrition. Other products are used to interrupt the spread of disease. Still others hold promise for improving the quality of life in the years ahead. As we shall see in this chapter, industrial microbiology is an extremely diversified field, in which inexpensive raw materials are converted to valuable commodities through the metabolism of microorganisms.

Microorganisms in Industry

Certain properties make microorganisms well suited for industrial processes. Microorganisms not only possess a broad variety of enzymes to make an array of chemical conversions possible, they also have a relatively high metabolic activity that allows conversions to take place rapidly. In addition, they have a large surface area for the quick absorption of nutrients and release of end-products. Moreover, they usually multiply at a high rate, as evidenced by the 20-minute generation time for *Escherichia coli* under ideal conditions.

In the industrial process, microorganisms act like **chemical factories**. To be effective, they should liberate a large amount of a single product that can be efficiently isolated and purified (MicroFocus 26.1). The organisms should be easy to maintain and cultivate, and should have genetic stability with infrequent mutations. Their value is enhanced if they can grow on an inexpensive, readily available medium that is a by-product of other industrial processes. For example, a large amount of whey is produced in cheese manufacturing, and microorganisms that convert whey components to lactic acid add to the overall profit of the cheese industry. FIGURE 26.1 displays some possible conversions from a single metabolic substance.

Whey:
the clear fluid remaining after protein curdles from milk.

THE PRODUCTION OF ORGANIC COMPOUNDS

Microorganisms are used in industry to produce a variety of organic compounds, including acids, growth stimulants, and enzymes. In some cases, the production

MicroFocus 26.1

ACETONE AND A HOMELAND

The situation in 1914 was desperate: Great Britain was at war with Germany, and the British supply of acetone was rapidly dwindling. Acetone was a solvent for cordite, the substance used to make explosives for naval guns. Before the war, German industrial firms were major suppliers of acetone, but to expect any more shipments was unrealistic.

At the end of 1914, the British war office invited scientists to report any of their discoveries that might be of military value. The following year David Lloyd George, then Minister of Munitions, learned of the work of Chaim Weizmann and arranged to meet him. Weizmann, a Russian chemist living in England, was interested in bacterial fer-

mentations. George explained the seriousness of the acetone situation and indicated that the usual wood distillation process was not working well enough to meet the demand. Weizmann's enthusiasm was fired; he resolved to do what he could.

Weizmann returned to his laboratory and worked relentlessly. Within a few weeks he had isolated an organism that transforms cornstarch to a mixture of acetone and several alcohols. The organism was the Gram-positive bacillus *Clostridium acetobutylicum*. Weizmann reported his success to Lloyd George, and with the help of Canadian and American corporations, the process was scaled up to industrial proportions. By 1917, the British had their acetone,

and cordite production resumed at full proportions.

Lloyd George (later Prime Minister of Great Britain) suggested that he would like to honor Weizmann for his work. Weizmann gracefully declined. Instead, he stepped up his political activity and lobbied for the recognition of a homeland for the Jewish people. The extent of Weizmann's influence has been debated, but on November 2, 1917, British Foreign Secretary David Balfour issued the famous Balfour Declaration, which states: "His Majesty's government views with favor the establishment in Palestine of a national home for the Jewish people." Thirty-one years later, the state of Israel was created. Its first president was Chaim Weizmann.

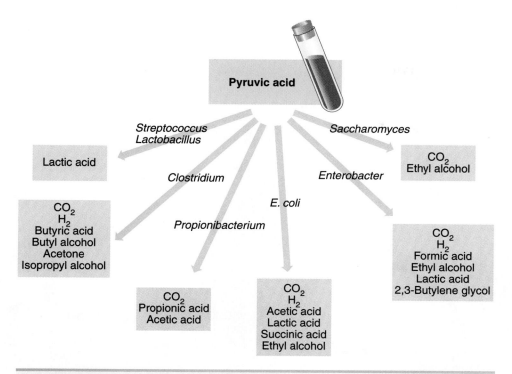

FIGURE 26.1

The Products of Fermentation

Industrial microbiology includes the metabolic conversions of organic compounds to other organic compounds by microorganisms. These conversions are called fermentations because they take place in the absence of oxygen. The process begins with the digestion of glucose (and other carbohydrates) by glycolysis, as explained in Chapter 5. The product of glycolysis is pyruvic acid, the starting point for the conversions shown here.

results from an apparent accident in nature in which an organism manufactures many thousands of times the amount necessary for its own metabolism.

One of the first organic acids to be made in bulk by microorganisms was **citric acid**. Manufacturers use this organic compound in soft drinks, candies, inks, engraving materials, and a variety of pharmaceuticals, such as anticoagulants and effervescent tablets (e.g., Alka-Seltzer). The organism most widely used in citric acid production is the mold ***Aspergillus niger***. Microbiologists inoculate the mold to a medium of cornmeal, molasses, salts, and inorganic nitrogen in huge shallow pans or fermentation tanks. The absence of a Krebs cycle enzyme in the mold prevents the metabolism of citric acid into the next component of the cycle, and the citric acid accumulates in the medium. FIGURE 26.2 outlines this chemistry.

Another important microbial product is **lactic acid**, a compound employed to preserve foods, finish fabrics, prepare hides for leather, and dissolve lacquers. Lactic acid is commonly produced by bacterial activity on the whey portion of milk. ***Lactobacillus bulgaricus*** is widely used in the fermentation because it produces only lactic acid from lactose.

Gluconic acid, another valuable organic acid, is useful in medicine as a carrier for calcium, because gluconic acid is easily metabolized in the body, leaving a store of calcium for distribution. This acid is produced from carbohydrates by *A. niger* and species of the bacterium ***Gluconobacter*** cultivated in fermentation tanks. Calcium

as'per-jil'us ni'jer

gloo'ko-no-bak'ter

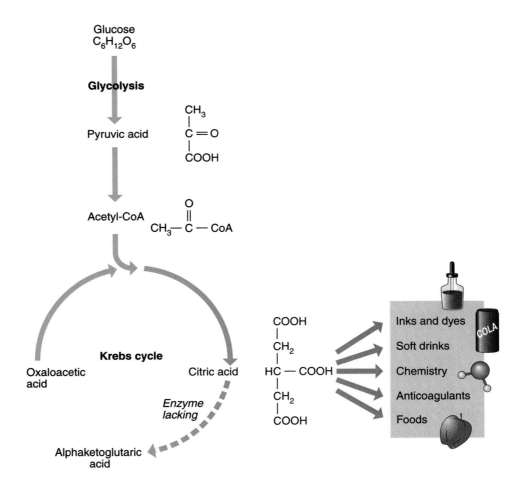

FIGURE 26.2

The Chemistry of Citric Acid Production

Aspergillus niger is grown in a mixture of nutrients, where it digests glucose into pyruvic acid. The pyruvic acid is then converted to acetyl-CoA, which condenses with oxaloacetic acid in the Krebs cycle to yield citric acid. However, the chemistry goes no further, because the next enzyme in the cycle is absent. Citric acid therefore accumulates and is isolated for use in various products, as shown.

gluconate is also added to the feed of laying hens to provide calcium that strengthens the eggshells.

When the amount of amino acid produced by a microorganism exceeds the need, the remainder is excreted into the environment. Such is the case with **glutamic acid** produced by certain species of *Micrococcus, Arthrobacter,* and *Brevibacterium.* Glutamic acid is a valuable food supplement for humans and animals, and its sodium salt, monosodium glutamate, is utilized in food preparations.

In the production of **lysine**, another amino acid, two organisms are involved. *E. coli* is first cultivated in a medium of glycerol, corn steep liquor, and other ingredients, and the compound diaminopimelic acid (DAP) accumulates. Several days later, *Enterobacter aerogenes* is added to the mixture. This organism produces an enzyme that removes the carboxyl group from DAP to produce the lysine used in breads, breakfast cereals, and other foods.

ar′thro-bak′ter
brev′e-bak-te′re-um

di-am′ĭ-no-pim-el′ik

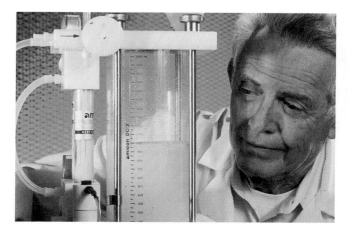

FIGURE 26.3

Enzyme Production, a Mainstay of the Industrial Microbiology Process

A chemist extracts an enzyme from a bacterium found in ship-worms that is a powerful new stain remover for laundry detergents.

Two important vitamins, riboflavin (vitamin B_2) and cyanocobalamin (vitamin B_{12}), are also products of microbial growth. **Riboflavin** is a product of ***Ashbya gossypii***, a mold that produces 20,000 times the amount it needs for its metabolism. **Cyanocobalamin** is produced by selected species of *Pseudomonas, Propionibacterium,* and *Streptomyces* grown in a cobalt-supplemented medium. The vitamin prevents pernicious anemia in humans and is used in bread, flour, cereal products, and animal feeds.

ash'be-ah go-sip'e-e

si'ah-no-ko-bal'ah-min
pro'-pe-on'e-bak-te're-um

ENZYMES AND OTHER PRODUCTS

The production of microbial enzymes for commercial exploitation has been an important industry since the emergence of industrial microbiology. Currently, over two dozen types of microbial enzymes are in use, and several others are in the research or developmental stage (**FIGURE 26.3**). Industrial enzymes have reached an annual market of $1.6 billion.

The important microbial enzymes include amylase, pectinase, and several proteases. **Amylase** is produced by the mold ***Aspergillus oryzae***. It is used as a spot remover in laundry presoaks, as an adhesive, and in baking, where it digests starch to glucose. **Pectinase**, a product of a ***Clostridium*** species, is employed to ret flax for linen. In this process, manufacturers mix the flax plant with pectinase to decompose the pectin "cement" that holds cellulose fibers together. The cellulose fibers are then spun into linen. MicroFocus 26.2 describes a more traditional process for retting. Pectinase is also used to clarify fruit juices.

o-ri'za

Retting:
the process by which enzymes remove the pectin that holds cellulose fibers together in flax plants.

Proteases are a group of protein-digesting enzymes produced by *Bacillus subtilis, Aspergillus oryzae,* and other microorganisms. Certain proteases are used for bating hides in leather manufacturing, a process in which organic tissue is removed from the skin to yield a finer texture and grain. Other proteases find value as liquid glues, laundry presoaks, meat tenderizers, drain openers, and spot removers.

Bating:
the process by which organic material is removed from hides in leather manufacturing.

One of the most appreciated but lesser known uses of a microbial enzyme is in making soft-centered chocolates. **Invertase**, an enzyme from yeast, is mixed with flavoring agents and solid sucrose, and then covered with chocolate. The enzyme converts some of the sucrose to liquid glucose and fructose, forming the soft center of the chocolate. In medical microbiology, doctors use another microbial enzyme, **streptokinase**, to break down blood clots formed during a heart attack. Still another enzyme, **hyaluronidase**, is used to facilitate the absorption of fluids injected under the skin.

hi'ah-lu-ron'ĭ-dās

MicroFocus 26.2

IT SMELLED BAD, BUT IT WORKED

In past centuries, industrial pectinase was not available for retting flax, nor was protease available for bating hides. Nevertheless, the processes were carried on efficiently and successfully.

The retting process began by bundling flax plants and drying them in stacks. The stacks were then placed in a long trench several feet deep, covered with water, and weighted down with stones to exclude as much air as possible. After a few days, the water turned black, and an unmistakable stench signaled that retting was taking place. Two weeks later the flax was so soft and pliable that the fibers could be easily removed by pounding with wooden blocks. Today's microbiologists point out that *Clostridium* species were probably producing pectinase in the trenches.

The method for treating hides was equally messy. Skins were mixed with dog or fowl manure and set aside to cure. Fragments of tissue and hair gradually dissolved in the muck, and soon the hide became soft and pliable. Apparently, the proteases from fecal bacteria were responsible for the digestion. Bating hides was another smelly process, to be sure, but like the method for retting, it was usually reliable.

gib-ber-el'in

gi-ber-el'ah fu'ji-kur'oi

Gibberellins are a series of plant hormones that promote growth by stimulating cell elongation in the stem. Botanists use the hormones to hasten seed germination and flowering, and agriculturalists find them valuable for setting blooms in the plant. This increases the yield of fruit and, in the case of grapes, enhances their size. Gibberellins are produced during the metabolism of the fungus *Gibberella fujikuroi* and may be extracted from these organisms for commercial use (MicroFocus 26.3).

Although most natural **food flavoring ingredients** are produced by traditional processes from plant origins, new biotechnology methods have made it possible to produce novel flavoring ingredients by converting relatively cheap starting materials into higher-value flavor and aroma additives. The latter are used in foods, beverages, cosmetics, and other consumer items. An example are the fruit, peach, and coconut flavoring agents called **lactones**. Although lactones can be generated from long-chain fatty acids from sweet potatoes, the fatty acids occur in limited quantity and are expensive to modify. To circumvent this problem, microbiologists use

MicroFocus 26.3

FOOLISH SEEDLINGS

During the 1890s, Japanese rice growers noticed that elongated seedlings sometimes appeared among their normal-sized seedlings in rice paddies. Although the elongated seedlings demonstrated vigorous early growth, the plants died before reaching maturity. After a time, growers began calling the condition "foolish seedling disease."

Little was known about the disease until 1926, when a Japanese botanist named Eiichi Kurosawa discovered an ascomycete fungus, *Gibberella fujikuroi*, growing on the plants. He isolated the fungus, transferred it to healthy seedlings, and found that they too developed elongated stems. In further studies, he reproduced the phenomenon with an extract made from the fungus and with samples of culture media in which the fungus grew. Kurosawa concluded that some chemical was involved and named the chemical gibberellin, after the fungus.

Gibberellin was isolated and identified by Japanese biochemists during the 1930s, but because of World War II, Western scientists did not learn of the work until 1950. That year, scientists from the United States and Great Britain read the scientific papers from Japan and began their own research. By 1956, they had isolated gibberellin from bean seeds and showed that it was really a mixture of plant substances. Today, 57 different gibberellins have been separated. The chemicals are known to be hormones that have dramatic effects on cell division, seed maturation, stem elongation, and numerous other activities in plants. Their function in the fungus *Gibberella*, however, still remains uncertain.

species of *Mucor* and other fungi to convert medium-chain fatty acids to compounds that other microorganisms can easily transform to lactones. Another example are **methylketones**, which confer strong cheese-associated flavors in dairy products. The flavoring agents are derived industrially from *Penicillium roqueforti* incubated in lipase-treated milk fats.

In addition to the major products we have surveyed, microorganisms provide a number of specialized materials. Typical of the miscellaneous microbial products is **alginate**, a sticky substance used as a thickener in ice cream, soups, and other foods. Another product of microbial origin is **perfume**. Musk oil, for example, is prepared from ustilagic acid, a product of the mold ***Ustilago zeae***, which, ironically, causes smut disease (Chapter 14). Moreover, there are numerous pharmaceutical products derived from the ergot poisons of the mold ***Claviceps purpurea***. These derivatives are prescribed to induce labor, treat menstrual disorders, and control migraine headaches.

us'ti-lah'jik
us'tĭ-la'go ze'a

To this point . . .

We have opened the study of industrial microbiology by outlining the properties of microorganisms that make them assets to manufacturing processes and by surveying the techniques used in industrial operations. We then discussed some of the organic compounds and products produced by microorganisms, emphasizing specific groups of compounds.

Among the important organic acids produced by microorganisms are citric acid, lactic acid, gluconic acid, and acetic acid. Microorganisms are also used to produce amino acids such as glutamic acid and lysine, and vitamins such as riboflavin and cyanocobalamin. The important enzymes from microorganisms include amylase, pectinase, and protease. Several additional classes of organic compounds can be more economically derived by microbial activity than by chemical synthesis. The text highlighted the panorama of applications for these organic substances.

In the next section, we shall discuss additional products from microorganisms. We shall begin with alcoholic beverages and examine the fermentation processes for beer, wine, and distilled spirits. These are among the most developed of all industrial processes, so much so that fermentation is considered by many people to be an art. We shall then move on to brief discussions of antibiotics and insecticides, and then explore the developing concept of bioremediation. We close with a survey of genetic engineering as an industrial process. Modern microbiologists are extremely optimistic about the future of genetic engineering. It is fitting, therefore, that we end our study of the microorganisms on this upbeat note.

26.2

Alcoholic Beverages

The fermentation of beer, wine, and other alcoholic beverages is one of the most venerable and universal of human domestic activities (FIGURE 26.4). The origin of beer fermentation, for example, has been traced as far back as 4000 B.C., when legend tells us that Osiris, the god of agriculture, taught Egyptians the art of brewing once they had learned how to farm the land. Wine production apparently has an equally long history because archaeologists have discovered evidence of grape cultivation in the Nile Valley during the same period. Furthermore, scientists have found

FIGURE 26.4

Ancient Wine Making

A Greek vase from the sixth century B.C. showing grapes being crushed for wine by two satyrs. In mythology, satyrs were part man, part goat creatures (note the horns, tails, and feet), who attended Dionysus, the Greek god of wine. Bacchus was the Roman counterpart of Dionysus.

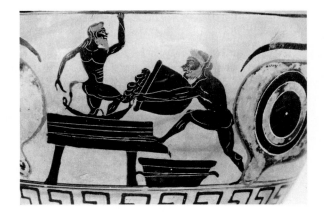

evidence of wine in jars excavated from an Iranian site 7000 years old. Thus, it is conceivable that the Egyptians, Sumerians, Assyrians, and other Near East peoples were among the earliest consumers, if not connoisseurs, of alcoholic beverages.

BEER

As early as 3400 B.C., a tax was placed on beer in the ancient Egyptian city of Memphis on the Nile. The Greeks later brought the art of brewing to Western Europe, and the Romans refined it. Indeed, the main drink of Caesar's legions was beer. During the Middle Ages, monasteries were the centers of brewing, and by the 1200s, breweries and taverns were commonplace in Great Britain. However, centuries passed before beer made its appearance in cans. That auspicious event took place in the United States in Newton, New Jersey, in 1935. The six-pack was a logical successor.

The word **beer** is derived from the Anglo-Saxon *baere*, meaning "barley." Thus, beer is traditionally a product of yeast fermentations of barley grains. However, yeasts are unable to digest barley starch, and therefore it must be predigested for them (FIGURE 26.5). This is accomplished in the process of **malting**, where barley grains are steeped in water while naturally occurring enzymes digest the starch to simpler carbohydrates, principally maltose (malt sugar).

At the brewery, the malt is ground with water to achieve further digestion of the starch. This process, called **mashing**, often includes corn as a starch supplement. Brewers then remove the liquid portion, or **wort**, and boil it to inactivate the enzymes. Dried petals of the vine *Humulus lupulus*, called **hops**, are now added to the wort, giving it flavor, color, and stability. Hops also prevent contamination of the wort, because the leaves contain at least two antimicrobial substances. At this point, the fluid is filtered, and yeast is added in large quantities.

The yeast usually employed in beer fermentation is one of two species of **Saccharomyces** developed for centuries by brewers. One species, *S. cerevisiae*, gives a uniform dark cloudiness to beer and is carried to the top of the fermentation vat by foaming carbon dioxide. This yeast is therefore called a **top yeast**. It is used primarily in English-type brews such as ale and stout. The second species, *S. carlsbergensis*, ferments the malt more slowly and produces a lighter, clearer beer, having less alcohol. This yeast sediments and is thus called a **bottom yeast**. Its product is pilsener or lager beer. Almost three-quarters of the world's beer is lager beer.

A normal fermentation requires approximately 7 days in a fermentation tank. The young beer is then transferred to vats for secondary aging, or **lagering**, which may take an additional 6 months. If the beer is intended for canning or bottling, it is pasteurized at 140°F for 55 minutes to kill the yeasts, or filtered through a membrane filter. Some

Malting:
the enzymatic process in which starch in barley grains converts to smaller carbohydrates, such as maltose.

hu'mu-lus loop'u-lus

sak'ah-ro-mi'sēz
ser'e-vis'e-ā

karls'berg-en'sis

lah'ger-ing

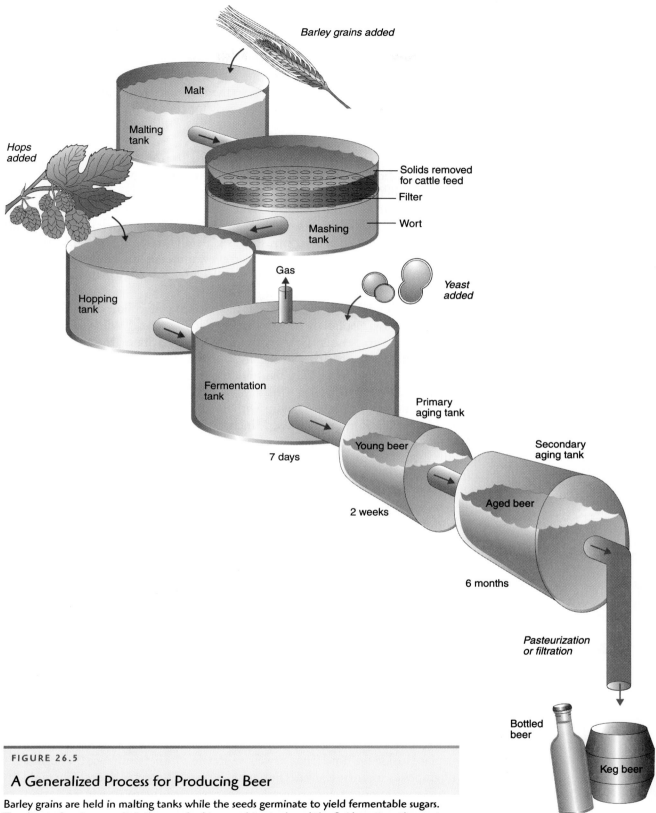

FIGURE 26.5

A Generalized Process for Producing Beer

Barley grains are held in malting tanks while the seeds germinate to yield fermentable sugars. The digested grain, or malt, is then mashed in a mashing tank and the fluid portion, the wort, is removed. Hops are added to the wort in the next step, followed by the yeast growth and alcohol production in fermentation. The young beer is aged in primary and secondary aging tanks. When it is ready for consumption, it is transferred to kegs, bottles, or cans.

yeast is used to seed new wort, and the remainder may be dried for animal feed or pressed to tablets for human consumption. The alcoholic content of beer is approximately 4 percent.

Although commonly referred to as rice wine, the Oriental beverage **sake** is more like a rice beer. It is produced by allowing **Aspergillus oryzae** to convert rice starch to fermentable sugar. *Saccharomyces* species then ferment the sugar until the alcohol level is about 14 percent. The sake is now ready for consumption.

Sake:
an Oriental beer derived from rice starch.

WINE

During the Middle Ages and the centuries thereafter, wine was called *aqua vitae*, the "water of life." The title was appropriate because wine was one of the few safe things to drink. Indeed, until the late 1800s, safe drinking water was virtually nonexistent in the Western world (note that the Bible makes no references to water for drinking purposes). Wine, by contrast, was generally free of pathogens due to its acidity and alcohol content, and it provided a few minerals and vitamins to the diet, while serving as a pain reliever. Of course, it also bred a society that was somewhat inebriated most of the time.

Essentially, all **wines** are derived from the natural conversion of grape or other fruit sugars to ethyl alcohol by the enzymes in *Saccharomyces*. Wild yeasts naturally occurring on the grapes may be used, but in the United States, the general trend is to use controlled cultures of yeast, usually *S. cerevisiae* variety *ellipsoideus*.

e'lip-soid'e-us

Wine may be made from fruit, fruit juice, or plant extracts such as dandelions. Among the grapes, the species *Vitis vinifera* is recognized as the highest-quality fruit. The winemaking process begins with crushing to produce the juice, or **must**. For **red wine**, black grapes are used, including skins and sometimes, the stems (MicroFocus 26.4). **White wine**, by contrast, is made from black or white grapes without their skins or stems. Yeasts begin to multiply immediately and initiate the fermentations. Anaerobic conditions are soon established as carbon dioxide evolves and takes up all the air space. The mixture froths with CO_2 and "ferments" in the original sense of the word.

Must:
fruit juice used to make wine.

Alcohol production requires only a few days, but the **aging process** in wooden casks may go on for weeks or months. During this time wine develops its unique flavor, aroma, and bouquet. These result from the array of alcohols, acids, aldehydes, and other organic compounds produced by the yeast during aging. (Wine is estimated to have thousands of components, most of which have not yet been identified.) Soil and climate conditions (the *terroir*, in French) also contribute to the wine because they determine what organic compounds are present in the grape. The type of yeast and nature of wood derivatives from the fermentation casks are other determining factors. Thus, there are "vintage years" and "poor years." FIGURE 26.6 shows some of the steps in the wine-making process.

The broad variety of available wines result from modifications of the basic fermentation process. In **dry wines**, for example, most or all of the sugar is metabolized, while in **sweet wines**, fermentation is stopped while there is residual sugar. **Sparkling wines**, including champagne, sparkle because of a second fermentation taking place inside the bottle. For a sweet **sauterne**, vintners enhance the sugar content of grapes by a controlled infection with the mold **Botrytis cinera**. The mold literally sucks water out of the grapes, thereby increasing the sugar concentration.

bo-tri'tis sin-er'a

The strongest natural wines measure about 15 percent alcohol because yeasts cannot tolerate alcohol above this level. Most table wines average about 10 to 12 percent alcohol, with **fortified wines** reaching 22 percent alcohol. In fortified wines, brandy or other spirits are added to produce such wines as Port, Sherry, and

MicroFocus 26.4

ANSWERING THE PARADOX

The medicinal properties of wine received a boost in 1996 with reports that wine, especially red wine, is the answer to a perplexing question that emerged some years before.

The story began in 1992 when researchers from the Bordeaux region of France did a population and epidemiological study and noted that French and other Mediterranean peoples eat large amounts of fatty foods, yet suffer a relatively low incidence of coronary artery disease. A *60 Minutes* report further pointed out that fatty meats, creams, butters, and sauces have little apparent effect on French hearts. The "French Paradox" was born.

In 1996, researchers pointed to an answer in phenol-based compounds in red wine. Studies at numerous research centers indicated that phenolics, as they are called, inhibit the oxidation of low-density lipoproteins (the LDLs in the

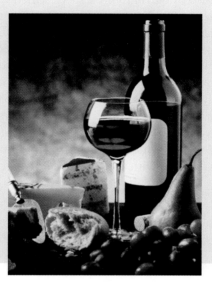

blood), and by doing so, they prevent the buildup of cholesterol and blood platelets in the arteries of the heart. Scientists point out that red wine contains more phenolics than white wine, and far more than beer. Indeed, the

most abundant phenolic in red wine, catechin (cat'ĭ-kin), is a well-known antioxidant. The phenolics are also present in other foods (e.g., raisins and onions), but not in the quantity found in the skins of grapes used for red wine. (And they concentrate even more after fermentation has taken place.)

But red wine is not for everyone. Indeed, alcohol should be avoided by pregnant women, people taking medication, those under the legal drinking age, and anyone with a family history of alcoholism. For these and for anyone else wishing to stay away from alcohol, the good news is "dealcoholized wines." These alcohol-free wines are now beginning to appear in the marketplace. They offer the opportunity to take advantage of a natural health ingredient while enjoying a glass of nature's bounty. "Ah, a glass of wine, thou, and a healthy heart."

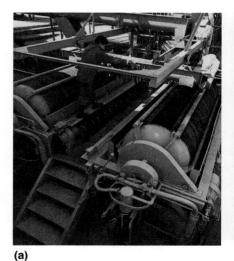

(a)

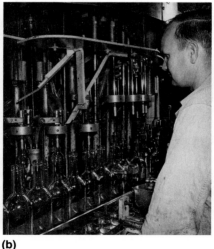

(b)

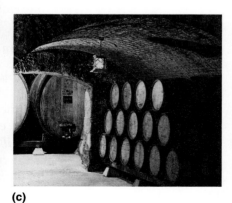

(c)

FIGURE 26.6

The Large-Scale Production of Wine

(a) A view of industrial model wine presses. The press on the right is open for loading with crushed grapes. Once loaded, a rubber bag is inflated in the center of the press to gently squeeze the grapes against the inside walls of the press. This extracts as much juice as possible from crushed grapes without breaking the seeds. (b) Bottles move along a conveyor belt and are mechanically filled with wine. (c) Wooden casks of wine aging in a cool cellar. The wine "ages" in casks for months or years.

Madeira. For mass production, wine is pasteurized to increase its shelf life, filtered, and bottled.

DISTILLED SPIRITS

Proof number:
twice the percentage of alcohol in a fermented product, such as distilled spirits.

Distilled spirits contain considerably more alcohol than beer or wine. Each is designated with a **proof number**, which is twice the percentage of the alcohol content. For example, a 90 proof product contains 45 percent alcohol.

The production of distilled spirits begins like a wine fermentation. A raw product is fermented by *Saccharomyces* species, then aged, and finally matured in casks. At this point, the process diverges as manufacturers concentrate the alcohol by a distillation apparatus using heat and vacuum. Next, they mature the product in wooden casks to introduce unique flavors from various chemicals, such as aldehydes and volatile acids. Finally, the alcohol is standardized by diluting it with water before bottling.

Four basic types of distilled spirits are produced: brandy, whiskey, rum, and neutral spirits. **Brandy** is made from fruit or fruit juice, while **rum** is produced from molasses. **Whiskey** is a product of various malted cereal grains, such as scotch from barley, rye from rye grain, and bourbon from corn. The final type, **neutral spirits**, includes vodka, which is made from potato starch and left unflavored, and gin, which is flavored with the oils of juniper berries.

26.3

Other Microbial Products

In addition to the products we have discussed, microorganisms are the sources of antibiotics and a number of valuable insecticides. Moreover, they are the producers of enzymes that break down natural and synthetic wastes in bioremediation. And they are the biological factories for the genetic engineering technology that has revolutionized industrial microbiology. In the final section of this text, we shall study the methods for antibiotic and insecticide production and bioremediation, and we discuss some details of the genetic engineering process.

ANTIBIOTICS

Penicillin:
an antibiotic that prevents cell wall synthesis primarily in Gram-positive bacteria.

krĭ-soj'en-um

Penicillin was the first antibiotic to be produced on an industrial scale. In 1941, Robert H. Coghill of the Fermentation Division of the USDA made the suggestion that the deep-tank method used to produce vitamins might be applied to penicillin. In the ensuing months, he offered several modifications to stimulate the growth of *Penicillium notatum* and increase the penicillin yield. For example, corn steep liquor in the culture medium increased the output 20 times, and the substitution of lactose for glucose made penicillin production still more efficient. Moreover, the search for a higher-yielding producer of the drug led researchers to *Penicillium chrysogenum*, a mold isolated from a rotten cantaloupe from a Peoria, Illinois, supermarket. Treatment with ultraviolet light resulted in a mutant with still higher penicillin yields. By 1943, the United States was producing enough penicillin for the Allied forces, and by 1945, sufficient amounts were available for the civilian population.

To the present time, over 5000 antibiotic substances have been described and approximately 100 such drugs are available to the medical practitioner. Although most antibiotics are produced by species of *Streptomyces* (FIGURE 26.7), a significant

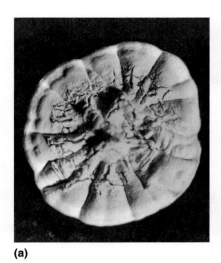

(a)

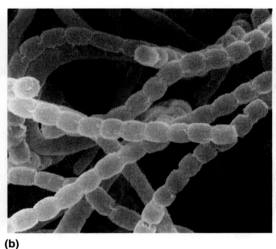

(b)

FIGURE 26.7

An Antibiotic Producer

Many modern antibiotics are produced by species of the soilborne rod *Streptomyces*. (a) A colony of *Streptomyces griseus*, the organism from which Selman Waksman isolated streptomycin in the 1940s. (b) A scanning electron micrograph of *S. griseus* grown on nutrient agar. This view displays the long chains of cells that characterize this organism.

number are products of *Penicillium* or *Bacillus* species. The worldwide production of antibiotics exceeded 25,000 tons in 1990, and two-thirds were penicillins.

Antibiotic production is carried on in huge, aerated tanks of stainless steel similar to those used in brewing. A typical tank may hold 30,000 gallons of medium. Older methods employed enormous mats of fungi or actinomycetes on the surface of the tank. Newer technology, however, employs small fragments of submerged hyphae or cells, rotated and agitated in the medium with a constant stream of oxygen. After several weeks of growth, the microorganisms are removed, and the antibiotic is extracted from the medium for further conversion to the desired product. The remaining brown mash of microorganisms may be dried and sold as an animal feed additive. Another alternative is to process it for use as human food.

INSECTICIDES

To be useful as an insecticide, a microorganism should be relatively specific for an insect pest and should act rapidly. It should be stable in the environment and easily dispensed, as well as inexpensive to produce. It helps if its odor is pleasant.

In the early part of this century, a scientist named G. S. Berliner found that sporulating cells of a *Bacillus* species were inhibitory to moth larvae. Berliner named the organism **Bacillus thuringiensis** after the European province Thuringia where he lived. The bacillus remained in relative obscurity until recent years, when scientists learned that *B. thuringiensis* produces **toxic crystals** in older cells during the process of sporulation (FIGURE 26.8). The toxic substance, an alkaline protein, is deposited on leaves and ingested by caterpillars (the larval forms of butterflies, moths, and related insects). In the caterpillar gut, the insecticide lyses the cells of the gut wall, possibly by inhibiting ATP phosphorylase or by forming pores in the microvilli membranes. As gut liquid diffuses between the cells, the larvae experience paralysis, and bacterial invasion soon follows.

thur'in-jen'sis

Alkaline: having basic properties.

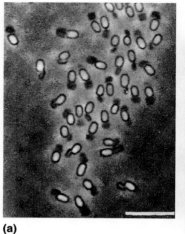

(a)

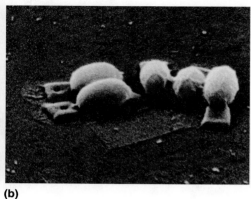

(b)

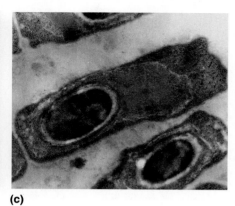

(c)

FIGURE 26.8

The Crystals and Spores of *Bacillus thuringiensis*

Photographs of a strain of the Gram-positive rod *Bacillus thuringiensis* showing its spores and the crystals associated with the insecticidal ability of this organism. (a) A phase-contrast photomicrograph of *B. thuringiensis* spores attached to the insecticidal crystals. (Bar = 5 μm.) (b) A scanning electron micrograph of the spore-crystal complex after isolation from the cells. (c) A transmission electron micrograph of a sporulating cell that contains a crystal-spore complex surrounded by a containing membrane called the exosporium.

ag′ro-bak-ter′ē-um
toom-e-fa′shens

Bacillus thuringiensis (Bt) appears to be harmless to plants and other animals. It is produced by harvesting bacteria at the onset of sporulation and drying them into a commercially available dusting powder. The product is useful on tomato hornworms and gypsy moth caterpillars. Its success encouraged further research and led to the discovery of a new strain called *B. thuringiensis israelensis* (Bti), first isolated in Israel.

But bacteria sprayed onto plants can soon wash off, so the protective effect of the insecticide can be limited. DNA technologists have realized that long-term protection can be provided by inserting the genes for toxin production directly into plants. To date, they have identified and isolated the gene for toxin production and have spliced it into plant genes using the Ti plasmid of *Agrobacterium tumefaciens* as the carrier (or vector), as noted in Chapter 6.

The first seeds with inserted *B. thuringiensis* (Bt) genes were added to the soil in 1996. Genetically engineered corn, cotton, seed potatoes, and other crops were planted on over 3 million acres in the United States. The crops displayed increased resistance to pests, but scientists noted an emerging resistance to Bt toxin in certain caterpillars. The resistance was thought to be related to a recessive gene passed along by typical Mendelian patterns. To prevent the development of resistance, scientists suggested planting adjacent fields without insecticide to dilute the gene. However, research reported in 1999 suggests that the resistance gene is dominant in certain pests, a factor that would work against the management strategy.

Another approach to gene-related plant resistance has been used in corn infested with corn borers. Researchers isolated the *B. thuringiensis* gene for toxin production and spliced it into a bacterium that lives harmlessly with corn plants. The researchers then forced a colony of gene-altered bacteria into corn seeds. When the seeds were sown, the toxin-producing bacteria flourished along with the plant, and when an insect ate the plant, it consumed the toxin. This approach is advantageous because only the insect attacking the plant is subjected to the toxin.

spher′i-cus

Another useful *Bacillus* species is **Bacillus sphaericus**, which kills at least two species of mosquitoes that ingest its poison. To increase the bacterium's efficiency, researchers inserted two of its genes to the bacterium **Asticcacaulis excentris** and achieved insecticidal activity against the mosquitoes that transmit malaria, filariasis, and St. Louis encephalitis. Using the gene carrier *A. excentris* is advantageous because it is easier to grow in large quantity; it tolerates sunlight better than *B. sphaericus*; and it floats in water, where mosquitoes feed (the heavier *Bacillus* species sinks because of its spores).

as'tic-ca-caul'is ex-cen'tris

In 1941, **Bacillus popilliae** was introduced as a control measure for Japanese beetles. The bacillus infects beetle larvae and causes **milky spore disease**, so named because the blood of the larvae becomes milky white. The larvae eventually die, and the bacillus spores remain in the soil to infect other larvae.

pop-il'e-ā

Many bacteriologists are also investigating the insecticidal abilities of the Gram-negative rod **Photorhabdus luminescens**. Its toxin, known as Pht, attacks the gut lining of larvae (as Bt does), and it is contained in large cytoplasmic crystals (also, as Bt); however, its spectrum of activity is wider than for Bt and includes numerous caterpillars as well as cockroaches. The Pht genes have been isolated, and efforts are underway to introduce them to plant cells. Normally, *P. luminescens* lives in the intestines of soilborne nematodes. The latter invade insect tissues in the soil, and the bacteria-derived toxin kills the insect. The bacteria also produce luciferase, an enzyme that induces a light-generating reaction and causes the nematode to glow. The significance of this reaction is currently unknown.

fo'to-rab'dus lum-in-es'cens

Viruses also show promise as pest-control devices, partly because they are more selective in their activity than bacteria. Once released in the field, the viruses spread naturally. It is also possible to harvest infected insects, grind them up, and use them to disseminate the virus to new locations. Among the insects successfully controlled with viruses are the cotton bollworm, cabbage looper, and alfalfa caterpillar. Chapter 6 explains experiments of this type.

Researchers can also develop insecticides by using a toxin from the venom of a scorpion. The toxin paralyzes the larvae of moths and other lepidopteran insects. It is attached to a **baculovirus**, a virus with a high affinity for lepidopteran tissues. Then the virus is sprayed on lettuce and cotton plants infested with moth larvae. At the conclusion of the field trial, the plot is sprayed with 1 percent bleach to destroy any remaining viruses.

Lepidopteran: relating to the order of insects that includes butterflies and moths.
bak'u-lo-virus

Viral genes have also been used to protect grapevines. In 1993, French biotechnologists announced the successful incorporation of genes from the **grape fan-leaf virus (GFLV)** to champagne grapevines. This virus is transmitted by a nematode and is endemic in the soils of many French regions. It causes malformation of the plant's leaf ("fan-leaf") and induces the plant to lose chlorophyll and become yellow. To protect the vines, researchers inserted the genes for viral capsids to *A. tumefaciens* and infected the plants with this bacterium. Soon the cells were producing viral capsid proteins, and they became resistant to the virus.

Even a fungus is being employed in the pesticide wars. California researchers have used **Lagenidium giganteum** to protect against crop-damaging mosquitoes in soybeans and rice, and in mosquito-infested nonagricultural settings such as wetlands. The fungus forces its spores into mosquito larvae, which die in a day or two. Marketed as Laginex, the fungal preparation has been approved for certain uses by the U.S. Environmental Protection Agency (EPA).

la-gen-id'i-um ji-gan'te-um

RECENT PRODUCTS

Industrial products of microbiology technology continue to emerge as the years unfold. In 1998, for instance, British scientists announced that they were using long strands of *Bacillus subtilis* to guide the assembly of such inorganic structures as **fibers** of magnetite, cadmium sulfide, and titanium dioxide. The researchers take advantage of a mutant whose cells fail to separate after binary fission, and soon elongate to form entangled chains and filaments that dry to a single hairlike structure almost a yard in length. The strands are used as templates (models), that is, a type of organic scaffold to which the inorganic materials cling. Such strands enable chemists to design materials in the micrometer range.

Another development allows chemists to obtain the dye **indigo** from leaves of a plant called woad. British biochemists discovered that a species of *Clostridium* ferments the carbohydrates in woad leaves and converts the indigo to a state where it is useful as a dye. This chemistry is valuable because the currently used synthetic versions of the dye tend to pollute waterways, while the naturally occurring dye is nontoxic. Denim garments of the future are prime candidates for the new dye.

Then there is the **bacterial cement** that South Dakota researchers have used to fix cracks in concrete blocks in the laboratory. Biochemists begin with urea-digesting strains of *Bacillus pasteurii* and *Sporosarcina ureae*, both found in the soil. They mix the two organisms with sand and add urea (the major waste product of urine), then add some calcium chloride. The bacteria digest the urea and produce ammonia, which reacts with water to form ammonium hydroxide. The latter converts calcium chloride to calcium carbonate, which crystallizes as limestone. Soon, the gaps between the sand have filled in with the solidifying limestone (the bacteria die within the solid material), and the bacterial cement has set. One observer has wryly noted that this is truly "a concrete use for bacteria."

BIOREMEDIATION

Recruiting bacteria and other microorganisms to break down synthetic waste is an immensely appealing idea. It signals a willingness to work with nature and adapt to its sophisticated sanitation systems, rather than trying to reinvent them. Putting microorganisms to work in this manner is the crux of **bioremediation**.

Although the term is recent and somewhat imposing, the concept of bioremediation is not new. In the 1800s, for example, night-soil men would, for a small fee, travel from house to house collecting sewage and excrement. After making their rounds, they would scatter their collections on fields, to be broken down by naturally occurring soil bacteria. Although modern waste-disposal systems have replaced the night-soil men, a new concern is the plethora of environmental pollutants contaminating the land. Bioremediation seeks to exploit microorganisms to degrade these pollutants.

The advantages of bioremediation were displayed following a major **oil spill** from the tanker *Exxon Valdez* in 1987 along the Alaska coastline (FIGURE 26.9). Previous studies showed that where oil is spilled, the bacteria that degrade oil (e.g., *Pseudomonas* species) are already present, and all technologists need to do is encourage their growth. Thus, when the oil spill occurred, technologists "fertilized" the oil-

FIGURE 26.9

The *Exxon Valdez* Oil Spill

In 1987, the oil tanker *Exxon Valdez* ran aground on the shoreline of Alaska. Numerous species of bacteria demonstrated their value in oil digesting during the ensuing cleanup efforts. This was one of the first large-scale attempts to use microorganisms in bioremediation.

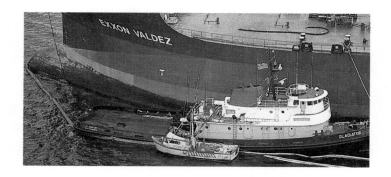

soaked water with nitrogen sources (e.g., urea), phosphorus compounds (e.g., laureth phosphate), and other mineral nutrients to modify the environment and stimulate the growth of indigenous (naturally occurring) microorganisms. Areas treated this way were cleared of oil significantly faster than nonremediated shorelines. Indeed, the oil degraded five times faster when microorganisms were put to work.

Bioremediation can also be applied to help eliminate **polychlorinated biphenyls** **(PCBs)** from the environment. PCBs were used widely in industrial and electrical machinery before their threat to environmental quality was realized. The compounds contain numerous chlorine atoms and chlorine-containing groups, and researchers have discovered that certain anaerobic bacteria remove the atoms and groups and reduce the compounds to smaller molecules. Aerobic bacteria now take over and reduce the molecular size still further. Field demonstrations in New York's Hudson River have shown the value of the combination anaerobic-aerobic degradation; and where there was an accumulation of PCBs, there now evolved carbon dioxide, water, and hydrogen chloride.

pol'i-chlor-in-ate'ed bi-fen'ils

Many years ago, **trichloroethylene (TCE)** was a much-used cleaning agent and solvent. At the time, scientists did not realize that TCE would diffuse through the soil and contaminate underground wells and water reservoirs (aquifers). To combat the problem, scientists are exploiting bacteria that grow on methane to degrade the TCE. During their metabolism, the bacteria produce a methane-digesting enzyme, which coincidentally breaks down TCE. Technologists pump methane and other nutrients into the TCE-contaminated water, and as the bacteria grow, they digest the TCE as well as the methane. The deliberate enhancement of microbial growth yields an environmental cleanup.

tri'klor-o-eth'i-lene

Among the big news stories of 1999 was a "superbug" able to withstand 3000 times more radiation than humans. The bacterium, a tetracoccus called ***Deinococcus radiodurans***, was found in a tin of irradiation-sterilized ground beef. Researchers are hoping to use it in the daunting task of cleaning up thousands of **toxic-waste sites** that include radioactive materials such as plutonium and uranium. Genetic engineering methods have produced a *D. radiodurans* strain that degrades ionic mercury compounds common to these sites. The strain utilizes a gene cluster from *E. coli* to reduce mercury to the less toxic form found in thermometers.

deen-o-kok'us ra'di-o-dur'ans

During the 1940s through the 1960s, a major component of weaponry was the explosive compound **2,4,6-trinitrotoluene (TNT)**. Like other synthetic wastes, this compound has contaminated the soil from residues deposited around weapons plants. Scientists have found that they can reduce the level of contamination by encouraging bacterial growth with molasses. In a pilot study, researchers mixed water with TNT-laced soil and added molasses at regular intervals. In a matter of weeks, the TNT concentration plummeted.

tri'ni-tro-tol'u-ene

Plants are apparently able to conscript bacteria for the task of environmental cleanup: Following the Gulf War of 1991, oily devastation remained in much of the Arabian Desert. Within 4 years, however, plant life returned, aided in large measure by *Arthrobacter* species. When researchers dug into oil-soaked desert, they found healthy plant roots surrounded by reservoirs of these oil-degrading Gram-negative rods.

For many years, the "haul-and-bury" technique was the prevailing method for disposing of synthetic waste. As the public becomes increasingly intolerant of that approach, the importance of bioremediation will become more apparent. Technologists are testing microorganisms for their ability to degrade flame-retardants, phenols, chemical warfare agents, and numerous other waste products of industry. Indeed, one prominent researcher has called bioremediation "a field with its own mass and momentum."

INDUSTRIAL GENETIC ENGINEERING

In 1973, **Herbert Boyer**, of the University of California at San Francisco, and **Stanley Cohen**, of Stanford University, performed the first practical experiment in genetic engineering. Working with *Escherichia coli*, they removed the genes for kanamycin resistance and spliced them to a plasmid that already carried genes for tetracycline resistance. The plasmids were then mixed with *E. coli* cells not resistant to either antibiotic. Finally, the cells were streaked on plates of culture medium containing both kanamycin and tetracycline. The bacteria that grew were ones that took up the plasmids and were now resistant to both antibiotics. Feats like these launched the modern era of biotechnology. As one observer later noted: "Biotechnology used to be BBC (before Boyer Cohen). Now, it is ABC (after Boyer Cohen)."

Genetic engineering based in plasmid technology has been hailed as the beginning of modern industrial microbiology. **Plasmids** are ultramicroscopic ringlets of double-stranded DNA that exist apart from the chromosome (**FIGURE 26.10**). A single plasmid may contain between 2 and 250 genes. The significance of **plasmid technology** lies in the fact that plasmids can be spliced with fragments of DNA from unrelated organisms and inserted into host organisms. The host organisms then produce the protein whose genetic message is carried by the foreign DNA. The mechanics of this reengineering process are explored in Chapter 6. Some contemporary products already obtained by plasmid technology include interferon, insulin, a vaccine for hoof-and-mouth disease, human growth hormone, and urokinase.

When microbiologists first developed the art of plasmid technology in the 1970s, the likely choice for the prototype "bacterial factory" was *E. coli*. Nonpathogenic strains had long been used as test organisms in the laboratory, and the genetics of *E. coli* was well understood. In the 1980s, however, attention shifted to *Bacillus subtilis* and yeasts as host organisms. Advocates of *B. subtilis* point out that this Gram-positive bacillus normally secretes the proteins it makes, while *E. coli* retains them. Also, *B. subtilis* is not regarded as a human pathogen, in contrast to *E. coli*, nor does it contain endotoxins in its cell wall. **Yeast** supporters point to the traditional role of their organism in fermentation processes and, therefore, the public acceptance of an organism without disease potential. One industrial firm has reengineered a *Saccharomyces* species to produce a synthetic vaccine for hepatitis B, while a second firm has used yeast to obtain rennin, the enzyme used to make cheese.

Plasmids:
loops of DNA apart from the chromosome that contain several genes and are used in genetic engineering experiments.

FIGURE 26.10

Plasmids

A transmission electron micrograph of bacterial plasmids. The large plasmid is from the intestinal organism *Bacteroides fragilis*. The smaller ones have been isolated from *Escherichia coli*. Both large and small plasmids contain genes that encode antibiotic resistance.

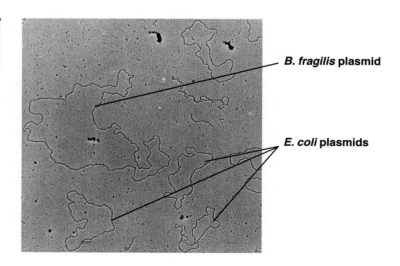

B. fragilis plasmid

E. coli plasmids

The implications of genetic engineering are far-reaching and thought-provoking. One group of biotechnologists has focused on the **antibiotic-producing genes** of plasmids and is attempting to remove the genes from *Streptomyces* species and insert them into more rapidly growing organisms. An allied group is trying to amplify the number of plasmids in antibiotic producers in order to obtain a higher yield of product.

In the 1960s, a "Green Revolution" took place in which high-yielding supergrains were exported to poor countries throughout the world to encourage self-sufficiency. However, the program stalled when stocks of essential petroleum fertilizers fell to high oil prices. Agriculturalists now hope for a second Green Revolution sparked by genetic engineering (FIGURE 26.11). They foresee the day when the genes for **nitrogen fixation** can be extracted from bacteria such as *Rhizobium* and inserted into grain plants such as wheat, rye, and barley. The most optimistic planners look to the future and foresee fertilizers becoming obsolete, plants using microbial toxins to drive off insects, grains growing in salty water, and crops living for weeks without water.

Another dream of biotechnologists is using **replacement organisms** to interrupt disease cycles in nature. For example, a transgenic snail that resists invasion of *Schistosoma* species could conceivably interrupt the life cycle of the parasite that causes schistosomiasis (Chapter 16). A slightly different strategy is being employed by DNA technologists who are attempting to produce transgenic bollworms by inserting a gene that activates a "suicide gene" in offspring of the cotton bollworm. And work continues to progress on the transgenic mosquito. Researchers have identified the critical genes that allow anopheline mosquitoes to harbor and transmit malarial parasites. Hopefully, those genes can be altered, and mutated insects can be produced. Released in large numbers, the mosquitoes could dilute or overwhelm native mosquito populations and break the chain of disease transmission.

Other research projects in genetic engineering have equally important goals. Biochemists at breweries are attempting to insert the starch-digesting enzyme **amylase** into yeasts to eliminate the malting process in beer production. At chemical companies, scientists are seeking to incorporate genes for **cellulase** activity into

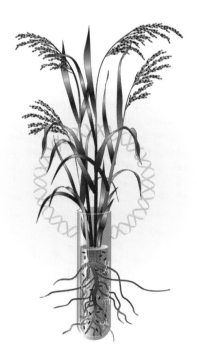

FIGURE 26.11

On the Horizon

An artist's fanciful conception of a futuristic superplant produced by genetic engineering.

microorganisms, to make cellulose a useful source of glucose. For the 20,000 hemophiliacs in the United States, new hope dawned when a genetic engineering company announced that it had isolated and cloned the genes for **Factor VIII**, an essential blood-clotting protein missing in people who have hemophilia. The next step was to splice the genes to bacteria and hope for an inexpensive, safe product.

Nor does it end here. Research in genetic engineering holds promise for new strategies for cancer prevention, new diagnostic procedures for microbial diseases and genetic abnormalities, new methods to correct genetic disorders, new hormones, antibiotics, and vaccines, and a generally improved quality of life. The discoveries and insights made possible by genetic engineering have been described as breathtaking. In the future, we can expect startling developments in medicine, agriculture, and the pharmaceutical and chemical industries. Indeed, it is an exciting time to be a microbiologist.

Note to the Student

It should be clear from this chapter that the microorganisms make a substantial contribution to the quality of life. Rather than gush with enthusiasm and rhetoric on the positive roles they play, I would prefer to paraphrase several concepts of applied microbiology set down by the late industrial microbiologist David Perlman of the University of Wisconsin. In a 1980 publication, Perlman wrote:

1. The microorganism is always right, your friend, and a sensitive partner;
2. There are no stupid microorganisms;
3. Microorganisms can and will do anything;
4. Microorganisms are smarter, wiser, and more energetic than chemists, engineers, and others; and
5. If you take care of your microbial friends, they will take care of your future.

Summary

Microorganisms occupy an important place in industry as the producers of many important products, such as organic compounds, alcoholic beverages, antibiotics, and insecticides. Among the organic compounds synthesized on an industrial scale are organic acids (such as citric, lactic, and gluconic acids), various amino acids and vitamins, and a series of enzymes such as amylase, pectinase, and proteases. Microorganisms also produce other key products and save much expense and tedium for the chemist. In addition, the plant hormones known as gibberellins can be produced on an industrial scale by microorganisms.

Beer, wine, and spirits are among the products for public consumption that yeast cells produce. Yeasts of the genus *Saccharomyces* ferment barley grains to beer under anaerobic conditions and grape juice to wine. Both processes require an aging step to develop the full flavor of the product. To produce spirits, the alcohol is distilled off to produce brandy, rum, whiskey, or neutral spirits.

Though antibiotics were originally a microbial product, most of these drugs are synthetically produced today. By contrast, the spores of *Bacillus thuringiensis* and *B. popilliae* are used in the live form as insecticides for plants. Both are successfully employed against the caterpillars of various insect pests. In addition, scientists are investigating the use of bacterial insecticides, such as *Photorhabdus*, because they have a broader spectrum of actitivy, as well as scorpion toxins carried into cells by viruses. Moreover, they have used microorganisms to guide the assembly of inorganic fibers, to obtain indigo dye from plants, and to cement cracks in concrete blocks.

Bioremediation is still another innovative use for industrial microorganisms. In this process, naturally occurring microorganisms are encouraged to grow in a polluted envirinment and break down the pollutants. Bioremediation has been successfully used to degrade the oil in oil spills and to help eliminate polychlorinated biphenyls and trichlorethylene from the environment. Researchers are hoping to use the process in the daunting task of cleaning toxic waste sites that contain radioactive materials.

The future of industrial microbiology will center on genetic engineering and plasmid technology. By inserting foreign genes into vector organisms such as bacteria and yeasts, biotechnologists can produce rare proteins on an industrial scale and provide treatments for such diseases as diabetes, hemophilia, and cancer. Genetic engineers forecast plants with inborn resistance to disease, animals that produce human proteins, and novel treatments for illness. Medicine, agriculture, and industry eagerly anticipate the fruits of modern biotechnology.

Questions for Thought and Discussion

1. The poet John Donne once wrote: "No man is an island, entirely of itself." This maxim applies not only to humans, but to all living things in the natural world. What are some roles the microorganisms play in the interrelationships among living things?

2. Certain beer companies have developed strains of yeasts that break down more of the carbohydrate in barley malt than traditional yeasts. What do you think their product is called?

3. In industrial microbiology, it is extremely helpful if the leftover product of one process can be fermented by microorganisms to produce a valuable product. Can you think of any leftover products that might be useful in industry?

4. When the *Mayflower* set sail for the New World, its intended destination was Virginia. Instead it landed at Plymouth, Massachusetts, because, as one diarist put it: "We could not now take time for further search or consideration, our victuals being much spent, especially our beer." What do these last few words tell you about the Pilgrims?

5. Bioremediation holds the key to solving numerous types of envirinmental problems in the future. Yet the process has been used for generations without our realizing it. How many instances can you point out where bioremediation is currently in use?

6. The discovery of the extremely high resistance of *Deinococcus radiodurans* to radioactivity has prompted hopes that this organism can be used in bioremediation. Suppose you were to go on a hunt for novel organisms that could be used for other envirinmental cleanups. Where might you look?

7. A product called Dipel contains *Bacillus thuringiensis*. It is used widely in the Northeast for destruction of the gypsy moth caterpillar. What dangers might result from extensive application of this product?

8. In Europe, in the month of March, it is customary to have a festival where the primary drink is bock beer. Bock beer is a very dark, lager beer that represents the dregs of the brewery. The word *bock* is German for "ram," the sign of Aries, which begins in March. How does this festival coincide with the brewing process, and why does it occur in March?

9. In several places in this text, we have noted how apparently harmless organisms have been later discovered to be dangerous in humans. Yeasts have been consumed in breads and alcoholic beverages for centuries, and still no pathogenic signs have been observed. Can you postulate why?

10. Certain bacteria produce many thousands of times their required amount of specific vitamins. Some biologists suggest that this makes little sense because the excess is wasted. Can you suggest a reason for this apparent overproduction in nature?

11. A biotechnologist suggests that one day it may be possible to engineer certain bacteria to produce antibiotics and then to feed the bacteria to diseased people. The bacteria would then serve as antibiotic producers within the body. Would you favor research of this type?

12. It was noted in this chapter that *Aspergillus oryzae* is used as a commercial source of amylase, and that the same organism is essential for the production of sake. How are the two processes related?

13. One of the side effects of the use of Bt toxin has been a reduction in the population of Monarch butterflies. Why do you think this may have happened, and what might you as a concerned citizen do about it?

14. The editors of *The Economist*, a British magazine, have referred to genetic engineering as "one of the biggest industrial opportunities of the late twentieth century." What evidence can you offer to support this contention, and why might you be inclined to reject it?

15. How many times in the last 24 hours have you had the opportunity to use or consume the industrial product of a microorganism?

16. The tale on the inside back cover of this book is adapted from a Middle Eastern story. It has been placed there for a particular reason. Can you guess why?

Review

Many different microorganisms find value in industrial microbiology. To test your knowledge of these organisms, match the microorganism on the right to the characteristic on the left by placing the correct letter in the space. A letter may be used once, more than once, or not at all. The answers are listed in Appendix D.

_____ 1. Used to ferment grapes.
_____ 2. Produces penicillin.
_____ 3. Used in riboflavin production.
_____ 4. Produces many antibiotics.
_____ 5. Enhances grape sugar content.
_____ 6. Lactic acid producer.
_____ 7. Used in lysine production.
_____ 8. Biological insecticide.
_____ 9. Source of musk oil.
_____ 10. Used for citric acid production.
_____ 11. Source of proteases.
_____ 12. Synthesizes acetic acid.
_____ 13. Produces amylase.
_____ 14. Produces plant growth hormones.
_____ 15. Yeast for making beer.
_____ 16. Ferments rice starch to sake.
_____ 17. Used for genetic engineering.
_____ 18. Causes milky spore disease.
_____ 19. Important to steroid synthesis.
_____ 20. Gluconic acid from carbohydrates.

A. *Aspergillus niger*
B. *Aspergillus oryzae*
C. *Bacillus subtilis*
D. *Bacillus popilliae*
E. *Clostridium* species
F. *Agaricus phalloides*
G. *Saccharomyces* species
H. *Ashbya gossypii*
I. *Staphylococcus aureus*
J. *Enterobacter aerogenes*
K. *Botrytis cinera*
L. *Claviceps purpurea*
M. *Streptomyces* species
N. *Penicillium chrysogenum*
O. *Lactobacillus bulgaricus*
P. *Ustilago zeae*
Q. *Acetobacter aceti*
R. *Gibberella fujikuroi*
S. *Corynebacterium diphtheriae*
T. *Rhizopus nigricans*

Appendix A: Metric Measurement

	SYMBOL	FUNDAMENTAL UNIT	QUANTITY	NUMERICAL UNIT	AMERICAN MEASUREMENT
Length		meter (m)			39.37 inches
	km		kilometer	1,000 m	0.62137 miles
	cm		centimeter	0.01 m	0.3937 inches
	mm		millimeter	0.001 m	
	μ		micrometer	0.000001 m	
	n		nanometer	0.000000001 m	
	Å		angstrom	0.0000000001 m	
Volume (liquids)		liter (l)			1.06 quarts
	ml		milliliter	0.001 l	
	μl		microliter	0.000001 l	
Mass		gram (g)			0.035 ounces
	kg		kilogram	1,000 g	2.2 pounds
	mg		milligram	0.001 g	
	μg		microgram	0.000001 g	

Appendix B: Temperature Conversion Chart

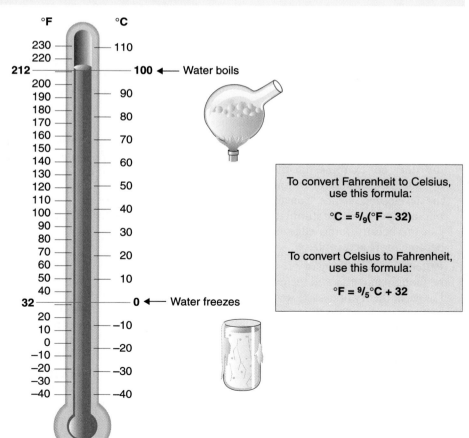

To convert Fahrenheit to Celsius, use this formula:

$$°C = \tfrac{5}{9}(°F - 32)$$

To convert Celsius to Fahrenheit, use this formula:

$$°F = \tfrac{9}{5}°C + 32$$

Appendix C: Answers to Selected Questions for Thought and Discussion

CHAPTER 1

3. Since measles is caused by a virus, and because the measles viruses cannot be seen or cultivated by methods that work for bacteria, your work would probably result in a series of dead-ends and your frustrations would mount quickly.

6. Spontaneous generation would hold that the microorganisms of infectious disease arise spontaneously in the body and are not obtained from outside the body. Thus, we could do little to interrupt the spread of microorganisms, and all the antimicrobial processes we employ (water purification, sanitation, care in food preparation) would be useless. The germ theory holds that disease agents enter the body from the outside. This means that transmission can be interrupted, and it brings an element of control to epidemics.

9. As I researched the material for Chapter 1, the year 1884 kept popping up and it soon became obvious that this was a remarkable year. Among the key events: cultivation of the typhoid bacillus by Gaffky, isolation of the diphtheria bacillus by Løeffler, description of phagocytosis by Metchnikoff, and announcement of the use of agar by Koch.

12. The improvements in microscopy that paralleled the interest in bacteria during the 1880s were probably not coincidental because one probably stimulated the other. For example, the interest in bacteria may have demanded that the technology be improved for the developing science. Conversely, the improved microscope may have stimulated interest in microorganisms because knowledge about microorganisms became more accessible.

15. Pasteur was something of a revolutionary in the way he thought and attacked the medical establishment. His germ theory of disease was severely at odds with prevailing ways of thinking, and his persistent hammering away at contemporary dogmas (e.g., the nature of fermentation, the cause and transmission of infectious disease, and the ability to interrupt epidemics) initiated a revolution that has carried through to the present day. In 1910, the French honored their "rebel" in connection with Mexican rebels. Pasteur was also a great patriot, as were the Mexicans.

CHAPTER 2

3. Detergents act on the lipid portions of bacterial membranes. They dissolve the membranes and cause leakage from the cytoplasm and subsequent death to the cell.

6. Wöhler showed that organic molecules could be synthesized, in effect demonstrating that living things could be synthetically produced. This finding stood in stark contrast to the pre-1800s belief that living things were something special and not within the ability of scientists to create. It also brought chemistry into the realm of biology, and made biologists begin thinking like chemists.

9. The organic matter of an individual consists of proteins, lipids, carbohydrates, and nucleic acids. Oxygen is a key component of each type of these groups of organic compounds. Also, there are large volumes of water in the body. It is not surprising, therefore, that a 120-pound individual contains 78 pounds of oxygen.

12. Carbon atoms have four electrons in their outer shell. They cannot lose their electrons easily, nor can they attract electrons from other atoms. Hence, they enter into covalent bonds, sharing their four electrons with four other atoms or radicals. This leads to enormous variations of chemical combination.

15. The proteins are not acidic because the acid (carboxyl) groups of the amino acid are used up to form the peptide bonds.

CHAPTER 3

2. The correct form is: "The famous bacterium *E. coli*."

5. The modern nomenclature establishes *meter* as the basic unit of measurement and uses prefixes for multiples of fractions. The older term *micron* was used as a basic unit, even though it was in fact a fraction of a meter. I recall using the word *millimicron* for one-thousandth of a micron. We now use the word *nanometer*.

9. You will receive an order of mushrooms because the Italian *fungi* (Italian pronunciation "foon-gee") translates to "mushroom."

13. Contrary to the belief of many, oil does not increase the magnification of the light microscope. It merely allows the gathering of enough light to make using the instrument possible. The magnification would be the same without the oil, but the resolution would be much reduced.

15. A class of artists or pseudoartists could have a field day with this project. Imagine all the shapes taken by protozoa, bacteria, fungi, algae, and the rest, and a rather diverse group of "patrons" would emerge. I am reminded of the famous bar scene in *Star Wars*.

CHAPTER 4

1. Various advantages derive from being able to form a spore, capsule, or flagellum. The answers may help you to see that the bacterium's life is not dramatically different than that of other creatures.

5. Boiling may kill the majority of bacteria, but bacterial spores survive 2 hours or more of boiling. It is wrong to believe the water is sterile after a few minutes of boiling. It has been disinfected, however, and is perfectly safe to drink under normal circumstances.

9. In the pre-electron microscope days, the chapter on bacterial anatomy would probably be very brief. Certainly there would be no discussion of pili, plasmids, magnetosomes, ribosomes, or the fluid mosaic model.

13. Bacteria may produce toxins that interfere with metabolic patterns in the body. Thus, the physical growth of bacteria may not be a necessary prerequisite to disease, but consuming food that contains toxins may be dangerous.

15. The stem *methano-* refers to "methane-loving" and *-halophilus* refers to "salt-loving." See the section on archaeobacteria for the conditions under which these organisms live.

CHAPTER 5

1. The cartoon in question appeared in a syndicated newspaper and was authored by Athelstan Spilhaus, former President of the AIBS. Spilhaus probably conjectured that the cellulose of newspapers would be broken down to units of glucose. The glucose would be metabolized by bacteria into metabolic intermediates which would then be converted to amino acids by adding amino groups to carbon skeletons in a reversal of deamination. The amino acids are fed to cattle, which would combine them to produce proteins.

6. One reason ATP is not supplied to the growth medium is that it probably could not be absorbed into the cytoplasm of a bacterial cell. You should speculate on other possible reasons.

8. A science fiction writer could have a field day with a story about how chlorophyll was altered and photosynthesis stopped on Earth. Perhaps you might like to try your hand at such a story.

10. You should recognize the *flavin* part of riboflavin and guess that it is used to make flavin adenine dinucleotide (FAD). Here is an example of how recognizing word stems helps one to make an intelligent guess. Without FAD, oxidative phosphorylation grinds to a halt, energy production ceases, and death is imminent.

15. This incident actually happened to me. I began writing at 9:00 A.M. and did not finish until 5:00 P.M. Essentially, the answer summarizes the chapter by showing how carbohydrates, fats, and proteins are digested and synthesized, and how the processes relate to one another. It is an excellent exercise in metabolism.

CHAPTER 6

1. Some ingenuity is required to explain genetic transformation as observed by Griffith in 1928. You might begin by assuming that a mistake was made and guessing how Griffith eliminated this possibility. From there, you will have to let your intuition work overtime.

4. Arguments can be offered for any of the three processes to be most common. For example, transformation might be common because local debris from dead bacteria is often encountered, but the ability of DNA to pass through the recipient's wall and membrane would mitigate against a high incidence of transformation. Pluses and minuses likewise exist for the other two types.

7. Several discoveries in this chapter have opened doors to other discoveries. Some examples: Avery's pointing to DNA as the transforming material; Berg's synthesis of a recombinant DNA molecule; Lederberg's work with conjugation. You should pick out other discoveries and understand why they were pivotal.

11. The label "second Industrial Revolution" has been widely applied to the development of genetic engineering, and to many observers, the label is justified because the process yields products that cannot be manufactured by other means. The manufacture of insulin, interferon, vaccines, and other products cited in the chapter are examples. Chapter 26 outlines multiple other offshoots of the process and delineates numerous products.

13. Why genetic variation exists in influenza viruses depends on the segments of RNA that make up the genome, but it is also conceivable that during replication, the viruses may acquire fragments of host

DNA, as in generalized transduction, and express these bits of DNA as new antigens unrecognized by circulating antibodies.

CHAPTER 7

1. Probably the most important factor was the introduction of the vaccine in 1887. Other factors might have been a strong surveillance system, the willingness of doctors to report cases, the establishment of a case definition to ensure that reports were accurate, using tests to assess continued vaccine effectiveness, and the willingness of public health departments to spend the necessary funds to help the eradication effort. Can you suggest any other public health measures that might have been used?

3. This question assumes that a pathogen is in an advantageous condition, a situation with which you might take issue. Perhaps the virus places the bacillus in a difficult position because pathogenicity is not always desirable, especially after the host dies. On the other hand, the virus permits active growth in the tissues, a situation not possible without the toxin.

4. This is a tough one, and I wouldn't be surprised if you didn't guess correctly. At the turn of the century, people believed that microorganisms hid in corners, so they built this hospital with rounded edges, carefully avoiding any corners. It was actually one of the first attempts at preventive medicine.

12. It would probably be a good idea to change the name to avoid confusion with the influenza virus. One choice is *Haemophilus meningitidis*. Perhaps you can come up with a more novel name.

14. Modern microbiological discoveries are the fruits of labor of many investigators, so it is unlikely that one or two will be immortalized in a common bacterial name. However, part of the scientific name may honor an investigator. For example, *Borrelia burgdorferi*, the Lyme disease spirochete, is named for Willy Burgdorfer, the investigator who isolated the spirochete from the tick in the early 1980s.

CHAPTER 8

8. This actually happened to me some years ago. I had intended to show how soilborne organisms contaminate food and cause the can to swell. A colleague pointed out that I would probably be cultivating *Clostridium botulinum* from the soil and asked whether I wanted to expose students to this organism. I cancelled the experiment.

11. Chickens and other forms of poultry may be infected with *Salmonella* serotypes. Evidence of this problem is often difficult to ascertain, and poultry manufacturers may unknowingly send infected chickens off to market. If the chicken is cut up on a carving board, the *Salmonella* cells can be deposited there and picked up by the salad ingredients. Old wooden carving boards are a particular problem because of numerous cracks and fissures. Thorough cooking kills the *Salmonella* in the poultry, but the salad is eaten raw and is a source of live bacteria. In this situation, the salad should be prepared before the chicken is cut up if the same carving board is used.

12. The public health official is probably asking a bit much to expect that doctors will recognize botulism symptoms. With about 50 cases per year, botulism is quite rare in the United States, and doctors who deal with botulism will probably be seeing their first and last case. Usually there is little to distinguish botulism from paralysis-associated disease such as a stroke. When the eating history of the patient is examined, however, the possibility of botulism arises.

13. The disease was brucellosis. All recovered and returned to work. The health department also made several recommendations to prevent further outbreaks, including the use of rubber gloves, face shields, and negative air pressure on the floor.

14. My knee-jerk reaction would be to select the frozen hamburger because there would be less opportunity for staphylococci or other bacteria to grow during the past 2 days. However, if you cooked the hamburgers for equal amounts of time, the frozen one would absorb less heat than the fresh one, and fewer internal bacteria would be destroyed. Therefore, the fresh one might be safer.

CHAPTER 9

2. The medical upheaval was bubonic plague. The town marks the farthest reach of the vast graveyard that the suburbs of London became after the plague.

9. Good-quality boots, preferably hip length, would be a wise suggestion.

12. The numerous soilborne diseases discussed in the chapter provide ample possibilities. Certainly tetanus and gas gangrene must be prime candidates for serious disease, but the list can also include anthrax, melioidosis, and leptospirosis. Since each disease has a different pathology, you should explore how each can be deadly in warfare.

13. When leaves and debris pile at the curbside, soilborne arthropods flourish, including ticks that commonly occur on grass and leaves. A child's chance playing in the leaves may bring it in contact with the ticks, and any of the three diseases indicated may follow.

15. Lice transmit typhus. Therefore, by reducing the louse population via head shaving, the people also reduced the opportunity for transfer of the rickettsiae of typhus. Accumulations of lice eggs are called nits. In past generations, nits were so common in the hair that people would habitually pick them out, a practice that resulted in the common expression "nit-picking."

CHAPTER 10

3. Impetigo is a skin disease often caused by staphylococci and occurring most commonly among children. Children tend to have more contact with one another during the summer months than during any other time of the year, and the skin is often unclothed at this time.

5. During douching, fluid is forcibly expelled into the vaginal tract to cleanse it. The fluid can force microorganisms in the vaginal tract up into the uterus and/or Fallopian tubes, where infection can occur. Pelvic inflammatory disease (PID) may result.

8. I can see pluses and minuses in this method. What do you think?

11. Organizations that help control the spread of leprosy point out that "leprosy" is a pejorative term and should be replaced by "Hansen's disease." This will probably take many years to accomplish, in view of the long history of leprosy. You might wish to focus on the modern methods for the detection and treatment of leprosy, and indicate that many diseases pose a greater threat to life. Thousands of leprosy patients are treated at centers throughout the U.S., often on an outpatient basis.

15. The disease is dental caries. You may be surprised that caries has a disease connotation, but a close look reveals that dental caries fulfills the prerequisites for an infectious disease.

CHAPTER 11

2. The concept certainly seems to be true. Then again, are viruses "organisms" or replicating entities that possess one but not all the properties of a living thing? And is "much" of their behavior or "all" of their behavior directed toward reproduction? And is it really "reproduction" as we generally mean the term? What do you think? Can you rephrase the concept to better suit the virus?

8. For bacterial disease, it is treatment; for viral disease, it is prevention. Think of all the vaccines available for various viral diseases, and compare that number with the limited number available for bacterial diseases.

11. It's simple—"prion" sounds better than "proin."

13. Dmitri Iwanowski did not discover viruses; he merely showed that something smaller than a bacterium was capable of causing disease. At the time it was a momentous discovery, because bacteria were believed to be the ultimate in simplicity. Iwanowski pointed out that a *filterable* virus caused tobacco mosaic disease. His key word was *filterable*, to show that whatever the agent was, it was able to pass through a filter that trapped bacteria.

15. Reproduction has a connotation in biology that implies the generation of new individuals by asexual or sexual processes. Although new individuals are generated in viral replication, the process is neither asexual nor sexual, but a completely separate process seen nowhere else in biology. Hence, virologists prefer "replicate" to "reproduce."

CHAPTER 12

2. Here is what transpired: Twice-daily reports were collected from delegations on whether any members had measles symptoms. All visitors to medical stations were observed for measles symptoms. Letters were sent to all participants, volunteers, and staff advising them of the situation and the control measures, signs, and symptoms. Daily telephone calls were made to all local hospital emergency rooms. State health departments of the competition participants were notified of the outbreak. Can you think of anything the epidemiologists missed? (P.S. No additional cases occurred.)

5. Children are easier to reach at 15 months for immunization, but after 20 years or so, the immunity has probably worn thin. By contrast, teenagers may be harder to reach and certify for immunization, but the level of immunity will be much higher. Additional discussion can lead from here. Avoiding common cold viruses effectively can be accomplished by several means: Keep hands away from the eyes; wash hands often; use disposable tissues, rather than handkerchiefs to cover coughs; and avoid people with colds. You should add to this list with other imaginative aproaches.

11. The evidence points to chickenpox. (You may notice that I use "chickenpox" as one word. This is for consistency with smallpox and cowpox, both of which are conventionally written as single words.)

12. It will certainly lead to a smelly shoe. It will also stop people from coming too close to you, which will decrease your possibility of coming in contact with disease organisms. Chapter 22 has a box on garlic that you might enjoy reading.

13. The incident helps prove that the agents of disease are transmissible. Pasteur and his supporters were right on target.

CHAPTER 13

4. Care to be a part of history? Then watch the continuing battle to eradicate polio from the world. Four strategies have been employed: (a) maintaining high vaccine coverage among children with at least three doses of oral vaccine; (b) developing sensitive systems of sur-veillance; (c) administering supplementary doses of vaccine during National Immunization Days; (d) instituting "mopping-up" vaccine campaigns in high-risk areas where wild polio virus is believed to exist.

9. Incidents such as these are the bane of laboratory instructors. The dangers that come to mind include AIDS and hepatitis B, but a case can be made for numerous other dangers such as staphylococcal disease. At this juncture, you might like to consider whether the pretreatment with alcohol is an effective safeguard against disease transfer.

12. Certainly, you should accept the offer. In fact if you work in any profession where blood is encountered (health-care or laboratory worker, mortician, police officer, corrections officer, fire-fighter), you should consider obtaining a hepatitis B immunization. Ask around. Your hospital, doctor's office, school, or other employer may offer it as a perk.

13. This is a palindrome, a phrase that can be read forward or backward. It is a unique palindrome because the only vowel used is A. Another palindrome you might find interesting is one that reflects the dilemma of Napoleon: ABLE WAS I ERE I SAW ELBA. This palindrome is a rare perfect palindrome because each word can be reversed.

15. Disease reflects a competition between host and parasite. If the parasite overcomes the body defenses, disease ensues; but if the body defenses overcome the parasite, the latter is driven away. In each case, the parasite and defenses compete until one wins out. AIDS is dramatically different. HIV eliminates body defenses by destroying portions of the body's immune system. Left defenseless, the body is subjected to marauding parasites in the form of opportunistic microorganisms. Few other diseases take this approach.

CHAPTER 14

3. There are several possible reasons for the small number of intestinal diseases of fungal origin. Perhaps the spores are destroyed by stomach acid, or perhaps intestinal nutrients for fungal growth are lacking, or perhaps receptor sites for tissue attachment are not present, or perhaps the oxygen supply is limited. Discussions like these are valuable because they help you focus on the requirements for infection to take place.

7. This student has an intriguing idea. The chitin will encourage chitin-digesting bacteria to emerge, and she may then isolate them to develop a natural fungicide.

8. A pizza with mushrooms.

10. Lots of luck.

12. It will be interesting to see which pronunciation your instructor prefers. I learned the second pronunciation and thought it was the only one until my colleagues told me about the other pronunciations. I suspect they evolved from various attempts to pronounce the word as it was written.

CHAPTER 15

3. The British found they could improve the taste of quinine by mixing it with gin. The drink came to be their "gin and tonic."

7. It will probably depend on whether the residents have suffered from intestinal disease due to protozoa. The residents of Milwaukee, Wisconsin, would probably favor a proposal, but other taxpayers would probably reject it until they experienced such an epidemic.

8. This is quite a bold statement, but it reflects the fact that dirty diapers are as capable of transmitting infectious disease as the open sewers of generations ago. Day-care center workers should take special note.

10. As the borders of Rome expanded, Romans ventured into far-off lands where mosquitoes thrived and where the malaria parasite was prevalent. Infected Romans probably brought the disease back to Rome, and the mosquito populations of the aqueducts and pools propagated the parasite and spread the disease.

11. Here's an example of how a name can reveal much: *Entamoeba histolytica* means intestinal-amoeba (*Entamoeba*) that digests (*lytic*) tissue (*histo-*). The amoeba lives in the intestine where it penetrates the tissue. Tissue penetration yields sharp appendicitis-like pain as the nerves are encountered and blood as the blood vessels are reached. We therefore expect bloody stools and sharp pain. For diagnosis, the physician will ask for a stool specimen (intestine) and the laboratory technician will hunt for amoebas. Transmission will probably be by fecal contamination of food or water.

CHAPTER 16

2. On a global scale, diseases as these "impede national and individual development, make fertile land inhospitable, impair intellectual and physical growth, and exact a huge cost in treatment and control programs." Solutions are straightforward: Develop new drugs, vaccines, diagnostic tests, and control methods. Can you suggest any novel approaches?

6. This question illustrates how knowing the stems of scientific words helps decipher their meaning. *Diphyllobothrium latum* is a very thin, broad tapeworm. It is associated with insanitary water, which the worm enters via human feces.

10. The threadlike body may have been an eyeworm, and the warmth of the fire may have brought it to the surface. A figure in this chapter portrays an eyeworm in the eye.

13. Improved sanitation methods would reduce mosquito populations and decrease the possibility of transmitting *Wuchereria*. By contrast, clearing forest lands for agriculture and installing drainage ditches would encourage mosquito populations and increase the possibility for filariasis. Now it's your turn to continue the comparisons.

15. The concept of studying parasitology to appreciate the web of life is intriguing and worthy of note. Hundreds of thousands of individuals are infected with multicellular parasites. The relationship is benign in huge numbers of cases but parasitical in many others, as this chapter shows. Perhaps a geographical summary of the parasites might help you appreciate how worldwide the parasites are.

CHAPTER 17

1. Consider how many people have handled a stamp and the conditions under which it was stored before it comes to you. Then think about whether you would want to place it in your mouth.

4. The salad bar remains one of the most common possibilities for disease transmission in the restaurant business. You should discuss how to limit microbial transmission by the chilling of foods, the selection of foods to be offered at the salad bar, the thorough washing of foods, cautions to patrons, the turnover of foods, the disinfection of salad bar areas, dust control, and other means.

7. This incident happened to me in 1982. At the emergency room, I was given a "tetanus shot," a preparation of tetanus toxoid to induce my immune system to produce tetanus antitoxins. These antitoxins would protect me against tetanus toxins, since tetanus spores had probably entered the wound from the soil.

12. Can you imagine how many people have handled a dollar bill before it gets into your hands? Wetting the fingers before touching the dollar bill brings whatever was on the bill into your mouth.

14. Few people realize how many bacteria are present under the fingernails. When the fingers are brought to the mouth, infection can take place. In a day-care center (or any situation) where fecal matter or blood or tissue is contacted, it is a good idea to brush under the fingernails regularly.

CHAPTER 18

2. Begin with the chemical signals that stimulate phagocytosis, and go from there. Remember that the heart and other organs are constantly "at work" but that the immune system lies at rest until it receives a signal to act. The signal can be an epitope; other signals are MHC molecules, interleukins, and antibody molecules.

6. Here is another intriguing possibility for microbiology research. The obvious advantage is freedom from tooth decay, but many problems must be solved. Is *S. mutans* the only agent of caries? Could the immune system be stimulated to produce enough IgA for protection? Would the IgA be delivered to and survive in the oral cavity? Would new organisms emerge as caries agents? Could IgA be used in a mouthwash or toothpaste?

7. The cockroach does appear to have an immune system, and the system apparently is a factor in its ability to survive. Far from being immunologically primitive, as suspected, the arthropods are able to produce antibodylike proteins. The next steps would be to identify and characterize these substances. How would you continue the experiments?

14. You can have a field day with this one. Would you write a letter correcting the statement?

15. You are encouraged to exercise imagination on your trip and consider the perils of phagocytosis, mechanical barriers, lysozyme, T-lymphocytes, and other protective measures in the body. An appreciation for resistance mechanisms should evolve from this discussion.

CHAPTER 19

1. In herd immunity, the immunizing agent can be spread in numerous ways. For example, day-care workers changing the diaper of a child recently immunized against polio may pick up the viruses on

their fingertips and inoculate themselves and other children they contact. Body secretions, such as saliva and respiratory droplets, may spread measles, mumps, or rubella viruses from children who recently received the MMR vaccine. These examples may serve as a starting point for the discussion.

4. The approach would seem favorable. In effect, the woman is being used as an "immunological factory" to produce antibodies for her newborn as well as herself. I cannot think of any negative effects other than the normal hazard of using a vaccine.

5. It would seem to be a good idea, but it will take lots of money to implement. And the willingness for the American taxpayer to part with the funds will depend in part on how serious the threat of disease is perceived to be. You should continue the debate from here.

7. With some insight and imagination, a case can be made for each type of immunity as being safest to obtain. Similarly, reasons may be offered for each type as being most helpful. Discussions such as these put immunity into perspective and help you make choices supported by what you have learned. Ultimately, I would think that the individual situation would dictate the choice.

14. Keeping a body alive for vaccine production is certainly possible, but the ethical implications must be considered. Strong arguments can be made pro and con. You may wish to set up a debate panel on a topic such as this one.

CHAPTER 20

3. Formaldehyde used for preservation of the animals is probably causing a contact dermatitis. The sensitivity began to develop during the first two exposures, and now, during the third exposure, it is manifesting itself. Rubber gloves would be helpful for protecting the hands.

7. The "he" is William J. Clinton; the condition is hay fever.

8. Athlete's foot usually occurs between the toes, while contact dermatitis occurs where the foot comes in contact with the shoe. Laboratory testing will reveal fungal cells if the condition is athlete's foot, but no cells if it is dermatitis. A patch test can be performed by the allergist to determine if a contact allergy exists.

11. The major histocompatibility complex codes for histocompatibility molecules, which exist on the cell surface. Over 50 versions of each gene have already been discovered, and the number of gene combinations and

histocompatibility molecules is enormous. Immunologically, there is probably no one else like you.

15. It is interesting to question whether the immune system is actually protecting the body during immune disorders. Allergies can be interpreted as protective mechanisms for ridding the body of antigens, and the theory can be extended to other types of hypersensitivity, as well as to transplants and tumors. Autoimmune diseases stand in stark contrast because the body appears to be attacking itself. An oxymoron is two terms that do not fit together (the dictionary definition is "two mutually exclusive juxtaposed words"). "Immune disorder" appears to be an oxymoron because *immune* means "free of" and a disorder is a problem. Therefore, how can you have a problem that you don't have? (For another oxymoron, see the MicroFocus on the enormous bacterium in Chapter 3.)

CHAPTER 21

3. A suspicious person might inquire what will happen within 30 days. Will spontaneous generation take place? Is it possible that the contents were sterilized at the manufacturing plant, but that the porous container is now permitting airborne microorganisms to enter? If so, then the product was once sterilized but is now contaminated, and evidence of contamination will appear by the expiration date.

4. Broiling of meat is done at extremely high heat. This heat would kill any surface organisms rapidly, and the meat would be safe for consumption.

10. In the laboratory, the Bunsen burner is used to sterilize loops, needles, and the tips of tubes and flasks. Some imagination might be needed to identify other uses.

12. Milk's taste apparently changes as the temperature becomes too high. Also, the protein will coagulate. The butterfat is another problem, because it will not pass through a filter. Recall that milk is a suspension rather than a true solution. A fruitful discussion could take place on the economic implications of a useful sterilization method for milk.

14. The autoclave is undoubtedly the first word to come to mind when we think of "sterilizer." However, the autoclave is merely a pressurized steam apparatus that can be used to achieve sterilization only under specific conditions. Unless these conditions are established in the machine, sterilization is not assured. Therefore, it would be incorrect to believe that "autoclave" and "sterilizer" are synonymous words.

CHAPTER 22

1. In selecting a laboratory disinfectant or sanitizing agent, it would be advisable to ask whether the agent was bactericidal or bacteriostatic under the desired conditions. Inquiry should also be made about its toxicity, solubility in water, shelf life, use in diluted form, penetrating ability, corrosiveness, temperature and pH of use, and cost. Many other avenues of inquiry are noted in the chapter.

4. Chlorhexidine is often used by dentists during treatments, but this chemical has not yet made its way into toothpastes. The up side is that it may reduce periodontal problems by reducing bacterial populations. The down side is that over a long period of time, the chemical may prove toxic to the tissues. Can you add to the list?

7. Some ways of reducing the spread of microorganisms in day-care centers are the disinfection of tabletops used for diaper changes, regular furniture and toy disinfection, and hand-washing and the use of an antiseptic after each diaper change. You should suggest other methods that are practical and useful.

9. *Bacteriostatic* is an adjective derived from the noun *bacteriostasis*. The adjective means essentially the same as the noun coined by Churchman; it applies to an agent that inhibits the further growth of bacteria without necessarily destroying them.

13. This advertisement was a nightmare. Some questions that occurred to me: Why wipe down or dunk a raw chicken? It's the inside that's a problem, not the outside—the cooking heat will take care of the outside. Why clean a raw pepper with Clorox? The skin is so smooth that ordinary water will probably wash away anything that's a problem. Why worry about the outsides of carrots? I always thought you peeled carrots before cooking them. Clean a red onion? Gimme a break! Exactly how big is a sinkful? And why worry about being so precise about the amount of Clorox (⅛ cup) when you have no idea of the sink size? Can you spot the other problems? How about ". . . germs and bacteria"; "salmonella . . ."; "*like* chicken . . ."?

CHAPTER 23

1. Pasteur and Joubert were probably observing the effects of an antibiotic produced by the contaminating microorganisms. It is clear that the concept of antibiosis was known over 100 years ago. You might enjoy speculating whether Pasteur and Joubert envisioned a therapeutic compound in the mixture of bacteria.

4. Sounds like an interesting idea. What do you think?

5. The arrival of antibiotics and modern medical practices in Nepal typifies how medical advances can disrupt the lives of a population. With more mouths to feed, forests had to be cleared, and great pressure was placed in preparing the land for crops. Living space soon became a premium, and natural resources, such as water supplies, were tapped to their limit. Greater populations also meant greater sanitation problems and, consequently, more opportunity for the spread of disease. Discussions such as these help us understand the negative aspects of medical advances.

8. Here are some origins of antibiotic names: Erythromycin is named after *Streptomyces erythraeus,* a red-pigmented actinomycete that produces it; tetracycline is named for the four benzene rings found in the molecule; and nystatin is named for New York State because it was discovered at the Department of Health laboratory in New York. The use of a dictionary, along with some imagination, should help reveal the origins of other antibiotic names in this chapter.

15. The antibiotic issue is one that can be argued for hours. Perhaps this might be a good question for a debate panel. Side effects, the emergence of antibiotic-resistant bacteria, the effect on human population growth, and human dependence on antibiotics would stimulate the anti-antibiotic side. The misery and death from disease, rising food costs, job impact in the pharmaceutical industry, and generally better quality of life might be discussed by the pro-antibiotic side.

CHAPTER 24

3. The correct sequence would be to prepare the salad before the chicken. *Salmonella* serotypes may be present in the chicken, and cross-contamination to the salad may take place. Cooking will eliminate *Salmonella* in chicken, but salad is eaten raw and is potentially dangerous. You should explore other precautions. A thorough cleaning of the knife and cutting board is a good place to begin.

5. This is another example of truth being stranger than fiction. The incident occurred as described, and the baked potato was superb. (I had it with crab cakes and a veggie.) The sour cream was preserved primarily by the acid present, and no symptoms of food poisoning or any other intestinal illness developed in the following days. This incident points up that the expiration date is merely a statistical guess on when the product will look or taste bad. It is not necessarily the date on which the product will begin posing a peril to health.

10. Some examples to ponder: Custard egg products, ice cream, fresh mayonnaise, meat loaf mixtures, many sauces, prepared cheese products, and on and on.

13. The calves liver would probably be the better choice because it will spoil more rapidly than the steak. Liver is an organ meat, with a looser tissue consistency and richer blood supply than muscle tissue. Contamination is therefore more probable in the liver.

CHAPTER 25

1. This idea of connecting storm and sanitary sewers was a poor one because it resulted in a huge body of water where storm runoff polluted sanitary waste, and vice versa. Separation probably would have made handling the waste considerably easier. However, you might present arguments for connecting the systems, the most obvious argument being the economic benefit.

5. Summertime pollution can be traced to many factors in addition to those cited: Animals are more active during the summer, and they tend to drink from and defecate in the water; summer thunderstorms cause substantial soil runoff of organisms from animal remains; bathers introduce intestinal organisms to the water; algae invade the water, inducing fish kills and bacterial growth during decomposition; and the heat, especially in a stagnant bay, leads to bacterial proliferation.

9. The presence of high coliform counts indicated that the water had been contaminated with sewage and that typhoid fever, bacterial dysentery, amoebiasis, hepatitis, or other serious diseases were imminent. Certainly the danger was equivalent to that posed by Legionnaires' disease.

12. The grass is greener over the septic tank because the organic-rich water flowing from it provides a natural lawn fertilizer. In the wintertime, the hot water from a cesspool or septic tank warms the soil and melts the snow over it. To locate a cesspool or septic tank in climates that have snow, one need only watch to see where the snow melts first.

13. The carbon, sulfur, and nitrogen cycles provide irrefutable evidence of the roles that microorganisms play in enhancing the quality of life. It is instructive to try and imagine a world where no microorganisms are available to recycle these elements.

CHAPTER 26

1. By the time you reach Chapter 26, you should have a firm understanding of how microorganisms contribute to the quality of life. Examples abound in this chapter. Combined with examples from Chapters 24 and 25, they are a formidable list that should help you see the positive roles of microorganisms in our lives.

3. You should explore a variety of industrial processes and identify useful end-products. Some examples might be waste from meat-packing plants and petroleum processes, wood by-products from paper manufacturing, residue from food-canning operations, and sewage-treatment end-products.

9. This is an intriguing question similar to that proposed for lactobacilli and streptococci in yogurt (Chapter 24). You might speculate about what factors might be necessary to establish pathogenicity in the yeast. The question also illustrates how we consume microorganisms regularly without a thought of dangerous consequences.

10. Why so much vitamin? Perhaps a defect in the enzyme system prevents the metabolism of the vitamin to the next step. Perhaps the organisms live in a symbiotic or synergistic relationship with other organisms that utilize the vitamin. As Pearlman suggests in the Note to the Student: "There are no stupid microorganisms."

16. The story on the inside back cover has been with me for years. Originally it involved cholera, a dervish, and the city of Baghdad. The idea is simple: An understanding of microorganisms can reduce the fear of microorganisms and enable individuals to better cope with disease. In writing this book, one of my hopes was that you would come to know the microorganisms and understand the role they play in disease. Fear arising from ignorance can be a terrifying experience. I trust that you have acquired sufficient knowledge to help dispel some of the fear.

Appendix D: Answers to Review Questions

CHAPTER 1

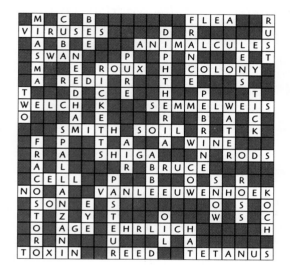

CHAPTER 2

1. IONIC 2. ORGANIC 3. HYDROGEN
4. GLUCOSE 5. FATS 6. ENZYMES
7. NUCLEOTIDES 8. PRIMARY 9. DEHYDRA-
TION 10. ACIDITY 11. ELEMENT 12. ISOTOPES
13. CARBOXYL 14. MALTOSE 15. HYDROGEN

CHAPTER 3

1. G 2. T 3. K 4. L 5. X 6. U 7. N 8. W 9. D 10. A
11. V 12. C 13. P 14. F 15. O 16. I 17. B 18. J 19. Z
20. Q

CHAPTER 4

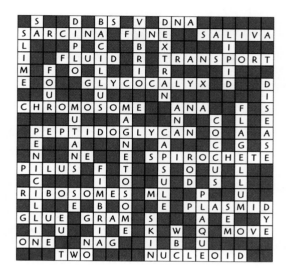

CHAPTER 5

1. metabolism; digestion; catabolism 2. protein;
speed up; substrate 3. glycolysis; energy; ATP
4. fermentation; oxygen; glucose; alcohol 5. electrons;
cytochromes; energy; ATP 6. pyruvic acid; carbon;
carbon dioxide; NAD 7. amino; amino; deamination
8. carbon dioxide; photosynthesis; glucose 9. chemical reactions; carbohydrates; *Nitrosomonas*
10. genetic; DNA; mRNA; transcription 11. ribosome; anticodon; an amino acid 12. repressor;
operator; structural

CHAPTER 6

1. PLASMIDS 2. SEXDUCTION 3. MUTATION
4. SALMONELLA 5. COMPETENCE 6. FERTILITY
7. BACTERIOPHAGE 8. ENDONUCLEASE
9. PNEUMOCOCCUS 10. PILI 11. LYSOGENY
12. CHIMERA 13. LIGASE 14. INTERFERON
15. TRANSPOSON 16. GRIFFITH 17. CONJUGA-
TION 18. MUTAGEN 19. VIRULENT 20. CHRO-
MOSOME

CHAPTER 7

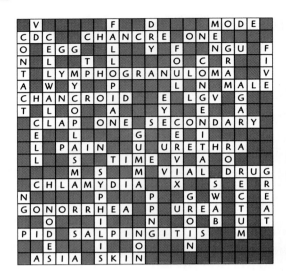

CHAPTER 8

1. ANTITOXIN 2. CHOLERA 3. UNDULANT
4. DYSENTERY 5. ROSE 6. STAPHYLOCOCCAL
7. CHICKENS 8. CARRIERS 9. NEGATIVE
10. CEREUS 11. CAMPYLOBACTER 12. ABORTION 13. PARALYSIS 14. NOSE 15. ACID
16. FLUID 17. RARE 18. VIBRIO 19. SALMONELLA 20. HEAT 21. ANAEROBIC 22. STOOL
23. SEAFOOD 24. MILK 25. ANIMALS

CHAPTER 9

1. G 2. B 3. K 4. L 5. O 6. N 7. C 8. J 9. M 10. G
11. A 12. N 13. L 14. F 15. I 16. A 17. G 18. E
19. M 20. C 21. L 22. F 23. B 24. M 25. G

CHAPTER 10

CHAPTER 11

1. CAPSID 2. HELIX 3. BACTERIOPHAGE
4. ANTIBODIES 5. NEGRI 6. ACYCLOVIR
7. INTERFERON 8. ATTENUATED 9. VIROID
10. TUMOR 11. ULTRAVIOLET 12. ONCOGENE
13. RECEPTOR 14. ICOSAHEDRON 15. GENOME
16. ENDERS 17. VIRION 18. LYSOGENY
19. AMANTADINE 20. ENVELOPE 21. STANLEY
22. FORMALDEHYDE 23. PRION 24. CAPSOMERES 25. INACTIVATED

CHAPTER 12

1. RNA; icosahedral; nose; mild 2. contact; blisters; emotional stress; acyclovir 3. in crops; teardrops; shingles; red; painful 4. measles; a skin rash; airborne droplets 5. Reye's; testes; orchitis; liver; SSPE
6. measles; Koplik spots; mouth; red rash 7. fifth, B19; parvovirus; DNA virus 8. airborne droplets; mumps; salivary 9. smallpox; cowpox; Jenner
10. influenza; vaccine; bacteria 11. RNA; lungs; children; clump together; syncytia 12. papilloma viruses; sexual contact; molluscum contagiosum 13. DNA; granules; common colds; eye; meninges 14. icosahedral; million; thin; weeks; stress 15. infectious; transplacental passage; newborns; rubella; herpes simplex 16. attenuated; children; long-term; measles; mumps; German measles

CHAPTER 13

1. F (RNA) 2. F (*Pneumocystis carinii*) 3. True
4. True 5. F (intestine) 6. True 7. F (rabies) 8. True
9. F (lymphocyte) 10. True 11. True 12. F (gastroenteritis) 13. F (eyes) 14. True 15. True 16. True
17. F (polio) 18. F (retrovirus) 19. F (Coxsackie)
20. True 21. F (liver) 22. F (inactivated viruses)
23. F (rotavirus) 24. True 25. True 26. F (infectious
mononucleosis) 27. F (high) 28. F (hantaviruses)
29. F (ctyomegalovirus) 30. F (arm)

CHAPTER 14

1. I 2. Q 3. W 4. M 5. K 6. U 7. A 8. S 9. C 10. E
11. P 12. S 13. U 14. G 15. O 16. Q 17. B 18. P
19. H 20. M 21. S 22. Z 23. M 24. K 25. P

CHAPTER 15

CHAPTER 16

1. a, b 2. c 3. a, c 4. c 5. a, b, c 6. b 7. a, c 8. a 9. b
10. a, b, c 11. a 12. a, b 13. c 14. b, c 15. c

CHAPTER 17

1. F (endemic) 2. True 3. True 4. F (infection) 5. F
(liver) 6. True 7. F (low) 8. F (acme) 9. F (mechanical) 10. True 11. F (carrier) 12. F (antitoxins)
13. True 14. F (coagulase) 15. True 16. True 17. F
(direct) 18. True 19. F (acute) 20. F (incubation)

CHAPTER 18

CHAPTER 19

1. innate, acquired 2. active; passive 3. measles;
mumps; rubella 4. diphtheria; pertussis, tetanus
5. natural; artificial 6. alum; mineral oil 7. hyperimmune serum; antiserum 8. IgG; IgM; IgA, IgE
9. transplacental passage; breast feeding 10. labored
breathing; swollen joints 11. capsule polysaccharides,
pilus protein 12. hepatitis B; foot-and-mouth disease
13. genetic factors; physiological factors; biochemical
factors 14. inactivated; attenuated 15. diphtheria;
tetanus 16. injection; oral consumption; nasal spray
17. gastrointestinal; respiratory 18. hepatitis B; chickenpox 19. therapy; prophylaxis 20. tetanus; diphtheria

CHAPTER 20

1. HISTAMINE 2. DIGEORGE 3. INDURATION
4. JOINTS 5. GRAVES 6. CYTOTOXIC 7. ATOPIC
8. ANTIGEN 9. PLASMA 10. TUBERCULOSIS
11. BASOPHILS 12. LYSIS 13. POSITIVE
14. KIDNEY 15. MHC 16. RASH 17. AUTOIM-
MUNE 18. CELLULAR 19. FACE 20. SMOOTH

CHAPTER 21

1. AUTOCLAVE 2. MEMBRANE 3. POWDER
4. DENATURATION 5. TYNDALL 6. DRYING
7. ULTRASONIC 8. GAMMA 9. SPORE
10. OXIDATION 11. PRESSURE 12. THIRTY
13. HOLDING 14. INSTRUMENTS 15. DIATOMS

16. ULTRAVIOLET 17. PLASTIC 18. TOXINS
19. SOLIDS 20. OSMOSIS 21. MICROWAVES
22. BACILLUS 23. BUNSEN 24. CLEANING
25. TUBERCULOSIS

CHAPTER 22

1. F 2. B 3. J 4. I 5. C 6. D 7. A 8. K 9. N 10. E
11. A 12. C 13. J 14. E 15. I 16. C 17. J 18. I 19. B
20. E 21. K 22. F 23. K 24. F 25. C

CHAPTER 23

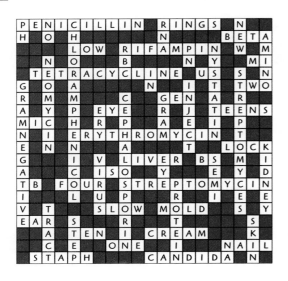

CHAPTER 24

1. SALMONELLA 2. LACTOBACILLUS
3. CLOSTRIDIUM 4. SERRATIA 5. CHLAMYDIA
6. PROTEUS 7. STREPTOCOCCUS 8. BACILLUS
9. ACETOBACTER 10. LEUCONOSTOC 11. CLAV-
ICEPS 12. CLOSTRIDIUM 13. PSEUDOMONAS
14. ENTEROBACTER 15. ASPERGILLUS

CHAPTER 25

1. a, c 2. b 3. b, c 4. a, b 5. a, b, c 6. a, b 7. b 8. a 9. b,
c 10. a, b 11. a, b, c 12. a, c 13. c 14. b, c 15. b

CHAPTER 26

1. G 2. N 3. H 4. M 5. K 6. O 7. J 8. D 9. P 10. A
11. B 12. Q 13. B 14. R 15. G 16. B 17. C 18. D
19. T 20. A

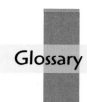

Glossary

This glossary contains concise definitions of approximately 1000 microbiological terms, along with pronunciations where appropriate. The numbers in parentheses indicate the chapters in which the terms are discussed.

A

abscess A circumscribed pus-filled lesion characteristic of staphylococcal skin disease. (10, 18)

abyssal zone The environment at the bottom of oceanic trenches. (25)

acid-fast technique A process in which certain bacteria resist decolorization with acid alcohol after staining with a primary dye. (3)

acidophilus (as´i-dof´i-lus) **milk** Milk in which *Lactobacillus acidophilus* has been cultivated, or milk to which the bacterium has been added. (24)

acquired immune deficiency syndrome (AIDS) A serious viral disease caused by human immunodeficiency virus (HIV) in which the T-lymphocytes are destroyed and opportunistic illnesses occur in the patient. (13)

Actinomyces (ak´ti-no-mi´sēz) *israelii* A Gram-positive funguslike bacterial rod that causes actinomycosis. (10)

actinomycetes (ak´ti-no-mi-se´tēz) A group of soil microorganisms that exhibit funguslike properties when cultivated in the laboratory (23, 25)

actinomycosis An endogenous bacterial disease caused by *Actinomyces israelii*, characterized by draining sinuses of the face and other organs. (10)

acute disease A disease that develops rapidly, exhibits substantial symptoms, and then comes to a climax. (17)

acute necrotizing ulcerative gingivitis (ANUG) A bacterial infection of the mucous membranes in the oral cavity; sometimes called Vincent's angina or trench mouth. (10)

acyclovir (a-si´klo-vir) A drug used as a topical ointment to treat herpes simplex and injected for herpes encephalitis. (11, 12)

adenosine triphosphate (ATP) A molecule that stores energy for use in chemical reactions; 1 mole of ATP liberates 7300 calories of energy when digested to adenosine diphosphate (ADP) and phosphate ions. (5)

adenovirus An icosahedral DNA virus involved in respiratory infections, viral meningitis, and viral conjunctivitis. (12)

adhesin A protein in bacterial pili that assists in attachment to the surface molecules of cells; a binding molecule that encourages parasites to hold firmly to the tissues of their host. (4, 17)

adjuvant (ad´ju-vant) A substance attached to a vaccine component that increases the efficiency of a vaccine. (19)

Aeromonas hydrophila (a´er-o-mo´nas hi-drof´i-lah) A Gram-negative bacterial rod transmitted by food and water and involved in intestinal disease. (8)

aflatoxin (af´lah-tok´sin) A toxin produced by *Aspergillus flavus* that may pass from contaminated grain to humans in grains, milk, or meat products and may induce tumors. (14, 24)

agar (ahg´ar) A derivative of marine seaweed used as a solidifying agent in many microbiological media. (1, 4)

agglutination (ah-gloo´tĭ-na´shun) A type of antigen-antibody reaction that results in visible clumps of organisms or other material. (18, 19)

agranulocytosis (a-gran´u-lo-si-to´sis) The destruction of neutrophils (granulocytes) resulting from the reaction of antibodies with antigens on the neutrophil surface; a type II hypersensitivity reaction. (20)

AIDS *See* acquired immune deficiency syndrome.

alga A plantlike organism that performs photosynthesis; algae differ structurally from mosses, ferns, and seed plants. (3)

alginate (al´gin-ate) A carbohydrate thickening agent used in ice cream, soups, and other foods; industrially produced by microorganisms. (24)

allergen An antigenic substance that stimulates an allergic reaction in the body. (20)

alloantigen A type of antigen that exists in certain but not all members of a given species; examples are the A, B, and Rh antigens in humans. (18)

allograft A tissue graft between two members of the same species, such as between two humans. (20)

alpha-hemolytic streptococci Streptococci that partially destroy red blood cells; when cultivated in blood agar, an olive green color forms around colonies of these streptococci. (7)

amantadine (ah-man´tah-dēn) A synthetic drug thought to block the penetration of influenza viruses to host cells. (11, 12)

Ames test A diagnostic procedure used to detect cancer agents by their ability to cause mutations in *Salmonella* cells. (6)

aminoglycosides (am´ĭno-gli´ko-sīdz) A group of antibiotics that contain amino groups bonded to carbohydrate groups; examples are gentamicin, streptomycin, and neomycin. (23)

amoebiasis (am´e-bi´ah-sis) A protozoal disease of the intestine caused by *Entamoeba histolytica*, transmitted by food and water; characterized by intestinal ulcers and the involvement of multiple internal organs. (15)

amoxicillin (ah-moks´ĭ-sil´in) A semisynthetic penicillin antibiotic related to ampicillin. (23)

amphitrichous (am´fi-trik´us) **bacteria** Bacteria that possess flagella at the opposite poles of the cell. (4)

amphotericin (am´fo-ter´ĭ-sin) **B** An antifungal drug used to treat serious fungal diseases, such as cryptococcosis, histoplasmosis, and blastomycosis. (14, 23)

ampicillin A semisynthetic penicillin derivative active against Gram-positive bacteria and certain Gram-negative bacteria. (23)

anabolism A chemical process involving the synthesis of organic compounds; usually an energy-utilizing process. (5)

anaerobic organism An organism that grows in an atmosphere free of oxygen. (4, 24)

analog A compound closely related to a naturally occurring compound. (11)

anaphylatoxin (an´ah-fĭ´lah-tok´sinz) A chemical substance that initiates a series of events leading to smooth muscle contraction. (18)

anaphylaxis (an´ah-fĭ-lak´sis) A life-threatening allergic reaction in which a series of mediators cause contractions of smooth muscle throughout the body. (20)

Ancylostoma duodenale (an´ki-los´to-mah du-od-in-al´e) A multicellular roundworm parasite of the intestine and other organs, transmitted by moist vegetation; commonly known as the Old World hookworm. (16)

anionic detergent A detergent that yields negatively charged ions in solution. (22)

anorexia (an´o-rek´se-ah) Loss of appetite.

anthrax A serious bacterial disease caused by *Bacillus anthracis*, characterized by severe blood hemorrhaging. Also called woolsorter's disease. (9)

antibiotic A product of the metabolism of a microorganism that is inhibitory to other microorganisms. (23)

antibody A highly specific protein molecule produced by plasma cells in the immune system in response to a specific chemical substance; antibodies function in antibody-mediated immunity. (11, 18, 19)

antibody-mediated immunity A type of immunity arising from the activity of antibodies directed against antigens in the tissues. Also called humoral immunity. (18)

anticodon A three-base sequence on the tRNA molecule that binds to the codon on the mRNA molecule during protein synthesis. (5)

antigen Any chemical substance that elicits a response by the body's immune system. (18)

antigenic determinant A section of an antigen molecule that stimulates a specific response and to which the response is directed; often consists of several amino acids or monosaccharides. Also called epitope. (18)

antigenic variation A process in which chemical changes occur periodically in antigens; known to take place in influenza viruses. (12)

antiglobulin antibody An antibody that reacts with a human antibody. (19)

antiseptic A chemical used to kill pathogenic microorganisms on a living object, such as the surface of the human body. (22)

antiserum Serum that is rich in a particular type or types of antibody. (19)

antitoxin An antibody that circulates in the bloodstream and provides protection against toxins by neutralizing them. (7, 17, 19)

aplastic (a-plas´tik) **anemia** A side effect of chloramphenicol therapy in which red blood cells are produced with little or no hemoglobin. (23)

apicomplexans A group of protozoa whose members contain a number of organelles used for host penetration at one end of the cell; no motion is observed in adult forms of the organisms. Also called sporozoa. (15)

arboviral encephalitis A type of encephalitis caused by a viral agent, transmitted by an arthropod. (13)

Archaea A domain of living things that includes the archaebacteria (archaea). (3)

archaebacteria (ar´ke-bac-tēr´-ē-ah) A group of bacteria believed to be of ancient origin. (4)

arsphenamine (ars-fen´ah-min) An arsenic-phenol compound synthesized by Ehrlich and Hata for use against syphilis spirochetes; the first modern chemotherapeutic agent. (23)

Arthropoda A large phylum of animals having jointed appendages and a segmented body; includes insects, such as lice, mosquitoes, and fleas, and spiderlike arachnids, such as ticks and mites. (17)

arthrospore A fungal spore formed by fragmentation of the hypha. (14)

artificially acquired active immunity Immunity resulting from the production of antibodies in response to antigens in a vaccine or toxoid. (19)

artificially acquired passive immunity Immunity resulting from an exposure to or injection of antibodies. (19)

Ascaris lumbricoides (as´ka-ris lum-bri-koid´ēz) A multicellular roundworm parasite of the intestine, commonly known as the roundworm. (16)

ascomycete (as´ko-mi-se´tē) A member of the fungal division Ascomycota. (14)

Ascomycota A division (phylum) of fungi whose members have septate hyphae and form ascospores within saclike asci, among other notable characteristics. (14)

ascospore A sexually produced spore formed by members of the fungal division Ascomycota. (14)

ascus A saclike structure that contains ascospores; formed by the ascomycetes group of fungi. (14)

aseptic (a-sep´tik) Free of microorganisms. (22)

aseptic meningitis A type of meningitis in which no bacterium or other agent can be readily identified; usually refers to meningitis caused by a virus. (13)

aspergilloma (as´per-jil-o´mah) A dense, round ball of mycelium often occurring in the lungs and commonly caused by *Aspergillus fumigatus*. (14)

Aspergillus flavus A fungus of the ascomycetes group that may produce toxins in certain consumable foods. (14, 24)

Aspergillus fumigatus A fungus of the ascomycetes group that may infect the lung and form a mass of hyphae called an aspergilloma. (14)

asthma (az´mah) A period of wheezing and stressed breathing resulting from a type I hypersensitivity reaction taking place in the respiratory tract. (20)

asymptomatic Without symptoms.

athlete's foot A fungal disease of the webs of the toes caused by various species of fungi. (14)

atopic (a-top´ik) **disease** A type I hypersensitivity reaction, characterized by limited production of IgE and a localized reaction in the body. Also called common allergy. (20)

attenuated (ah-ten´u-a´ted) **virus** A weakened variant of a virus that emerges during successive transfers of the virus in tissue cultures; used in immunizations because of its reduced virulence. Sometimes called live virus. (11, 19)

autoantigens A person's own proteins and other organic compounds that elicit a specific response in the body. (18)

autoclave A laboratory instrument that sterilizes microbiological materials by means of steam under pressure. (21)

autograft Tissue taken from one part of the body and grafted to another. (20)

autoimmune disease A disease in which antibodies react with an individual's own chemical substances and cells. (18, 20)

avirulent organism An organism that is normally without pathogenicity. (17)

axial filament A microscopic fiber located along cell walls in certain species of spirochetes; contractions of the filaments yield undulating motion in the cell. (9)

azathioprine (a´za-thī´o-prēn) An antimitotic drug used to treat cancer. (20)

azithromycin A macrolide antibiotic that inhibits protein synthesis in Gram-negative and Gram-positive bacteria. (23)

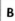 **B**

B19 disease An alternate name for fifth disease. (12)

Babesia microti (bah-be´ze-ah mi-cro´ti) A protozoan of the apicomplexan group that causes babesiosis. (15)

babesiosis A tickborne protozoal disease of the red blood cells caused by *Babesia microti*, characterized by periods of high fever, anemia, and blood clotting. (15)

bacille Calmette Guérin (BCG) (bah-sil´ā kal-met´ ga-ran´) A strain of attenuated *Mycobacterium bovis* used for immunization against tuberculosis and, on occasion, leprosy. (7, 19, 20)

bacillus A bacterial rod. (4)

Bacillus cereus A Gram-positive sporeforming bacterial rod, transmitted by food and water; a cause of intestinal disease. (8)

bacitracin (bas´ĭ-tra´sin) An antibiotic derived from a *Bacillus* species, effective against Gram-positive bacteria when used topically. (23)

bacterial dysentery An alternate name for shigellosis. (8)

bactericidal agent An agent that kills bacteria. (22)

bacteriochlorophyll (bak-te´re-o-klo´ro-fil) A pigment located in bacterial membrane systems that upon excitement by light, loses electrons and initiates photosynthetic reactions. (5)

bacteriocins (bak-te´re-o´sinz) A group of bacterial proteins toxic to other bacteria. (6)

bacteriophage (bak-te´re-o-faj´) A type of virus that attacks and replicates within bacteria. (6, 11)

bacteriorhodopsin (bak-te´re-o-ro-dop´sin) A photosynthetic pigment found in archaebacteria. (5)

bacteriostatic agent An agent that prevents the multiplication of bacteria without killing them. (22)

baculovirus A virus with a high affinity for lepidopteran tissues; used as a carrier for genes that encode pesticides. (26)

balantidiasis A waterborne and foodborne protozoal disease of the intestine caused by *Balantidium* coli, characterized by mild to severe diarrhea. (15)

Balantidium (bal´an-tid´e-um) ***coli*** A ciliated protozoan that causes balantidiasis. (15)

Bang's disease An alternate name for brucellosis. (7)

barophilic (bar´o-fil´ik) **microorganism** A microorganism that lives under conditions of high pressure. (25)

Bartonella bacilliformis A rickettsia that causes bartonellosis.

bartonellosis A relatively mild sandfly-transmitted disease of the blood, caused by *Bartonella bacilliformis*, characterized by fever and a skin rash.

basal body A structure at the base of a bacterial flagellum having a central rod and set of enclosing rings. (4)

basidiomycete A member of the fungal division Basidiomycota. (14)

Basidiomycota A division (phylum) of fungi whose members have septate hyphae and form basidiospores on supportive basidia, among other notable characteristics. (14)

basidiospore A sexually produced spore formed by members of the basidiomycetes group of fungi. (14)

basidium A clublike structure that contains basidiospores; formed by the basidiomycetes group of fungi. (14)

basophil (ba´so-fil) A type of leukocyte that functions in allergic reactions and, possibly, other reactions not yet established. (17, 20)

bejel A mild syphilislike disease occurring in remote parts of the world, caused by a species of *Treponema*. (10)

benthic zone The environment of the ocean floor. (25)

Bergey's Manual of Systematic Bacteriology The official manual of bacteriology that lists the names and characteristics of the known bacteria and presents a classification scheme for these organisms. (3)

beta-hemolytic streptococci Streptococci that destroy red blood cells completely; when cultivated in blood agar, a clearing forms around the colonies of the streptococci. (7)

beta-lactam nucleus The chemical group central to all penicillin antibiotics. (23)

beta-lactamase An alternative name for penicillinase, the enzyme that converts penicillin to penicilloic acid. (23)

bilharziasis (bil´har-zi´ah-sis) An alternate name for schistosomiasis. (16)

binary fission An asexual process by which a cell divides to form two new cells; specifics of the process vary among organisms. (4)

binomial system The system of nomenclature that uses the genus and specific modifier to refer to organisms. (3)

biochemical oxygen demand (BOD) A number referring to the amount of oxygen utilized by the microorganisms in a sample of water during a 5-day period of incubation. (25)

biofilm A series of encased microcolonies of bacteria attached to a surface, such as a catheter or industrial pipeline. (4, 10, 17, 25)

biological vector An infected living organism that transmits disease agents. (17)

bioremediation The use of naturally occurring biofilm populations to degrade toxic wastes and other synthetic products of industry. (25, 26)

biphasic (bi-fāz´ik) **fungus** A fungus that grows in two different patterns depending on growth conditions. Also known as dimorphic fungus. (14)

bipolar staining A characteristic of *Yersinia* and *Francisella* species in which stain gathers at the poles of the cells, yielding the appearance of safety pins. (9)

bisphenol (bĭs-phe´nol) A combination of two phenol molecules used in disinfection. (22)

blackwater fever An alternate name for malaria. (15)

blanching A process in which food is subjected to steam for 3 to 5 minutes in order to destroy cellular enzymes and enhance preservation. (24)

blastomycosis A fungal disease caused by Blastomyces dermatiditis, characterized by infection of the lungs and other systemic organs. Also called Gilchrist's disease. (14)

blastospore A fungal spore formed by budding. (14)

B-lymphocyte A lymphocyte formed in the bursa of Fabricius in embryonic chicks and possibly in the fetal bone marrow in humans; responsible for antibody-mediated immunity. Also called B-cell. (18)

boil A raised pus-filled lesion. (8, 10, 18)

Bordetella pertussis A Gram-negative bacterial rod transmitted by droplets that causes pertussis (whooping cough). (7)

Borrelia burgdorferi (bo-rel´e-ah burg-dorf´er-i) A spirochete transmitted by ticks that causes Lyme disease. (9)

Borrelia recurrentis A spirochete transmitted by arthropods that causes relapsing fever. (9)

botulism A foodborne disease of the nervous system characterized by paralysis. (8)

boutonneuse (boo-ten-ez´) **fever** A tickborne rickettsial disease due to *Rickettsia conori*, characterized by fever and a skin rash. (9)

bovine spongiform encephalopathy (BSE) A viral disease of cows and other large animals in which infected brain tissue becomes soft and spongy; accompanied by neurological defects. Also called mad cow disease. (13)

bradykinin (brad´e-ki´nin) A peptide that functions in type I hypersensitivity reactions by contracting smooth muscles. (20)

breakbone fever A term applied to dengue fever, reflecting sensations that the bones are breaking. (13)

broad-spectrum antibiotic An antibiotic useful for treating many groups of microorganisms, including Gram-positive and Gram-negative bacteria, rickettsiae, fungi, and protozoa. *See also* narrow-spectrum antibiotic. (23)

bronchopneumonia A disease characterized by scattered patches of pneumonia, especially in the bronchial tree. (7)

Brucella abortus A Gram-negative bacterial rod, transmitted by food and water, that causes brucellosis in animals and undulant fever in humans. (7)

brucellosis A foodborne bacterial disease of the blood caused by *Brucella* species and accompanied in humans by blood involvement and undulating fever; in large animals, a disease of the reproductive organs. Also known as Malta fever, Bang's disease, and undulant fever; called contagious abortion in animals. (7)

Bruton's agammaglobulinemia (a-gam´ah-glob´u-lĭ-ne´me-ah) An immune deficiency disease in which the body fails to produce plasma cells from B-lymphocytes. (20)

bubo A swelling of the lymph nodes. (9)

budding An asexual process of reproduction in fungi, in which a new cell forms at the border of the parent cell and then breaks free to live independently. (14)

Burkitt's lymphoma A type of lymphoid cancer occurring in the connective tissues of the jaw. (11, 20)

bursa of Fabricius A lymphoid organ of the gastrointestinal tract of the embryonic chick in which B-lymphocytes are formed. (18)

C

calcivirus An RNA virus appearing as a six-pointed star with abundant calcium in the capsid; calciviruses include the Norwalk virus. (9, 13)

Calymmatobacterium (kah-lim´mah-to-bak-te´re-um) ***granulomatis*** A Gram-negative rod that causes granuloma inguinale. (10)

Campylobacter (kam´pi-lo-bak´ter) ***jejuni*** A Gram-negative curved bacterial rod transmitted by food and water and involved in campylobacteriosis of the intestine. (8)

campylobacteriosis (kam´pi-lo-bac´ter-i-o´sis) A foodborne and waterborne bacterial disease of the intestine caused by *Campylobacter jejuni*, characterized by diarrhea. (8)

cancer A disease characterized by the radiating spread of cells that reproduce at an uncontrolled rate. (11, 20)

Candida albicans A fungus that causes candidiasis; also, an opportunistic fungus that infects immune-compromised individuals, such as AIDS patients. (14)

candidiasis (kan-di-di´ah-sis) An infection due to *Candida albicans* that manifests as a yeast infection of the intestine, the vaginal tract, or the mucous membranes of the mouth (thrush). (14)

capsid The surrounding layer of protein that encloses the genome of a virus. (11)

capsomere A protein subunit of the capsid on the surface of a virus; the number of capsomeres varies among different viruses. (11)

capsule A layer of polysaccharides and small proteins that adheres to the surface of certain bacteria; serves as a buffer between the cell and its environment. (4)

carbenicillin (kar´ben-i-sil´in) A semisynthetic penicillin antibiotic used to treat urinary tract infections caused by certain Gram-negative bacteria. (23)

carbuncle An enlarged abscess formed from the union of several smaller abscesses. (18)

carcinogen A cancer-causing substance. (11)

cardiolipin (kar´de-o-lip´in) An alcoholic extract of beef heart used as an antigen in the VDRL test. (19)

carrier An individual who has recovered from a disease but retains live organisms in the body and continues to shed them. (8, 17)

Carrion's disease An alternate name for bartonellosis. (10)

casein (ka´sēn) A mixture of three long chains of amino acids; the major protein in milk. (24)

catabolism A chemical process in which organic compounds are digested; usually an energy-liberating process. (5)

cationic detergent A detergent that yields positively charged ions in solution. (22)

cat-scratch disease An infectious disease of the lymph channels accompanied by lymph node swellings. Also called cat-scratch fever. (10)

cavitation The formation and implosion of bubbles in a liquid in which ultrasonic vibrations are propagated. (21)

cefoxitin (se-foks´i-tin) A semisynthetic derivative of a *Streptomyces* species used as a penicillin substitute where penicillin resistance is encountered. (23)

cell-mediated immunity Immunity arising from the activity of cytotoxic T-lymphocytes on or near the body cells. Also called tissue immunity. (18, 20)

cephalosporins (sef´ah-lo-spōr´inz) A group of antibiotics derived from the mold *Cephalosporium* and used against Gram-positive bacteria and certain Gram-negative bacteria. (23)

cercaria (ser-ka´re-ah) A tadpolelike intermediary stage in the life cycle of a fluke. (16)

cestode A type of flatworm, commonly known as a tapeworm. (16)

Chagas' disease An alternate name for American trypanosomiasis. (15)

chancre (shag´ker) A circular, purplish hard ulcer with a raised margin that occurs during primary syphilis. (10)

chancroid A sexually transmitted bacterial disease of the external genital organs caused by *Haemophilus ducreyi*, characterized by soft, spreading chancres and swollen lymph nodes. Also called soft chancre. (10)

Chediak-Higashi syndrome An immune disorder characterized by delayed killing of phagocytized microorganisms. (20)

chemically defined medium A medium in which the nature and quantity of each component are identified. Also called synthetic medium. (4)

chemoautotroph (ke´mo-aw´to-troph) An organism that derives energy from chemical reactions and uses the energy to synthesize nutrients from carbon dioxide. (5)

chemoheterotroph (ke´mo-het´er-o-troph) An organism that derives energy from chemical reactions and uses the energy to synthesize nutrients from carbon compounds other than carbon dioxide. (5)

chemotactic factor A lymphokine that draws phagocytes to the antigen site in cell-mediated immunity. (18)

chemotaxis A chemical attraction. (18)

chemotherapeutic agent A synthetic or semisynthetic chemical compound that is inhibitory to microorganisms and is used in the body for therapeutic purposes; includes antibiotics synthetically manufactured. (23)

chickenpox A communicable skin disease caused by a DNA icosahedral virus, characterized by teardrop-shaped, highly infectious, skin lesions. Also called varicella. (12)

chimera (ki-mer´-ah) A plasmid engineered to contain a fragment of foreign DNA. (6)

chitin (kī´tin) A polymer of acetylglucosamine units found in the cell walls of fungi that provides rigidity. (14)

chlamydia (klah-mid´e-ah) A sexually transmitted bacterial disease of the urethra and reproductive organs caused by *Chlamydia trachomatis*; accompanied by urinary tract symptoms and possible pelvic inflammatory disease, leading to sterility. (10)

chlamydiae (klah-mid´e-e) A subgroup of rickettsiae visible only with the electron microscope and cultivated within living tissue medium. (3, 7, 10)

chlamydial ophthalmia (kla-mid´e-al of-thal´me-ah) An infection of the eye tissues caused by *Chlamydia trachomatis*; may occur in newborns from exposure to chlamydiae during birth. (10)

chlamydial pneumonia An influenzalike disease of the lungs caused by *Chlamydia pneumoniae*. (7)

Chlamydia pneumoniae A chlamydia that causes chlamydial pneumonia; formerly known as TWAR. (7)

Chlamydia psittaci (sit´a-si) A chlamydia that causes psittacosis. (7)

Chlamydia trachomatis (tra-ko´mah-tis) A chlamydia that causes chlamydia as well as trachoma. (10)

chloramine (klo´rah-mēn) A chlorine derivative formed by adding a chlorine to an amino group on a carrier molecule. (22)

chloramphenicol (klo´ram-fen´ĭ-kol) A broad-spectrum antibiotic derived from a *Streptomyces* species, used to treat typhoid fever and various other diseases; interferes with protein synthesis. (23)

chlorhexidine (klor-hexs´ĭ-dēn) A bisphenol compound widely used as an antiseptic and disinfectant. (22)

chlorophyll A pigmented molecule that functions in photosynthesis; exists free in the cytoplasm of prokaryotes and within the chloroplasts of eukaryotes. (3, 5, 15)

chloroquine (klor´o-kwin) A synthetic drug used to treat malaria in the clinical phase. (15)

chocolate agar A bacteriological medium consisting of a nutritious base and whole blood; the medium is heated to disrupt the blood cells and release the hemoglobin. (4)

cholera A foodborne and waterborne bacterial disease of the intestine caused by *Vibrio cholerae*, characterized by massive diarrhea, fluid and electrolyte imbalance, and severe dehydration. (8)

chronic disease A disease that develops slowly, tends to linger for a long time, and requires a long convalescence. (17)

cilium A hairlike appendage in eukaryotic cells; cilia assist motion in certain protozoa and are used for filtering air by respiratory epithelial cells. (15, 17)

Ciliophora (sil-e-of´o-rah) A group of protozoa whose members move by means of cilia. (15)

clarithromycin A macrolide antibiotic that inhibits protein synthesis in Gram-negative and Gram-positive bacteria. (23)

Claviceps purpurea A fungus that infects rye and other grains and produces toxins with hallucinatory properties that may be consumed. (24)

clindamycin An antibiotic used as a penicillin substitute and for certain anaerobic bacterial diseases. (23)

clinical disease A disease in which the symptoms are apparent. (17)

clonal selection hypothesis A theory that shows how certain lymphocytes are selected out from the mixed population of B-lymphocytes when stimulated by processed antigens. (18)

clone A collection, or colony, of identical cells arising from a single cell. (18)

Clonorchis sinensis (klo-nor´kis si-nen´sis) A multicellular flatworm parasite of the liver; commonly known as the Chinese liver fluke. (16)

clostridial myonecrosis (mi´o-nĕ-kro´sis) An alternate name for gas gangrene, referring to the death of muscle cells following an invasion of certain *Clostridium* species. (9)

Clostridium botulinum A Gram-positive anaerobic sporeforming rod that causes botulism. (8)

Clostridium perfringens A Gram-positive anaerobic sporeforming rod that causes gas gangrene and a form of food poisoning. (8, 9)

Clostridium tetani A Gram-positive anaerobic sporeforming rod that causes tetanus. (9)

clotrimazole (klo-trī´mah-zōl) An imidazole drug used in the treatment of fungal diseases, such as candidiasis. (23)

coagulase An enzyme that catalyzes the formation of a fibrin clot; produced by virulent staphylococci. (17)

Coccidioides (kok-sid´e-oi´dēz) *immitis* A fungus transmitted by dust that causes coccidioidomycosis. (14)

coccidioidomycosis (kok-sid´e-oi´do-mi-ko´sis) A fungal disease of the lungs caused by *Coccidioides immitis*, characterized by cough, malaise, and other respiratory symptoms. (14)

coccobacillus A form of bacteria characterized by rods with rounded edges. (4)

coccus A spherical bacterium. (4)

codon A three-base sequence on the mRNA molecule that specifies a particular amino acid in the protein molecule. (5)

coenocytic fungus (se´no-sit´ik) A fungus containing no septa (cross-walls) in the hyphae. (14)

coenzyme An organic molecule that forms the nonprotein part of an enzyme molecule. (5)

cold agglutinin screening test (CAST) A laboratory procedure in which *Mycoplasma* antibodies agglutinate human red blood cells at cold temperatures. (7)

cold sore A herpes-induced blister that may occur on the lips, gums, nose, and adjacent areas. (12)

coliform (kol´ĭ-form) **bacteria** Gram-negative nonsporeforming bacilli usually found in the human and animal intestine; they ferment lactose to acid and gas. (25)

Colorado tick fever A tickborne disease caused by an RNA virus, occurring in the western United States; characterized by high fever and joint pains. (13)

colostrum (kŏ-los´trum) The first milk secreted from the mammary glands of animals or humans. (18, 24)

commensalism A close and permanent association between two populations of organisms in which only one population benefits. (4, 17)

common allergy An allergic reaction taking place in a localized area of the body. Also called atopic disease. (20)

communicable disease A disease that is transmissible among various hosts. (17)

competent cell A bacterium that can take up DNA in the recombination process of transformation. (6)

complement A group of proteins that functions in a cascading series of reactions during the response by the body to certain antigens; the complement cascade is stimulated by antigen-antibody activity. (18)

congenital rubella syndrome A condition in which rubella viruses pass across the placenta of an infected woman and cause damage in the fetus. (12)

conidium (ko-nid´e-um) An asexually produced fungal spore formed on a supportive structure without an enclosing sac. (14)

conidiophore (ko-nid´e-o-fōr) The supportive structure on which conidia form. (14)

conjugation A type of bacterial recombination in which genetic material passes from a live donor cell into a live recipient cell during a period of contact. (6)

conjunctivitis (kon-junk´tĭ-vi´tis) A general term for disease of the conjunctiva, the thin mucous membrane that covers the cornea and forms the inner eyelid. Also called pinkeye. (10)

contact dermatitis A type IV hypersensitivity in which the immune system responds to allergens such as clothing materials, metals, and insecticides; the reaction is usually characterized by an induration. (20)

contagious abortion An alternate name for brucellosis in animals. (7)

contagious disease A communicable disease whose agent passes with particular ease among hosts. (17)

continuous flow technique An industrial process in which medium is continually added to a fermentation tank to replace that which has been used. (25)

convalescent serum Antibody-rich serum obtained from a convalescing patient. (19)

Coombs test An antibody test used to detect rh antibodies involved in hemolytic disease of the newborn.

copepod (ko´pĕ-pod) A small aquatic arthropod that serves as an intermediary host for the fish tapeworm. (16)

Corynebacterium (ko-ri-ne´bac-te´re-um) **diphtheriae** A Gram-positive club-shaped bacterial rod that causes diphtheria. (7)

covalent bond A chemical bond created by the sharing of electrons between atoms. (2, 5)

cowpox A mild viral disease of the skin tissues that occurs in humans and bovine species. Also called vaccinia. (12)

Coxiella (kok´se-el´lah) **burnetii** A rickettsia transmitted by food, water, arthropods, or contact; the cause of Q fever. (7)

Coxsackie (cook-sak´e) **virus** An RNA virus of the enterovirus group transmitted by food and water and involved in intestinal disease; also, the cause of disease of the heart muscle (myocarditis) and the chest wall (pleurodynia). (13)

cresol (kre´sol) A derivative of phenol that contains one or more methyl groups on the benzene ring. (22)

Creutzfeldt-Jakob disease (CJD) A nervous system disorder in humans believed to be caused by a prion and possibly related to bovine spongiform encephalopathy. (13)

croup (kroop) A collective name for upper respiratory tract infections often caused by adenoviruses, characterized by hoarse coughing. (12)

cryptococcosis (krip´to-kok-o´sis) A fungal disease of the lungs and spinal cord that occurs as an opportunistic disease in immune-compromised individuals, such as AIDS patients. (14)

Cryptococcus neoformans (krip´to-kok´us ne-o-form´anz) The fungus that causes cryptococcosis; also, an opportunistic fungus that infects immune-compromised individuals, such as AIDS patients. (14)

cryptosporidiosis (krip´to-spor-id´e-o´sis) A waterborne protozoal disease of the intestine caused by *Cryptosporidium coccidi* and *C. parvum*, characterized by intense diarrhea; often occurs in immune-compromised individuals, such as AIDS patients. (15)

Cryptosporidium (krip´to-spor-id´e-um) **coccidi** An opportunistic protozoan that infects the intestines and causes cryptosporidiosis. (15)

Cryptosporidium parvum An opportunistic protozoan that infects the intestines and causes cryptosporidiosis. (15)

cyanobacteria (si´ah-no-bak-tēr´e-ah) A group of pigmented microorganisms occurring in unicellular and filamentous forms; formerly called blue-green algae. (3, 5, 25)

Cyclospora cayetanensis An apicomplexan protozoan responsible for outbreaks of cyclosporiasis; a coccidian parasite. (15)

cyclosporiasis A protozoal disease of the intestine, characterized by vomiting, nausea, and watery diarrhea. (15)

cyclosporin A A drug that suppresses cell-mediated immunity and encourages the body's acceptance of transplanted tissue. (20)

cyst A dormant and very resistant form of a microorganism, such as a protozoan or multicellular parasite. (15, 16)

cystic fibrosis A genetic disease characterized by a buildup of sticky mucus in the respiratory tract and often accompanied by bacterial infection. (8, 10)

cytokine A glycoprotein secreted by helper and other types of T-lymphocytes; stimulates the activity of immune system cells. Also known as lymphokine. (18)

cytomegalovirus (CMV) (si´to-meg´ah-lo-vi´rus) An icosahedral DNA virus that causes infected cells to enlarge. (13)

cytomegalovirus (CMV) disease A viral disease of multiple organs accompanied by nonspecific symptoms an malaise; transmissible to the fetus of a pregnant woman; an opportunistic disease in AIDS patients. (13)

cytotoxic hypersensitivity A cell-damaging or cell-destroying hypersensitivity that develops when IgG reacts with antigens on the surfaces of cells. (20)

D

dalton A unit of weight equal to the mass of one hydrogen atom; used to measure molecular weights. (2)

dalfopristin A streptogramin antibiotic used with quinupristin to inhibit reproduction in *Staphylococcus aureus*. (23)

dander Particles of animal skin, hair, or feathers that may contain materials that cause allergic reactions. (20)

dapsone A chemotherapeutic agent used to treat leprosy patients. (10, 23)

Darling's disease An alternative name for histoplasmosis. (14)

deamination (de-am'-ĭ-na'shun) A biochemical process in which amino groups are enzymatically removed from amino acids and hydroxyl groups are substituted, thereby allowing the carbon skeleton to be used for energy purposes. (5)

decline phase The final portion of a bacterial growth curve in which environmental factors overwhelm the population and induce death. (4)

degerm To mechanically remove organisms from a surface. (22)

dehydration synthesis A process of bonding two molecules together by removing the products of water and joining the open bonds. (2)

Deinococcus radiodurans A bacterium able to repair its chemical damage after exposure to an extremely high level of radiation.

delavirdine An antiviral drug that binds to and inhibits reverse transcriptase; used against HIV in AIDS patients. (11, 23)

denaturation A process in which proteins change from the tertiary structure to the secondary structure; heat and certain chemicals may induce denaturation. (2, 21)

dendritic cell A cell having long fingerlike extensions, found within all tissues; they phagocytize infected cells. (18)

dengue (deng'e) **fever** A viral disease transmitted by the *Aedes aegypti* mosquito, characterized by bone-breaking sensations. Also called breakbone fever. (13)

Dermacentor andersoni A tick that transmits Rocky Mountain spotted fever and other infectious diseases. (9)

dermatomycosis (der-mah'to-mi-ko'sis) A fungal disease of the skin tissues. (14)

desensitization A process in which minute doses of antigens are used to remove antibodies from the body tissues to prevent a later allergic reaction. (20)

desquamation (des'kwah-ma'shun) Peeling of the skin of the fingertips and toes; associated with toxic shock syndrome and Kawasaki disease. (12)

deuteromycete A member of the fungal division Deuteromycota. (14)

Deuteromycota A division (phylum) of fungi whose members have no known sexual cycle of reproduction. (14)

diarrhea Excessive loss of fluid from the gastrointestinal tract.

diatomaceous (di'ah-to-ma'shus) **earth** Filtering material composed of the remains of diatoms. (21, 25)

diatom (di'ah-tom) A eukaryotic marine microorganism that performs photosynthesis; a type of unicellular alga. (3, 21, 25)

differential medium A growth medium in which different species of microorganisms can be distinguished. (4)

differential technique A staining or other procedure intended to separate organisms into different categories. (3)

DiGeorge syndrome An immunodeficiency disease in which the thymus fails to develop, thereby leading to a reduced number of T-lymphocytes. (20)

dimorphic fungus A fungus that takes a yeast form in the human body, and a hyphal form when cultivated in the laboratory. Also called biphasic fungus. (14)

dinoflagellates A group of photosynthetic marine flagellates that form one of the foundations of the food chain in the ocean. (3, 25)

diphtheria (dif-the're-ah) A bacterial disease of the respiratory tract caused by toxin-producing *Corynebacterium diphtheriae*, characterized by tissue destruction and the accumulation of pseudomembranes. (7)

Diphyllobothrium (di-fil'o-both're-um) *latum* A multicellular flatworm, a parasite of the intestine and other organs; transmitted by contaminated seafood; commonly known as the fish tapeworm. (16)

dipicolinic (di'pik-o-lin'ik) **acid** An organic substance that helps stabilize the proteins in a bacterial spore, thereby increasing spore resistance. (4, 21)

diplococcus A pair of cocci. (4, 7)

disease Any change from the general state of good health. (17)

disinfectant A chemical used to kill pathogenic microorganisms on a lifeless object such as a tabletop. (22)

DNA ligase An enzyme that binds together DNA fragments; important in genetic engineering experiments. (6)

DNA polymerase An enzyme that forms DNA by combining fragments during DNA replication. (6)

double helix The spiral staircase arrangement of the chromosome, in which two strands of DNA sit opposite each other, with the nitrogenous bases forming the rungs of the staircase. (2, 5)

Downey cell A swollen lymphocyte with foamy cytoplasm and many vacuoles that develops as a result of infection with infectious mononucleosis viruses. (11, 13)

Dracunculus medinensis (drah-kung'ku-lus med-i-nen'sis) A multicellular roundworm parasite of the intestine and other organs, transmitted by food; commonly known as the Guinea worm. (16)

droplets Airborne particles of mucus and sputum from the respiratory tract that contain disease organisms. (7, 12, 17)

dysentery A condition marked by frequent, watery stools, often with blood and mucus. (8, 15)

E

Eaton agent An alternate name for *Mycoplasma pneumoniae*. (7)

Ebola virus An RNA virus existing in Africa that causes a type of hemorrhagic fever called Ebola fever. (13)

Echinococcus granulosus (e-ki'-no-kok'us gran-u-lo'sis) A multicellular roundworm parasite of the liver that causes hydatid disease; commonly known as the dog tapeworm. (16)

echovirus An RNA virus transmitted by food and water and involved in diseases of the intestine and the skin. (13)

E. coli O157:H7 A virulent strain of *Escherichia coli* that causes bloody diarrhea and kidney hemorrhaging after transmission by contaminated food and water. (8, 17)

edema A swelling of the tissues brought about by an accumulation of fluid. (16, 20)

Ehrlichia (er-lik´e-ah) *chaffeensis* The rickettsia that causes ehrlichiosis. (9)

ehrlichiosis (er-lik-e-o´sis) A tickborne rickettsial disease caused by *Ehrlichia chaffeensis*, characterized by fever, headache, and malaise. (9)

electrophoresis (e-lek´tro-fo-re´sis) A laboratory technique involving the movement of charged organic molecules through an electrical field; used to separate DNA fragments in diagnostic procedures. (19)

elementary body An infectious form of a chlamydia in the early stage of reproduction. (10)

elephantiasis (el´ah-fan-tī´ah-sis) A condition of swelling and distortion of the tissues, especially the legs and scrotum, commonly caused by infection with *Wuchereria bancrofti*. Also called filariasis. (16)

encephalitis Inflammation of the tissue of the brain or infection of the brain. (13)

endemic typhus A relatively mild fleaborne disease of the blood caused by *Rickettsia typhi*, characterized by fever and a skin rash. Also called tabardillo. (9)

endogenous (en-doj´ĕ-nus) **disease** A disease caused by organisms commonly found within the body.

endonuclease An enzyme that cleaves a DNA molecule at the sugar-phosphate bond; used in genetic engineering techniques. (6)

endotoxin A metabolic poison produced chiefly by Gram-negative bacteria; endotoxins are part of the bacterial cell wall and consequently are released on cell disintegration; composed of lipid-polysaccharide-peptide complexes. (17)

Entamoeba histolytica An amoeboid protozoan, transmitted by food and water, that causes amoebic dysentery. (15)

enteritis A synonym for gastrointestinal illness; commonly, an alternate name for salmonellosis. (8)

Enterobius vermicularis (en´ter-o´be-us ver´mik-u-la´ris) A multicellular roundworm parasite of the intestine, commonly known as the pinworm. (16)

enterotoxin A toxin that is active in the gastrointestinal tract of the host. (8, 17)

enterovirus A virus that infects intestinal cells. (13)

envelope The flexible membrane of protein and lipid that surrounds many types of viruses. (11)

enzyme A reusable protein molecule that brings about a chemical change while remaining unchanged itself; the molecule may include a nonprotein part. (5)

enzyme-linked immunosorbent assay (ELISA) A serological test in which an enzyme system is used to detect test material linked to antigens or antibodies on a solid surface. (19)

eosinophil (e´o-sin´o-fil) A type of leukocyte whose functions are not clearly established but may involve phagocytosis. (17)

epidemic parotitis An alternate name for mumps. (12)

epidemic typhus A relatively serious louseborne disease of the blood caused by *Rickettsia prowazecki*, characterized by high fever and a skin rash beginning on the body trunk. (9)

Epidermophyton (ep´e-der-mof´i-ton) **species** A fungus spread by contact; one of the causes of athlete's foot and ringworm. (14)

episome A plasmid attached to the chromosome of a bacterium. (6)

Epstein-Barr (EB) virus An icosahedral DNA virus thought to cause infectious mononucleosis; also associated with Burkitt's lymphoma. (13)

ergot disease A toxemia transferred to humans from rye grain; the toxin is produced by the fungus *Claviceps purpurea*. (14, 24)

erythema A zone of redness in the skin due to an accumulation of blood.

erythema chronicum migrans (ECM) An expanding circular red rash that occurs on the skin of patients with Lyme disease. (9)

erythema infectiosum An alternate name for fifth disease. (7)

erythrogenic toxin A streptococcal toxin that leads to the rash in scarlet fever. (7)

erythromycin (ĕ-rith´ro-mi´sin) An antibiotic derived from a *Streptomyces* species; used against Gram-positive bacteria, mycoplasmas, and certain other organisms. (23)

Escherichia (esh-er-ik´e-ah) *coli* A Gram-negative bacterial rod, transmitted by food and water, that causes traveler's diarrhea and infantile diarrhea (8); also used widely in genetic engineering techniques (6) and as an indicator of water pollution (25).

estivo-autumnal malaria A type of malaria in which the attacks occur at widely spaced intervals. (15)

Eubacteria A domain of nonbacterial living things that includes all organisms not classified as Archaea or Eukarya.

Eukarya A domain of living things encompassing the true bacteria. (3)

eukaryote (u-kar´e-ōt) A relatively complex organism whose cells contain organelles as well as a nucleus with multiple chromosomes and a nuclear membrane; reproduction involves mitosis. *See also* prokaryote. (3)

exanthem (eg-zan´them) A maculopapular rash occurring on the skin surface. (12)

exotoxin A metabolic poison produced chiefly by Gram-positive bacteria; exotoxins are released to the environment on production; composed of protein and affect various organs and systems of the body. (7, 17)

extremophile A type of prokaryote that lives in extreme environments, such as high acid, high salt, or high temperature. (4)

 F

F factor A fragment of DNA in the cyptoplasm of an F⁺ bacterial cell that may pass to a recipient bacterial cell in conjugation and change the recipient into an F⁺ cell. (6)

Fab fragment The portion of an antibody molecule that combines with the determinant site of the antigen. (18)

facultative organism An organism that grows in the presence or absence of oxygen. (4)

farmer's lung A condition that results from a type III immune complex hypersensitivity following exposure to antigens. (20)

Fasciola (fas-e-o´lah) ***hepatica*** A multicellular flatworm parasite of the liver; commonly known as the liver fluke. (16)

Fasciolopsis (fas´e-o-lop´sis) ***buski*** A multicellular flatworm parasite of the intestine and other organs, transmitted by water; commonly known as the intestinal fluke. (16)

Fc fragment The portion of an antibody molecule that combines with phagocytes, viral receptor sites, and complement. (18)

fermentation Anaerobic respiration in which intermediaries in the process are used as electron acceptors; also refers to the industrial use of microorganisms. (5,25)

fifth disease A communicable skin disease caused by a DNA virus and accompanied by a fiery red rash especially on the checks of the face. Also called B19 disease and erythema infectiosum. (12)

filariform (fi-lār´i-form) **larva** A hairlike intermediate form of the hookworm. (16)

fimbriae (fim´bre-ā) Short, hairlike structures used by bacteria for attachment; sometimes used as an alternative term for pili. (4)

flaccid (flak´sid) **paralysis** Paralysis in which the limbs have little tone and become flabby. (8)

flagellum A long, hairlike appendage composed of protein and responsible for motion in microorganisms; found in bacteria and protozoa. (4, 15)

flare A spreading zone of redness around a wheal that occurs during an allergic reaction. (20)

flash method A process of pasteurization in which milk is heated at 71.6°C for 15 to 17 seconds and then cooled rapidly. Also known as the HTST method, for "high temperature, short time." (21, 24)

flatworm A common name for a member of the phylum Platyhelminthes. (16)

flavin adenine dinucleotide (FAD) A coenzyme that functions in electron transport during oxidative phosphorylation. (5)

flocculation (flok´u-1a´shun) The formation of jellylike masses of coagulated material in the water-purification process; also, a serological reaction in which particulate antigens react with antibodies to form visible aggregates of material. (19, 25)

flucytosine (flu-si´to-sēn) An antifungal drug that interrupts nucleic acid synthesis in cells. (23)

fluid mosaic structure The model for the cell membrane in microorganisms where protein globules "float" within two parallel layers of phospholipid. (4)

fluke A flatworm belonging to the phylum Platyhelminthes. Also known as trematode. (16)

folic acid The organic compound in bacteria whose synthesis is blocked by sulfonamide drugs. (5, 23)

fomite (fo´mit) An inanimate object, such as clothing or a utensil, that carries disease organisms. (17)

foraminifera (fo-ram´i-nif´er-ah) A group of shell-containing amoeboid protozoa having chalky skeletons with windowlike openings between sections of the shell. (15)

formalin A solution of formaldehyde used as embalming fluid, in the inactivation of viruses, and as a disinfectant. (22)

Francisella tularensis A Gram-negative rod that displays bipolar staining and causes tularemia. (9)

Friedländer's bacillus An alternate name for *Klebsiella pneumoniae.* (7)

fruiting body The general name for an asexual reproductive structure of a fungus. (14)

functional group A group of atoms functioning as a unit. (2)

fungemia The dissemination of fungi through the circulatory system. (17)

Fungi (fun´jī) One of the five kingdoms in the Whittaker classification of living things, composed of nongreen eukaryotic microorganisms. (14)

fungicidal agent An agent that kills fungi. (22)

fungus A mold or yeast microorganism within the kingdom Fungi. (14)

fusospirochetal (fu´so-spi´ro-ke´tal) **disease** An alternate name for trench mouth. (10)

G

gamma globulin A general term for antibody-rich serum. (19)

gamma-hemolytic streptococci Streptococci that have no effect on red blood cells. (7)

gangrene A physiological process in which the enzymes from wounded tissue digest the surrounding layer of cells, whose enzymes digest the next layer of cells, and so on, thereby inducing a spreading death to the tissue cells; often called dry gangrene. *See also* gas gangrene. (9)

Gardnerella (gard-ner-el´ah) ***vaginalis*** A Gram-negative bacterial rod, transmitted by sexual contact, that causes vaginitis. (10)

gas gangrene A serious soilborne bacterial disease caused by *Clostridium perfringens,* characterized by gas accumulation in the muscle tissues and gangrene; often called wet gangrene. (9)

gastroenteritis Infection of the intestinal tract often due to a virus. (13)

gene A segment of a DNA molecule that provides the biochemical information for protein synthesis and inherited traits. (6)

generalized transduction A type of transduction in which the prophage accidentally incorporates bacterial DNA into its own DNA while replicating during the lytic cycle; the bacterial DNA is then carried into the next cell by the virus. *See also* specialized transduction. (6)

generation time The time interval between bacterial divisions; varies among bacteria and can be as brief as 20 minutes. (4)

genome (je´nom) The nucleic acid component of a virus or an organism. (11)

gentamicin (jen´tah-mi´sin) An aminoglycoside antibiotic often used to treat infections caused by Gram-negative bacteria. (23)

genus A rank in the classification system of organisms composed of two or more species; a collection of genera constitute a family. (3)

germ theory of disease The theory that holds that microorganisms are responsible for infectious diseases. (1)

germicidal agent An agent that kills microorganisms. (22)

Giardia (je-ar´de-ah) ***lamblia*** A flagellated protozoan transmitted by food and water that causes giardiasis. (15)

giardiasis (je-ar-di´ah-sis) A foodborne and waterborne protozoal disease of the intestine caused by *Giardia lamblia*, characterized by mild to severe diarrhea. (15)

gibberellins (gib-ber-el´inz) A series of plant hormones that promote growth by stimulating cell elongation in the stem. (25)

Gilchrist's disease An alternate name for blastomycosis. (14)

glomerulonephritis (glo-mer´u-lo-ne-fri´tis) A complication of streptococcal disease involving the inflammation of blood vessels in the kidneys due to reactions between antigens and antibodies. (7, 20)

glycocalyx (gli´ko-ka´liks) A layer of capsule or slime around certain bacteria that assists in attachment to a surface and imparts resistance. (4)

glycolysis (gli-kol´i-sis) A series of enzyme-catalyzed chemical reactions in which glucose is broken down into two molecules of pyruvic acid with a net gain of two ATP molecules. (5)

Golden Age of Microbiology The approximately 60-year period from 1857 to 1914 during which microorganisms were related to infectious disease. (1)

gonococcal ophthalmia (off-thal´mē-ah) Infection of the eye by *Neisseria gonorrhoeae*; may occur in newborns exposed during birth. (10)

gonococcus A colloquial name for *Neisseria gonorrhoeae*. (10)

gonorrhea A sexually transmitted bacterial disease of the urethra and reproductive organs caused by *Neisseria gonorrhoeae*; accompanied by urinary tract symptoms and possible pelvic inflammatory disease, leading to sterility. (10)

Goodpasture syndrome A type II hypersensitivity reaction in which antibodies are directed against antigens on the membranes of kidney cells, often resulting in kidney failure. (20)

graft-versus-host reaction (GVHR) A phenomenon in which a tissue graft produces immune substances against the host. (20)

Gram stain technique A technique used for differentiating bacteria into two groups, Gram-positive and Gram-negative, depending upon their ability to retain a crystal violet iodine complex on treatment with an alcohol solution. (3)

granuloma inguinale A sexually transmitted bacterial disease of the external genital organs caused by *Calymmatobacterium granulomatis*, characterized by bleeding ulcers and swollen lymph nodes. (10)

Graves' disease A type II hypersensitivity reaction in which antibodies react with receptors on thyroid gland cells, resulting in an overabundant secretion of thyroxine. (20)

gray syndrome A side effect of chloramphenicol therapy, characterized by a sudden breakdown of the cardiovascular system. (23)

green rot Spoilage in eggs due to the production of a green, fluorescent pigment by *Pseudomonas* species. (24)

griseofulvin (gris´e-o-ful´vin) An antifungal drug used against tinea infections of the skin, hair, and nails. (14, 23)

Guillain-Barré syndrome (GBS) (ge-yan´bar-ra´) A complication of influenza and chickenpox, characterized by nerve damage and poliolike paralysis. (12)

Guinea worm The common name for *Dracunculus medinensis*, a multicellular roundworm parasite of the human blood and subcutaneous tissues. (16)

gumma (gum´ah) A soft, granular lesion that forms in the cardiovascular and/or nervous systems during tertiary syphilis. (10)

H

Haemophilus (he-mof´i-lus) ***aegyptius*** A Gram-negative bacterial rod, transmitted by contact, that causes bacterial conjunctivitis. (10)

Haemophilus ducreyi A Gram-negative bacterial rod, transmitted by sexual contact, that causes chancroid. (10)

***Haemophilus influenzae* b (Hib)** A Gram-negative bacterial rod, transmitted by respiratory droplets, that causes *Haemophilus* meningitis. (7)

Haemophilus (he-mof´i-lus) **meningitis** An airborne bacterial disease caused by *Haemophilus influenzae* b, characterized by respiratory distress followed by inflammation of the meninges. (7)

halogen A chemical element whose atoms have seven electrons in their outer shell; examples are iodine and chlorine. (22)

halophilic (hal´o-fil´ik) **microorganism** An organism that lives in environments with high concentrations of salt. (25)

Hansen's disease An alternate name for leprosy. (10)

hapten A small molecule that combines with tissue proteins or polysaccharides to form an antigen. (18)

Hashimoto's disease A type II hypersensitivity reaction in which antibodies react with thyroid gland cells, leading to a deficiency of thyroxine. (20)

hay fever A type I hypersensitivity reaction resulting from the inhalation of tree and grass pollens. (20)

Hazard Analysis Critical Control Points (HACCP) A set of federally enforced regulations to ensure the dietary safety of seafood, meat, and poultry. (24)

Helicobacter pylori A spiral bacterium involved in the majority of cases of gastric ulcers. (8)

helix A figure resembling a tightly wound coil such as a corkscrew or spring; one of the major shapes of viral capsids. (3, 11)

helminth A term referring to a multicellular parasite; includes roundworms and flatworms. (16)

helper T-lymphocyte A T-lymphocyte that enhances the activity of B-lymphocytes. (18, 20)

hemagglutination (hem´ah-gloo´tĭ-na´shun) The agglutination of red blood cells. (11, 19)

hemagglutinin (hem´ah-gloo´tin-in) An enzyme on the surface spikes of certain influenza viruses that enables the viruses to bind to red blood cells. (12)

hemoglobin The red oxygen-carrying pigment in erythrocytes. (19)

hemolysin (he-mol´ĭ-sin) An enzyme that dissolves red blood cells; produced by streptococci, staphylococci, gas gangrene, bacilli, and other microorganisms. (17)

hemolytic disease of the newborn A disease in which rh antibodies from a pregnant woman combine with Rh antigens on the surface of fetal erythrocytes and destroy them; a type II hypersensitivity reaction. Also known as Rh disease and erythroblastosis fetalis. (20)

hemolytic uremic syndrome (HUS) A disease characterized by the formation of hemorrhages in the kidney and often resulting in kidney failure; associated with *E. coli* O157:H7. (3, 8)

hemorrhagic colitis Bloody diarrhea associated with infection by *E. coli* O157:H7. (8)

hemorrhagic fever Any of a series of viral diseases characterized by high fever and hemorrhagic lesions of the throat and internal organs. (13)

hepatitis A A foodborne and waterborne disease of the liver caused by a highly resistant RNA virus, characterized by jaundice, abdominal pain, and degeneration of the liver tissue. (13)

hepatitis B A bloodborne disease of the liver caused by a fragile DNA virus, characterized by jaundice, abdominal pain, and degeneration of the liver tissue. (13)

hepatitis B core antigen (HBcAG) An antigen located in the inner lipoprotein coat enclosing the DNA of a hepatitis B virus. (13)

hepatitis B surface antigen (HBsAg) An antigen located in the outer surface coat of a hepatitis B virus; previously known as the Australia antigen. (13)

hepatitis C A bloodborne disease of the liver caused by a virus, characterized by jaundice, abdominal pain, and degeneration of the liver tissue. (13)

hepatocarcinoma (hep-at´o-car-cin-o´mah) Cancer of the liver tissue. (13)

hermaphroditic (her-maf´ro-dit´ik) **organism** An organism that possesses both male and female reproductive organs.(16)

herpes simplex A viral disease of the skin and nervous system, often characterized by blisterlike sores. (11)

heterophile (het´er-o-fil) **antigen** An antigen that occurs in apparently unrelated species of organisms. (9, 13, 18)

heterotrophic (het´er-o-trof´ik) **organism** An organism that feeds on preformed organic matter and obtains energy from this matter. (4)

hexachlorophene (hek´sah-klo´ro-fēn) A bisphenol compound containing six chlorine atoms; used in disinfectants and antiseptics. (22)

histamine (his´tah-mēn) A mediator in type I hypersensitivity reactions; released from the granules in mast cells and basophils, causing the contraction of smooth muscles. (20)

histocompatibility (his´to-kom-pat´ĭ-bil´ĭ-te) **molecule** A molecule on the surface of animal tissue cells involved in transplant acceptance and rejection. (20)

Histoplasma capsulatum A fungus often found in the human lung that causes histoplasmosis. (14)

histoplasmosis A fungal disease of the lungs and other systemic organs caused by *Histoplasma capsulatum*, often occurring in immune-compromised individuals, such as AIDS patients. (14)

His-Werner disease An alternate name for trench fever. (9)

holding method A process of pasteurization in which milk is heated at 62.9°C for 30 minutes. Also known as the LTLT method, for "low temperature, long time." (21, 24)

human granulocytic ehrlichiosis (HGE) A tickborne form of ehrlichiosis in which the causative agent infects the body's neutrophils. (9)

human monocytic ehrlichiosis (HME) A tickborne form of ehrlichiosis in which the causative agent infects the body's monocytes. (9)

humoral immunity Immunity arising from the activity of antibodies directed against antigens in the tissues. Also called antibody-mediated immunity. (18)

Hutchinson's triad Deafness, impaired vision, and notched, peg-shaped teeth; may accompany congenital syphilis. (10)

hyaluronidase (hi´ah-lu-ron´ĭ-dās) An enzyme that digests hyaluronic acid and thereby permits the penetration of parasites through the tissues; known as the spreading factor. (17)

hydatid cyst A thick-walled body formed in the human liver by *Echinococcus granulosus*. (16)

hydrogen bond A weak chemical bond that forms between protons and adjacent pairs of electrons. (2, 5)

hydrophobia "Fear of water," an emotional condition arising from the inability to swallow as a consequence of rabies. (13)

Hymenolepis (hi´me-nol´e-pis) ***nana*** A multicellular flatworm, a parasite of the intestine; commonly known as the dwarf tapeworm. (16)

hyperimmune serum Serum that contains a higher than normal amount of a particular antibody. (19)

hypha (hi´fah) A microscopic filament of cells that represents the basic unit of a fungus. (14)

I

icosahedron A symmetrical figure composed of 20 triangular faces and 12 points; one of the major shapes taken by the viral capsid. (11)

idoxuridine (i-doks-ur′ĭ-dēn) The drug 5-iodo-2-deoxyuridine (IDU) that replaces thymine in DNA molecules; useful in treating herpes simplex. (12)

IgA An antibody in humoral immunity; present in the respiratory and gastrointestinal tracts and in body secretions such as milk. (18)

IgD An antibody of uncertain function believed to act as a receptor site on B-lymphocytes. (18)

IgE The antibody involved in type I hypersensitivity reactions; fixes to the surface of mast cells and basophils. (18, 20)

IgG The major circulating antibody in antibody-mediated immunity; passes across the placental barrier; principal component of the secondary antibody response. (18, 19)

IgM The largest antibody formed in antibody-mediated immunity; remains in the circulation; principal component of the primary antibody response. (18, 19)

imidazoles (im-id′ah-zolz) A group of antifungal drugs that interfere with sterol synthesis in fungal cell membranes; examples are miconazole and ketoconazole. (23)

imipenem A beta-lactam antibiotic used again Gram-positive bacteria. (23)

immune adherence phenomenon Increased phagocytosis of a cell resulting from the attachment of certain complexes to the cell surface. (18)

immune complex hypersensitivity Type III hypersensitivity, in which antigens combine with antibodies to form aggregates that are deposited in blood vessels or on tissue surfaces. (20)

immune complexes Aggregates of antigen-antibody material that are deposited in body tissues; characteristic of type III hypersensitivity reactions. (20)

immunoelectrophoresis (im′mu-no-e-lek′tro-fo-re′sis) A laboratory technique in which antigen molecules move through an electric field and then diffuse to meet antibody molecules to form a precipitation line; used in diagnostic procedures. (19)

immunoglobulin An alternate term for antibody. (18)

imperfect fungi Fungi that are known to multiply only by asexual processes. (14)

impetigo contagiosum An infectious skin disease usually caused by staphylococci or streptococci, characterized by abscesses and boils. (10)

inactivated virus A weakened virus that results from treatment with physical or chemical agents; used in immunizating agents because of its reduced virulence; sometimes called a dead virus. (11, 19)

inclusion A granulelike body that forms in cellular cytoplasm infected with certain organisms; an inclusion represents accumulations of organisms such as chlamydiae or viruses. (10, 11)

incubation period The time that elapses between the entry of a parasite to the host and the appearance of symptoms. Also called period of incubation. (17)

induced mutation A mutation arising from a mutagenic agent used under controlled laboratory conditions. (6)

induration A thickening and drying of the skin tissue that occurs in type IV hypersensitivity reactions. (20)

infarction A blockage of the blood vessels.

infection The relationship between two organisms and the competition for supremacy that takes place between them. (17)

infection allergy A type IV hypersensitivity reaction in which the immune system responds to the presence of certain microbial agents. (20)

infectious mononucleosis A disease of the white blood cells caused by an icosahedral DNA virus, characterized by sore throat, mild fever, and malaise. (13)

inflammation A nonspecific defensive response to injury; usually characterized by red color from blood accumulation, warmth from the heat of blood, swelling from fluid accumulation, and pain from injury to local nerves. (18)

influenza A disease of the lungs caused by a helical RNA virus, characterized by cough and malaise. (13)

initial body A noninfectious form of chlamydia in the later stage of reproduction. (10)

innate immunity An inborn capacity for resisting disease. (19)

insect An arthropod having six legs; examples are fleas, mosquitoes, and lice.

insertion sequence A segment of DNA that forms a copy of itself, after which the copy moves into areas of gene activity to interrupt the genetic coding sequence. (6)

interferon (in′ter-fēr′on) An antiviral protein produced by body cells on exposure to viruses; interferons trigger the production of a second protein that binds to mRNA coded by the virus, thereby inhibiting viral replication. (11)

interleukin (in′ter-loo′kin) A lymphokine produced by white blood cells that acts on other white blood cells; important in immune processes. (18)

interleukin-2 A lymphokine found to have value in cancer therapy by activating natural killer cells among other activities. (20)

intermediary host The host in which the larval or other intermediary stage of a multicellular parasite is found. (16)

invasiveness The ability of a parasite to invade the tissues of the host and cause structural damage to the tissues. (17)

iodophor (i-o′do-for) A complex of iodine and detergents that releases iodine over a long period of time; used as an antiseptic and disinfectant. (22)

ionizing radiation A type of radiation such as gamma rays and X rays, that causes the formation of ions. (21)

isograft Tissue taken from an identical twin and grafted to the other twin. (20)

isomers (i′so-merz) Molecules with the same molecular formula but different structural formulas. (2)

isoniazid (i′so-ni′ah-zid) A chemotherapeutic agent effective against the tubercle bacillus. (7, 23)

isopropyl alcohol A two-carbon alcohol compound widely used as a disinfectant; commonly known as rubbing alcohol. (22)

isotopes Variants of an atom in which the numbers of neutrons differ. (2)

Ixodes (iks-o′dez) The genus of tick that transmits Lyme disease. (9)

J

jaundice A condition in which bile seeps into the circulatory system, causing the complexion to have a dull yellow color. (13, 17)

Job syndrome An immune disorder characterized by defective chemotaxis between phagocyte and microorganism. (20)

K

kala-azar An alternate name for leishmaniasis. (15)

kanamycin An aminoglycoside antibiotic derived from a *Streptomyces* species; used to treat infections caused by Gram-negative bacteria. (23)

Kaposi's sarcoma A type of skin cancer that affects immune-compromised individuals, such as AIDS patients. (13)

kappa factor A nucleic acid particle produced by species of *Paramecium*; appear responsible for the production of toxins by these protozoa. (15)

Kawasaki disease A disease of undetermined origin characterized by a skin rash and desquamation and often involving the cardiovascular system. (12)

kefir (ke-fir′) A fermentation product of goat's milk that contains acid and alcohol. (24)

keratitis Infection of the cornea of the eye.

keratoconjunctivitis (ker′ah-to-kon-junk′tĭ-vi′tis) Eye inflammation accompanied by infection of the cornea and conjunctiva; the condition is characterized by tearing, swelling, and sensitivity to light. (12)

ketoconazole (ke-te-kon′ah-zōl) An imidazole drug often used in the treatment of various fungal diseases. (23)

killer T-lymphocyte A type of T-lymphocyte that attacks and destroys cells altered by the presence of antigens; important in the destruction of cancer cells. Also called killer cell. (18, 20)

Kirby-Bauer test An agar diffusion test used to determine the antibiotic concentration effective against a test organism. (23)

Klebs-Löffler bacillus An alternate name for *Corynebacterium diphtheriae*. (7)

Klebsiella (klebs-e-el′ah) ***pneumoniae*** A Gram-negative encapsulated bacterial rod transmitted by contact, involved in diseases of the respiratory tract and intestine. (7, 10)

Koch's postulates A set of procedures by which a specific organism can be related to a specific disease. (1)

Koch-Weeks bacillus An alternate name for *Haemophilus aegyptius*. (10)

Koplik spots Red patches with white central lesions that form on the gums and walls of the pharynx during the early stages of measles. (11, 12)

Krebs cycle A cyclic series of enzyme-catalyzed reactions in which carbon from acetyl-CoA is released as carbon dioxide; the reactions also yield protons and high-energy electrons that are transported among coenzymes and cytochromes as their energy is released. (5)

kumiss (koo′mis) A fermentation product of mare's milk that contains acid and alcohol. (25)

kuru A disease characterized by slow degeneration of the brain tissue, possibly caused by a prion. (13)

L

lactalbumin A protein occurring in minor quantities in cow's milk. (24)

lactose A milk sugar composed of one molecule of glucose and one molecule of galactose. (2, 5, 24)

lag phase A portion of a bacterial growth curve encompassing the first few hours of the population's history; minimal reproduction occurs. (4)

larva A preadult immature stage in the life cycle of certain eukaryotic organisms; also, a tiny worm in the life cycle of a multicellular parasite. (16)

Lassa fever A hemorrhagic fever disease of the blood caused by an RNA virus, characterized by severe throat lesions. (13)

lecithinase (les′ĭ-thĭ-nās) A toxin produced by gas gangrene bacilli that dissolves the membranes of tissue cells. (9)

Legionella (lĕg-on-el′ah **nu-mof′i-lah**) ***pneumophila*** A Gram-negative bacterial rod, transmitted by droplets, that causes Legionnaires' disease. (7)

legionellosis An alternate name for Legionnaires' disease. (7)

Legionnaires' disease A bacterial disease of the lungs caused by *Legionella pneumophila*, characterized by pneumonia, fever, and malaise. Also called legionellosis. (7)

legume A plant that bears seeds in pods; examples are beans, soybeans, and alfalfa. (26)

Leishmania (lĕsh-ma′ne-ah) **species** Flagellated protozoa transmitted by sandflies; the causes of leishmaniasis; examples are *L. donovani* and *L. tropica*. (15)

leishmaniasis (lĕsh-ma-ni′ah-sis) A protozoal disease of the white blood cells caused by *Leishmania* species, transmitted by sandflies; characterized by fever, sores, and emaciation; occurs in visceral and cutaneous forms. Also called kala-azar. (15)

leproma A tumorlike growth on the skin associated with leprosy. (10)

lepromin (lep-ro′min) **test** A skin test used in the screening and diagnosis of leprosy. (10)

leprosy A bacterial disease transmitted by contact and caused by *Mycobacterium leprae*; characterized by destruction of the skin tissues and the peripheral nerves, leading to local anesthesia. (10)

Leptospira interrogans A spirochete; the cause of leptospirosis. (9)

leptospirosis A soilborne bacterial disease caused by *Leptospira interrogans*, characterized by mild fever. (9)

leukemia Cancer of the white blood cells.

leukocidin (loo´ko-si´din) A bacterial enzyme that destroys phagocytes, thereby preventing phagocytosis. (17)

leukocyte An alternate name for white blood cell. (17)

leukopenia A condition characterized by a drop in the normal number of white blood cells.

leukotriene (loo´ko-tren) A substance that acts as a mediator during type I hypersensitivity reactions; formed from arachidonic acid after the antigen-antibody reaction has taken place. (20)

lichen An organism composed of a fungal mycelium within which are embedded photosynthetic algae. (14)

lincomycin An antibiotic used as a penicillin substitute for diseases caused by Gram-positive bacteria. (23)

lipase A fat-digesting enzyme produced by certain contaminating bacteria in milk. (24)

lipid An organic compound that dissolves in organic solvents; composed of carbon, hydrogen, and oxygen; lipids include fats and are used in energy metabolism and structural compounds. (2, 4, 5)

lipopolysaccharide A molecule composed of lipid and polysaccharide, found in the outer membrane of Gram-negative bacteria, where it functions as an endotoxin. (4)

Lipschütz body An inclusion that forms in the nucleus of cells infected with herpesviruses. (11)

Listeria monocytogenes (lis-ter´e-ah mon´o-si-toj´e-nez) A small Gram-positive rod that causes listeriosis. (8)

listeriosis A soilborne and foodborne bacterial disease caused by *Listeria monocytogenes* and accompanied by mild symptoms, except in pregnant women where miscarriage may occur. (8)

littoral zone The environment along the shoreline of an ocean.(25)

Loa loa A multicellular roundworm parasite of the eye, commonly known as the eyeworm. (16)

lobar pneumonia Pneumonia that involves an entire side or lobe of the lung. (7)

local disease A disease restricted to a single area of the body, usually the skin. (17)

lockjaw A common name for tetanus, based on the spasms of the jaw muscles. (9)

locus An individual site on a bacterial chromosome where genetic activity can be located. (6)

logarithmic (log) phase The second portion of a bacterial growth curve, in which active growth leads to a rapid rise in numbers of the population. (4)

long incubation hepatitis An alternate name for hepatitis B. (13)

louse A type of insect of the genus *Pediculus* that transmits epidemic typhus and other diseases. (9)

lumpy jaw A common name for actinomycosis in the jaw, characterized by hard nodules in the tissue. (10)

Lyme disease A serious arthropodborne bacterial disease transmitted by ticks, caused by *Borrelia burgdorferi*; characterized by a skin rash (ECM) and malaise, and later a swelling and degeneration of the large joints. (9)

lymph node A bean-shaped organ located along lymph vessels, involved in the immune response; the major cells of lymph nodes are phagocytes and lymphocytes. (17)

lymphocyte A type of leukocyte that functions in the immune system. (17, 18, 20)

lymphocytic choriomeningitis (lim-fo-sit´ik kor´e-o-men-in-gi´tis) A disease of the brain tissue possibly caused by a virus, characterized by headache, drowsiness, and stupor, as well as large numbers of lymphocytes in the meninges. (13)

lymphogranuloma (lim´fo-gran-u-lo´mah) **venereum** A sexually transmitted bacterial disease of the external genital organs, caused by *Chlamydia trachomatis* and characterized by swollen lymph nodes. (10)

lymphokine (lim´fo-kīn) A glycoprotein that increases the efficiency of immune system reactions, such as at the antigen site. Also called cytokine. (18)

lymphopoietic (lim-fo´poi-et´ik) **cells** Primitive cells that arise from stem cells, modified to form B-lymphocytes or T-lymphocytes, (18)

lyophilization (li-of´i-li-za´shun) A process in which food or other material is deep frozen, after which its liquid is drawn off by a vacuum. (24)

lysogenic bacterium A bacterium that carries a prophage. (6)

lysogeny (li-soj´e-ne) The process by which a virus remains in the cell cytoplasm as a fragment of DNA or attaches to the chromosome, but fails to replicate in or destroy the cell. (6, 11)

lysosome A microscopic organelle found in eukaryotic cells; contains digestive enzymes. (3, 15, 18)

lysozyme (li´so-zīm) A nonspecific enzyme found in tears and saliva that digests the peptidoglycan of Gram-positive bacteria and leads to their destruction. (4, 17)

lytic cycle A process by which a virus replicates within a host cell and ultimately destroys the host cell. (11)

M

Machupo A type of viral hemorrhagic fever occurring primarily in South America. (13)

mad cow disease A common name for bovine spongiform encephalopathy. (10)

macrophage A large cell derived from monocytes and found within the tissues; macrophages actively phagocytize foreign bodies and comprise the reticuloendothelial system. (17, 18)

macule A pink-red skin spot associated with infectious disease. (12)

maculopapular (mak´u-lo-pap´u-lar) **rash** A rash consisting of pink-red spots that later become dark red before fading; occurs in rickettsial diseases. (9)

Madura foot Substantial swelling of the tissues of the foot due to *Nocardia asteroides*. (10)

magnetosome A cytoplasmic body in certain bacteria that assists orientation to the environment by aligning with the magnetic field. (4)

major histocompatibility complex (MHC) A set of genes that controls the expression of MHC proteins; involved in transplant rejection. (20)

major histocompatibility (MHC) protein Any of a set of proteins at the surface of all body cells that identify the uniqueness of the individual. (20)

malaria A serious protozoal disease of the red blood cells caused by *Plasmodium* species, transmitted by mosquitoes, and characterized by periods of high fever, anemia, and blood clotting. (15)

mannitol salt agar An enriched medium that encourages the growth of staphylococci; contains a high percentage of salt, a feature that makes it inhibitory to most other organisms. (4)

Marburg disease A viral disease caused by an RNA virus and characterized by fever and hemorrhaging. (13)

mast cell A connective tissue cell to which IgE fixes in type I hypersensitivity reactions; mast cells degranulate and release histamine during allergic attacks. (20)

Mastigophora (mas´ti-gof´o-rah) A group of protozoa whose members move by means of flagella. (15)

maternal antibodies Type IgG antibodies that cross the placenta from the maternal to the fetal circulation and protect the newborn for the first few months of life. (18)

measles A communicable respiratory disease, caused by an RNA helical virus, characterized by respiratory symptoms and a blushlike skin rash. Also called rubeola. (12)

mechanical vector A living organism, or an object, that transmits disease agents on its surface. (17)

melioidosis (me´le-oi-do´sis) A soilborne bacterial disease, caused by *Pseudomonas pseudomallei*; characterized by lung abscesses. (9)

memory cell A cell derived from B-lymphocytes or T-lymphocytes that reacts rapidly upon the future recurrence of antigens in the tissues. (18)

meninges The covering layers of the brain and spinal cord; the three meninges are the dura mater, arachnoid, and pia mater. (7, 13)

meningitis A general term for inflammation of the meninges due to any of several bacteria, fungi, viruses, or protozoa. (7, 13, 14, 15)

meningococcemia (me-ning´go-kok-se´me-ah) A type of endotoxic shock caused by *Neisseria meningitidis*. (7)

meningococcus A common name for *Neisseria meningitidis*. (7)

merozoite (mer´o-zo´it) A stage in the life cycle of *Plasmodium* species; parasites invade the red blood cells in this form. (15)

mesophile An organism that grows in temperature ranges of 20°C to 40°C. (4)

metabolism The sum of all biochemical processes taking place in a living cell. (5)

metacercaria (met´ah-cer-cār´e-ah) An encysted intermediary stage in the life cycle of a fluke. (16)

metachromatic granule A phosphate-storing granule that stains deeply with methylene blue; commonly found in *Corynebacterium diphtheriae*. Also called volutin granule. (4, 7)

methanogen A bacterium that lives on simple compounds in anaerobic environments and produces methane during its metabolism. (4)

metronidazole (me´tro-ni´dah-zōl) A chemotherapeutic agent used to treat trichomoniasis and other protozoal diseases. (14, 23)

miasma (mi-az´mah) An ill-defined entity generally referring to an altered chemical quality of the atmosphere; believed to cause disease before the establishment of the germ theory of disease. (1)

miconazole (mi-kon´ah-zōl) An imidazole drug used in the treatment of topical and systemic fungal diseases. (23)

microaerophilic (mi´kro-a-rō-fil´ik) **organism** An organism that grows best in an oxygen-reduced environment. (4)

microfilaria An intermediate eellike form of *Wuchereria bancrofti*. (16)

micrometer A unit of measurement equivalent to one millionth of a meter; the unit is abbreviated as μm and is commonly used in measuring the size of microorganisms. (3)

microorganism A microscopic form of life including bacteria, viruses, fungi, protozoa, and some multicellular parasites.

miliary tuberculosis Tuberculosis that spreads through the body. (7)

miracidium (mi-rah-sid´e-um) A ciliated larva representing an intermediary stage in the life cycle of a fluke. (16)

mite A spiderlike arthropod that transmits such diseases as rickettsialpox and tsutsugamushi. (9)

mold A type of fungus that consists of chains of cells and appears as a fuzzy mass. (14)

molecule The smallest part of a compound that retains the properties of the compound. (2)

molluscum (mŏ-lus´kum) **body** A cytoplasmic inclusion that occurs in cells infected with the viruses of molluscum contagiosum. (12)

molluscum contagiosum A viral skin disease caused by a DNA virus and accompanied by firm, waxy, wartlike lesions with a depressed center. (13)

Monera One of the five kingdoms in the Whittaker classification of living things, composed of prokaryotes, such as bacteria and cyanobacteria. (3)

monoclonal antibody A type of antibody produced by a clone of hybridoma cells, consisting of antigen-stimulated plasma cells fused to myeloma cells. (18)

monocyte A leukocyte with a large bean-shaped nucleus; functions in phagocytosis. (17)

monotrichous (mon´o-trik´us) **bacterium** A bacterium that has a single flagellum. *See also* peritrichous bacterium. (4)

Montauk knee A form of Lyme disease named for a town near New York City. (9)

mortality rate The percentage of victims of a disease who succumb to the disease.

most probable number (MPN) A laboratory test in which a statistical evaluation is used to estimate the number of bacteria in a sample of fluid; often employed in determinations of coliform bacteria in water. (25)

moxalactam (mox-ah-lac´tam) A monobactam antibiotic used against Gram-negative bacteria. (23)

M protein A protein that enhances the pathogenicity of streptococci by allowing organisms to resist phagocytosis and adhere firmly to tissue. (7)

μm The symbol for micrometer, a millionth of a meter. (4)

multidrug-resistant *Staphylococcus aureus* (MRSA) A strain of *S. aureus* displaying resistance to a multitude of available antibiotics. (10, 23)

mumps A communicable disease caused by an icosahedral DNA virus, characterized by swelling of the parotid and other salivary glands. (12)

mutation A change in the characteristic of an organism arising from an alteration of a chromosome. (6)

mutualism A close and permanent association between two populations of organisms in which both benefit from the association. (4)

myasthenia gravis A type II hypersensitivity reaction in which antibodies react with acetylcholine receptors on the membranes of muscle fibers. (20)

mycelium (mi-se´le-um) A visible mass of tangled filaments of fungal cells. (14)

Mycobacterium avium-intracellulare An acid-fast bacterial rod that causes lung infection in immune-compromised individuals, such as AIDS patients. (7)

Mycobacterium leprae An acid-fast bacterial rod that causes leprosy. (10)

Mycobacterium tuberculosis An acid-fast bacterial rod that causes tuberculosis. (7)

mycologist One who studies fungi. (14)

mycology The study of fungi. (14)

mycoplasma One of a group of tiny submicroscopic bacteria that lack cell walls and are visible only with an electron microscope. (3, 7, 10)

Mycoplasma hominis An extremely tiny submicroscopic bacterium that causes mycoplasmal urethritis. (10)

Mycoplasma pneumoniae An extremely tiny submicroscopic bacterium that causes mycoplasmal pneumonia (7).

mycoplasmal pneumonia An airborne primary pneumonia transmitted by droplets, caused by *Mycoplasma pneumoniae*; characterized by lung tissue destruction and respiratory symptoms. Also called primary atypical pneumonia and walking pneumonia. (7)

mycoplasmal urethritis A sexually transmitted disease caused by *Mycoplasma hominis* and characterized by urinary tract discomfort. (10)

mycotoxin A fungal toxin. (14)

myocarditis Infection of the heart muscle, often due to Coxsackie virus. (13)

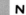

N

Naegleria fowleri (na-gle´ri-ah fow-ler´i) A flagellated protozoan, transmitted by water, that causes primary amoebic meningoencephalitis. (15)

nalidixic (nal-ĭ-diks´ik) **acid** A chemotherapeutic agent that blocks protein synthesis in certain Gram-negative bacteria that cause urinary tract infections. (23)

nanometer A unit of measurement equivalent to one billionth of a meter; the unit is abbreviated as nm and is often used in measuring viruses and the wavelength of energy. (3)

narrow-spectrum antibiotic An antibiotic that is useful for a restricted group of microorganisms. *See also* broad-spectrum antibiotic. (23)

natural killer cell A type of defensive body cell that attacks and destroys cancer cells and infected cells without the involvement of the immune system. (18)

naturally acquired active immunity Immunity resulting from the immune system's response to disease antigens. (9)

naturally acquired passive immunity Immunity resulting from the passage of antibodies to the fetus via the placenta or the milk of a nursing mother. Also called congenital immunity. (19)

Necator americanus A multicellular roundworm parasite of the intestine and other organs, transmitted by moist vegetation; commonly known as the New World hookworm. (16)

necrosis Cell death.

negative stain technique A staining process that results in clear bacteria on a stained background when viewed with the light microscope. (3)

Negri body A cytoplasmic inclusion that occurs in brain cells infected with rabies viruses. (11)

Neisseria gonorrhoeae (ni-se´re-ah gon´o-re´ā) A Gram-negative bacterial diplococcus, transmitted by sexual contact, that causes gonorrhea. (10)

Neisseria meningitidis (ni-se´re-ah men-in´gi-ti´dis) A Gram-negative bacterial diplococcus, transmitted by droplets, that causes meningococcal meningitis. (7)

nematode A common name for the roundworm, a member of the phylum Nematoda, or Nemathelminthes. (16)

neomycin An aminoglycoside antibiotic derived from a *Streptomyces* species; used topically for infections caused by Gram-negative bacteria, especially in the eye. (23)

neoplasm An uncontrolled growth of cells; often called a tumor. (11)

Neufeld quellung reaction A laboratory test used to distinguish strains of *Streptococcus pneumoniae*. (7)

neuraminidase (nūr-ah-min´ĭ-dās) An enzyme on the surface spikes of certain viruses that dissolves the cell membrane when the virus attaches to a cell during replication. (12)

neurotoxin A toxin that is active in the nervous system of the host. (17)

neutralization A type of antigen-antibody reaction in which the activity taking place between reactants is not visible. (18, 19)

neutrophil A type of polymorphonuclear cell that functions chiefly as a phagocyte. (17)

nevirapine An antiviral drug that binds to and inhibits the action of reverse transcriptase; used against HIV. (11, 23)

nicotinamide adenine dinucleotide (NAD) A coenzyme that transports electrons during oxidative phosphorylation and fermentation reactions. (5)

night soil Human feces sometimes used as an agricultural fertilizer. (16)

nitrogen fixation A general term for the chemical process in which organisms trap atmospheric nitrogen and use it to form organic compounds. (25)

nitrogenous (ni-troj´en-us) **base** Any of five nitrogen-containing compounds found in nucleic acids, including adenine, guanine, cytosine, thymine, and uracil. (2, 4, 5)

Nocardia asteroides An acid-fast funguslike bacterial rod that causes endogenous infections of the lungs and other internal organs characterized by abscesses; the cause of Madura foot. (10)

non-A non-B (NANB) hepatitis A type of hepatitis caused by an as-yet unidentified virus. (13)

noncommunicable disease A disease whose causative agent is acquired from the environment and is not easily transmitted to the next host. (17)

normal flora The populations of organisms that infect various pails of the body without usually causing disease. (17)

Norwalk virus A virus transmitted by food and water and involved in intestinal diseases. (13)

nosocomial (nos´o-ko´me-al) **disease** A disease acquired during an individual's stay at a hospital. (10)

nucleocapsid The combination of genome and capsid in a virus. (11)

nucleoid The chromosomal region of a bacterium. (4)

nucleotide A component of a nucleic acid consisting of a carbohydrate molecule, a phosphate group, and a nitrogenous base. (2, 5)

nutrient agar A common bacteriological growth medium consisting of beef extract, peptone, water, and agar. (4)

nutrient broth A common bacteriological growth medium consisting of beef extract, peptone, and water. (4)

nystatin (nis´tah-tin) An antifungal drug effective against *Candida albicans*. (14, 23)

O

Okazaki (o-ka-zak´e) **fragments** Segments of DNA that combine with one another to form a DNA molecule during chromosomal duplication. (6)

oncofetal antigen An antigen in tumor cells thought to be expressed during differentiation of the tissues in the embryonic stage. (20)

oncogene (ong´ko-jēn) A region of DNA in human cells thought to induce uncontrolled growth of the cell if permitted to function. (11)

oncology The study of tumors and cancers. (11, 20)

oocyst (o´o-sist) An oval body in the reproduction cycle of certain protozoa that develops by a complex series of asexual and sexual processes. (15)

oospore (o´o-spōr) A sexually produced spore that is formed by members of the oomycetes group of fungi. (14)

operon The unit of gene activity that expresses a particular trait; also, the unit that controls protein synthesis. (5)

ophthalmia Severe inflammation of the eye. (10)

opportunist An organism that invades the tissues when body defenses are suppressed. (13, 17)

opsonins (op´so-ninz) Antibodies or complement components that encourage phagocytosis. (18)

opsonization Enhanced phagocytosis due to the activity of antibodies or complement. (18)

orchitis (or-ki´tis) A condition caused by the mumps virus in which the virus damages the testes. (12)

organelle A membrane-enclosed compartment in eukaryotic cells; the site of various cellular functions. (3, 14, 15)

Oriental sore A cutaneous form of leishmaniasis characterized by skin sores. (15)

ornithosis An alternate name for psittacosis. (7)

osmosis The flow of water from a region of low concentration of chemical substance through a semipermeable membrane to a region of high concentration of the same chemical substance. (24)

oxidase An enzyme that catalyzes oxidation-reduction reactions. (5)

oxidation A chemical change in which electrons are lost by an atom; also, the union of oxygen with a chemical substance. (2)

oxidative phosphorylation A series of sequential steps in which energy is released from electrons as they pass among coenzymes and cytochromes, and ultimately, to oxygen; the energy is used to combine phosphate ions with ADP molecules to form ATP molecules. (5)

P

pandemic A worldwide epidemic. (17)

papilloma (pap´ĭ-lo´mah) A tumor of the skin tissue. (11)

papilloma virus An icosahedral DNA virus and one of the causes of skin warts. (13)

papule A pink pimple on the skin. (12)

Paragonimus westermani (par´ah-gon´i-mus wes´ter-man-i) A multicellular flatworm parasite of the lung transmitted by seafood; commonly known as the lung fluke. (16)

parainfluenza A disorder caused by an RNA helical virus, characterized by mild upper respiratory illness. (12)

parasite A type of heterotrophic organism that feeds on live organic matter such as another organism. (4, 17)

parasitemia The spread of protozoa and multicellular worms through the circulatory system. (15, 16)

parasitism A close and permanent association between two organisms in which one feeds on the other and may cause injury to the other organism. (4, 17)

parasitology The discipline of biology concerned with pathogenic protozoa. (15)

paromomycin (par´o-mo-mi´sin) A drug used in the treatment of amoebiasis and balantidiasis. (15)

paroxysm (par-ok´sizm) A sudden intensification of symptoms, such as a severe bout of coughing. (7)

parvovirus An icosahedral DNA virus that causes disease in dogs and fifth disease in humans. (12)

passive agglutination An immunological procedure in which antigen molecules are adsorbed to the surface of latex spheres or other carriers that agglutinate when combined with antibodies. (19)

Pasteurella multocida (pas-tur-el´ah mul-toc´i-dah) A Gram-negative bacterial rod that causes pasteurellosis. (10)

pasteurellosis (pas´tur-el-lo´sis) A bacterial disease transmitted by animal bites, caused by *Pasteurella multocida*; characterized by abscess formation at the bite site. (10)

pasteurization A heating process that destroys pathogenic bacteria in a fluid such as milk and lowers the overall number of bacteria in the fluid. (21, 24)

pathogen A type of parasite that causes disease in the host organism. (4, 17)

pathogenicity The ability of a parasite to gain entry to a host and bring about a physiological or anatomical change interpreted as disease. (17)

Paul-Bunnell test A diagnostic procedure for infectious mononucleosis in which a sample of a patient's serum is combined with sheep red blood cells; the cells agglutinate in a positive test. (13)

pebrine (pa-brēn´) A protozoal disease of silkworms studied by Louis Pasteur. (1)

Pediculus (ped-ik´u-lus) The genus of lice that transmit epidemic typhus and other diseases. (9)

pellicle A rigid covering layer of certain protozoa composed in part of chitinlike material. (15)

pelvic inflammatory disease (PID) A disease of the pelvic organs; often a complication of a sexually transmitted disease. (10)

penicillin Any of a group of antibiotics derived from *Penicillium* species or produced synthetically; effective against Gram-positive bacteria and several Gram-negative bacteria by interfering with cell wall synthesis. (23)

penicillinase An enzyme produced by certain microorganisms that converts penicillin to penicilloic acid and thereby confers resistance against penicillin. (23)

peptidoglycan (pep´tĭ-do-gli´kan) A complex molecule of the bacterial cell wall composed of alternating units of *N*-acetylglucosamine and *N*-acetylmuramic acid; formation of the molecule is prevented by the use of penicillin. (4, 23)

perforin A protein secreted by cytotoxic T-lymphocytes to dissolve the cell membrane attacked during cell-mediated immunity. (18)

period of acme The phase of a disease during which specific symptoms occur and the disease is at its height. (17)

period of convalescence The phase of a disease during which the body's systems return to normal. (17)

period of decline The phase of a disease during which symptoms subside. (17)

period of incubation *See* incubation period.

period of prodromal symptoms The phase of a disease during which general symptoms occur in the body. (17)

peritrichous (per´e-trik´us) **bacterium** A bacterium that has flagella over the entire surface of the cell. *See also* monotrichous bacterium. (4)

pertussis A bacterial disease of the upper respiratory tract in which an accumulation of mucus causes a narrowing of the tubes and a characteristic "whoop" on inhalation, thus the common name, whooping cough. (7)

Pfiesteria piscicida A dinoflagellate protozoan linked to fish kills in waters along the eastern U.S. coast. (15)

pH An abbreviation for the negative logarithm of the amount of hydrogen ions in 1 liter of solution; the pH scale extends from 1 to 14 and indicates the degree of acidity or alkalinity of a solution. (2)

phagocyte A cell that performs phagocytosis. (18)

phagocytosis (fag´o-sī-to´sis) A process in which solid particles are taken into the cell; important in nutritional processes and in defense against disease. (18)

phagosome A vesicle that contains particles of phagocytized material. (18)

phenol coefficient A number that indicates the effectiveness of an antiseptic or disinfectant compared to phenol. (22)

phosphatase (fos´fah-tās) An enzyme normally found in milk; it is destroyed by pasteurization processes, and its absence indicates that the pasteurization has been successful. (24)

photoautotroph (fo´to-aw´to-troph) An organism that uses light energy to synthesize nutrients from carbon dioxide. (5)

photoheterotroph (fo´to-het´er-o-troph) An organism that uses light energy to synthesize nutrients from carbon compounds other than carbon dioxide. (5)

photophobia Sensitivity to bright light.

photosynthesis A biochemical process in which light energy is converted to chemical energy and used in carbohydrate synthesis. (5)

picornavirus (pi-kor´nah-vir´us) A small virus containing RNA in its genome. (13)

pigeon fancier's disease A condition that develops from a type III hypersensitivity reaction following exposure to antigens from a pigeon. (20)

pilin A protein subunit found in the bacterial pilus. (4)

pilus One of many short, hairlike appendages of bacteria that anchor the cell to a surface; pili are also involved in conjugations between bacteria. (4, 6, 8)

pinkeye A disease of the conjunctival membranes of the eye usually caused by bacteria or viruses and accompanied by red, swollen eyes. Also called conjujnctivitis. (10)

pinocytosis A type of phagocytosis in which materials dissolved in fluid are taken into the cell. (18)

pinta A mild syphilislike disease of the skin occurring in remote parts of the world, caused by a species of *Treponema*. (10)

pinworm The common name for *Enterobius vermicularis*, a multicellular roundworm parasite that infects the intestine. (16)

plague A serious arthropodborne bacterial disease transmitted by the flea, caused by *Yersinia pestis* and characterized by severe blood hemorrhaging. (9)

plaque A clear area on a lawn of bacteria where viruses have destroyed the bacteria; also, the gummy layer of gelatinous material consisting of bacteria and organic matter on the teeth. (10, 11)

plasma The fluid portion of blood remaining after the cells have been removed; serum plus the clotting agents. (17)

plasma cell The cell derived from B-lymphocytes; plasma cells produce antibodies. (18)

plasmid A small, closed-loop molecule of DNA apart from the chromosome; plasmids carry genes for drug resistance and pilus formation and are used in genetic engineering techniques. (4, 6, 25)

Plasmodium species Protozoa of the Sporozoa group, transmitted by mosquitoes, that infect human red blood cells and cause malaria; examples are *P. vivax*, *P. malariae*, and *P. falciparum*. (15)

pleomorphic (ple´o-mor´fik) **organism** An organism that occurs in a variety of shapes. (9)

Plesiomonas shigelloides A Gram-negative, facultatively anaerobic rod commonly found in the gut of tropical fish; the cause of human intestinal disease.

pleurodynia (ploo´o-din´e-ah) Infection of the chest wall commonly due to Coxsackie virus. (13)

pneumococcus A common name for *Streptococcus pneumoniae*. (7)

Pneumocystis carinii (nu´mo-sis´tis car-in´e-e) An opportunistic protozoan that infects the lungs and causes pneumonia in immune-compromised individuals, such as AIDS patients. (15)

Pneumocystis carinii pneumonia (PCP) A lung infection caused by *Pneumocystis carinii*, characterized by consolidation of the lung and suffocation; occurs primarily in immune-compromised individuals, such as AIDS patients. Also called pneumocystosis. (15)

pneumonia An infectious disease of the lower respiratory tract. (7)

pneumonic plague A form of plague in which *Yersinia pestis* invades the lung tissues and causes severe respiratory symptoms. (9)

polymorphonuclear (pol´e-mor´fo-nu´kle-ar) **cell** A type of white blood cell with a multilobed nucleus. (17)

polyvalent serum Serum that contains a mixture of antibodies. (19)

Pontiac fever A form of Legionnaires' disease. (7)

porin A protein in the outer membrane of Gram-negative bacteria that acts as channels for the passage of biomolecules. (4)

portal of entry The site at which a parasite enters the host. (17)

portal of exit The site at which a parasite leaves the host. (17)

Pott's disease Tuberculosis of the spine. (7)

pox Pitted scars remaining on the skin of individuals who have recoverered from smallpox. (12)

precipitation A type of antigen-antibody reaction in which thousands of molecules of antigen and antibody cross-link to form particles of precipitate. (18, 19)

prednisone (pred´nih-sōn) A steroid hormone that suppresses the inflammatory response; used to retard transplant rejection. (20)

primaquine (prim´a-kwin) A synthetic drug used to treat malaria in the dormant phase. (15)

primary antibody response The initial response by the immune system to an antigen, characterized by an outpouring of IgM. *See also* secondary antibody response. (18)

primary atypical pneumonia (PAP) An airborne bacterial disease of the lungs caused by *Mycoplasma pneumoniae*, characterized by degeneration of the lung tissue. Also called mycoplasmal pneumonia and walking pneumonia. (7)

primary disease A disease that develops in an otherwise healthy individual. (17)

prion (prē´on) An infectious particle of protein, possibly involved in human diseases of the brain. (11)

proctitis Infection of the rectum. (10)

proglottid (pro-glot´id) One of a series of segments that make up the body of a tapeworm. (16)

prokaryote (pro-kar´e-ōt) A relatively simple organism composed of single cells having a single chromosome but no intracellular organelles, nucleus, or nuclear membrane; reproduction does not involve mitosis. *See also* eukaryote. (3)

prontosil (pron'to-sil) A red dye found by Domagk to have significant antimicrobial activity when tested in live animals, and from which sulfanilamide was later isolated. (23)

properdin (pro'per-din) A protein that functions in the alternative pathway of complement activation. (18)

prophage The DNA fragment of a temperate phage. (6)

prophylactic serum (pro'fi-lak'tic) Antibody-rich serum used to protect against the development of a disease. (19)

prostaglandins Substances resulting from interactions involving arachidonic acid and acting as mediators in type I hypersensitivity reactions. (20)

protein A chain of amino acids used as a structural material or enzyme in living cells; all proteins have primary and secondary structures, and some have a tertiary structure. (2, 5)

Protista One of the five kingdoms in the Whittaker classification of living things, composed of the protozoa and various other simple forms; also, the term used by Haeckel to denote single-celled organisms of microscopic size. (3)

proto-oncogene A region of DNA in the chromosome of human cells; they are altered by carcinogens into oncogenes that transform cells. (11)

pruritus Itching sensations. (12)

pseudomembrane An accumulation of mucus, leukocytes, bacteria, and dead tissue in the respiratory passages of diphtheria patients. (7)

pseudomembranous colitis A condition of the wall of the small intestine, characterized by membranous lesions; believed to be caused by *Clostridium difficile*. (10, 23)

Pseudomonas aeruginosa (soo'do-mon'as a'er-jin-o'sa) A Gram-negative bacterial rod, transmitted by contaminated materials, that causes disease in the burned tissue of burn victims; also causes urinary tract infections. (10)

Pseudomonas pseudomallei A Gram-negative bacterial rod, transmitted by soilborne materials, that causes melioidosis. (9)

pseudopodium (soo'do-po'de-um) One of many projections of the cell membrane that allow movement in members of the Sarcodina group of protozoa. (15)

psittacosis An airborne bacterial disease of the lung caused by *Chlamydia psittaci*, characterized by respiratory discomfort and influenzalike symptoms; occurs in birds of the psittacine group (parrots, etc.) and in humans. Also called ornithosis. (7)

psychrophile (si'kro-fil) An organism that lives at cold temperature ranges of 0°C to 20°C. (4, 24)

psychrotrophic (si'kro-troph'ik) **organism** An organism that normally live at medium temperatures but tolerate and grow at cold temperatures. (4, 24)

ptomaine (tō'mān) A nitrogen compound having a strong odor; once thought responsible for food poisoning. (8, 24)

pure culture A culture or colony of microorganisms of one type. (1)

pus A mixture of serum, dead tissue cells, leukocytes, and bacteria that accumulates at the site of infection. (18)

Q

Q fever A rickettsial disease characterized by flulike symptoms. (17)

quartan malaria A type of malaria in which attacks occur at 4-day intervals. (15)

quinine A drug derived from the bark of the *Cinchona* tree; used to treat malaria. (15, 23)

quinupristin A streptogramin antibiotic used with quinupristin to inhibit reproduction in *Staphylococcus aureus*. (23)

R

R factor A plasmid that occurs frequently in Gram-negative bacteria and carries genes for drug resistance. (6, 8)

rabbit fever An alternate name for tularemia. (9)

rabies A serious nervous system disease due to a helical RNA virus, transmitted by an animal bite; characterized by the destruction of brain tissue, leading to paralysis and death. (13)

racial immunity Immunity present in one race of people but not in another. (18)

radioallergosorbent test (RAST) A type of radioimmunoassay in which antigens for the unknown antibody are attached to matrix particles. (19)

radioimmunoassay (RIA) An immunological procedure that uses radioactive-tagged antigens to determine the identity and amount of antibodies in a sample. (19)

rat-bite fever A bacterial disease of the skin and blood due to either *Aspergillum minor* or *Streptobacillus moniliformis* and transmitted by a rat bite. (10)

reagin An alternate name for the IgE that stimulates anaphylaxis in the body. (20)

real image An image that can be projected onto a screen; formed by the objective lens in light microscopy. (3)

recombinant DNA molecule A DNA molecule that carries foreign genes. (6)

recombination An alteration in the genetic information in a microorganism arising from the acquisition of DNA; in bacteria, recombination occurs by transformation, conjugation, and transduction. (6)

red rot Spoilage in milk and eggs due to the production of red pigment by *Serratia marcescens*. (24)

redia (re'de-ah) An intermediary stage in the life cycle of a fluke. (16)

relapsing fever A serious arthropodborne bacterial disease transmitted by ticks and lice, caused by *Borrelia recurrentis*; characterized by periods of fever. (9)

rennin An enzyme that accelerates the curdling of protein in milk. (24)

reservoir A human or other animal that retains disease organisms in the body but has not experienced disease and shows no evidence of illness. (17)

resolving power The numerical value of a lens system indicating the size of the smallest object that can be seen clearly when using that system. (3, 11)

respiration Any biochemical process in which energy is liberated; respiration may occur in the presence of oxygen (aerobic respiration) or in its absence (anaerobic respiration). (5)

respiratory syncytial (RS) disease An airborne viral disease occurring in young children, characterized by pneumonia in the lung tissues. (12)

respiratory syncytial (RS) virus A helical RNA virus that causes lung infections primarily in young children. (12)

restriction enzyme A type of endonuclease that splits open a DNA molecule at a specific restricted point; important in genetic engineering techniques. (6)

reticuloendothelial system (RES) A collection of large, monocyte-derived cells that perform phagocytosis within the tissues, Also known as mononuclear phagocyte system. (18)

retrovirus An RNA virus that uses reverse transcriptase to synthesize DNA using RNA as a template. (13)

reverse transcriptase An enzyme that synthesizes a DNA molecule from the code supplied by an RNA molecule. (6, 11, 13)

Reye syndrome A complication of influenza and chickenpox, characterized by vomiting and convulsions as well as liver and brain damage. (12)

rhabditiform larva (rab-dit´ī-form) An elongated intermediate form of the hookworm. (16)

rheumatic fever A complication of streptococcal disease in which damage to the heart valves develops from the reactions between antigens and antibodies. (7, 20)

rheumatoid arthritis An autoimmune disease characterized by immune complex formation in the joints. (20)

rhinovirus An icosahedral RNA that causes diseases of the upper respiratory tract commonly known as head colds. (12)

ribosome A cellular component of RNA and protein that participates in protein synthesis. (3, 4, 5, 11)

rice-water stool A colorless, watery diarrhea containing particles of intestinal tissue in cholera patients. (7)

rickettsiae (rik-et´se-e) A group of small bacteria generally transmitted by arthropods; most rickettsiae are cultivated only within living tissue medium. (3, 7, 9)

Rickettsia prowazecki A species of rickettsia transmitted by a louse that causes epidemic typhus. (9)

Rickettsia rickettsii A species of rickettsia transmitted by a tick that causes Rocky Mountain spotted fever. (9)

Rickettsia tsutsugamushi (soot´soo-ga-moosh´e) A species of rickettsia transmitted by a mite that causes tsutsugamushi. (9)

Rickettsia typhi A species of rickettsia transmitted by fleas that causes endemic typhus. (9)

rickettsialpox A relatively mild miteborne disease of the blood caused by *Rickettsia akari*, characterized by fever and a skin rash. (9)

rifampin (rif-am´pin) An antibiotic prescribed for tuberculosis and leprosy patients and for carriers of *Neisseria* and *Haemophilus* species. (23)

rifapentine A drug related to rifampin, used to treat tuberculosis.

Rift Valley fever A disease caused by an RNA virus, occurring primarily in the Rift Valley of Africa, characterized by intense fever and joint pains. (13)

ringworm A fungal disease caused by numerous species of fungus, characterized by scaly, circular patches of infection, usually on the head; ringworm of the feet is athlete's foot; ringworm of the groin, nails, face, and other body regions also occurs. (14)

ritonavir An antiviral drug that inhibits the activity of protease in the formation of the viral capsid; belongs to a group known as protease inhibitors. (11, 23)

Ritter's disease A type of impetigo contagiosum of the skin caused by *Staphylococcus aureus*. (10)

Rocky Mountain spotted fever A relatively serious tickborne disease of the blood caused by *Rickettsia rickettsii*, characterized by high fever and a skin rash beginning on the body extremities and proceeding toward the body trunk. (9)

rolling circle mechanism A type of DNA replication in which the broken strand of DNA "rolls off" the loop and serves as a template for the synthesis of a complementary strand of DNA. (6)

ropy bread Bread that has become soft and stringy due to the depositing of glycocalyx material by a bacterium such as *Bacillus subtilis*. (4, 24)

ropy milk Milk that has become thick and viscous due to an accumulation of capsular material deposited by a bacterium such as *Alcaligenes viscolactis*. (4, 24)

roseola A condition marked by fever and body rash. (12)

rose spots Bright red skin spots associated with diseases such as typhoid fever and relapsing fever. (8, 9)

rotavirus An RNA virus transmitted by food and water, involved in intestinal diseases. (13)

rubella A communicable skin disease caused by an icosahedral RNA virus, characterized by mild respiratory symptoms and a measleslike rash; can cause damage in the fetus if contracted by a pregnant woman. (12)

rubeola An alternate name for measles. (12)

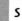

S

Sabia virus An arenavirus that causes hemorrhagic illnesses. (13)

Sabin vaccine A type of polio vaccine prepared with attenuated viruses; the vaccine is taken orally. (13)

Sabouraud (sab´oo-rō) **dextrose agar** A growth medium for fungi. (14)

saddleback fever A condition characterized by fluctuations of fever. (13)

Salk vaccine A type of polio vaccine prepared with viruses inactivated with formaldehyde; the vaccine is injected into the body. (13)

Salmonella enteritidis (en´ter-it´i-dis) A Gram-negative bacterial rod transmitted by food and water, involved in intestinal diseases. (8)

Salmonella typhi A Gram-negative bacterial rod transmitted by food and water that causes typhoid fever, a disease of the intestines. (8)

salpingitis (sal´pin-ji´tis) Blockage of the Fallopian tubes; a possible complication of a sexually transmitted disease. (10)

sandfly fever A sandfly-transmitted viral disease occurring in Mediterranean regions, characterized by high fever and joint pains. (13)

sanitize To reduce microbial populations to a safe level as determined by public health standards. (22)

saprobe A type of heterotrophic organism that feeds on dead organic matter, such as rotting wood or compost; formerly called a saprophyte. (4)

saquinavir An antiviral drug that inhibits the activity of protease in the formation of the viral capsid; belongs to a group known as protease inhibitors. (11, 23)

sarcina (sar´sĭn-ah) A cubelike packet of eight cocci. (4)

Sarcodina (sar´ko-di´nah) A group of protozoa whose members move by means of pseudopodia. (15)

sarcoma A tumor of the connective tissues. (11)

scalded skin syndrome A staphylococcal skin disease in infants characterized by a red, wrinkled surface with a sand-paper texture. (10)

scarification A method of inoculating an immunizing agent by scratching the skin.

scarlatina A mild case of scarlet fever.

Schick test A skin test used to determine the effectiveness of diphtheria immunization. (7)

Schistosoma (shis-to-so´mah) **species** A group of multicellular flatworm parasites of the blood transmitted by contact with water, commonly known as blood flukes; examples are *S. mansoni* and *S. japonicum.* (16)

schistosomiasis A waterborne blood disease caused by *Schistosoma* species and characterized by fever, chills, and liver damage. (16)

schmutzdecke (shmoots´dek-ĕ) A slimy layer of microorganisms that develops in a slow sand filter. (25)

sclerotium (skle-ro´she-um) A hard purple body that forms in grains contaminated with *Claviceps purpurea.* (14)

scolex The head region of a tapeworm where the attachment organ is located. (16)

scrapie A disease of sheep and other animals in which nerve damage causes the animal to scratch the skin. (10)

scrofula A bacterial disease of the lymph nodes of the neck caused by *Mycobacterium scrofulaceum.* (7)

secondary anamnestic response A vigorous immune response stimulated by a second or subsequent entry of antigens to the body. (19)

secondary antibody response The second response by the immune system to an antigen; characterized by an outpouring of IgG. *See also* primary antibody response. (19)

secondary disease A disease that develops in a weakened individual. (17)

Seitz (sĭtz) **filter** A filter composed of a pad of porcelain or ground glass. (21)

selective medium A growth medium that contains ingredients to inhibit certain microorganisms while encouraging the growth of others. (4)

septicemia A generalized bacterial infection of the bloodstream due to any of several organisms, including streptococci and staphylococci; once known as blood poisoning. (7, 17)

septum A cross-wall in the hypha of a fungus. (14)

serological reaction An antigen-antibody reaction studied under laboratory conditions and involving serum. (19)

serology A branch of immunology that studies serological reactions. (19)

serotonin (ser´o-to´nin) A derivative of tryptophan that functions in type I hypersensitivity reactions to contract smooth muscles. (20)

serotype A rank of classification below the species level based on an organism's reaction with antibodies in serum; used for several bacteria, especially *Salmonella.* (3, 8)

Serratia marcescens (se-ra´she-ah mar-ses´ens) A Gram-negative red-pigmented bacterial rod involved as an opportunist in diseases of the respiratory and urinary tracts. (7)

serum The fluid portion of the blood consisting of water, minerals, salts, proteins, and other organic substances; contains no clotting agents. (9, 17, 19)

serum sickness A type of hypersensitivity reaction in which the body responds to proteins contained in foreign serum. (19, 20)

severe combined immunodeficiency (SCID) An immune disease in which the lymph nodes lack both B-lymphocytes and T-lymphocytes. (20)

sexduction A process of recombination in which chromosomal genes pass from a donor cell to a recipient cell while attached to the F factor. (6)

Shigella **species** A group of Gram-negative bacterial rods, transmitted by food and water, that cause shigellosis. (7)

shigellosis A foodborne and waterborne bacterial disease of the intestine caused by *Shigella* species, characterized by extensive diarrhea, often with blood and mucus. (7)

shingles An alternate name for herpes zoster; a condition of the nerves and skin due to varicella-zoster virus. (12)

short incubation hepatitis An alternate name for hepatitis A. (13)

silage A type of animal feed produced by fermenting grains and other plants in silos, the huge cylindrical structures that often stand next to barns. (24)

slime layer A thinner, flowing, and less tightly bound form of a glycocalyx. (4)

slapped-cheek disease An alternate name for fifth disease. (12)

slow virus disease A slow-developing viral disease in which the effects appear after a long time period. (13)

smallpox An extinct viral disease of the skin and body organs caused by a complex DNA virus and accompanied by bleeding skin pustules, disfigurements, and multiple organ involvements. Also called variola. (12)

smut A fungal disease of agricultural crops, so named because of the sooty black appearance of infected plants. (14)

sodium hypochlorite (NaOCl) A derivative of chlorine used in disinfection practices; also known as bleach. (22)

sodoku (so´do-koo) An alternate name for rat-bite fever caused by a spirillum. (10)

soft chancre An alternate name for chancroid. (10)

sorbitol An alcoholic carbohydrate fermented slowly by *E. coli* O157:H7 and used in the medium to identify this organism. (8)

specialized transduction A transduction in which the prophage carries some bacterial genes when it breaks free from the chromosome; the bacterial genes are then replicated and carried into the next cell by the virus. *See also* generalized transduction. (6)

species The fundamental rank in the classification system of organisms; two or more species are grouped together as a genus. (3)

species immunity Immunity present in one species of organisms but not another species. (18)

specific immunologic tolerance A phenomenon in which a person's own proteins and polysaccharides contact and inactivate cells that might later respond to them immunologically (as "nonself"). (18)

spectinomycin An antibiotic used as a substitute for penicillin in cases of gonorrhea that are caused by penicillinase-producing *Neisseria gonorrhoeae*. (23)

spherule (sfer´ūl) A stage in the life cycle of the fungus *Coccidioides immitis*. (14)

spike A functional projection of the viral envelope. (11, 12)

spirillum A bacterium characterized by twisted or curved rods, generally with a rigid cell wall and flagella. (4)

Spirillum minor A spiral bacterium; one of the causes of rat-bite fever. (10)

spirochete (spi´ro-ket) A twisted bacterial rod with a flexible cell wall containing axial filaments for motility. (4)

spontaneous generation A theory suggesting that lifeless objects give rise to living things in their present form. (1)

spontaneous mutation A mutation that arises from chance events in the environment. (6)

sporangiospore An asexually produced fungal spore formed within a sporangium. (14)

sporangium (spo-ran´je-um) A protective sac that contains asexually produced fungal spores. (14)

spore A highly resistant structure formed from vegetative cells in several genera of bacteria, including *Bacillus* and *Clostridium*; also, a reproductive structure formed by a fungus. (4, 14)

sporicidal agent An agent that kills bacterial spores. (22)

sporocyst An intermediary stage in the life cycle of a fluke; usually occurs in the snail. (16)

Sporothrix schenkii A fungus that causes sporotrichosis. (14)

sporotrichosis A soilborne fungal disease of the lymph channels caused by *Sporothrix schenkii*, characterized by knotlike growths under the skin surface and occasional skin lesions. (14)

Sporozoa A group of protozoa whose members have no means of locomotion in the adult form. (15)

sporozoite A stage in the life cycle of *Plasmodium* species; the parasite enters the human body in this form. (15)

sputum (spu´tum) Thick, expectorated matter from the lower respiratory tract. (7)

staphylococcus (stafi-lo-kok´us) A bacterium characterized by spheres in a grapelike cluster. (4, 24)

Staphylococcus aureus A Gram-positive grapelike cluster of cocci that can be the cause of food poisoning and/or infections of the skin (boils, abscesses), lungs, meninges, or other organs. (8, 10)

stationary phase The third portion of a bacterial growth curve in which the reproductive and death rates of cells are equal. (4)

stem cell A primordial cell of bone marrow from which hematopoietic and lymphopoietic cells develop. (18)

sterilization The removal of all life forms, especially bacterial spores. (21)

stormy fermentation Fermentation and curdling of milk accompanied by gas accumulation that forces the curds apart. (24)

streptobacillus A chain of bacterial rods. (4)

Streptobacillus moniliformis A rod-shaped bacterium in chains; one of the causes of rat-bite fever. (10)

streptococcus A chain of bacterial cocci. (4, 24)

Streptococcus mutans A Gram-positive chain of cocci that causes dental caries. (10)

Streptococcus pneumoniae A Gram-positive chain of cocci that causes bacterial pneumonia. Also called pneumococcus. (7)

Streptococcus pyogenes A Gram-positive chain of cocci that causes streptococcal diseases, such as scarlet fever. (7)

streptokinase (strep´to-ki´nās) An enzyme that dissolves fibrin clots; produced by virulent streptococci. (17)

streptomycin An antibiotic derived from *Streptomyces griseus* that is effective against Gram-negative bacteria and the tubercule bacillus; interferes with protein synthesis. (23)

Strongyloides stercoralis (stron′ji-loi′dēz ster-ko-ral′is) A multicellular roundworm parasite of the intestines and lungs. (16)

subacute sclerosing panencephalitis (SSPE) A rare complication of measles that affects the brain, characterized by a loss of cortical functions and a decrease in cognitive skills. (12)

subclinical disease A disease in which there are few or inapparent symptoms. (17)

substrate The substance upon which an enzyme acts. (5)

subunit vaccine A vaccine that contains parts of microorganisms, such as capsular polysaccharides or purified pili. (19)

sulfamethoxazole (sul′fah-meth-oks′ah-zōl) A sulfonamide compound used to treat vaginal infections, conjunctivitis, and other diseases. (23)

sulfanilamides (sul′fah-nil′ah-mīds) A group of sulfur-containing compounds used as antimicrobial agents. (23)

sulfur granule A small, hard granule found in tissue infected with *Actinomyces israelii*; they resemble the sulfur granules used in a pharmacy. (10)

superantigen An antigen that stimulates an immune response without any prior processing.

suppressor T-lymphocyte A T-lymphocyte that interferes with the activity of the immune system. (18, 20)

swimmer's itch Dermatitis of the skin caused by the body's reaction to certain species of schistosomes. (16)

symbiosis (sim′bi-o′sis) An interrelationship between two populations of organisms where there is a close and permanent association for mutual benefit. (4)

syncytium (sin-sish′um) A giant tissue cell in culture formed by the fusion of cells infected with respiratory syncytial viruses. (12)

syndrome A collection of symptoms.

synergism (sin′er-jizm) A close and permanent association between two populations of organisms such that the populations are able to accomplish together what neither could otherwise accomplish alone. (4)

synthetic vaccine A vaccine that contains chemically synthesized parts of microorganisms, such as proteins normally found in viral capsids. (19)

syphilis A sexually transmitted bacterial disease of multiple organs, caused by *Treponema pallidum* and occurring in three stages, characterized by extensive skin lesions, multiple organ involvements, and complications of the nervous and cardiovascular systems. (10)

systemic disease A disease that has disseminated to the deeper organs and systems of the body. (17)

systemic lupus erythematosus (SLE) An autoimmune disease in which antibodies form against nuclear components of the individual's cells and then unite with the antigens to form immune complexes in the skin and body organs. (20)

T

tabardillo (tab′ar-dēl′yo) An alternate name for endemic typhus. (9)

Taenia saginata A multicellular flatworm parasite of the intestine, transmitted by contaminated beef; commonly known as a beef tapeworm. (16)

Taenia solium A multicellular flatworm parasite of the intestine, transmitted by contaminated pork; commonly known as a pork tapeworm. (16)

tapeworm A ribbonlike flatworm belonging to the phylum Platyhelminthes; also called cestode. (16)

taxonomy The science dealing with the systematized arrangements of related living things in categories. (3)

teichoic (ti-ko′ik) **acid** A polysaccharide found in the cell wall of Gram-positive bacteria. (4)

temperate phage A bacteriophage that enters a bacterium but does not replicate; the phage DNA may remain in the bacterial cytoplasm or attach to the bacterial chromosome. (6)

tertian malaria A type of malaria in which the attacks occur every 48 hours. (15)

tetanospasmin An exotoxin produced by *Clostridium tetani*; acts at synapses, thereby stimulating muscle contractions. (9)

tetanus A soilborne bacterial disease of the muscles and nerves, caused by toxins produced by *Clostridium tetani*; characterized by uncontrolled muscle spasms. (9)

tetracyclines A group of antibiotics, each of which is characterized by four benzene rings with attached side groups; used for many diseases caused by Gram-negative bacteria, rickettsiae, and chlamydiae; inhibit protein synthesis in bacteria. (9, 23)

T-dependent antigen An antigen that requires the assistance of T-lymphocytes to stimulate antibody-mediated immunity.

therapeutic serum Antibody-rich serum used to treat a specified condition. (19)

thermal death point The temperature required to kill an organism in a given length of time. (21, 24)

thermal death time The length of time required to kill an organism at a given temperature. (21, 24)

thermoacidophile A prokaryote living under high temperature conditions. (4)

thermoduric (ther′mo-du′rik) **organism** An organism that normally lives at medium temperatures but may tolerate and live at high temperatures. (24)

thermophile An organism that lives at high temperature ranges of 40°C to 90°C. (4, 24)

thioglycollate (thi′o-gli′ko-lāt) **medium** A bacteriological medium that contains thioglycollic acid; the latter binds oxygen from the atmosphere and creates an environment suitable for anaerobic growth. (4)

three domains The system of classification established by Carl Woese and his coworkers based on their studies of ribosomal RNA. (3)

thrombocytopenia (throm′bo-si′to-pe′ne-ah) A reduced count of blood platelets (thrombocytes) resulting from the reaction of antibodies with antigens on the platelet surface; a type II hypersensitivity reaction. (20)

thrush Oral candidiasis. (14)

thymus A flat, bilobed organ that lies in the neck below the thyroid; T-lymphocytes are modified in the thymus. (18)

ticarcillin A semisynthetic penicillin antibiotic used against Gram-positive bacteria. (23)

tincture of iodine An iodine solution consisting of 2 percent iodine plus iodide in ethyl alcohol. (22)

T-independent antigen An antigen that does not require the assistance of T-lymphocytes to stimulate antibody-mediated immunity; found in bacterial flagella and capsules. (18)

tinea Any of a group of fungal infections of the skin, including tinea pedis (athlete's foot) and tinea capitis (ringworm of the scalp). (14)

tinidazole (ti-nid′ah-zōl) A chemotherapeutic agent used to treat trichomoniasis. (15)

tissue immunity An alternate term for cell-mediated immunity. (18, 20)

titer (ti′ter) The most dilute concentration of antibody that will yield a positive reaction with a specific antigen; a method of expressing the amount of antibody in a sample of serum. (19)

T-lymphocyte A lymphocyte modified in the thymus gland, associated with cell-mediated immunity. Also called T-cell. (13, 18)

topoisomerase An enzyme that prevents excessive coiling of DNA molecules. (3)

TORCH An acronym for four diseases that pass from the mother to the unborn child: toxoplasmosis, rubella, cytomegalovirus disease, and herpes simplex; the O stands for other diseases. (12, 13, 15)

toxic shock syndrome A bacterial disease of the blood caused by toxins produced by *Staphylococcus aureus*; characterized by shock and circulatory collapse. (10)

toxin A poisonous substance produced by a species of microorganism; bacterial toxins are classified as exotoxins or endotoxins. (17)

toxoid An immunizing agent produced from an exotoxin that elicits antitoxin production by the body. (7, 9, 17, 19)

Toxoplasma gondii A protozoan of the Sporozoa group that causes toxoplasmosis. (15)

toxoplasmosis A protozoal disease of the blood caused by *Toxoplasma gondii,* transmitted by contact with cats or the consumption of beef, characterized by malaise and nonspecific symptoms; a serious disease in immune-compromised patients; may cause fetal injury in pregnant women. (15)

trachoma A contact disease of the eye caused by *Chlamydia trachomatis*; characterized by tiny, pale nodules on the conjunctiva, and possibly leading to blindness. (10)

transcription The biochemical process in which RNA is synthesized according to a code supplied by the bases of the DNA molecule. (5)

transduction A type of bacterial recombination in which a virus transports fragments of DNA from a donor cell to a recipient cell. (6)

transfer RNA (tRNA) A molecule of RNA that unites with amino acids and transports them to the ribosome in protein synthesis. (5)

transformation A type of bacterial recombination in which competent bacteria acquire fragments of DNA from disintegrated donor cells and incorporate the DNA into their chromosomes. (6)

translation The biochemical process in which the code on the mRNA molecule is translated into a sequence of amino acids in the protein molecule. (5)

transposon A segment of DNA that moves from one site on a DNA molecule to another site, carrying information for protein synthesis. Also known as jumping gene. (6)

traveler's diarrhea A foodborne and waterborne bacterial disease of the intestine often caused by *Escherichia coli*, characterized by diarrhea. (8)

trematode A flatworm, commonly known as a fluke. (16)

trench fever A louseborne rickettsial disease due to *Rochalimaea quintana*, characterized by fever and a skin rash. Also called His-Werner disease. (9)

Treponema pallidum A spirochete that causes syphilis. (10)

Treponema pertenue A spirochete that causes yaws. (10)

Trichinella spiralis (trik′i-ne′ah spir-al′is) A multicellular roundworm parasite of the muscles, transmitted by contaminated pork, that causes trichinosis. (16)

trichinosis A foodborne disease of the muscles caused by the parasite *Trichinella spiralis*, contracted from poorly cooked pork, characterized by muscle pains. (16)

trichlosan A bisphenol antiseptic incorporated into a wide variety of household products.

trichocyst (trik′o-sist) An organelle of *Paramecium* species that discharges filaments used to trap the organism's prey. (15)

Trichomonas vaginalis A flagellated protozoan, transmitted by sexual contact, that causes trichomoniasis. (15)

trichomoniasis A protozoal disease of the reproductive tract caused by *Trichomonas vaginalis*, transmitted by sexual contact, characterized by discomfort in the urinary and lower reproductive tracts. (15)

Trichophyton (tri-kof′i-ton) **species** A fungus spread by contact; one of the causes of athlete's foot and ringworm. (14)

Trichuris trichiura (trik-u′ris trik-e-u′rah) A multicellular roundworm parasite of the intestine, commonly known as a whipworm. (16)

trivalent vaccine A vaccine consisting of three components, each of which stimulates immunity.

Trombicula (trom-bik´u-lah) **species** Species of mite, a spiderlike arthropod. (9)

trophozoite (trof´o-zo´īt) The feeding form of a microorganism, such as a protozoan. (13)

Trypanosoma brucei (tri-pan-o-so´mah bru´ce-i) A flagellated protozoan, transmitted by tsetse flies, that causes African trypanosomiasis. (15)

Trypanosoma cruzi A flagellated protozoan, transmitted by the triatomid bug, that causes South American trypanosomiasis. (15)

trypanosomiasis A protozoal disease of the blood caused by *Trypanosoma* species, transmitted by arthropods, and characterized by periods of high fever and coma. Also called sleeping sickness. (15)

tsutsugamushi (soot´soo-ga-moosh´e) A relatively mild miteborne disease of the blood caused by *Rickettsia tsutsugamushi*, characterized by fever and a skin rash. Also called scrub typhus. (9)

tubercle A hard nodule that develops in tissue infected with *Mycobacterium tuberculosis*. (7)

tuberculin test A skin test used for the early detection of tuberculosis; performed by applying purified protein derivative to the skin and noting a thickening of the skin with a raised vesicle in a few days. (7, 20)

tuberculosis An airborne bacterial disease of the lungs caused by *Mycobacterium tuberculosis*, characterized by degeneration of the lung tissue and spreading to other organs.(7)

tularemia A mild arthropodborne bacterial disease, transmitted by the tick and by contact, caused by *Francisella tularensis*; characterized by mild fever and vague symptoms of malaise. (9)

tumor An abnormal functionless mass of cells. (11, 20)

tyndallization (tyn´dal-i-za´shun) A sterilization method in which materials are heated in free-flowing steam for 30 minutes on each of three successive days. (21)

typhoid fever A foodborne and waterborne bacterial disease of the intestine and blood caused by *Salmonella typhi*; characterized by intestinal ulcers, high fever, and red skin spots. (7)

U

ultrapasteurization A pasteurization process in which milk is heated at 82°C for 3 seconds. (24)

undulant fever An alternate name for brucellosis in humans, due to the undulating nature of the fever. (8)

Ureaplasma urealyticum (u-re´ah-plaz´mah u-re´ah-lit´i-kum) A species of mycoplasma that causes ureaplasmal urethritis. (10)

ureaplasmal urethritis A sexually transmitted bacterial disease of the urinary and genital organs caused by *Ureaplasma urealyticum*, characterized by urinary tract symptoms. (10)

urticaria (ur´tĭ-ka´re-ah) A hivelike rash of the skin. (20)

urushiol (u-roo´she-ol) A chemical substance on the leaves of certain plants that induces poison ivy. (20)

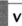
V

vaccination Originally, the process by which Jenner introduced vaccinia (cowpox) to volunteers; currently, any immunization procedure involving an injection. (12)

vaccinia (vak-sin´e-ah) An alternate name for cowpox, a mild form of smallpox. (12)

vaginitis A general term for infection of the vagina. (10)

vancomycin An antibiotic used in treating diseases caused by Gram-positive bacteria, especially staphylococci. (23)

varicella An alternate name for chickenpox; means "little vessel," a reference to small chickenpox lesions. (12)

varicella-zoster (VZ) virus The virus that causes varicella (chickenpox) and herpes zoster (shingles). (12)

variola An alternate name for smallpox. (12)

VDRL test A precipitation test used in the detection of syphilis antibodies. (19)

vector A living organism that transmits the agents of disease. (9, 17)

vesicle A fluid-filled skin lesion, such as that occurring in chickenpox. (12)

vibrio A form of bacterium occurring as a curved rod; resembles a comma. (4, 7)

Vibrio cholerae A Gram-negative curved bacterial rod, transmitted by food and water, that causes cholera. (8)

Vibrio parahaemolyticus (par´ah-he-mo-lit´i-kus) A Gram-negative curved bacterial rod, transmitted by food and water, involved in intestinal diseases. (8)

Vibrio vulnificus A marine bacterium known to cause intestinal infection when ingested in water. (8)

vidarabine A drug useful in treating herpes zoster and herpes encephalitis. (11, 12)

Vincent's angina Bacterial infection of the tonsil and soft palate areas due to several species of bacteria; a form of acute necrotizing ulcerative gingivitis. (10)

viremia The spread of viruses through the circulatory system. (17)

virion A completely assembled virus outside its host cell. (11)

viroid A tiny fragment of nucleic acid associated with certain plant diseases; possibly associated with animal disease. (11)

virucidal agent An agent that inactivates viruses. (22)

virulence The degree of pathogenicity of a parasite. (17)

virulent phage A bacteriophage that replicates within a bacterium and destroys the bacterium. (6)

virus A particle of nucleic acid (either DNA or RNA) surrounded by a protein sheath, and, in some cases, a membranous envelope; neither prokaryotic nor eukaryotic; highly infectious. (3, 6, 11)

W

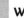

walking pneumonia A colloquial expression for a mild case of pneumonia. (7, 12)

wart A small, usually benign skin growth commonly due to a virus. (12)

Waterhouse-Friderichsen syndrome The formation of hemorrhagic lesions in the adrenal glands; thought to be an allergic reaction with immune complex formation; associated with meningococcal meningitis. (7, 20)

Weil-Felix test A diagnostic procedure for rickettsial diseases, performed by combining serum from a patient and *Proteus OX-19* on a slide; in a positive test, the *Proteus* cells clump together. (9)

wetting agent An agent that emulsifies and solubilizes particles clinging to a surface; an example is soap. (22)

wheal An enlarged, hivelike zone of puffiness on the skin, often due to an allergic reaction. (20)

whey The clear liquid remaining after protein has curdled out of milk. (24)

whipworm A common name for *Trichuris trichiura*. (16)

whooping cough An alternate name for pertussis. (7)

Widal (ve-dahl´) **test** An immunological procedure used for diagnostic purposes in which *Salmonella* antibodies agglutinate *Salmonella* antigens. (8, 19)

woolsorter's disease An alternate name for anthrax, derived from the fact that people who work with wool inhale the spores of the causative agent. (9)

Wuchereria bancrofti A multicellular roundworm parasite of the lymph channels, transmitted by mosquitoes, that causes elephantiasis. (16)

X

xenograft (zen´o-graft) A tissue graft between members of different species, such as between an animal and a human. (20)

Xenopsylla (zen´op-sil´ah) **cheopis** The rat flea, the vector in plague. (9)

Y

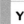

yaws A mild syphilislike disease occurring in remote parts of the world, caused by a species of *Treponema*. (10)

yeast A type of fungus that is unicellular and resembles bacteria in culture. (5, 14)

yellow fever A highly fatal viral disease transmitted by the *Aedes aegypti* mosquito, characterized by intense fever and jaundice. (13)

Yersinia enterocolitica A Gram-negative bacterial rod, transmitted by food and water, involved in intestinal diseases. (8)

Yersinia pestis A Gram-negative rod that displays bipolar staining and causes plague. (9)

Z

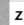

zoonosis (zo´o-no´sis) An animal disease that may be transmitted to humans. (9, 17)

zoospore (zo´o-spōr) A flagellated spore produced asexually by members of the Oomycota fungi. (14)

zygomycete A member of the fungal division Zygomycota. (14)

Zygomycota A division (phylum) of fungi whose members have coenocytic hyphae and form zygospores, among other notable characteristics. (14)

zygospore A sexually produced spore formed by members of the Zygomyca fungi. (14)

Index

NOTE: A *t* following a page number indicates tabular material, an *f* following a page number indicates a figure, and a *b* following a page number indicates a MicroFocus box. Drugs are listed under their generic names. When a drug trade name is listed, the reader is referred to the generic name.

G

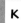

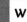
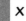

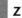

Photograph Acknowledgments

Note: Photographs from *ASM News*, *Journal of Bacteriology*, *Journal of Clinical Microbiology*, *Infection and Immunity*, *Applied and Environmental Microbiology*, and *Antimicrobial Agents and Chemotherapy* are used with permission from the American Society of Microbiology.

CDC = Centers for Disease Control and Prevention, Public Health Service, U.S. Department of Health and Human Services, Atlanta, Georgia.

COVER

Background photo of *Aspergillus niger:* Courtesy of Drs. Z. Yoshii, J. Tokunaga, and J. Tawara, *Atlas of Scanning Electron Microscopy in Microbiology*, IGAKU-SHOIN, Ltd., 1976. Test tube and pipette: PhotoDisc.

WEB SITE

Background photo of mixed bacteria: David M. Phillips, Photo Researchers, Inc.

PART 1 OPENER

Dennis Kunkel, University of Hawaii.

PART 1 MICROBIOLOGY PATHWAYS

Corbis.

CHAPTER 1

1.1a: From Parke-Davis Series "Great Moments in Medicine." 1.2: Courtesy Royal Society, London. 1.3a: Bettman/Corbis. 1.4: Courtesy of L. Tao from *J. Bacteriol.* **169**:2543 (1987). 1.5a: Courtesy of Institut Pasteur, Paris. 1.5b: From Parke-Davis Series. 1.7a: Courtesy of National Library of Medicine. 1.7b: Bettmann/Corbis. 1.8 Courtesy of the CDC. 1.9: Courtesy of Institut Pasteur, Paris. Box 1.1: Bettman/Corbis. Box 1.3: National Library of Medicine. Box 1.4: National Library of Medicine. Box 1.6: AP/World Wide Photos. Box 1.7: PhotoDisc.

CHAPTER 2

Box 2.1: Courtesy of L. Tao, from *J. Bacteriol.* **169**:2543 (1987).

CHAPTER 3

3.2: From R.E. Mueller, et al. *AEM* **47**:715 (1984). 3.3a: From John, Cole, & Marciano-Cabral. *AEM* **47**:12–14 (1984). 3.3b: Scanning micrograph by L. Tetley, from K. Vickeman, *Nature* **273**:613 (1978). 3.3c: Courtesy of Robert L. Owen, *Gastroenterology* **76**:759–769 (1979). 3.5a: Courtesy of E.M. Peterson, R.J. Hawlay, and R.A. Calerone. 3.5b: Courtesy of Ilan Chet, from *J. Bacteriol.* **154**:1431 (1983). 3.5c: USDA/ARS Information Staff. 3.10: Leonard Lessin/Peter Arnold, Inc. 3.14: Visuals Unlimited/David M. Phillips. 3.16: "Isolation of the Outer Membranes from *Treponema pallidum* and *Treponema vincentii*," by Blanco, Reimann, Skare, et al. *J. Bacteriol.* **176(19)**: 6088–6099 (1994) ASM fig. 3a. 3.17: Courtesy of N. Gotoh, from *J. Bacteriol.* **171**:983 (1989). Box 3.1: PhotoDisc. Box 3.4: Courtesy of N. Pace and E. Angert, from *ASM News* **58**:419 (1992).

PART 2 OPENER

Corbis.

PART 2 MICROBIOLOGY PATHWAYS

Agricultural Research Service, USDA.

CHAPTER 4

4.2a: Courtesy of D.L. Shungu, J.B. Cornett, and G.D. Schockman, *J. Bacteriol.* **138**:601 (1979). 4.2b: Courtesy of K. Amako. 4.2c: Courtesy of Dr. M. Matsuhashi, from Yamada et al., *J. Bacteriol.* **129**:1513–1517 (1977), Figure 2A. 4.3a and b: D.L. Balkwill, D. Maratean, and R.P. Blakemore, from *J. Bacteriol.* **141**:1399–1408 (1980). 4.4d: Photograph by Gary Gaard. Courtesy of Dr. A. Kelman (Department of Plant Pathology, University of Wisconsin-Madison). 4.5a: Courtesy of G. Biwas, from *J. Bacteriol.* **171**:657 (1989). 4.5b: Courtesy of Dr. B. Sugarman, Houston Veterans Administration Medical Center. 4.7: Courtesy of S.D. Acres, VIDO, University of Saskatchewan, and J.W. Costeron, University of Calgary. From *Infect. Immun.* **37**(3):1170 (1982). 4.10: With permission of Victor Lorian, M.D., Bronx Lebanon Hospital Center, Bronx, NY. 4.11a: Courtesy of E. Kellenberger, from *J. Bacteriol.* **173**:3149 (1992). 4.11b: Courtesy of Dennis A. Bazylinski, Iowa State University. 4.13a: Courtesy of Dr. C. Robinow, from *The Bacteria*, Vol. 1, Academic Press, New York (1960), Fig. 7, p. 214. 4.13b: Courtesy Gerhardt, Pankrants, and Scherrer, *Appl. Environ. Microbiol.* **32**:438–439 (1976). 4.13c: Courtesy of Drs. Yoshii, J. Tokunaga, and J. Tawara, *Atlas of Scanning Electron Microscopy in Microbiology*, IGAKU-SHOIN, Ltd., 1976. 4.16a: Courtesy of P. Scherer, from *ASM NEWS* **56**:569 (1990). 4.16b: Courtesy of Drs. Z. Yoshii, J. Tokunaga, and J. Tawara, *Atlas of Scanning Electron Microscopy in Microbiology,* IGAKU-SHOIN, Ltd., 1976. 4.17: "Isolation of Thermus Strains from Hot Composts (60 to 80° C)" by Trello Beffa, M. Blanc, et al. *Appl. Environ. Microbiol.* **62**: 1772–1727 (1996) ASM fig. 2, page 1725. 4.19b: Jack Bostrack/Visuals Unlimited. 4.20e: John Durham/ Science Photo Library/Photo Researchers, Inc. 4.21: Courtesy of J. Kwaik, from *Appl. Environ. Microbiol.* **62(6)**: 2022–2028 (1996), fig. 1H, page 2025. 4.22: Courtesy of R.E. Mueller et al., *AEM* **47**:715 (1984). 4.23: Beth Davidow/Visuals Unlimited. Box 4.2: John Mitchell/Photo Researchers, Inc. Box 4.3: Dennis Bazylinski. Box 4.7a: David McKay, NASA. Box 4.7b: Courtesy John Bradley.

CHAPTER 5

5.1: "The *Candida boidinii* Peroxisomal Membrane Protein Pmp30 Has a Role in Peroxisomal Proliferation and Is Functionally Homologous to Pmp27 from *Saccharomyces cerevisiae*" by Y. Sakai, PA. Marshall, et al. *J. Bacteriol.* **177(23)**: 6773-6781 (Dec. 1995), ASM fig. 4a&b, page 6778. 5.9 Courtesy of L. Tao, from *J. Bacteriol.* **169**:2543 (1987). 5.10: Elizabeth Gentt/Visuals Unlimited. 5.12a: Courtesy of H.W. Jannasch, from *Appl. Environ. Microbiol.* **41**:528–538 (1981). 5.12b: News Office, Woods Hole Oceanographic Institute. Box 5.4: Corbis.

CHAPTER 6

6.2a: H. Potter-D. Dressler/Visuals Unlimited. 6.4: Courtesy of C. Nombela, from *J. Bacteriol.* **172**:2384 (1990). 6.11a: Courtesy of CDC. 6.11b: Oliver Meckes, Photo Researchers, Inc. 6.17: Courtesy Celera Genomics. 6.18: "Usefulness of Leifson Staining Method in Diagnosis of *Helicobacter pylori* Infection," by R. Piccolomini, G. Di Bonaventura, et al. *J. Clin. Microbiol.* **37(1)**: 199–200 (Jan.1999), ASM fig.1, page 200. Box 6.4: Corbis. Box 6.7 PhotoDisc.

PART 3 OPENER

© James A. Sullivan, CELLS alive!

PART 3 MICROBIOLOGY PATHWAYS

PhotoDisc.

CHAPTER 7

7.1: Courtesy of Frederick Quinn, CDC. 7.2a: Courtesy of L. Tao, from *J. Bacteriol.* **169**:2543 (1987). 7.2b: Courtesy of U. Fluckiju and V.A. Fischetti, from *Infect. and Immun.* **66**:974–979 (1998). 7.2c: Courtesy of V. Fischetti, from *ASM News* **57**:619 (1991). 7.3: Ken Greer/Visuals Unlimited. 7.4b: Courtesy Professor Mumtaz Virji and Dr. David J.P. Ferguson from cover of *ASM News* **64(7)**, 1998. 7.7: "Portrait of a Woman," by Franz Hals. The Detroit Institute of Arts, City of Detroit Purchase. 7.8: PhotoDisc. 7.9a: Courtesy of Gourley, Leach, and Howard, *J. Gen. Microbiol.* **81**:475 (1974), with permission from ASM. 7.9b: Courtesy of Respiratory Disease Laboratory Section, DCDP, from *Appl. Environ. Microbiol.* **47(3)**:467 (1984). 7:10: Courtesy of Dr. B. Sugarman, Houston Veterans Administration Medical Center. 7.11a: S. Ito and A.R. Flesher, Harvard Medical School. 7.11b: Courtesy of J. Kwaik, from *Appl. Environ. Microbiol.* **62(6)**: 2022–2028 (1996), fig. 1E p. 2025. 7.13: Courtesy of Dr. Edgar Ribi and William R. Brown, Ribi ImmunoChem Research, Inc., Hamilton, Montana. 7.15: Courtesy of Arking, Appelt, and Balin, from *Science News* **154**: 325 (1998). Box 7.1: Chinch Gryniewicz/Ecoscene/Corbis. Box 7.5: Courtesy Stephanie Torta. Box 7.7: AP/Wide World Photos.

CHAPTER 8

8.1: "Characterization of a Region of the IncH12 Plasmid R478 Which Protects *Escherichia coli* from Toxic Effects Specified by Components of the Tellurite, Phage and Colicin Resistance Cluster," by K.F. Whelan, R.K. Sherburne and D.E. Taylor, *J. Bacteriol.* Vol. **179(1)**: 63–71 (Jan. 1997), ASM fig. 6c, page 69. 8.3a: Courtesy of Drs. Z. Yoshii, J. Tokunaga, and J. Tawara, *Atlas of Scanning Electron Microscopy in Microbiology,* IGAKU-SHOIN, Ltd., 1976. 8.3b: Courtesy of CDC. 8.5a: Courtesy of D.J. Thomas and T.A. McMeekin, University of Tasmania, Tasmania, Australia. 8.5b: Courtesy of Dr. W.L. Dentler. 8.6a and b: Courtesy of Drs. Z. Yoshii, J. Tokunaga, and J. Tawara, *Atlas of Scanning Electron Microscopy in Microbiology,* IGAKU-SHOIN, Ltd., 1976. 8.7: Corbis. 8.8: Courtesy of N. Schifferli, from *J. Bacteriol.* **173**:1230 (1991). 8.11 a and b: Courtesy of Diane E. Taylor, from *J. Bacteriol.* **164(1)**:338–343 (1985). 8.12: Courtesy of Tilney, from *Trends in Microbiol.* **1(1)** (1993). 8.13: USDA-ARS Information Staff. 8.14: Courtesy of Chai, from *Appl. Environ. Microbiol.* **62**:1300–1305 (1996). 8.15: Courtesy of V. Miller, from *ASM News* **58**:26 (1992) with permission of American Society for Microbiology. Box 8.1: Bettmann/Corbis. Box 8.3: PhotoDisc. Box 8.4: USDA-ARS Information Staff.

CHAPTER 9

9.1a and b: Courtesy of Drs. Z. Yoshii, J. Tokunaga, and J. Tawara, *Atlas of Scanning Electron Microscopy in Microbiology.* IGAKU-SHOIN, Ltd., 1976. 9.2: Charles W. Stratton/Visuals Unlimited. 9.3: Courtesy of The Royal College of Surgeons, Edinburgh. 9.4: Courtesy of CDC. 9.5a and b: Courtesy of Drs. Z. Yoshii, J. Tokunaga, and J. Tawara, *Atlas of Scanning Electron Microscopy in Microbiology,* IGAKU-SHOIN, Ltd., 1976. 9.6: Bettman/Corbis. 9.8a and b: Courtesy of Armed Forces Institute of Pathology (a) Neg. No. N-85837-2, and (b) Neg. No. AN1147-1A. 6.9: Courtesy of National Library of Medicine. 9.10a: Courtesy of A. Garon, Rocky Mountain Laboratory, Hamilton, Montana. 9.10b: Courtesy of J. Radolf, from *J. Bacteriol.* **173**:8004 (1991). 9.11: Science VU/ Visuals Unlimited. 9.14a: CDC Photo by James Gathany. 9.14b: Oliver Meckes/Photo Researchers, Inc. 9.14c: John Burbidge/SPL/Photo Researchers, Inc. 9.15: Armed Forces Institute of Pathology. 9.16: Armed Forces Institute of Pathology. Box 9.1: S & G Press Agency, Ltd. Box 9.7: Grant Heilman/Grant Heilman Photography.

CHAPTER 10

10.1a: Corbis. 10.1b: Ken Greer, Visuals Unlimited. 10.1c: Courtesy of CDC. 10.2a: Courtesy of the CDC. 10.2b: Courtesy of the CDC. 10.4a and b: Courtesy of Drs. Z. Yoshii, J. Tokunaga, and J. Tawara, *Atlas of Scanning Electron Microscopy in Microbiology,* IGAKU-SHOIN, Ltd., 1976. 10.4c: Biofoto Associates/Photo Researchers, Inc. 10.5b: Courtesy of Dr. L.A. Page. From *Bergey's Manual of Determinative Bacteriology,* 8th ed., Williams and Wilkins Co.: Baltimore (1974). 10.7: Courtesy of D. Krause from *J. Bacteriol.* **173**:1041 (1991). 10.8a and b: Courtesy of American Leprosy Mission, 1 Broadway, Elmwood Park, NJ. 10.9b: Courtesy of CDC. 10.10: Courtesy of CDC. 10.11: "Plaque Formation by and Plaque Cloning of *Chlamydia trachomatis* Biovar Trachoma," by Akira Matsumoto, H. Izutsu, N. Miyashita and M. Ohuchi, *J. Clin. Microbiol.* Vol. **36(10)**: 3013–3018 (Oct. 1988), ASM Fig. 4a, page 3016. 10.12: David M. Phillips/Visuals Unlimited. 10.13a and b: Armed Forces Institute of Pathology. 10.14b: Courtesy of the Naval Dental Research Institute, Naval Training Center, Great Lakes, Illinois. 10.15: Courtesy of Gobel, from *J. Clin. Microbiol.* **36**: 1399 (1998). 10.16a: Courtesy of K.F. Whelan, R.K. Sherburne, and D.E. Taylor, from *J. Bacteriol.* **179(1)**: 63–71 (1997). 10.16b: Courtesy M. Robert Belas, Center of Marine Biotechnology, Maryland Biotechnology Institute. 10.17: Courtesy of Z. Samara, Rabin Medical Center, Israel. 10.19: Courtesy of N. Gotoh, from *J. Bacteriol.* **171**:983 (1989). 10.20: Courtesy of Gerald Pier. Box 10.2: Courtesy of National Hansen's Disease Programs, Carville, LA. Box 10.4 Ken Cavanagh/Photo Researchers, Inc.

PART 4 OPENER

Corbis.

PART 4 MICROBIOLOGY PATHWAYS

Courtesy Anne Simon.

CHAPTER 11

11.1a: Courtesy of National Library of Medicine. 11.1b and c: Courtesy of the American Type Culture Collection. 11.4: Courtesy of C.K.Y. Fong, from *J. Clin. Microbiol.* **30**:1612 (1992). 11.5b: Courtesy of Dr. Glenn Howard, Pall Biomedical Products Corporation, Glen Cove, NY. 11.7: PhotoDisc. 11.8: Courtesy of the CDC. 11.9: Courtesy of Dr. Sara Miller, Duke University Medical Center. 11.11a and b: Courtesy of Drs. Z. Yoshii, J. Tokunaga, and J. Tawara, *Atlas of Scanning Electron Microscopy in Microbiology,* IGAKU-SHOIN, Ltd., 1976. 11.16: Courtesy of Fisher Scientific Company. 11.17a: Courtesy of J. Smit, from *J. Bacteriol.* **173**:5677 (1991). 11.17b: Courtesy of J. Smit, from *J. Bacteriol.* **173**:5568 (1991). 11.22: Hank Morgan/Science Source/Photo Researchers, Inc. 11.24a: AFP/Corbis. 11.24b: Courtesy Dr. Stanley Prusiner. Box 11.5: PhotoDisc. Box 11.7: PhotoDisc.

CHAPTER 12

12.1a: Courtesy of the CDC. 12.1b: Bettmann/CDC. 12.3: Courtesy of Dr. Sara Miller, Duke University Medical Center. 12.6a: St. Bartholomew's Hospital/SPL/Photo Researchers, Inc. 12.6b: Corbis. 12.7: Courtesy of Spotswood L. Spruance, from *J. Clin. Microbiol.* **22(3)**:366–368 (1985). 12.9a: Biofoto Associates/Photo Researchers, Inc. 12.9b: Science Photo Library/Photo Researchers, Inc. 12.10: Courtesy of J. Vreeswijk, from *J. Clin. Microbiol.* **30**:2487 (1992). 12.13: Dr. P. Marazzi/SPL/Photo Researchers, Inc. 12.14a: Hans Gelderblom/ Visuals Unlimited. 12.14b: Courtesy of V. Murphy, from *ASM News* **57**:579 (1991). 12.15: Courtesy of the CDC. 12.16: Courtesy of Parke-Davis, Division of Warner-Lambert Company, Morris Plains, NJ. 12.17: Courtesy of the CDC. Box 12.1: Science VU. Box 12.7: Courtesy of Gertrude B. Elion.

CHAPTER 13

13.1: Sinclair Stammers/SPL/Photo Researchers, Inc. 13.2a: London School of Hygiene and Tropical Medicine/ SPL/Photo Researchers, Inc. 13.2b: CDC Photo by James Gathany. 13.4: Courtesy of Dr. E.H. Cook, Jr., Hepatitis and Viral Enteritis Division, CDC, Phoenix, AZ. 13.6 a and b: Courtesy of Fred B. Williams, Jr., U.S. Environmental Protection Agency, Cincinnati, OH 45268. 13.9a and b: Scott Camazine/Photo Researchers, Inc. 13.14 : Courtesy of Drs. F.A. Murphy and A.K. Harrison, in *Rhabdoviruses,* D.H.L. Bishop, ed., Vol. I, pp. 66–106, CRC Press, 1979. 13.16: Courtesy of the CDC. 13.18: EM Unit, VLA/SPL/Photo Researchers, Inc. Box 13.1: Courtesy of Parke-Davis, Division of Warner-Lambert Company, Morris Plains, NJ. Box 13.9: S. Nagandra, Photo Researchers, Inc.

CHAPTER 14

14.1: Courtesy of R. Simmons, from *ASM News* **57**:400 (1991). 14.2: Courtesy of C. Nombela, from *J. Bacteriol.* **172**:2384 (1990). 14.3 "Disseminated Invasive Infection Due to *Metarrhizium anisopliae* in an Immunocompromised Child," by D. Burgner, G. Eagles, M. Burgess, P. Procopis, M. Rogers, D. Muir, R.Pritchard, A. Hocking and M. Priest. *J. Clin. Microbiol.* **36**: 1146-1150 (Apr.1998) ASM Fig. 1a, page 1147. 14.4: Courtesy of Drs. L.F. Ellis and

S.W. Queener. Reproduced by permission of the National Research Council of Canada, from the *Canadian Journal of Microbiology,* Vol. 21, pp. 1982–1996. 14.5a and b: Courtesy of Drs. Z. Yoshii, J. Tokunaga, and J. Tawara, *Atlas of Scanning Electron Microscopy in Microbiology,* IGAKU-SHOIN, Ltd., 1976. 14.6a–f: Courtesy of Northern Regional Research Center, Peoria, IL 61604. 14.7a: Bob Evans, Peter Arnold, Inc. 14.7b: Richard Gross. 14.7c: Jack Bostrack/Visuals Unlimited. 14.8: Courtesy of K.J. Kwon-Chung, from *J. Clin. Microbiol.* 30:3290 (1992). 14.9: Courtesy of T. Sewall, from *ASM News* 54:657 (1988). 14.10b: Richard Gross. 14.13a: Courtesy of Joseph Schlitz Brewery. 14.13b: David M. Phillips/Visuals Unlimited. 14.14a: Stuart Levitz, Boston University School of Medicine from *ASM News* Vol. 64(12): 693–698, Fig. 2. 14.14b: Courtesy of M.A. Kydstra, from *Infect. Immun.* 16:129 (1977). 14.15: Photograph by Marion J. Balish. Courtesy of Edward Balish, from *AEM* 47(4):647 (1984). 14.16a and b: Courtesy of CDC. 14.18a and b: "Case of Onychomycosis Caused by *Microsporum racemosum*" by P. Garcia-Martos, J. Gene, et al. *J. Clin. Microbiol.* 37(1): 258–260 (Jan.1999) ASM fig. 1, page 258, fig. 2a, page 259. 14.20a: Courtesy of J.D. Raj, California State University, Long Beach, and S.S. Sekhon, Veterans Administration Hospital, Long Beach, from *ASM News* 49(4), April 1983. 14.20b: Courtesy of CDC. Box 14.4: PhotoDisc. Box 14.5: Courtesy of Dr. Gary Strobel, University of Montana. Box 14.6: Courtesy Fleishmann's Yeast. Box 14.7: Courtesy, Block Drug Company, Inc. Box 14.8: USDA-ARS Information Staff.

CHAPTER 15

15.1: Courtesy of D. White, from *ASM News* 54:583 (1988). 15.3: From John, Cole, & Marciano-Cabral *AEM* 47:12–14 (1984). 15.4a–f: Courtesy of Carolina Biological Supply Company. 15.5: Diana Laulaien-Schein. 15.6: Courtesy of E. Bottone, from *J. Clin. Microbiol.* 30:2447 (1992). 15.8a and b: Courtesy of Govinda S. Visvesvara, Division of Parasitic Diseases, CDC. 15.10a–c: Courtesy of Robert L. Owen and the editors of *Gastroenterology* 76:759–769 (1979). 15.11a and b: Courtesy of C. Chetty, A. Armstrong, and M. Miller, Abbott Laboratories. 15.12a: Courtesy of Armed Forces Institute of Pathology, Neg. No. 74–5195. 15.12b: Courtesy of Steven T. Brentans and John E. Donelson, University of Iowa. 15.13: Courtesy of T. Minnick, from *ASM News* 51:239 (1985). 15.14: Courtesy of CDC. 15.16a and b: Courtesy of Chiappino, Nichols, and O'Connor, *J. Protozool.* 31:228 (1984). 15.19: Courtesy of Saul Tzipori, from *Microbiological Review* 47(1):84–96 (March 1983). 15.20a: PhotoDisc. 15.20b: Courtesy of Michael Arrowood, Ph.D., Division of Parasitic Diseases, CDC. Box 15.1: AP/ Wide World Photos. Box 15.5: Portrait of Charles Darwin, 1840 by George Richmond (1809–96). Down House, Downe, Kent, UK/Bridgeman Art Library. Box 15.7: PhotoDisc.

CHAPTER 16

16.1a: Courtesy of Armed Forces Institute of Pathology, Neg. No. 69-77765-2. 16.1b: Courtesy of Dr. Clive E. Bennet, Jr., *Parasitology* 61:892 (1975). 16.4a–c: Courtesy of Dr. J. Jujino. 16.7: Courtesy of B. Schieven, from *ASM News* 57:566 (1991). 16.8: Courtesy of Dr. K.A. Wright, Jr., *J. Parasitology* 65(3):441 (1979). 16.10a and b: Courtesy of Armed Forces Institute of Pathology, (a) Neg. No. 69-3584, and (b) Neg. No. 60-3583. 16.12: Courtesy of Armed Forces Institute of Pathology, Neg. No. 74-11349. 16.13: R. Umesh Chandran, WHO/SPL/Photo Researchers, Inc. 16.14a and b: Courtesy of Armed Forces Institute of Pathology, (a) Neg. No. 73-6654, and (b) Neg. No. 75-11789-4.

PART 5 OPENER

© James A. Sullivan, CELLS alive!

PART 5 MICROBIOLOGY PATHWAYS

PhotoDisc.

CHAPTER 17

17.1: Courtesy of Drs. Z. Yoshii, J. Tokunaga, and J. Tawara, *Atlas of Scanning Electron Microscopy of Microbiology,* IGAKU-SHOIN, Ltd., 1976. 17.4: Courtesy Segal, et al. *J. Clin. Microbiol.* 36: 1772 (1998). 17.12a and b: Courtesy of Drs. D.C. Savage and R.V.H. Blumershine, *Infect. Immun.* 10:240–250 (1974). 17.16a: Courtesy of J.A. Dowsett and J. Reid, from *Mycologia* 71:329 (1979). 17.16b: Courtesy of D. Corwin and S. Falkow, Rocky Mountain Laboratory, NIAID, NIH, Hamilton, Montana. 17.17: Courtesy of B. Finlay, from *ASM News* 58:486 (1992). 17.18: "Reciprocal Exchange of Minor Components of Type and 1 and F1C Fimbriae Results in Hybrid Organelles with Changed Receptor 19.3 Specificities, " by P. Klemm, G. Christiansen, B. Kreft, R. Marre and H. Bergmans *J. Bacteriol.* Vol. 176(8): 2227–2234 (Apr.1994) ASM fig. 2a&b, page 2231. 17.19: Courtesy of Jose Galan, SUNY, Stony Brook. 17.20: Courtesy of Tilney, from *Trends in Microbiology* 1(1) (1993)17.21 "Tobramycin Resistance of *Pseudomonas aeruginosa* Cells Growing as a Biofilm on Urinary Catheter Material," by J.C. Nickel, I. Ruseska, J.B. Wright, and J.W. Closterton *Antimicrobial Agents and Chemotherapy* 27(4): 619–624 (Apr.1985) ASM fig. 2, page 620, fig. 3, page 621. 17.22: Courtesy of Howard J. Faden. Box 17.1: Steve Chenn/Corbis. Box 17.6: PhotoDisc. Box 17.7: Courtesy Paul Ewald/Amherst College. Box 17.8: London School of Hygiene & Tropical Medicine /SPL/Photo Researchers, Inc. Box 17.9: Art Wolfe/Photo Researchers, Inc.

CHAPTER 18

18.2: Courtesy of Drs. D.F. Bainton and M.G. Farquhar. 18.8: Juergen Berger/Max-Planck Institute/Photo Researchers, Inc. 18.11: SPL/Photo Researchers, Inc. Box 18.1: Courtesy of David Pfennig.

CHAPTER 19

19.3: Courtesy of G. Christiansen, *J. Bacteriol.* **176**:2227–2234 (1994). 19.7a: Courtesy of CDC. 19.7b: From Razin et al., *Infect. Immun.* **30**:538–546 (1980). 19.9: "Phylogeny of Not-Yet-Cultured Spirochetes from Termite Guts," by B.J. Paster, F.E. Dewhirst, S.M. Cooke, V.Fussing, L.K. Poulsen and J.A. Breznak *Appli. Environ. Microbiol.* Vol. **62(2)**: 347–352. (Feb. 1996) ASM fig. 2 a-c, page 350. Box 19.1: Corbis. Box 19.6: Corbis. Box 19.7: Photo Researchers, Inc.

CHAPTER 20

20.4a and b: Photos by Scott T. Clay-Poole. 20.5: David M. Grossman/Photo Researchers, Inc. 20.9a and b: Courtesy of Dr. Robert A. Marcus. 20.10: Ken Greer/Visuals Unlimited. 20.12: SIU/Photo Researchers, Inc. 20.13: Corbis. 20.15: Larry Mulvehill/Photo Researchers, Inc. Box 20.1: Ed Reschke. Box 20.3: USDA-ARS Information Staff. Box 20.5: Visuals Unlimited. Box 20.8: David Young-Wolff/PhotoEdit.

PART 6 OPENER

orbis

PART 6 MICROBIOLOGY PATHWAYS

PhotoDisc.

CHAPTER 21

21. Courtesy of J. Moran, from *J. Bacteriol. Vol.* **176**: 2003–2012. (Apr. 1994) ASM fig. 4, page 2007. 21.1b: Courtesy of the CDC. 21.2: "Salt-Mediated Multicell Formation in *Deinococcus radiodurans*," by F.I. Chou and S. T.n *J. Bacteriol.* Vol. **173(10)**: 3184–3190 (May,1991) ASM fig. 1e, page 3185, 2A, page 3187. 21.3: Lester V. Bergn/Corbis. 21.4: Bettmann/Corbis. 21.8: Courtesy of AMSCO/American Sterilizer Company, Erie, PA 1651.1.9: Larry Lefever/Grant Heilman Photography. 21.10b: Courtesy of Glenn Howard, Pall Biomedical Prodt Corporation, Glen Cove, NY. 21.11a and b: Courtesy of Pall Biomedical Products Corporation, Glen Cove, 21.12a–d: Courtesy of Millipore Corporation, Bedford, MA. 21.15: Nordion/Visuals Unlimited. Box 21.5: Ctesy Panasonic Consumer Products. Box 21.6: Snack Food Association.

CHAP 22

22.1: Co.sy Parke-Davis, Division of Warner-Lambert Company, Morris Plains, NJ. 22.3: Courtesy of the CDC. 22 ourtesy C.J. Thomas and T.A. McMeekin, University of Tasmania, Tasmania, Australia. 22.6: CDC Photo by ce Carr. 22.8: Courtesy of T.J. Marrie and J.W. Costerton, from *Appl. Environ. Microbiol.* **42(6)**:1093 (1981). 2. and b: Courtesy of American Sterilizer Company. Box 22.1: Courtesy of Parke-Davis, Division of Warner-L.rt Company, Morris Plains, NJ. Box 22.2: PhotoDisc. Box 22.3: PhotoDisc.

CHAPTER

23.1: The C.er Collection, New York. 23.2: Courtesy of Parke-Davis, Division of Warner-Lambert Company, Morris Plai. 23.4a and b: Courtesy of the National Library of Medicine. 23.5: Courtesy of Parke-Davis, Division of 'er-Lambert Company, Morris Plains, NJ. 23.7: James Webb, Phototake. 23.9a and b: Courtesy of H. Konish.n *J. Bacteriol.* **168**:1476 (1986). 23.10: Courtesy of Dr. D.R. Zusman. 23.11b: Kenneth E. Greer/Visual.mited. 23.13a: Miles/Visuals Unlimited. 23.13b and c: Courtesy, bioMerieux, Inc. Box 23.1: Holt Studios ational/Photo Researchers, Inc. Box 23.2: Vanni Archive/Corbis. Box 23.5: Courtesy of S. Horinuchi, *. Bacteriol.* **172**:3003 (1990) with permission of American Society for Microbiology.

PART 7 OPEN

Corbis.

PART 7 MICRO GY PATHWAYS

Corbis.

CHAPTER 24

24.5: "Bacterial Pl.sis as a Physical Indicator of Viability," by D.R. Korber, A. Choi, G.M. Wolfaardt and D.E. Caldewell. *A.iron. Microbiol.* **62(11)**: 3939-3947 (Nov. 1996) ASM fig. 6a, page 3944. 24.6a and b: Courtesy of the Na.ood Processors Association, Washington, DC. 24.8: Courtesy of C.J. Thomas and R.A. McMeekin, Ur. of Tasmania, Tasmania, Australia, from *Appl. Environ. Microbiol.* **41(2)**:492–503. 24.9: Robert Longuehaye./SPL/Photo Researchers, Inc. 24.11: Corbis. 24.12: Courtesy of Paul Gustafson. 24.13: Courtesy of M.A. D.and H.P. Flemming, USDA-ARS, Raleigh, NC. 24.14: Courtesy of Kikkoman Foods, Inc., Walworth, WI. .urtesy of the Switzerland Cheese Association. Box 24.3: Corbis. Box 24.6: Courtesy Snack Food Associati

CHAPTER 25

25.1a: Biophoto Assoc.to Researchers, Inc. 25.1b: Courtesy of Tomio Kawata. 25.3: Robert Brons, BPS, Tony Stone Images. 25. provided by A.C. Scott, Central Veterinary Laboratory, Wexbridge, U.K., British Crown Copyright 1982. d b: Courtesy of J. Kwaik, from *Appl. Environ. Microbiol.* **62(6)**: 2022–2028 (1996), fig. 1D, page 202 page 2025. 25.6a: Courtesy, Florida Fish & Wildlife Conservation Commission.

25.6b: AP/Wide World Photos. 25.7: Courtesy of Robert L. Owen, et al., from *Gastroenterology* **76**: 757–769 (1979). 25.10 "Resistance of *Pseudomonas aeruginosa* Cells Growing as a Biofilm on Urinary Catheter Material," by J.C. Nickel, I. Ruseska, J.B. Wright, and J.W. Closterton *Antimicrobial Agents and Chemotherapy* **27**(**4**): 619–624 (Apr.1985) ASM fig. 2, page 620, fig. 3, page 621. 25.11: Corbis. 25.13: Allan R.J. Eaglesham, Boyce Thompson Institute. 25.15a and b: Courtesy of Louis Sherman, used with permission of the ASM. 25.16a: Runk/Schoenberger/Grant Heilman Photography. 25.16b "Generation of Buds, Swellings, and Branches instead of Filaments after Blocking the Cell Cycle of *Rhizobium meliloti*," by J. N. Latch and William Margolin. *J. Bacteriol*. Vol. **179**(**7**):2373–2381 (Apr.1997) ASM fig. 4E, page 2378.

CHAPTER 26

26.3: USDA-ARS Information Staff. 26.4: Photo ACL, Bruxelles. Prière de verser 1000 FB au compte 000-0343629-55 du Patrimoine des Muscès royaux d'art et d'histoire. 10 parc du Cinquantenaire B-1040 Bruxelle 26.6a and b: Courtesy of Wine Institute of California. 26.6c: Courtesy of Wine Institute of California. 26.7a: Courtesy of Pfizer, Inc. 26.7b "Cloning and Characterization of a Gene Involved in Aerial Mycelium Formaðn in *Streptomyces griseus*," by N. Kudo, M. Kimura, T. Beppu, and S. Horinuchi *J. Bacteriol*. Vol. **177**(**22**): 640 6410 (Nov.1995) ASM fig.2a, page 6404. 26.8 a–c: "Characterization of a Novel Strain of *Bacillus thuringiensis*, "y J. E. Lopez-Mesa & J. E. Ibarra *Appl. Environ. Microbiol*. Vol. **62**(**4**): 1306–1310 (Apr.1996) ASM Fig. 1 a-cage 1307. 26.9: Michael Baytoff. Box 26.4: PhotoDisc. 26.10: Courtesy of the CDC.

Fundamentals of Microbiology depends on two major opinion sources: professional reviewers and individuals like you, the ones actually using the book. Please help us and the users of the next edition by completing this postage-paid questionnaire and returning it to us at your convenience.

Many thanks,
E. Alcamo

1. What do you like *most* about *Fundamentals of Microbiology*? _____

_____

2. What do you like *least* about the book? _____

_____

3. Which sections, if any, were particularly difficult to understand? _____

_____

4. How interesting and informative were the **MicroFocus** features? _____

5. How useful were the **Thought Questions** and **Review** sections? _____

6. Are all the chapters used in your microbiology course? (Please list those not used.)

_____

7. Can you offer any suggestions for improving the quality of the book? _____

_____

8. Any closing comments you care to make would be very appreciated: _____

_____

_____

_____

_____

_____

_____

_____

_____

_____

Name _____ Instructor? _____ Student? _____

School Name _____

Personal Address _____

City_____State_____Zip Code _____

May we contact you for editorial input? _____ May we quote you? _____

Please remove this page, fold it on the dotted lines, and seal it so that the return address is displayed. No postage is necessary if mailed in the United States.

NO POSTAGE
NECESSARY
IF MAILED
IN THE
UNITED STATES

BUSINESS REPLY MAIL

FIRST-CLASS MAIL   PERMIT NO. 40   SUDBURY MA

POSTAGE WILL BE PAID BY ADDRESSEE

Attn: I. Edward Alcamo PhD
Jones and Bartlett Publishers Inc
40 Tall Pine Drive
Sudbury MA 01776-9849